THE TRANSPLANTATION AND REPLACEMENT OF THORACIC ORGANS

The Present Status of Biological and Mechanical Replacement
of the Heart and Lungs

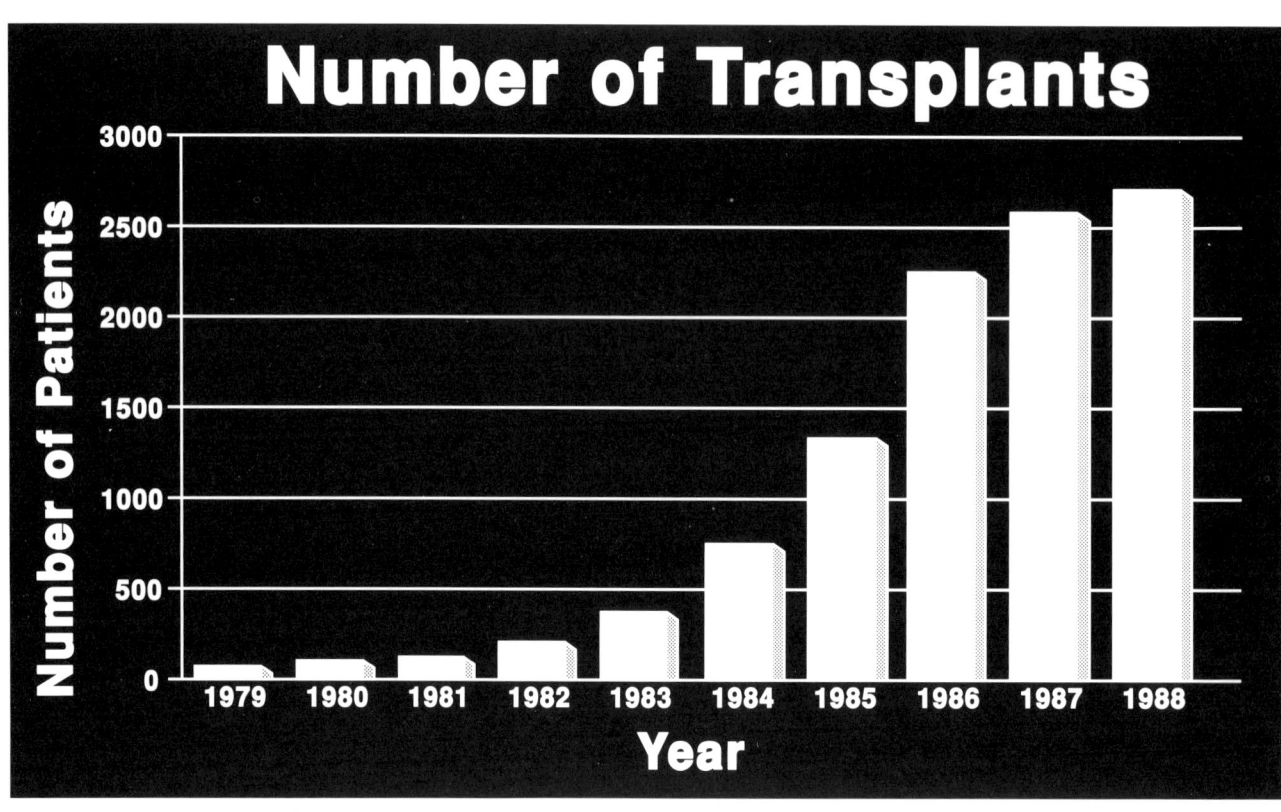

Growth in the number of heart transplants performed annually 1979–1988 as reported to the International Society for Heart Transplantation Registry (Courtesy ISHT Registry, 1989). There was no further expansion in heart transplantation in 1989.

THE TRANSPLANTATION AND REPLACEMENT OF THORACIC ORGANS

The Present Status of Biological and Mechanical Replacement of the Heart and Lungs

Edited by

DAVID K.C. COOPER, MA, MD, PhD, FRCS

*Cardiothoracic Surgeon and Director of Research and Education,
Oklahoma Transplantation Institute, Baptist Medical Center,
Oklahoma City, Oklahoma, USA
Formerly, Associate Professor of Cardiothoracic Surgery,
University of Cape Town Medical School and Groote Schuur Hospital,
Cape Town, South Africa*

and

DIMITRI NOVITZKY, MD, FCS (SA)

*Cardiothoracic Surgeon
Oklahoma Transplantation Institute, Baptist Medical Center,
Oklahoma City, Oklahoma, USA
Formerly, Specialist in Cardiothoracic Surgery,
Groote Schuur Hospital, Cape Town, South Africa*

with a Foreword by **Christiaan Barnard** and **Nazih Zuhdi**

KLUWER ACADEMIC PUBLISHERS
DORDRECHT / BOSTON / LONDON

British Library Cataloguing in Publication Data

The transplantation and replacement of thoracic organs.
 1. Man. Heart. Transplantation 2. Man. Lungs. Transplantation
 I. Cooper, D. K. C. (David K C), 1939–   II. Novitzky, Dimitri
 617'. 4120592

 ISBN 0-7923-8909-3

Library of Congress Cataloging in Publication Data

The Transplantation and replacement of thoracic organs: the present status of biological and mechanical replacement of the heart and lungs / edited by David K.C. Cooper and Dimitri Novitzky : with a foreword by Christiaan Barnard and Nazih Zuhdi.
   p. cm.
   Includes bibliographical references.
   ISBN 0-7923-8909-3 (U.S.) : £90.00 (est.)
   1. Heart—Transplantation. 2. Lungs—Transplantation.
 I. Cooper, D. K. C. (David K. C.), 1939– . II. Novitzky, Dimitri.
   [DNLM: 1. Heart Transplantation. 2. Lung Transplantation. WG 169 T772]
 RD598.35.T7T73 1990
 617.4' 120592—dc20
 DNLM/DLC
 for Library of Congress   89-71707
                                                              CIP

Distributors

for the United States and Canada: Kluwer Academic Publishers, PO Box 358, Accord Station, Hingham, MA 02018-0358, USA
for all other countries: Kluwer Academic Publishers Group, Distribution Center, PO Box 322, 3300 AH Dordrecht, The Netherlands

Copyright

© 1990 by Kluwer Academic Publishers

All rights reserved. No part of this publication may be reproduced, stored in a retrieval system, or transmitted in any form or by any means, electronic, mechanical, photocopying, recording or otherwise, without prior permission from the publishers, Kluwer Academic Publishers BV, PO Box 17, 3300 AA Dordrecht, The Netherlands.

Published in the United Kingdom by Kluwer Academic Publishers, PO Box 55, Lancaster, UK

Kluwer Academic Publishers BV incorporates the publishing programmes of D. Reidel, Martinus Nijhoff, Dr W. Junk and MTP Press.

Printed in Great Britain by Butler and Tanner Ltd., Frome and London.

Typeset by Lasertext Ltd., Thomas Street, Stretford, Manchester.

The Transplantation and Replacement of Thoracic Organs

Edited by:

DAVID K.C. COOPER AND DIMITRI NOVITZKY

With contributions by:
M.A. Acker, W.A. Anderson, G.R. Barnhart, E.D. Bateman, E. Becerra, D.W. Bethune, R.M. Bolman III, R.S. Bonser, C.R. Bridges Jr., C. Cabrol, J.S. Chaffin, F.A. Chapman, I.Y. Christlieb, P.J. Commerford, D.K.C. Cooper, J.D. Cooper, P.K. Davis, W.A.P. DeMajo, J.C. de Villiers, J.S. Dummer, J.M. Dunn, E.D. du Toit, D.M. Eich, R.W. Evans, A.A. Forder, L.S. Fragomeni, A.E. Frost, R.F. Grossman, J.D. Hardy, A. Hastillo, A. Haverich, C.F. Heck, A. Heroux, M.L. Hess, T.W. Higenbottam, A.R. Horak, S.W. Jamieson, J. Kaplan, M.P. Kaye, G.L.G. Kempeneers, W.J. Kolff, R.R. Lower, G.J. Magovern, L. Makowka, J.R. Maurer, C.G.A. McGregor, C.A. Miller, A.G. Mitchell, D.L. Modry, J.S. Muchmore, C. Muneretto, E.S. Nash, T.D. Noakes, D. Novitzky, M. Oudshoorn, W.E. Pae Jr., S.A. Parascandola, W.D. Paris, G.A. Patterson, I. Penn, D.G. Pennington, W.S. Pierce, J. Prop, S. Qian, R.J. Quigg, D. Ragsdale, A.G. Rose, S.S. Sanbar, R. Shapiro, S.J. Shumway, L.S. Smith, E. Solis, T.E. Starzl, L.W. Stephenson, M.T. Swartz, R.Y. Tarazi, J. Theodore, J. Thompson, T.R. Todd, A.G. Tzakis, C.J. Uys, J. Wallwork, R.W. Welch, A.L. Westra, D.R. Wheeldon, W.N. Wicomb, S.A. Yousem.

Contents

Foreword: *Christiaan Barnard and Nazih Zuhdi*   xi

Preface   xiii

Contributing authors   xv

Acknowledgements – Personal   xix

Acknowledgements – Journals   xx

SECTION I: ORTHOTOPIC AND HETEROTOPIC HEART TRANSPLANTATION

1. Experimental development and early clinical experience   3
   D.K.C. Cooper

2. Indications, selection and management of the recipient   11
   P.J. Commerford

3. The concept and diagnosis of brain death   19
   J.C. de Villiers

4. Medico-legal aspects   27
   L.S. Smith and S.S. Sanbar

5. Donor organ availability and transplant coordination   33
   J.S. Chaffin

6. Selection and management of the donor   41
   D.K.C. Cooper and D. Novitzky

7. Storage of the donor heart   51
   W.N. Wicomb and D.K.C. Cooper

8. Pretransplant immunological considerations   63
   E.D. du Toit, M. Oudshoorn and D.K.C. Cooper

9. Anesthetic management including cardiopulmonary bypass   71
   D.W. Bethune and D.R. Wheeldon

10. Surgical technique of orthotopic heart transplantation   75
    D.K.C. Cooper and D. Novitzky

11. Surgical technique of heterotopic heart transplantation   81
    D. Novitzky and D.K.C. Cooper

12. Immediate postoperative care and maintenance immunosuppressive therapy   89
    D.K.C. Cooper

13. Physiology and pharmacology of the transplanted heart   101
    A.R. Horak

14. Immunobiology of allograft destruction   109
    D. Novitzky and D.K.C. Cooper

15. Pathology of acute rejection   115
    A.G. Rose and C.J. Uys

16. Diagnosis and management of acute rejection   127
    D.K.C. Cooper

17. Infectious complications   143
    E.D. Bateman and A.A. Forder

18. Pathology of graft atherosclerosis (chronic rejection)   161
    A.G. Rose and C.J. Uys

19. Diagnosis and management of graft atherosclerosis (chronic rejection)   169
    D.M. Eich, R.J. Quigg, A. Heroux, A. Hastillo, J. Thompson, G.R. Barnhart, R.R. Lower and M.L. Hess

20. Retransplantation   177
    D.K.C. Cooper and D. Novitzky

#	Title	Page
21	Malignant neoplasia in the immunocompromised patient *I. Penn*	183
22	Other complications of transplantation and immunosuppressive therapy *D.K.C. Cooper, J.S. Muchmore and R.W. Welch*	191
23	Heterotopic heart transplantation – indications and special considerations *D.K.C. Cooper*	203
24	Heart transplantation in infants and children – indications and special considerations *J.M. Dunn*	209
25	Psychiatric aspects *E.S. Nash*	217
26	Medico-social aspects *W.D. Paris*	223
27	Nutrition and diet *D. Ragsdale*	227
28	Exercise rehabilitation *T.D. Noakes and G.L.G. Kempeneers*	233
29	Non-cardiac surgery in patients with heart transplants – anesthetic and operative considerations *E. Becerra and D.K.C. Cooper*	241
30	Non-cardiac autopsy findings in patients with heart (or heart–lung) transplants *A.G. Rose*	245
31	Results of cardiac transplantation and factors influencing survival. 1. International Society for Heart Transplantation Registry *C.F. Heck, L.S. Fragomeni, S.J. Shumway and M.P. Kaye*	251
32	Results of cardiac transplantation and factors influencing survival. 2. Collaborative Heart Transplant Study *D.K.C. Cooper*	257

SECTION II: TRANSPLANTATION OF THE HEART AND BOTH LUNGS

#	Title	Page
33	Experimental background and early clinical experience *E. Becerra, J. Kaplan and D.K.C. Cooper*	261
34	Indications, selection, and management of the recipient *A.G. Mitchell*	267
35	Selection of the donor; excision and storage of donor organs *A. Haverich, D. Novitzky and D.K.C. Cooper*	273
36	Anesthetic management *D.W. Bethune and D.R. Wheeldon*	283
37	Surgical technique of the recipient operation *D. Novitzky and D.K.C. Cooper*	289
38	Postoperative management, surgical complications, diagnosis and management of acute rejection *T.W. Higenbottam and J. Wallwork*	299
39	Immunological aspects *A.L. Westra and J. Prop*	307
40	Pathology of heart–lung transplantation *S.A. Yousem*	315
41	Infectious complications *J.S. Dummer*	325
42	Physiology and pharmacology of the transplanted lungs *J. Theodore*	333
43	Diagnosis and management of bronchiolitis obliterans (chronic rejection): retransplantation *R.S. Bonser, R.Y. Tarazi and S.W. Jamieson*	341
44	Results of heart–lung transplantation and factors influencing survival *D.L. Modry*	349

SECTION III: SINGLE AND DOUBLE LUNG TRANSPLANTATION

#	Title	Page
45	Experimental background and early clinical experience *J.D. Hardy*	357
46	Indications, selection and management of the recipient *A.E. Frost, R.F. Grossman and J.R. Maurer*	363
47	Selection of the donor: excision and storage of the lungs *T.R. Todd*	369

48	Anesthesia for single lung transplantation W.A.P. DeMajo	375
49	Surgical technique of single lung transplantation J.D. Cooper	381
50	Surgical technique of double lung transplantation J.D. Cooper and G.A. Patterson	385
51	Postoperative management C.G.A. McGregor	391
52	Complications G.A. Patterson	399
53	Results of lung transplantation D.K.C. Cooper, G.A. Patterson and J.D. Cooper	407

SECTION IV: THE ROLE OF MECHANICAL SUPPORT DEVICES IN CARDIAC TRANSPLANTATION

54	Indications and selection of cardiac support device D.G. Pennington and M.T. Swartz	413
55	Non-pulsatile centrifugal pumps R.M. Bolman III	417
56	Pulsatile ventricular assist devices P.K. Davis, W.E. Pae, Jr. and W.S. Pierce	423
57	Total artificial hearts E. Solis, C. Muneretto and C. Cabrol	431
58	Results of mechanical circulatory support as a 'bridge' to cardiac transplantation – Combined Registry Report W.E. Pae, Jr., S.A. Parascandola, C.A. Miller and W.S. Pierce	445

SECTION V: PERMANENT CARDIAC REPLACEMENT BY THE TOTAL ARTIFICIAL HEART

| 59 | Experimental background and current problems
W.J. Kolff | 453 |

| 60 | Clinical experience
D.K.C. Cooper | 463 |

SECTION VI: CARDIAC XENOTRANSPLANTATION

61	Xenotransplantation: overview D.K.C. Cooper	471
62	Pathology of xenograft rejection A.G. Rose	479
63	Mechanisms and possible management of hyperacute (vascular, humoral) or xenograft rejection L. Makowka, R. Shapiro, F.A. Chapman, S. Qian, A.G. Tzakis and T.E. Starzl	485
64	Clinical experience D.K.C. Cooper	493

SECTION VII: CARDIAC AUGMENTATION WITH SKELETAL MUSCLE

| 65 | Cardiomyoplasty
G.J. Magovern and I.Y. Christlieb | 497 |
| 66 | Blood pumps constructed from skeletal muscle
C.R. Bridges, Jr., W.A. Anderson, M.A. Acker and L.W. Stephenson | 503 |

SECTION VIII: THE FUTURE OF THORACIC ORGAN REPLACEMENT

67	Some ethical and logistic issues in transplantation R.W. Evans	515
68	Heart and lung replacement: future perspectives D.K.C. Cooper	523
	Index	535

Foreword

It gives us great pleasure to contribute a short introduction to this important volume.

The transplantation of thoracic organs – heart, heart–lung, lung – is a field of surgery that is expanding annually. The use of mechanical assist devices and artificial hearts to support patients awaiting transplantation is also developing rapidly, and further advances in this field may eventually lead to a totally implantable device that will function successfully for many years.

It is therefore timely that such a volume as this should be made available to those who wish to be brought up-to-date with the current state of knowledge in these related fields. The editors have done us all a great service in bringing together experts in every aspect of heart and lung transplantation and replacement to contribute to this outstanding book. This comprehensive work provides an immense fund of information, and will be an invaluable source of knowledge to physicians, surgeons, and scientists for many years to come.

April 1990

Christiaan Barnard
Cape Town, South Africa

Nazih Zuhdi
Oklahoma City, USA

Preface

The fields of the transplantation and replacement of thoracic organs have expanded immensely since the first human-to-human heart transplant was performed in 1967. This expansion has possibly been most rapid since the predecessor to this current volume was published in 1984. This previous volume, *Heart Transplantation*, co-edited by one of us with Robert Lanza, contained only one short chapter on heart–lung transplantation, a bare mention of mechanical 'bridging' devices, and essentially nothing on clinical lung transplantation. When the publishers requested a second edition, it was clear that an attempt would have to be made to cover the widening interests and activities of those involved in this field of transplantation.

The introduction of cyclosporine and increasing experience in the management of patients with heart transplants have enabled cardiac transplantation to become an accepted form of therapy with steadily improving clinical results. Improved immunosuppression and further experimental work on aspects of surgical technique have led to both heart–lung and lung transplantation becoming clinical realities. Refinements in bioengineering have enabled mechanical assist devices and the total artificial heart to support patients successfully until a suitable donor becomes available.

Already, surgeons are looking to new methods of overcoming the inadequate supply of donor hearts; the permanent placement of a mechanical device (of which there has already been a clinical trial), xenotransplantation, and myocardial augmentation by skeletal muscle are all receiving increasing attention.

With the help of a large number of experts, we have tried to put together a comprehensive review that we hope will keep the interested physician or scientist abreast of current knowledge in these various fields.

April 1990

David K.C. Cooper
Dimitri Novitzky
Oklahoma Transplantation Institute
Baptist Medical Center
Oklahoma City, Oklahoma, USA

Contributing Authors

Acker, Michael A., MD,
Instructor in Surgery, The Harrison Department of Surgical Research, Department of Surgery, University of Pennsylvania, Philadelphia, Pennsylvania, USA

Anderson, William A., MD,
Post-Doctoral Research Fellow, The Harrison Department of Surgical Research, Department of Surgery, University of Pennsylvania, Philadelphia, Pennsylvania, USA

Barnhart, Glenn R., MD,
Assistant Professor of Cardiothoracic Surgery, Medical College of Virginia, Richmond, Virginia, USA

Bateman, Eric D., MD, DCH, FRCP,
Associate Professor, Respiratory Clinic, Department of Medicine, University of Cape Town Medical School and Groote Schuur Hospital, Cape Town, South Africa

Becerra, Eduardo, MD,
Cardiothoracic Surgeon, Hospital Gustavo Fricke, Vina del Mar, Chile. Formerly, Senior Registrar, Department of Cardiothoracic Surgery, Groote Schuur Hospital, Cape Town, South Africa

Bethune, Donald, MB, BS, FFARCS,
Consultant Anesthetist, Cardiothoracic Surgical Unit, Papworth Hospital, Cambridge, UK

Bolman, R. Morton III, MD,
C. Walton and Richard C. Lillehei Professor of Cardiovascular and Thoracic Surgery, Department of Surgery, and Director, Minnesota Heart and Lung Institute, University of Minnesota Hospitals and Clinic, Minneapolis, Minnesota, USA.
Formerly, Associate Professor of Surgery, Director of Cardiac Transplantation, Washington University School of Medicine, St. Louis, Missouri, USA

Bonser, Robert S., MB, BCh, MRCP, FRCS,
Senior Registrar in Cardiothoracic Surgery, National Heart and Chest Hospitals, London, UK.
Formerly, British Heart Foundation — American Heart Association Reciprocal Fellow, Minnesota Heart and Lung Institute, University of Minnesota, Minneapolis, Minnesota, USA

Bridges, Charles R., Jr., MD, ScD,
Research Associate, The Harrison Department of Surgical Research, Department of Surgery, and Visiting Scientist, Department of Bioengineering, University of Pennsylvania, Philadelphia, Pennsylvania, USA

Cabrol, Christian, MD,
Professor and Head, Department of Cardiovascular Surgery, Hopital La Pitie–Salpetriere, Paris, France

Chaffin, John S., MD,
Cardiothoracic Surgeon, Oklahoma Transplantation Institute, Baptist Medical Center, Oklahoma City, Oklahoma, USA

Chapman, Frances A., AHT,
Research Associate, Department of Surgery, Cedars-Sinai Medical Center, Los Angeles, California.
Formerly, Research Specialist, Department of Surgery, University Health Center of Pittsburgh, University of Pittsburgh, Pittsburgh, Pennsylvania, USA

Christlieb, Ignacio Y., MD,
Director, Thoracic Surgical Research, Allegheny-Singer Research Institute, Pittsburgh, Pennsylvania, USA

Commerford, Patrick J., MB, ChB, FCP (SA),
Helen and Morris Mauerberger Professor of Cardiology, Department of Medicine, University of Cape Town Medical School and Groote Schuur Hospital, Cape Town, South Africa

Cooper, David K.C., MA, MD, PhD, FRCS,
Cardiothoracic Surgeon and Director of Research and Education, Oklahoma Transplantation Institute, Baptist Medical Center, Oklahoma City, Oklahoma, USA.
Formerly, Associate Professsor of Cardiothoracic Surgery, University of Cape Town Medical School and Groote Schuur Hospital, Cape Town, South Africa

Cooper, Joel D., MD, FRCS(C),
Professor of Surgery, and Head of the Section of Thoracic Surgery, Division of Cardiothoracic Surgery, Washington University School of Medicine, St. Louis, Missouri, USA.
Formerly, Professor of Surgery and Head of the Department of Thoracic Surgery, Toronto General Hospital, Toronto, Ontario, Canada

Davis, Paul K., MD,
Resident in Cardiothoracic Surgery, Division of Cardiothoracic Surgery, Department of Surgery, College of Medicine, Milton S. Hershey Medical Center, The Pennsylvania State University, Hershey, Pennsylvania, USA

DeMajo, Wilfred A.P., MD,
Anesthesiologist, Department of Anesthesiology, Toronto General Hospital, Toronto, Ontario, Canada

de Villiers, J.C., MD, FRCS, FRCS(Ed),
Helen and Morris Mauerberger, Professor and Head, Department of Neurosurgery, University of Cape Town Medical School and Groote Schuur Hospital, Cape Town, South Africa

Dummer, J. Stephen, MD,
Associate Professor of Medicine and Surgery, Department of Infectious Diseases and Microbiology, University of Pittsburgh, Pittsburgh, Pennsylvania, USA

Dunn, Jeffrey M., MD,
Professor of Surgery and Director, Pediatric Heart Institute, St. Christopher's Hospital for Children and Temple University School of Medicine, Philadelphia, Pennsylvania, USA

du Toit, Ernette D., MD,
Head, Provincial Laboratory for Tissue Immunology, Cape Town, South Africa

Eich, David M., MD,
Fellow, Division of Cardiology, Medical College of Virginia, Richmond, Virginia, USA

Evans, Roger W., PhD,
Senior Research Scientist, Health and Population Research Center, Battelle Human Affairs Research Centers, Seattle, Washington, USA

Forder, Arderne A., MB, ChB, MMed(Path),
Wernher and Beit Professor and Head, Department of Medical Microbiology, University of Cape Town Medical School and Groote Schuur Hospital, Cape Town, South Africa

Fragomeni, Luis S., MD,
Visiting Professor, Minnesota Heart and Lung Institute, University of Minnesota, Minneapolis, Minnesota, USA

Frost, Adaani E., MD,
Clinical Research Fellow, Toronto Lung Transplant Group, University of Toronto, Toronto, Ontario, Canada

Grossman, Ronald F., MD, FRCP(C),
Associate Professor of Medicine, University of Toronto, and Head, Respiratory Division, Mount Sinai Hospital, Toronto, Ontario, Canada

Hardy, James D., MD,
Veterans Administration Distinguished Physician, Professor Emeritus of Surgery, and formerly Chairman, Department of Surgery, University of Mississippi Medical Center, Jackson, Mississippi, USA

Hastillo, Andrea, MD,
Associate Professor, Division of Cardiology, Medical College of Virginia, Richmond, Virginia, USA

Haverich, Axel, MD,
Cardiothoracic Surgeon, Department of Cardiothoracic Surgery, Hannover Medical School, Hannover, West Germany

Heck, Christopher F., MD,
Senior Surgical Resident, University of California, San Francisco, California, USA.
Formerly, Medtronic Research Fellow, University of Minnesota Cardiovascular Research Laboratory, Minneapolis, Minnesota, USA

Heroux, Alain, MD,
Cardiac Transplant Fellow, Division of Cardiology, Medical College of Virginia, Richmond, Virginia, USA

Hess, Michael L., MD,
Professor of Medicine, Division of Cardiology, Medical College of Virginia, Richmond, Virginia, USA

Higenbottam, Tim W., BSc, MD, FRCP,
Consultant Physician and Co-director, Heart–lung Transplant Research Unit, Papworth Hospital, Cambridge, UK

Horak, Adrian R., MB., ChB, FCP(SA),
Cardiologist, Department of Medicine, Groote Schuur Hospital, Cape Town, South Africa

Jamieson, Stuart W., MB, BS, FRCS,
Professor and Head, Division of Cardiothoracic Surgery, University of California, San Diego, California, USA.
Formerly, Professor of Thoracic and Cardiovascular Surgery, Minnesota Heart and Lung Institute, University of Minnesota, Minneapolis, Minnesota, USA

Kaplan, Jorge, MD,
Cardiothoracic Surgeon, Hospital Gustavo Fricke, Vina del Mar, Chile

Kaye, Michael P., MD,
Professor, Division of Cardiothoracic Surgery, University of California, San Diego, California, USA.
Formerly, Professor of Cardiothoracic Surgery, Minnesota Heart and Lung Institute, University of Minnesota, Minneapolis, Minnesota, USA

Kempeneers, Gerrit L.G., B.Sc. (Hons),
Research Student, Medical Research Council/University of Cape Town Bioenergetics of Exercise Research Unit, Department of Physiology, University of Cape Town Medical School, Cape Town, South Africa

Kolff, Willem J., MD, PhD,
Distinguished Professor of Medicine and Surgery, Department of Surgery, Division of Artificial Organs, University of Utah, Salt Lake City, Utah, USA

Lower, Richard R., MD,
Formerly, Professor and Chairman, Department of Cardiac Surgery, Medical College of Virginia, Richmond, Virginia, USA

Magovern, George J., MD,
Chairman, Division of Thoracic Surgery, Department of Surgery, Allegheny General Hospital, and Professor of Surgery, Medical College of Pennsylvania, Pittsburgh, Pennsylvania, USA

Makowka, Leonard, MD, PhD, FRCS(C),
Director of Surgery and Transplantation Services, Department of Surgery, Cedars-Sinai Medical Center, Los Angeles, California, USA.
Formerly, Associate Professor of Surgery, University of Pittsburgh School of Medicine, Pittsburgh, Pennsylvania, USA

Maurer, Janet R., MD, ABIM, FRCP(C),
Assistant Professor of Medicine, University of Toronto, Toronto, Ontario, Canada

McGregor, Christopher G.A., MB, BS, FRCS(Ed and Glas),
Consultant Surgeon, Section of Thoracic and Cardiovascular Surgery, Mayo Clinic, and Associate Professor of Surgery, Mayo Medical School, Rochester, Minnesota, USA

Miller, Cynthia A., BS,
Senior Research Technician, Division of Cardiothoracic Surgery, Milton S. Hershey Medical Center, The Pennsylvania State University, Hershey, Pennsylvania, USA

Mitchell, Andrew G., BA, BM, BCh, MRCP,
Cardiologist, Harefield Hospital, Middlesex, UK

Modry, Dennis L., MD, MSc, FRCS(C),
Cardiovascular and Thoracic Surgeon, and Director, Division of Cardiovascular and Thoracic Surgery, Faculty of Medicine, University of Alberta, Edmonton, Alberta, Canada

Muchmore, John S., MD, PhD,
Endocrinologist, Baptist Medical Center, Oklahoma City, Oklahoma, USA

Muneretto, Claudio, MD,
Resident, Department of Cardiovascular Surgery, Hopital La Pitie-Salpetriere, Paris, France

Nash, Eleanor S., MB, ChB, FRCP(Ed), DPM, FFPsych(SA),
Associate Professor, Department of Psychiatry, University of Cape Town Medical School and Groote Schuur Hospital, Cape Town, South Africa

Noakes, Timothy D., MD,
Associate Professor and Director, Medical Research Council/University of Cape Town Bioenergetics of Exercise Research Unit, Department of Physiology, University of Cape Town Medical School, Cape Town, South Africa

Novitzky, Dimitri, MD, FCS(SA),
Cardiothoracic Surgeon, Oklahoma Transplantation Institute, Baptist Medical Center, Oklahoma City, Oklahoma, USA.
Formerly, Specialist in Cardiothoracic Surgery, Groote Schuur Hospital, Cape Town, South Africa

Oudshoorn, Machteld, M.Sc.,
Senior Medical Natural Scientist, Provincial Laboratory for Tissue Immunology, Cape Town, South Africa

Pae, Walter E., Jr., MD,
Associate Professor of Surgery, Division of Cardiothoracic Surgery, Milton S. Hershey Medical Center, The Pennsylvania State University, Hershey, Pennsylvania, USA

Parascandola, Salvatore A., MD,
Research Fellow, Division of Cardiothoracic Surgery, Milton S. Hershey Medical Center, The Pennsylvania State University, Hershey, Pennsylvania, USA

Paris, Wayne D., MSW,
Clinical Social Worker, Baptist Medical Center, Oklahoma City, Oklahoma, USA

Patterson, G. Alexander, MD,
Thoracic Surgeon and Director, Lung Transplantation, Toronto General Hospital, Toronto, Ontario, Canada

Penn, Israel, MD,
Professor of Surgery, College of Medicine, University of Cincinnati Medical School, Cincinnati, Ohio, USA

Pennington, D. Glenn, MD,
Cardiothoracic Surgeon and Director, Heart Replacement Service, Department of Surgery, St. Louis University, St. Louis, Missouri, USA

Pierce, William S., MD,
Evan Pugh and Jane A. Fetter Professor of Surgery and Chief, Division of Artificial Organs, Department of Surgery, Milton S. Hershey Medical Center, The Pennsylvania State University, Hershey, Pennsylvania, USA

Prop, Jochum, MD, PhD,
Staff Member, Cardiopulmonary Surgery Research Division, Thoraxcentrum, University Hospital, Groningen, The Netherlands

Qian, Shiguang, MD,
Transplant Research Fellow, Department of Surgery, University Health Center of Pittsburgh, University of Pittsburgh, Pittsburgh, Pennsylvania, USA

Quigg, Rebecca J., MD,
Assistant Professor of Medicine, Division of Cardiology, Medical College of Virginia, Richmond, Virginia, USA

Ragsdale, Deanna, MS, RD,
Dietician, Department of Nutrition and Dietetics, Methodist Hospital of Indiana, Indianapolis, Indiana, USA

Rose, Alan G., MD, MMed(Path), MRCPath,
Wernher and Beit Professor and Head, Department of Pathology, University of Cape Town Medical School and Groote Schuur Hospital, Cape Town, South Africa

Sanbar, S. Sandy, MD, PhD, JD, FCLM,
Cardiologist, Baptist Medical Center, Oklahoma City, Oklahoma, USA.
President, American College of Legal Medicine

Shapiro, Ron, MD,
Assistant Professor of Surgery, Department of Surgery, University Health Center of Pittsburgh, University of Pittsburgh, Pittsburgh, Pennsylvania, USA

Shumway, Sara J., MD,
Assistant Professor of Cardiothoracic Surgery, Minnesota Heart and Lung Institute, University of Minnesota, Minneapolis, Minnesota, USA

Smith, L.S., MB, BCh, DPH, DBact, FRCPath,
Professor, Faculty of Law, University of Southern Africa.
Formerly, Professor and Head, Department of Forensic Medicine and Toxicology, University of Cape Town Medical School, Cape Town, South Africa

Solis, Eduardo, MD,
Resident, Department of Cardiovascular Surgery, Hopital La Pitie-Salpetriere, Paris, France

Starzl, Thomas E., MD, PhD,
Professor of Surgery, Department of Surgery, University Health Center of Pittsburgh, University of Pittsburgh, Pittsburgh, Pennsylvania, USA

Stephenson, Larry W., MD,
Professor and Chief, Division of Cardiothoracic Surgery, Harper Hospital, Wayne State University, Detroit, Michigan, USA.
Formerly, J. William White Professor of Surgery, Harrison Department of Surgical Research, Department of Surgery, Division of Cardiothoracic Surgery, University of Pennsylvania, Philadelphia, Pennsylvania, USA

Swartz, Marc T., BA,
Division of Circulatory Support, Department of Surgery, St. Louis University, St. Louis, Missouri, USA

Tarazi, Riyad Y., MD,
Assistant Professor of Thoracic and Cardiovascular Surgery, Minnesota Heart and Lung Institute, University of Minnesota, Minneapolis, and Chief, Cardiac Surgery, St. Paul-Ramsey Hospital, St. Paul, Minnesota, USA

Theodore, James, MD,
Pulmonologist and Associate Professor, Department of Medicine, Stanford University Medical School, Palo Alto, California, USA

Thompson, James, MD,
Assistant Professor of Medicine, Division of Cardiology, Medical College of Virginia, Richmond, Virginia, USA

Todd, Thomas R., MD, FRCS(C),
Associate Professor, Department of Thoracic Surgery, University of Toronto and Toronto General Hospital, Toronto, Ontario, Canada

Tzakis, Andreas G., MD,
Assistant Professor of Surgery, Department of Surgery, University Health Center of Pittsburgh, University of Pittsburgh, Pittsburgh, Pennsylvania, USA

Uys, Cornelius J., MD, DClinPath, FRCPath,
Formerly, Wernher and Beit Professor and Head, Department of Pathology, University of Cape Town Medical School and Groote Schuur Hospital, Cape Town, South Africa

Wallwork, John, BSc, MB, BS, FRCS(Ed),
Cardiothoracic Surgeon and Co-director, Heart-lung Transplant Research Unit, Papworth Hospital, Cambridge, UK

Welch, Richard W., MS, MD,
Gastroenterologist, Baptist Medical Center, Oklahoma City, Oklahoma, USA

Westra, Albertine L., MD,
Research Fellow, Cardiopulmonary Surgery Research Division, Thoraxcentrum, University Hospital, Groningen, The Netherlands

Wheeldon, Derek R., MIBiol.,
Senior Research Technician, Cardiothoracic Surgical Unit, Papworth Hospital, Cambridge, UK

Wicomb, Winston N., PhD,
Director, Organ Preservation, Medical Research Institute, Pacific Presbyterian Medical Center, San Francisco, California, USA

Yousem, Samuel A., MD,
Assistant Professor of Pathology, Presbyterian-University Hospital, Pittsburgh, Pennsylvania, USA

Acknowledgements–Personal

Firstly, we record our appreciation to our mentors and friends, Chris Barnard and Nazih Zuhdi, both men of great vision, for honoring us by contributing the *Foreword* to this volume, and for the stimuli they have provided for our own work in the field of transplantation.

We should like to couple their names with those of Kenneth Bonds and Stanley Hupfeld, respectively Chairman and President of the Oklahoma Healthcare Corporation, and Thomas Lynn, Vice-President of Medical Staff Affairs, Baptist Medical Center, who have supported our clinical and research activities so strongly since we joined the Oklahoma Transplantation Institute at Baptist Medical Center in early 1987.

We wish to express our appreciation to our co-authors, who have contributed their knowledge, experience, and time in the preparation of this book.

Several of our colleagues at Baptist Medical Center in Oklahoma City have advised us on aspects of this work, amongst them Janita Ardis, Charles Barton, Carol Blackwell Imes, Merle Carter, Mel Clark, J.W. Greenawalt, Jay Harolds, Tommy Hewitt, John Huff, Marilyn Kanoski, Neil Kimerer, William Lanehart, Dennis Parker and Vadakepat Ramgopal. Jack Kolff, MD, of Philadelphia, USA, David White, PhD, of Cambridge, UK, and Fritz Bach, MD, of Minneapolis, USA, have also kindly advised on certain sections of the book, and a visiting fellow at our center, Chiara Liguori, MD, helped check several points in the text. We extend our thanks to all of them (and to any others we may have inadvertently omitted).

The excellent surgical drawings are the work of Jenny Kukielski, and the equally fine charts and graphs that of Carolyn Martel. The photographic work was shared by John Philbin of the Department of ProGraphics of Baptist Medical Center and Carolyn Martel. We gratefully acknowledge their respective expertise and skills.

The entire manuscript was typed or re-typed most efficiently and accurately by Crystal Taylor, of CompOne Services, Oklahoma City, to whom we are greatly indebted. Much secretarial help was given to us by Sue Colliver and Kelly Ward of the Oklahoma Transplantation Institute, and Pattie King of CompOne Services. Joyce Metzer, medical library assistant at Baptist Medical Center, kindly took responsibility for ensuring the accuracy of the numerous references cited, and Bill Jackson, one of our heart transplant recipients, contributed invaluable assistance by checking the order of the references, figures and tables quoted in the text. We thank them all for the many hours they have put into this project.

Finally, we take this opportunity to thank the many members of the medical, nursing and paramedical staff of Baptist Medical Center, who have provided the immense help and expertise that have been invaluable to the establishment of our thoracic organ transplantation program.

April 1990

David K.C. Cooper
Dimitri Novitzky
Oklahoma Transplantation Institute
Baptist Medical Center
Oklahoma City, Oklahoma, USA

Acknowledgements–Journals

We gratefully acknowledge permission to reproduce tables and illustrations either previously published in, or modified from, the following journals: *Annals of Thoracic Surgery, Archives of Pathology and Laboratory Medicine, British Journal of Clinical Practice, Journal of the American Medical Association, Journal of Heart Transplantation, Medicine and Science in Sports and Exercise, New England Journal of Medicine, South African Medical Journal, Thorax, Transplantation.*

Section I

Orthotopic and heterotopic heart transplantation

1
Experimental Development and Early Clinical Experience

D.K.C. COOPER

INTRODUCTION

Clinical heart transplantation was made possible by the considerable experimental work carried out earlier this century which embraced mainly the technical, physiological and immunological aspects of the procedure. This chapter endeavours to review briefly the evolution and results of experimental surgical techniques utilized by cardiac transplant research workers; a comprehensive review appears elsewhere[1].

Experimental work on cardiac transplantation evolved through several overlapping phases. In the earliest experiments animals were given a second, often parasatic, heart which enabled certain physiological, pharmacological and pathological studies to be made. Initially, the neck was chosen as the locus, though the abdomen and inguinal regions were occasionally used. The subsequent evolution of surgical techniques permitted the insertion of the donor heart into the chest as an auxiliary pump in circuit with the recipient organ. With the advent of hypothermia and the pump-oxygenator, total excision and replacement of the recipient heart became more feasible. Finally, after technical and physiological problems had been studied and minimized, efforts were made to combat the immune response with immunosuppressive agents.

TRANSPLANTATION OF AN ACCESSORY HEART

The first reported attempts at experimental heart transplantation were by Carrel (Figure 1.1) and Guthrie in 1905[2,3]. The principal technique they used is inadequately described as 'anastomosing the cut ends of the jugular vein and the carotid artery to the aorta, the pulmonary artery, one of the vena cava and a pulmonary vein'. Although contractions of the donor atria appeared immediately, effective contractions of the ventricles did not begin for approximately 1 hour. The experiment was interrupted after a further 2 hours when coagulation occurred in the cavities of the heart.

The crucial factor of donor coronary perfusion (viviperfusion) was simplified in 1933 when Mann and his colleagues developed a technique of cervical transplantation[4] (Figure 1.2). Numerous investigators have subsequently used modifications of the Mann technique to study problems of heart transplantation and the response of the denervated heart to

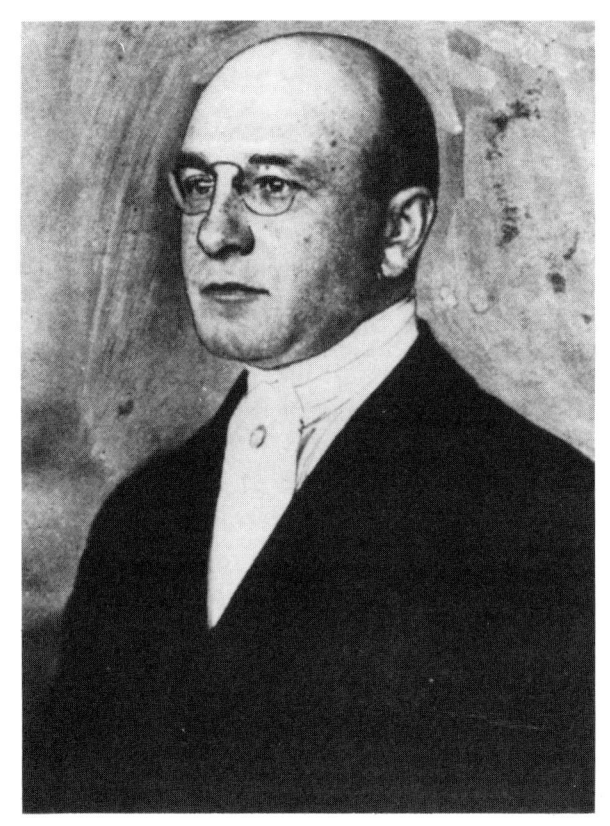

Figure 1.1 Alexis Carrel was awarded the Nobel Prize for Physiology and Medicine in 1912, primarily for his work on the anastomosis of blood vessels

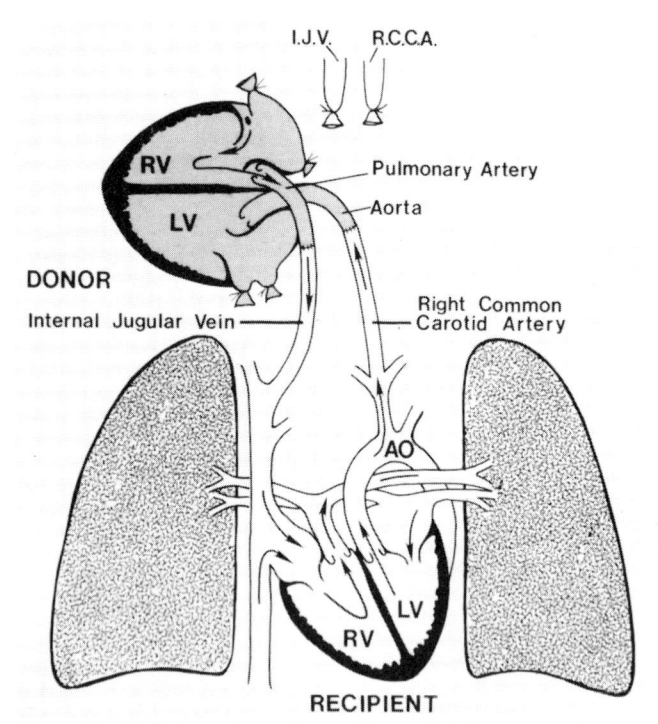

Figure 1.2 Technique of experimental heterotopic heart transplantation in the neck (Mann et al., 1933)[4]. I.J.V. = internal jugular vein; R.C.C.A. = right common carotid artery

pharmacological agents and physiological stresses[1]. One such modification remains a standard model in many laboratories, including our own, for experimental animal studies on acute rejection and immunosuppression (Figure 1.3).

From their results, Mann and his co-investigators concluded that a functioning cardiac allograft was no less 'resistant' than a renal allograft, the graft failing to survive due to the same 'biologic factor' which also prevented survival of other homo (allo) transplanted tissues and organs. Such a transplanted heart, however, proved a valuable test object for the investigation of various physiological problems. For example, the effect of the intravenous administration of thyroxine to the host animal was investigated; the denervated donor heart was demonstrated to be more sensitive to the accelerating influence of the drug, since central nervous system influence was inhibitory.

In more recent years, techniques for transplanting the auxiliary donor heart into the abdomen of the recipient have been described, principally for the study of the immune response and its modification by therapeutic agents (Figure 1.4); using microsurgical techniques, it remains an important experimental model in rats[5,6].

THE TRANSPLANTED HEART AS AN AUXILIARY INTRATHORACIC PUMP

In 1946, Demikhov (Figure 33.1) began extensive studies on transplantation of the heart into the thorax. These involved the addition of a second heart (occasionally with an attached lobe of a lung) as an auxiliary pump, as well as orthotopic transplantation of the heart with and without both lungs[7]. The ambitious nature of Demikhov's attempts can be appreciated best when it is remembered that supportive techniques, such as hypothermia and cardiopulmonary bypass, had not yet been developed.

In all, Demikhov described 24 variants of his technique to place an additional heart within the thorax, performing 250 operations on dogs utilizing most of the major vessels within the chest cavity. Few animals survived more than a few days, most of the early deaths being associated with

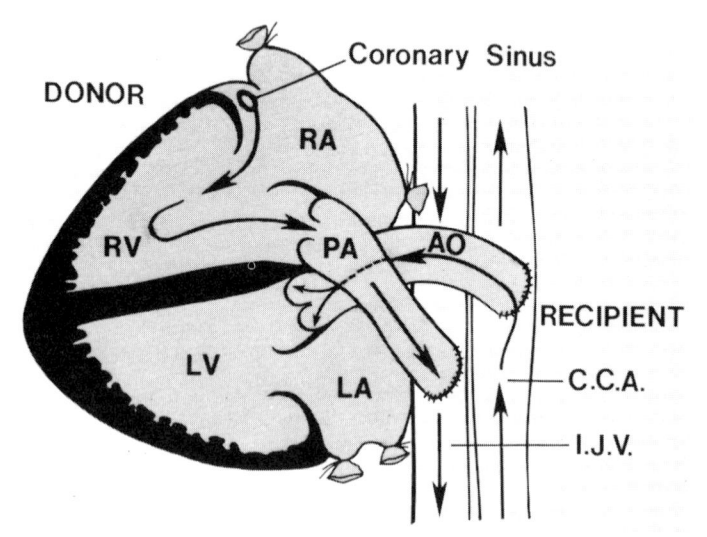

Figure 1.3 Modification of the Mann experimental cervical heterotopic heart transplantation technique[4] as used in our own laboratory

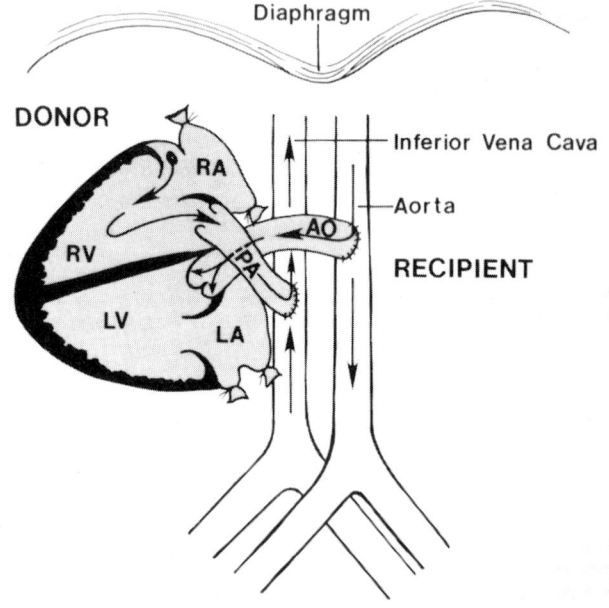

Figure 1.4 Technique of experimental heterotopic heart transplantation in the abdomen (Abbott et al., 1964)[5]

technical problems. The best results with regard to functional activity of the transplanted heart and preservation of its structure were obtained after operations using the technique illustrated in Figure 1.5. Physiologically, the transplanted heart was distinguished by the comparative constancy of its rhythm and by its greater resistance to the action of toxic doses of various cardiac glycosides. The physiological and pharmacological responses of the denervated, transplanted heart are discussed more fully in Chapter 13.

In 1964, Reemtsma[8] described a method of inserting an additional intrathoracic heart as an auxiliary pump, which was similar in principle to that later developed and used clinically in the heterotopic heart transplant program in Cape Town[9,10]. The donor inferior vena cava was anastomosed to the recipient's right atrial appendage, followed by anastomosis of the two left atrial appendages, and end-to-side anastomoses of the two pulmonary arteries and aortae. Function as an auxiliary pump was maintained for a maximum period of 72 hours.

One year later, Sen and his colleagues described a further technique in which the transplanted heart supported only the systemic circulation of the recipient[11]. This auxiliary heart functioned in one animal for 48 hours, when it was surgically excised and the animal supported solely by its own heart once again, thus demonstrating the heterotopic heart transplant as a temporary left ventricular assist device.

ORTHOTOPIC TRANSPLANTATION OF THE HEART

On 25 December 1951 – a date which surely tells us a great deal about this surgeon – Demikhov made the first recorded attempt to replace the heart alone[7]. Without the availability of hypothermia or pump-oxygenator support, the technique was necessarily complicated. The procedure consisted of end-to-side anastomoses between the corresponding thoracic aortae, superior and inferior venae cavae, and pulmonary arteries. The two inferior pulmonary veins of the donor were joined together and connected to the recipient's left atrial appendage. After these anastomoses, the ascending part of the recipient's thoracic aorta and pulmonary artery were ligated, and the recipient's left atrium was indrawn at its border with the ventricle by means of a purse-string suture. The entire segment of the recipient's heart thus excluded from the circulation was then excised.

Demikhov performed this procedure on 22 occasions, and in 1955 was successful in obtaining good cardiac function in two cases for periods of just over 11 and 15 hours, respectively. In all but one case, death resulted from technical problems. These were amongst the first reported experiments, however, where animals survived for a few hours solely on the activity of a transplanted heart.

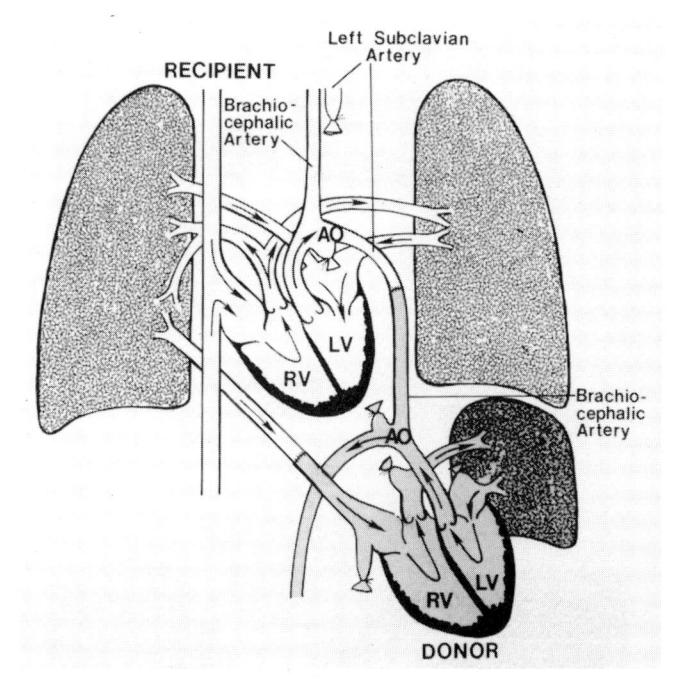

Figure 1.5 Technique of insertion of the heterotopic heart in the chest as an auxiliary pump (Demikhov, 1962)[7]

ADVENT OF SUPPORTIVE TECHNIQUES

With the advent of methods of supporting the recipient during the operative procedure, workers in this field became more ambitious. Significant early attempts were made by Neptune and his colleagues, using hypothermia[12], by Webb and Howard[13,14] and by Goldberg and Berman[15,16], both using mechanical pump-oxygenator support.

In 1959, Cass and Brock reported six attempts at autotransplantation and homotransplantation using a modification of Goldberg's technique, where both atria were left intact in the recipient, thus simplifying the procedure[17]. Anastomoses of the atria, aorta and pulmonary artery were now all that were required. This procedure was described independently 1 year later at Stanford Medical School by Lower (Figure 1.6) and Shumway (Figure 1.7), who obtained the first consistently successful results[18]. With further modifications made by Barnard[19], the technique is now used in the clinical operation of orthotopic heart transplantation and is described in detail in Chapter 10.

It was, therefore, not until 1960 that the major experimental advance was made, when Lower and Shumway reported that five out of eight consecutive dogs undergoing transplantation had lived for 6–21 days[18,20]. During convalescence the dogs eat and exercised normally, the pulse rate was variable and increased moderately with exercise, and only a few hours before death the ECG remained virtually normal, showing no evidence of arrhythmia or conduction defects. After death, microscopical examination of sections of myocardium demonstrated severe myocarditis, with massive round cell infiltration, patchy necrosis, interstitial hemor-

USE OF PROFOUND HYPOTHERMIA

Orthotopic transplantation performed in puppies under profound hypothermia, rather than with a pump-oxygenator, was described by Kondo and his colleagues in 1965[31]. Total body cooling by iced water immersion of both recipient (to 16–17°C rectally) and donor (to 27–29°C) was carried out, allowing complete circulatory arrest of the recipient for the 45-minute operation. Heart massage was begun immediately after the anastomoses were completed. After being warmed to 26–28°C by body immersion and flushing of the chest cavity with warm saline, the heart was electrically defibrillated, and rewarming continued until the temperature returned to normal. One animal remained alive and well 112 days after operation.

PROLONGATION OF GRAFT SURVIVAL BY IMMUNOSUPPRESSION

When many of the technical and physiological problems had been overcome, investigators turned their attention

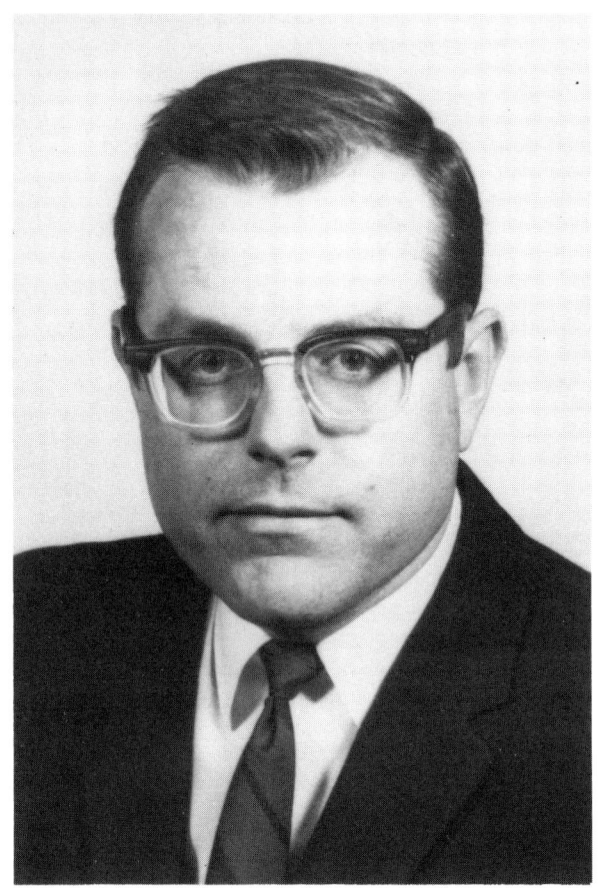

Figure 1.6 Richard Lower, who worked with Norman Shumway at Stanford Medical School over many years, and performed much of the early experimental work on heart transplantation. He subsequently set up the heart transplant program at the Medical College of Virginia

rhage, and edema. The authors concluded that in all likelihood the graft would have continued to function for the normal life span of the animal if the immunologic mechanisms of the host had been suppressed.

These investigators and their colleagues subsequently studied autotransplantation[21,22] and allotransplantation[23,25] of the heart, achieving long-term survival, and contributing extensively to our knowledge of this subject[26-28]. In the experimental animal the transplanted heart was found to have the capacity to increase cardiac output under a variety of physiological stresses; a normal cardiac output was demonstrated 1 year after allotransplantation and 5 years 6 months after autotransplantation; evidence of autonomic reinnervation of the heart after autotransplantation was obtained.

Beginning in 1962, Willman and his colleagues produced the first of several papers on the subject of myocardial structure and function following autotransplantation of the heart[29], including autotransplantation in the primate[30].

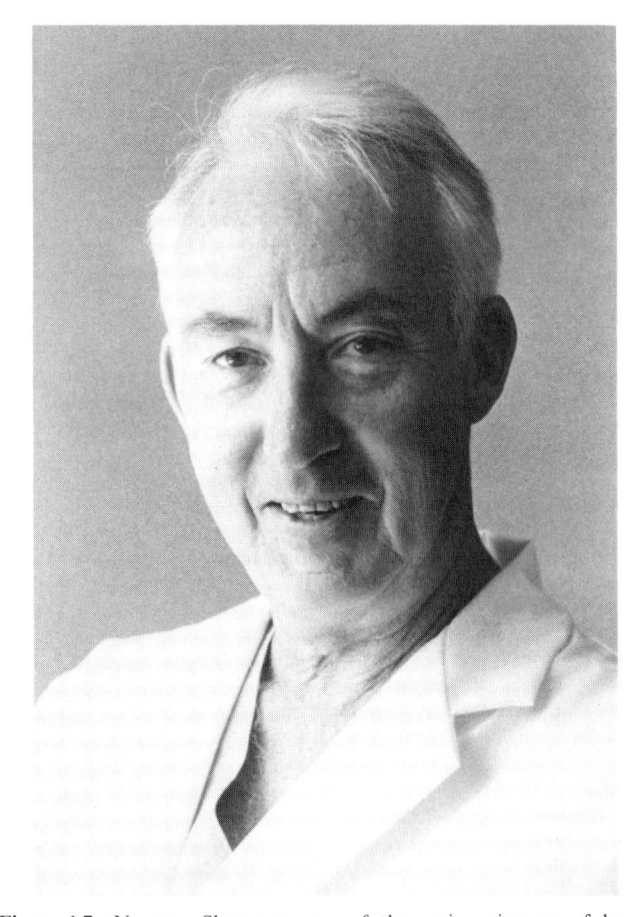

Figure 1.7 Norman Shumway, one of the major pioneers of heart transplantation. Much of the experimental work that led to the initiation of clinical heart transplantation was carried out in Shumway's laboratory at Stanford Medical School

EXPERIMENTAL DEVELOPMENT

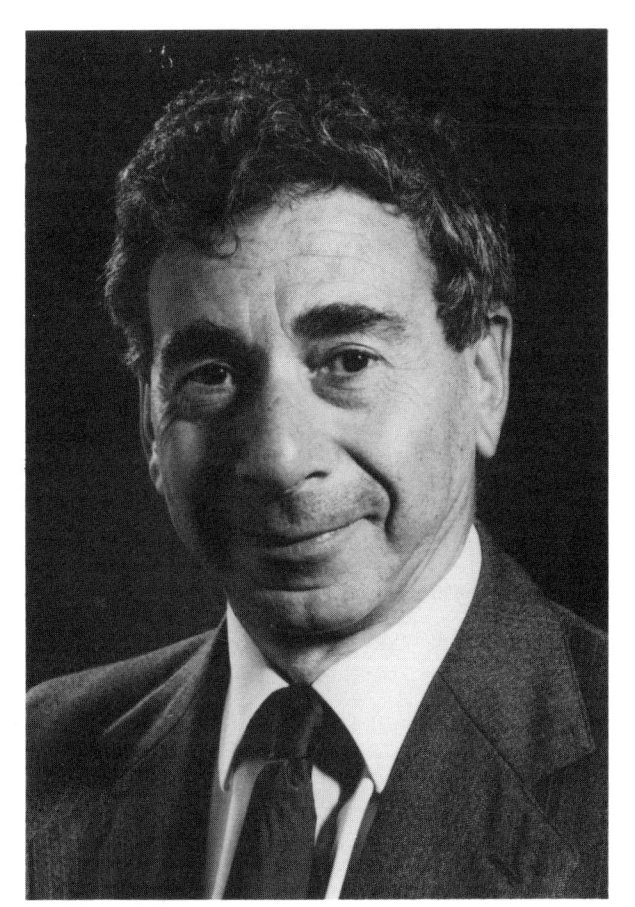

Figure 1.8 Sir Roy Calne, of Cambridge University, who was responsible for the introduction of azathioprine as an immunosuppressive agent in transplantation. Later, with David White, he carried out much of the experimental work on cyclosporine, and was the first to use this drug in a clinical transplant program

to the problem of combating the immune response by chemotherapy. Reemtsma and his colleagues used Mann's cervical transplantation technique to study the effect of methotrexate, a folic acid antagonist[32]. In a control series of untreated dogs, cardiac activity continued for a maximum of only 10 days, whereas in the methotrexate-treated group maximal survival extended to 27 days. When the recipient was given azathioprine, a drug introduced as an immunosuppressive agent by Calne (Figure 1.8), the maximal survival was 32 days[8]. Blumenstock and his colleagues, using methotrexate in dogs with orthotopic transplants, obtained five dogs that survived from 12 to 42 days[33].

The Stanford group reported its experience with a combination of steroids (hydrocortisone or methylprednisolone) and azathioprine or mercaptopurine, achieving a mean survival of 17 days, in comparison to 7 days in control dogs[25]. Six further dogs were given immunosuppressant drugs only during threatened rejection, as demonstrated by diminution of the R-wave voltage in all leads of the ECG, which had previously been found to accompany immune rejection of the cardiac allograft; five of the six dogs survived for over a month, and three for over 3 months.

CARDIAC TRANSPLANTATION IN MAN – FIRST ATTEMPT USING A XENOGRAFT

By the mid-1960s a considerable fund of knowledge had been acquired. The increasing success of experimental cardiac transplantation led Hardy (Figure 1.9) and his colleagues at the University of Mississippi to consider heart transplantation in man. This group had considerable experience of cardiac and lung transplantation in animals, and had carried out the first lung transplant in man[34] (Chapter 45).

In 1964, they reported their attempt to transplant the heart of a large chimpanzee into the chest of a 68-year-old man with hypertensive cardiovascular disease, widespread atheroma, and evidence of previous myocardial infarction[35]. Before operation the patient deteriorated suddenly and passed into terminal shock. He was taken to the operating room and supported by a pump-oxygenator just as effective heart action ceased. As no human donor was available, and as some of the members of the group had been impressed

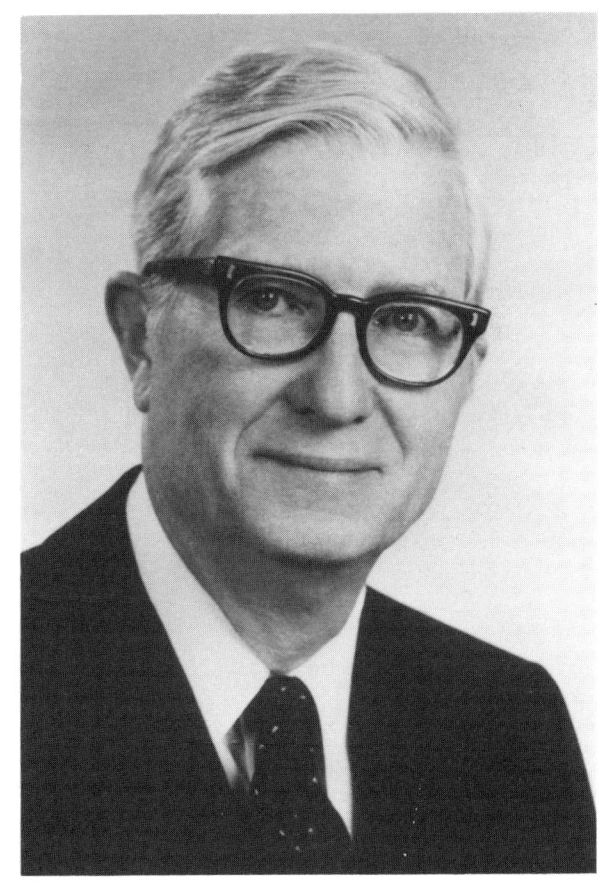

Figure 1.9 James Hardy, who, in 1963, led the team that performed the world's first single lung transplant, and, in the following year, the first heart transplant. In this latter operation, he used a chimpanzee as donor

by the early results of kidney xenografts from chimpanzees to man reported by Reemtsma et al.[36], the heart of a 96 lb (43.6 kg) chimpanzee was used for orthotopic transplantation. After defibrillation, the donor heart beat regularly and forcefully, but it soon became apparent that the rather small heart would not be able to support the circulation unless its rate were increased. The heart was paced at 100 beats per minute to maintain a systolic blood pressure of 60–90 mmHg. About 1 hour after the removal of the bypass catheters, however, the heart was judged incapable of accepting a large venous return without intermittent decompression by manual massage. Further support was abandoned.

THE FIRST HUMAN-TO-HUMAN HEART TRANSPLANT

After nearly 4 years and much further experimental work, another attempt was reported. Barnard (Figure 1.10) and his colleagues performed the first human-to-human heart transplantation on a 57-year-old man with ischemic heart disease at Groote Schuur Hospital in Cape Town on the

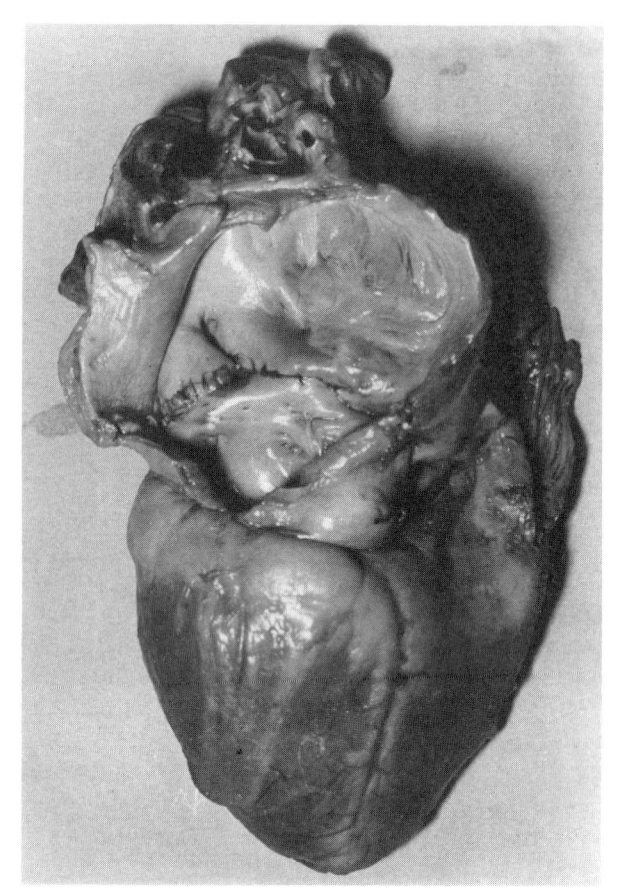

Figure 1.11 Postmortem appearance of the donor heart from the first human-to-human heart transplant. The atrial suture line can clearly be seen. Histopathologic features of mild to moderate acute rejection were present on microscopic examination

night of the 2nd–3rd December 1967[37]. The operative procedure was successful, and the patient's orthotopically transplanted heart functioned satisfactorily throughout the early postoperative course. Immunosuppression was with azathioprine and corticosteroids. Like many patients who followed, however, he developed pneumonia, and died on the 18th postoperative day. At autopsy his transplanted heart showed features of mild to moderate acute rejection (Figure 1.11)[38].

The first patient who could realistically be acclaimed as a 'long-term' survivor was operated on in Cape Town 1 month later. This 60-year-old patient lived an active and full life for over 1 1/2 years until he died from the hitherto undescribed complication of chronic rejection[39].

EARLY CLINICAL PROGRESS

The initial enthusiasm for heart transplantation waned as the problems of acute rejection and infection became apparent to those who had embarked upon a transplant program without a full understanding of the complications

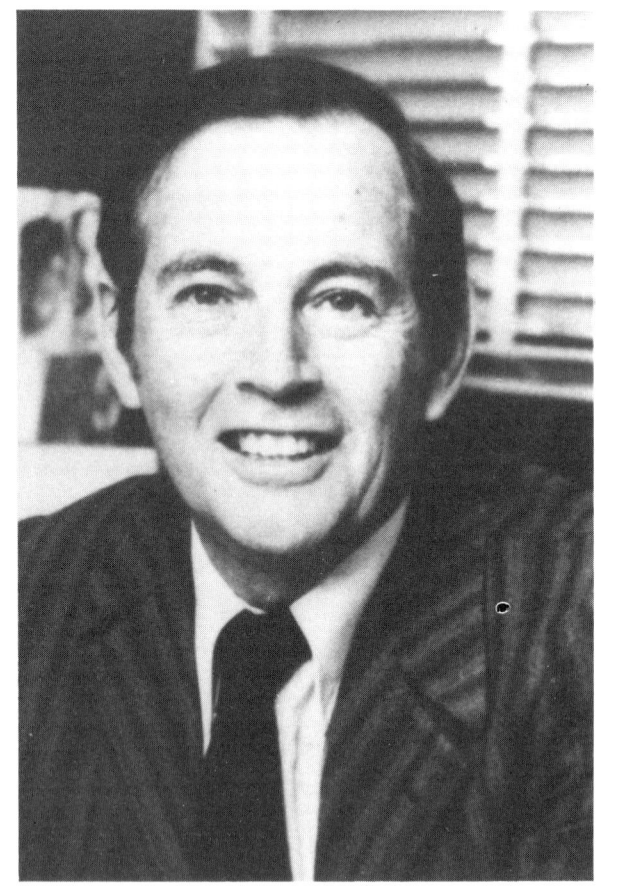

Figure 1.10 Christiaan Barnard, who led the team that performed the first human-to-human heart transplant at Groote Schuur Hospital in Cape Town in December 1967

which might be involved. Four centers, those of Stanford University[40] and the Medical College of Virginia[41] in the USA, Hopital La Pitie in Paris[42] and Groote Schuur Hospital in Cape Town[43], continued with planned programs of heart transplantation.

With improved patient selection based on experience, and improved postoperative care, in particular with regard to the administration of immunosuppressive drugs and the prevention, diagnosis and treatment of infectious complications, the results in these centers slowly improved. The introduction of the technique of percutaneous transvenous endomyocardial biopsy to diagnose acute rejection by Caves and his colleagues in 1973[44,45] contributed much to the successful management of patients with cardiac allografts, allowing timely increases in immunosuppression or, of equal importance, the avoidance of over-immunosuppression.

The introduction of the operation of heterotopic heart transplantation by Barnard and Losman in 1975[9] added a further surgical technique, with some advantages and some disadvantages over orthotopic transplantation, which could be used by those treating patients with terminal myocardial disease.

During the late 1970s cardiac transplantation came to be accepted as a definitive form of therapy rather than as a clinical research program. As a result, in the late 1970s and early 1980s several other groups in North America and Europe initiated clinical heart transplant programs.

INTRODUCTION OF CYCLOSPORINE

Following the discovery of the immunosuppressive effects of cyclosporine A by Borel (Figure 1.12) and colleagues in 1976[46], and extensive experimental studies at several centers, notably Cambridge in the United Kingdom[47] and Stanford in the USA[48], cyclosporine was introduced into a clinical cardiac transplantation program in 1980[49]. Until this time, immunosuppression had been achieved with a combination of azathioprine[50], corticosteroids[51], and antilymphocyte globulin[40], which was probably first used in cardiac transplantation in 1968 (Barnard, C.N., personal communication).

Prolonged survival of heart and heart–lung transplants in non-human primates was achieved using immunosuppressive regimens in which cyclosporine played a major role[48]. Based on these studies, the initial clinical programs suffered from incorporating an excessively high dose of cyclosporine in the pre- and early post-transplant period, and many patients suffered morbidity or even death from complications of cyclosporine therapy, in particular, renal failure. With experience, however, the dose of cyclosporine was gradually reduced, and the potential complications minimized.

The subsequent good results obtained with a combination

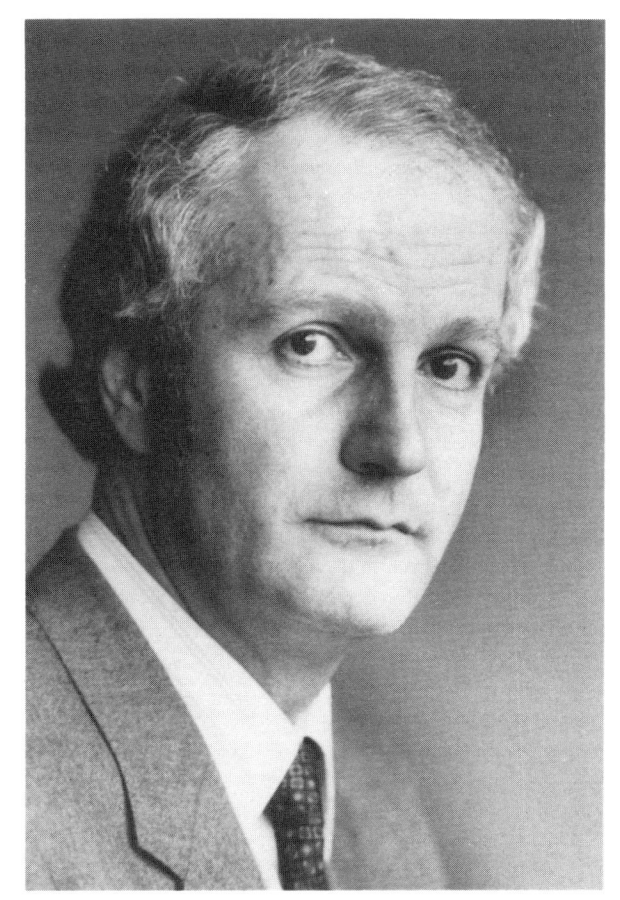

Figure 1.12 Jean Borel, of Sandoz Ltd., Basel, Switzerland, who discovered the immunosuppressive properties of the drug, cyclosporine A

of a lower dose of cyclosporine with azathioprine and low-dose corticosteroids, reserving antilymphocyte globulin and, more recently, the monoclonal antibody OKT3[52] primarily as treatment for rejection episodes, have encouraged many centers worldwide to embark on heart transplantation programs. In 1988, more than 170 centers performed almost 2500 heart transplants[53] (Chapter 31).

References

1. Cooper, D.K.C. (1968). Experimental development of cardiac transplantation. *Br. Med. J.*, **4**, 174
2. Carrel, A. and Guthrie, C.C. (1905). The transplantation of veins and organs. *Am. Med. (Philadelphia)*, **10**, 1101
3. Carrel, A. (1907). The surgery of blood vessels. *Bull. Johns Hopkins Hosp.*, **18**, 18
4. Mann, F.C., Priestley, J.T., Markowitz, J. and Yater, W.M. (1933). Transplantation of the intact mammalian heart. *Arch. Surg.*, **26**, 219
5. Abbott, C.P., Lindsey, E.S., Creech, O.Jr. and De Witt, C.W. (1964). A technique for heart transplantation in the rat. *Arch. Surg.*, **89**, 645
6. Abbott, C.P., De Witt, C.W. and Creech, O.Jr. (1965). The transplanted rat heart; histologic and electrocardiographic changes. *Transplantation*, **3**, 432
7. Demikhov, V.P. (1962). *Experimental Transplantation of Vital Organs.* Authorized translation from the Russian by Haigh, B. (Consultants Bureau, New York)

8. Reemtsma, K. (1964). The heart as a test organ in transplantation studies. *Ann. N.Y. Acad. Sci.*, **120**, 778
9. Barnard, C.N. and Losman, J.G. (1975). Left ventricular bypass. *S. Afr. Med. J.*, **49**, 303
10. Losman, J.G. and Barnard, C.N. (1977). Hemodynamic evaluation of left ventricular bypass with a homologous cardiac graft. *J. Thorac. Cardiovasc. Surg.*, **74**, 695
11. Sen, P.K., Parulkar, G.B., Panday, S.R. and Kinare, S.G. (1965). Homologous canine heart transplantation; a preliminary report of 100 experiments. *Indian J. Med. Res.*, **53**, 674
12. Neptune, W.B., Cookson, B.A., Bailey, C.P., Appler, R. and Rajkowski, F. (1953). Complete homologous heart transplantation. *Arch. Surg.*, **66**, 174
13. Webb, W.R. and Howard, H.S. (1957). Cardiopulmonary transplantation. *Surg. Forum*, **8**, 313
14. Webb, W.R., Howard, H.S. and Neely, W.A. (1959). Practical methods of homologous cardiac transplantation. *J. Thorac. Surg.*, **37**, 361
15. Goldberg, M., Berman, E.F. and Akman, L.C. (1958). Homologous transplantation of the canine heart. *J. Int. Coll. Surg.*, **30**, 575
16. Berman, E.F., Goldberg, M. and Akman, L. (1958). Experimental replacement of the heart in the dog. *Transplant. Bull.*, **5**, 10
17. Cass, M.H. and Brock, R. (1959). Heart excision and replacement. *Guy's Hosp. Rep.*, **108**, 285
18. Lower, R.R. and Shumway, N.E. (1960). Studies on orthotopic homotransplantation of the canine heart. *Surg. Forum*, **11**, 18
19. Barnard, C.N. (1968). What we have learned about heart transplants. *J. Thorac. Cardiovasc. Surg.*, **56**, 457
20. Lower, R.R., Stofer, R.C., Hurley, E.J. and Shumway, N.E. (1961). Complete homograft replacement of the heart and both lungs. *Surgery*, **50**, 842
21. Hurley, E.J., Dong, E. Jr., Stofer, R.C. and Shumway, N.E. (1962). Isotopic replacement of the totally excised canine heart. *J. Surg. Res.*, **2**, 90
22. Dong, E.Jr., Hurley, E.J., Lower, R.R. and Shumway, N.E. (1964). Performance of the heart two years after autotransplantation. *Surgery*, **56**, 270
23. Lower, R.R., Stofer, R.C. and Shumway, N.E. (1961). Homovital transplantation of the heart. *J. Thorac. Cardiovasc. Surg.*, **41**, 196
24. Lower, R.R., Stofer, R.C., Hurley, E.J., Dong, E.Jr., Cohn, R.B. and Shumway, N.E. (1962). Successful homotransplantation of the canine heart after anoxic preservation for seven hours. *Am. J. Surg.*, **104**, 302
25. Lower, R.R., Dong, E.Jr. and Shumway, N.E. (1965). Long-term survival of cardiac homografts. *Surgery*, **58**, 110
26. Shumway, N.E. and Lower, R.R. (1964). Special problems in transplantation of the heart. *Ann. N.Y. Acad. Sci.*, **120**, 773
27. Lower, R.R., Dong, E.Jr. and Glazener, F.S. (1964). Electrocardiograms of dogs with heart homografts. *Circulation*, **33**, 455
28. Angell, W.W., Dong, E.Jr. and Shumway, N.E. (1967). Four-day storage of the canine cadaver heart. *Surg. Forum*, **18**, 223
29. Willman, V.L., Cooper, T., Cian, L.G. and Hanlon, C.R. (1962). Autotransplantation of the canine heart. *Surg. Gynecol. Obstet.*, **115**, 299
30. Willman, V.L., Cooper, T., Kaiser, G.C. and Hanlon, C.R. (1965). Cardiovascular response after cardiac autotransplant in primate. *Arch. Surg.*, **91**, 805
31. Kondo, Y., Gradel, F. and Kantrowitz, A. (1965). Heart homotransplantation in puppies: long survival without immunosuppressive therapy. *Circulation*, **31**, (Suppl. 1), 181
32. Reemtsma, K., Williamson, W.R.Jr., Iglesias, F., Pena, E., Sayegh, S.F. and Creech, O.Jr. (1962). Studies in homologous canine heart transplantation; prolongation of survival with a folic acid antagonist. *Surgery*, **52**, 127
33. Blumenstock, D.A., Hechtman, H.B., Jaretzki, A., Hosbein, J.D., Zingg, W. and Powers, J.H. (1963). Prolonged survival of orthotopic homotransplants of the heart in animals treated with methotrexate. *J. Thorac. Cardiovasc. Surg.*, **46**, 616
34. Hardy, J.D., Webb, W.R., Dalton, M.L.Jr. and Walker, G.R.Jr. Lung homotransplantation in man; report of the initial case. *J. Am. Med. Assoc.*, **186**, 1065
35. Hardy, J.D., Chavez, C.M., Kurrus, F.E., Neely, W.A., Webb, W.R., Eraslan, S., Turner, M.D., Fabian, L.W. and Labecki, J.D. (1964). Heart transplantation in man; developmental studies and report of a case. *J. Am. Med. Assoc.*, **188**, 1132
36. Reemtsma, K., McCracken, B.H., Schlegel, J.U., Pearl, M.A., De Witt, C.W. and Creech, O.Jr. (1964). Reversal of early graft rejection after renal heterotransplantation in man. *J. Am. Med. Assoc.*, **187**, 691
37. Barnard, C.N. (1967). The operation. A human cardiac transplant: an interim report of a successful operation performed at Groote Schuur Hospital, Cape Town. *S. Afr. Med. J.*, **41**, 1271
38. Thompson, J.G. (1968). Heart transplantation in man – necropsy findings. *Br. Med. J.*, **2**, 511
39. Thompson, J.G. (1969). Atheroma in a transplanted heart. *Lancet*, **2**, 1297
40. Baumgartner, W.A., Reitz, B.A., Oyer, P.E., Stinson, E.B. and Shumway, N.E. (1979). Cardiac homotransplantation. *Curr. Probl. Surg.*, **61**, 1
41. Lower, R.R., Szentpetery, S., Thomas, F.T. and Kemp, V.E. (1976). Clinical observations on cardiac transplantation. *Transplant. Proc.*, **8**, 9
42. Cabrol, C., Gandjbakhch, I., Guiraudon, G., Pavie, A., Villemot, J.P., Viars, P., Cabrol, A., Mattei, M.F. and Rottembourg, J. (1982). Cardiac transplantation; our experience at La Pitie' Hospital in Paris. *Heart Transplant.*, **1**, 116
43. Barnard, C.N., Barnard, M.S., Cooper, D.K.C., Curcio, C.A., Hassoulas, J., Novitzky, D. and Wolpowitz, A. (1981). The present status of heterotopic cardiac transplantation. *J. Thorac. Cardiovasc. Surg.*, **81**, 433
44. Caves, P.K., Stinson, E.B., Graham, A.F., Billingham, M.E., Grehl, T.M. and Shumway, N.E. (1973). Percutaneous transvenous endomyocardial biopsy. *J. Am. Med. Assoc.*, **225**, 288
45. Caves, P.K., Billingham, M.E., Stinson, E.B. and Shumway, N.E. (1974). Serial transvenous biopsy of the transplanted human heart – improved management of acute rejection episodes. *Lancet*, **1**, 821
46. Borel, J.F., Feurer, C., Gubler, H.U. and Stahelin, H. (1976). Biological effects of cyclosporin-A: a new antilymphocytic agent. *Agents Actions*, **6**, 468
47. Calne, R.Y., White, D.J., Rolles, K., Smith, D.P. and Herbertson, B.M. (1978). Prolonged survival of pig orthotopic heart grafts treated with cyclosporin-A. *Lancet*, **1**, 1183
48. Reitz, B.A., Bieber, C.P., Raney, A.A., Pennock, J.L., Jamieson, S.W., Oyer, P.E. and Stinson, E.B. (1981). Orthotopic heart and combined heart and lung transplantation with cyclosporin-A immune suppression. *Transplant Proc.*, **13**, 393
49. Oyer, P.E., Stinson, E.B., Jamieson, S.W., Hunt, S., Reitz, B.A., Bieber, C.P., Schroeder, J.S., Billingham, M. and Shumway, N.E. (1982). One year experience with cyclosporin A in clinical heart transplantation. *Heart Transplant.*, **1**, 285
50. Calne, R.Y. (1961). Inhibition of the rejection of renal homografts in dogs by purine analogues. *Transplant Bull.*, **28**, 65
51. Goodwin, W.E., Kaufman, J.J., Mims, M.M., Turner, R.D., Glassock, R., Goldman, R. and Maxwell, M.M. (1963). Human renal transplantation. I. Clinical experiences with six cases of renal homotransplantation. *J. Urol.*, **89**, 13
52. Bristow, M.R., Gilbert, E.M., Renlund, D.G., De Witt, C.W., Burton, N.A. and O'Connell, J.B. (1988). Use of OKT3 monoclonal antibody in heart transplantation: review of the initial experience. *J. Heart Transplant.*, **7**, 1
53. Heck, C.F., Shumway, S.J. and Kaye, M.P. (1989). The Registry of the International Society for Heart Transplantation: sixth official report – 1989. *J. Heart Transplant.*, **8**, 271

2
Indications, Selection and Management of the Recipient
P.J. COMMERFORD

INTRODUCTION

Cardiac transplantation offers an attractive alternative form of therapy for the physician caring for a patient with intractable heart failure in whom symptoms are poorly controlled. The option of referring patients for cardiac transplantation, however, presents the physician with several difficult questions:

(1) Should cardiac transplantation be performed at all?

(2) Considering the variable and unpredictable natural history of congestive heart failure, when is the optimum time for the procedure to be performed in the individual patient?

(3) Which patient will benefit from transplantation, and who should be referred?

(4) How best may the recipient be maintained prior to surgery?

The answer to the first of these questions is clearer now than it was during preparation of the predecessor to this book in 1984[1]. The success of heart transplantation in the treatment of patients with severe intractable heart failure has changed our perception of the procedure from experiment to an accepted form of therapy for which there is currently a far greater demand than supply.

SHOULD PHYSICIANS REFER PATIENTS FOR CARDIAC TRANSPLANTATION?

A heart transplant program has a major impact on patient care. It commits scarce and costly resources to a procedure that, at best, will benefit only a very small number of patients. The argument that such resources should be kept available for the benefit of many is strong. A heart transplant program further loads the already overburdened intensive care facilities, not only with postoperative patients, but with potential transplant recipients, some of whom will die while awaiting a donor heart[2,3]. Some 20% of those patients selected as possible candidates will die while awaiting transplantation[4].

Thus the questions of cost and potential benefit arise. It is not an accurate economic and social analysis of the cost of end-stage cardiac disease to simply compute the cost of providing medical and surgical treatment for such patients. The emphasis should be on the cost of treating end-stage cardiac disease by conventional medical and surgical therapy versus heart transplantation[5]. Some authors have concluded that both methods are in the same range of cost to society[6]. The true cost of heart transplantation, however, is not simply what appears on the bottom line when all the bills come in; it must also include the value of what must be sacrificed to make room for transplantation[7]. Some argue that resources allocated to heart transplantation would be better spent on preventive health care. Gains associated with preventive health care measures, however, are by no means clear, and remain controversial[8]. The issues are complex, and estimates of the true costs and benefits vary. The estimates of Casscells[9] and Evans and colleagues[10] of the cost per added year of life are in the same range as the costs of hemodialysis for end-stage renal disease and screening and treatment of mild hypertension. These relevant issues and existing dilemmas are clearly reviewed by Evans[11] (Chapter 67).

With the expansion of heart transplantation programs, important ethical and moral issues have been raised and voiced. Concerns have been expressed about perceived inequities in the distribution of hearts for the purpose of transplantation, the apparent complexity of allocation decisions, and the fact that financial consideration or media publicity may influence selection of individual recipients[12]. These considerations apply to all solid organ transplants but achieve particular prominence in heart transplantation because of the symbolic significance of the heart in our culture and its perception as being a special organ imbued with mystical properties[13].

It is difficult to separate society's interest in a fair distribution of resources from the individual patient's right to treatment. Most physicians are uncomfortable when called on to withhold treatment from an individual patient on the grounds that prescribing such therapy may jeopardize the treatment of others. In an ideal world such decisions would not be necessary. With the improving results of heart transplantation, and the dramatic improvement in the quality of life[14] offered by the procedure in suitable recipients, physicians will continue to refer patients for transplantation as long as the procedure is available.

Informed consent

Having taken the decision to refer a patient for transplantation, the procedure must be explained to the patient and informed consent must be obtained. Patients who have undergone an acute cardiac catastrophe, such as acute myocardial infarction, or who are in severe heart failure, are usually placed in intensive care units, treated with drugs that may impair judgement, surrounded by formidable-looking equipment, and subjected to the psychological stress of their diminished state of health. Under these conditions, truly informed consent is difficult, if not impossible, to obtain[15]. The physician has a responsibility to ensure that the patient and his family understand the nature of the treatment offered and the potential benefits, as well as the necessity of prolonged postoperative hospitalization, follow-up, and the hazards associated with immunosuppression.

WHEN SHOULD THE PROCEDURE BE PERFORMED?

The prognosis of patients in severe left ventricular failure is variable, and prediction of life expectancy is extremely difficult. Most experienced physicians indicate that they often misjudge the duration of survival of patients with chronic congestive heart failure[15]. This renders the timing of the intervention difficult.

Selection of the optimum time for surgery is, however, extremely important. Although one does not wish to subject a patient who still has a reasonable prognosis to an operation that carries a significant postoperative mortality, it is equally important not to delay the operation until permanent non-cardiac organ damage has occurred. As the patient reaches the terminal stages of his cardiac disease, other organs, particularly the kidneys, lungs and liver, may deteriorate. If transplantation is delayed until death is imminent, the patient may not survive, regardless of how successful the transplant operation is. While the availability of donor hearts will always be the final factor determining the time of transplantation, it is important that patients be referred for consideration for transplantation before irreversible organ damage has occurred.

A prognostic study of patients in New York Heart Association (NYHA) functional Class III or IV, who were treated optimally with vasodilators and antiarrhythmics, showed overall 1- and 2-year survival of 52% and 32%, respectively for the whole group[16]; patients in NYHA Class IV had an even lower 1-year survival. The annual mortality rate was lower (20%) in those patients with 'stable' heart failure, and considerably higher (approximately 50%) in those with progressively worsening heart failure. These findings are similar to those of others[17–19]. Placebo-controlled trials of drug therapy of congestive cardiac failure confirm the gloomy prognosis, but also demonstrate that both combinations of vasodilators (isosorbide dinitrate and hydralazine)[20] and angiotensin-converting enzyme inhibitors[21] improve survival. The reduction in total mortality brought about by such therapy is found among patients with progressive heart failure, whereas no difference is seen in the incidence of sudden death[21].

It is the inability to predict sudden cardiac death (within 1 hour of the onset of symptoms), and rapid deterioration leading to death within 24 hours of the onset of symptoms, which renders the timing of cardiac transplantation so difficult. Such deaths account for approximately half of all cardiovascular deaths in patients with severe heart failure[21]. Because of the shortage of donors[22] and the 10–20% 3-month mortality following transplantation[23] (Chapter 31), current practice is to defer transplantation until symptoms are severe.

Even the most experienced centers have difficulty in the timing of the transplant. Of 30 patients seen at Stanford with dilated non-ischemic cardiomyopathy, who were denied transplantation solely because of the absence of severe symptoms, 46% survived 1 year without transplantation[24]. Nine of the 14 who did not survive 1 year without transplantation died suddenly; hemodynamic decompensation developed in five, of whom three underwent emergency transplantation and two died. In this group of patients with poor left ventricular function, but relatively mild symptoms, the authors identified a high-risk group who had either a low stroke volume or an arrhythmia history. Low-risk status was associated with short duration of symptoms.

Further studies, which will provide useful information of this nature, will hopefully assist in the decision as to the timing of surgery. At the moment, evaluation of the rate of clinical decline, response to medical therapy, and the risk of death in Class III or IV patients, is best made by the cardiologist closely involved in caring for the patient over a period of time.

The clinician will be guided by objective evidence of decline. Major events, such as recurrent hospital admissions for episodes of decompensation, the occurrence of life-threatening arrhythmias, and the development of cardiac cachexia, are indicators that it is appropriate to proceed to transplantation, as is progressively declining renal or hepatic function[25].

Patients in Class IV heart failure are potential candidates for assessment for transplantation, as are patients in Class III with progression of symptoms over the preceding weeks or months.

There is a small, but possibly increasing, number of patients being referred as potential candidates for transplantation who do not fit into the above categories. These are patients with severe and widespread coronary artery disease, who experience angina on light exertion or even at rest, despite maximal medical and conventional surgical therapy; myocardial function, however, remains surprisingly good, with left ventricular ejection fractions sometimes approximating 50%. Further revascularization procedures have been ruled out by coronary arteriography. Although the patient is not limited by dyspnea, and may show no signs of heart failure, he is at high risk from sudden death, and many physicians would put him forward as a candidate for heart transplantation, which might be his best opportunity for prolonged survival.

WHICH PATIENT WILL BENEFIT FROM HEART TRANSPLANTATION?

The substantial improvement in survival that has occurred following transplantation is the result, primarily, of improvement in survival during the first 3 postoperative months. This reflects improvement not only in management but also in patient selection. Restrospective analysis has aided recognition of recipient-related factors that influence survival after transplantation[26]. Selection of appropriate recipients for cardiac transplantation may be the most important factor determining long-term survival, yet it remains difficult and controversial, and guidelines for patient selection vary. With the widespread availability of cyclosporin since 1983, there has been a relaxation in selection criteria, and both older and younger patients and diabetics are being offered transplantation. With greater experience with the new immunosuppressive regimens, it is likely that there will be still further changes in selection criteria.

Contraindications

There are a number of 'absolute' and 'relative' contraindications to cardiac transplantation (Table 2.1), though, increasingly, what was 'absolute' last year may become 'relative' this year[2,25-29]. The weight given to the relative contraindications will differ in different centers, depending on the availability of donor hearts and the number of recipients waiting.

Table 2.1 Absolute and relative contraindications to cardiac transplantation

Absolute	Relative
Active infection	Advanced age
Untreated malignancy	*Unresolved* pulmonary infarction
Co-existing systemic illness that may limit life expectancy	Insulin-requiring diabetes mellitus
	Active peptic ulcer disease
Irreversible and severe dysfunction of any other major organ (kidney, liver, lungs)	Significant peripheral vascular or cerebrovascular disease
Fixed pulmonary vascular resistance (PVR) (> 5 Wood units) Heterotopic heart transplantation may be possible in the presence of a higher PVR	Drug addiction, alcoholism, mental illness or psychological instability

Active infection

Patients with active infection must generally be excluded because of the risk of exacerbation by postoperative immunosuppression. When the infecting organism is known, however, correct treatment initiated, and the patient seen to be responding well, then it may be considered acceptable to proceed with transplantation if the cardiac status of the patient is critical. The high risk of death from the underlying cardiac disorder may outweigh the risk of transplantation carried out in the presence of persisting infection.

Pre-existing malignancy

Pre-existing malignancy may progress rapidly in the immunocompromised patient (Chapter 21). A history of successfully treated malignancy may represent a relative contraindication as immunosuppression may impair the body's ability to control residual malignant cells; renal transplant recipients have experienced recurrences of neoplasms[30].

Co-existing systemic disease

The decision to include a condition under the broad general category of co-existing systemic illness is clearly subjective. The degree of rigidity with which the condition will be used as a reason for withholding the possibility of transplantation may vary depending on the availability of donor hearts. Many physicians may wish to exclude patients with collagen vascular disease and other systemic illnesses. A report of the demonstration of amyloid protein deposition in a cardiac allograft 14 weeks after transplantation has reaffirmed the theoretical concern that amyloidosis is a contraindication to heart transplantation[31].

Dysfunction of other major organs

It is frequently difficult to determine whether dysfunction of other major organs will be reversible once myocardial function has returned to normal. Correction of the underlying circulatory state often results in a surprising degree of recovery of organ dysfunction. In the patient with chronic congestive cardiac failure, therefore, every effort must be made to demonstrate whether renal, hepatic, or respiratory insufficiency is reversible or not. Significant chronic obstructive pulmonary disease, resulting from chronic bronchitis and emphysema, must be differentiated from the features of left ventricular failure, but if clearly demonstrated, may contraindicate cardiac transplantation; active chronic bronchitis and emphysema predispose to postoperative pulmonary infection. Cyclosporine is metabolized in the liver and induces significant nephrotoxicity; its use, therefore, means that great care must be taken to ensure that irreversible renal and/or hepatic dysfunction are not already present.

Elevated pulmonary vascular resistance

In the early days of cardiac transplantation, it became obvious that a greatly elevated pulmonary vascular resistance (PVR) was a contraindication to orthotopic transplantation. An increased post-transplant mortality of patients with even a moderately raised PVR has been documented recently[32,33]. The procedure of heterotopic transplantation was introduced in part to deal with this problem. A fixed high PVR of above 5 or 6 Wood units (400–480 dynes $s^{-1}cm^{-5}$) is therefore thought by most to be an absolute contraindication to orthotopic transplantation. After heterotopic transplantation, the recipient's right ventricle remains functional and, unless right-sided failure has occurred, has adapted to the pressure overload, and will continue to support the pulmonary circulation (Chapter 23).

However, a high PVR in patients with advanced myocardial disease may be reversible, at least in part, and a significant fall in resistance may be observed after transplantation[34]. It is said that the degree of reversibility can be predicted before transplantation by recording the PVR both before and during the administration of 100% oxygen or sodium nitroprusside, which may bring about a marked fall in resistance in patients with a large reactive component[35]. The same authors suggest that correcting the pulmonary vascular resistance for body size more accurately predicts those patients at risk of postoperative right ventricular failure[36]. We have noted variability in pulmonary resistance in several patients, and emphasize the importance of making the assessment after the patient is stabilized on optimal vasodilator therapy. (Further experience with cardiac transplantation in the presence of a high PVR is discussed in Chapter 23.)

Advanced age

The first transplants performed were in older patients. Using conventional immunosuppressive therapy with azathioprine and methylprednisolone, our local experience was that mortality rose in patients over the age of 40 years; no recipient aged 50 or over at the time of transplantation survived beyond his second year[26]. Early experience elsewhere was similar. More recently, even before cyclosporine became available, improved survival was found in carefully selected patients over the age of 50[14]. There are now several reports of successful transplantation in older patients (even to the mid-sixties)[37–39], and, indeed, of decreased frequency of rejection episodes in this group[40], which is attributed to an age-associated decline in immune function; obviously this might well represent an advantage to this group. Clearly, absolute age limits are no longer applicable. Attention must be paid to the general condition of the patient, and physiologic rather than chronologic age. One study suggests that the likelihood that a patient over age 55 is a suitable recipient decreases as age increases, and reaches zero at age 67[25].

Unresolved pulmonary infarction

A patient with recent unresolved pulmonary infarction should probably be excluded because of the risk of cavitation and secondary infection. This is a temporary condition and, when resolution and scarring has occurred, the patient once again becomes eligible.

Insulin-requiring diabetes mellitus

A major contraindication to transplantation in the pre-cyclosporine era was insulin-requiring diabetes mellitus, because of the exacerbation of diabetes by high-dose corticosteroids. Therapy with cyclosporine and azathioprine alone (or with added low-dose corticosteroids) has been successful, thus allowing transplants in patients with diabetes mellitus. Those with significant diabetic complications, however, including microvascular disease (e.g. retinopathy) and neuropathy, would probably not be suitable candidates; unstable brittle diabetes would similarly exclude some patients[25]. Those with Type II diabetes and impaired glucose tolerance are warned that they may require insulin therapy whilst taking corticosteroids post-transplantation.

Active peptic ulcer disease

Active peptic ulcer disease is a contraindication because of the risk of bleeding, perforation, and infection in the immunosuppressed patient. This too is temporary, and healed ulceration is not a contraindication.

Peripheral or cerebrovascular disease

The presence of significant peripheral or cerebrovascular disease will prevent the patient obtaining maximum benefit from the procedure and/or increase the short-term risks.

Psychological instability

Patients addicted to drugs, or who consume excessive amounts of alcohol, or who are otherwise emotionally unstable or suffer from acute mental illness are not suitable candidates for cardiac transplantation. The drug-addicted or alcoholic patient is unlikely to comply during the postoperative period, when compliance with a complex drug regimen and regular attendance for follow-up visits are important.

Patient non-compliance

As with many major cardiac surgical procedures, the success of the operation depends on the patient's ability to understand fully the life-long treatment and follow-up program that is an essential part of his management. A strong supportive family may be of great value in seeing the patient through the perioperative and early post-transplant periods[41,42].

These last non-medical criteria are, by their very nature, difficult to define and to some extent subjective. Inevitably, they arouse more controversy than the relatively straightforward medical criteria[12,43]. Family support, job stability, and an assessment of the patient's will to live, to comply with medical therapy, and to undergo possibly repeated admissions and biopsies after transplantation are difficult to assess, and are best evaluated by a team consisting of the physician responsible for the care of the patient, a psychiatrist, and social worker experienced in the problems associated with heart transplantation. Not infrequently, an initial evaluation that a patient is unsuitable for transplantation because of inadequate family support or emotional instability is shown to be incorrect. Observation and evaluation over a period of time may, in fact, show that some such patients, initially judged to be unsuitable, are in fact capable of adhering to complex medical regimens involving multiple diagnostic tests, clinical visits, and medications[44].

Financial considerations

Perhaps the most important practical difficulty is to ensure that the patient has sufficient financial resources to pay for those expenses not covered by the State, insurance, or a medical aid agency. Whilst the State or other organization may bear the cost of the operation and postoperative care, the facilities available to maintain the recipient awaiting transplantation and his family may be inadequate. In planning transplantation, care is needed to ensure that the patient and his family do not incur unnecessary expense by needlessly traveling great distances in the hope of a life-saving procedure, only for the patient to die while awaiting a donor.

In summary, the ideal transplant recipient should have severe cardiac failure untreatable by conventional surgery or medical therapy. He should be free of any condition likely to predispose to the complications of immunosuppression, be psychologically stable, and have sufficient resources to support himself and his family through the perioperative period prior to full rehabilitation.

FURTHER ASSESSMENT

Screening of the recipient begins with a full history and physical examination, including a chest radiograph and electrocardiogram; at this stage, any major contraindications should be evident. Many patients will be rejected at this early, informal evaluation, as they are seen to be completely unsuitable. Usually this is on the grounds of age, co-existent disease in other organ systems, or an unsuitable social or psychological background.

Once having passed this informal assessment, candidates undergo systematic and extensive medical screening. This includes hemodynamic evaluation, including cardiac catheterization and angiography, if recent results are not available. Once the patient is judged to be a candidate for transplantation on the basis of clinical status and cardiac catheterization, then further screening is performed to ensure that major contraindications to the use of immunosuppression are not present.

This screening process is obviously guided by clinical judgement, but includes a full blood count, biochemical screening of blood and urine, a glucose tolerance test, respiratory function tests, dental examination and radiography, and bacteriological screening where indicated. Further investigation of major systems, such as barium studies and intravenous pyelography, are performed where appropriate. Based on the results of these investigations, specific therapy may be indicated, or the patient may be deemed unsuitable for transplantation. If no contraindication is detected, then the patient becomes a candidate and awaits a suitable donor.

MAINTENANCE OF THE SELECTED RECIPIENT

These patients are all seriously ill, and have short life expectancies, usually measured in weeks. The mean survival of patients accepted as recipients but who died while awaiting a donor at our own institution was 26 days[2]. Maintenance of such a patient prior to transplantation poses a formidable problem. The management of chronic congestive heart failure in the transplant recipient is no different from that in other patients. A few points, however, deserve emphasis.

Anti-failure therapy

At the time of referral for consideration, many patients are not optimally treated. They will benefit from intensive therapy, guided by monitoring of the left ventricular filling pressure after placement of a pulmonary arterial catheter. Intravenous diuretics, nitroprusside, and inotropic agents can be administered to optimize hemodynamics rapidly, usually within 24–48 hours. Angiotensin-converting enzyme inhibitors (e.g. captopril, enalapril) and oral diuretics are then introduced to maintain the hemodynamics. Intensive medical therapy, guided by hemodynamic monitoring, allows safe and rapid determination of optimal filling pressures[45], and is superior to empiric therapy. Many patients may be stabilized, enabling them to be ambulant and to be managed as outpatients, where they incur fewer financial and psychological costs while awaiting transplantation[46]. This approach also allows for urgent priority status to be reserved for patients demonstrated to have truly refractory heart failure.

Inotropic support

Some patients will temporarily require aggressive management with intravenous inotropic agents, and a few will become dependent on them. In the absence of an adequate supply of donor hearts, this is an unfortunate situation, since many such patients will not survive until operation, and many that do will have such severe non-cardiac organ dysfunction (e.g. renal, hepatic) that, in our experience, a successful outcome from transplantation is less likely.

Mechanical support

Initial reports of transplantation in patients dependent on mechanical support suggested that, unless donor hearts were freely available, patients with end-stage heart failure should not be submitted to this procedure[47]. More recent reports, however, are encouraging[46,48,49] (Section IV). Total experience is still limited to a relatively small number of patients, and each of the mechanical devices available is associated with morbidity related to trauma of insertion, hemolysis, infection, thromboembolic complications, and bleeding, which are additive to the morbidity resulting from transplantation and immunosuppression. A recent review of the role of mechanical support suggested that it should only be used if non-cardiac organs are free of major dysfunction[50].

Arrhythmias

Prevention of fatal ventricular arrhythmias remains a major concern in patients awaiting transplantation. A prime aim must be to ensure that the therapy prescribed in the treatment of heart failure does not promote arrhythmias by, for example, diuretic-induced electrolyte imbalance, the use of sympathomimetic agents or digoxin, or by the development of drug interactions with digoxin[51]. It is important to try and identify patients at highest risk from sudden death, and thus likely to benefit from antiarrhythmic therapy. Those with the lowest ejection fraction and a previous history of sustained ventricular tachycardia are at highest risk[24,52] and should be aggressively treated. Patients who have not experienced sustained symptomatic ventricular arrhythmias are less easy to manage. Their risk is less clear, and not well stratified by ambulatory electrocardiography. The use of antiarrhythmic agents, which may themselves be pro-arrhythmic[53] and further impair left ventricular function, is controversial. Our practice is to treat only those patients who have had sustained or symptomatic ventricular arrhythmias.

COMMENT

The availability of heart transplantation has provided physicians with a novel form of therapy for heart failure. At the same time, however, it has posed difficult questions related to allocation of resources, selection of patients for therapy, and maintenance of the dying patient.

References

1. Commerford, P.J. (1984). Selection and management of the recipient. In Cooper, D.K.C., Lanza, R.P. (eds.) *Heart Transplantation.* p. 15 (Lancaster: MTP Press Ltd.)
2. Cooper, D.K.C., Charles, R.G., Beck, W. and Barnard, C.N. (1982). The assessment and selection of patients for heterotopic heart transplantation. *S. Afr. Med. J.*, **61**, 575
3. Leaf, A. (1980). The MGH trustees say no to heart transplants. *N. Engl. J. Med.*, **302**, 1087
4. Copeland, J. G., Emery, R. W. and Levinson, M.M. (1985). The role of mechanical support and transplantation in treatment of patients with end-stage cardiomyopathy. *Circulation*, **72**, II–7
5. Evans, R.W. (1982). Economic and social costs of heart transplantation. *Heart Transplant.*, **1**, 243
6. Thomas, F.T. and Lower, R.R. (1978). Heart transplantation – 1978. *Surg. Clin. North Am.*, **58**, 335
7. Centerwall, B.S. (1981). Cost–benefit analysis and heart transplantation. *N. Engl. J. Med.*, **304**, 901
8. Russel, L. B. (1986). *Is Prevention Better than Cure?* (Washington, DC: The Brookings Institution)
9. Casscells, W. (1986). Special report: heart transplantation. Recent policy developments. *N. Engl. J. Med.*, **315**, 1365
10. Evans, R.W., Manninen, D.L., Overcast, T.D., Garrison, L.P., Yagi, J., Merrikin, K. and Jonsen, A.R. (1984). *The National Heart Transplantation Study: Final Report.* (Seattle: Batelle Human Affairs Research Centers)
11. Evans, R.W. (1987). The economics of heart transplantation. *Circulation*, **75**, 63
12. Caplan, A.L. (1987). Equity in the selection of recipients for cardiac transplants. *Circulation*, **75**, 10

13. Commerford, P.J. (1987). Cardiology: recent advances and their implications. Inaugural lecture, University of Cape Town Press
14. Copeland, J.G., Manwara, R.B., Fuller, J.K., Campbell, D.W., McAleer, M.J. and Sailer, J.A. (1984). Heart transplantation; four years experience with conventional immunosuppression. *J. Am. Med. Assoc.*, **251**, 1563
15. Woolley, F.R. (1984). Ethical issues in the implantation of the total artificial heart. *N. Engl. J. Med.*, **310**, 292
16. Wilson, J.R., Schwartz, S., St. John Sutton, M., Ferraro, N., Horowitz, L.N., Reichek, N. and Josephson, M.E. (1983). Prognosis in severe heart failure: relation to hemodynamic measurements and ventricular ectopic activity. *J. Am. Coll. Cardiol.*, **2**, 403
17. Massie, B., Ports, T., Chatterjee, K., Parmley, W., Ostland, J., O'Young, J. and Haughom, F. (1981). Long-term vasodilator therapy for heart failure: clinical response and its relationship to hemodynamic measurements. *Circulation*, **63**, 269
18. Franciosa, J.A., Wilen, M., Ziesche, S. and Cohn, J.N. (1983). Survival in men with severe chronic left ventricular failure due to either coronary heart disease or idiopathic dilated cardiomyopathy. *Am. J. Cardiol.*, **51**, 831
19. Fuster, V., Gersh, B.J., Giuliani, E.R., Tajik, A.J., Brandenburg, R.O. and Frye, R.L. The natural history of idiopathic dilated cardiomyopathy. *Am. J. Cardiol.*, **47**, 525
20. Cohn, J.N., Archibald, D.G., Ziesche, S., Franciosa, J.A., Harston, W.G., Tristani, F.E., Dunkman, W.B., Jacobs, W., Francis, G.S., Flohr, K.H., Goldman, S., Cobb, F.R., Shah, P.M., Saunders, R., Fletcher, R.D., Loeb, H.S., Hughes, V.C. and Baker, B. (1986). Effect of vasodilator therapy on mortality in chronic congestive heart failure: results of a Veterans Administration cooperative study. *N. Engl. J. Med.*, **314**, 1547
21. The CONSENSUS Trial Study Group (1987). Effects of enalapril on mortality in severe congestive heart failure. *N. Engl. J. Med.*, **316**, 1429
22. Evans, R.W., Manninen, D.L., Garrison, L.P. and Maier, A.M. (1986). Donor availability as the primary determinant of the future of heart transplantation. *J. Am. Med. Assoc.*, **255**, 1892
23. Solis, E. and Kaye, M.P. (1986). Registry of the International Society for Heart Transplantation: third official report. *J. Heart Transplant.*, **5**, 2
24. Stevenson, L.W., Fowler, M.B., Schroeder, J.S., Stevenson, W.G., Dracup, K.A. and Ford, V. (1987). Poor survival of patients with idiopathic cardiomyopathy considered too well for transplantation. *Am. J. Med.*, **83**, 871
25. Copeland, J.G., Emery, R.W., Levinson, M.M., Icenogle, T.B., Carrier, M., Ott, R.A., Copeland, J.A., McAleer-Rhenman, M.J. and Nicholson, S.M. (1987). Selection of patients for cardiac transplantation. *Circulation*, **75**, 1
26. Cooper, D.K.C., Lanza, R.P., Boyd, S.T. and Barnard, C.N. (1983). Factors influencing survival following heart transplantation. *Heart Transplant.*, **3**, 86
27. Thompson, M.E. (1983). Selection of candidates for cardiac transplantation. *J. Heart Transplant.*, **3**, 65
28. Oyer, P.E., Stinson, E.B., Bieber, C.P. and Shumway, N.E. (1982). Cardiac transplantation. In Chatterjee, S.N. (ed.) *Organ Transplantation*, p. 347. (Boston: P.S.G. Wright)
29. Lower, R.R., Szentpetery, S., Quinn, J. and Thomas, F.T. (1979). Selection of patients for cardiac transplantation. *Transplant Proc.*, **11**, 293
30. Penn, I. (1982). Problems of cancer in organ transplantation. *J. Heart Transplant.*, **2**, 71
31. Conner, R., Hosenpud, J., Norman, D., Cobanoglu, A., Floten, S., Niles, N., Ray, J., Maricle, R. and Starr, A. (1986). Recurrence of amyloidosis in a cardiac allograft. *J. Heart Transplant.*, **5**, 385
32. Kirklin, J.K., Naftel, D.C., Kirklin, J.W., Blackstone, E.H., White-Williams, C. and Bourge, R.C. (1988). Pulmonary vascular resistance and the risk of heart transplantation. *J. Heart Transplant.*, **7**, 331
33. Costard, A., Hill, I., Schroeder, J. and Fowler, M. (1989). Response to nitroprusside – predictor of early post-transplant mortality. *J. Am. Coll. Cardiol.*, **13**, 62A
34. Pucillo, A.L., Reison, D.S., Rose, E.A., Drusin, R.E., Reemtsma, K. and Powers, E.R. (1983). Reversibility of elevated pulmonary vascular resistance after cardiac transplantation. *J. Am. Coll. Cardiol.*, **1**, 722 (Abstract)
35. Addonizio, L.J., Robbins, R.C., Reison, D.S., Drusin, R.E., Smith, C.R., Reemtsma, K. and Rose, E.A. (1986). Transplantation in patients with high pulmonary vascular resistance. *J. Heart Transplant.*, **5**, 394
36. Addonizio, L.J., Gersony, W.M., Robbins, R.C., Drusin, R.E., Smith, C.R., Reison, D.S., Reemtsma, K. and Rose, E.A. (1987). Elevated pulmonary vascular resistance and cardiac transplantation. *Circulation*, **76**, V52
37. Carrier, M., Emery, R.W., Riley, J.E., Levinson, M.M. and Copeland, J.G. (1986). Cardiac transplantation in patients over 50 years of age. *J. Am. Coll. Cardiol.*, **8**, 285
38. Miller, L.W., Pennington, D.G., Kanter, K. and McBride, L. (1986). Heart transplantation in patients over 55 years of age. *J. Heart Transplant.*, **5**, 367
39. Olivari, M., Antolick, A., Kaye, M., Jamieson, S. and Ring, W.R. (1986). Heart transplantation in the elderly. *J. Heart Transplant.*, **5**, 366
40. Renlund, D.G., Gilbert, E.M., O'Connell, J.B., Gay, W.A., Jones, K.W., Burton, N.A., Doty, D.B., Karwande, S.V., De Witt, C.W., Menlove, R.L., Herrick, C.M. and Bristow, M.R. (1987). Age-associated decline in cardiac allograft rejection. *Am. J. Med.*, **83**, 391
41. Lunde, D.T. (1969). Psychiatric complications of heart transplants. *Am. J. Psychiatry*, **126**, 369
42. Cooper, D.K.C., Lanza, R.P., Nash, E.S. and Barnard, C.N. (1984). Non-compliance in heart transplant recipients: The Cape Town experience. *J. Heart Transplant.*, **3**, 248
43. Robertson, J.A. (1987). Supply and distribution of hearts for transplantation: legal, ethical and policy issues. *Circulation*, **75**, 81
44. Henrick, C.M., Mealey, P.C., Tischner, L.L. and Holland, C.S. (1987). Combined Heart Failure Transplant Program: advantages in assessing medical compliance. *J. Heart Transplant.*, **6**, 141
45. Pierpont, G.L. and Francis, G.S. (1982). Medical management of terminal cardiomyopathy. *Heart Transplant.*, **2**, 18
46. Stevenson, L.W., Donohue, B.C., Tillisch, J.G., Schulman, B., Dracup, K.A. and Laks, H. (1987). Urgent priority transplantation: when should it be done. *J. Heart Transplant.*, **6**, 267
47. Bregman, D., Drusin, R., Lamb, J., Reemtsma, K. and Rose, E. (1982). Heart transplantation in patients requiring mechanical circulatory support. *Heart Transplant.*, **1**, 154
48. Griffith, B.P., Hardesty, R.L., Kormos, R.L., Trento, A., Borovetz, H.S., Thompson, M.E. and Bahnson, H.T. (1987). Temporary use of the Jarvik-7 total artificial heart before transplantation. *N. Engl. J. Med.*, **316**, 130
49. Bolman, R.N., Spray, T.L., Cance, L., Saffitz, J., Genton, R.E. and Eisen, H. (1986). Heart transplantation in patients requiring pre-operative mechanical support. *J. Heart Transplant.*, **5**, 374
50. Copeland, J.G., Emery, R.W. and Levinson, M.M. (1987). The role of mechanical support and transplantation in treatment of patients with end-stage cardiomyopathy. *Am. Coll. Cardiol. Learning Center Highlights*, **5**, 11
51. Opie, L.H. (1987). Drug-related arrhythmias during therapy of congestive heart failure. *Cardiovasc. Drugs Therapy*, **1**, 195
52. Swerdlow, C.D., Winkle, R.A. and Mason, J.W. (1983). Determinants of survival in patients with ventricular tachyarrhythmias. *N. Engl. J. Med.*, **308**, 1436
53. Ruskin, J.N., McGovern, B., Garan, H., DiMarco, J.P. and Kelly, E. (1983). Antiarrhythmic drugs: a possible cause of out-of-hospital cardiac arrest. *N. Engl. J. Med.*, **309**, 1302

3
The Concept and Diagnosis of Brain Death

J.C. DE VILLIERS

INTRODUCTION

The concept of brain death or coma dépassé as opposed to clinical death, which is the absence of all vital signs, was first formulated by Mollaret and Goulon in 1959[1]. As could be expected, this new concept of death evoked considerable controversy both in medical and lay circles. It is, however, not an academic cor philosophical question but a common one of very real practical importance, and one with wide ethical, legal and economic implications.

The almost universal availability of efficient resuscitation facilities after injury or acute organ failure has created a situation where patients may be mechanically ventilated and the circulatory volume and blood pressure artificially maintained without any possibility of recovery of cerebral function. This state has come to be known as cerebral death. That cerebral death means death of the individual is now virtually universally accepted in the Western World, but there are countries where this is not so[2]. The high cost of maintaining such patients in intensive care units has led to financial evaluation by those who have to foot the bill for health care, individuals, insurance companies, and the State. The fact that other patients with treatable conditions may be precluded from curative care by prolonged management of 'brain dead' patients, the workload for nursing and medical staff, the emotional toll taken of relatives, and distress caused to nursing staff, are all very real considerations[3].

These patients may be potential donors of essential organs such as kidneys, heart and liver, so that their care has also acquired medico-legal and ethical significance[4]. It is not the task of the neurosurgeon or, for that matter, of any other medical practitioner to provide organs for donation, but neither can any doctor, on the basis of insufficient evidence or mere prejudice, deny patients in need of transplant surgery this chance of a cure.

CLINICAL DEATH

The classical features of clinical death have been accepted for centuries, and can be simply stated as the absence of spontaneous heart beat and respiration. In most countries, legislators have steered clear of any definition of death for very understandable reasons; in the Republic of South Africa, a patient is legally regarded as dead when he has been certified to be so by a qualified medical practitioner.

BRAIN DEATH

That irreversible loss of function of the brain must inevitably lead to progressive deterioration in function and death of the rest of the body, is universally accepted. The next step, i.e. to equate brain stem death with brain death and death of the individual, came later, but few would question this concept today[5-7]. The practical problem which arose in the beginning was that there was need of a system of diagnosing brain stem death with such certainty that there could be no reasonable doubt that this diagnosis was unquestionably correct and that further resuscitative or sustaining activities were pointless and could be terminated. This has, however, been overcome and the diagnosis is now an acceptable clinical exercise[8-10].

PATHOPHYSIOLOGY OF IRREVERSIBLE BRAIN STEM DAMAGE

In order to produce coma, pathological processes must either affect the brain diffusely or directly encroach upon its deep central structures. Three major groups of lesions can be differentiated:

(1) Supratentorial lesions, such as subdural, subarachnoid or intracerebral hematoma, or cerebral infarction, tumor or abscess.

(2) Infratentorial masses or destructive lesions which directly damage the brain stem, e.g. brain stem-cerebellar hemorrhage, abscess, brain stem infarction or tumor.

(3) Metabolic disorders which widely depress or interrupt brain stem function, including anoxia, ischemia, infec-

tions such as meningitis or encephalitis, exogenous toxins and deficiencies.

The end-result of major trauma, whether physical or chemical, which leads to progressive brain swelling is progressive herniation of the para-hippocampal gyri with lateral compression and downward displacement of the brain stem, eventually resulting in loss of brain stem function. Unless relieved in time, any expanding lesion will increase intracranial pressure until it is equal to systemic arterial pressure, at which point there will be complete arrest of cerebral circulation. Cerebral circulatory arrest can therefore be confidently used as a criterion of irreversible cerebral injury.

Functional disintegration, following on the conditions mentioned, leads to cessation of spontaneous respiration, which in turn results in hypoxic cardiac arrest. If gaseous exchange and circulation are maintained artificially, the heart, kidneys and liver may continue to function for some hours or days, but after brain stem death has occurred, cardiac arrest will follow within 2 weeks[11].

DIAGNOSIS OF BRAIN DEATH

Before a patient can be considered as being in a state of brain stem death, a positive diagnosis of the structural alterations in the brain which have caused this damage must have been made. All investigations necessary to come to this diagnosis, and efforts to reverse this process, if at all reversible, should be instituted. Conditions which may simulate brain stem death have to be excluded, such as depressant drugs, hypothermia or metabolic and endocrine disorders (e.g. hypo- or hyperglycemia, acid–base or electrolyte disturbances), although the latter three may have resulted from extensive brain damage or the patient's subsequent management.

In the early phase of declining brain stem function, the clinician should be concerned with diagnostic and resuscitative measures and not with speculations about irreversible coma. Three questions, therefore, have to be answered:

(1) What is the cause of the deterioration?

(2) Can it be reversed?

(3) Can this state be simulated by any other benign condition?

CLINICAL FEATURES OF BRAIN STEM DEATH

Level of consciousness

A patient can only be considered to be cerebrally dead if, due to an irremediable cause, he is in absolutely non-responsive coma with bilaterally fixed, non-reacting pupils, and makes no spontaneous respiratory effort. This has also been called coma stage 4. To consider any patient with a level of activity higher than this as having a dead brain stem reveals a lack of understanding of the condition, and may consequently lead to serious errors.

The patient with a supratentorial space-demanding lesion may show progressive rostro-caudal disintegration of brain stem function during which he descends irretrievably from a normal level of consciousness to the stage of irreversible coma. In the established case there is little diagnostic difficulty; the patient is totally unresponsive as far as brain stem reactivity is concerned, and is artificially respired because spontaneous respiration had become inadequate during the clinical decline. After 24 hours, the patient is often hypothermic and may develop diabetes insipidus.

The real problem is to know how soon this diagnosis can be established with incontrovertible certainty.

Respiratory function

A patient may have all the signs of severe cerebral and upper brain stem injury but, as long as he breathes spontaneously, he may still recover[12]. Obvious as this may seem, it does bear repetition and, if this is remembered, the embarrassing situation of the patient who has been considered for organ donation recovering consciousness, will not occur.

The reason for maintaining the patient on a mechanical ventilator must be because spontaneous respiration had previously become inadequate or had ceased altogether[12]. Neuromuscular blocking agents as a cause of respiratory inadequacy must be excluded. The necessity for artificial ventilation may be determined when the patient is seen to make no respiratory effort throughout a 5-minute period of observation (off the ventilator). The partial arterial carbon dioxide pressure ($PaCO_2$) should be within the normal range (5.3–6.1 kPa) at the beginning of the period of observation, and must be allowed to rise above the threshold for stimulating respiration (6.7 kPa). In order to prevent hypoxemia, oxygen is delivered at a rate of at least 6 liters per minute (l/min) via an endotracheal catheter throughout the test period.

If blood gas analysis is not available to measure the $PaCO_2$, an alternative procedure is to supply the ventilator with pure oxygen for 10 minutes (pre-oxygenation), then with 5% carbon dioxide in oxygen for 5 minutes to avoid hypocarbia, and then to disconnect the ventilator for 10 minutes, while delivering oxygen at 6 l/min via an endotracheal catheter. This establishes diffusion oxygenation and ensures that hypoxia will not occur during the 10 minutes that artificial ventilation is interrupted.

During apnea-testing, abnormal respiratory-like movements may be observed. These movements comprise shoulder elevation and adduction, back arching and slight intercostal movement, but no abdominal respiratory action or clavicular elevation[13]. These movements occur at adequate CO_2 pressures, are not effective for ventilation and rapidly disappear.

Brain stem reflexes

Because of the anatomical position of the brain stem nuclei and their known connections, the integrity of these nuclei and their connections can be assessed, level by level, by utilizing standard clinical reflex responses. In this way, the progressive deterioration in neurological function which follows on irreversible cerebral damage can be followed fairly accurately. Some of these reflexes can be assessed electrophysiologically and yield more reliable and measurable results, but such sophistication is not essential for the clinical diagnosis to be made with certainty.

Pupillary response (second/third nerve interaction)

For an effective test of pupillary function, the room should be darkened, a strong light used, and the pupil observed through a magnifying glass. If a diagnosis of non-reactivity is to be made, the pupil must remain fixed on testing its reaction to a strong light. Depending on the cause of the cerebral damage, there may be pupillary inequality, where the one pupil enlarges first and the other follows later. On the other hand, with central massive downward herniation of the brain stem, both pupils may be small initially and dilate later. The pupils are not only fixed to light, but obviously also do not react to painful stimulation, either locally or distantly. In some patients there is no pupillary dilation, the pupils being small or mid-sized; in these instances, it is presumed that there is associated central damage to the sympathetic system with inability to effect mydriasis.

Corneal reflex (fifth/seventh nerve interaction)

Light touch with a wisp of cotton wool is not enough; a firm contact with the cornea should be made with a soft object, such as a tuft of cotton wool. If this evokes not only a direct and consensual blink (fifth/seventh interaction), but also upward movement of the eyes (Bell's phenomenon), it indicates integrity of the third nerve/seventh nerve connections.

The corneo-mandibular reflex (deviation of the jaw to the opposite side) on firm touching of the cornea is an intratrigeminal response and is seen in upper brain stem injury, particularly in the early stages of rostro-caudal disintegration.

Grimace response (fifth/seventh nerve interaction)

Painful stimulation or irritation in the field of the fifth nerve will evoke a grimace response in the normal individual. In the deeply unconscious patient, supraorbital stimulation is used, but a more sensitive test is irritation of the nasal mucosa with a vibration fork, tickling, or *light* pin-prick. This response disappears in brain stem death.

Lower brain stem responses such as coughing and gagging on stimulation of the throat will usually have been noted by the nursing staff during suctioning, but should be tested by the physician himself.

Oculo-cephalic reflex

In a normal alert person, turning the head from side to side is followed by virtual instantaneous adjustment of the eye position to that of the head. This is a cortical response, which diminishes with progressive loss of cortical control in the presence of an intact brain stem. In this situation, the eyes lag behind the head movement, and then rapidly adjust their position again. When the brain stem centers which integrate the vestibulo-cervical input with ocular position have been destroyed, these responses are lost and there is no movement of the eye independently from that of the head. This test should not be performed where there is a suspicion of a cervical spinal injury.

Vestibulo-ocular reflexes (cold caloric tests)

This response involves pathways almost identical to those subserving the oculo-cephalic response but, because of the stronger stimulus needed to evoke it, it disappears later. In an awake person lying supine, irrigation of the external auditory meatus with 20 ml of ice water will elicit slight deviation of the eyes towards the irrigated side followed by nystagmus with the coarse beat to the opposite side.

In the unconscious patient with an intact brain stem and loss of cortical control the eyes will deviate towards the irrigated ear and remain immobile for 2–3 minutes before they gradually return to the initial resting position. With progressive decline in consciousness, the sequence of response is as follows:

(1) Conjugate ocular deviation with nystagmus,

(2) Conjugate ocular deviation without nystagmus,

(3) Dysconjugate ocular deviation o possibly response only from the ipsilateral eye,

(4) Loss of caloric response in the presence of coma stage 4.

It must be stressed that cold caloric responses are also lost completely in patients in deep barbiturate coma: accordingly, this test is of decisive importance only in the determination of brain stem death in patients who have suffered structural cerebral lesions. In patients with neocortical death, vestibulo-ocular reflexes may be retained as may be the case with other brain stem reflexes in the presence of an isoelectric electroencephalogram (EEG)[14].

SPINAL SEGMENTAL REFLEXES

These reflexes often cause confusion because they may be retained for a long period of time after all evidence of cerebral activity has ceased, or may even reappear after the initial loss of all neural activity. Reflexes which may remain present for a long time are the superficial abdominal, the cremasteric and plantar flexion withdrawal responses, as well as an isolated knee or ankle jerk. The persistent plantar response is usually in the nature of a very slow flexion withdrawal reaction. The upper limb may display a slow extension/internal rotation movement elicitable from a limited skin area on the arm and chest[15]. It is a localized response and indicates a high transection of the spinal cord.

These reflexes are subserved by local arcs through the spinal cord and occur independently of suprasegmental influences from the brain[16]. Similarly, the spinal sympathetic outflow may remain intact for a considerable time. Fluctuations in intensity of these responses are probably dependent on fluctuations in spinal cord perfusion. Physiologically, one is dealing with a peculiar form of acute transection with spinal shock, which is modified by the fact that previous destruction of the brain stem has occurred. It must be emphasized that persistent spinal cord function has nothing to do with irretrievable loss of cerebral or brain stem function and need not interfere with the diagnosis of brain stem death. Indeed, spinal cord areflexia is the exception in brain death, as demonstrated by central cerebral circulatory arrest[15,16].

HYPOTHALAMIC PITUITARY DYSFUNCTION

Diabetes insipidus occurs commonly, but not invariably, in brain death, while loss of diurnal temperature fluctuations and a progressive drop in body temperature are constant features. Hall *et al.*[17] found that hypothalamic pituitary action is maintained for at least 24 hours after brain death has occurred, so that hormonal evaluation is of no value in early diagnosis.

It bears repetition that the clinical diagnosis of the irreversible loss of brain stem function is the mainstay in establishing brain stem death. If reversible causes of brain stem dysfunction have been excluded and the basic criteria of functional loss have been satisfied, this clinical conclusion is as valid as any other absolute clinical observation.

Before a final diagnosis can be made, one further question must be answered. Could this state be simulated by other conditions – drugs, hypothermia, metabolic or endocrine disturbance, electrical injury? The latter is particularly important in countries where lightning injury is common, and can cause cessation of respiration and fixed dilated pupils which can be reversed after prolonged resuscitation[18]. All these causes are theoretically reversible and should have been considered right at the outset, but, if not, it is worthwhile to ask the question at this stage, because patients should not have been considered as brain stem dead if any one of these conditions were in evidence earlier on[19].

ANCILLARY TESTS

Ever since the concept of brain death first arose, efforts have been made to find electrophysiological ways of diagnosing brain stem death. The reason for this was probably the search for an 'objective' and absolute non-clinical mode of diagnosis. These tests are not available in all hospitals, and not one of them has proved to be an indisputable indicator of brain or brain stem death. These tests are therefore indicated for reasons of interest and not because they replace clinical evaluation; at most they assist or confirm such evaluation. Apart and aside from these correlations, many of these tests, although they have contributed greatly to the understanding and definition of brain stem death, have little place in clinical practice because of unavailability, cost, invasiveness, and inappropriateness in the setting of accident units and intensive care wards.

Electroencephalography

The EEG was the obvious means for diagnosing brain death and formed one of the earliest criteria for this diagnosis. Despite extensive research into the methods of recording and safeguards to be observed, this investigation rapidly fell into disuse. In 1969, a year after the publication of the Harvard criteria[20], it was recommended that the EEG was not essential for the diagnosis of irreversible coma. Beecher[21] and Hughes[22] indicated the limitations of the EEG in coma and diagnosis of brain death. That EEG activity may occur following brain death, and that reliance on the EEG to confirm brain death may be unwarranted, were shown by Grigg *et al.*[23].

The practical reality is that the EEG has been dropped by most clinicians from the criteria for determining brain stem death, and the fact that it is not available does not debar anyone from making the diagnosis clinically with confidence[19].

Scalp electromyograms

The electromyograms (EMGs) which appear spontaneously during EEG recordings of some patients who are clinically brain stem dead are considered to be artefacts. They have, however, been considered by some as evidence of residual brain stem function[24]. Such motor neuron survival may be an over-sensitive measure of brain stem function which does not correlate with the potential for brain stem recovery. It does not yield additional information not provided by clinical and EEG examinations[25].

Evoked potentials

After the EEG, these electrophysiological tests have probably been the most widely explored methods for establishing the diagnosis of brain death. Theoretically, they offer distinct advantages because clinical and EEG evaluation of patients under the influence of depressant drugs or therapeutic neuromuscular paralyzing agents cannot be relied upon. It is in this setting that auditory brain stem responses (ABR) may be particularly useful, as they are not significantly influenced by depressant agents[26]. These tests can be performed in an intensive care unit, provided adequate clinical skill and apparatus are available[27]. Despite earlier uncertainty due to technical difficulties in recording, and remaining uncertainties about the interpretation of certain wave forms, brain stem auditory evoked potentials (BAEPs) have acquired a place in the diagnosis of brain death, although not a pre-eminent one.

All patients, who on a previous recording had revealed medullary, pontine or midbrain potentials, but who later lost all peaks beyond P2 on repeated recordings, have been found to demonstrate EEG silence and clinical signs of brain death. Recovery of BAEP after disappearance of P2 has also not been observed[28]. There is, however, a difficulty with the interpretation of absent BAEPs after severe head injury due to the possibility of local trauma (petrous fractures, hemotympanum, meatal injury) being present, and there is frequently an absence of information about prior auditory function in the patient. Clinical skill in recording is required, as well as attention to recording minutiae, and some patients cannot be studied due to excessive ambient artefact[29].

There is no absolute agreement between various experts on the value of cord latency in somatic evoked responses (SER), and this method will therefore remain in abeyance until such time as contradictory findings have been clarified[30].

Lower esophageal contractility

Monitoring of lower esophageal contractility as a method of early identification of brain death has recently been suggested[31]. Loss of spontaneous lower esophageal contractility was thought to identify early brain death. This was not confirmed by Aitkenhead and Thomas[32], and the test is probably no more than another mechanism for assessing lower brain stem function, which may be lost early or late in the process leading to brain stem death.

Carotid and vertebral angiography

Often, these studies would have been done as part of the initial diagnostic procedure (subarachnoid hemorrhage). Where computerized tomographic scanning is not available, angiography will probably be the first method of investigation of a severely head-injured patient. In the patient with an expanding intracranial lesion, the rising intracranial pressure will eventually be equal to systemic arterial pressure. Cerebral circulatory arrest will be shown on the arteriogram, a feature which can confidently be used as a criterion of irreversible cerebral injury[33]. Isotope angiography has also been utilized to show complete cerebral circulatory arrest effectively[34]. Braunstein et al.[35] introduced a bedside evaluation of cerebral blood flow using a radio-isotope injected intravenously as a bolus; these isotope studies were found to agree with EEG findings to a high degree.

The metabolic disturbances which follow cerebral circulatory arrest, i.e. arterio-venous differences in oxygen, glucose, lactate and pyruvate, may be highly sensitive indicators of cerebral death. Again, one has a problem with the invasiveness of the investigations to prove this[36].

TIMING

One must return to the clinical examination to establish a final conclusive diagnosis. The questions which remain are first, how soon can this diagnosis be established with incontrovertible certainty, and second, if there is uncertainty, at what time interval does one have to repeat the examination? Only by allowing time to pass can one have absolute proof of irreversibility and of further downward progression. The clinician's judgement is important because rapidity of decline in the neurological status may vary from patient to patient, depending on the basic pathology and progression prior to the initial clinical examination. When all the criteria outlined above have been fulfilled, and the patient has already deteriorated for a period of 6 or more hours prior to testing, there would be little point in waiting for longer than 3 hours before essential tests are repeated. To wait for 24 hours would be pointless.

In order to facilitate and clarify the examination of patients on whom the diagnosis of brain death is being considered, a simple form based on that of Searle and Collins[37] (Appendix 3.1), abbreviating the above points, is provided at Groote Schuur Hospital for completion by the examining doctor. Legally (in South Africa), two registered doctors must certify the fact of brain death and it would seem wise for each one to examine the patient independently and draw his or her own conclusions, thus minimizing the risk of mutual influence and observer error. In situations where the observers disagree, repeated examination after a few hours becomes imperative. No further investigative procedure is necessary to make a confident diagnosis of brain death, and the patient may be declared dead if the above criteria have been met, safeguards have been observed, and an adequate examination has been performed. Mechanical ventilation may be discontinued at this point.

If the viability of certain organs is to be maintained for possible subsequent transplantation, mechanical ventilation can be continued and the circulation supported artificially, but with a clear understanding that these measures are not therapeutic but are continued in order to maintain a cadaver in a perfused condition. A member of the transplantation team is informed of the state of affairs. (In the Cape Town area, if the referring physician so requests, all subsequent medical and administrative care of the potential donor will be carried out by the transplant team.)

The doctor who takes care of the patient from the time of admission has a special responsibility towards the relatives who are passing through an extremely anxious time. For the layman it is still a macabre concept that the heart can be beating yet the doctors speak of death. They may not be able to grasp this concept, and this possibility should be respected, particularly when such understanding has to occur across cultural dividing lines. Continued small 'progress' reports to the relatives, informing them of the patient's deterioration, help to prepare them for the inevitable blow which must follow. In our experience, however, the request for organ donation must come from the transplant team, and not from those who have been treating the primary pathology.

References

1. Mollaret, P. and Goulon, M. (1959). Le coma dépassé (mémoire préliminaire). *Rev. Neurol.*, **101**, 3
2. Stuart, F.P., Veith, F.J. and Cranford, R.E. (1981). Brain death laws and patterns of consent to remove organs for transplantation from cadavers in the United States and 28 other countries. *Transplantation*, **31**, 238
3. Clark, G.P., Kahuho, S.K. and Ayim, E.N. (1979). Brain death. Some medical, ethical, legal, socio-economic and diagnostic considerations. A review. *East Afr. Med. J.*, **56**, 362
4. Jennett, B. (1975). The donor doctor's dilemma: observation on the recognition and management of brain death. *J. Med. Ethics*, **1**, 63
5. Conference of Medical Royal Colleges and their Faculties in the United Kingdom (1976). Diagnosis of brain death. *Br. Med. J.*, **2**, 1187
6. Wikler, D. (1984). Brain death (Correspondence). *J. Med. Ethics*, **10**, 101
7. Lamb, D. (1984). Correspondence. *J. Med. Ethics*, **2**, 102
8. Black, P. McL. (1978). Brain death. *N. Engl. J. Med.*, **299**, 338
9. Jennett, B. (1982). Brain death. *Intensive Care Med.*, **8**, 1
10. Pallis, C. (1983). ABC of brain stem death. The arguments about the EEG. *Br. Med. J.*, **286**, 284
11. Legg, N. (1981). Brain death. (Correspondence). *Lancet*, **1**, 107
12. Brendler, S.J. and Selverstone, B. (1970). Recovery from decerebration. *Brain*, **93**, 381
13. Ropper, A.H., Kennedy, S.K. and Russell, L. (1981). Apnea testing in the diagnosis of brain death. *J. Neurosurg.*, **55**, 942
14. Nayyar, M., Strobos, R.J., Singh, B.M., Brown-Wagner, M. and Pucillo, A. (1987). Caloric-induced nystagmus with isoelectric electroencephalogram. *Ann. Neurol.*, **21**, 98
15. Ivan, L.P. (1973). Spinal reflexes in cerebral death. *Neorology*, **23**, 650
16. Jorgensen, E.O. (1973). Spinal man after brain death. The unilateral extension-pronation reflex of the upper limb as an indication of brain death. *Acta Neurochir.* (*Wien*), **28**, 259
17. Hall, G.M., Mashiter, K., Lumley, J. and Robson, J.G. (1980). Hypothalamic pituitary function in the 'brain dead' patient. *Lancet*, **2**, 1259
18. Hanson, G.C. and McIlwraith, G.R. (1973). Lightning injury: two case histories and a review of management. *Br. Med. J.*, **4**, 271
19. Pallis, C. (1982). ABC of brain stem death. Pitfalls and safeguards. *Br. Med. J.*, **285**, 1720
20. Report of the ad hoc committee of Harvard Medical School to examine the definition of brain death (1968). Definition of irreversible coma. *J. Am. Med. Assoc.*, **205**, 337
21. Beecher, H.K. (1969). After the 'definition of irreversible coma'. (editorial). *N. Engl. J. Med.*, **281**, 1070
22. Hughes, J.R. (1978). Limitations of the EEG in coma and brain death. *Ann. N.Y. Acad. Sci.*, **315**, 121
23. Grigg, M.M., Kelly, M.A., Celesia, G.G., Ghobrial, M.W. and Ross, E.R. (1987). Electroencephalographic activity after brain death. *Arch. Neurol.*, **44**, 948
24. Arfel, G. (1975). Brain death – evidence contributed by laboratory studies other than surface EEGs. In Remond, A. (ed.) *Handbook of Electroencephalography and Clinical Neurophysiology.*, p. 116 (Amsterdam: Elsevier)
25. Wee, A.S. (1986). Scalp EMG in brain death electroencephalogram. *Acta Neurol. Scand.*, **74**, 128
26. Hall, J.W., Mackey-Hargadine, J.R. and Kim, E. (1985). Auditory brain stem response in determination of brain death. *Arch. Otolaryngol.*, **111**, 613
27. Stohr, M., Trost, E., Ullrich, A., Riffel, B. and Wengert, P. (1986). Bedeutung der fruhen akustisch evozierten Potentiale bei der Feststellung des Hirntodes. *Dtsch. Med. Wochenschr.*, **111**, 1515
28. Klug, N. (1982). Brain stem auditory evoked potentials in syndromes of decerebration, the bulbar syndrome and cerebral death. *J. Neurol.*, **227**, 219
29. Goldie, W.D., Chiappa, K.H., Young, R.P. and Brooks, E.B. (1981). Brainstem auditory and short latency somatosensory evoked responses in brain death. *Neurology*, **31**, 248
30. Plum, F. and Posner, J.B. (1980). *The Diagnosis of Stupor and Coma.* 3rd ed. (Philadelphia: F.A. Davis)
31. Sinclair, M.E. and Suter, P.M. (1987). Lower oesophageal contractility as an indicator of brain death in paralysed and mechanically ventilated patients with head injury. *Br. Med. J.*, **294**, 935
32. Aitkenhead, A.R. and Thomas, D.I. (1987). Lower oesophageal contractility as an indicator of brain death in paralysed and mechanically ventilated patients with head injury. (Correspondence). *Br. Med. J.*, **294**, 1287
33. Bergquist, E. and Bergstrom, K. (1972). Angiography in cerebral death. *Acta Radiol. (Diag.)*, **12**, 283
34. Goodman, J.M., Mishkin, F.S. and Dyken, M. (1969). Determination of brain death by isotope angiography. *J. Am. Med. Assoc.*, **209**, 1869
35. Braunstein, P., Korein, J., Kricheff, I., Corey, K. and Chase, N. (1973). A simple bedside evaluation of cerebral blood flow in the study of cerebral death: a prospective study on 34 deeply comatose patients. *Am. J. Roentgenol.*, **118**, 757
36. Smith, A.J. and Walker, A.E. (1973). Cerebral blood flow and brain metabolism as indicators of cerebral death. *Johns Hopkins Med. J.*, **133**, 107
37. Searle, J. and Collins, C. (1980). A brain death protocol. *Lancet*, **1**, 641

APPENDIX 3.1

Minimum criteria for a diagnosis of brain death

THE DIAGNOSIS OF BRAIN DEATH CAN ONLY BE MADE IF THE ANSWER TO ALL THE QUESTIONS IS NO.

(1) *Respiration**
   (a) Is there spontaneous ventilation within 5 minutes of disconnecting the ventilator (with $PaCO_2$ normal before the ventilator was disconnected)?

   OR

   (b) Is there any spontaneous ventilation within 10 minutes of disconnecting the ventilator?

(2) *Brain stem reflexes*
   (a) Do the pupils react to light?
       Do the pupils react to painful stimulation?
   (b) Are doll's eye movements present?
   (c) Does nystagmus occur when each ear is in turn irrigated with ice-cold water for 1 minute?
   (d) Is there any movement in the head and neck, either spontaneous or in response to stimulation?
   (e) Is there a gag or a reflex response following bronchial stimulation by a suction catheter passed down the trachea?

(3) *Body temperature*
   Is the rectal temperature below 35°C?

(4) *Drugs*
   Have any drugs which may affect ventilation or the level of consciousness been administered during the past 12 hours?

(5) *Cerebral state*
   Have you any doubt that this patient's cerebral state is due to an irreversible cause?

DATE _____

DOCTOR _____

*Methods of testing for spontaneous respiration

(a) *If arterial blood-gas analysis can be performed*:
   (i) Ventilate the patient with 100% oxygen for 15 min.
   (ii) Check $PaCO_2$ – must be within normal limits (5.3–6.1 kPa).
   (iii) Disconnect the patient from the ventilator.
   (iv) Administer oxygen (6 l/min) through a catheter in the trachea.
   (v) Check $PaCO_2$ – must be greater than 6.7 kPa.

(b) *If arterial blood-gas analysis cannot be performed*:
   (i) Ventilate the patient with 100% oxygen for 10 min.
   (ii) Ventilate the patient with 5% carbon dioxide for a further 5 min.
   (iii) Disconnect the patient from the ventilator.
   (iv) Administer oxygen (6 l/min) through a catheter in the trachea.

4
Medico-legal Aspects
L.S. SMITH AND S.S. SANBAR

INTRODUCTION

The law of human organ donation varies from country to country, although in broad terms the legal requirements, both by statute and at common law, denote substantial similarities. This chapter provides an overview principally of the statutory requirements relating to heart transplantation in the United States of America (USA), the United Kingdom (UK), and the Republic of South Africa (RSA) in comparison with the relevant laws in other countries. Comments will also be made pertaining to medical malpractice. Professional ethical codes and issues relating to civil litigation in general will not be discussed.

CERTIFICATION OF THE FACT OF DEATH

The certification of the *fact* of death must not be confused with other legal requirements where the doctor attending the patient is required to certify forthwith the *cause* of death (or his inability to do so where death is not solely and exclusively due to natural causes). In the issuing of such a death (cause) certificate, the purpose is the registration of the death and the disposal of the body by burial or cremation. In the case of an organ donation, both certifications are required to be completed.

In the USA and the RSA, the *fact* of death must be certified by two registered medical practitioners, who may not be members of the transplant team. What constitutes 'death' is left to the discretion of the two doctors concerned (Chapter 3). The grounds for so certifying would have to be justified by these doctors should this become an issue of litigation. The 1961 British Human Tissues Act allows removal of tissue once a registered medical practitioner has satisfied himself by personal examination of the body that life is extinct.

There has generally been opposition to making provision in the law that would define the moment of death because the *moment* of death cannot be defined. The solution to this problem would seem to be to define those who should be qualified to determine death, for, in the final analysis, it is the opinion of the physician that determines the time of death regardless of what instruments or methods he uses to assess the condition[1].

The 22nd World Medical Assembly, at the meeting in Sydney, Australia, in 1963, issued a statement that 'the determination of death should be based on clinical judgement supplemented, if necessary, by a number of diagnostic aids, of which electroencephalography is currently most helpful'. In the case of those persons kept alive by artificial means of resuscitation (in use or contemplated), or in which the transplantation of an organ is being considered, it emphasized that the moment of irreversibility of the processes leading to death must be determined rather than the moment of death. This declaration further states that, while the electroencephalograph is the most useful diagnostic aid, 'no single technological criterion is entirely satisfactory in the present state of medicine, nor can any one technological procedure be substituted by the overall judgement of the physician'[1].

While many may recoil from the suggestion of removal of organs from a body whilst the heart is still beating, it is clear that there is substantial support for the view that cerebral death is an acceptable criterion. The difficulty, however, is that absolute unanimity as to what constitutes irreversible cerebral death has so far not been fully achieved[2].

In general, the determination of time or moment of death has always been placed with the attending or certifying physician, provided the determination is based on accepted medical procedures. In addition to the traditional criteria of cessation of heart beat and respiration, brain death is now recognized by law in most USA states. In 1975, a New York court addressed the legal definition of time of death as used in provision of the Anatomical Gift Act. The court held that the term 'death' implies a definition consistent with the generally accepted medical practices of doctors, who in this case were primarily concerned with effectuating the purposes of the 1968 Uniform Anatomical Gift Act. It also noted that the intent of the Act was to provide a systematic procedure of implementing the public policy of New York State, which is to encourage anatomical gifts on death. To avoid the potential for conflict of interest in the determination of death, Section 7B of the Uniform Anatomical Gift Act requires that the physician determining death should not be a part of the transplant team.

By 1979, 25 states in the USA had recognized brain death as a basis for declaring the fact of death. The 1978 Uniform Brain Death Act specifies that: 'For legal and medical purposes, an individual who has sustained irreversible cessation of all functioning of the brain, including the brain stem, is dead. A determination under this section must be made in accordance with reasonable medical standards.' The law is, however, silent on the actual criteria to be used for determining death. The time of death is determined by the physician who attends the death, or, if none, by the physician who certifies the death. By this law too, this physician may not participate in the procedures for removing or transplanting a part of the deceased's body[3].

In contrast, most other countries have no specific laws relating to brain death as evidence of the fact of death, and generally rely on acceptable medical criteria. A Working Party on behalf of the Health Departments of Great Britain and Northern Ireland has prepared a quasilegal Code of Practice, intended for hospital staff and medical administrators relating to 'Cadaveric Organs for Transplantation' (1983)[4]. In the section dealing with brain death, it states: 'There is no legal definition of death. Death has traditionally been diagnosed by the irreversible cessation of respiration and heart beat. This Working Party accepts the view held by the Conference of Royal Colleges that death can also be diagnosed by the irreversible cessation of brain-stem function – "brain death". In diagnosing brain death, the criteria laid down by the Colleges[5] should be followed.'

In an attempt to seek clarity in regard to 'reasonable medical standards', a US report was issued by 'The Medical Consultants on the Diagnosis of Death to the President's Commission for the Study of Ethical Problems in Medicine and Biomedical Behavioral Research', entitled 'Guidelines for the Determination of Death'[6]. In this report, attention is directed towards: (1) eliminating errors in classifying a living individual as dead, (2) minimizing errors in classifying a dead body as alive, (3) allowing a determination of death to be made without unreasonable delay, (4) making the guidelines adaptable to a variety of clinical situations, and (5) explicit and accessible to verification. These guidelines are advisory, in the authors' words, 'representing a distillation of current practice tending to be too inflexible to be mandatory'.

Subsequently, the American Bar Association, the American Medical Association, and the National Conference of Commissions of Uniform State Laws, together with the aforementioned Commission, proposed a model statute to replace the Uniform Brain Death Act by a Uniform Determination of Death Act[6]. The relevant section reads: 'An individual who has sustained either (1) irreversible cessation of circulatory and respiratory functions, or (2) irreversible cessation of all functions of the entire brain, including the brain stem, is dead. A determination of death must be made in accordance with *accepted* medical standards.' The changed emphasis is italicized and tends to give legal standing to a decision made in terms of 'good medical practice', i.e. accepted standards, rather than reasonable medical standards.

Although recommendations and codes of practice regarding the criteria for death certification are not statutory prescriptions, they carry such evidential weight as to be read almost as a rider to what the laws would generally consider to constitute 'good medical practice'. (The clinical diagnosis of brain death is discussed in detail in Chapter 3.)

DONATIONS AND THE ACQUISITION OF TISSUE

There is legislation in several countries that permits the donation of a human heart to be made in one of three ways.

By any individual prior to death

Any person may make such a donation to be implemented after his death: (1) in his will, if he is competent to make such a will, (2) in any document attested to by two competent witnesses, (3) by an oral statement made by the deceased during life in the presence of two persons of at least 18 years of age, and (4) by wearing a prescribed identity tag issued by an approved institution (e.g. driving license). Any such donation may be revoked prior to death by the donor.

In the USA, the Uniform Anatomical Gift Act of 1968 allows any individual of sound mind who is over 18 years of age to make a gift during his life by will (to be effective immediately upon death without waiting for probate), or by a card or other document. If the donor is incapable of signing for any reason, including sickness, then the document can be signed on his behalf, if validated by two witnesses.

The system of donor cards has the merit of simplicity and portability. A typical example is the Uniform Card developed in the USA following the Uniform Anatomical Gift Act. This card, which can be carried easily in a pocket or wallet, states in simple words the donor's desire to make an anatomical gift to take effect upon death. On the reverse side the card contains provisions for signature, witnessing and personal details. Similar cards are available in several other countries, including Australia, Canada and Britain. In Britain, under the Human Tissues Act, 1961, a patient may carry a signed donor card or record his wishes 'in writing at any time or orally in the presence of two or more witnesses during his last illness'.

By a relative of the deceased

In the absence of specification by the individual while alive (as above), permission to donate organs at death may be obtained from certain specified next of kin of the deceased, i.e. the adult or legally competent spouse, child, parent, brother or sister, provided the deceased donor had not forbidden such a donation. Prior to actual organ removal, any donation by a relative may be revoked by the next of kin who made it. In this context, legal competency refers to a person of sound mind who is over the age of 18 or 21 years, depending on the legally specified age of majority for the country.

In the USA, relatives of a deceased may also legally donate by document, telegraph, recorded telephone or other recorded message; in order of legal priority, the next of kins are the spouse, adult children, parents and adult siblings.

In many countries 'relative' is not defined.

By an authority empowered to donate

The acquisition of hearts in the absence of a donation (as above) may be possible in some countries. If a relative authorized at law to consent to a donation cannot be traced, the law of some countries may allow for a designated official to authorize under certain prescriptions the removal of tissue from a deceased person for purposes of a donation, e.g. the District Surgeon in South Africa, and the Coroner in England and Wales. In the USA, however, the law makes no actual reference to the deposition in use of an unclaimed cadaver. A few states allow transplantation of certain organs (such as corneas) if a reasonable effort has been made to trace the relatives; authorization must be given by the Medical Examiner.

This official can only authorize removal of organs if he has satisfied himself on certain points. For example, in South Africa the District Surgeon must be clear that: (1) two doctors have stated in writing that in their opinion the use of the tissue in the body of another person is immediately necessary to save the life or restore the sight of the envisaged recipient, and (2) all reasonable steps have been taken to trace the relatives of the deceased. This second provision is difficult to implement, and District Surgeons are loath to give such consent where the identity of the deceased is not known, as it is argued, if this be the case, that it is impossible for any meaningful effort to have been made to trace the relatives of such a deceased.

Where the body is to become the subject of a medicolegal examination, in many countries certain authorities are empowered under certain circumstances to remove tissue (e.g. a heart) and donate such tissue to an authorized institution. Such removal or donation is not subject to the consent of the relatives. The medical practitioner who gives this authority must, however, satisfy himself that removal of the organ will in no way affect the outcome of the autopsy, and is not contrary to a direction of the deceased made before death.

In the USA, the State is given an overriding power to conduct legally required autopsies, and the exercise of this power cancels out the 'anatomical gift' (i.e. the donation for purposes of transplantation). When death occurs under suspicious, violent or unusual circumstances, the Medical Examiner or Coroner assumes jurisdiction and control of the body immediately; he may, however, give permission for transplantation (in the absence of statutory language to the contrary).

There are certain circumstances in the USA where the Medical Examiner may not approve organ donations, including homicide, poisoning, industrial accidents, and car accidents involving other persons where there is a question of liability.

For unclaimed bodies, statutes generally require a 48-hour waiting period after the death of the patient, during which time the hospital in possession of the body must make a reasonable search for the next of kin. Additionally, the physician who wishes to use the unclaimed body in a transplant procedure is required to obtain clearance from the Medical Examiner.

Stuart and his colleagues analyzed patterns of consent to remove cadaveric organs for transplantation in 29 different countries[3]. Their findings were based on their own experience in the USA and on a mailed questionnaire sent to renal transplant programs in 40 countries; replies were forthcoming from 28. A system of donor card disc, prepared before death, was used in 19 countries; in 16 consent to remove organs had to be obtained from the donor or a family member, whilst 13 countries used 'presumed consent' as a basis for removal of organs for transplantation, though in six of the 13 the family was approached before proceeding with organ removal. Some countries provided for both card donations and presumed consent. In the USA, in no state is consent presumed.

PURPOSE OF DONATION

In most countries each donation or 'removal' must be for the purposes of medical and dental education, research, therapy (including use in any other living person) or for any other scientific purpose; such purpose need not be specifically expressed and may include the production of a therapeutic, diagnostic, or prophylactic substance.

THE DONEE

In the USA, state statutes vary with regard to permissible recipients of donated tissue. In general, licensed hospitals, teaching institutions, colleges, medical schools, universities, storage banks, state public health and anatomy boards and institutes approved by the State Department of Health may be donees. Unless the donee has been previously indicated during life by the deceased, the attending physician becomes the donee. If he so desires, he can transfer his ownership to another person. Although he is not permitted to participate personally in removing and transplanting organs or parts, he is allowed to communicate with other relevant donees or transplant teams.

In South Africa, a donee may be any hospital, medical practitioner, dentist, university or technikon, authorized institution or any person. The donee may upon delivery of the tissue have exclusive right over it subject to the prohibition of the sale of the tissue. Except in the case of a donation of a whole body, the donee has 24 hours after death of a donor to have the tissue removed, since the relatives may claim the body for burial or cremation 24 hours after death.

AUTHORIZATION FOR THE REMOVAL OF ORGANS

Once a donation has been made in South Africa, a donee specified, and the fact of death certified, the transplant surgeon or a member of the team must request authority from the appropriate medical practitioner (for example, the medical superintendent of the hospital in which the donor is being cared for, or his authorized medical deputy) to remove the donated organ, which removal may only be undertaken by or on the authority of a medical practitioner or dentist. The person authorizing removal must satisfy himself that the body is not required for examination in terms of other legislation which has a higher ranking claim on the body, e.g. the Inquest Act.

Authority to remove a valid donation in the United Kingdom is not essentially different from the above provisions, with the noticeable exception that the person lawfully in possession of the body of a deceased may so authorize, after practicable inquiries, providing that the deceased had not expressed objection to his body being so dealt with, or the surviving spouse or any relative of the deceased expressed objection. Normally, the 'person' lawfully in possession of a dead body is a National Health Service hospital until such time as the body is claimed by the person with the right to possession, i.e. the Coroner, executor, or the next of kin[4].

CONFIDENTIALITY

Disclosure to any other person of any fact whereby the identity of the deceased donor or donee may be established is prohibited by statute in some countries. In the United Kingdom, confidentiality is not prescribed, but the staff of hospitals and organ procurement organizations 'must respect the wishes of the donor, the recipient, and the families with respect to anonymity'[4]. There appear to be no specific statutory laws regarding transplantation confidentiality in the USA. However, the constitutionally protected right of privacy and general statutes governing medical care in the USA preclude unpermitted disclosure.

At common law, the privacy of the individual may not normally be intruded upon. The legal and ethical obligations of a medical practitioner to treat patient information as confidential appears to be based also on contract[7]. Experience has shown that breaches in confidentiality in regard to heart transplantation have generally had their origin beyond the medical profession.

IMPORTATION/EXPORTATION OF TISSUE

In most countries the importation or exportation of tissues is subject to permission being obtained from a government authority.

SALE OF TISSUE

An authorized institution or the importer of tissue may receive payment for providing tissue to any person for therapeutic or scientific purposes. If any other person receives payment for such tissue, he shall refund such payment to the person who made it. The object of this and the aforementioned provision is to prohibit trading in tissue, which ethically and scientifically is unacceptable. This prohibition, however, does not prevent a medical practitioner from being paid for his services in the collecting or use of such tissue as a part of therapy.

In the USA, the sale of organs is prohibited by the National Organ Transplant Act of 1984, as amended in 1986 by the fiscal 1987 budget Reconciliation Legislation, setting a uniform policy in this area following a private attempt to establish an organ brokerage firm in Virginia during 1983[7,8]. A reasonable charge for removal costs is allowed. While questions have been raised concerning the constitutionality of the non-sales provision under the 'right of privacy' doctrine, the better position is that the provision is constitutional under the commerce power, and does not properly fall within the sphere of constitutional privacy.

TRANSPLANT MALPRACTICE

With regard to medical malpractice involving transplantation, the reasons for malpractice as a cause of action are the same in transplant cases as in any other medical situation: negligence, lack of informed consent, battery, invasion of privacy, fraud, abandonment, breach of fiduciary duty, etc. To date, there have been relatively few cases of medical malpractice involving transplant patients, probably because transplantation is still relatively new and experimental. Also, expectations for success are low, and there has usually been a cultivated personal relationship and good communication between the transplant surgeon and the patient and relatives. What suits have occurred have generally turned on the question of informed consent, rather than the applicable standard of care[9].

An area of developing concern, in light of current AIDS malpractice litigation, is that of liability on the part of the physician, hospital, and donor's estate for the transplantation of AIDS-infected organs. A cause of action could also arise on the part of the donor's family, if they became involved in an active concealment of the donor's health status prior to death.

This is, in reality, an extension of the general question of strict liability for body tissues raised previously in the areas of blood and blood products. While early cases allowed the plaintiff to hold the blood supplier strictly liable for contaminated blood products, the clear trend of later cases has been to reject strict liability, considering blood as a 'service'. This is in keeping with provisions of the Federal Act preventing the sale of organs. Thus, the major impact of the increase in AIDS cases will most likely be to limit the number or organs available for transplant, rather than produce a significant risk of malpractice to the practitioner (in the absence of negligence).

At the state level, the Uniform Anatomical Gift Act of 1968 was adopted in all 50 USA states. Under this Act, the physician may incur possible liability for making an errant determination of the time of death in the transplant donor, resulting in premature harvesting of the organ(s). (The time of death of the patient must be determined by a 'treating' physician.) However, when the physician removes an organ from a donor patient in 'good faith', the physician is not liable in a civil action under the terms of the Act or an applicable state law.

While not yet tested, the Act will most likely protect the physician from criminal liability, particularly as regards a question concerning the determination of the time of death. However, the surgeon who removes the desired organ prematurely may not be protected from wrongful death action, even though the Act may prevent the filing of charges of mutilation or mayhem. Liability for medical malpractice prior to death is also not exempted by the Act.

Failure to comply with the Anatomical Gift Act is evidence of 'bad faith' *per se*. A physician who makes an honest effort to determine the time of death based on reasonable and well-recognized medical standards, and who acts in the best interest of the patient, would probably be considered to be exhibiting good faith.

COMMENT

Jeddeloh, in a review of legal aspects of transplantation[10], emphasizes that the law today is for the purpose of *inter alia* protecting individual rights in a complex technological society which has the capability to transplant tissue from one person to another as a form of medical treatment. This poses new, ever-changing challenges with regard to the rights and obligations of, and relationships between, the donor, whether living or dead, and the donee of human body tissue.

'Presently these issues have not been fully settled. While the law recognizes that the transplantation of human body tissue is an important, and in many cases, highly successful means of treatment which should be encouraged, it also seeks vigorously to protect potential donors from exploitation in all forms. In most recent decisions and cases, courts have struggled to balance societal needs and rights of individual donors. The law is only beginning to consider matters such as facile procurement and easy distribution of various body parts, right of minor and incompetent donors, proper standards of informed consent for giving a human body part, liability for injury caused to a donee by the transplantation procedure itself, the time at which a necessary human body part may be removed from a deceased donor, the legitimate scope of protection which ought to be afforded the transplant surgeon and other questions'[10].

References

1. Report: Select Committee (1968). *The Anatomical Donations and Post Mortem Examinations Bill*. (Republic of South Africa: Government Printer)
2. Strauss, S.A. (1980). *Doctor, Patient and the Law.*, p. 125. (Pretoria: Van Schaik)
3. Stuart, F.P., Veith, F.J. and Crawford, R.E. (1981). Brain death laws and patterns of consent to remove organs for transplantation from cadavers in the United States and 28 other countries. *Transplantation*, **31**, 238
4. Working Party of the Health Departments of Great Britain and Northern Ireland (1983). *Cadaveric Organs for Transplantation*. (London: HMSO)
5. Conference of Medical Royal Colleges and Their Faculties in the United Kingdom (1976). *Br. Med. J.*, **2**, 1187
6. Report of the Medical Consultants on the Diagnosis of Death to the President's Commission for the Study of Ethical Problems in Medicine and Biomedical Behavioral Research; Guidelines for the determination of death (1981). *J. Am. Med. Assoc.*, **246**, 2184
7. Johnson, K.L. (1987). The sale of human organs: implicating a privacy right. *Valparaiso Law Rev.*, **21**, 741

8. Denise, S.H. (1985). Regulating the sale of human organs. *Virginia Law Rev.*, **71**, 1015
9. Sanbar, S.S. (1984). Medicolegal aspects of human organ transplantation. *Legal Aspects Med. Practice*, **12**, 1
10. Jeddeloh, N.P. (1980). Legal aspects of transplantation. In Chatterjee, S.N. (ed.) *Renal Transplantation – A Multi-disciplinary Approach.* (New York: Raven Press)

5
Donor Organ Availability and Transplant Coordination

J.S. CHAFFIN

INTRODUCTION

Organ donation is a process that begins with a need. The need is a patient suffering from failure of an essential organ. To satisfy that need, organ procurement agencies (OPAs) have developed mechanisms for identification, referral, and equitable distribution of organs that are made available. The primary function of most OPAs is education, not only of the general public, but, more importantly, of the professional community, regarding the need for organs and tissue for transplantation. Unfortunately, most OPAs are still haunted, not by lack of money or surgical skills, but rather by the lack of suitable donor referrals[1].

'Harvesting organs' is not a phrase transplant surgeons commonly use or enjoy hearing used in public. But, with rare exceptions, we use it routinely in work, journals, and at medical meetings unattended by the press. In today's climate of ever expanding demand for organs, the mounting pressure to find viable organs is felt by all transplant units. Nowhere is the pressure felt more greatly than by the retrieval team, whose job it is to locate, evaluate, prepare, and 'harvest' the organ(s).

REASONS FOR INADEQUACY OF DONOR ORGAN SUPPLY

Gallup polls have determined that more than 80% of Americans state that they are willing to donate their organs and tissue for transplantation after death. Only about 17%, however, carry organ donor cards[2]. Currently, in the USA, 30% of patients approved for cardiac transplantation die awaiting a donor organ. If 80% of Americans actually donated postmortem organs for transplantation, more than enough would be available to supply current needs. Personal experience demonstrates that grieving families frequently welcome an opportunity to consider organ and tissue donation. The knowledge that other lives have been enhanced through the gift of organs is generally a strong solace for a family struggling to accept what they feel is a 'meaningless' death. Statistically, fewer than 30% of those asked turn down the request for donaton. The majority do not donate either because they were not approached, or because the personnel involved in the care of the patient were not aware of the suitability of the patient as a donor of organs. Well-coordinated public and professional education programs must continue to be developed[3].

In 1968, the National Conference of Commissioners on Uniform Law and the American Bar Association drafted the Uniform Anatomical Gift Act, an attempt to provide the states within the USA with a model for recognizing and formalizing methods through which individuals or famiies could make a gift of their organs or those of a relative. The Act authorizes an individual 18 years of age or older, in the presence of two witnesses, to record his wishes regarding organ donation by will, donor card, or other written document, or orally in the presence of two witnesses, and authorize the next of kin to consent to organ donation in the absence of the deceased's known objection. Space has been made available on the back of all drivers' licenses for recording the wishes of potential organ donors. Less than 10% of those eligible, however, actually mark their license[4].

While it may not seem to be healthy or 'natural' to anticipate one's own death or the death of a family member, such anticipation is not infrequent – we buy life insurance to provide benefits upon death, we prepare wills, trusts, and even buy cemetery plots in anticipation of death. In a similar manner, we must convince the members of the public to accept consent for organ donation as a logical preparatory step for their own demise.

Trust in the system is imperative, and lack of knowledge or understanding of organ donation procedures may instill fear or lack of trust (Table 5.1). Common sources of concern or mistrust include: (1) lack of awareness of religious or moral propriety of invasion of the body or removal of parts

Table 5.1 Questions frequently asked by the family of a potential organ donor

Is there anything more that can be done?
Is he really dead?
Why does his heart still beat?
What organs or tissue will be used?
Who will remove the organs?
Who will receive the organs?
What will surgery be like?
How long will surgery take?
Will an autopsy be necessary?
Will the body be picked up by the funeral home?
Will the Medical Examiner be involved?
When can a funeral be held?
How will he look, after donation?
Who will pay the cost of organ donation?
Will anyone know we donated?
Will the media be involved?
Will we be able to make contact with the recipient?
When will we know if the organs were used?

for transplantation, (2) concern over the care of or proper respect for a body after donation, (3) concern that organs may be sold for profit of others, (4) superstition that talk of death or signing a donor card might accelerate their own death, and finally (5) fear that organs might be removed from a person before death has occurred[5]. It is the responsibility of the transplant community to alleviate such fears and concerns through proper education. Historically, mankind responds with altruism when called upon to meet needs it understands and trusts.

Our own personal experience has been largely in the USA, where organization of organ retrieval is now well advanced at a national level. Most of our comments will therefore relate to the system of organ retrieval as it is in the USA, though the underlying principles are relevant in all countries where organ transplantation is performed.

ORGAN PROCUREMENT NETWORKS

USA

At one time there were over 120 separate organ procurement agencies in the United States, and another eight in Canada. These were either hospital-based agencies serving the parent hospital, or independent organ procurement agencies serving one or several transplant centers in a given area[5].

In 1982 the demand became so great for organizations that could expedite procurement, preservation, and distribution of vital organs that the North American Transplant Coordinators Organization (NATCO) established a computer registry called '24-Alert' to facilitate the distribution of organs other than kidneys. This system coordinated more than 80% of the hearts transplanted in the USA from September, 1982 through June, 1986.

The National Organ Transplant Act, signed into law in 1984, called for the design and implementation of a national computerized network that would include transplant centers, procurement agencies, voluntary health organizations, and the public. The United Network for Organ Sharing (UNOS), which has been active with kidney programs since 1976, now coordinates organ donation nationally, lists all vital organs required and available, and produces a printout of the listing. This system cannot be activated without a computer terminal[6]. The computer data base includes information on all potential recipients, including age, sex, name, blood type, lymphocytotoxic antibody status, medical status, and identification of unacceptable HLA antigens.

Western Europe

Western Europe now has a number of regional organ matching services, the first of which was set up in the Netherlands, which is now the base of the European Transplantation Service (Eurotransplant) (Table 5.2). Spain as yet does not have a national organ matching service, although organization in the northern Catalonian region is well developed[7]. Most of these units were set up originally for kidney placement. Although most fulfill their functions primarily in their own areas, should there be no suitable local recipient, the organ will then be offered to another transplant service. In this way, there has been progress towards an international organization. Since 1984, there has been a marked increase in multiple organ donation throughout Europe, although this is still hampered to some extent by laws concerning the definition of brain death, cultural differences, and the lack of transplant coordinators in some regions. Each region and country retains the right to service its own population first; only if there is no suitable recipient will that organ be offered to another country.

With multiple organ retrieval, the potential for chaos in the operating room seems great when perhaps four separate surgical teams, possibly unknown to each other and speaking different languages, may gather for organ removal. One possible solution, pioneered in Cambridge, England, is to provide one surgical team trained to remove and preserve all organs and tissues for transplantation[7]. It is possible that, in the future, such teams will become available throughout Europe to expedite multiple organ retrieval.

Table 5.2 Major international, national and regional organ procurement agencies

Organ procurement agency	Countries served
United Network for Organ Sharing	USA
Eurotransplant	Netherlands, Belgium, Luxemburg, Germany, Austria
UK Transplant Services	United Kingdom, Ireland
France Transplant	France
Rhone-Mediteranee	France
Scandia Transplant	Norway, Sweden, Denmark, Finland
Italy Transplant	Northern Italy

The future development of transplantation services in Europe depends on the allocation of financial resources by the individual governments, increasing cooperation between medical and nursing professionals in the referral of potential donors across national borders, and the support of the general public, who must be able to make informed decisions on organ donation in the event of a tragic or untimely death.

Elsewhere

In most other countries, such as South Africa, organ retrieval networks are not as yet well organized. Major transplant centers tend to rely on organs in their immediate vicinity, and on direct referral from physicians at other hospitals who are aware of their requirements. In South Africa, for example, there is no central unified organ retrieval network, though organs are exchanged from center to center depending on need.

ORGANIZATION OF ORGAN RETRIEVAL

The transplant coordinator

With the evolution of transplantation has come a number of new health-care professionals, none more important than the transplant coordinator. In the USA, coordinators are organized under the North American Transplant Coordinators Organization (NATCO) for credentialling and certification. Large centers will have both donor and recipient coordinators on their staff. In smaller centers, the combined duties may be performed by a single coordinator. The donor coordinator provides expertise in the management of the brain-dead potential donor, and in the procurement, preservation, and distribution of transplantable organs. The recipient coordinator is responsible for coordination of the pretransplant assessment and preparation of the recipient, together with post-transplant care and follow-up.

For the purposes of this review, we will consider that, at each center, the transplant coordinator carries out the combined duties.

Transplant coordination

Recipients are listed on computer by their individual criteria through the United Network for Organ Sharing (UNOS). Once an organ has been identified for transplantation, the chain of events may be lengthy, but, in practice, the system works efficiently (Figure 5.1).

A member of the medical or nursing team caring for the potential donor will contact the local organ procurement agency, either directly or through the hospital transplant coordinator. A member of the local procurement agency will generally go to the hospital to assess the donor personally, and initiate therapy to maintain the donor in as stable a hemodynamic state as possible (Figure 5.2). A number of essential blood tests will also be requested (Chapter 6).

When basic data, such as blood group, weight, and age, are known, the procurement agency will enter this information into the computer, and search for a compatible recipient. With regard to heart transplantation, a potential recipient is generally located within the geographical region in which the donor hospital is situated, but a recipient in a distant region may on occasion be identified as the most suitable.

If the recipient is at a distant center, communications will be via the procurement agency serving that area. This agency will, in turn, contact the transplant coordinator or a member of the transplant team in the hospital on whose waiting list the potential recipient is listed. If the donor appears a suitable match for the potential recipient, a number of activities is set in motion.

Transplant coordination at the recipient center

The transplant coordinator at the recipient center notifies the operating room team of the planned transplant,

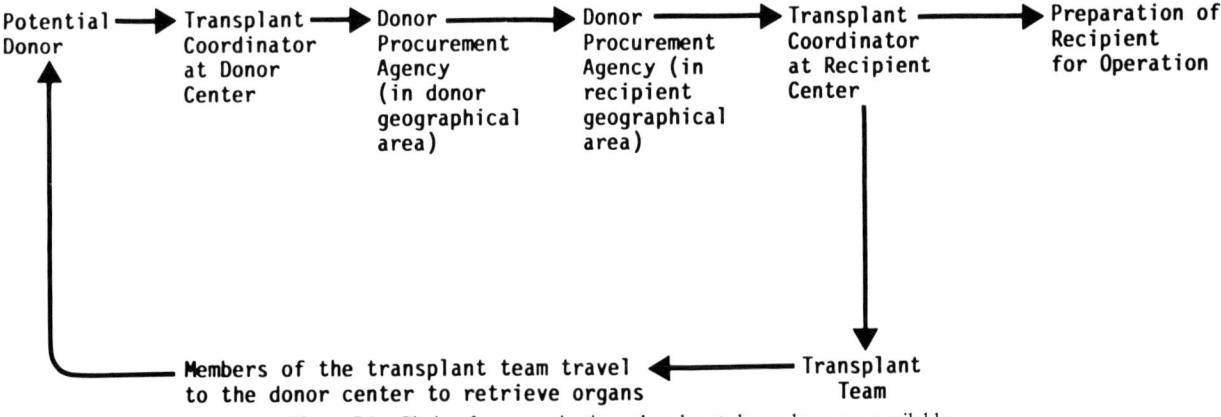

Figure 5.1 Chain of communication when heart donor becomes available

THE TRANSPLANTATION AND REPLACEMENT OF THORACIC ORGANS

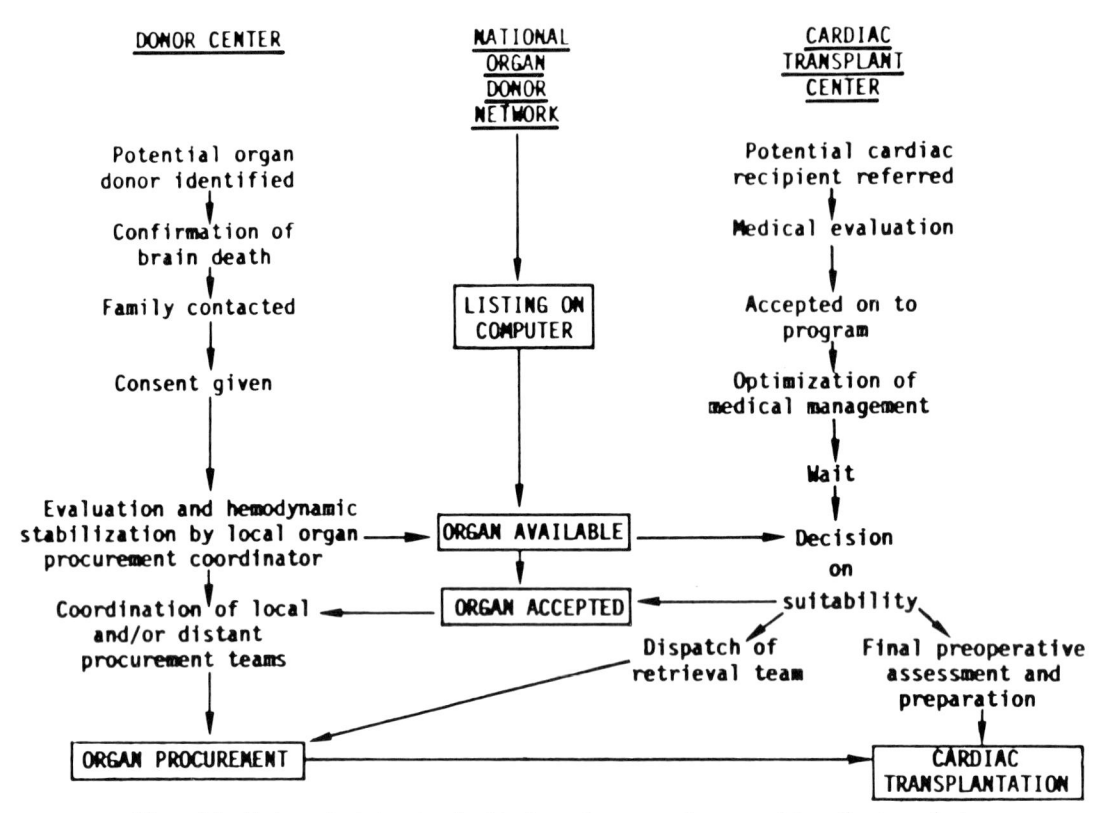

Figure 5.2 Pretransplant steps involved in the performance of a successful cardiac transplant

organizes the retrieval team (who will travel to the donor center) to include at least one surgeon, one operating room nurse, a hospital transplant coordinator (or a member of the local donor procurement agency), and the necessary equipment (Table 5.3). The most expedient transportation (ambulance for short, helicopter for medium range, and private jet for longer distances) is organized. If the recipient is not an inpatient, he is notified, arrangements are made to transport him to the hospital, and he is prepared for surgery. All potential recipients waiting as out-patients carry radiopagers so that they may be easily contacted.

Transplant coordination at the donor center

Simultaneously, the coordinator at the donor center confirms information on both donor and recipient to insure acceptable matching of size and blood type. It is not unusual in the USA to have retrieval teams arriving from at least three different locations to harvest heart, kidneys, and liver, and possibly lungs and/or pancreas also. It is important that the local coordinator arranges ground transportation from the airport for the teams. It is the donor coordinator's responsibility to insure that the donor is properly cared for prior to arrival of the retrieval teams, and that on-site arrangements are made for operating room personnel to assist in the retrieval. This would include anesthesia personnel, as they do not usually travel with the harvest teams.

Table 5.3 Equipment required by the cardiac retrieval team

Supplied generally by donor hospital	Supplied and transported by retrieval team
Esophageal temperature probe	Necessary drugs
Blood warmers	Sternal saw
Steri-drape	Special clamps or retractors
Cautery	Cannulas (for cardioplegic infusion)
Suction	Sterile tubing
Sternal retractors – several sizes	Cardioplegic solution
Vascular instruments	Cold (4°C) saline or ice slush
Vascular clamps (e.g. Cooley)	Intestinal bags (for transport of heart)
Pedicle clamps	
Satinski clamps	
DeBakey forceps	
Umbilical tapes, vessel loops	
Hemoclips	
Ties: silk (0000, 000, 00, 0, #1, #2)	
Sutures: silk retention sutures (0)	
Cold (4°C) normal saline for irrigation	
Large basin	
Extra poles for supporting i.v. infusion fluids and cardioplegic bags	
Table covers – towels	
Cysto tubing	
Ice and ice bucket	
Specimen bottles for lymph nodes	

An added burden in the European community might be to insure a translator is present to overcome any language barrier that might exist between the retrieval teams.

Since we believe that, whenever possible, the heart should not be ischemic for more than approximately 4 hours, and as 30–60 minutes of this time must be allowed to sew in the transplanted heart, the time of donor aortic cross-clamp should be arranged so that the heart can be delivered to the transplant center within 3 hours. It is essential that close communication be maintained between the retrieval team and the team preparing the recipient to insure that the ischemic period is not unnecessarily prolonged. The liver and kidney retrieval teams are usually cooperative, as they appreciate that the heart has the shortest ischemic survival time of any of the solid organs.

It is vitally important that coordination between the heart retrieval team and colleagues at the recipient center be well organized at this point, because unnecessary delays of the other retrieval teams do not go unnoticed; a poorly coordinated team may find that it is not invited a second time! Multi-organ procurement etiquette requires being able to work professionally with multiple surgical teams from other programs without creating turbulence. Factors causing friction include arriving late, being unnecessarily demanding with regard to investigations and/or operating room personnel support, and discourteous behavior.

The ideal scenario is when all teams arrive before the donor is taken to the operating room. The procurement surgeons can each examine the donor, review the relevant charts, chest radiographs, and electrocardiogram. The retrieval transplant coordinators can copy appropriate chart information, and speak with the family, if desired. The procurement surgeons and coordinators can call their respective transplantation centers to confirm the donor's suitability and coordinate the final stages of preoperative care for the recipients. Before the surgical recovery begins, the surgeons from each of the procurement teams should agree on an order of organ excision which is acceptable to all concerned[6].

While the surgeon and his assistant are completing the 'packaging' of the heart for transportation, the coordinator should confirm that ground and air transportation are available. One last call is made to inform the recipient surgeon that the donor team is ready to leave the donor center; the estimated time of arrival at the recipient center is communicated, so that the recipient surgeon can plan his operation to coincide with the heart's arrival in the operating room.

COMMENT

As heart transplantation matures medically, a number of ethical and policy issues demand attention. A central fact about organ transplantation, and heart transplantation in particular, is the scarcity of organs for transplantation. The National Heart Transplant Study in the USA found that 14 000–15 000 people a year could benefit from heart transplantation; the recent relaxation of some of the criteria for recipients makes the number even greater[8]. An estimated 17 000–26 000 persons annually are declared brain-dead while on respirators, making them potential donors[9]. It is further estimated that 12 000–14 000 persons in this group would qualify medically as heart donors. Evidence from kidney donation suggests that only 20–40% of this medically qualified group will actually become donors[10], this number being far short of the 14 000–15 000 needed. The chronic shortage of hearts for transplantation raises a number of issues which must be considered if we are to meet the growing demands of our patients.

The essential need to continue a program of making both the public and the medical profession aware of the requirements of the patient awaiting transplantation has already been discussed. There are, however, several other ways in which the number of organs made available for transplantation could be significantly increased. Several involve possible changes in the laws concerning donation, and some of these will be discussed below. Furthermore, attention must be paid to the efficient use of such organs; unnecessary wastage must be eliminated whenever possible.

Alternatives to the 'family consent' requirement

The present system of family consent for donation from brain-dead, heart-beating cadavers does not result in donation of all the organs that are medically acceptable for transplantation. It is likely that more hearts could be retrieved if the need for family consent were modified or even eliminated. The argument in favor of doing this rests on the assumption that the harm that might be inflicted on a (potential donor's) non-consenting family is of less concern than that suffered by a transplant candidate (and his family) who dies from lack of a suitable donor organ.

An alternative to family consent is 'presumed consent', in which the consent of the family (or deceased) to donate is assumed unless they come forward and object. Some states currently have such laws covering the donation of corneas, and have seen a significant increase in the supply of corneal tissue[9]. A more radical option would be the elimination of consent altogether, allowing the routine salvage of organs in every suitable brain-dead patient. Routine salvage would treat the deceased's organs or body as a community resource, and permit organs and tissue to be excised as needed. This may not be as radical a solution as it seems. The military 'draft', or the conscription of young men into the armed forces, which is or has been legal in many countries, demonstrates the community's willingness to accept jurisdiction of the live body when an important public purpose – the safety of the community – is at stake. Saving the lives of persons with end-stage organ failure is arguably as important as saving lives by raising armies, and may justify overriding the family's traditional control of the deceased's remains[11].

Relaxation of brain death requirements

Some persons have proposed relaxing the requirement for brain death, which at present includes death of the brain stem, to permit organ retrieval from persons who lack cortical function only[12]. Such a re-definition of death would allow organ retrieval from irreversibly comatose and anencephalic patients. While such a change is not likely to increase significantly the supply of adult hearts, it may prove to be an important factor in the expansion of pediatric heart transplantation.

Routine inquiry or required request policies

Perhaps our best immediate hope for increasing the organ supply lies with implementing 'routine inquiry' or 'required request' policies. Such policies maintain respect for family wishes, and address the main flaw in the present organ procurement system, namely the reluctance of some physicians to discuss brain death and organ donation with grieving families. This reluctance to broach the subject of organ donation is due to many factors, including lack of knowledge about transplantation, misunderstanding of brain death, fears about legal liability, fears that discussions will be upsetting to families, and a general distaste for the subject. As a result, many families are not asked to donate, and potential donors are lost. Routine request laws have been recommended by many organizations, including the Federal Task Force on Organ Donation, and have been enacted into law in most states in the USA. These laws place a duty on hospitals to identify all potentials donors and counsel the next of kin on the possibility of organ donation.

The sale and purchase of organs

A 'market' in organs has been proposed as a way to increase the supply. In the USA, however, it is now a federal crime, punishable by 5 years in prison, to 'acquire, receive, or otherwise transfer any human organ for valuable consideration'[13]. Opponents of the sale of organs point out the adverse effect it would have on voluntary organ donation and on donors' families, and its dehumanizing symbolic connotation. Proponents of such a market feel that these concerns can be minimized and are outweighed by the benefits to recipients of a market-driven increase in the supply of organs. If organ transplant operations are 'sold' by surgeons, in as much as the recipient pays the surgeon, the proponents see no harm in selling the organs that make the operations possible[12]. It is our hope that if more families are informed of donation options through routine inquiry policies, there will be no need to offer financial incentives.

Xenografts

The Baby Fae case, in which a baboon heart was transplanted into a 2-week-old baby with hypoplastic left heart syndrome, showed that a human could survive with a baboon heart for 20 days[14]. Ethical problems raised by this case concern respect for both human and non-human animals. Given our current rudimentary knowledge of cross-species transplantation, the chances of significantly prolonging meaningful life seem, at present, relatively remote (Section VI). Killing a primate to retrieve its heart for transplantation might be accepted by many people if efficacy were established. Without a clearer demonstration of lasting benefit, however, sacrificing primates for experimental use of their organs will continue to generate controversy.

Modifications in recipient selection

The scarcity of hearts for transplantation inevitably requires a rationing of the hearts that do become available. The basis for selecting recipients involves a balance between efficiency and equity in the use of organs. Efficiency is clearly favored at the candidacy evaluation stage, while equity plays a larger role in deciding which candidate on the waiting list receives the heart. The cardiologist's attitude in referring patients for evaluation for candidacy plays an important role in the selection of patients for transplant, and will draw greater scrutiny in the future. The frequency of referral for evaluation varies with the knowledge and attitudes of each individual cardiologist treating patients with end-stage heart disease. Physicians who are unaware of transplant options, or who neglect to refer patients for evaluation, may be denying their patients a viable therapy. Although malpractice suits challenging referral decisions have not yet been brought, negligence may soon be claimed in cases of non-referral of patients to transplant centers for evaluation.

The current selection system gives priority to those candidates on the list whose poor physical condition makes them most urgent, including those who are rejecting a transplant and frequently those who have received a temporary mechanical assist device or artificial heart as a bridge to transplantation. A strict concern for the efficacious use of donated hearts might argue against such an allocation, for the most urgent cases are frequently less likely to do as well as healthier candidates[9].

While efficiency is important, a strong equity consideration is to avoid abandonment of critically ill patients. Once in the candidate list, one could argue that there is a special commitment not to abandon those in greatest need. Retransplantation after rejection of a heart also appears to conflict with efficiency by allocating a second heart to a patient who may not have as good a chance of survival as a healthier candidate. Aggressive efforts on behalf of a recipient in acute rejection, however, are viewed by some physicians as essential to demonstrate commitment. Transplantation of a third heart, after a second rejection, would appear to be even more controversial, and policy in this situation is divided between the major centers.

A similar situation arises with the use of the total artificial heart or ventricular assist device as a bridge to transplantation. Since 30–40% of candidates die awaiting transplantation, mechanical hearts and assist devices have been used experimentally in some programs to act as a bridge until a donor heart becomes available[8]. This actually exacerbates rather than relieves the supply problem for the entire group of potential recipients, although it benefits the individual involved. It increases the number of patients awaiting a transplant, thus increasing the pool of patients from which selection for the next available heart must be made[15]. Moreover, these patients will almost all be urgent cases, since the risk of thromboembolism and infection increases, and the likelihood of a successful transplant decreases, with the duration of the artificial implant. Though the results of subsequent transplantation in this group are inferior, they tend to gain priority in the allocation of the scarce resource of the donor heart. This may become a significant source of inefficiency in the use of donor hearts.

Official designation of transplant centers

Now that heart transplantation has achieved accepted status, a major issue is whether there should be limits on the number of centers doing heart transplants. There were 12 centers performing heart transplants in the USA in 1983, but it is estimated that there will be over 200 in 1990. Only one-third of the 17 centers functioning in 1985 performed more than 10 transplants during that year[9].

The Federal Task Force on Organ Transplantation recommended that heart transplants be carried out only at those centers meeting certain criteria, including a minimum volume of 12 transplants a year[9]. The Medicare coverage decision, announced in July 1986, also limits reimbursement to centers meeting certain requirements for volume and survival. The purpose of permitting only those centers that meet volume and survival criteria to perform heart transplants includes the protection of recipients and the efficient use of scarce organs. Since neither physicians, patients, nor institutions have an inherent right to the use of scarce organs, the community is free to limit heart transplants to designated centers if it deems this limitation essential to the efficient use of this resource.

Physicians in centers unable to meet criteria will argue that access to transplantation in one's own community is a distinct advantage, or that the local community should receive first priority for the organ donations it generates. They should be aware, however, that poor outcomes in centers that do not meet volume or other designated standards may be vulnerable to malpractice claims. It is arguably negligent to conduct a transplant program when components that are reasonably deemed essential to good outcome are missing. In any event, it is essential that transplant candidates be informed of a local center's compliance with or deviation from volume or other accepted standards. In addition, the referring physician should be aware of the standards of a specific center and realize that referral to a center not meeting public criteria for center designation could lead to malpractice claims.

Finally, organ procurement agencies must consider whether it is wise to provide organs to programs that do not meet minimum criteria for safe and efficacious use of donated organs. Presumably, a national network that controlled the distribution of organs would not permit supply to unqualified centers.

The medical and legal constraints on organ supply result in a chronic shortage of hearts for transplantation. It seems that the demand for hearts will always out-strip the supply. How donated hearts are distributed, how recipients are selected, etc. are now emerging as issues of public concern, with demands voiced for public accountability in rationing organs. Medical efficacy plays a major role in selecting recipients, but a variety of equitable and other concerns also enters into the picture. More public scrutiny and debate about conflicts between efficiency and equity are likely, as is a reduction in the freedom now held by medical professionals to resolve these questions[11].

References

1. Broznick, B.A. (1988). Organ procurement: fulfilling a need. *Transplant Proc.*, **20**, 1010
2. Casscells, W. (1986). Heart transplantation: recent policy development. *N. Engl. J. Med.*, **315**, 1365
3. Corry, R.J. (1988). Public policy and organ distribution. *Transplant Proc.*, **20**, 1011
4. Miller, M. (1987). A proposed solution to the present organ donation crisis based on a hard look at the past. *Circulation*, **75**, 20
5. Davis, F.D., Lucier, J.S. and Logerfo, F.W. (1986). Organization of an organ donation network. *Surg. Clin. North Am.*, **66**, 641
6. Davis, F.D. (1987). Coordination of cardiac transplantation: patient processing and donor organ procurement. *Circulation*, **75**, 29
7. Wight, C. (1988). Organ procurement in Western Europe. *Transplant Proc.*, **20**, 1003
8. Evans, R.W., Manninen, D.L., Garrison, L.P. Jr., Overcast, T.D., Yagi, J., Merriken, K. and Jonsen, A.R. (1984). The National Heart

Transplant Study: final report. *Batelle Human Affairs Research Centers*, Vols. 2–4
9. Department of Health and Human Services (1986). *Task Force on Organ Transplantation.* pp. 28–125
10. Evans, R.W., Manninen, D.L., Garrison, L.P. and Maier, A.M. (1986). Donor availability as the primary determinant of the future of heart transplantation. *J. Am. Med. Assoc.*, **255**, 1892
11. Robertson, J.A. (1987). Supply and distribution of hearts for transplantation: legal, ethical, and policy issues. *Circulation*, **75**, 77
12. Green, M.B. and Wikler, D. (1980). Brain death and personal identity. *Philosophy Publ. Affairs*, **9**, 389
13. 42 U.S.C. 274 (e); P.L. 98–507, 98 stat 2346
14. American Medical Association Council on Scientific Affairs (1985). Xenografts: review of the literature and current status. *J. Am. Med. Assoc.*, **254**, 3353
15. Annas, G.A. (1983). Consent to the artificial heart: the lion and the crocodiles. *Hastings Cent. Rep.*, **13**, 20

6
Selection and Management of the Donor

D.K.C. COOPER AND D. NOVITZKY

INTRODUCTION

The importance of a well-functioning donor heart cannot be overemphasized; it is clearly crucial to the success of the heart transplant procedure, particularly if orthotopic transplantation is to be performed. Early donor heart failure accounts for approximately 25% of the deaths of heart transplant patients today (Chapter 31), and is therefore an area where significant improvements can still be made. Careful selection and meticulous management of a potential donor therefore remain essential.

SELECTION OF DONOR HEART

Donor age

As the incidence of coronary atheroma in Caucasian men increases markedly after the age of 40–45, it had until recently been our policy to exclude men above this age from donation of hearts. Similarly, women over the age of 45–50 were also excluded. The shortage of donor hearts has become so acute, however, that we now consider hearts of both men and women up to the age of 60 years as long as left ventriculography, coronary angiography, and basic pressure measurements, such as left ventricular end-diastolic pressure or pulmonary artery 'wedge' pressure, reveal no significant disease.

Should coronary angiography not be available at the donor center, then, if it is essential to find a heart for a desperate recipient, we believe that, under these circumstances, the heart can be used if certain conditions are fulfilled: (1) echocardiography should show normal left ventricular wall movement; (2) direct coronary palpation and inspection should reveal no significant signs of atheromatous disease; (3) the heart rate should be increased by infusion of isoproterenol whilst an electrocardiogram (ECG) is being recorded – there should be no significant ECG changes suggestive of ischemia with the heart rate increased to above 140 beats/minute.

Though these studies provide only a crude assessment, we believe that such hearts can be used, but we would attempt to confine such use to recipients of 60 years or older. This policy of using older hearts for older recipients is now followed by several centers, and, though controversial, we believe is justified (in view of the extreme shortage of suitable donors) in critically ill, older patients.

Potential donors of certain ethnic groups may be considered to an older age without the need for coronary angiography. For example, black patients in South Africa have an extremely low incidence of coronary atheroma, and may be acceptable as donors up to the age of approximately 60 years without coronary angiography.

Donor size

It is generally accepted that hearts taken from donors whose body mass is within approximately 25% of that of the potential recipient will support the circulation after orthotopic transplantation. The relative heights and the muscle masses of the two subjects should also be taken into consideration in assessing the suitability of a donor heart for a specific recipient; the heart may prove inadequate if the recipient is much taller and has little fat when compared with the donor. If the need of the recipient for transplantation is urgent, and yet the body mass of the donor is 25% less than that of the recipient, then heterotopic heart transplantation should be performed.

Donor blood group

It is essential to have ABO blood group compatibility between donor and recipient (Chapter 8). There is an estimated approximate 60% risk of early hyperacute or accelerated acute rejection if ABO incompatibility is present[1]. A recent report has suggested that a recipient who receives a heart from an ABO-identical donor (e.g. O to O, or A to A) will survive longer than one who receives a heart from an ABO non-identical, yet compatible, donor (e.g. O to A)[2], though this has not been confirmed by a multi-center trial (Chapter 32). The shortage of donors is such, however, that most groups will transplant if there is ABO compatibility. Rhesus compatibility is not thought to be of importance.

Presence of lymphocytotoxic antibodies in the recipient

Whenever lymphocytotoxic (LCT) antibodies have been demonstrated to be present in the recipient serum (by prior screening against a panel of lymphocytes), the results of a donor lymphocyte–recipient serum cross-match should be obtained (see also Chapter 8). In the presence of a positive cross-match (demonstrating antibodies to be present in the recipient serum against the donor cells), the risk of hyperacute rejection of the transplanted heart is high, and that donor should not be used for that specific recipient.

Exclusion of cardiac disease

Patients with pre-existing cardiac disease are obviously unsuitable for heart donation. Severe or long-standing diabetes mellitus and hypertension may also preclude donation. The presence of a cardiac disorder can be excluded by taking, whenever possible, a clinical history from the patient's relatives or his/her own medical practitioner, by clinical examination, by study of a chest radiograph and a 12-lead ECG. If murmurs or added sounds are not to be missed, it is essential that the clinical examination be performed when a normal arterial pressure is present. Intracranial damage itself may cause ST and T wave changes on the ECG[3,4]. Hypothermia leads to bradycardia and/or the presence of J waves, which are of no pathological significance, but can be confused with electrocardiographic changes suggestive of ischemia. Rarely, cardiac catheterization and angiography may be indicated to exclude suspected cardiac disease.

Echocardiography to determine ventricular wall shortening fraction should also be carried out to give some indication of the quality of myocardial contractility. Septal motion is often paradoxical in brain-dead subjects, though the cause of this is unclear; in our experience, its presence does not appear to be associated with impaired ventricular function in the post-transplant period.

Ideally, there should be no history of severe hypotension or cardiac arrest at any time. Recovery from such episodes, however, with return of an adequate blood pressure and diuresis, suggests that myocardial function remains satisfactory.

Many cardiac surgeons believe that the most reliable means of assessing donor heart function is by direct inspection of the organ at the time of procurement, and we concur that this is a most important part of donor selection. It is therefore essential that an experienced surgeon should assess each donor heart on an individual basis. Donor heart assessment and retrieval is not a procedure that can be left to an unsupervised junior member of the surgical team.

Transferable disease

Hearts should not be transplanted from donors with transferable disease, such as a malignant lesion (other than a primary tumor of the central nervous system) or certain serious infections.

The presence of pyrexia in the hours or days before death may be related to the brain injury itself, and may not necessarily indicate serious infection, although every effort must be made to exclude this possibility; once brain death has occurred, body temperature usually falls to subnormal levels over the course of a few hours. The length of time that the patient has been ventilated mechanically is equated with an unavoidable degree of infection, overt or otherwise; not more than 3 days is desirable, and longer than 7 is usually unacceptable.

The presence of acute pulmonary infection almost certainly precludes donation of the lungs, but does not rule out heart donation. Infection in the renal tract of the donor is also not a contraindication to use of the heart. Many hearts have been transplanted successfully from donors with positive blood cultures; the decision to use a heart from such a donor is a difficult one, and not without risk, but, if the infected organism is known, the recipient can be administered the appropriate antibiotics. Our own policy is liberal in regard to the chance finding of a positive blood culture; if the patient has overwhelming sepsis, however, then organs should not be excised for transplantation.

Positive human immunodeficiency virus (HIV) antibody serology should preclude transplantation, and, whenever possible, this test should be performed before donor heart excision. When positive, the test should be repeated as false-positive results can occur. If the donor is believed to be at 'high risk' for HIV positivity (e.g. homosexuals, intravenous drug abusers, hemophiliacs), and yet the HIV antibody serology remains negative, the decision whether to use the organ must be based on the urgency of the recipient's condition, after full discussion with the patient and/or his or her family. When making such a decision, the possible risks to operating room, intensive care unit and laboratory staffs must also be taken into consideration. HIV transmission by kidney transplantation has been reported[5–7], and the present evidence is that organs from 'high risk' donors should not be used[8].

Blood specimens are taken for bacterial culture and serological tests for syphilis, cytomegalovirus, and hepatitis B surface antigen (HBsAg, Australia). Although the results may not be available before the organ is transplanted, they may, if positive, be of considerable importance in the subsequent care of the recipient.

The presence of a positive test for venereal disease in the donor need not preclude donation, but it would seem wise to give the recipient a course of antibiotic therapy to prevent transfer of the disease. An IgM level suggestive of recent cytomegalovirus infection would not preclude use of the heart for transplantation, though many groups would not use such a donor for a heart–lung transplantation in a cytomegalovirus-negative recipient. When the presence of hepatitis B antigen is strongly suspected, the result of the serological investigation must be awaited; it remains our policy not to transplant organs taken from patients in whom a positive result is obtained. When the need of the recipient is urgent, however, a strongly positive hepatitis antibody reaction possibly should not prevent donation as long as the recipient is covered by a course of gamma globulin.

THE BRAIN-DEAD DONOR

The effects of the agonal period and brain death on myocardial function and structure

The major source of donor hearts has been, and would appear to continue to be, persons dying of head injury or spontaneous intracranial hemorrhage. The adverse effect of brain dysfunction on the heart was demonstrated as early as 1954[9-13]. Electrocardiographic changes have been reported clinically in association with subarachnoid hemorrhage, intracranial infections, and cerebral tumors. Subendocardial hemorrhage and even myocardial necrosis have been reported in association with intracranial lesions. Electrocardiographic changes can be produced in animals by midbrain stimulation, and chronic stimulation produces myocardial necrosis; excessive sympathetic discharge may be etiologically responsible.

Although Griepp and his colleagues[14] found no evidence of central nervous system-mediated cardiac damage in a series of 22 patients evaluated as potential cardiac donors, more recent studies in both the experimental animal and potential clinical donors have suggested that brain death has major histopathological and functional effects[15-23].

Two major effects of brain death have been observed in experimental studies. The first is a series of major electrocardiographic, hemodynamic, and histopathological changes which take place during and immediately following the agonal period[15,16,18,20,22]. The second consists of significant changes in circulating levels of certain hormones, which in turn result in major changes in body metabolism[15-17,21].

'Autonomic (sympathetic) storm'

In an experimental model of brain death, a sudden increase in intracranial pressure or the sudden onset of ischemia of the brain lead to a series of major pathophysiological changes which may collectively be referred to as the 'autonomic storm'[15,17,18,20]. Though there is a brief initial period of excessive parasympathetic activity, evidenced by a marked bradycardia, most of the effects are brought about by the sympathetic nervous system[17,18,20]; the terms 'sympathetic storm' or 'catecholamine storm' have also been used to describe these events.

There is a large increase in circulating and endogenous catecholamines in the early few minutes after induction of brain death, which is associated with an increase in myocardial activity, together with the appearance on the ECG of ventricular arrhythmias[15]. Within 5 minutes of a sudden rise in intracranial pressure, circulating epinephrine, norepinephrine, and dopamine concentrations rise markedly, though they return to control levels within 10–15 minutes[15].

Electrocardiographic effects

When intracranial pressure is increased acutely (or the brain made acutely ischemic), an immediate bradycardia, progressing to sinus standstill with occasional junctional escape beats and a short period of atrioventricular dissociation, is rapidly followed by a sinus tachycardia and, subsequently, ventricular ectopic activity of multifocal origin[15] (Figure 6.1). A further period of sinus tachycardia follows, but, on this occasion, with marked ischemic changes.

Factors which contribute to ischemia possibly include endogenous catecholamine release, spasm of coronary arteries (indicated by contraction band necrosis in the major coronary arterial walls), and a high systemic vascular resistance from increased sympathetic activity which

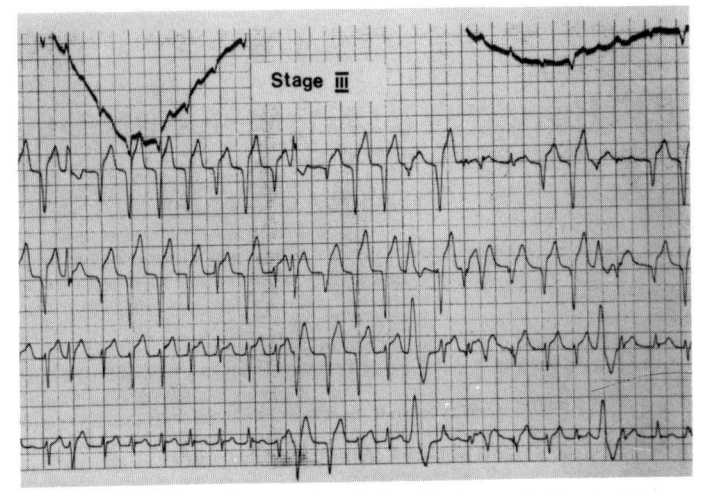

Figure 6.1 Electrocardiogram taken during development of brain death in an experimental animal showing multifocal ventricular extrasystoles

increases afterload and results in acute temporary myocardial oxygen supply–demand imbalance. This ischemia not infrequently results in myocardial histopathological damage, especially in the subendocardium, though this is rarely significant enough to exclude use of the heart for transplantation.

Finally, there is a reduction in rate to the pre-agonal level or below, with a regular rhythm. A total of 50% of experimental animals, however, continue to show abnormalities of the QRS complex and/or ST segment, including pseudo-infarct patterns. These ECG changes rarely indicate severe ischemic injury, and are believed to be due to loss of energy within the cell. In the clinical subject, such changes are commonly reversible following hormonal therapy (see later).

Hemodynamic effects

The hemodynamic changes observed in such experimental animals reflect the body's attempts to compensate for the intracranial changes taking place during 'coning' (Cushing's reflex)[17]. Significant and often massive increases in systemic vascular resistance (SVR) and mean arterial pressure (MAP) occur (Figures 6.2 and 6.3), and are almost certainly the direct result of a great increase in sympathetic nervous activity, which produces an extreme degree of peripheral vasoconstriction. Blood is therefore re-distributed into the capacitance vessels, leading to a rapid accumulation within the great veins and right atrium. Due to a combination of low pulmonary vascular resistance (PVR), high pulmonary vessel compliance, and pulmonary capillary reserve recruitment, associated with a higher degree of right ventricular compliance compared to the left ventricle, the right ventricle is able to adjust to this increased venous return, and increase its output, demonstrated by an increase in pulmonary artery flow compared with aortic flow at this time[18].

The left atrial pressure may actually exceed the pulmonary artery pressure for a matter of seconds during the period of peak peripheral vasoconstriction[18]. This remarkable and surprising observation implies that the pulmonary capillary blood flow temporarily ceases entirely. The extreme rise in SVR which occurs during the agonal period almost certainly results in transient mitral regurgitation following temporary failure of the left ventricle. It would seem likely that it is during this period that disruption of the normal pulmonary capillary anatomy can occur. As the peak left atrial pressure far exceeds the normal hydrostatic pulmonary capillary pressure, capillary integrity within the lungs may be disrupted, resulting in pulmonary edema with high protein content and interstitial hemorrhage.

Histopathological effects

In approximately 75% of experimental animals undergoing brain death, histopathological changes develop in the left ventricular wall[15,17]. These consist of contraction bands, focal coagulative necrosis, and myocytolysis, with edema formation and interstitial mononuclear cell infiltration (Fig-

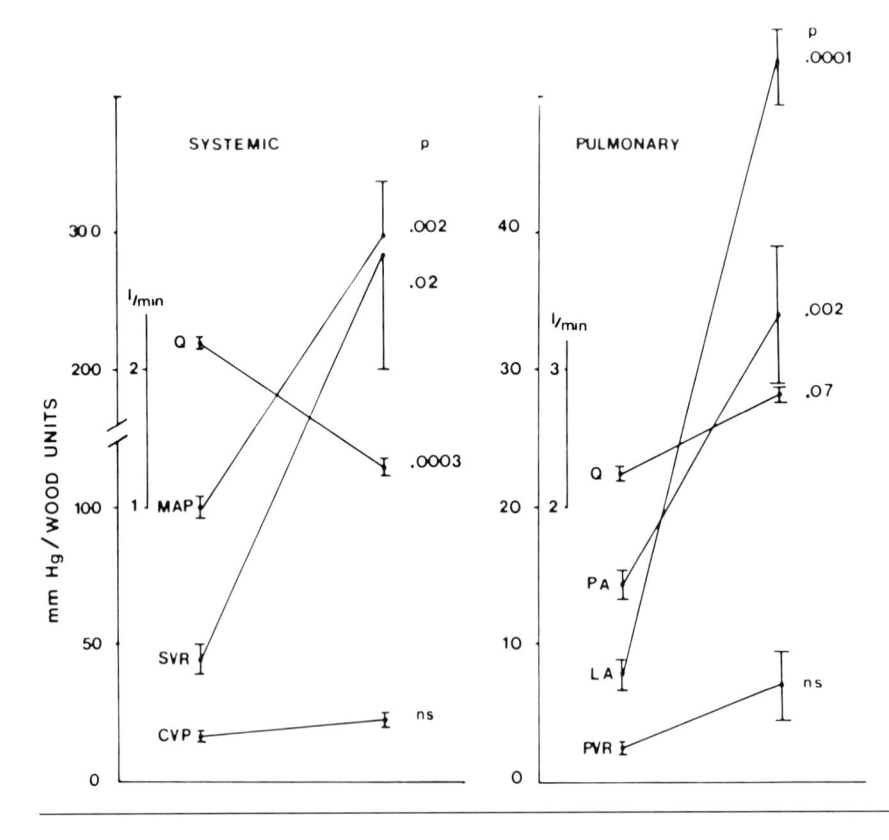

Figure 6.2 Mean changes in systemic and pulmonary hemodynamic data during the induction of brain death in eight baboons. The left-hand graph shows changes in systemic hemodynamics between control levels and those recorded at the peak of systemic vascular resistance. (MAP = mean arterial pressure (mmHg); SVR = systemic vascular resistance (Wood units); CVP = central venous pressure (mmHg); Q = aortic blood flow (l/min)). The changes in MAP, SVR and Q reached statistical significance. The right-hand graph shows changes in pulmonary hemodynamics between control levels and those recorded at the peak of systemic vascular resistance. (PA = pulmonary artery pressure (mmHg); LA = left atrial pressure (mmHg); PVR = pulmonary vascular resistance (Wood units); Q = pulmonary artery blood flow (l/min)). The changes in PA and LA reached statistical significance

SELECTION AND MANAGEMENT OF THE DONOR

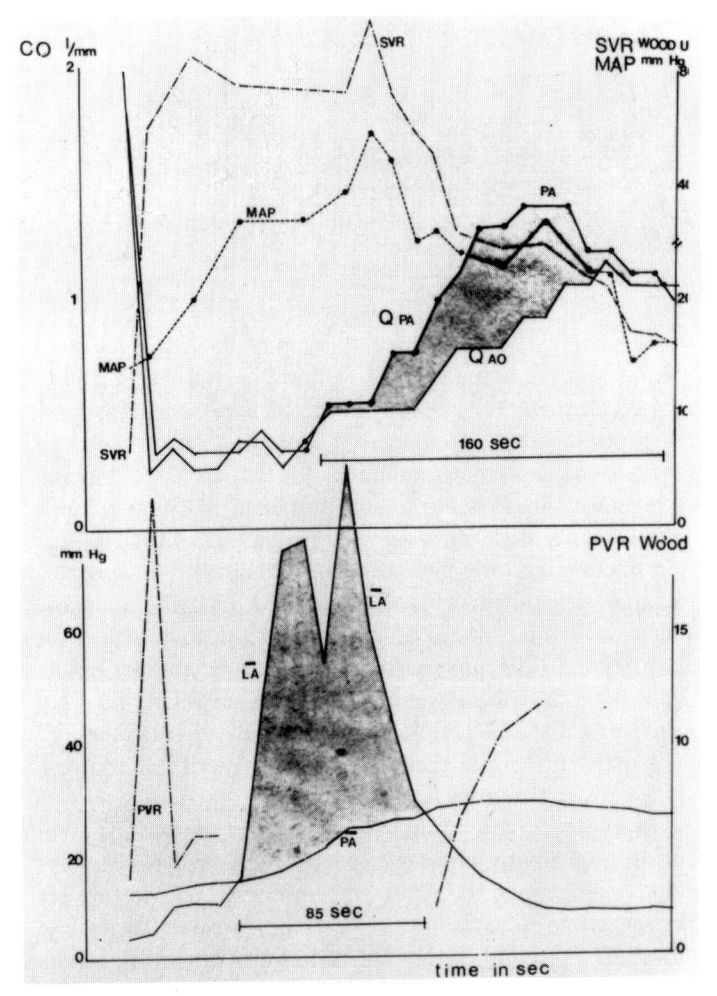

Figure 6.3 Systemic and pulmonary hemodynamic data during induction of brain death in a baboon. The upper graph shows changes in systemic vascular resistance (SVR) (Wood units), mean arterial pressure (MAP (mmHg), pulmonary artery blood flow (PA) (l/min) and aortic blood flow (AO) l/min. The discrepancy between pulmonary artery and aortic blood flows (shaded area) represents the period and extent of blood pooling within the lungs; in this case, blood pooling extended for a period of 160 s. In the lower graph, changes in mean left atrial pressure (LA) (mmHg), mean pulmonary artery pressure (PA) (mmHg) and pulmonary vascular resistance (PVR) (Wood units) are shown. The shaded area represents the period of 85 s during which the left atrial pressure exceeded the pulmonary artery pressure

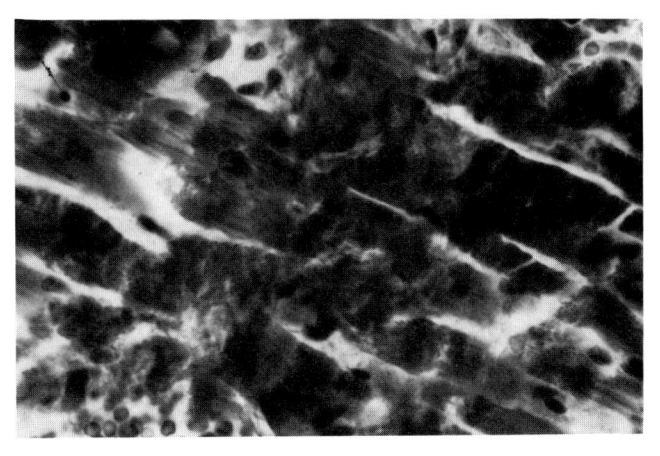

Figure 6.4 Light micrograph section of myocardium showing widespread contraction bands and edema (H & E × 310)

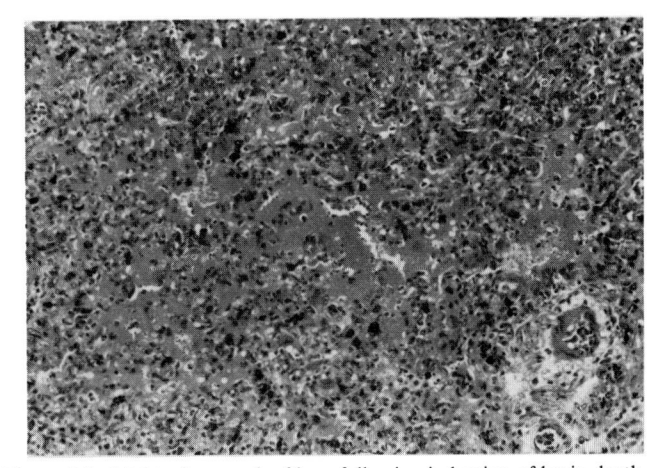

Figure 6.5 Light micrograph of lung following induction of brain death. Alveolar wall hemorrhage due to disruption of capillary integrity can be seen, as well as considerable pulmonary edema. The heavy eosinophilic staining of the edema fluid demonstrates it to be an exudate rich in protein (H & E × 100)

ure 6.4). Contraction band necrosis may even develop in conduction tissue and in coronary arterial smooth muscle.

In addition, over a third of the animals show pulmonary edema with an exudate rich in proteins (Figure 6.5); there is also evidence of capillary endothelial damage, and, on occasion, diffuse hemorrhage, both in the alveolar walls and into the alveolar spaces[18].

All of these changes are believed to be the result of the catecholamine excess which occurs during the development of brain death, and are thought to be related to cytosolic calcium overload. Similar myocardial structural damage has been clearly documented in human potential organ donors[19]. Various combinations of the three forms of acute myocardial necrosis have been described, namely contraction bands, coagulative myocytolysis, and coagulative necrosis (colliquative myocytolysis). Focal mononuclear cellular infiltration has also been described surrounding areas of myocyte necrosis.

A majority of human donor hearts show mild (or occasionally more severe) degrees of myocardial injury (Figure 6.6), such as subendocardial hemorrhage, presumably once again due to the high catecholamine output during the period of brain injury and the development of brain death.

Endocrine changes and metabolic responses

In the baboon, the thyroid hormones plasma free triiodothyronine (T3) and thyroxine (T4), together with plasma cortisol and insulin, fall significantly within a few hours of the onset

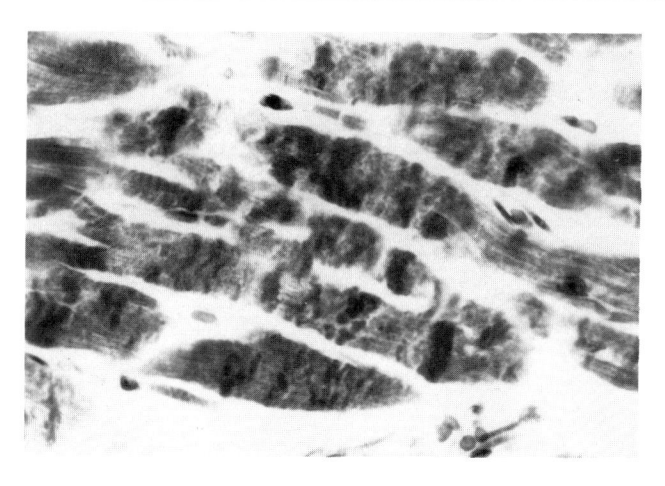

Figure 6.6 Light micrograph of a human donor heart which failed 2 h after operation, showing extensive contraction bands (H & E × 320)

of brain death[15]. Antidiuretic hormone also disappears from the plasma within a few hours. These changes in circulating hormones are associated with a reduction in myocardial energy stores (adenosine triphosphate (ATP), creatine phosphate (CP) and glycogen), as well as a significant increase in myocardial lactate[15,16,24]. These myocardial tissue changes suggest that there is impairment of aerobic metabolism following brain death.

The functional testing of hearts taken from brain-dead animals demonstrates a deterioration in myocardial function, as evidenced by significant reductions in cardiac output, stroke volume, and left ventricular pressure[16,24]. There is also evidence that brain death leads to functional deterioration of the kidney[25].

Plasma free T3 levels have also been shown to be reduced in human potential donors, and there would appear to be some correlation between the level of T3 with the time interval that has elapsed since brain death took place[23]. Cortisol and insulin have also been shown to be in the low normal range.

Further experimental work in the baboon, studying the kinetics following single bolus injection of 14-carbon labeled metabolites (glucose, pyruvate, and palmitate) confirms that there is a major change in metabolic oxidative processes following brain death, involving the entire animal[21]. The rates of glucose, pyruvate and palmitate utilization are markedly reduced, and there is an accumulation of lactate and free fatty acids in the plasma. These findings indicate a change from aerobic metabolism affecting the body as a whole, and correlate well with the previous findings relating to metabolism in the heart and kidney alone. High energy phosphates are rapidly depleted under this changed metabolic environment, almost certainly leading to deterioration in function of all organs.

MANAGEMENT OF THE DONOR

Care of the donor can be a time-consuming activity. If the patient is to be maintained in an ideal state for organ donation, as much care has to be taken over his management as would be given to any patient in an intensive care unit. When brain death has been confirmed, interest in the care of the subject by the primary medical and nursing personnel may wane, and support by the retrieval team is often called for.

Mechanical ventilation will already be employed, and blood gases are maintained within the normal range. A urinary catheter may already be *in situ*; if not, one is inserted. A central venous pressure (CVP) monitoring catheter is essential if the volemic state of the patient is to be well controlled. An arterial pressure line is an advantage, but is not essential if monitoring by sphygmomanometer cuff is satisfactory; its presence, however, facilitates the frequent estimation of arterial blood gases. (The femoral artery and vein, or jugular vein, can be utilized for easy access for arterial and CVP monitoring.) At least one, and preferably two, other peripheral venous infusions are set up for fluid and drug administration. Care is taken to introduce all vascular and urinary catheters under sterile conditions, especially if the groin is used.

Brain-dead patients frequently pass large quantities of urine, and rapidly become hypovolemic and hypotensive if fluid is not replaced. Fluid, preferably warmed to prevent hypothermia, is administered in the form of electrolyte solution or colloid. If the patient has bled significantly, e.g. from a head or other injury, whole blood (or packed cells) is given to maintain the hemoglobin above 8 g/dl. The serum sodium may rise to high levels in patients with impairment of production of antidiuretic hormone, and the administration of sodium chloride as a replacement fluid is therefore avoided. Potassium is lost in the urine and may require replacement on a large scale; 30 mEq potassium chloride are added to each liter of intravenous fluid given. Further supplements of 15–40 mmol/l administered in 30–100 ml of intravenous fluid over periods of 15–60 minutes may be necessary to maintain the serum potassium level above 3.5 mmol/l.

A systemic mean arterial pressure (MAP) of between 60 and 80 mmHg would appear sufficient to provide an adequate coronary flow. Such a pressure may be best obtained by a combination of fluids, to maintain a moderate preload, and an intravenous infusion of vasopressin (or small increments of intramuscular vasopressin) to increase the afterload. Excessive increases in either preload or afterload may be damaging to the myocardium[15,16]. The CVP, therefore, should not be increased to high levels if the systemic arterial pressure is adequate. If the kidneys are also to be excised for the purpose of transplantation, as is usually the case, an MAP of much below 60 mmHg may, however, prove inadequate to maintain renal perfusion.

If urinary output is excessive, making adequate fluid replacement difficult, vasopressin given intravenously or intramuscularly is of value in reducing this loss. Since vasopressin acts by peripheral (including renal) vasoconstriction, great care is required in its administration if the kidneys are to remain suitable for donation. (Similarly, phenylephrine is contraindicated, although neither of these agents is harmful if the heart alone is to be donated.) We have found the intramuscular administration of vasopressin to be particularly effective, only small doses being required (0.1–0.25 U/kg), repeated as necessary. For intravenous infusion, vasopressin (100 U/250 ml normal saline, administered initially at approximately 0.25 ml (0.1 U)/min) usually results in a decrease in urine flow and/or increase in blood pressure.

Brain-dead patients lose thermoregulation and rapidly cool to low temperatures if not actively warmed with an electric warming blanket. Although a mild degree of hypothermia may, in fact, be beneficial to the preservation of organs in a satisfactory condition, ventricular fibrillation can occur at temperatures below 30°C. Our policy has been to maintain the central temperature at approximately 35°C.

If the PaO_2 and $PaCO_2$ are maintained within normal limits by mechanical ventilation, and if the central venous and arterial pressures are also maintained within the desired range, acid–base balance may remain within normal limits. If acidosis occurs, as a result of a combination of increasing anaerobic metabolism and peripheral vasoconstriction associated with hypothermia, sodium bicarbonate should be administered to correct the base deficit (base deficit × body weight (kg) × 0.3/2 = ml 8.4% sodium bicarbonate).

A suitable wide-spectrum, non-nephrotoxic antibiotic (e.g. chloramphenicol or a cephalosporin) is initially administered at the dose of 2 g intravenously, and at 1 g 6-hourly thereafter until the donor is taken to the operating room for organ excision.

By the measures outlined above, the hearts of most brain-dead donors can be maintained in a viable state for several hours, occasionally up to 24 hours. In our experience, however, increasing instability of the circulation is the rule, and every effort should be made to organize the transplant operation as soon as possible.

Hormonal therapy

Noting both the deterioration in cardiac function and depletion of myocardial energy stores that can occur after brain death, consideration was given as to whether these effects resulted from the depletion in circulating hormones, such as T3, cortisol, and insulin.

Experimental observations

Brain-dead experimental animals treated with these hormones showed a return towards control level in respect to cardiac output, though left ventricular pressure remained slightly reduced[24]. Myocardial ATP, CP, glycogen (which had been depleted) and lactate (which had been increased) did, however, return to control values[24]. Similarly, there was a return to normal renal function following hormonal therapy to the brain-dead animal[25].

When T3 was administered to a brain-dead baboon (2 μg at hourly intervals), there was a dramatic increase in the rate of metabolite (glucose, pyruvate, and palmitate) utilization, and reductions in plasma lactate and free fatty acids[21]. These changes indicate stimulation of aerobic metabolism in the body as a whole, resulting in a reversal from anaerobic to aerobic metabolism in the brain-dead animal. These observations correlated well with the earlier studies which showed replacement of myocardial energy stores and improvement in myocardial function.

Clinical observations

A group of potential donors was treated with intravenous T3 (3 μg), cortisol (100 mg), and insulin (10–20 international units) when first seen, and the therapy repeated at hourly intervals, depending on the condition of the donor and his response to the treatment, until the heart was excised. Observations in this group of potential donors were compared with those in potential donors who did not receive any form of hormonal therapy[23] (Table 6.1).

The hormonally-treated group showed a marked improvement in cardiac performance, as measured by significant increases in MAP and heart rate and a fall in CVP, despite a significant reduction in inotropic requirements. This was in contradistinction to the donors who did not receive hormonal therapy, in whom there was no improvement in cardiac function, despite a significant increase in the level of inotropic support. In the hormonally-treated donors, there was a reduction in the bicarbonate requirement, and falls in serum lactate and pyruvate; in those who did not receive hormonal therapy, the need for bicarbonate administration increased by 100% over the same period of time.

Of the donor hearts in the untreated group 19% were eventually considered unsuitable for subsequent transplantation on the basis of poor or deteriorating hemodynamic performance, whereas all of the hormonally-treated donors were considered suitable for transplantation, and all showed immediate good function following transplantation, and good long-term performance except where affected by acute or chronic rejection.

These observations provide further evidence of the impairment of aerobic metabolism which occurs in brain-dead

Table 6.1 Initial and final hemodynamic and metabolic observations in brain-dead donors at Groote Schuur Hospital

Group	Timing of observations	Temperature (°C)	MAP (mmHg)	CVP (cmH$_2$O)	Heart rate (beats/min)	Dopamine requirement (μg/kg/min)	Base deficit (mmol/l)	Bicarbonate requirement (ml (8.4%))	Serum lactate (mmol/l)	Serum pyruvate (mmol/l)
A (n = 26) (received no hormonal therapy)	initial final p*	33.7 (0.64) 33.3 (0.70) NS	79.9 (6.81) 82.4 (3.26) NS	9.1 (2.70) 11.8 (2.24) NS	72.5 (6.30) 83.6 (7.40) NS	14.4 (3.71) 19.3 (2.90) < 0.05	−12.0 (2.03) −7.4 (1.40) < 0.005	113 (31) 225 (33) < 0.0003	— — —	— — —
B (n = 21) (received hormonal therapy)	initial final p	32.5 (0.71) 35.6 (0.80) < 0.05	56.1 (14.4) 86.1 (3.60) < 0.02	11.3 (6.36) 7.3 (3.77) < 0.02	67.4 (10.61) 35.6 (0.80) < 0.003	27.0 (10.36) 13.0 (2.73) < 0.005	−10.6 (3.60) −2.4 (1.64) < 0.0002	191 (77) 100 (7) < 0.0001	5.1 (0.97) 2.4 (0.32) < 0.02	0.29 (0.300) 0.16 (0.020) < 0.005

*p = statistical difference between initial and final observation
Figures in parentheses refer to standard error; MAP = mean arterial pressure; CVP = central venous pressure

donors. Increasing anaerobic metabolism (as evidenced by low pH, large base deficit, rise in serum lactate, pyruvate and free fatty acids, and repeated and increasing need for bicarbonate administration) appears to be associated with diminished myocardial function (as evidenced by low cardiac output, low MAP, high CVP, the appearance of abnormalities on the ECG, and the need for inotropic support).

We have now treated over 70 consecutive potential donors with hormonal therapy; no donor has proved unsuitable for transplantation, and no recipient has died from low output cardiac failure within the first few days after operation. The optimum dosage of T3, which is considered the most important of the replacement hormones, is still uncertain, but may be more than the 2 μg/hour given in the above studies. Unpublished data from the Papworth group in the United Kingdom suggest that, to achieve and maintain normal blood levels of T3, an initial bolus of 4 μg is required, followed by an infusion of 4 μg/hour (Wheeldon, D., personal communication).

These findings from both the brain-dead experimental animal and human potential organ donors suggest that, after brain death, inhibition of a common oxidative pathway for carbohydrates and fatty acids takes place in the mitochrondria, which are the main site of oxygen utilization. In the absence of T3, aerobic metabolism in the mitochondria is inhibited, and anaerobic cellular metabolism takes place. Following T3 therapy, the rapid increase in glucose, pyruvate, and palmitate utilization and in CO_2 production, and the normalization of lactate and free fatty acid metabolism, indicate reactivation of the mitochondria, resulting in aerobic energy generation.

The roles of corticosteroid and insulin therapy in the improvement of donor heart, or other organ, function are less clear, and have been discussed elsewhere[23,26].

It should be stressed that hormonal therapy remains controversial and is not yet fully accepted by the transplant community[27]. There are increasing data, however, to suggest that it may prove a most physiological way of maintaining donor organs in a viable state before excision and transplantation[27].

References

1. Cooper, D.K.C. (1989). A clinical survey of cardiac transplantation between ABO-blood group incompatible recipient and donors. *J. Heart Transplant.*, In press
2. Nakatani, T., Aida, H., Macris, M.P. and Frazier, O.H. (1988). Effect of ABO blood type on survival of CSA-treated cardiac transplant patients (abstract). *J. Heart Transplant.*, **7**, 81
3. Fentz, V. and Gormsen, J. (1962). Electrocardiographic patterns in patients with cerebrovascular accidents. *Circulation*, **25**, 22
4. Cooper, D.K.C. (1976). The donor heart; the present position with regard to resuscitation, storage, and assessment of viability. *J. Surg. Res.*, **21**, 363
5. L'Age-Stehr, J., Schwarz, A., Offermann, G., Langmaack, H., Bennhold, I., Niedrig, M. and Koch, M.A. (1985). HTLV-III infection in kidney transplant recipients. *Lancet*, **2**, 1361
6. Prompt, C.A., Reis, M.M., Grillo, F.M., Kopstein, J., Kraemer, B., Manfro, R.C., Maia, M.H. and Comiran, J.B. (1985). Transmission of AIDS virus at renal transplantation. *Lancet*, **2** 672
7. Schwarz, A., Hoffman, F., L'Age-Stehr, J., Tegzess, A.M. and Offermann, G. (1987). Human immunodeficiency virus transmission by organ donation. *Transplantation*, **44**, 21
8. Rubin, R.H., Jenkins, R.L., Shaw, B.W., Shaffer, D., Pearl, R.H., Erb, S., Monaco, A.P. and Van Thiel, D.H. (1987). The acquired immunodeficiency syndrome and transplantation. *Transplantation*, **44**, 1
9. Burch, G.E., Meyer, R. and Abildskov, J. (1954). A new electrocardiographic pattern observed in cerebrovascular accidents. *Circulation*, **9**, 719
10. De Pasquale, N.P. and Burch, C.E. (1969). How normal is the donor heart? *Am. Heart J.*, **77**, 719
11. Greenhoot, A.H. and Reichenbach, D.D. (1969). Cardiac injury and subarachnoid hemorrhage. *J. Neurosurg.*, **30**, 521
12. Heggtveit, H.A. (1970). The donor heart; brain death and pathological changes in the heart. *Laval Med.*, **41**, 178
13. Smith, R.P. and Tomlinson, B.E. (1954). Subendocardial hemorrhages associated with intracranial lesions. *J. Pathol. Bacteriol.*, **68j**, 327
14. Griepp, R.B., Stinson, E.B., Clark, D.A., Dong, E.Jr. and Shumway, N.E. (1971). The cardiac donor. *Surg. Gynecol. Obstet.*, **133**, 792
15. Novitzky, D., Wicomb, W.N., Cooper, D.K.C, Rose, A.G., Fraser, R.C. and Barnard, C.N. (1984). Electrocardiographic, hemodynamic and endocrine changes occurring during experimental brain death in the Chacma baboon. *J. Heart Transplant.*, **4**, 63
16. Wicomb, W.N., Cooper, D.K.C., Lanza, R.P., Novitzky, D. and Isaacs, S. (1986). The effects of brain death and 24 hours storage by hypothermic perfusion on donor heart function in the pig. *J. Thorac. Cardiovasc. Surg.*, **91**, 896
17. Novitzky, D., Wicomb, W.N., Cooper, D.K.C., Rose, A.G. and Reichart, B. (1986). Prevention of myocardial injury during brain

death by total cardiac sympathectomy in the Chacma baboon. *Ann. Thorac. Surg.*, **41**, 520
18. Novitzky, D., Wicomb, W.N., Rose, A.G., Cooper, D.K.C. and Reichart, B. (1987). Pathophysiology of pulmonary edema following experimental brain death in the Chacma baboon. *Ann. Thorac. Surg.*, **43**, 288
19. Novitzky, D., Cooper, D.K.C., Rose, A.G., Wicomb, W.N., Becerra, E. and Reichart, B. (1987). Early donor heart failure following transplantation – the possible role of myocardial injury sustained during brain death. *Clin. Transplantation*, **1**, 108
20. Novitzky, D., Cooper, D.K.C., Rose, A.G. and Reichart, B. (1987). Prevention of myocardial injury by pre-treatment with verapamil hydrochloride following experimental brain death; efficacy in a baboon model. *Am. J. Emerg. Med.*, **15**, 11
21. Novitzky, D., Cooper, D.K.C., Morrell, D. and Isaacs, S. (1988). Change from aerobic to anaerobic metabolism after brain death, and reversal following triiodothyronine (T3) therapy. *Transplantation*, **45**, 32
22. Novitzky, D., Rose, A.G. and Cooper, D.K.C. (1988). Injury of myocardial conduction tissue and coronary artery smooth muscle following brain death in the baboon. *Transplantation*, **45**, 964
23. Novitzky, D., Cooper, D.K.C. and Reichart, B. (1987). Hemodynamic and metabolic responses to hormonal therapy in brain-dead potential organ donors. *Transplantation*, **43**, 852
24. Novitzky, D., Wicomb, W.N., Cooper, D.K.C. and Tjaalgard, M.A. (1987). Improved cardiac function following hormonal therapy in brain-dead pigs: relevance to organ donation. *Cryobiology*, **24**, 1
25. Wicomb, W.N., Cooper, D.K.C. and Novitzky, D. (1986). Impairment of renal slice function following brain death, with reversibility of injury by hormonal therapy. *Transplantation*, **41**, 29
26. Toledo-Pereyra, L.H. and Jara, F.M. (1979). Myocardial protection with methylprednisolone. *J. Thorac. Cardiovasc. Surg.*, **77**, 619
27. Cooper, D.K.C., Novitzky, D. and Zuhdi, N. (eds.) Hormonal therapy – a new concept in the management of organ donors. *Transplant. Proc.*, **20**, 1

7
Storage of the Donor Heart
W.N. WICOMB AND D.K.C. COOPER

INTRODUCTION

The development of successful methods of myocardial protection during open heart operations has been one of the major advances in cardiac surgery. At present, cardioplegic arrest followed by simple storage in ice-cold saline provides good protection of the myocardium against ischemic damage for up to 4 hours, possibly a little longer. This allows for transport of a donor heart from one hospital to another over distances of up to approximately 2000 km (1250 miles), but necessitates highly organized and expensive forms of communication and transportation between these centers.

Methods of storage of the heart for periods longer than 4 hours are still in their infancy. Improved techniques of preservation must be devised, however, if cardiac transplantation is to develop fully as a routine therapeutic procedure. The essential gain from storing the isolated heart is, of course, time. This includes time to transport the donor heart to the recipient, time to tissue type the donor and perform donor–recipient lymphocytotoxic cross-matching, time to do an elective operation, and time, possibly, to resuscitate a heart too damaged by antemortem changes to transplant immediately.

Today, in most countries involved in cardiac transplantation, the law allows the patient to be certified dead once the brain has undergone total and irreversible death. This enables the heart to be excised while still beating within the donor, which therefore gives some indication of its viability. The effects of brain death on subsequent myocardial function have already been discussed briefly (Chapter 6). Unprotected anoxic or ischemic arrest of the heart leads to significant damage of the organ[1], and no major group involved in cardiac transplantation is at present attempting to resuscitate and transplant hearts which have already ceased functioning under less than ideal cardioplegic conditions.

MYOCARDIAL CELL METABOLISM

The myocardium is composed of highly specialized cells, which function satisfactorily only within the narrow limits of a defined, regulated, biochemical environment. The cells of both the vascular and cellular compartments of the myocardium require specific osmotic pressures, pH and inorganic ions to function adequately, and metabolic substrates for their energy requirements. A change in any one or more of these factors results in a change in energy production. The pathways involved in the conversion of chemical energy from nutrient substrates into a form which can be utilized by the myocardium for useful work, that is, the normal metabolic pathways, are fully described in standard biochemical texts[2].

In outline, under normothermic conditions, four major pathways are operative in the myocardial cell in the oxidation of glucose: (1) glycolysis, (2) the hexosemonophosphate shunt, (3) the Krebs' cycle, and (4) the electron transport chain. The former two can operate under aerobic or anaerobic conditions and are functional in the cytoplasm of the cell, whereas the latter two take place in the mitochondria only under aerobic conditions. The metabolic activity of these four pathways is interrelated. This unity will be disturbed if the supply of any essential factor, such as oxygen or glucose, is inadequate.

In the absence of an adequate oxygen supply, there is significant depression of the Krebs' cycle and of electron transport, and myocardial energy is derived from the anaerobic glycolytic pathway. Anaerobic glycolysis is a much less efficient system of energy supply compared with the oxidation of glucose under aerobic conditions; the efficiency of energy conservation in anaerobic glycolysis is only 3%, whereas that of aerobic metabolism is 50%[3].

The stability of myocardial metabolic activity is interrupted as soon as a period of *in situ* or *in vitro* preservation intervenes, whether it be by pharmacological arrest, simple ice storage, or by a form of continuous myocardial perfusion. Satisfactory myocardial preservation will only be achieved if compensation is made for the altered myocardial environment, either by efficient metabolic inhibition or by metabolic support.

DONOR PRETREATMENT

Studies on the rat kidney have shown that if the donor animal is treated variously with methylprednisolone, phenoxybenzamine, chlorpromazine or heparin before the organ is removed, subsequent function after a period of warm ischemia can approximate that in control experiments[4]. The steroid, α-receptor blocker and phenothiazine are believed to function by 'stabilizing membranes', by which it is inferred that the cell and intracellular organelle membranes retain a greater degree of control over the exchange of ions across them, particularly the intracellular compartments; the α-blocker and chlorpromazine reduce agonal vascular spasm, and heparin prevents intravascular clotting. In addition, phenoxybenzamine maintains both the intracellular concentrations of adenosine triphosphate (ATP) and the electron microscopic structure of the organ. There is also evidence that donor pretreatment with methylprednisolone improves subsequent myocardial function if a period of preservation intervenes[5,6].

In our own experimental laboratory, a combination of triiodothyronine, cortisol and insulin, if administered to brain-dead animals before excision of the organ, has been shown to have a beneficial effect in stored hearts[7] and kidneys[8]. The significant reduction in myocardial energy stores (ATP, CP and glycogen) and increase in lactate seen after storage of hearts taken from brain-dead baboons was prevented by such pretreatment, as was the associated deterioration in myocardial function[7]. Similarly, renal parenchymal function (as measured by the sodium–potassium ratio) did not deteriorate following 24-hour storage in ice of kidneys which had been pretreated with such hormones[8]; marked deterioration occurred in untreated kidneys.

In the clinical situation, most cardiac donors receive heparin (and some a corticosteroid) immediately before cardiectomy. The observed beneficial effects of T3 and insulin in human donors have been discussed in Chapter 6.

METHODS OF ORGAN STORAGE

Organ preservation can be achieved in two fundamental ways: (1) by reducing the metabolic demands of the tissues, increasing the organ's resistance to injury, and (2) by increasing the supply of vital substances such as oxygen and nutrients to the organ. Several techniques combine a method of increasing resistance to injury with maintenance of a supply of vital substances to the organ.

Whatever method is employed, most research workers in this field have felt that it is desirable to prevent intravascular thrombosis in the coronary vessels by heparinizing the donor before excision of the heart. Our own experimental observations would suggest, however, that, though desirable, this may not be absolutely essential[9].

Preservation methods which have been explored in the laboratory can be divided into two basic groups – those which utilize some form of perfusion system and those which do not (Table 7.1). In the clinical setting, only a combination of simple ice storage with or without pharmacological inhibition is used extensively in heart transplantation programs, though extracorporeal hypothermic perfusion has been used in a small number of cases in Cape Town[10]. (In clinical heart–lung transplantation, however, total body perfusion using a pump-oxygenator is being utilized as a method of cooling all organs (Chapter 35), though transportation of the heart–lung block is again by simple ice storage. The autoperfusing heart–lung preparation has been in vogue recently, but has proved to be a difficult system to manage (Chapter 35).)

Non-perfusion methods

Hypothermia

The simplest method of preservation is hypothermia, which has been used in renal transplantation since 1956[11]. Much of the early work on preservation of the heart by simple hypothermia resulted from studies devoted to arrest of the heart during intracardiac surgical procedures[12,13]. Webb and Howard were the first to study heart preservation by refrigeration[14]. In 1962 the Stanford group was the first to report successful orthotopic transplantation of the dog heart after 7 hours of preservation in cold saline[15].

The physiological basis for the efficiency of hypothermia as a cell protectant during ischemia is its effect on reducing the metabolic demands of the organ[16]. Decreasing the temperature by 10°C decreases the metabolic rate by a factor of 2–3. Metabolic activity still continues at temperatures of −60°C and, as a result, tissue stored at 0°C by simple ice storage is still subject to the relatively fast onset of ischemic damage. During hypothermic storage, oxygen depletion, increased lactate production, and acid–base imbalance all occur, demonstrating that all the enzymes of the glycolytic pathway are still functional at reduced temperatures. Unless these three features are continually corrected during the preservation period, tissue damage will occur following reperfusion (reperfusion injury), and, in the case of the heart, result in arrhythmia, gross edema formation, and inadequate function. Similar damage will follow any inadequate storage technique.

Table 7.1 Major methods of storage of the heart which have been investigated experimentally

Non-perfusion methods	Perfusion methods
Simple ice storage	Total body perfusion using a pump-oxygenator
Pharmacological inhibition	Autoperfusion (biological oxygenation)
Combined hypothermia and pharmacological inhibition	Intermediate host perfusion (parabiosis)
Combined hypothermia and hyperbaric oxygenation	Extracorporeal normothermic perfusion
Supercoolin	Extracorporeal hypothermic perfusion
Freezing	

Continuing metabolic activity in an ischemic organ will result in exhaustion of its oxygen supply and glycogen reserves, during which time the organ resorts to anaerobic glycolysis as its major energy contributor. The pH progressively decreases, predominantly from ATP hydrolysis[17]. The low pH inhibits the glycolytic regulatory enzyme phosphofructokinase (PFK)[18], and energy production by glycolysis is thereafter reduced. The low oxygen tension that develops results in a decreased formation of calcium chelating agents (ATP and citrate), predisposing the myocardium to inadequate calcium homeostasis. It is also likely that leakage from the sarcoplasmic reticulum and the extracellular space results in a net increase in cytoplasmic ionized calcium[19]. This may result in an increased resting myocardial tension, which increases the metabolic demands of the cell. The ultimate effect of an increase in intracellular calcium will be a 'stone heart'. Tissue lactate has already reached high levels, though a further rise may be somewhat inhibited by the continuing fall in pH.

In the case of the myocardium, the reversibility of injury is limited to a maximum ice storage period of approximately 12 hours at 4°C. The injury occurs during storage, but it is only during the phase of reperfusion that the effects of the injury become evident (see later), when normothermia increases the metabolic rate of the organ. The replenishment of oxygen, of which the organ was starved, has a paradoxical effect, because ionized calcium is now rapidly taken up by the mitochondria[20]. This is followed by explosive cell swelling, mitochondrial and myofibrillar damage, and the appearance of contraction bands and intramitochondrial calcium phosphate deposits[21].

Pharmacological inhibition

During the early years of open heart surgery, surgeons experimented with various methods of inducing cardiac arrest; of the chemical agents tested, potassium citrate is perhaps the best known[22]. In the correct doses potassium is a safe, reversible agent, and today is a constituent of many cardioplegic solutions[23]. High potassium solutions act as metabolic inhibitors by depolarizing cell membranes; intracellular-based solutions attempt to maintain intracellular K^+ close to normality; thus at reperfusion the tissue is in an ionic state that can resume functioning immediately. The metabolic inhibition achieved by magnesium sulfate, used singly or in combination with chlorpromazine, has been shown to maintain the anoxic normothermic heart at virtually its antemortem functional state for at least 3 hours[24]. A number of other pharmacological agents has been shown to have some metabolic inhibitory effect on the myocardium, among them phenothiazines, phenoxybenzamine, and procaine hydrochloride in high concentrations. Combinations of various agents in perfusion solutions were tested at normothermia by Hearse *et al.*[25].

Combined hypothermia and pharmacological inhibition

The combination of some pharmacological cardioplegic agents with hypothermia appears to be synergistic. For example, the combination of magnesium sulfate and hypothermia extends more than two-fold the effects of either alone in the preservation of the rat heart[26]. Hearts have been stored at 4°C in intracellular-like solutions containing a high potassium content for periods of 18–26 hours without oxygen or perfusion[27]. To date, 26 hours is the longest reported period of anoxic arrest which has been followed by indubitably viable heart function.

Combined hypothermia and hyperbaric oxygenation/supercooling/freezing

These three methods have been extensively studied in the laboratory[1,28], but the results have not justified clinical application. From the results reported to date, it must remain doubtful whether the addition of hyperbaric oxygen produces more successful preservation of the heart than hypothermia alone. Although a method of preservation based on the techniques of supercooling or freezing may offer the prospect of successful long-term storage in the future, at the present time cryobiological techniques of preservation are not clinically applicable.

Perfusion methods

Total body perfusion using a pump-oxygenator

The donor heart can be preserved for relatively long periods of time in the brain-dead subject by pump-oxygenator support[28,29]. The donor is cooled until the esophageal temperature has fallen to approximately 16–20°C, at which point the heart and other organs are excised, and perfusion discontinued. Additional cardioplegic arrest may or may not be induced, after which the intermittent application of cold (4°C) saline to the heart to maintain a low myocardial temperature is sufficient protection during transportation and implantation.

Total body perfusion allows protection during preparation for heart (and other organs) excision, but entails a large team of staff and may not prove possible at small peripheral hospitals (and therefore may necessitate transfer of the donor to a major center). Its major advantage is in achieving and maintaining a state of whole body hypothermia during which multiple organ excision can be carried out. This may be important in a donor who has become hemodynamically unstable and in whom cardiac arrest or severe hypotension seem imminent.

If excision of the heart alone is being considered, it would seem that this technique has few advantages and several disadvantages over cardioplegic arrest and simple ice storage. With storage of the heart and both lungs, however, where efficient storage techniques are less well developed, it has been used with success (Chapter 35). Small, simple pump-oxygenators, which are therefore easily portable, have been utilized.

Autoperfusion (biological oxygenation)

The use of an autoperfusing heart–lung preparation as a means of short-term preservation of the heart during its insertion into the recipient must be credited to Demikhov[30], who initially published his work in 1948. The essential feature of the Demikhov preparation is that the systemic circulation is represented by the coronary vessels alone. With artificial maintenance of respiration and temperature, the heart could function normally for many hours.

In 1959, as a method of heart preservation, Robicsek and his colleagues[31] developed a modification in which the coronary perfusion pressure was kept stable and the blood volume was self-adjusting. Progressive metabolic deterioration of the heart and lungs occurs within a few hours[32–34], however, limiting the period in which cardiac (or pulmonary) viability can be maintained. As a method of preservation, the system can be unstable if hypovolemia occurs, but it has been used with success as a means of protecting the heart and lungs during transportation (Chapter 35).

Intermediate host perfusion (parabiosis)

Experimental experience with this method has been reviewed previously[1,28]. Although it is difficult to see a homologous intermediate host storage system being used in man, xenogeneic storage, using an immunosuppressed animal[35], might prove to be a potential answer to short-term storage of human organs. As with other aspects of this experimental field, such a procedure may not be aesthetically acceptable to many members of the lay and medical communities.

Extracorporeal normothermic perfusions

No major success has been obtained[1,28]. Using only moderate hypothermia (perfusion with modified blood at 32°C), Solis et al. stored hearts for 12 to 24 hours[36]. After 12 hours storage, high energy phosphates were found to be significantly reduced, but tissue norepinephrine and epinephrine remained within normal ranges.

The addition of more profound hypothermia has led to improved results.

Extracorporeal hypothermic perfusion

Progress here has been substantial[28], and at Groote Schuur Hospital in Cape Town advanced to the point of clinical application in 1981[10]. One of the first major advances in this field came from Proctor and Parker[37], who managed to preserve the isolated canine heart for 72 hours with hypothermic perfusion (5°C) using filtered modified Krebs' solution. Using a technique based on that of Proctor, Copeland and his colleagues[38] successfully preserved hearts for 24 hours followed by orthotopic transplantation, with three dogs surviving for 4 days or more and dying of rejection. Recent work by Kioka et al.[39] achieved some success when dog hearts were continuously perfused with a cold modified Collins' solution containing albumin and perfluorochemicals for 24 hours. Only one out of eight hearts could not be weaned from cardiopulmonary bypass following transplantation. Heart function, however, was only monitored for 2 hours, and therefore the degree of recovery of the stored hearts cannot be conclusively ascertained.

At the University of Cape Town, baboon hearts were stored for 24 or even 48 hours with immediate good function after orthotopic transplantation[40–42]. When storage and autotransplantation of the baboon's own heart was carried out – the baboon being kept alive during the storage period by an allograft – long-term survival was achieved with no significant demonstrable functional or morphological injury to the heart[43].

An initial clinical trial of this system in four patients undergoing heterotopic heart transplantation was successful after donor heart ischemic periods of approximately 7–17 hours (Figure 7.1)[10]. In two of these patients, however, satisfactory donor heart function was delayed for periods of approximately 19 hours, during which time the recipient's own heart, supported by inotropic agents, maintained the circulation. Such delayed recovery had not been seen in any of the experimental studies. Subsequent work suggests that it was associated with the depletion of myocardial energy stores which occurs during brain death, and which is further amplified when a period of ischemic storage is added[7,44].

Hypothermic perfusion has the advantage over ice storage in that the former provides a continuous supply of oxygen and substrates and a continuous removal of waste products from the organ. Over short periods of time of up to 4 hours, the need for perfusion is not critical, but over longer periods perfusion is to be preferred. Its success or failure depends on the chemical components, the redox control, and the degree of oxygenation of the perfusate.

Although hypothermia allows perfusion to be successful, its addition actually complicates perfusion preservation in homeotherms (mammals) by its inhibition of the sodium-potassium ATPase[45], and by leading to a change in the saturated membrane lipids, thus altering the normal physiology of the mitochondrial membrane[46]. The mitochondrial membrane ADP–ATP translocator function is also impaired, limiting the supply of high energy phosphates for metabolic needs[47,48]. Though hypothermia reduces cellular

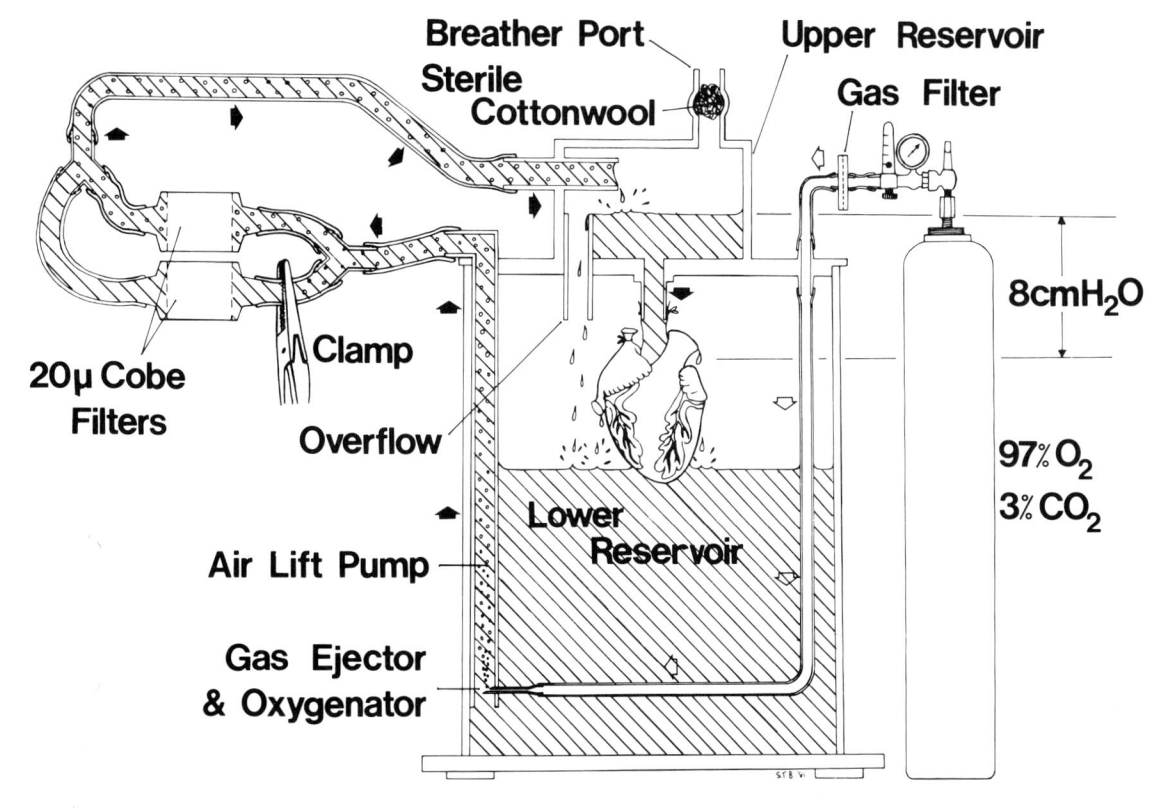

Figure 7.1 Portable hypothermic perfusion apparatus used clinically at Groote Schuur Hospital, Cape Town, in 1981

energy consumption, it still remains essential to stimulate sufficient energy production to continue essential cell functions and thus maintain viability.

The regulation of calcium distribution is a major factor if successful hypothermic perfusion preservation is to be achieved. In the hypothermic myocardium ($> 20°C$), any absence of calcium can lead to the so-called calcium paradox[48]. At temperatures below $20°C$, protection from calcium paradox is offered by hypothermia[49]. However, despite this protection, the initial ischemic insult to the myocardial cells can result in enhanced resting myocardial tension (stone heart), followed by poor or no function at reperfusion[50]. The choice of the chemical components for a perfusate must therefore ensure that calcium distribution is kept under stringent control. Five basic factors are considered important: (1) perfusate calcium concentration, (2) degree of oxygenation, (3) pH, (4) redox control, and (5) edema formation. Some of these factors have been discussed previously[28]; oxygenation and redox control are intimately involved in reperfusion injury (see later).

The routine clinical use of extracorporeal hypothermic perfusion still appears to be limited by the state of the myocardium at the onset of the preservation period. Studies of the influence of donor heart pretreatment on subsequent function of stored hearts are continuing. These aspects of myocardial preservation are close to resolution, which may enable such storage systems to be introduced once again into the clinical arena, greatly extending the ischemic period available.

One such new technique of hypothermic perfusion, termed microperfusion ($3-6\,ml/g/24\,h$), has recently been developed for 24-hour storage of the myocardium using a modified University of Wisconsin solution. This method appears to have potential to resuscitate hearts, as 121% of control function can be obtained following 24-hour storage[51].

REPERFUSION INJURY AND OXYGEN FREE RADICAL SCAVENGERS

Much attention has been given recently to the so-called 'reperfusion injury' of the myocardium, as it is believed that, if this can be prevented or reversed, successful storage of organs for prolonged periods will be more likely. An attempt will be made here to clarify the nature of reperfusion injury.

The injury is an amplification at normothermia of an event (or events) that occurred during the ischemic phase, whether normothermic or hypothermic[52]. During normothermic ischemia, the injury can be measured as it develops by various parameters, such as a decrease in substrate or oxygen, or altered serum enzyme concentrations. Under hypothermic storage conditions, however, there is no reliable method of detecting or quantitating the sustained injury; only when reperfusion has occurred does the injury become manifest. On reperfusion (and the return of normothermia), an ideal milieu is created for the generation of toxic species (oxygen free radicals) that result in the classical features of reperfusion injury. Whether excessive oxygen free radicals are produced, or the oxygen scavenging system is impaired, is not known. Although it is during the reperfusion phase that any impaired metabolic mechanisms are operative and become detected, it is not implied that reperfusion is the primary cause of the injury.

At the time of the development of the injury there are many biochemical systems within the organ that operate in a relatively uncontrolled manner, including an imbalance of ionic fluxes. These deranged mechanisms can be discussed under two main headings, namely the 'calcium cascade' and 'oxygen free radicals'.

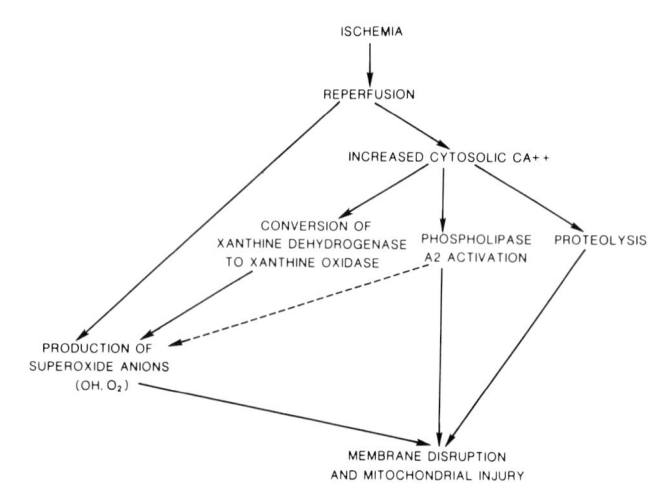

Figure 7.2 Initial events in the development of reperfusion injury

Calcium (Ca^{2+}) cascade

Changes in myocardial intracellular Ca^{2+} homeostasis occur during the early stages of ischemia[53]. The total myocardial tissue Ca^{2+} remains constant during this period, suggesting the redistribution of intracellular Ca^{2+} ions, with an increased cytosolic concentration. It is this raised cytosolic Ca^{2+} level that results in the so-called Ca^{2+} 'cascade' after reperfusion. Upon reoxygenation at reperfusion, the extracellular–intracellular Ca^{2+} gradient (10^{-3}–10^{-7} M) is altered, with an increased flux of Ca^{2+} into the cell. Jennings and Ganote[54] reported minor Ca^{2+} fluxes after coronary ligation, but reperfusion led to a 10-fold increase in myocardial cytosolic calcium. This increase is accompanied by intramitochondrial Ca^{2+} phosphate deposits, swelling and structural damage[55].

The initial events in the cascade are shown schematically in Figure 7.2. The first phase following reperfusion is that the elevated cytosolic Ca^{2+} levels result in the conversion of xanthine dehydrogenase (XD) to xanthine oxidase (XO), which leads to the generation of cytotoxic oxygen radicals. Cytosolic Ca^{2+} is usually elevated due to energy (ATP) depletion, and McCord proposes that the conversion of XD to XO is mediated by Ca^{2+}-activated proteases[56]. During reperfusion, hypoxanthine serves as an oxidizable substrate for XD and XO and, in the catalysis, cytotoxic superoxide anions (O_2^-) and hydrogen peroxide (H_2O_2) are formed[57]. The original pathophysiology of oxygen free radicals in ischemic tissue reperfusion injury was described in detail by Hess et al.[58].

The final results of the elevated cytosolic Ca^{2+} are depressed mitochondrial function, and activation of phospholipases, proteases and ATPases, impairing membrane structural components[59-62]. Phospholipase A_2 activation by Ca^{2+} has been demonstrated in mitochondria from the liver, and is associated with mitochondrial swelling and altered Ca^{2+} flux[63]. Other destructive effects of a raised Ca^{2+} level, such as proteolysis, have been documented or postulated[64-67].

Inhibition of the calcium cascade

Inhibition of this catabolic pathway has been demonstrated by trifluoperazine, an inhibitor of calmodulin, which slows the conversion of XD to XO, and by allopurinol which inhibits formation of XO[56]. The benefit derived from the use of allopurinol may also be due to its metabolite oxypurinol, which appears to be an hydroxyl radical scavenger[68,69]. In another study, however, allopurinol was shown to be less effective than other scavengers in protecting the myocardium[70]. Inhibitors of this proteolytic pathway, if given during the cold ischemic period, may be effective in preventing the injury on reperfusion. Ca^{2+} chelators (such as acetate, citrate, and ATP-$MgCl_2$) have been reported to chelate ionized Ca^{2+}[71,72].

The injury associated with mitochondrial respiration can be reversed by pretreatment with verapamil, which inhibits slow channel Ca^{2+} accumulation and subsequent phospholipase A_2 activation, thus maintaining the total phospholipid content of the mitochondria at control levels[73]. Another effective phospholipase A_2 inhibitor is chlorpromazine[74].

Oxygen free radicals

A free radical is a molecule or atom that possesses an unpaired electron. When molecular oxygen accepts an electron from a reducing agent, the primary product generated is the superoxide anion ($O_2^- \cdot$). $O_2^- \cdot$ can also reduce H_2O_2 directly, yielding the hydroxyl radical ($OH \cdot$)[75].

The reduction of oxygen to water in living tissues usually proceeds by two pathways.

(1) Mitochondrial enzymes have the capability of reduc-

ing O_2 to H_2O by tetravalent reduction without the production of any intermediates; this pathway usually accounts for 95% of the oxygen consumption of tissues.

(2) The remaining 5% consumption proceeds by a univalent pathway in which the above reactive species of oxygen radicals are produced[76].

Superoxide anions are produced in the mitochondrial internal membrane during electron transport, and appear to be a product of autoxidation of semiquinones[77]. Other sources of superoxide anions include the autoxidation of low molecular weight molecules, by-products of enzyme substrate reactions (e.g. XO, as discussed earlier), and auto-oxidizable electron carriers, such as NADH dehydrogenase[78,79].

Several potential sources of free radicals exist within the plasma membranes of cells; these have been discussed elsewhere[80-83]. At reperfusion the destructive features of the calcium cascade become evident, and the introduction of oxygen results in increased production of superoxide anions and hydroxyl radicals (Figure 7.2). This excessive production overloads the oxygen free radical scavenger system, which itself is impaired. The destructive effects of oxygen radicals on the cell are several, and are believed to play a major role in the development of reperfusion injury by attacking polyunsaturated fatty acids. This results in lipid hydroperoxides and hence further structural changes in membranes and membrane components[84-87].

At the time of reperfusion, the immune system may also play a role in the development of further tissue injury, as phagocytes have the capacity to produce large quantities of oxygen-derived free radicals. They also promote inflammation, and recruit more cells as the generated $O_2^-\cdot$ and H_2O_2 promote formation of chemotactic lipids[88]. These activated phagocytes can inflict acute vascular injury by the cytotoxic metabolites $OH\cdot$ and hypochlorous acid.

The effect of oxygen provided to the tissues during the ischemic period remains uncertain. It is unlikely that oxygen exerts an obvious toxic effect during a 2-hour period of ischemia, but severe toxicity has been demonstrated during a 24-hour period of continuous hypothermic perfusion (Wicomb et al., unpublished data). Some groups encourage the use of oxygen in cardioplegic solutions[89-91], but others emphasize the risks of oxygen toxicity[57,92,93]. In the case of myocardial preservation by hypothermic perfusion, oxygen is essential, but the P_{O_2} must not exceed 300–700 mmHg, and the volume of O_2 required to maintain the P_{O_2} must remain at a minimum (Wicomb et al., unpublished data).

Oxygen free radical scavengers

The effects of the administration of oxygen free radical scavengers (OFRS) to ischemic tissues remain controversial, with some investigators showing effectiveness in protecting the myocardium from injury[69,70,73] and others showing no obvious benefit[94,95]. Vitamins E and C have been shown to be effective OFRS, protecting cell membranes against lipid peroxidation; vitamin E has been shown to be a constituent of cellular and mitochondrial membranes[96,97].

The primary mechanism of OFRS in mammalian tissues is by the action of superoxide dismutase (SOD), which catalyzes the dismutation of $O_2^-\cdot$ to $H_2O_2 + O_2$[80,98,99]. The generated H_2O_2 can be metabolized either (1) by the cytoplasmic heme enzyme catalase by divalent reduction to water, or (2) by the selenium-dependent glutathione peroxidase to water[100]. These enzymes are found in the cytoplasm of cells. The copper-transporting globulin, ceruloplasmin, also has antioxidant activity, scavenging $O_2^-\cdot$, singlet O_2, and hydroxyl radicals[101].

The number of OFRS used in research is rapidly increasing and includes deferoxamine[70], dimethyl sulfoxide (DMSO), glycerol[102], propylene glycol[103], horseradish peroxidase[104], mannitol[105], reduced glutathione[106] and taurine[107].

Another approach to combat reperfusion injury is to maintain an optimum oxidation–reduction state throughout the ischemic period; this results in less injury during reperfusion[108].

In conclusion, the destructive role of oxygen free radicals in reperfusion injury is adequately supported by experimental findings, and, in recent years, there have been great advances in the understanding of the basic mechanisms involved. Although the use of OFRS is still in its infant stages, there are rapidly accumulating data illustrating the effectiveness of OFRS. In some cases, the specific oxygen free radical species have been identified.

Reperfusion injury following global hypothermic ischemia of the heart (24 hours of ice storage or hypothermic perfusion) is still severe, and hence storage for clinical purposes is limited to a maximum of 8 hours[109]. This injury could be reversed if (1) scavengers were available at the site of injury, and (2) the correct scavengers could be selected for the type of oxygen radical involved.

THE ASSESSMENT OF MYOCARDIAL VIABILITY

Ideally, the transplanted heart must be capable of full function immediately after its insertion into the recipient. A test of functional viability of the organ would therefore be a great advantage if storage systems are to become a clinical reality[1]. A simple, reliable, in vitro test of organ viability would similarly save a great deal of time (and a large number of experimental animals) in the assessment of any new preservation technique. The ultimate measure of viability of the preserved heart is its capacity to fully support the circulation after orthotopic transplantation. Ethically this cannot be a test of function in the clinical situation and, ideally, the viability should be known at all times throughout the storage period and also at the time of transplantation.

Any such test of organ viability should be simple, rapid and reproducible. The search for such a test has explored two main routes[1].

The first of these is a simple, single measurement or observation that confirms that the tissues under study are not irreversibly damaged. This may take the form of, for example, a visual assay of a myocardial enzyme system, a histochemical change, or the monitoring of a fundamental metabolic event such as anaerobic glycolysis or lactic acid production.

The second is a functional evaluation of the isolated heart. At present, this involves multiple hemodynamic and biochemical observations of myocardial function while the heart is perfused. Such methods are frequently elaborate and time-consuming, but it is possible that, with further experience, a single measurement will be found which will indicate the functional state of the myocardium.

The single, simple observation can be classified as a 'tissue viability test', whereas the hemodynamic and biochemical studies carried out on the isolated, perfused heart can be considered methods of 'functional evaluation' of the organ. Whatever the method used, it is crucial that the results obtained correlate closely with the function of the whole organ after storage and orthotopic transplantation.

Tissue viability tests

At the present time there is no completely satisfactory viability test which will give an immediate answer regarding the viability of the myocardium. Quantitative birefringence assessment is being explored as a possible test, and initial results are encouraging[110-115]. Quantitative birefringence measurements assess the response of muscle fibers in myocardial biopsies to adenosine triphosphate (ATP) and calcium. In normal cardiac muscle there is a great increase in birefringence following the addition of ATP and calcium, due to increased orientation of the myosin micelles as the muscle fibers contract. In damaged or ischemic muscle this response is diminished[110-114]. Birefringence assessment has been shown to correlate with physiologic measurements of function at cardiac catheterization, and with measurements of contractility[112].

Since such a measurement can be made on small biopsy specimens and may be completed within 30 minutes of sampling, the technique can provide a sensitive index of the functional status of the donor heart before, during and after transplantation. In one study of 160 human donor hearts, dysfunction of a group of hearts when assessed by quantitative birefringence was subsequently confirmed by the high proportion that required inotropic agents before cardiopulmonary bypass could be withdrawn after implantation (Figure 7.3)[115].

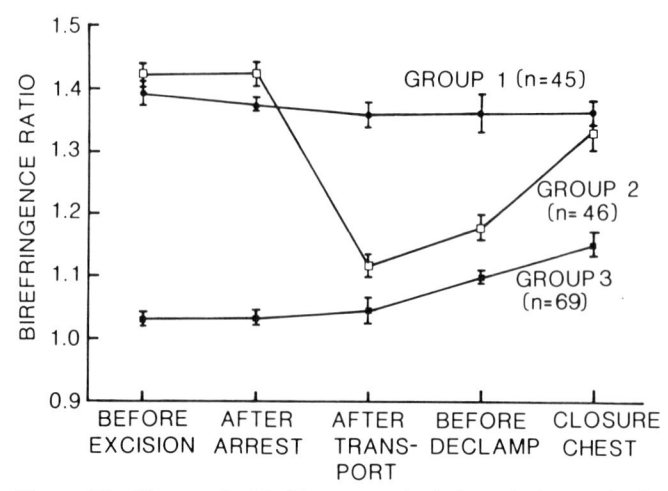

Figure 7.3 Changes in birefringence ratio before, during, and after transplantation in 160 donor hearts. Ninety-one had good initial birefringence values; 45 remained good throughout the procedure (Group 1), but 46 deteriorated during cold storage and transplantation (Group 2). Sixty-nine hearts had a poor birefringence ratio throughout (Group 3). (Courtesy of Dr S. Čanković Darracott)

Functional evaluation of the heart

Several complex systems for functional evaluation of isolated hearts have been designed, and have successfully demonstrated the capabilities of hearts after varying methods and periods of storage[116,117]. None is ideal as a rapid test of function of a donor heart about to be implanted into a recipient. In the hypothermic perfusion system developed by Proctor, changes in coronary resistance were found to be a reliable indicator of the subsequent functional capability of the myocardium[37], though we have not found this parameter entirely reliable.

A successful outcome of the search for a simple, yet reliable, viability test would not only allow the rapid evaluation of a cadaver donor organ, but would also greatly facilitate the search for reliable methods of resuscitation and preservation; the necessity of demonstrating the efficiency of such a technique by orthotopic transplantation of the organ would be removed. To date, however, no single test has satisfied all of the criteria necessary, though the results of quantitative birefringence assessment are encouraging.

References

1. Cooper, D.K.C. (1976). The donor heart; the present position with regard to resuscitation, storage and assessment of viability. *J. Surg. Res.*, **21**, 363
2. Lehninger, A.L. (1975). Catabolism and generation of the phosphate bond energy. In *Biochemistry: The Molecular Basis of Cell Structure*

and Function, 2nd ed., p. 361. (New York: Worth)
3. Pegg, D.E. (1981). The biology of cell survival *in vitro*. In Karow, A.M. and Pegg, D.E. (eds.) *Organ Preservation for Transplantation*, 2nd ed., p. 31. (New York and Basel: Dekker)
4. Leading article (1973). Reporting the proceedings of the first international symposium on organ preservation. Cambridge. *Lancet*, **2**, 715
5. Kirsh, M.M., Behrendt, D.M. and Jockim, K.E. (1979). Effects of methylprednisolone in cardioplegic solution during coronary bypass grafting. *J. Thorac. Cardiovasc. Surg.*, **77**, 896
6. Fox, A.C., Hoffstein, S. and Weissmann, G. (1976). Lysosomal mechanisms in production of tissue damage during myocardial ischemia and the effects of treatment with steroids. *Am. Heart J.*, **91**, 394
7. Novitzky, D., Cooper, D.K.C., Wicomb, W.N. and Reichart, B. (1986). Improved function of stored hearts following hormonal therapy after brain death in pigs. *Transplant Proc.*, **18**, 1419
8. Wicomb, W.N., Cooper, D.K.C. and Novitzky, D. (1986). Impairment of renal slice function following brain death, with reversibility of injury by hormonal therapy. *Transplantation*, **41**, 29
9. Cooper, D.K.C. (1976). Resuscitation of the cadaver donor heart in the dog. III. The influence of the agonal period on the success of resuscitation. *Guy's Hosp. Rep.*, **123**, 363
10. Wicomb, W.N., Cooper, D.K.C., Novitzky, D. and Barnard, C.N. (1984). Cardiac transplantation following storage of the donor heart by a portable hypothermic perfusion system. *Ann. Thorac. Surg.*, **37**, 243
11. Bogardus, G.M. and Schlosser, R.J. (1956). The influence of temperature upon ischemic renal damage. *Surgery*, **39**, 970
12. Gott, V.L., Bartlett, M., Johnson, J.A., Long, D.M. and Lillehei, C.W. (1960). High energy phosphate levels in the human heart during potassium citrate arrest and selective hypothermic arrest. *Surg. Forum*, **10**, 544
13. Greenberg, J.J., Edmunds, L.H. and Brown, R.B. (1960). Myocardial metabolism and post-arrest function in the cold and chemically arrested heart. *Surgery*, **48**, 31
14. Webb, W.R. and Howard, H.S. (1957). Cardiopulmonary transplantation. *Surg. Forum*, **8**, 313
15. Lower, R.R., Stofer, R.C., Hurley, E.J., Dong, E.Jr., Cohn, R.B. and Shumway, N.E. (1962). Successful homotransplantation of the canine heart after anoxic preservation for seven hours. *Am. J. Surg.*, **104**, 302
16. Bigelow, W.G., Mustard, W.T. and Evans, J.G. (1954). Some physiological concepts of hypothermia and their application to cardiac surgery. *J. Thorac. Surg.*, **28**, 480
17. Gevers, W. (1977). Generation of protons by metabolic processes in heart cells. *J. Mol. Cell Cardiol.*, **9**, 867
18. Hand, S.C. and Somero, G.N. (1982). Urea and methylamine effects on rabbit muscle phosphofructokinase. *J. Biol. Chem.*, **257**, 734
19. Parr, D.R., Wimshurst, J.M. and Harris, E.J. (1975). Calcium-induced damage of rat heart mitochondria. *Cardiovasc. Res.*, **9**, 366
20. Ganote, C.E., Worstell, J. and Kaltenbach, J.P. (1976). Oxygen-induced enzyme release irreversible myocardial injury; effects of cyanide in perfused rat hearts. *Am. J. Pathol.*, **84**, 327
21. Jennings, R.B. and Ganote, C.E. (1976). Mitochondrial structure and function in acute myocardial ischemic injury. *Circ. Res.*, **38**, (Suppl. 1), 80
22. Melrose, R.G., Dreyer, B., Bentall, H.H. and Baker, J.B.E. (1955). Elective cardiac arrest. *Lancet*, **2**, 21
23. Hearse, D.J., Stewart, D.A. and Chain, E.B. (1974). Recovery from cardiac bypass and elective cardiac arrest. The metabolic consequences of various cardioplegic procedures in the isolated rat heart. *Circ. Res.*, **35**, 448
24. Nakae, S., Webb, W.R., Salyer, K.E., Unal, M.O., Cook, W.A., Dodds, R.P. and Williams, C.T. (1957). Extended survival of the normothermic anoxic heart with metabolic inhibitors. *Ann. Thorac. Surg.*, **3**, 37
25. Hearse, D.J., Stewart, D.A. and Braimbridge, M.V. (1976). Cellular protection during myocardial ischemia. *Circulation*, **54**, 193
26. Kamiyama, T.M., Webb, W.R. and Baker, R.R. (1970). Preservation of the anoxic heart with a metabolic inhibitor and hypothermia. *Arch. Surg.*, **100**, 596
27. Reitz, B.A., Brody, W.R., Hickey, P.R. and Michaelis, L.L. (1974). Protection of the heart for 24 hours with intracellular (high K^+) solution and hypothermia. *Surg. Forum*, **25**, 149
28. Wicomb, W.N. and Cooper, D.K.C. (1984). Donor heart storage. In Cooper, D.K.C. and Lanza, R.P. (eds.) *Heart Transplantation*. p. 51, (Lancaster: MTP Press)
29. Barnard, M.S., Van Heerden, J., Hope, A., O'Donovan, T.G. and Barnard, C.N. (1969). Total body perfusion for cardiac transplantation. *S. Afr. Med. J.*, **43**, 64
30. Demikhov, V.P. (1962). *Experimental Transplantation of Vital Organs*. Authorized translation from the Russian by Haigh, B. (New York: Consultants Bureau)
31. Robicsek, F., Stam, R.E., Rees, T.T., Taylor, F.H. and Sanger, P.W. (1959). Transplantation of the heart. 2. Haemodynamic observations of the isolated heart. *Heineman Laboratories Collected Works on Cardiopulmonary Disease*, **1-2**, 96
32. Yamada, T., Bosher, L.R.Jr. and Richardson, G.M. (1965). Observations on the autoperfusing heart–lung preparation. *Trans. Am. Soc. Artif. Intern. Organs*, **11**, 192
33. Robicsek, F., Lesage, A., Sanger, P.W., Daugherty, H.K., Moore, M. and Bagby, E. (1968). The maintenance of function of the donor heart in the extracorporeal stage and during transplantation. *Ann. Thorac. Surg.*, **6**, 331
34. Cooper, D.K.C. (1975). Hemodynamic studies during short-term preservation of the autoperfusing heart–lung preparation. *Cardiovasc. Res.*, **9**, 753
35. Dupree, E.L., Mills, M., Clark, R. and Sell, K.W. (1969). Xenogeneic storage of primate hearts. *Transplant. Proc.*, **1**, 840
36. Solis, E., Tyce, G.M., Bianco, R., Mahoney, J. and Kaye, M.P. (1986). High energy phosphates and catecholamine stores after prolonged *ex vivo* heart preservation. *J. Heart Transplant.*, **5**, 444
37. Proctor, E. and Parker, R. (1968). Preservation of isolated heart for 72 hours. *Br. Med. J.*, **4**, 296
38. Copeland, J.G., Jones, M., Spragg, R. and Stinson, E.B. (1973). *In vitro* preservation of canine heart for 24 to 48 hours followed by successful orthotopic transplantation. *Ann. Surg.*, **178**, 687
39. Kioka, Y., Tago, M., Bands, K., Seno, S., Shinozaki, Y., Murakami, T., Nawa, S., Senoo, Y. and Teramoto, S. (1986). Twenty-four hours isolated heart preservation by perfusion method with oxygenated solution containing perfluorochemicals and albumin. *J. Heart Transplant.*, **5**, 437
40. Cooper, D.K.C., Wicomb, W.N. and Barnard, C.N. (1983). Storage of the donor heart by a portable hypothermic perfusion system: experimental development and clinical experience. *J. Heart Transplant.*, **2**, 104
41. Cooper, D.K.C., Wicomb, W.N., Rose, A.G. and Barnard, C.N. (1983). Orthotopic allotransplantation and autotransplantation of the baboon heart following twenty-four hours storage by a portable hypothermic perfusion system. *Cryobiology*, **20**, 385
42. Wicomb, W.N., Novitzky, D., Cooper, D.K.C. and Rose, A.G. (1986). Forty-eight hours hypothermic perfusion storage of pig and baboon hearts. *J. Surg. Res.*, **40**, 276
43. Wicomb, W.N., Rose, A.G., Cooper, D.K.C. and Novitzky, D. (1986). Hemodynamic and myocardial histological and ultrastructural studies in baboons three to twenty-seven months following autotransplantation of hearts stored by hypothermic perfusion for 24 or 48 hours. *J. Heart Transplant.*, **5**, 122
44. Wicomb, W.N., Cooper, D.K.C., Lanza, R.P., Novitzky, D. and Isaacs, S. (1986). The effects of brain death and 24 hours storage by hypothermic perfusion on donor heart function in the pig. *J. Thorac.*

Cardiovasc. Surg., **91**, 896

45. Martin, C.D., Scott, D.F., Downes, G. and Belzer, F.O. (1972). Primary cause of unsuccessful liver and heart preservation; cold sensitivity of the ATPase system. *Ann. Surg.*, **175**, 111
46. Lyons, J.M. and Raison, J.K. (1970). A temperature-induced transition in mitochondrial oxidation; contrasts between cold- and warm-blooded animals. *Comp. Biochem. Physiol.*, **37**, 405
47. Kemp, A., Groot, G.S.P. and Reemtsma, H.J. (1969). Oxidative phosphorylation as a function of temperature. *Biochem. Biophys. Acta*, **180**, 28
48. Zimmerman, A.N.E., Daems, W., Huismann, W.C., Snijder, J., Wisse, E. and Durrer, D. (1967). Morphological changes of heart muscle caused by successive perfusing with Ca^{++}-free and Ca^{++}-containing solutions (Calcium paradox). *Cardiovasc. Res.*, **1**, 201
49. Alto, L.E. and Dhalla, N.S. (1981). Role of changes in microsomal calcium uptake on the effects of reperfusion of Ca^{++}-deprived rat hearts. *Circ. Res.*, **48**, 17
50. Katz, A.M. and Tada, M. (1972). The 'stone heart'; a challenge to the biochemist. *Am. J. Cardiol.*, **29**, 578
51. Wicomb, W.N. and Collins, G.M. (1989). Twenty-four hour rabbit heart storage with UW solution: effects of low flow perfusion, colloid, and shelf storage. *Transplantation*, **48**, 6
52. Toledo-Pereyra, L.H. (1987). Definition of reperfusion injury in transplantation. *Transplantation*, **43**, 931
53. Naylor, W.G., Poole-Wilson, P.A. and William, A. (1979). Hypoxia and calcium. *J. Mol. Cell Cardiol.*, **11**, 683
54. Jennings, R.B. and Ganote, C.E. (1976). Mitochondrial structure and function in acute myocardial ischemic injury. *Circ. Res.*, **38**, (Suppl. I), 80
55. Opie, J.C., Taylor, G., Ashmore, P.G. and Kalousek, D. (1981). "Stone heart" in the neonate. *J. Thorac. Cardiovasc. Surg.*, **81**, 459
56. McCord, J.M. (1985). Oxygen derived free radicals in post-ischemic tissue injury. *N. Engl. J. Med.*, **312**, 159
57. Ytrehus, K., Myklebust, R. and Mjos, O.D. (1986). Influence of oxygen radicals generated by xanthine oxidase in the isolated perfused rat heart. *Cardiovasc. Surg.*, **20**, 597
58. Hess, M.L., Warner, M.R., Roblins, A.D., Crute, S. and Greenfield, L.J. (1981). Characterization of the excitation–contraction coupling system of the hypothermic myocardium following ischemia and reperfusion. *Cardiovasc. Res.*, **15**, 380
59. Jennings, R.B., Ganote, C.E. and Reimer, K.A. (1975). Ischemic tissue injury. *Am. J. Pathol.*, **81**, 197
60. Trump, B.F. and Berezesky, I.K. (1983). The role of Ca^{++} deregulation in cell injury and cell death. *Surv. Synth. Path. Res.*, **2**, 165
61. Naylor, W.G. (1983). Calcium and cell death. *Eur. Heart. J.*, **4**, (Suppl.), 33
62. Shen, A.C. and Jennings, R.B. (1972). Myocardial calcium and magnesium in acute ischemic injury. *Am. J. Pathol.*, **67**, 417
63. Beatrice, M.C., Stiers, D.L. and Pfeiffer, D.R. (1984). The role of glutathione in the retention of Ca^{++} by liver mitochondria. *J. Biol. Chem.*, **259**, 1279
64. Rodemann, H.P., Waxman, L. and Goldberg, A.L. (1982). The stimulation of protein degradation in muscle by Ca^+ is mediated by PGE_2 and does not require the calcium activated protease. *J. Biol. Chem.*, **257**, 8716
65. Etlinder, J.D., Kameyama, T., Toner, K., Van der Westhuyzen, D. and Matsumoto, K. (1980). In Pette, D. (ed.) *Plasticity of Muscle.*, p. 541. (New York: Walter de Gruyter)
66. Goldberg, A.L. and St. John, A.C. (1974). Intracellular protein degradation in mammalian and bacterial cells. *Ann. Rev. Biochem.*, **45**, 747
67. Lee, S. L. and Dhalla, N.S. (1976). Subcellular calcium transport in failing hearts due to calcium deficiency and overload. *Am. J. Physiol.*, **231**, 1159
68. Moorhouse, P.C., Grootveld, M., Halliwell, B., Quinlan, J.E. and Gutteridge, J.M.C. (1987). Allopurinol and oxypurinol are hydroxyl radical scavengers. *FEBS. Lett.*, **213**, 23
69. Bergsland, J., Lobalsamo, L., Lajos, P., Feldman, M.J. and Mookerjee, B. (1987). Allopurinol in prevention of perfusion injury of hypoxically stored rat hearts. *J. Heart Transplant.*, **6**, 137
70. Myers, C.L., Weiss, S.J., Kirsch, M.M., Shephard, B.M. and Shlafer, M. (1986). Effects of supplementing hypothermic crystalloid cardioplegic solution with catalase superoxide dismutase, allopurinol, or deferoxamine on functional recovery of globally ischemic and reperfused isolated hearts. *J. Thorac. Cardiovasc. Surg.*, **91**, 281
71. Christoffersen, G.R.J. and Skibsted, L.H. (1975). Calcium ion activity in physiological salt solutions: influences of anions substituted for chloride. *Comp. Biochem. Physiol.*, **52A**, 317
72. Kopf, G.S., Chaudry, I., Condos, S. and Baue, A.E. (1987). Reperfusion with $ATP-MgCl_2$ following prolonged ischemia improves myocardial performance. *J. Surg. Res.*, **43**, 114
73. Kajiyama, K., Pauly, D.F., Hughes, H., Yoon, S.B., Entman, M.L. and McMillan-Wood, J.B. (1987). Protection by verapamil of mitochondrial glutathione equilibrium and phospholipid changes during reperfusion of ischemic canine myocardium. *Circ. Res.*, **61**, 301
74. Chien, K.R., Abrams, J., Pfau, R.G. and Farber, J.L. (1977). Prevention by chlorpromazine of ischemic liver cell death. *Am. J. Pathol.*, **88**, 539
75. Pryor, W.A. (1976). The role of free radical reactions in biological systems. In Pryor, W.A. (ed.) *Free Radicals in Biology.* p. 1. (New York: Academic Press)
76. Fridovich, I. (1978). The biology of oxygen radicals. *Science*, **201**, 875
77. Fridovich, I. (1970). Quantitative aspects of the production of superoxide anion radical by milk xanthine oxidase. *J. Biol. Chem.*, **245**, 4053
78. Fee, J.A. and Valentine, J.S. (1977). Chemical and physical properties of superoxide. In Michelson, A.M., McCord, J.M. and Fridovich, I. (eds.) *Superoxide and Superoxide Dismutase.* p. 19. (New York: Academic Press)
79. Nilsson, R., Pick, F.M. and Bray, R.C. (1969). EPR studies on reduction of oxygen to superoxide by some biochemical systems. *Biochem. Biophys. Acta*, **192**, 145
80. Estabrook, R.A. and Werringloer, J. (1977). Cytochrome P450: its role in oxygen activation for drug metabolism. In Gould, R.F. (ed.) *Drug Metabolism Concepts.* p.1. (Washington, DC: American Chemical Society)
81. Masters, C. and Holmes, R. (1977). Peroxisomes: new aspects of cell physiology and biochemistry. *Physiol. Rev.*, **57**, 816
82. Samuelson, B. (1983). Leukotrines: mediators of immediate hypersensitivity reactions and inflammation. *Science*, **220**, 568
83. Klebanoff, S.J. (1980). Oxygen metabolism and the toxic properties of phagocytes. *Ann. Intern. Med.*, **93**, 480
84. Mead, J.F. (1976). Free radical mechanisms of lipid damage and consequences of cellular membranes. In Pryor, W.A. (ed.) *Free Radicals in Biology.* Vol. I, p. 51. (New York: Academic Press)
85. Maridonneau, I., Braquet, P. and Garay, R.P. (1983). Na^+ and K^+ transport damage induced by oxygen free radicals in human red cell membranes. *J. Biol. Chem.*, **258**, 3107
86. Moody, C.S. and Hasson, H.M. (1982). Mutagenicity of oxygen free radicals. *Proc. Natl. Acad. Sci. USA*, **79**, 2855
87. Fligiel, S.E.G., Lee, E.C. and McCoy, J.P. (1984). Protein degradation following treatment with hydrogen peroxide. *Am. J. Pathol.*, **115**, 418
88. Perez, H.D., Wedsler, B.B. and Goldstein, I.M. (1980). Generation of a chemotactic lipid from arachidonic acid by exposure to a superoxide generating system. *Inflammation*, **4**, 313
89. Oguma, F., Imai, S. and Eguchi, S. (1986). Role played by oxygen in myocardial protection with crystalloid cardioplegic solution. *Ann. Thor. Surg.*, **42**, 172
90. Coetzee, A., Kotze, J., Law, J. and Lochner, A. (1986). Effect of oxygenated crystalloid cardioplegia on the functional and metabolic recovery of the isolated perfused rat heart. *J. Thorac. Cardiovasc.*

Surg., **91**, 259

91. Rousou, J.A., Engelman, R.M., Anisimowicz, L., Lemeshow, S., Dobbo, W.A., Breyer, R.H. and Das, D.K. (1986). Metabolic enhancement of myocardial preservation during cardioplegic arrest. *J. Thorac. Cardiovasc. Surg.*, **91**, 270
92. Otani, H. Engelman, R.M., Rousou, J.A., Breyer, R.H., Lemeshow, S. and Das, D.K. (1986). Cardiac performance during reperfusion improved by pretreatment with oxygen free radical scavengers. *J. Thorac. Cardiovasc. Surg.*, **91**, 290.
93. Prodjian, A.K., Levitsky, S., Krukenkamp, I., Silverman, N.A. and Feinberg, H. (1987). Developmental changes in reperfusion injury. *J. Thorac. Cardiovasc. Surg.*, **93**, 428
94. Mak, I.T., Misra, H.P. and Weglicki, W.B. (1983). Temporal relationship of free radical-induced lipid peroxidation and loss of latent enzyme activity in highly enriched hepatic lysosomes. *J. Biol. Chem.*, **258**, 13733
95. Kramer, J.H., Mak, I.T. and Weglicki, W. B. (1984). Differential sensitivity of canine cardiac sarcolemmal and microsomal enzymes to inhibition by free radical-induced lipid peroxidation. *Circ. Res.*, **55**, 120
96. Lucy, J.A. (1972). Functional and structural aspects of biological membranes: a suggested structural role of vit. E in the control for membrane permeability and stability. *Ann. NY Acad. Sci.*, **203**, 4
97. Packer, J.E., Slater, T.F. and Willson, R.L. (1979). Direct observation of a free radical interaction between vit. E and vit. C. *Nature (London)*, **278**, 737
98. Frank, L. and Massaro, D. (1980). Oxygen toxicity. *Am. J. Med.*, **69**, 117
99. Halliwell, B. (1982). Superoxide and superoxide-dependent formation of hydroxyl radicals are important in oxygen toxicity. *Trends. Biochem. Sci.*, **Aug.**, 271
100. Laurence, R.A. and Burk, R.F. (1978). Species tissue and subcellular distribution of non-selenium dependent glutathione peroxidase activity. *J. Nutr.*, **108**, 211
101. Al-Timini, D.J. and Dormandy, T.L. (1977). The inhibition of lipid autoxidation by human ceruloplasmin. *Biochem. J.*, **168**, 283
102. Miller, J.S. and Cornwell, D.G. (1978). The role of cryoprotective agents as hydroxyl radical scavengers. *Cryobiology*, **15**, 585
103. Collins, G.M., Wicomb, W.N. and Halasz, N.A. (1984). Beneficial effect of low concentrations of cryoprotective agents on short-term rabbit kidney perfusion. *Cryobiology*, **21**, 246
104. Menasche, P., Grousset, C., Gauduel, Y. and Piwnica, A. (1986). A comparative study of free radical scavengers in cardioplegic solutions. *J. Thorac. Cardiovasc. Surg.*, **92**, 264
105. McCord, J. and Fridovich, I. (1980). Superoxide dismutase: threat and defense. *Acta Physiol. Scand.* (Suppl.), **492**, 9
106. Belzer, F.O. and Southard, J. (1988). Principles of solid-organ preservation by cold storage. *Transplantation*, **45**, 673
107. Houpert, Y. (1976). Comparison of procedures for extracting free amino acids from polymorphonuclear leukocytes. *Clin. Chem.*, **22**, 1618
108. Jellinek, M., Castaneda, M., Garvin, P.J., Nichoff, M. and Codd, J.E. (1985). Oxidation–reduction maintenance in organ preservation. *Arch. Surg.*, **120**, 439
109. Wicomb, W.N., Hill, J.D., Avery, J. and Collins, G.M. (1989). Comparison of cardioplegic and UW solutions for short-term rabbit heart preservation. *Transplantation*, **47**, 733
110. Čanković-Darracott, S., Braimbridge, M.V., Williams, B.T., Bitensky, L. and Chayen, J. (1977). Myocardial preservation during aortic valve surgery. *J. Thorac. Cardiovasc. Surg.*, **73**, 699
111. Braimbridge, M.V., Chayen, J., Bitensky, L., Hearse, D.J., Jynge, P. and Čanković-Darracott, S. (1977). Cold cardioplegia or continuous coronary perfusion? *J. Thorac. Cardiovasc. Surg.*, **74**, 900
112. Čanković-Darracott, S. (1982). In Engelman, R.M. and Levitsky, D. (eds.) *A Handbook of Clinical Cardioplegia.* p. 43. (New York: Futura)
113. Bull, C., Cooper, J. and Stark, J. (1984). Cardioplegic protection of the child's heart. *J. Thorac. Cardiovasc. Surg.*, **88**, 287
114. Chayen, J., Bitensky, L. and Čanković-Darracott, S. (1985). Increased myosin orientation during muscle contraction: a measure of cardiac contractility. *Cell Biochem. Funct.*, **3**, 101
115. Čanković-Darracott, S., Hutter, J., Wallwork, J., Wheeldon, D. and English, T.A.H. (1988). Biopsy assessment of myocardial preservation in 160 human donor hearts. *Transplant. Proc.*, **20** (5 Suppl. 17), 44
116. Pitzele, S., Sze, S. and Dobell, A.R.C. (1971). Functional evaluation of the heart after storage under hypothermic coronary perfusion. *Surgery*, **70**, 569.
117. Levitsky, S., Williams, W.H., Hetmer, D.E., McIntosh, C.L. and Morrow, A.G. (1970). A functional evaluation of the preserved heart. *J. Thorac. Cardiovasc. Surg.*, **60**, 625

8
Pretransplant Immunological Considerations

E.D. DU TOIT, M. OUDSHOORN AND D.K.C. COOPER

INTRODUCTION

Since numerous detailed accounts of transplantation immunology appear elsewhere in the literature[1-3] and the mechanism of allograft destruction is outlined in Chapter 14, this chapter will concentrate only on those pretransplant immunological aspects that are of practical clinical importance before a cardiac transplant is performed. Four topics will be discussed: (1) the necessity for donor-recipient ABO blood group compatibility, (2) the role of human leukocyte antigen (HLA) matching, (3) the lymphocytotoxic crossmatch test and the problem of preformed antibodies, and (4) the effect of pretransplant blood transfusions in recipients of cardiac allografts.

RED BLOOD CELL GROUPS

ABO groups

ABO blood group compatibility between donor and recipient is a prerequisite in patients undergoing organ transplantation, with the possible exception of the liver[4,5]. Incompatibility nearly always leads to rapid destruction of the allograft[6,7], although there have been very occasional reports of successful A to O, or B to A kidney grafts[8]. Opelz, in 59 cases, verified that ABO incompatible cadaver kidney transplants showed poor results[9]; a similar poor graft survival was observed in a subset of these patients treated with cyclosporine. However, the importance of ABO incompatibility has been questioned following the observation that a proportion of ABO-incompatible liver transplants continue to function[4]. In a recent survey, the incidence of irreversible hyperacute or accelerated acute rejection in patients receiving incompatible ABO hearts was approximately 60%[10]. The mechanism of rejection is thought to be due to antibodies directed against incompatible A or B antigens present on the vascular endothelium of the allograft[11], and may be immediate[8].

Several transplant centers have shown that group O recipients survive longer after renal[12,13] and cardiac[14] transplantation than non-O recipients, particularly in the presence of HLA-DR mismatching. Early in our series of cardiac transplants at Groote Schuur Hospital in Cape Town (with patients immunosuppressed with azathioprine, corticosteroids, and antithymocyte globulin), we observed poor survival of recipients with the B antigen (blood groups B and AB)[15]. It was presumed that those with blood group B antigen might elicit a greater immune response. This observation, however, remains controversial[16,17]. Data collected for the Collaborative Heart Transplant Study by Opelz shows no major influence of recipient-donor ABO blood type on graft survival[18] (Chapter 32).

There is some evidence that patients receiving ABO-identical hearts (e.g. A to A) have significantly improved survival and less fatal rejection episodes than those receiving ABO-non-identical hearts (e.g. O to A)[17,19,20]. Similar results have been clearly documented in large studies of renal transplants[21]. Opelz' data, however, showed no evidence that ABO-compatible (as opposed to ABO-identical) cardiac transplants have an inferior success rate[18] (Chapter 32).

Rhesus group

Rhesus (Rh) antigens are weak immunogens with regard to organ transplantation and are not considered important[22]. A few studies have found improved renal allograft survival in Rh-positive recipients when compared with Rh-negative recipients[23].

THE HUMAN LEUKOCYTE ANTIGEN (HLA) SYSTEM

The immune response to an allograft is determined primarily by the major histocompatibility complex (MHC), known in man as the human leukocyte antigen (HLA) system. The genes coding for the HLA antigens are located on the short arm of chromosome 6. Molecular data have now identified many of the genes in the HLA region, and their arrangement, and to date nine closely linked HLA loci have been described, designated HLA-A, B, C, E, DR, DQ, DO, DN and DP[24]. HLA-A, B and C antigens have been designated MHC Class I, and the HLA-D system of antigens MHC Class II. Both groups of antigens, but particularly Class II, play a role in the mechanism of allograft rejection (Chapter 14).

HLA-A, B and C antigens (MHC Class I)

HLA-A, B and C antigens have been shown to be expressed on the surface of nucleated cells in the body. A new locus called HLA-E, which cannot be detected by serology, has been defined by molecular techniques in this region of the chromosome[24]. To determine an individual's HLA-A, B and C phenotype, the T-lymphocytes are set up in a complement dependent lymphocytotoxic test against a large number of known antisera. The lymphocytes are lysed if the HLA antigen is recognized by specific antibodies. For example, if the antiserum known to contain antibodies against HLA-A1 lyse the lymphocytes, then those lymphocytes are coded as HLA-A1.

At the HLA-A locus there are 24 known alleles (different genes that may occupy the same position or locus on a specific chromosome), at the HLA-B 50 alleles, and at the HLA-C 11; each allele produces a gene product which is expressed on the cell surface as an antigen (Table 8.1)[24]. Each individual has two chromosomes 6, one inherited from each parent, and therefore has two of the 24 HLA-A antigens (for example, A1 and A2), two of the 50 HLA-B antigens, and 2 of the 11 HLA-C antigens. If the recipient and donor are not HLA-identical, the immune response of the recipient following organ transplantation is directed primarily against those antigens on the surface of the donor organ that are not shared by the two individuals.

The exact role of HLA-A, B and C matching between recipient and donor in allograft survival remains controversial, but analyses from large regional and national centers in Europe and North America have found a consistent correlation between HLA-A and B matching and improved renal graft survival[2,3]. The survival rate of recipients of well-matched renal allografts is approximately 10–20% higher than that of recipients of poorly-matched allografts. The only major analysis of the effect of HLA-C matching on renal allograft survival did not show any significant difference in transplant outcome between well-matched and poorly-matched donor–recipient groups[25].

Several reports have demonstrated no evidence for an improved outcome of cardiac allograft survival with HLA-A and B matching[19,25–28]. However, in a study of 164 consecutive cyclosporine-treated cardiac transplant patients, the Stanford group found that the degree of mismatching for HLA antigens at the A and B loci correlated with long-term survival in their patients[29]. A limited study on the effect of HLA-A and B locus antigen matching in 40 consecutive heart–lung transplant patients also showed that HLA–A locus matching may have a beneficial effect on long-term graft survival[30].

In a previous study they observed that patients with HLA-A2 or A3 incompatibilities had a significantly higher incidence of graft arteriosclerosis (chronic rejection) than patients with other A locus incompatibilities[31]. These results could not be shown to be valid in cyclosporine-treated heart–lung transplant patients[30]. In an early review of our own cardiac transplant recipients, we also did not find this association[32].

HLA-DR, DQ and DP antigens (MHC Class II)

All the HLA loci prefixed by the letter D form part of the HLA-D region. The products of these D-region loci are expressed on the surface of B-lymphocytes, macrophages, and dendritic cells, all of which are involved in interaction with helper T-lymphocytes during normal immune responses (Chapter 14). They are also expressed on other cell types including vascular endothelial cells, thymic epithelium, and Langerhans cells. No protein products have been demonstrated for the DO and DN sub-regions to date.

The HLA-DR and DQ antigens are determined by a serological test, as are HLA-A, B and C antigens, though B-lymphocytes rather than T-lymphocytes are used as the target cells. Cellular typing reagents are capable of identifying HLA-D region specificities, which may not be detectable using alloantisera, or for which appropriate serological reagents have not yet been identified.

HLA-Dw specificities have been identified traditionally with HLA-D homozygous typing cells (HTCs) in primary *in vitro* mixed lymphocyte cultures (MLCs). The MLC can be considered as the *in vitro* homologue of the *in vivo* immune respose to an allograft[33]. Up to 6 days, however, are required to complete the MLC test, which is therefore of no practical importance with regard to cardiac transplantation. Though the HLA-Dw specificities of the recipient can be identified, the recipient–donor HLA-Dw matching can only be known retrospectively. There is evidence, however, that matching for HLA-Dw specificities greatly improves the outcome of kidney allografts from living related donors[34,35].

HLA-DP antigens are also detected with cellular reagents although a few allo- and monoclonal antibodies are now available for DP typing. HLA-DP antigens do not appear to be of clinical significance in heart and kidney transplantation. It has been suggested, however, that disparity at this locus may be important in the pathogenesis of graft-versus-host disease[36].

Table 8.1 Complete listing of recognized HLA specificities (1987)*

HLA-A	B	C	D	DR	DQ	DP
A1	B5	Cw1	Dw1	DR1	DQw1	DPw1
A2	B7	Cw2	Dw2	DR2	DQw2	DPw2
A3	B8	Cw3	Dw3	DR3	DQw3	DPw3
A9	B12	Cw4	Dw4	DR4	DQw4	DPw4
A10	B13	Cw5	Dw5	DR5	DQw5(w1)	DPw5
A11	B14	Cw6	Dw6	DRw6	DQw6(w1)	DPw6
Aw19	B15	Cw7	Dw7	DR7	DQw7(w3)	
A23(9)	B16	Cw8	Dw8	DRw8	DQw8(w3)	
A24(9)	B17	Cw9(w3)	Dw9	DR9	DQw9(w3)	
A25(10)	B18	Cw10(w3)	Dw10	DRw10		
A26(10)	B21	Cw11	Dw11(w7)	DRw11(5)		
A28	Bw22		Dw12	DRw12(5)		
A29(w19)	B27		Dw13	DRw13(w6)		
A30(w19)	B35		Dw14	DRw14(w6)		
A31(w19)	B37		Dw15	DRw15(2)		
A32(w19)	B38(16)		Dw16	DRw16(2)		
Aw33(w19)	B39(16)		Dw17(w7)	DRw17(3)		
Aw34(10)	B40		Dw18(w6)	DRw18(3)		
Aw36	Bw41		Dw19(w6)			
Aw43	Bw42		Dw20	DRw52		
Aw66(10)	B44(12)		Dw21			
Aw68(28)	B45(12)		Dw22	DRw53		
Aw69(28)	Bw46		Dw23			
Aw74(w19)	Bw47		Dw24			
	Bw48		Dw25			
	B49(21)		Dw26			
	Bw50(21)					
	B51(5)					
	Bw52(5)					
	Bw53					
	Bw54(w22)					
	Bw55(w22)					
	Bw56(w22)					
	Bw57(17)					
	Bw58(17)					
	Bw59					
	Bw60(40)					
	Bw61(40)					
	Bw62(15)					
	Bw63(15)					
	Bw64(14)					
	Bw65(14)					
	Bw67					
	Bw70					
	Bw71(w70)					
	Bw72(w70)					
	Bw73					
	Bw75(15)					
	Bw76(15)					
	Bw77(15)					
	Bw4					
	Bw6					

* From Dupont, B. (ed.) (1989). *Immunobiology of HLA. Volume 1, Histocompatibility Testing, 1987.* (New York: Springer-Verlag). p. 77.

It has been said that HLA-DR incompatibility between donor and recipient may well be the major stimulus for the generation of the immune response against a transplanted kidney[37]. A number of large studies report evidence favoring an important role for HLA-DR antigens in renal transplantation[38,39]. Matching for HLA-DR appears to improve cardiac allograft survival[19,26,27,40,41]. Because donor hearts are not allocated according to HLA match, most heart transplants are HLA-incompatible. It is therefore difficult for any one group to obtain sufficient data to make valid analyses possible. In a multicenter study of over 1000 heart transplants by Opelz[28], however, mismatching for HLA-DR antigens was associated with reduced graft survival (86% versus 76% at 1 year). The greater the mismatch for both HLA-B and DR antigens, the greater the deleterious effect (91% versus 77%). A similar result with regard to HLA-DR matching has been demonstrated at a single center (Harefield)[40]. HLA Class II matching also appeared to influence survival after combined heart–lung transplantation[42].

At the present time, there are insufficient data on the relationship between HLA-DQ matching and renal, as well as cardiac, allograft survival to arrive at any meaningful conclusions.

In view of data showing some evidence of improved cardiac allograft survival in patients with HLA antigen matching, our policy with regards to recipient–donor HLA matching has been to offer the heart to the patient with the greatest number of antigens matched with the donor, if this information is available at the time of surgery. If the critical physical state of one patient necessitates urgent transplantation, then this patient is given priority regardless of the results of recipient–donor HLA matching.

THE LYMPHOCYTOTOXIC CROSS-MATCH TEST AND THE PROBLEM OF PREFORMED ANTIBODIES

As soon as a potential recipient is selected for transplantation, the patient's serum is set up against a panel of 30 or more T-lymphocytes and a similar panel of B-lymphocytes, representing the major antigenic stimuli. These tests are performed to detect preformed HLA antibodies in the recipient. Donor-specific HLA-A, B and C antibodies (Class I) are identified by reactivity (cytotoxic effect in the presence of complement) with donor T-lymphocytes. Donor-specific HLA-DR antibodies (Class II) are identified by reactivity with donor B-lymphocytes. Preformed antibodies may be present in the recipient following previous organ transplantation, pregnancy, or blood transfusion.

Should the recipient's serum be shown to contain preformed lymphocytotoxic antibodies against T-cells, difficulty may be met in finding a compatible donor for that particular recipient. If there are no preformed antibodies, selection of a suitable donor should in all likelihood be easy. We believe that a donor-specific lymphocytotoxic cross-match should be performed in every case whenever preformed lymphocytotoxic antibodies have been identified, and that it is preferable (though perhaps not essential) in cases where no antibodies have been detected. When the donor is at a distant center, shortage of time may make a prospective cross-match inconvenient, and it can be performed retrospectively in patients without preformed antibodies.

When a possible donor becomes available, the lymphocytotoxic cross-match test is performed using recipient serum and donor T- and B-cells. From data obtained from large series of kidney transplants, Ting has pointed out that a number of factors require consideration in the interpretation of a positive cross-match[43]. These include:

(1) The specificity of the antibody; lymphocytotoxic antibodies can be HLA Class I, Class II, or autoantibody (against T- and B-cells or B-cells alone);

(2) The time interval between the date of the last serum giving a positive cross-match and the date of transplantation; the peak reactive serum and current serum or only the peak serum can give a positive cross-match;

(3) The immunoglobulin (Ig) class of antibody; this can be IgG or IgM.

Autoantibodies (which are IgM) do not cause graft rejection even if present at the time of transplantation[43]. Class I IgM antibodies giving a positive peak and yet negative current sera cross-match are not damaging, whereas a positive peak and negative current cross-match due to Class I IgG antibodies are associated with graft failure. Where the peak and current sera are both positive on cross-match due to Class I IgG antibodies, hyperacute and acute rejection may occur. There appear to be no published data on the outcome of transplants performed with a positive peak and positive current sera on cross-match due to Class I IgM antibodies.

For practical purposes, if the recipient serum is shown to contain antibodies that react against the donor T-lymphocytes[44,45], the recipient is said to be 'presensitized', and there is a strong chance of hyperacute rejection after transplantation. In one series, 24 out of 30 renal transplant recipients who were presensitized to their donors had immediate and irreversible rejection of the allograft[46].

Although the importance of T-cell lymphocytotoxic antibodies in the subsequent destruction of an allograft is accepted, that of B-cell lymphocytotoxic antibodies remains uncertain. The role of B-cell antibodies in clinical transplantation has received much attention following the first reports of a successful graft outcome in the presence of a positive B-cell lymphocytotoxic cross-match[47,48]. Donor-specific B-cell lymphocytotoxic antibodies, when present in a potential recipient before transplantation, have been variously reported to: (1) lead to early graft rejection[49,50], (2) bear no relationship to the subsequent transplant outcome[51,52], and (3) correlate with improved graft survival[53]. Furthermore, a distinction has been made according to the temperature at which the test is performed. Antibodies reacting at 37°C are said to correlate with a poor prognosis, whilst those reacting at 5°C correlate with an improved prognosis[54]. It has been established, however, that preformed donor-specific B-cell lymphocytotoxic antibodies do not lead to the immediate or early allograft failure from hyperacute or accelerated graft rejection which may occur when preformed donor-specific T-cell lymphocytotoxic antibodies are present in the recipient serum[54,55], although an isolated case has been reported[56].

The influence of preformed, non-donor-specific T-cell lymphocytotoxic antibodies (that is, when non-donor-specific T-cell lymphocytotoxic antibodies have been demonstrated against a panel of T-lymphocytes) on the subsequent survival of an allograft remains uncertain. There is some evidence that patients with broadly reactive antibodies (antibodies with a high frequency of lymphocytotoxicity against a random panel) have impaired renal[57-59] and heart–lung[42] graft survival rates.

The evidence that antibody formation following rejection of a renal allograft confers a less favorable prognosis on subsequent graft survival is supported by our own observations in one patient following cardiac retransplantation[60]. This patient developed strong multispecific antibodies against T-lymphocytes after rejection at 5 weeks of an HLA non-identical heterotopic cardiac transplant. The heterotopic allograft was excised, and the patient remained alive supported by his own heart. After some months the antibodies could not be detected, though they recurred following a test transfusion of 500 ml of HLA non-identical blood. When another donor heart became available, the donor-specific T-cell lymphocytotoxic cross-match test using both stored and fresh recipient sera was negative. A second heterotopic heart transplant was performed, but the donor heart failed within 5 days, following the onset of a severe irreversible acute rejection episode. At that time, a 32-fold increase in lymphocytotoxic antibodies against donor T-cells was demonstrated in the patient's blood.

In a more recent retrospective analysis of 304 cardiac allografts, Kormos et al. also showed that preformed antibodies reactive against a panel of T-lymphocytes significantly decreased the long-term survival rate[19]. The Harefield group, however, showed no such correlation in patients undergoing heart transplantation, demonstrating a 72% graft survival at 2 years for those with a positive lymphocytotoxic antibody screen compared with 74% survival in those with a negative screen[41]. The presence of a positive lymphocytotoxic cross-match between donor and recipient, however, did significantly reduce 2-year survival (52% versus 78%). In patients undergoing heart–lung transplantation at Harefield, however, the presence of cytotoxic antibodies on pretransplant screening against a panel of lymphocytes was associated with significantly reduced survival at 2 years (50% versus 76%).

PRETRANSPLANT BLOOD TRANSFUSION

For a number of years blood transfusions were avoided whenever possible in potential transplant recipients in order to minimize the risk of presensitization. It was thought that the development of cytotoxic antibodies to HLA alloantigens would reduce the number of potential donors compatible with the particular recipient[61,62]. In 1973, however, it was demonstrated in a large renal transplant series that transplant recipients who had never received blood transfusions before transplantation had a significantly lower allograft survival rate than their counterparts who had been transfused[63]. These results have been confirmed by most renal transplant centers[64-67], though the magnitude of the effect varies markedly from center to center.

The beneficial effect of pretransplantation blood transfusion in cyclosporine-treated patients is controversial. Several studies have reported that, in patients transplanted without prior transfusion, graft survival is no longer substantially lower than that in transfused patients[68-71], while others still report a beneficial effect[72]. As mentioned by Cecka et al.[72], these controversial reports (coupled with the public awareness that recipients of blood transfusions may be at higher risk for acquired immunodeficiency syndrome (AIDS)), present a serious impediment to the physician who must justify recommending blood transfusions to a potential transplant recipient.

Although one major center has reported that favorable renal allograft outcome is directly related to the number of pretransplant transfusions received[73], other groups have not confirmed this, and have instead reported that a single transfusion is as effective as several transfusions and lessens the risk of the potential recipient developing antibodies against HLA antigens[74,75].

One possible explanation for the favorable effect of blood transfusions on allograft survival is that the transfusions differentiate between 'high responders', who would have a high rate of rejection after subsequent organ transplantation, and 'low responders', who would have a low rate. As the high responders develop antibodies following blood transfusion, subsequent transplantation may prove impossible, as no donor can be found against whom the recipient does not have a positive cross-match. Only the low responders are transplanted, with good results[76]. An alternative explanation is that the transfusions induce a state of unresponsiveness similar to immune enhancement[63].

Any beneficial effect of blood transfusion on patients undergoing cardiac transplantation is even less certain. A beneficial, though not statistically significant, effect was observed and reported by the Stanford group as early as 1973[77]. In an early review of the patients in our series, pretransplant blood transfusions were related to improved survival, though this reached statistical significance only at the 3-year time interval[32].

In experimental work in baboons we have found that pretransplant transfusion, whether given as one or more large transfusions or as small transfusions at frequent intervals, does not result in any significant prolongation of cardiac allograft survival[78]. These results, however, are at variance with those reported by Van Es et al., who observed an increase in survival of kidney allografts in rhesus monkeys following transfusion[79]. Furthermore, Van Es observed that the length of survival was greater in the monkeys in whom transplantation was performed sooner rather than later after the last transfusion. Unless this is a species or organ-related difference, the lack of correlation between our own results and those of Van Es and his colleagues cannot be adequately explained.

It has already been pointed out that pretransplant transfusion can sensitize some patients to HLA antigens, and thus decrease the chances of finding a donor with a negative cross-match for those patients. The major limiting factor to the number of transplants performed in most centers is the availability of donor organs. Thus, any manipulation that might further reduce the number of donors available to any potential recipient should be avoided unless it imparts a clearly beneficial effect which overrides this consideration. There would, therefore, appear to be no indication at the present time to electively transfuse patients awaiting cardiac transplantation.

There is, however, some evidence that the administration of immunosuppressive drugs at the time of blood transfusion reduces or eliminates sensitization[80,81]. There is also some evidence that the state of sensitization, if not severe, may be reversed. Observations of two cardiac transplant patients in our institution would suggest that the administration of cyclosporine to a sensitized patient may lead to the loss of these circulating antibodies[82], though this observation has not been generally confirmed.

Subsequently, pretransplant donor-specific blood transfusion has been shown to correlate with improved graft survival following kidney transplantation from genetically disparate living-related donors[83,84]. Transplantation from living-related donors is clearly impossible in patients requiring heart transplantation, and therefore pretransplant transfusion from the potential donor is not applicable. However, it is possible to administer a donor-specific transfusion at the time of cardiac transplantation, though in baboons we have not found this to be related to any improved survival[78].

COMMENT

In summary, therefore, before cardiac transplantation is performed, donor-recipient ABO compatibility and a negative cross-match using donor T-lymphocytes and recipient serum must be assured. A transplant between ABO-identical recipient and donor may lead to improved graft survival compared with that between ABO-compatible recipient and donor. Recipients with non-O blood groups may be at some disadvantage. There is evidence to show that HLA compatibility and, in particular, matching for HLA-B plus HLA-DR, improves graft survival. Patients with high levels of circulating T-lymphocytotoxic antibodies are at higher risk of losing graft function from acute rejection, despite a negative donor-specific cross-match at the time of transplantation. There would appear to be no indication to transfuse electively patients awaiting heart transplantation.

References

1. Hamburger, J. (1982). Transplantation immunology. In Hamburger, J. Crosnier, J., Bach, J.F. and Kreis, H. (eds.) *Renal Transplantation: Theory and Practice*. 2nd ed. (Baltimore/London: Williams & Wilkins)
2. Carpenter, C.B. and Strom, T.B. (1980). Transplantation immunology. In Parker, C.W. (ed.) *Clinical Immunology*. (Philadelphia: W.B. Saunders)
3. Thomas, F. and Thomas, J. (1980). Transplantation immunology. In Chatterjee, S.N. (ed.) *Renal Transplantation – A Multidisciplinary Approach*. (New York: Raven Press)
4. Gordon, R.D., Iwatsuki, S., Esquivel, C.O., Tzakis, A., Todo, S. and Starzl, T.E. (1986). Liver transplantation across the ABO blood groups. *Surgery*, **100**, 342
5. Fischel, R.J., Ascher, N.L., Payne, W.D., Freese, D.K., Stock, P., Fasola, C. and Najarian, J.S. (1989). Pediatric liver transplantation across ABO blood group barriers. *Transplant. Proc.*, **21**, 2221
6. Dausset, J. and Rapaport, F.T. (1966). The role of blood group antigens in human histocompatibility. *Ann. NY Acad. Sci.*, **129**, 408
7. Murray, J.E. and Harrison, J.H. (1963). Surgical management of fifty patients with kidney transplants, including eighteen pairs of twins. *Am. J. Surg.*, **105**, 205
8. Starzl, T.E., Marchioro, T.L., Holmes, J.H., Hermann, G., Brittain, R.S., Stonington, O.H. and Talmage, D.W. (1964). Renal homografts in patients with major donor-recipient blood group incompatibilities. *Surgery*, **55**, 195
9. Opelz, G. (1988). A Collaborative Transplant Study. *Newsletter*, **2**, 2
10. Cooper, D.K.C. (1989). A clinical survey of cardiac transplantation between ABO-blood group incompatible recipients and donors. *J. Heart Transplant.*, in press
11. Wilbrandt, R., Tung, K.S.H., Deodhar, S.R. and Waddell, W.R. (1969). ABO blood incompatibility in human renal homotransplantation. *Am. J. Clin. Pathol.*, **51**, 15
12. Opelz, G. and Terasaki, P.I. (1977). Effect of blood group on relation between HLA match and outcome of cadaver kidney transplants. *Lancet*, **1**, 220
13. Joysey, V., Roger, J.H. and Evans, D.B. (1973). Kidney graft survival and matching for HLA and ABO antigens. *Nature (London)*, **246**, 163
14. Hendriks, G.F.J., Wenting, G.J., Mochzar, B., Bos, E., Simoons, M.L., Balk, A.H.M.M., Laird-Meeter, K., Essed, C.E. and Weimar, W. (1989). The influence of ABO blood groups on the incidence of cardiac allograft rejection in males. *Transplant. Proc.*, **21**, 803
15. Lanza, R.P., Cooper, D.K.C. and Barnard, C.N. (1982). Effect of ABO blood group antigens on long-term survival after cardiac transplantation. *N. Engl. J. Med.*, **397**, 1275
16. Shumway, S.J., Baumgartner, W.A., Soule, L.M., Gardner, T.J. and Reitz, B.A. (1987). Lack of effect of ABO blood-group antigens on survival after cardiac transplantation. *N. Engl. J. Med.*, **317**, 772
17. Nakatani, T., Aida, H., Macris, M.P. and Frazier, O.H. (1989). Effect of ABO blood type on survival of heart transplant patients treated with cyclosporine. *J. Heart Transplant.*, **8**, 27
18. Opelz, G. (1989). Collaborative Heart Transplant Study. *Newsletter*, **2**,
19. Kormos, R.L., Colson, Y.L., Hardesty, R.L., Griffith, B.P., Trento, A., Vanek, M., Duquesnoy, R.J. and Zeevi, A. (1988). Immunologic and blood group compatibility in cardiac transplantation. *Transplant. Proc.*, **20** (Suppl. 1), 741
20. McKenzie, F.N., Tadros, N., Stiller, C., Keown, P., Sinclair, N. and Kostuk, W. (1987). Influence of donor-recipient lymphocyte crossmatch and ABO status on rejection risk in cardiac transplantation. *Transplant. Proc.*, **19**, 3439
21. Stock, P.G., Sutherland, D.E.R., Fryd, D.S., Ascher, N.L., Payne, W., Simmons, R.L. and Najarian, J.S. (1987). ABO-compatible mismatching decreases five year actuarial graft survival after renal transplantation. *Transplant. Proc.*, **19**, 4522

22. Van Hooff, J.P., Hendriks, G.F.J. and Van Rood, J.J. (1976). The influence of a number of immunogenic and non-immunogenic factors on the graft prognosis. The relative importance of HLA matching in kidney transplantation. *Academic Thesis*, University of Leiden, p. 69
23. Opelz, G. and Terasaki, P.I. (1979). Cadaver kidney transplants in North America: analysis 1978. *Dial. Transplant.*, **8**, 167
24. Nomenclature for factors of the HLA system, 1987 (1989). In Dupont, B. (ed.) *Immunobiology of HLA. Vol. 1. Histocompatibility Testing*, 1987. p. 77. (New York: Springer-Verlag)
25. Solheim, B.G., Flatmark, A., Enger, E., Jervell, J. and Thorsby, E. (1977). Influence of HLA-A, B, C and D matching on the outcome of clinical kidney transplantation. *Transplant. Proc.*, **9**, 475
26. Yacoub, M., Festenstein, H., Doyle, P., Martin, M., McCloskey, D., Awad, J., Gamba, A., Khaghani, A. and Holmes, J. (1987). The influence of HLA matching in cardiac allograft recipients receiving cyclosporine and azathioprine. *Transplant. Proc.*, **19**, 2487
27. Opelz, G. (1988). Collaborative Heart Transplant Study. *Newsletter*, **1**, 1
28. Opelz, G. for the Collaborative Heart Transplant Study (1989). Effect of HLA matching in heart transplantation. *Transplant. Proc.*, **21**, 794
29. First, W.H., Oyer, P.E., Baldwin, J.C., Stinson, E.B. and Shumway, N.E. (1987). HLA compatibility and cardiac transplant recipient survival. *Ann. Thorac. Surg.*, **44**, 242
30. Harjula, A.L.J., Baldwin, J.C., Glanville, A.R., Tazelaar, H., Oyer, P.E., Stinson, E.B. and Shumway, N.E. (1987). Human leukocyte antigen compatibility in heart-lung transplantation. *J. Heart Transplant.*, **6**, 162
31. Bieber, C.P., Hunt, S.A., Schwinn, D.A., Jamieson, S.A., Reitz, B.A., Oyer, P.E., Shumway, N.E. and Stinson, E.B. (1981). Complications in long-term survivors of cardiac transplantation. *Transplant. Proc.*, **13**, 207
32. Cooper, D.K.C., Boyd, S.T., Lanza, R.P. and Barnard, C.N. (1983). Factors influencing survival following heart transplantation. *Heart Transplant.*, **3**, 86
33. Fournier, C. (1982). Mixed lymphocyte reaction and cell-mediated lympholysis techniques. In Hamburger, J., Crosnier, J., Bach, J.F. and Kreis, H. (eds.) *Renal Transplantation: Theory and Practice*. p.361. (Baltimore/London: Williams & Wilkins)
34. Cochrum, K.C., Perkins, H.A., Payne, R., Kountz, S. and Belzer, F.O. (1973). The correlation of MLC with graft survival. *Transplant. Proc.*, **5**, 391
35. Walker, J., Opelz, G. and Terasaki, P.I. (1978). Correlation of MLC response with graft survival in cadaver and related donor kidney transplants. *Transplant. Proc.*, **10**, 949
36. Odum, N., Platz, P., Jakobsen, B.K., Munck Petersen, C., Jacobsen, N., Moller, J., Ryder, L.P., Lamm, L. and Svejgaard, A. (1987). HLA-DP and bone marrow transplantation: DP-incompatibility and severe acute graft versus host disease. *Tissue Antigens*, **30**, 213
37. Ting, A. (1982). HLA and organ transplantation. In Morris, P.J. (ed.) *Tissue Transplantation*. p. 28. (New York: Churchill Livingstone)
38. Cicciarelli, J., Terasaki, P.I. and Mickey, M.R. (1987). The effect of zero HLA Class I and II mismatching in cyclosporine-treated kidney transplant patients. *Transplantation*, **43**, 636
39. Opelz, G. (1987). Effect of HLA matching in 10,000 cyclosporine-treated cadaver kidney transplants. *Transplant. Proc.*, **19**, 641
40. Khaghani, A., Yacoub, M., McCloskey, D., Awad, J., Burden, M., Fitzgerald, M., Hawes, R., Holmes, J., Smith, J., Banner, N. and Festenstein, H. (1989). The influence on survival of HLA matching, donor/recipient sex and incidence of acute rejection in cardiac allograft recipients receiving cyclosporine and azathioprine. *Transplant. Proc.*, **21**, 799
41. McCloskey, D., Festenstein, H., Banner, N., Hawes, R., Holmes, J., Khaghani, A., Smith, J. and Yacoub, M. (1989). The effect of HLA lymphocytotoxic antibody status and HLA cross-match result on cardiac transplant survival. *Transplant. Proc.*, **21**, 804
42. Festenstein, H., Banner, N., Smith, J., Awad, J., Burden, M., Fitzgerald, N., Holmes, J., Khaghani, A., McCloskey, D. and Yacoub, M. (1989). The influence of HLA matching and lymphocytotoxic status in heart-lung allograft recipients receiving cyclosporine and azathioprine. *Transplant. Proc.*, **21**, 797
43. Ting, A. (1989). What crossmatches are required in organ transplantation? *Transplant. Proc.*, **21**, 613
44. Kissmeyer-Nielsen, F., Olsen, S., Peterson, V.P. and Fjeldborg, O. (1966). Hyperacute rejection of kidney allografts associated with pre-existing humoral antibodies against donor cells. *Lancet*, **2**, 662
45. Weil, R., Clarke, D.R., Iwaki, Y., Porter, K.A., Koep, L.J., Paton, B.C., Terasaki, P.I. and Starzl, T.E. (1981). Hyperacute rejection of a transplanted human heart. *Transplantation*, **32**, 71
46. Patel, R. and Terasaki, P.I. (1969). Significance of the positive crossmatch test in kidney transplantation. *N. Engl. J. Med.*, **280**, 735
47. Ettinger, R.B., Terasaki, P.I. and Opelz, G. (1976). Successful renal allografts across a positive crossmatch for donor B-lymphocyte alloantigens. *Lancet*, **2**, 56
48. Lobo, P.I., Werterwelt, F.B. and Rudolf, L.E. (1977). Kidney transplantability across a positive crossmatch. Crossmatch assays and distribution of B-lymphocytes in donor tissue. *Lancet*, **1**, 925
49. Ayoub, G., Min Sik Park, Terasaki, P.I., Iwaki, Y. and Opelz, G. (1980). B-cell antibodies and crossmatching. *Transplantation*, **29**, 227
50. Buckingham, J.M., Geis, W.P., Giacchinoo, J.L., Subhash, R., Hano, J.E., Chejfec, G. and Jonasson, O. (1979). B-cell directed antibodies and delayed hyperacute rejection: a case report. *J. Surg. Res.*, **27**, 268
51. Coxe-Gilliland, R. and Cross, D.E. (1979). Warm B-cell antibodies and DRW matching: their influence on transplant outcome at a single center. *Transplant. Proc.*, **11**, 945
52. Morris, P.J. (1978). Histocompatibility antigens in human organ transplantation. *Surg. Clin. North Am.*, **58**, 233
53. D'Apice, A.J.F. and Taits, B.D. (1979). Improved survival and function of renal transplants with positive B-cell crossmatches. *Transplantation*, **27**, 324
54. Cross, D.E., Coxe-Gilliland, R. and Weaver, P. (1978). DRW antigen matching and B-cell antibody crossmatching: their effect on clinical outcome in renal transplants. *Transplant. Proc.*, **11**, 1908
55. Morris, P.J., Ting, A. and Oliver, D. (1978). Renal transplantation in the presence of positive crossmatch. *Transplant. Proc.*, **10**, 476
56. Dejelo, C.L. and Williams, T.C. (1977). B-cell crossmatch in renal transplantation. *Lancet*, **2**, 241
57. Van Hooff, J.P., Schippers, H.M.A., Van der Steen, G.J. and Van Rood, J.J. (1972). Efficiency of HLA matching in Eurotransplant. *Lancet*, **2**, 1385
58. Salvatierra, O., Perkins, H.A., Amend, W., Feduska, N.J., Duca, R.M., Potter, D.E. and Cochrum, K.C. (1977). The influence of presensitization on graft survival rate. *Surgery*, **81**, 146
59. Opelz, G. (1987). Kidney transplantation in sensitized patients. *Transplant. Proc.*, **19**, 3737
60. Lanza, R.P., Campbell, E.M., Cooper, D.K.C., Du Toit, E. and Barnard, C.N. (1983). The problem of the presensitized heart transplant recipient. *Heart Transplant.*, **2**, 151
61. Curtoni, E.S., Scudeller, P.I., Mattiuz, G., Savi, M. and Ceppellini, R. (1972). Anti-HLA antibody evaluation in recipients of planned transfusions. *Tissue Antigens*, **2**, 415
62. Terasaki, P.I., Mickey, M.R. and Krasler, M. (1971). Presensitization and kidney transplant failures. *Postgrad. Med.*, **47**, 89
63. Opelz, G., Sengar, D.P.S., Mickey, M.R. and Terasaki, P.I. (1973). Effect of blood transfusions on subsequent kidney transplants. *Transplant. Proc.*, **5**, 253
64. Festenstein, H., Sachs, J.A., Paris, A.M.I., Pegrum, G.D. and Moorhead, J.F. (1976). Influence of HLA matching and blood transfusion on outcome of 502 London transplant group renal-graft recipients. *Lancet*, **1**, 157
65. Fuller, T.C., Demanico, T.L., Cosimi, A.B., Huggins, C.E., King, M.

and Russell, P.S. (1977). Effects of various types of RBC transfusions on HLA alloimmunization and renal allograft survival. *Transplant. Proc.*, **9**, 117
66. Svejgaard, A. and Solheim, B.G. (1977). Blood transfusion and kidney transplantation. In *Proceedings of the North Scandinavian Transplantation Meeting. Scand. J. Urol. Nephrol.* (Suppl.), **42**, 79
67. Van Hooff, J.P., Kalff, M.W., Van Poelgeest, A.E., Lansbergen, Q., Hendriks, G.F.J., Castelli, M. and MacKenzie, C.L.S. (1976). Blood transfusion and kidney transplantation. *Transplantation*, **22**, 306
68. Kerman, R.H., Van Buren, C.T., Fletchner, S.M., Lorber, M.I. and Kahan, B.D. (1985). The beneficial effect of cyclosporine on renal transplantation at a single US transplant center. *Transplant. Proc.*, **17**, 2193
69. Groth, C.G. (1987). There is no need to give blood transfusions as pretreatment for renal transplantation in the cyclosporine era. *Transplant. Proc.*, **19**, 153
70. Opelz, G. (1987). Improved kidney graft survival in non-transfused recipients. *Transplant. Proc.*, **19**, 149
71. Opelz, G. for the Collaborative Transplant Study (1989). The role of HLA matching and blood transfusions in the cyclosporine era. *Transplant. Proc.*, **21**, 609
72. Cecka, J.M., Cicciarelli, J., Mickey, M.R. and Terasaki, P.I. (1988). Blood transfusions and HLA matching – an either/or situation in cadaveric renal transplantation. *Transplantation* **45**, 81
73. Opelz, G. and Terasaki, P.I. (1978). Improvement of kidney-graft survival with increased number of blood transfusions. *N. Engl. J. Med.*, **299**, 799
74. Persijn, G.G., Van Hooff, J.P., Kalff, M.W., Lansbergen, Q. and Van Rood, J.J. (1977). Effects of blood transfusions and HLA matching on renal transplantation in the Netherlands. *Transplant. Proc.*, **9**, 503
75. Williams, K.A., Ting, A., Cullen, P.R. and Morris, P.J. (1979). Transfusions: their influence on human renal graft survival. *Transplant. Proc.*, **11**, 175
76. Van Es, A.A. and Balner, H. (1979). Effects of pretransplant transfusions on kidney allograft survival. *Transplant. Proc.*, **11**, 127
77. Dong, E., Stinson, E.B., Griepp, R.B., Coulson, A.S. and Shumway, N.E. (1973). Cardiac transplantation following failure of previous cardiac surgery. *Surg. Forum.*, **24**, 150
78. Cooper, D.K.C., Rose, A.G., Du Toit, E., Langman, E. and Wicomb, W.N. (1985). Failure of pretransplant third party and per-operative donor-specific blood transfusion to improve heterotopic cardiac allograft survival in baboons. *Transplantation*, **40**, 569
79. Van Es, A.A., Marquet, R.L., Van Rood, J.J., Kalff, M.W. and Balner, H. (1977). Blood transfusions induce prolonged kidney allograft survival in rhesus monkeys. *Lancet*, **1**, 506
80. Monaco, A.P., Clarke, A.W., Wood, M.L., Sahyoun, A.I., Codish, S.D. and Brown, R.W. (1976). Possible active enhancement of a human cadaver renal allograft with antilymphocyte serum (ALS) and donor bone marrow: case report of an initial attempt. *Surgery*, **79**, 384
81. Anderson, C.B., Sicard, G.A., Rodey, G.E., Anderman, C.K., and Etheredge, E.E. (1983). Renal allograft recipient pretreatment with donor-specific blood and concomitant immunosuppression. *Transplant. Proc.*, **15**, 939
82. Novitzky, D., Cooper, D.K.C., Du Toit, E., Oudshoorn, M., Langman, E. and Jacobs, P. (1985). Preformed lymphocytotoxic antibodies following cyclosporine therapy. *J. Heart Transplant.*, **4**, 362
83. Salvatierra, O., Vincenti, E., Amend, W., Potter, D., Iwaki, Y., Opelz, G., Terasaki, P.I., Duca, R., Cochrum, K., Hanes, D., Stoney, R.J. and Feduska, N.J. (1980). Deliberate donor-specific blood transfusion prior to living related renal transplantation. *Ann. Surg.*, **192**, 543
84. Salvatierra, O., Vicenti, E., Amend, W., Potter, D., Garovoy, M., Iwaki, Y., Terasaki, P.I., Duca, R., Hopper, S., Slemmer, T. and Feduska, N. (1983). Four years' experience with donor-specific blood transfusions. *Transplant. Proc.*, **15**, 924

9
Anesthetic Management Including Cardiopulmonary Bypass

D.W. BETHUNE AND D.R. WHEELDON

INTRODUCTION

Following the first reports of a successful cardiac transplantation over 20 years ago[1] there was an initial surge of activity in many centers, but it is only in the past 10 years that successful cardiac transplant programs have become widely established. Several of the centers have reported details of the anesthetic techniques they have used[1-9], and, not surprisingly, most of these have been closely related to those used for conventional cardiac surgery. Examination of these reports and the results of a multicenter survey[10] reveal interesting differences between the techniques we use at our own center (Papworth Hospital, United Kingdom), and those used in the majority of North American centers.

PRE-ANESTHESIA MANAGEMENT

In our practice it is rare for the recipient to be in our hospital when the donor call is received. The recipient is contacted either in his local hospital or at home, and then removed to Papworth and prepared for operation. Most patients will therefore not have had any oral intake for 5-6 hours before induction of anesthesia. On admission, a period of intense activity follows. The patient is bathed and shaved, bacteriological swabs are obtained, and a final surgical and anesthetic assessment undertaken.

After transfer to the anesthetic room, an arterial, a peripheral venous, and two right internal jugular lines are inserted under local anesthesia. In our early experience, we avoided the right internal jugular route to leave this approach unsullied for subsequent endomyocardial biopsies. More recently, we have routinely used the right side without causing any problem in the postoperative period.

Sedation is administered as necessary, using either midazolam in 1-2 mg increments or similar increments of papaveretum. Prophylactic antibiotics and methylprednisolone (500 mg) are administered i.v. Azathioprine is normally given orally, but may be administered intravenously at this time. We no longer give cyclosporine preoperatively, as studies have demonstrated that withholding this drug until the postoperative period results in significantly less early renal dysfunction without any apparent increase in early rejection. Until mid-1987 we commenced the infusion of equine antithymocyte globulin (ATG) before the induction of anesthesia, but, as even a minor reaction to this equine preparation in a decompensated cardiac patient can cause a catastrophic hemodynamic collapse, we now administer the ATG while on cardiopulmonary bypass (CPB). The hypotension that can occasionally result can be controlled with a vasopressor more easily on CPB; the T-cell suppression has been found to be just as effective.

At this stage, if time permits, the patient's relatives are allowed to join him in the anesthetic room until we have a definite time for the return of the donor team.

INDUCTION OF ANESTHESIA

Immediately prior to the induction of anesthesia, sedation is increased (5-10 mg of papaveretum, and possibly some additional midazolam). Anesthesia is then induced with an inhalational technique using nitrous oxide, oxygen, and trichloroethylene. When light hypnosis has been obtained, a muscle relaxant is administered. Pancuronium, despite its tendency to cause tachycardia, is well-tolerated and does not cause hypotension. Vecuronium, tracrium, and alcuronium are also used, but occasional episodes of hypotension and/or bradycardia have required treatment.

An orotracheal tube is inserted and the patient connected to the ventilator, using a Pall BB50 bacteria filter as a heat and moisture exchanger[11]. We believe that the use of a bacterial filter to isolate the airway represents a major advance in the management of the immunosuppressed patient. We do not insert a nasogastric tube. We routinely insert a urinary catheter, and have not noted problems related to urinary tract infection. Nitrous oxide is discontinued 10 min before CPB is initiated to minimize the effects of any gaseous microemboli arising from the pump-oxygenator[12].

As far as possible the patient is kept in a sitting position, apart from a brief period when the internal jugular lines are being inserted. This is important as many of the recipients are close to (or in) cardiac failure even when sitting up. When they are laid flat the increased venous return may push them over the top of the Frank–Starling curve into the unstable state where increased filling pressure causes a fall in cardiac output[13], and results in a further rise in filling pressures and a rapid downwards hemodynamic spiral.

Infusion of inotropes at this time seems to be inappropriate (despite their almost universal use in the 46 North American centers surveyed in 1986[10]). Our practice is to reduce preload by venesection (0.5–1.0 l) and to reduce the afterload, and to a lesser extent the preload, by using nitroprusside. It is not uncommon to see a paradoxical response to nitroprusside in such patients, where high doses of the vasodilator result in an increase in the systolic and pulse pressures, as well as an invariable increase in cardiac output. This approach to the patient with intractable heart failure is similar to that widely used for the management of heart failure in general medical practice[14,15].

We do not insert a pulmonary artery catheter as we consider the risks of inducing arrhythmias during insertion, and the need to remove the catheter before the heart is excised, while not absolute contraindications, are sufficient to make the benefit marginal. Once the chest is open, visualization of the heart is the best possible monitor; the effect of reducing the preload and afterload can be observed in the action of the ventricles. (Following transplantation, an electromagnetic flow probe placed around the aorta allows continuous monitoring of cardiac output.)

CARDIOPULMONARY BYPASS

Following heparinization, which is checked by confirming an activated clotting time (ACT) longer than 350 s, the aorta, superior and inferior venae cavae are cannulated and connected to the extracorporeal circuit (Figure 9.1). The routine at Papworth is to use a membrane oxygenator and to provide non-pulsatile perfusion with moderate hypothermia (30°C). The machine is primed with crystalloid solution to which 6000 IU of heparin are added. Pump flow is 2.4 l min^{-1} m^{-2} at normothermia, reducing to 2.0 l min^{-1} m^{-2} at 30°C.

Facilities are always available for hemofiltration and/or hemodialysis[16] should either prove necessary.

Pressure on bypass is controlled to give a perfusion pressure between 40 and 60 mmHg. This almost invariably involves the use of vasodilators; diazoxide was our preferred

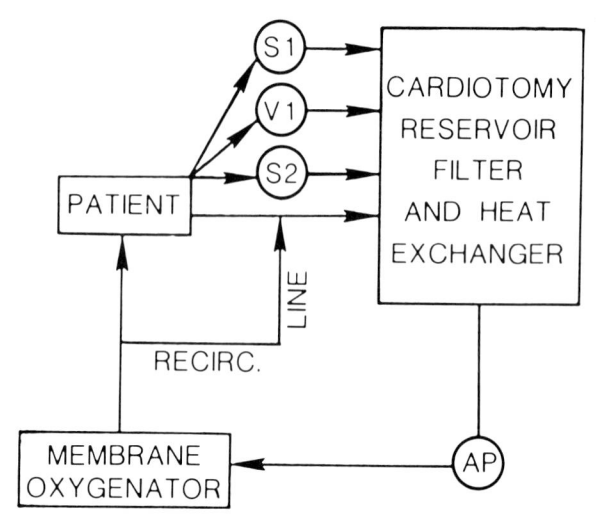

Figure 9.1 Cardiopulmonary bypass circuit as used in cardiac transplant operations at Papworth Hospital. (Abbreviations: S = sucker; V = vent; AP = arterial roller pump; Recirc. Line = recirculation line)

dilator until its interaction with the phosphodiesterase-inhibiting inotropic agents was established. Phentolamine is useful, as its main site of action is on the arterioles, therefore resulting in little volume shift between patient and oxygenator. Nitroprusside can be used, but its venodilating effect will move a significant volume of perfusate from the circuit into the patient. At the initiation of CPB, various factors combine to produce a fall in peripheral resistance. This is normally self-limiting, and vasoconstrictors are not administered unless the pressure is below 40 mmHg, and there is dilation of the pupils, which could be interpreted as evidence of inadequate cerebral circulation.

Rewarming is initiated during the aortic or pulmonary artery anastomosis, the aim being to achieve a blood temperature of 37°C by the time of release of the aortic clamp. Mannitol (20 g) is added to the perfusate immediately before aortic clamp removal. Potassium is also added at this time to ensure a serum level above 4.5 mmol/l. We have not observed the reported abnormal sensitivity of the transplanted heart to potassium[7]; in our experience, low potassium levels have been associated with an increased incidence of arrhythmias.

Pump flow is reduced to attain an initial coronary perfusion pressure of 30–40 mmHg, and subsequently increased to normal flow over the next few minutes. Supportive bypass is continued for at least 15 min following removal of the aortic cross-clamp, maintaining a pulsatile output, but with the heart decompressed.

Cardiopulmonary bypass is discontinued, with particular care being taken to avoid over-distension of the ventricles. Methylprednisolone 500 mg is administered at this time. An aortic electromagnetic flow probe is helpful in monitoring (and therefore optimizing) the patient's hemodynamic status; a relatively low systemic vascular resistance is common in such patients. It is our experience that the heart will usually support the circulation without the need for inotropic agents, though isoproterenol may be required for its chronotropic action. Temporary pacing wires are placed to allow correction of any postoperative bradycardia.

IMMEDIATE POSTOPERATIVE MANAGEMENT (see also Chapter 12)

With the assurance of an adequate cardiac output, a mean systemic pressure of 50 mmHg can be accepted. The systemic vascular resistance usually increases in the early postoperative period, and nitroprusside is frequently required to control the rise in systemic pressure.

In a small number of patients, we have experienced problems with a raised pulmonary vascular resistance (PVR) after discontinuation of CPB. This has usually been related to a deterioration in the recipient's condition that occurred between the date of assessment and that of operation. In some patients the rise in PVR has been associated with the development of pulmonary edema, which will acutely raise PVR. Though the deleterious effect of a raised PVR on long-term prognosis has recently been recognized[17], we have found that in the immediate post-bypass period, once a reasonable hemodynamic state has been achieved, progress is satisfactory. In two patients, a prostacycline infusion (epoprostenol flolan, Wellcome, UK) was required to lower the PVR before pump-oxygenator support could be satisfactorily discontinued.

Following completion of the operation, the patient is transferred to the intensive care unit, and lung ventilation is continued until the patient is awake. It is rarely necessary for the relaxant to require reversal before extubation 3–6 h later.

References

1. Ozinsky, J. (1967). Cardiac transplantation – the anesthetist's view: a case report. *S. Afr. Med. J.*, **41**, 1268
2. Harrison, G.A., Bailey, R.J. and Thomson, P.G. (1969). A heart transplantation. 4. Anesthesia and cardiopulmonary bypass. *Med. J. Aust.*, **1**, 670
3. Keats, A.S., Strong, J.M., Girigis, K. and Goldstein, A. (1969). Observations during anesthesia for cardiac homotransplantation in ten patients. *Anesthesiology*, **30**, 192
4. Paiement, B., Wielhorski, W.A., Grondin, P., Lepage, G. and Dytda, I. (1970). Anesthetic management in nine heart transplantations. *Laval. Med.*, **41**, 100
5. Fernando, N.A., Keenan, R.L. and Boyan, C.P. (1978). Anesthetic experience with cardiac transplantation. *J. Thorac. Cardiovasc. Surg.*, **75**, 531
6. Garman, J.K. (1981). Anesthesia for cardiac transplantation. *Cleve. Clin.*, **48**, 442
7. Grebenik, C.R. and Robinson, P.N. (1985). Cardiac transplantation at Harefield. *Anaesthesia*, **40**, 131
8. Demas, K., Wyner, J., Mihm, F.G. and Samuels, S. (1986). Anaesthesia for heart transplantation. *Br. J. Anaesth.*, **58**, 1357
9. Bethune, D.W., Collis, J.M., Hardy, I. and Latimer, R.D. (1988). Anesthesia for cardiac transplantation. In Farman, J. (ed.) *Transplant Surgery: Anesthesia and Perioperative Care.* p. 335. (Amsterdam: Elsevier Science)
10. Hensley, F.A., Martin, D.E., Larach, D.R. and Romanof, M.E. (1987). Anesthetic management for cardiac transplantation in North America – 1986 survey. *J. Cardiothoracic Anesth.*, **1**, 429
11. Shelley, M.P., Bethune, D.W. and Latimer, R.D. (1986). A comparison of five heat and moisture exchangers. *Anaesthesia*, **41**, 527
12. Bethune, D.W. (1976). Organ damage after open heart surgery. *Lancet*, **2**, 1410
13. Forester, J.S. and Waters, D.D. (1978). Hospital treatment of congestive heart failure. *Am. J. Med.*, **65**, 173
14. Braunwald, E. (1981). Heart failure: pathophysiology and treatment. *Am. Heart J.*, **102**, 486
15. Zelis, R., Flaim, S.F., Moskowitz, R.M. and Nellis, S.H. (1979). How much can we expect from vasodilator therapy in congestive heart failure? *Circulation*, **59**, 1092
16. Hakim, M., Wheeldon, D., Bethune, D.W., Milstein, B.B., English, T.A.H. and Wallwork, J. (1985). Hemodialysis and hemofiltration on cardiopulmonary bypass. *Thorax*, **40**, 101
17. Kirklin, J.K., Naftel, D.C., Kirklin, J.W., Blackstone, E.H., White-Williams, C. and Bourge, R.C. (1988). Pulmonary vascular resistance and the risk of heart transplantation. *J. Heart Transplant.*, **7**, 331

10
Surgical Technique of Orthotopic Heart Transplantation

D.K.C. COOPER AND D. NOVITZKY

INTRODUCTION

There are two standard operations for performing heart transplantation – orthotopic, in which the recipient heart is excised and replaced in the correct anatomical position by the donor heart, and heterotopic (the so-called 'piggyback' heart transplant), in which the donor heart is placed in the right chest alongside the recipient organ, and anastomosed in such a way to allow blood to pass through either or both hearts (Chapter 11).

With either transplant technique, we believe that the recipient operation should not be begun until the donor has been carefully assessed by the transplant surgeon, and found to be suitable for transplantation. Whenever there is doubt, e.g. when there is the possibility of cardiac injury from chest trauma, the recipient operation should be delayed until the donor chest has been opened and the heart inspected.

The basic technique of orthotopic heart transplantation was developed in the research laboratory in the late 1950s and early 1960s[1] (Chapter 1). It was the work of Lower and Shumway in 1960[2] which established the operation as a successful procedure in the experimental animal. The operation was first attempted clinically by Hardy and his colleagues in 1964[3] and by Barnard in 1967[4]. In 1968, Barnard[5] contributed a small but significant modification to the operative technique whereby the incision in the right atrium of the donor heart was extended from the opening of the inferior vena cava (IVC) into the base of the right atrial appendage, and not into the superior vena cava (SVC), thus avoiding the region of the sinoatrial node. The operation has remained essentially unchanged since then, and is the operation of choice in the majority of centers performing heart transplantation today.

DONOR HEART EXCISION

With the subject supine, a median sternotomy is performed and the pericardium opened longitudinally. The heart is inspected, in possible cases, for external signs of major injury caused by trauma or external cardiac massage; the coronary arteries should be palpated to exclude obvious coronary disease. The ascending aorta is dissected from the pulmonary artery to allow subsequent application of a cross-clamp. The SVC is mobilized up to the azygos vein to allow SVC ligation cephalad to the sinus node. Two heavy ties are placed around the SVC, but not ligated at this stage. The IVC is mobilized. The donor is fully heparinized. A cannula or needle for infusion of cold cardioplegic agent is inserted into the ascending aorta.

The SVC is doubly ligated (or suture ligated) and divided between the ligatures. (Any indwelling central venous pressure cannula must be withdrawn high into the SVC before this vessel is ligated and divided.) The IVC is clamped at the diaphragm, completing inflow occlusion, and divided immediately central to the clamp, thus decompressing the right side of the heart. One or more pulmonary veins are incised or divided to decompress the left side of the heart. As no left ventricular vent has been inserted, we believe that adequate decompression of the heart in this way is essential before the aorta is cross-clamped. If an arterial line is in place, the pulse wave should be lost, indicating that the left ventricle has emptied. The ascending aorta is then cross-clamped at the level of the brachiocephalic (innominate) artery, and cardioplegic solution (approximately 10 ml/kg at 4°C) infused into the root of the aorta. At least 1–2 l of cold saline (at 4°C) are poured over the heart to cool it rapidly.

Infusion pressure in the aorta should not exceed approximately 100 mmHg. This can be achieved by placing the bag containing the cardioplegic agent in a pressure bag, pressurized to 300 mmHg; experience has shown that this results in an aortic pressure in the desired range. During infusion, the heart should be gently massaged at intervals to ensure that adequate decompression is maintained. Cardioplegic infusion is usually complete within 3–5 min.

During the ischemic period in which the heart is transferred to the recipient, there will be no cardioplegic washout from collateral blood flow (as occurs in a cardioplegically arrested heart during open-heart surgery). It is theoretically, therefore, only necessary to give sufficient cardioplegic agent to bring about arrest of the heart. The cardioplegic infusion, however, also contributes towards a rapid cooling of the myocardium, and it is our policy, therefore, to infuse approximately 10 ml/kg (500–1000 ml) unless the anticipated ischemic period is expected to be very short.

Once the cardioplegic agent has been administered, the topical cold saline is sucked out of the pericardial cavity, and section of the four pulmonary veins is completed. Division of the aorta as high as possible, immediately proximal to the cross-clamp, and of the pulmonary artery at its bifurcation (or of its main right and left branches) completes division of the major vessels.

The apex of the heart is then lifted anteriorly, and the mediastinal tissue posterior to the atria and major vessels is divided by sharp dissection, allowing the heart to be removed from the pericardial cavity.

The approximate time taken from ligation of the SVC to completion of excision of the heart is 5–10 min.

Multiple organ excision

Donor heart excision is frequently combined with removal of both kidneys and liver. After the initial preparation of the donor heart, the liver and kidneys are mobilized. While cardioplegic arrest and local cooling of the heart are being induced, the liver and kidneys are also perfused. Finally, excision of the cold arrested heart is completed. If the liver is to be removed, it is helpful to the liver team to apply the IVC clamp approximately 1.5 cm above the diaphragm (or to apply no clamp at all), thus leaving a cuff of IVC to be excised with the liver.

Should the liver transplant surgeon request decompression of the IVC, this vessel can be incised either immediately caudal to the clamp within the chest or within the abdomen, and a sucker placed in it to evacuate the hepatic infusion fluid. As this fluid is also mixed with blood, which may warm the heart, we believe it is important to exclude it from the pericardial cavity until the heart has been excised. Alternatively, if the liver transplant surgeon wishes to decompress the liver via the IVC into the chest, the IVC need not be clamped; in such cases, the right pleuropericardium should be incised vertically down from the sternum to the junction of IVC with right atrium. This allows the IVC to drain directly into the right pleural cavity, thus insuring that the liver perfusion solution and/or warm blood do not contaminate the heart, or interfere with the surgical field in which the cardiac surgeon is working. It is convenient to introduce a suction catheter into the right pleural cavity to insure that the collected fluid does not overflow into the pericardial cavity.

PREPARATION OF DONOR HEART

The heart is placed in a bowl of cold (4°C) saline while it is prepared for insertion into the recipient.

The right atrial cavity is opened, beginning posterolaterally at the IVC orifice and continuing the incision into the base of the right atrial appendage, thus avoiding the areas of the coronary sinus and the sinoatrial node[5] (Figure 10.1). The tissue between the orifices of the four pulmonary veins on the posterior aspect of the left atrium is excised, leaving one large opening (Figure 10.2). (The aorta and pulmonary

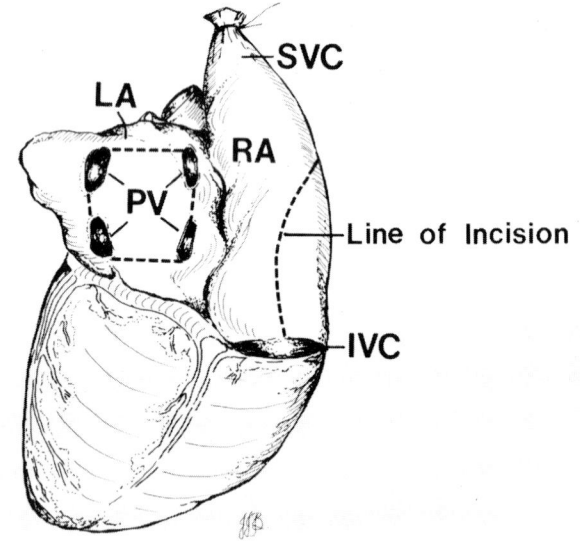

Figure 10.1 Excised donor heart (posterior view), showing lines of incision. (Abbreviations used in figures in this chapter are: LA = left atrium; RA = right atrium; SVC = superior vena cava; IVC = inferior vena cava; PV = pulmonary vein; RV = right ventricle; PA = pulmonary artery; AO = aorta; LV = left ventricle)

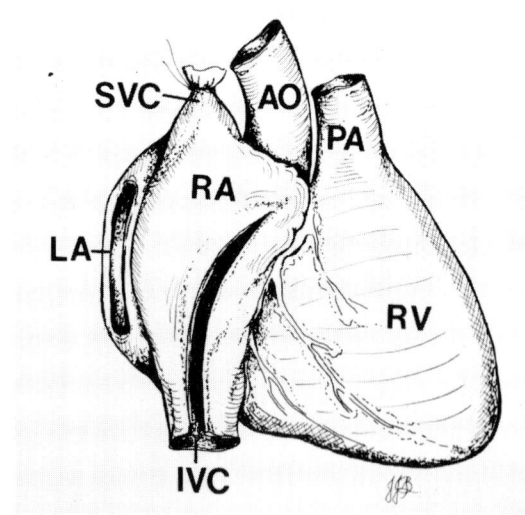

Figure 10.2 Donor heart (right anterolateral view) prepared for implantation

artery should not be trimmed to the ideal lengths until the atrial anastomoses have been completed during insertion into the recipient.

The heart can then be transferred to the surgical team preparing the recipient.

THE RECIPIENT OPERATION

With the patient lying supine, a median sternotomy is performed, the pericardium opened longitudinally, and its edges retracted.

Initiation of cardiopulmonary bypass

After heparinization, cardiopulmonary bypass is initiated via cannulae inserted into the ascending aorta, at the level of the brachiocephalic artery, and into the SVC and IVC via the lateral wall of the right atrium (Figure 10.3). Snares (snuggers) or clamps are placed around the SVC and IVC to bring about total cardiopulmonary bypass. Body cooling to at least 28°C, and possibly lower (26°C), helps prevent early rewarming of the donor heart as it lies in the pericardial cavity during insertion. The aorta is then cross-clamped immediately proximal to the aortic cannula.

Excision of recipient heart

The heart is excised by dividing the right and left atrial walls (close to the atrioventricular groove) and atrial septum, leaving a cuff of atrial wall to allow easy suture of the donor heart. Both atrial appendages should be excised to prevent thrombus formation occurring in these cavities subsequently. The aorta and main pulmonary artery are divided as close to their respective valves as possible (Figure 10.3). Subsequently, these vessels may be trimmed before being sutured to their counterparts of the donor heart.

The chronological order of division of these structures is unimportant, but a simple and accepted sequence is (1) free wall of right atrium, (2) free wall of left atrium, excluding the superior wall posterior to the origins of the aorta and pulmonary artery, (3) pulmonary artery, (4) aorta, (5) (after retracting the proximal aorta and pulmonary artery anteriorly) the remaining superior wall of the left atrium, and (6) the atrial septum.

Anastomosis of left atria

The donor heart is then placed (or held by an assistant) over the left side of the divided sternum, parallel to the remnants of the excised recipient heart. The donor heart is rotated 90–180° to the left so that its posterior surface faces anteromedially (towards the surgeon if he is standing to the right side of the table); the free walls of both recipient and donor left atria will then lie adjacent to each other (Figure 10.4). Using a double-ended 4/0 polypropylene suture, the left atrial walls are anastomosed by a continuous suture, beginning at the base of the donor left atrial appendage and at a point close to the caudal end of the recipient left superior pulmonary vein (Figure 10.4). At a convenient stage, the donor heart is drawn down into the pericardium

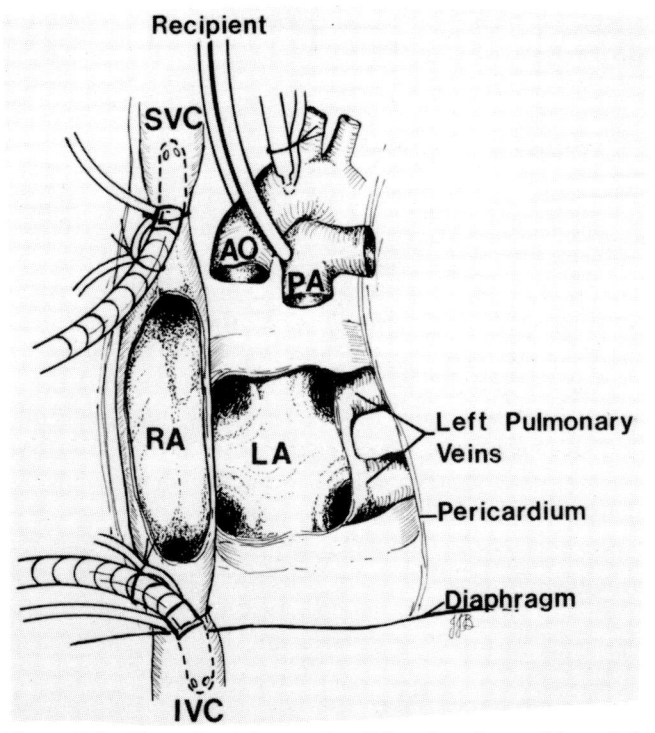

Figure 10.3 View of recipient pericardial cavity after excision of the recipient heart

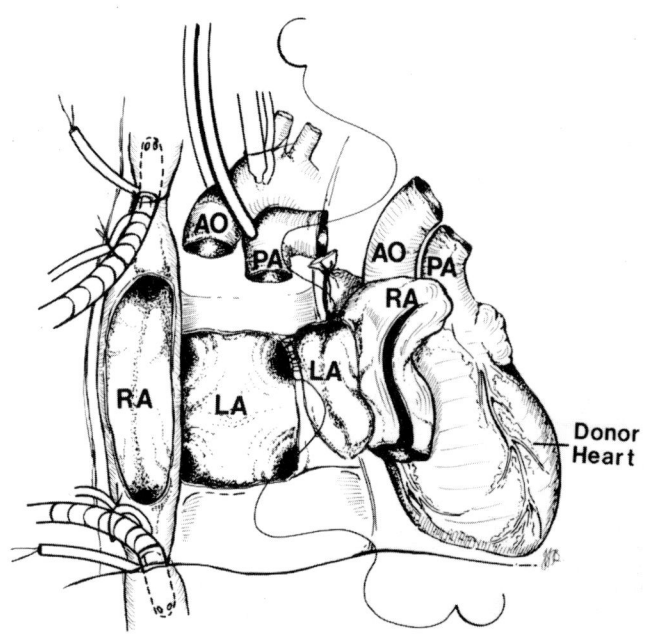

Figure 10.4 Donor and recipient hearts, showing the beginning of the anastomosis between the two left atria

and the suture tightened. The suture is continued around the superior and inferior borders of the left atrium on to the atrial septum, and tied in the middle of the septum (Figure 10.5).

It is essential to maintain myocardial temperature as low as possible, preferably below 15°C, throughout the ischemic period, though tissue damage from freezing must be avoided. Between the performance of each suture line, therefore, the pericardium should be temporarily irrigated with cold saline to maintain a low myocardial temperature, or, ideally, a system of continuous myocardial cooling should be utilized. (Signs of ventricular myocardial activity rarely occur, but if such activity is seen or detected on the electrocardiogram, then further cardioplegic agent should be administered.)

Anastomosis of right atria

The two right atria are anastomosed using a double-ended suture of 5/0 polypropylene (or of 4/0 polypropylene if the right atrial walls are particularly thick). The suture is initially placed at the mid-point of the donor septum and at a convenient point in the posterior lip of the incision in the recipient right atrium (usually slightly caudal to the mid-point). The anastomosis is continued first inferiorly, as this is the more difficult area, in view of the small cuff of recipient right atrium which remains in the region of the IVC. Subsequently, the superior anastomosis is completed, and the two ends of the suture (inferior and superior) tied at the mid-point of the right atrial free wall (Figure 10.6). The

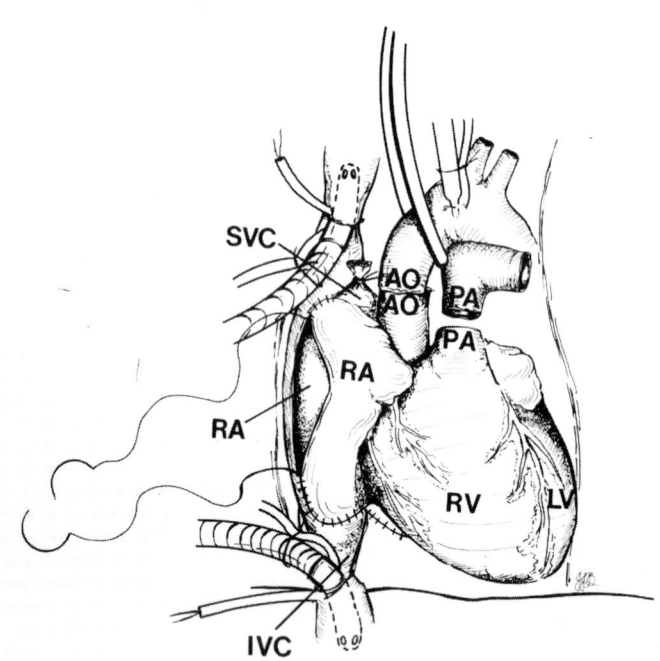

Figure 10.6 The septal anastomosis has been completed; the free walls of the two right atria are being anastomosed

atrial septum has therefore been sutured twice, once on the left atrial side and once on the right.

Anastomosis of pulmonary arteries

The two pulmonary arteries are then trimmed to their ideal lengths and anastomosed using a continuous suture of 4/0 polypropylene (Figure 10.7).

Anastomosis of aortae

The aortae are similarly trimmed and anastomosed by continuous suture using 4/0 polypropylene (Figure 10.7).

Air needles are then placed in the apex of the left ventricle, anterior wall of the right ventricle, ascending aorta and main pulmonary artery. (Additionally, the left atrial appendage can be incised.) The SVC and IVC snares or clamps are released and the heart is gently massaged to expel air from the ventricles and major vessels. The lungs should be gently ventilated to increase the venous return to the left side of the heart, thus expressing further air, though care must be taken to ensure that the heart is not over-distended.

The aortic cross-clamp is then released, allowing the coronary arteries of the donor heart to be perfused once again with oxygenated blood (Figure 10.8). Further efforts are made to expel air from both ventricles and major arteries.

Total body rewarming can now begin. Soon vigorous ventricular fibrillation or spontaneous coordinated myocardial contractions should occur. If ventricular fibrillation is

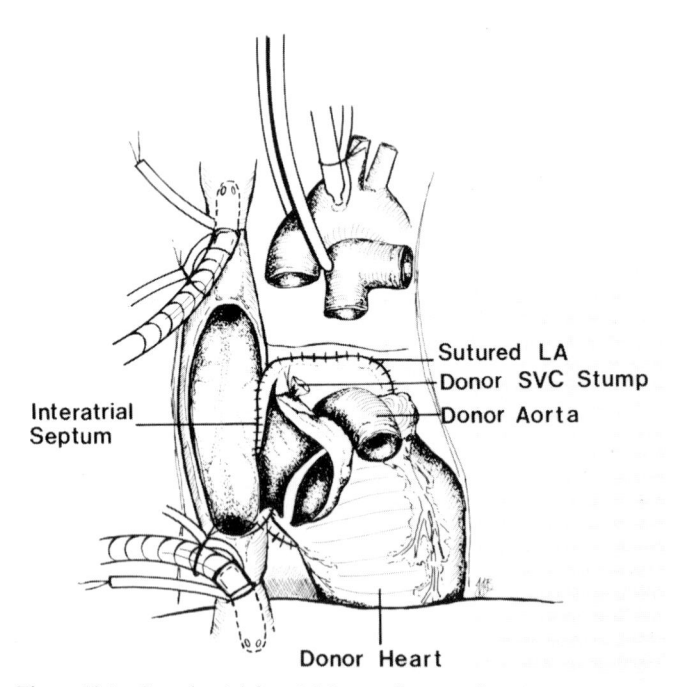

Figure 10.5 Completed left atrial free wall suture line; the anastomosis between the two septa is being performed

ORTHOTOPIC HEART TRANSPLANTATION

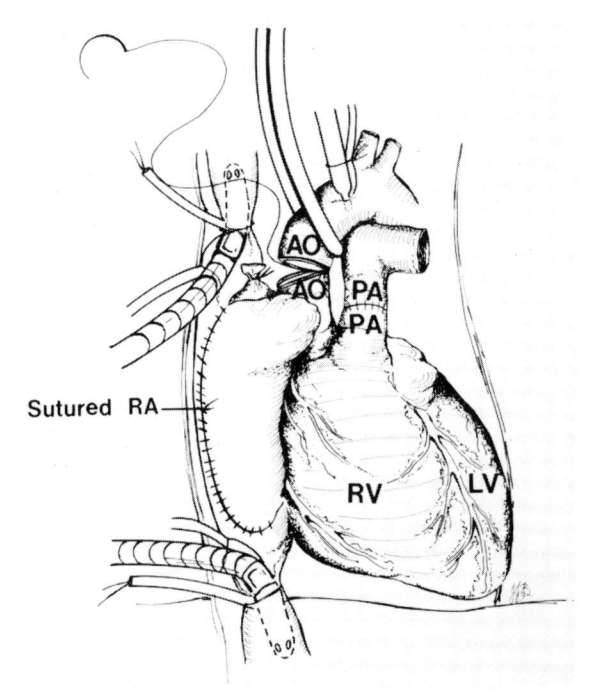

Figure 10.7 The right atrial and pulmonary artery suture lines have been completed; beginning of aortic anastomosis

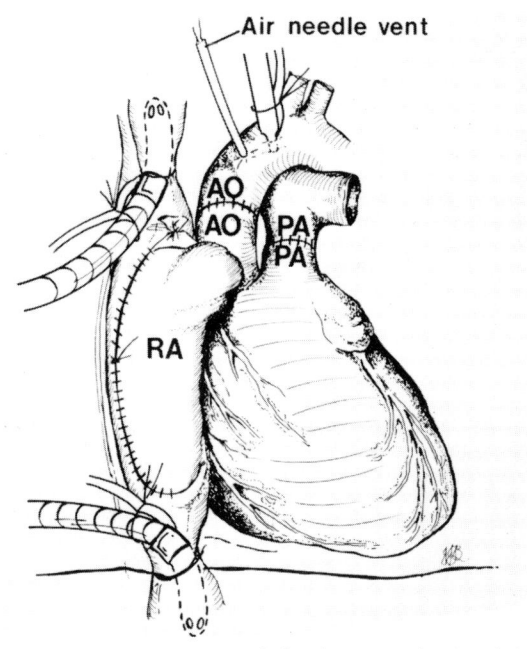

Figure 10.8 The aortic anastomosis has been completed and the aortic cross-clamp removed. An aortic air needle vent has been inserted. Similar needle vents should be placed in both ventricles and main pulmonary artery

present, electrical defibrillation should be attempted. Further vigorous efforts to expel air from the cavities of the heart should then be repeated.

Until coordinated contractions occur, and are sufficient to eject blood and thus decompress the ventricles, the heart should be gently manually decompressed at intervals if distention occurs. Ventricular pacing wires are routinely applied, in case temporary heart block or bradycardia ensues; in such cases, the ventricles are paced to stimulate ejection of blood and ventricular decompression.

It has been our policy to provide at least 30–60 min of pump-oxygenator support after release of the aortic clamp to allow full recovery of the donor heart from its ischemic episode, before challenging it with responsibility for support of the circulation. During this period a careful check for bleeding is made on all suture lines, and further sutures inserted if necessary.

Discontinuation of pump-oxygenator support

When myocardial function is clearly satisfactory, and adequate rewarming has taken place, the ventricular and pulmonary artery air needles are removed, and their insertion sites oversewn with 4/0 polypropylene. The SVC cannula is withdrawn into the right atrium, and the IVC cannula removed. Cardiopulmonary bypass is discontinued, and the aortic air vent removed, and its site oversewn. If cardiac performance is satisfactory, then the aortic and SVC cannulae are removed and protamine sulfate administered (Figure 10.9).

Two drains are inserted, one into the pericardial cavity posterior to the heart and the other into the anterior mediastinum; the pericardium may be left entirely open, though it has been our policy to close it partially. Complete closure, even when the pericardial cavity is very large, should probably be avoided as a safeguard to help ensure that early or late tamponade does not occur. The sternum is reunited with at least six stainless steel wire or other

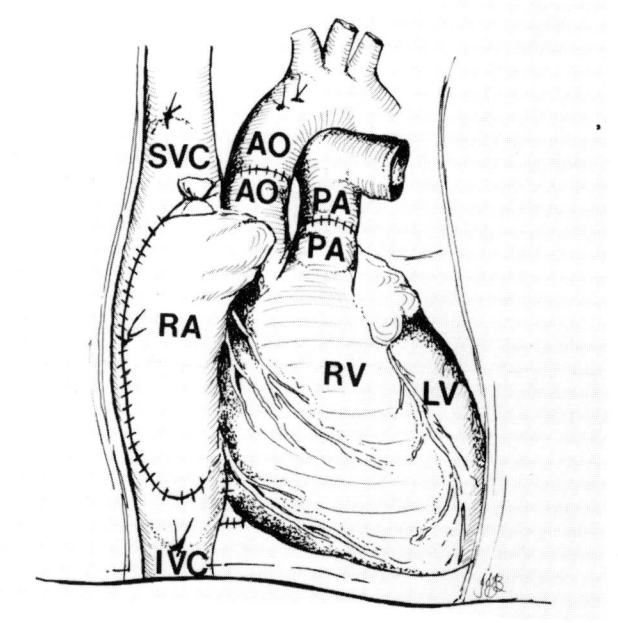

Figure 10.9 Completed operation. Arterial and venous cannulae have been removed

strong sutures, and the tissues anterior to the sternum repaired.

COMMENT

The two potential major complications of this operation are bleeding, in view of the extensive areas of anastomosis, and systemic air emboli. Great care must be taken to dispel all air from the left atrial and ventricular cavities before the donor heart resumes coordinated contractions after reperfusion.

Every effort must be made to maintain donor myocardial temperature as low as possible (yet avoid freezing injury) during transfer of the heart from donor to recipient, and this should be continued until blood reperfusion is commenced. The limitations of simple hypothermia and other storage methods in maintaining myocardial viability are discussed elsewhere (Chapter 7).

Inadequate donor heart function, or even non-function, is still reported[6] (Chapter 31), and may be due to the effects of the agonal period or brain death on the myocardium, or from inadequate preservation during transportation. If inotropic support fails to retrieve the situation, then the only options open are to continue pump-oxygenator support or provide some other form of mechanical assistance until a second donor heart becomes available. We have found the intravenous administration of triiodothyronine (T3) to the recipient to be helpful in several such cases where donor heart function was less than adequate[7]; the background to such therapy is discussed in Chapter 6.

References

1. Cooper, D.K.C. (1968). Experimental development of cardiac transplantation. *Br. Med. J.*, **4**, 174
2. Lower, R.R. and Shumway, N.E. (1960). Studies on orthotopic transplantation of the canine heart. *Surg. Forum*, **11**, 18
3. Hardy, J.D., Chavez, C.M., Kurrus, F.E., Webb, W.R., Neely, W.A., Eraslan, S., Turner, M.D., Fabian, L.W. and Labecki, J.D. (1964). Heart transplantation in man; developmental studies and report of a case. *J. Am. Med. Assoc.*, **188**, 113
4. Barnard, C.N. (1967). A human cardiac transplant; an interim report of a successful operation performed at Groote Schuur Hospital, Cape Town. *S. Afr. Med. J.*, **41**, 1271
5. Barnard, C.N. (1968). What we have learnt about heart transplants. *J. Thorac. Cardiovasc. Surg.*, **56**, 457
6. Fragomeni, L.S. and Kaye, M.P. (1988). The Registry of the International Society for Heart Transplantation: fifth official report, 1988. *J. Heart Transplant.*, **7**, 249
7. Novitzky, D., Human, P.A. and Cooper, D.K.C. (1988). Inotropic effect of triiodothyronine (T3) following myocardial ischemia and cardiopulmonary bypass: an experimental study in pigs. *Ann. Thorac. Surg.*, **45**, 50

11
Surgical Technique of Heterotopic Heart Transplantation

D. NOVITZKY AND D.K.C. COOPER

INTRODUCTION

Heterotopic heart transplantation has a long history in the experimental laboratory[1] (Chapter 1), but was not attempted clinically until 1974[2]. Based on extensive experimental work by Losman and Barnard[3], a form of heterotopic transplantation was carried out whereby the donor heart acted solely as a left ventricular assist device[2]. This operation involved anastomoses between the donor and recipient left atria and aortae; donor coronary sinus venous return was drained via the donor right atrium and right ventricle into the recipient circulation by anastomosing the donor pulmonary artery to the recipient right atrium. Two such operations were performed. Both patients suffered recurrent attacks of recipient heart dysrhythmias, including ventricular fibrillation, during which time the donor heart supported the circulation alone, though with significant loss of blood pressure. As a result of this experience, the technique was modified to allow bypass and support of both recipient ventricles[2,4].

Today, heterotopic heart transplantation has specific indications, and both advantages and disadvantages over orthotopic transplantation (Chapter 23).

DONOR HEART EXCISION

Donor heart excision is very similar to that described previously for orthotopic transplantation (Chapter 10), but a greater length of superior vena cava (SVC) should be retained. The SVC is, therefore, mobilized along the whole of its length and two ligatures passed around it cranial to the azygos vein, which itself is doubly ligated and divided. Otherwise, excision is as described for orthotopic transplantation.

PREPARATION OF DONOR HEART

The heart is placed in a bowl containing saline or cardioplegic solution at 4°C, where it is prepared for implantation into the recipient (Figure 11.1).

The orifices of both right pulmonary veins and of the inferior vena cava (IVC) are closed with a continuous, double-layered suture of 5/0 polypropylene, care being taken to ensure that coronary sinus drainage is not obstructed during closure of the IVC.

The bridge of tissue between the left superior and inferior pulmonary veins is excised to make a single opening into the left atrium; this opening may need to be extended to achieve a diameter of approximately 3.5–4.0 cm or the equivalent of a normal mitral valve orifice. The midpoint of the posterior wall of this may be marked with a suture to act as a reference during subsequent implantation into the recipient.

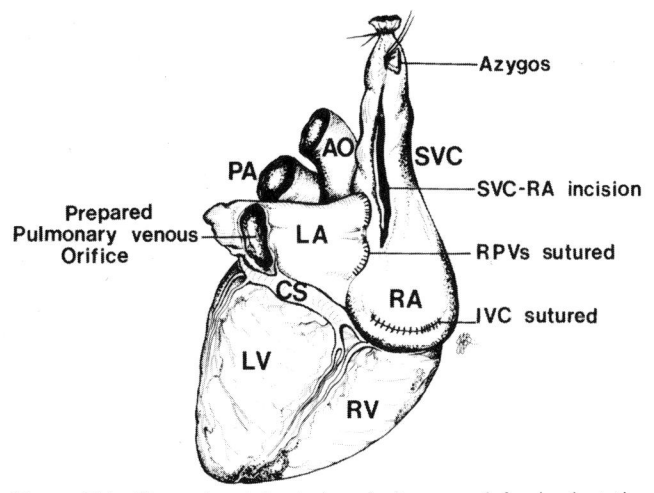

Figure 11.1 Donor heart (posterior view) prepared for implantation. (Abbreviations used in figures in this chapter are: LA = left atrium; RA = right atrium; SVC = superior vena cava; IVC = inferior vena cava; PV = pulmonary vein; RV = right ventricle; PA = pulmonary artery; AO = aorta; LV = left ventricle; CS = coronary sinus)

THE TRANSPLANTATION AND REPLACEMENT OF THORACIC ORGANS

A longitudinal incision is made in the posterior aspect of the SVC, beginning immediately caudal to the ligated azygos vein, and extended down just to the right of the interatrial septum into the right atrium. At least half the length of this 5 cm incision must involve the right atrial wall. It is essential to ensure that the incision is posteriorly sited in order to avoid injury to the sinoatrial node.

Approximately 10 min are required to prepare the heart in this way. The organ is then transferred to the recipient surgical team.

THE RECIPIENT OPERATION

With the patient supine, a midline sternotomy is performed and the pericardium opened longitudinally. A right-sided pleuropericardial flap is created (Figure 11.2), first by dividing the mediastinal pleura immediately posterior to the sternum and then by extending this incision posteriorly at the level of the diaphragm to a point 2 cm from the right phrenic nerve; a similar reflection of the pleuropericardium is made superiorly, extending the incision toward the SVC at the level of the azygos vein, again taking care to avoid the phrenic nerve. In this way a rectangular flap is created that comprises the parietal pericardium and mediastinal pleura. Hemostasis of the edges of this flap must be carried out carefully as no further opportunity to do this will arise. The flap is allowed to fall back over the hilum of the right lung (Figure 11.3) (or can be resected), creating a single large right pleuropericardial cavity.

Initiation of cardiopulmonary bypass

The patient is fully heparinized. An aortic cannula is inserted at least at the level of the origin of the brachiocephalic artery, and preferably higher, between the brachiocephalic and left common carotid arteries. Venous cannulae are placed in the SVC (either directly or through the right atrial appendage) and IVC (low in the lateral wall of the right atrium) (Figure 11.4). Cardiopulmonary bypass is initiated and the patient cooled.

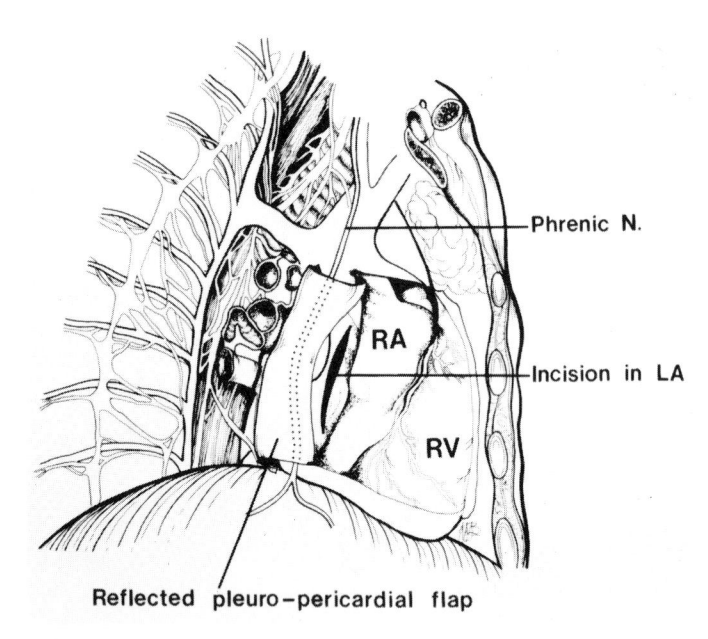

Figure 11.3 Recipient; reflection of pleuropericardial flap to lie anterior to the hilum of the right lung

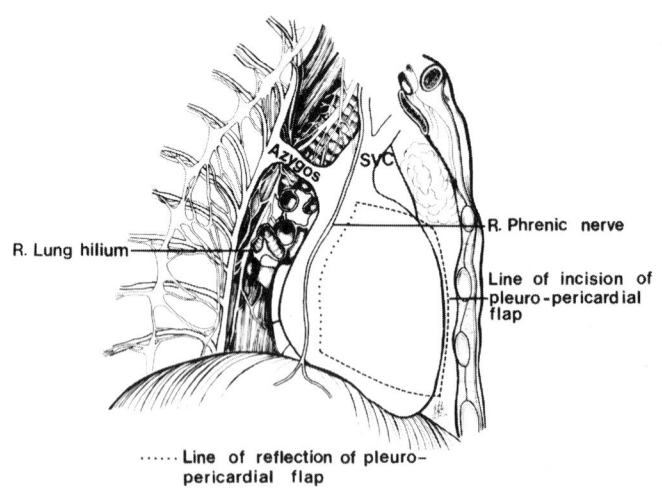

Figure 11.2 Recipient; right-sided view of mediastinum; the line of the pleuropericardial incision is indicated

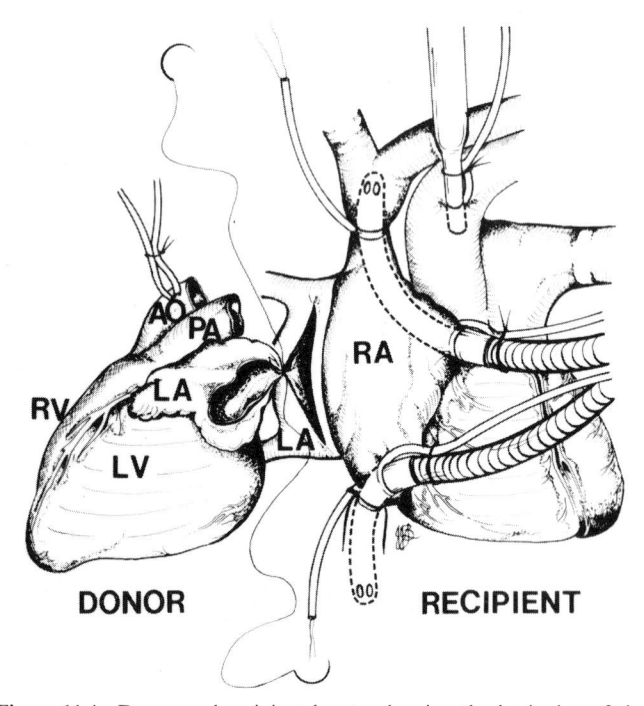

Figure 11.4 Donor and recipient hearts, showing the beginning of the posterior suture line of the left atrial anastomosis

For most open heart procedures, our cardiopulmonary bypass system includes two cardiotomy suction catheters which return blood to the pump-oxygenator; for heterotopic heart transplantation we have available three such suction catheters.

Myocardial protection of recipient and donor hearts

The recipient heart can be continuously perfused by the pump-oxygenator, and therefore allowed to beat throughout the period of insertion of the donor heart. If the recipient heart is to remain beating, however, the temperature of the circulating blood must not be lowered much below 32°C, or ventricular fibrillation is likely to occur, which may result in less satisfactory myocardial protection.

Alternatively, the recipient aorta can be cross-clamped and the recipient heart protected by the infusion of cardioplegic agent and by the topical application of cold saline throughout the operation. Cross-clamping of the recipient aorta facilitates the technical steps of the operation by preventing recipient coronary sinus blood return to the operating field, and also allows the blood temperature to be reduced to lower levels, thus facilitating the maintenance of a low donor myocardial temperature. Systemic hypothermia of 26–28°C is maintained, largely to diminish rewarming of the donor heart by its proximity to the recipient organs during its ischemic period. Our own preference at present is for cardioplegic arrest and hypothermic protection of the recipient heart, as this allows rather better myocardial protection of the donor heart, which we feel has a high priority.

The operation will therefore be described with the recipient heart arrested throughout (although for simplicity the aortic cross-clamp is not indicated in the accompanying figures).

A catheter for cardioplegic solution infusion is placed high in the root of the recipient aorta, which is then cross-clamped immediately proximal to the pump-oxygenator cannula at the level of the brachiocephalic artery. Cardioplegic solution is rapidly infused into the root of the aorta, and cold saline poured over the heart to irrigate the entire pleuropericardial cavity. Irrigation with cold saline of both the pericardial cavity (to cool the recipient heart) and right pleural cavity (to cool the donor heart) must be carried out. Clamps or snuggers (snares) are placed around the SVC and IVC.

Until the donor heart is revascularized, between each anastomosis cold saline (4°C) is poured over both hearts to help maintain an adequate state of myocardial hypothermia. If there is evidence of ventricular activity in either heart, either mechanical or electrocardiographic, then further increments of cold cardioplegic solution should be infused into one or both recipient and donor ascending aortae as necessary. The cannula inserted into the donor aorta for the initial infusion of cardioplegic agent before excision can be used again for this purpose; once cardioplegic infusion has begun and all air displaced from the aorta, a cross-clamp is applied to occlude the distal end of this vessel, thus ensuring that the donor coronary arteries are adequately perfused.

Anastomosis of left atria

An incision, as for mitral valve surgery, is made into the recipient left atrium immediately posterior to the interatrial groove, extending from the superior to the inferior extremes of the groove (Figure 11.4).

The donor heart is then placed in the right thoracic cavity anterior to the collapsed right lung and lying alongside the recipient heart. It is frequently necessary to lie the heart on a sponge or swab, soaked in cold (4°C) saline, to support the donor organ and thus facilitate performance of the left atrial anastomosis. Using double-ended 4/0 polypropylene, the midpoint of the posterior lip of the incision in the recipient left atrium is sutured to the midpoint of the posterior lip of the opening in the donor left atrium. The two atria are anastomosed by a continuous suture, first along the posterior aspect and then along the anterior aspect. The completed anastomosis will be totally inaccessible at the end of the operation and therefore it it essential that it be hemostatic.

A wide communication between the two left atria has been created, forming a common atrium from which blood can enter either donor or recipient left ventricles.

Anastomosis of right atria

A 5 cm longitudinal incision is made into the lateral aspect of the recipient SVC and right atrium just anterior to the interatrial groove, beginning 2–3 cm above the vena caval–right atrial junction and continued 2–3 cm into the right atrium (Figure 11.5). It is essential that the SVC–right atrial incision should be at least 5 cm in length, and that it be made posteriorly to avoid the region of the sinoatrial node.

The donor SVC is extended alongside its counterpart. An eyelid retractor is used to retract the anterior lip of the incision in the recipient right atrium. The midpoint of the posterior lip of the incision in the recipient atrium is sutured to the *most caudal point of the incision in the donor atrium*, using a double-ended 4/0 polypropylene suture (Figure 11.6). The two right atria are then anastomosed by a continuous suture carred in each direction (superiorly and inferiorly), first to complete the posterior wall anastomosis (Figure 11.7), and then to complete the anterior wall

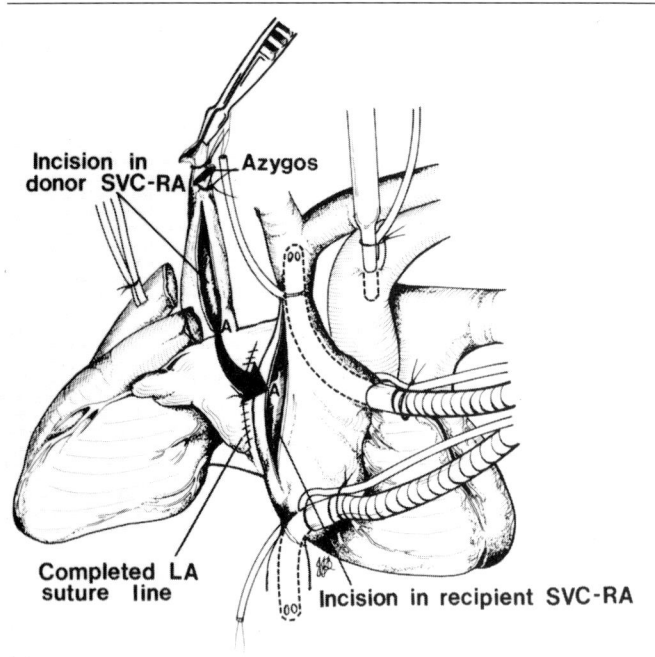

Figure 11.5 Completed anterior left atrial suture line. The SVC–RA incision in each heart is shown; note that the inferior point of the incision in the donor SVC–RA (A) will be sutured to the midpoint of the posterior lip of the incision in the recipient SVC–RA (A)

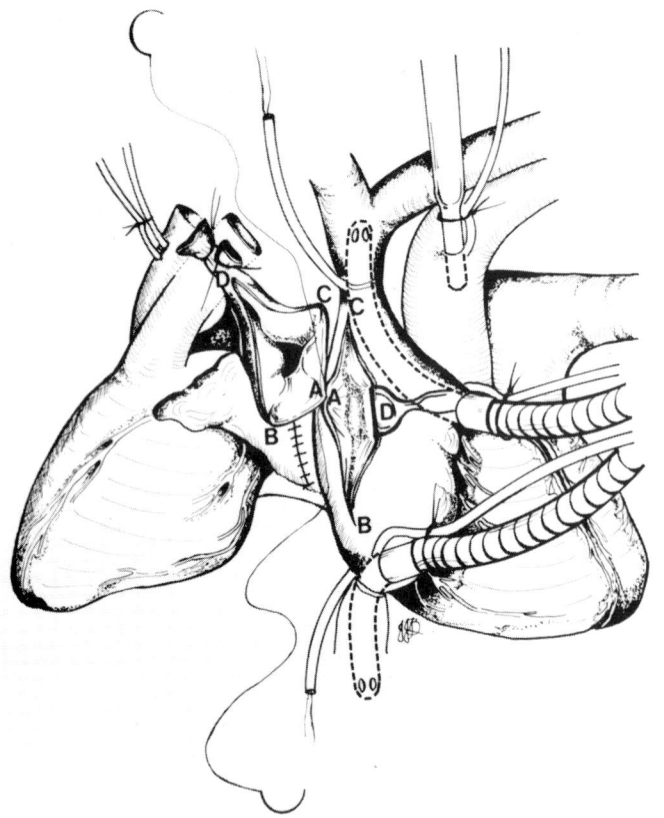

Figure 11.6 The first suture in the anastomosis between the donor and recipient SVC–RA has been inserted (A:A)

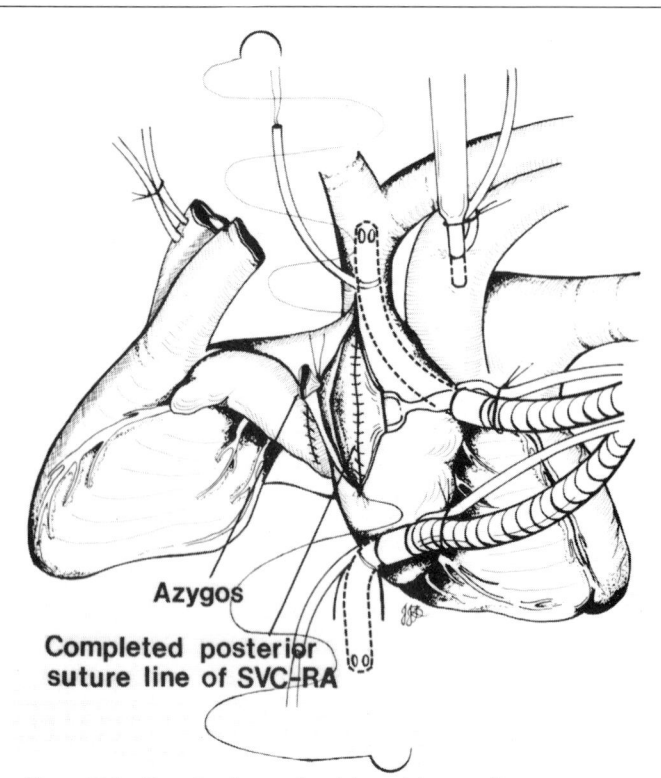

Figure 11.7 Completed posterior right atrial suture line

anastomosis. At the completion of this anastomosis, the ligated donor azygos vein remnant will lie anterior to the midpoint of the anterior suture line (Figure 11.7), over which a small metal ring is tied down as a fluoroscopic reference for the passage of endomyocardial biopsy forceps into the donor heart during the postoperative period.

The maneuver of suturing the midpoint of the posterior lip of the recipient atrial wall to the most inferior aspect of the incision in the donor atrium, thus creating a diamond-shaped opening, ensures that this anastomosis will remain wide, allowing free flow of blood from one chamber to the other, and permitting the easy passage of endomyocardial biopsy forceps.

Anastomosis of aortae

The donor aorta is trimmed to the minimum length required to allow anastomosis to the recipient aorta and yet avoid distortion or kinking of the left or right atrial anastomoses. An unnecessarily long donor aorta will allow the donor heart to drop back into the right pleural cavity, compressing the right lung. A short donor aorta will lift the donor heart anteriorly and superiorly, and allow for maximal expansion of the right lung posterior to the transplant organ. Temporary inflation of the lungs at this stage will help in estimating optimal length.

A longitudinal incision, equal in length to the diameter of the donor aorta, is made into the *right lateral wall* of the

HETEROTOPIC HEART TRANSPLANTATION

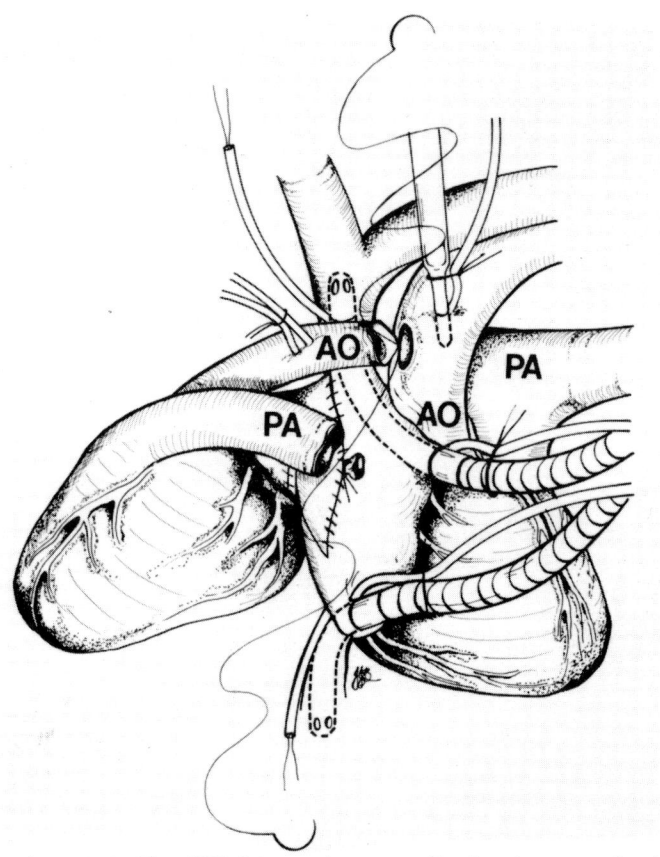

Figure 11.8 The SVC–RA anterior suture line has been completed; beginning of aortic anastomosis. (When the recipient heart is continuously perfused throughout the operation, a side-biting clamp is applied to the aorta for the performance of this anastomosis)

recipient ascending aorta. Correct siting of this incision is essential to ensure that the donor aorta lies satisfactorily without kinking, and is not compressed when the sternum is reunited. End-to-side anastomosis of donor to recipient aorta is made using a continuous suture of 4/0 polypropylene (Figure 11.8).

Anastomosis of pulmonary arteries

In our experience, the donor pulmonary artery (PA) will not adequately reach to the recipient PA without undue tension or distortion of the other anastomoses; a conduit of pre-clotted woven Dacron is therefore inserted. The diameter of the conduit chosen will depend largely on the diameter of the donor PA; this is usually of the order of 20–22 mm. (With a similarly sized polytetrafluorethylene ('Gore-tex') graft, difficulty has been found in positioning it to configurate with the surrounding anatomy without kinking.)

A longitudinal incision of suitable length is made in the recipient main PA. This incision should be slightly shorter than the diameter of the Dacron conduit, as stretching will inevitably occur during anastomosis. The Dacron graft is anastomosed end-to-side to the recipient PA using continuous 4/0 polypropylene, the first stitch being placed at the distal end of the incision (Figure 11.9). The graft is tailored to the correct length to bridge the gap between the two pulmonary arteries. The end-to-end anastomosis to the donor PA is again performed using continuous 4/0 polypropylene (Figure 11.10). To ensure a bloodless field during this procedure, it is sometimes necessary to insert a flexible cardiotomy sucker along the lumen of the Dacron graft into the recipient PA; any recipient and donor PA suckers are removed before completion of the final anastomosis. The Dacron conduit will be the most anteriorly placed structure in the pericardial cavity, crossing the recipient ascending aorta, and will lie immediately behind the sternum.

All anastomoses have now been completed. The cardioplegic catheters in both aortae are converted to use as air vents, and air needles placed in both donor and recipient left and right ventricles and pulmonary arteries; the caval cannulae are unsnugged and each heart is gently massaged to expel air. The cross-clamp is removed from the recipient aorta and from this point both donor and recipient myocardiums are continuously perfused with blood from the pump-oxygenator. Further efforts are made to remove air from the cavities of both hearts. The patient is rewarmed to 37°C.

As rewarming occurs, each heart will either begin spontaneous sinus rhythm or lapse into vigorous ventricular fibrillation, requiring electrical defibrillation. Both hearts

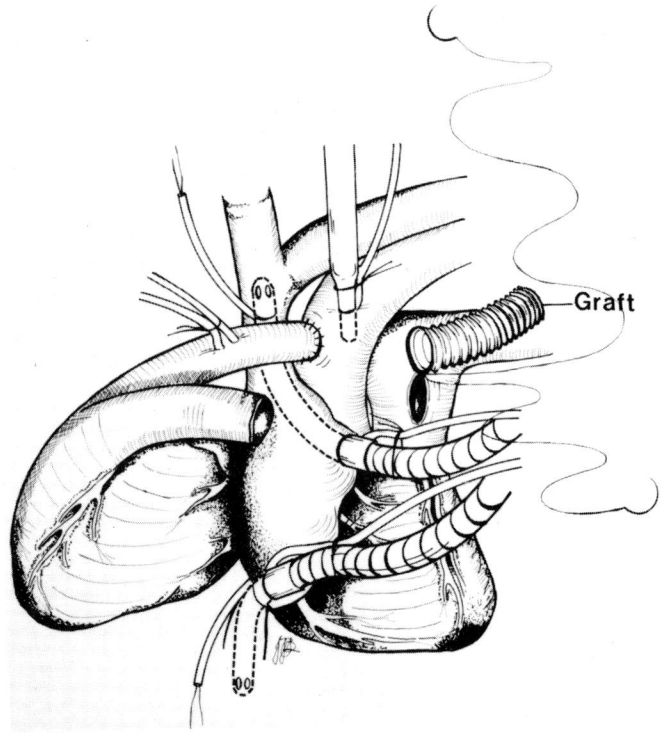

Figure 11.9 The aortic anastomosis has been completed; recipient pulmonary artery (PA) incision and beginning of anastomosis of Dacron graft

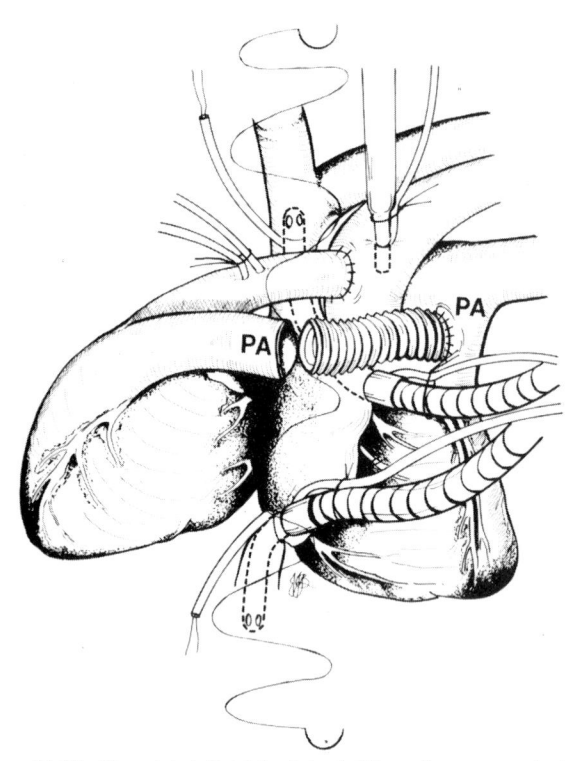

Figure 11.10 Completed distal (recipient) PA–graft anastomosis; beginning of proximal (donor) PA–graft anastomosis. A suction catheter is usually inserted through the pulmonary valve into the donor right ventricle to insure a relatively bloodless field while this anastomosis is being performed; the catheter is removed before completion of the anastomosis

must be gently manually compressed if they show any sign of over-distention. Further attempts to expel air from both hearts are made, and then all air needles are removed and their sites of insertion oversewn.

Discontinuation of pump-oxygenator support

As with orthotopic transplantation, it has been our policy to allow at least 30–60 min for donor heart recovery, especially if the ischemic time has been long. During this period a careful inspection is made of the accessible suture lines to confirm hemostasis; the PA and aortic anastomoses can usually be inspected satisfactorily, though the posterior aortic suture line may be difficult to see. The anterior right atrial suture line can usually be inspected without difficulty, but it is impossible to see the deeper suture lines (posterior right atrial and both left atrial). The venous cannula in the SVC is withdrawn into the right atrium, the IVC cannula removed, and, if the hemodynamic status of the patient is stable, cardiopulmonary bypass is discontinued and the patient decannulated (Figure 11.11). (Frequently, at this stage, it is the recipient's own heart that provides the major support of the circulation; the donor heart may take several hours for full recovery.) The heparin is neutralized with protamine sulfate. At least three drains are inserted, one into the pericardial cavity inferoposterior to the recipient heart, a second anterior to this heart, and a third (and possibly a fourth) inserted preferably directly though the right chest wall, to ensure adequate drainage of the right pleural cavity basally (and apically).

Before closure of the chest, the anesthesiologist is required to ventilate both lungs fully to ensure expansion of the right lung, particularly of the lower lobe, which has been compressed by the donor heart throughout the procedure. The sternum is united with at least six wire or other strong sutures.

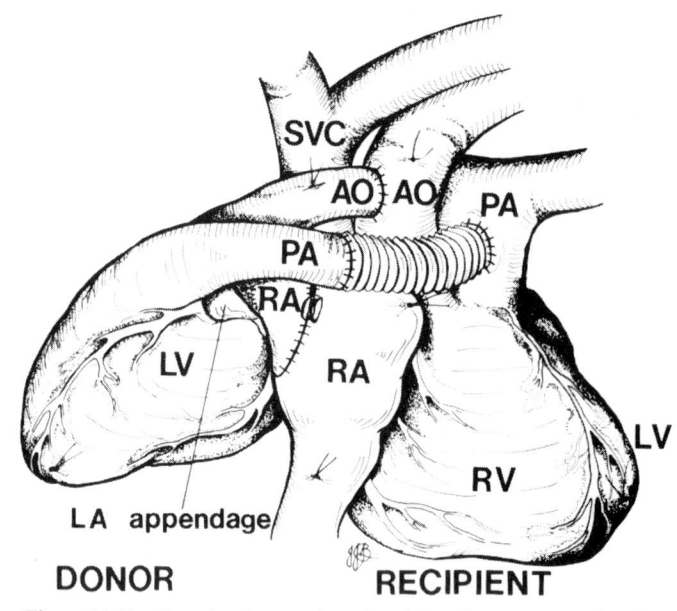

Figure 11.11 Completed operation. Arterial and venous cannulae have been removed

COMMENT

This operation has been combined on occasion with other procedures to the recipient heart, such as resection of a left ventricular aneurysm, coronary artery bypass graft, or mitral annuloplasty. Free or friable thrombus within the recipient left ventricle can be sucked out through the left atrial incision before anastomosis of the donor heart. Although this technique involves the inclusion of a vascular prosthesis into a patient who will subsequently be heavily immunosuppressed, we have seen no infectious complications related to the presence of this graft.

Neither the left nor the right atrial anastomosis must be restrictive. If the right atrial anastomosis is confined to the superior venae cavae, then inadequate flow into the donor right atrium may result. Any subsequent contraction at the suture line may lead to difficulty in manipulating biopsy forceps into the donor right ventricle; in such cases, left ventricular biopsies must be obtained by the arterial route.

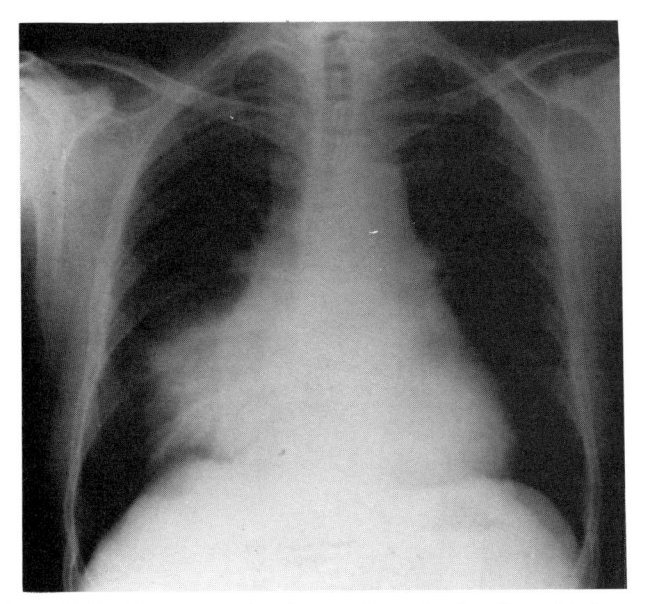

Figure 11.12 Postero-anterior chest radiograph of patient with heterotopic transplant; the donor heart lies in the right chest

The incision in each heart must, therefore, be extended well down the atrial wall.

Heterotopic heart transplantation by the technique described above connects the donor heart in parallel with the recipient heart. Preferential flow to donor or recipient ventricle will be directly related to the respective ventricular compliance and contractility (Chapter 13). Ejection of blood is asynchronous, depending on the different heart rates, but does not substantially interfere with the performance of either heart[5]. Pacing of the two hearts to coordinate ejection, either synchronously or asynchronously, has not been found to be beneficial, and is not advocated. Pacing of either heart may, of course, be necessary if there is a definite indication, such as atrioventricular dissociation or bradycardia.

Though the right middle lobe is often displaced superiorly by the donor heart, some collapse of the right lower lobe is nearly always present at the end of the operation, but with adequate physiotherapy this lobe expands over the course of the next few days; this has not increased the incidence of postoperative pulmonary infection in this lobe. The presence of the heterotopic allograft in the right chest (Figures 11.12 and 11.13) leads to a slight reduction in right lung volume, but in no case has this been associated with symptoms of impaired ventilatory capacity. We have transplanted large adult hearts into two 14-year-old boys without problems in this respect.

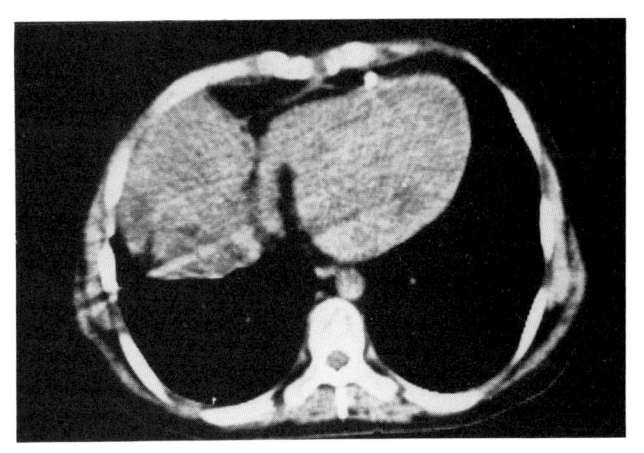

Figure 11.13 Computerized axial tomographic scan of the chest (viewed from below) showing the donor heart in the right chest anteriorly

References

1. Cooper, D.K.C. (1968). Experimental development of cardiac transplantation. *Br. Med. J.*, **4**, 174
2. Barnard, C.N. and Losman, J.G. (1975). Left ventricular bypass. *S. Afr. Med. J.*, **49**, 303
3. Losman, J.G. and Barnard, C.N. (1977). Hemodynamic evaluation of left ventricular bypass with a homologous cardiac graft. *J. Thorac. Cardiovasc. Surg.*, **71**, 695
4. Novitzky, D., Cooper, D.K.C. and Barnard, C.N. (1983). The surgical technique of heterotopic heart transplantation. *Ann. Thorac. Surg.*, **36**, 476
5. Beck, W. and Gersh, B.J. (1976). Left ventricular bypass using a heterotopic cardiac allograft; hemodynamic studies. *Am. J. Cardiol.*, **37**, 1007

12
Immediate Postoperative Care and Maintenance Immunosuppressive Therapy

D.K.C. COOPER

IMMEDIATE POSTOPERATIVE CARE

The immediate postoperative care of a patient who has undergone heart transplantation, whether it be orthotopic or heterotopic, is similar to that of any patient who has undergone open heart surgery. Precautions need to be taken, however, to minimize the risk of infection. Maintenance immunosuppressive therapy is begun immediately before the operation and is continued afterwards.

Patient monitoring

The patient will return from the operating room intubated and ventilated with a volume-cycled ventilator capable of providing intermittent mandatory ventilation and positive end-expiratory pressure. *In situ* arterial and central venous (CVP) cannulae allow monitoring of pressures, and other intravenous lines allow replacement of blood and fluid as well as administration of vasoactive drugs if necessary. A urinary catheter, central temperature probe (blood, bladder or rectal), and electrocardiogram (ECG) electrodes are also in position. If heterotopic heart transplantation has been performed, the ECG electrodes are positioned to allow clear monitoring of complexes from both hearts. *In situ* drainage catheters will drain both the pericardial cavity and anterior mediastinum in the case of an orthotopic transplant, as well as the right pleural cavity in the case of a heterotopic transplant.

A Swan-Ganz catheter to monitor cardiac output and pulmonary capillary 'wedge' pressure (or an oxymetric catheter to give additional continuous information on the SVO_2) is an advantage, but not essential. Following orthotopic transplantation, if donor heart function is clearly satisfactory, we do not feel that measurements of left heart pressures or cardiac output are necessary. Such observations may be essential, however, if donor heart function is poor, requiring intravenous inotropic drug therapy, or if there is significant pulmonary vascular disease. The complex anatomy of heterotopic heart transplants renders measurement of cardiac output difficult, but information gained on pulmonary artery and 'wedge' pressures may prove valuable.

The nursing staff will monitor arterial and central venous pressures, central temperature, respiratory and ventilator parameters, the heart rate(s), and peripheral pulse rate. They will also keep careful records of blood loss from the drains, urinary output, and blood, plasma, and fluid input.

Most centers involved in heart transplantation consider it an advantage to extubate the patient as soon as possible to minimize the risk of lung infection. It is argued that the presence of an indwelling endotracheal tube, which prevents the normal cough reflex, and the intermittent introduction of tracheal suction catheters are factors that predispose to infection. Extubation should be carried out as soon as the patient is awake enough to cooperate with the nursing and physiotherapy personnel and can cough when requested, as long as his or her hemodynamic state is satisfactory. We have not seen any early postoperative chest infections, however, in patients in whom, for one reason or another, there has been a delay in extubation until 24 or even 48 hours have elapsed. There would appear to be an increased risk of pulmonary infection should the patient require ventilation beyond this time.

Chest drains are removed when there is no risk of further bleeding and, in heterotopic heart transplant patients, in the absence of a right pneumothorax or significant pleural effusion. Removal can generally be carried out within 48 hours, but we have experienced no complications from leaving the drains in longer, if indicated.

Initially, chest radiographs are taken at frequent intervals until the chest drains have been removed and the patient is being mobilized, and then at daily intervals to augment the clinical examination of the chest. The radiographs are taken primarily to confirm bilateral lung re-expansion and absence of pleural effusion, particularly after heterotopic transplantation, and also to exclude the presence of areas of consolidation that might suggest infection. Frequent chest radiographs are obtained throughout the hospital stay of the patient to exclude early changes suggestive of infection.

Precautions to prevent infection

Meticulous attention to sterility is required by the nursing staff for all procedures affecting the patient. All personnel attending the patient should wash their hands on entering the room, and it is probably advisable for them to wear face masks.

Several specimens are taken each day for laboratory study to monitor possible early infection. Tracheal aspirate or sputum, blood, urine, and swabs from the throat and from around the various drains and cannulae are sent daily for the first few days for culture to exclude significant bacterial growth. Urine and throat swabs (or gargle culture media) are sent for virological studies. Blood cytomegalovirus titers are estimated weekly.

All arterial and intravenous cannulae are removed as soon as possible to reduce the risk of introducing infection into the blood either through or alongside the cannulae. A CVP line can be kept *in situ* for several weeks, if required, in patients who require such a line for any purpose, such as the daily intravenous administration of antithymocyte globulin, but meticulous care of the skin entry site must be maintained. The surrounding skin should be cleaned with iodine or other effective antiseptic, and a new sterile dressing applied at least daily and preferably 8-hourly.

The patient should preferably be nursed in a clean-air environment. The number of hospital personnel entering the room should be kept to a minimum, and at this stage only close relatives should be permitted to visit the patient. We no longer believe that it is essential for personnel to change into operating room garments or cover their outer clothing with a clean surgical gown, but frequent hand washing is essential, and the use of masks probably helpful.

Respiratory and physical therapy

To ensure early re-expansion of the lungs, and to keep the airways clear of secretions, physiotherapy is commenced within 2 hours of operation, and continued every 4 hours for 2 days, and then as often as necessary until the patient is fully mobilized, at which time it may be reduced or discontinued altogether. In the intubated patient this takes the form of vibration of the thoracic cage, postural drainage, and hyperinflation of the lungs by manual Ambu bagging to expand the lungs and loosen secretions, followed by tracheobronchial suction. A mucolytic agent may be injected into the airways of patients with viscid secretions. In the extubated patient, nebulization of the airways by a Bird ventilator, together with positive end-expiratory pressure, followed by assisted expectoration, should be carried out every 4 hours to prevent atelectasis and to keep the airways free from excessive secretions.

Within 6 hours of operation, passive muscular exercises are introduced, particularly to the legs to prevent deep vein thrombosis and to strengthen the musculature. Active exercises are introduced as soon as the patient can cooperate. As soon as possible, usually within 48 hours, the patient should be assisted to sit and stand out of bed at intervals of a few hours, and encouraged to become fully mobile over the next few days.

These patients have frequently been relatively inactive, or even bedridden, for some weeks or months before transplantation due to their underlying myocardial failure. Their muscles may have become weak and wasted. Furthermore, the steroid drugs, which may be given to prevent rejection, particularly if given in large doses, contribute in most patients to a further wasting of the musculature that is so extreme in some to warrant the description of 'steroid myopathy'. A similar myopathy is believed to occur in hypomagnesemic patients receiving cyclosporine. Frequent and regular attention is required from the physiotherapist if this muscle wasting is to be kept to a minimum and eventually reversed. Each patient is prescribed a program of exercises which he is expected to perform every 2 hours throughout the waking hours. This exercise program concentrates on strengthening the arms and legs. Static dynamic bicycle riding is generally begun under the physiotherapist's supervision within the first 3 or 4 days, as long as the patient's general condition does not contraindicate this more vigorous form of exercise. Initially, the bicycle work-load is set low, and the period of time the patient spends on it restricted to 2 minutes, but both factors are steadily increased as the patient's recovery continues. Bicycle riding is carried out four times each day, and the period of exercise increased up to 15 minutes per session.

During a severe acute rejection episode, when the myocardium is edematous and undergoing cellular infiltration and myofiber injury, we believe it is only sensible to restrict the exercise of the patient in an effort to minimize permanent myocardial damage. Vigorous exercise, such as bicycle riding, should be omitted, though gentle exercise and walking may continue.

Prevention of psychological isolation and boredom

It is rare today for a patient to require isolation in an intensive care unit for more than a few days, but should the patient need physical isolation for longer, it is important to prevent boredom by providing such facilities as television and/or video, which the patient may make use of if he feels inclined. The occupational therapist may play an important role at this stage.

DRUG THERAPY OTHER THAN IMMUNOSUPPRESSION

Antibiotic therapy

Prolonged prophylactic antibiotic therapy is to be avoided in the immunosuppressed patient, as there is a greater risk of this leading to the growth of resistant bacteria or fungi. Patients should receive a suitable antibiotic (e.g. a cephalosporin) at the time of induction of anesthesia, with further doses after operation to cover the first 24 hours. Further antibiotics should be given only when signs of clinical infection are present and when the causative organism(s) has been identified, if this proves possible. Further guidelines on infection and antibiotic policy are given in Chapter 17.

Vasoactive drug therapy

If inotropic support is indicated, we prefer dobutamine hydrochloride, though isoproterenol hydrochloride is administered if an increase in donor heart rate is considered desirable. Intravenous vasodilator therapy with, for example, sodium nitroprusside or nitroglycerine may be indicated in the early postoperative period to reduce afterload, as in any patient who has undergone open heart surgery. Cyclosporine therapy may result in hypertension, though it is relatively unusual for this to be a problem within the initial hospital stay of the patient.

The role of prostaglandins (eicosanoids) in the treatment of pathophysiologic states of the cardiovascular system is being increasingly appreciated. Their metabolism, physiology, and pharmacology in relation to the cardiovascular system have been reviewed[1]. If severe right heart failure is present after orthotopic transplantation, and if this failure is secondary to a high PVR, prostaglandin E_1 (PGE_1) has been shown to have a beneficial effect, often dramatic, when given through a central venous catheter[2,3]. PGE_1 can be administered as an infusion of 500 μg in 100 ml of normal saline at a rate sufficient to bring about a reduction in systemic pressure. The patient should also be receiving 100% inspired oxygen. Pulmonary hypertension is relieved in large part by the vasodilating properties of the drug. As up to 95% of injected prostaglandins is extracted by the lungs in a single pass through the pulmonary circulation[4], systemic hypotension requiring high-dose vasopressors can usually be avoided. PGE_1 inhibits the release of thromboxane, a potent vasoconstrictor and potentiator of platelet aggregation[5], and has several other effects which make it of value in this situation[6]. If PGE_1 is to be used, the insertion of a Swan-Ganz catheter is essential.

It has long been known that plasma free triiodothyronine (T3) is reduced in patients on cardiopulmonary bypass[7,8]. As recent laboratory research has confirmed an inotropic effect of T3 following a period of myocardial ischemia on cardiopulmonary bypass[9], it is now our policy to administer T3 to patients receiving heart transplants, though the value of such therapy is still under clinical study. An initial dose of 1.5–2.0 μg/10 kg body weight is given at the time of donor heart reperfusion, and further doses (0.75–1.0 μg/10 kg) are given subsequently at 4- or 8-hourly intervals, depending on hemodynamic response, for 24 hours.

If vasoactive drug therapy fails to support either right or left circulations, then some form of mechanical assistance will be required. This may take the form of an intra-aortic balloon pump in patients with predominant left ventricular failure, or a pneumatically-driven assist device for either left or right ventricular failure (Section IV). If a period of such support is unsuccessful in allowing donor heart recovery, then retransplantation may be the only remaining alternative.

Pain relief

Large doses of morphine and other central nervous system or respiratory depressant drugs should be avoided; intravenous doses of 2.5 mg of morphine given when necessary rarely cause significant respiratory depression. After extubation, adequate pain relief or, preferably, pain avoidance is essential if the patient is to be encouraged to cough adequately to prevent secretion accumulation in his airways.

Dysrhythmias

Rhythm disturbances are relatively uncommon in donor hearts that have not suffered damage from prolonged ischemia during implantation. Following heterotopic heart transplantation, dysrhythmias of the recipient heart may occur, though these can often be ignored, unless they lead to hemodynamic embarrassment of the donor heart, which is rare.

When prescribing therapy, it should be remembered that the response of the denervated donor heart to therapeutic agents that have an effect in correcting dysrhythmias may differ from that of an innervated heart (Chapter 13). Calcium antagonists, such as verapamil hydrochloride, and β-blocking agents have a greater effect on the denervated heart than on an innervated heart, whereas the donor heart is less sensitive to some other drugs, for example, digoxin. After heterotopic transplantation, the effect of such drugs on each heart should be monitored, and the dosage carefully balanced to prevent unwanted effects on either heart.

When ventricular fibrillation of donor or recipient heart

occurs after heterotopic heart transplantation, care must be taken in defibrillating, as this may lead to fibrillation of the other heart. If both hearts fibrillate, positioning the defibrillating paddles over the respective lateral walls of the chest (i.e. just below each axilla) is often successful in defibrillating both organs.

Fluid retention

A diuretic is frequently necessary during the first few postoperative days, particularly in patients who were in severe cardiac failure before operation. The fluid-retention effect of corticosteroids may be a factor in some patients. A temporary loss of right ventricular compliance immediately after transplantation also leads to a raised jugular venous pressure. Intravenous furosemide therapy is preferable in the early post-transplant period, oral furosemide or other diuretic if such therapy is indicated for a longer period of time.

Cyclosporine (CsA), particularly if given intravenously, may be associated with an acute oliguria, which may respond to furosemide therapy, though, in addition, reduction in the CsA dosage or omission of this drug is required for a period of time. It may be difficult to distinguish between oliguria from CsA toxicity and acute tubular necrosis from other causes.

Prevention of peptic ulceration

Patients undergoing major surgical procedures and receiving corticosteroids are clearly at risk of developing peptic ulceration. An H_2 antagonist, such as ranitidine, or antacid, such as aluminum hydroxide or magnesium trisilicate, is begun immediately after operation to help prevent gastric erosion or stress ulcer, and should be continued at least during the first 3 months after transplantation, by which time steroid dosage should have been substantially reduced. Therapy should be continued in those considered at high risk (e.g. previous history of peptic ulceration) until steroids have been discontinued.

Anticoagulation

Full anticoagulation is unnecessary in patients with orthotopic heart transplants unless there are other specific indications. Some groups prescribe an antiplatelet agent for the first 6 weeks, and others continue such agents indefinitely in the hope of delaying or preventing the development of graft arteriosclerosis (chronic rejection) (Chapter 19).

Patients with heterotopic heart transplants, however, are at risk from thrombus formation in the left ventricle of the recipient heart. Thrombus may be present or may form in the poorly functioning recipient left ventricle, and be ejected through the aortic valve. Furthermore, left ventricular thrombus may spread retrogradely through an incompetent mitral valve into the common left atrium, from where it may be ejected by the donor left ventricle as an embolus. It is essential, therefore, to fully anticoagulate patients in whom the recipient heart remains *in situ*. Coumadin administration is begun once the chest drains have been removed, and is continued for the lifetime of the patient. An antiplatelet agent such as sulphinpyrazone or dipyridamole, may also be administered, but is not essential; aspirin or other salicylates. have been avoided in view of the risk of gastric erosion, which is already increased in patients receiving corticosteroids.

Prevention of chronic rejection

It is generally considered that a diet low in lipids may reduce the rate of progression of chronic rejection (accelerated graft arteriosclerosis), particularly in patients with hyperlipidemia (Chapter 19). This diet should be initiated as soon as practicable in the postoperative period (Chapter 27).

Hypercholesterolemia

In patients with underlying ischemic heart disease who are known to be hypercholesterolemic, therapy with a cholesterol-reducing agent, such as cholestyramine or probucol, may reduce the rate of progress of atheroma in peripheral vessels; in patients at risk, this therapy is begun in the early postoperative period. The new drug lovastatin, however, should be used with extreme caution in view of the risk of rhabdomyolysis which has been reported when it has been used in association with cyclosporine[10,11]. Whether such therapy slows the development of graft arteriosclerosis remains in doubt, and is discussed further in Chapter 19.

Antituberculous therapy

Long-term antituberculous therapy is essential in patients who have contracted this disease in the past. In patients with features on chest radiographs of previous tuberculosis infection, it has become our policy to administer isoniazid for at least the first 6 months as prophylaxis against recurrence.

Mineral replacement therapy

Many patients who undergo heart transplantation have osteoporosis induced by inactivity and diuretic therapy. Further bone loss may occur from corticosteroid therapy.

An attempt should be made to prevent or reduce such loss by dietary supplements of calcium. Cyclosporine neurotoxicity is associated with a low serum magnesium[12,13]. Hypomagnesemia is common in heart transplant patients receiving cyclosporine, and dietary supplements of magnesium should be administered if necessary.

MAINTENANCE IMMUNOSUPPRESSIVE THERAPY

The various pharmacological immunosuppressive agents available to those involved in transplantation have been discussed by a number of authors, notably by Salaman[14], and detailed accounts of their structure and mode of action can be found elsewhere[15-19]. The number of immunosuppressive regimens used is many, and consists of various combinations and dosages of the drugs available. The majority of centers today, however, utilize triple or quadruple drug therapy with cyclosporine, azathioprine, corticosteroids, and antithymocyte (ATG) or antilymphocyte (ALG) globulin.

Cyclosporine

Cyclosporine (CsA) was initially isolated from the fermentation broth of a soil fungus, *Trichoderma polysporum Rifai*[20]. The cyclosporines have a narrow spectrum of antibiotic activity[21], reducing the growth rate of a few yeasts and fungi. Full reviews of the immunosuppressive properties of this drug, which were first documented by Borel (Figure 1.12), have been published elsewhere[22-24]. The drug is lipid-soluble, metabolized in the liver and excreted mainly in the bile as metabolites. CsA acts primarily, by inhibition of interleukin-2, a growth factor for T-lymphocytes (Chapter 14). It does not depress the bone marrow as do cytotoxic agents.

Ideally, CsA should be begun before operation, the dose, administered orally, being based on the physical condition of the patient. A patient in good condition (no overt signs of cardiac failure, good renal and hepatic function) may receive 4–6 mg/kg body weight. A patient in extremely poor condition (severe cardiac failure with secondary renal and/or hepatic failure) should receive no or very little CsA before operation. Rather, the patient should be immunosuppressed with the other available drugs until postoperative progress has been assessed. A perioperative period of hypotension or severe liver dysfunction in a patient receiving CsA may result in nephrotoxicity, which may greatly complicate management.

Whenever in doubt, it has been our experience that it is wiser to administer less rather than more CsA in the pre- or early post-transplant period. The drug level in the blood or serum should be monitored daily (or more frequently) and the dose gradually increased (by perhaps 1 or 2 mg/kg per day) until a safe therapeutic range has been reached. It is usually possible to immunosuppress a patient adequately with a combination of azathioprine, corticosteroids (and antithymocyte globulin (ATG) where necessary) for the first few post-transplant days, whilst the CsA level is being slowly increased.

In regimens where ATG is not used, the dose of CsA must be carefully modified in the light of the renal function of the patient. The University of Minnesota group, who have obtained excellent results using such a regimen[25], calculate the initial pretransplant dose of CsA on the basis of the serum creatinine (Table 12.1). No further CsA is administered for 24 hours, at which time a second dose equal to half of the initial dose is administered, again taking into consideration any change in serum creatinine. This dose is given twice daily until kidney function is clearly normal, at which time the dosage is adjusted to obtain a whole blood trough level by HPLC of 200 ng/ml.

For oral administration, the drug comes in liquid form, and is commonly given in a chocolate drinking solution that the pharmaceutical company (Sandoz Ltd., Basle, Switzerland) provides. Though less palatable, CsA can be administered in any other drink, such as orange juice, but ideally it should be mixed in a glass rather than a soft plastic container as the drug may adhere to the plastic. CsA in a soft gelatin capsule is now available in some countries.

If the patient is unable to take oral drugs, then CsA can be given intravenously, but in much reduced dosage of approximately 0.5–2 mg/kg, given continuously over a 24-hour period. The intravenous dose is diluted in normal saline (100 mg/CsA in 100 ml saline) and administered continuously to reduce its renal toxic effect. Both the oral and intravenous forms can induce oliguria from toxicity on the proximal renal tubules. In our experience, the intravenous administration of CsA appears to be more readily followed by acute oliguria, and therefore we initiate intravenous therapy with small doses (0.25 mg/kg per 24 hours) and steadily increase over 2 or 3 days until the therapeutic level is achieved. Though absorption of the drug when given orally is usual (though erratic) in patients recovering from cardiac transplantation, achievement of a stable therapeutic blood level may be difficult. In recent months, therefore, it has been our policy to administer the drug intravenously to all patients for the first few days until the patient is eating and drinking normally, at which time oral therapy is initiated. Intramuscular administration is not recommended since the drug is poorly absorbed.

Whether CsA is given orally or intravenously, it is essential to measure the blood levels frequently (at least daily) until the dosage has been adjusted to achieve the correct therapeutic blood level. Blood levels are then estimated at intervals of a few days for one further month and on a less frequent basis thereafter. Blood should be drawn

Table 12.1 Recent immunosuppressive protocol used at the University of Minnesota for heart transplant patients

Cyclosporine (oral)
Pretransplant	6 mg/kg if serum creatinine < 1.5 mg/dl (< 133 μmol/l)
	4 mg/kg if serum creatinine 1.5–2.0 mg/dl (133–177 μmol/l)
	2 mg/kg if serum creatinine > 2 mg/dl (> 177 μmol/l)
Early post-transplant	3 mg/kg, 2 mg/kg, or 2 mg/kg twice daily depending on serum creatinine level
When renal function satisfactory	dosage adjusted to maintain whole blood CsA level (by HPLC) at 200 ng/ml
6 months post-transplant	reduce blood level to 150 ng/ml
12 months post-transplant	reduce blood level to 100–125 ng/ml

Azathioprine (i.v. or oral)
Pretransplant	2.5 mg/kg
Post-transplant	2.5 mg/kg per day (maintain WBC > 4000 cells/mm^3)

Corticosteroids
Methylprednisolone	500 mg i.v. during cardiopulmonary bypass
	125 mg i.v. every 8 hours for 24 hours
Prednisone	1 mg/kg per day (divided into four doses/day) for 3 days, reducing at 3-day intervals to approximately 0.4 mg/kg per day at 12 days
	Thereafter monthly reductions (giving the drug in two divided doses/day) until a dosage of 0.125–0.15 mg/kg per day is reached after 6 months. This dose is maintained indefinitely

immediately before administration of the drug to give a 'trough' level.

CsA levels can be measured by radioimmunoassay (RIA)[26,27], fluorescent polarization immunoassay (TDx)[28], or by a high pressure liquid chromatography (HPLC) technique[29]. As several metabolites of CsA are measured by RIA and TDx, but not by HPLC, the therapeutic range differs depending on the technique used, and is generally 50–70% lower when measured by HPLC. The therapeutic activity and significance of some of the metabolites are uncertain, and, therefore, the method of choice (RIA and HPLC) remains in doubt. The most commonly used method today is possibly fluorescent polarization immunoassay, which offers rapid sample turn-around times without putting great demands on the laboratory[28]. Some groups believe, however, that only the parent cyclosporine should be measured, without the metabolites, and therefore the HPLC technique should be the method of choice.

Immunoassay methodology involves labeling an antibody with either a radioactive molecule or a fluorescent molecule; the antibody, which can be monoclonal or polyclonal, is then bound to the CsA. The monoclonal form shows little or no cross-reactivity with metabolites of CsA[30], and the results correlate well with those obtained by HPLC. Monoclonal techniques therefore offer a simpler alternative to HPLC.

A number of other drugs affect the blood level of CsA (Table 12.2)[31], in particular ketoconazole and erythromycin, which increase its concentration, and phenytoin, phenobarbitone, and rifampicin, which decrease its concentration. Major changes in CsA dosage may be required if these other drugs are being administered simultaneously. (Caution must also be exerted in the presence of a low serum cholesterol, as neurotoxicity has been reported (Chapter 22).)

For reasons that remain uncertain, the blood or serum level which is considered adequate therapeutically differs substantially from center to center, even when the same method of measurement is utilized. Each center should ascertain for itself its own therapeutic and toxic ranges. In many centers, a whole blood trough level by RIA or TDx of between 500 and 800 ng/ml is considered adequate in the early post-transplant period, whilst the level in plasma would be approximately one-fifth to one-third of this. When HPLC is used to measure CsA level, whole blood trough levels of 200 ng/ml are generally considered adequate in the early post-transplant period, reducing to 150 ng/ml at 6 months and 100–125 ng/ml at 1 year[25].

The level that may be considered therapeutic varies considerably, of course, depending on the other therapy

Table 12.2 Selected drugs which influence blood levels and toxicity of cyclosporine*

Increase blood levels	Decrease blood levels	Potentiate nephrotoxicity
Diltiazem	Phenobarbitone	Aminoglycosides (gentamicin)
Erythromycin	Phenytoin	Amphotericin B
Ketoconazole	Rifampicin	Melphalan
Corticosteroids	Sulfatrimethoprim	Sulfonamides
Metoclopramide	(i.v. only)	Trimethoprim

* Only well-substantiated drugs have been included. Data provided by Sandoz Pharmaceuticals, USA. An extensive survey has been conducted by Lake[47].

being given. For example, if large daily doses of ALG are being administered, the patient may remain very adequately immunosuppressed whilst receiving only small doses of CsA. If no ALG or azathioprine are being administered, then the patient may require a high CsA level if acute rejection is to be prevented.

Maintenance oral CsA therapy should consist of twice daily doses (rarely it may be necessary to give three doses per day) sufficient to maintain the therapeutic level in the blood or plasma. When triple therapy (CsA, azathioprine and corticosteroids) is being administered, CsA dosage is generally between 4 and 10 mg/kg per day.

In view of the toxic effect of CsA on the proximal tubules, careful monitoring of the blood urea, serum creatinine, urine electrolytes, and creatinine clearance is essential. The most sensitive test would appear to be the creatinine clearance, which falls when toxicity occurs, though this does not differentiate CsA toxicity from acute tubular necrosis. Certain other drugs, if given concomitantly, increase the risk of nephrotoxicity (Table 12.2).

Hepatotoxic effects of CsA have been reported with increasing levels of various liver enzymes, though we have not found this to be a significant problem in administering the drug. The potential complications of use of CsA are discussed more fully in Chapter 22.

Azathioprine

Azathioprine (AZA) is one of the large group of antimetabolite compounds that compete for and block specific receptors, thus affecting DNA and RNA synthesis, and interfering with protein synthesis. AZA was introduced into experimental and clinical practice with regard to renal transplantation by Calne (Figure 1.8) in 1961[32]. Specifically, it is a purine antagonist that is similar in structure to 6-mercaptopurine. Since these agents are effective only against proliferating cells, they are most effective when given after antigen exposure[33]. All immune responses requiring cell proliferation may be inhibited by the drug, including antibody production and graft rejection. It is rather ineffective when used as a sole immunosuppressant following human renal transplantation[34,35]. It has not been used alone after cardiac transplantation.

AZA's main toxic effect is on the bone marrow, which results in leukopenia, thrombocytopenia and, occasionally, anemia, though leukopenia has rarely proved a problem following cardiac transplantation. Following withdrawal or reduction of the drug, recovery of the bone marrow is usually rapid in patients with cardiac allografts. AZA not infrequently results in minor abnormalities of liver function, but rarely leads to clinical hepatic dysfunction; substitution of AZA with cyclophosphamide is recommended in such cases.

It has been our policy to begin AZA immediately before operation with a loading dose of approximately 3–5 mg/kg intravenously. After transplantation, it is given initially intravenously and subsequently orally at the maximal tolerable level as judged by the absence of bone marrow and hepatic toxicity. The intravenous and oral doses are identical. In our experience the average maintenance dose for adults ranges between 0.5 and 3.0 mg/kg per day; the total white blood count should be maintained in the range of 5000–8000 cells/mm^3.

Corticosteroids

Steroids were introduced into clinical renal transplant practice in 1963[36]. It is the glucocorticoids, rather than the mineralocorticoids, which possess immunosuppressive activity. Prednisone or prednisolone have been most commonly used in transplantation. They inhibit a variety of intracellular enzymes that depress protein, RNA, and DNA synthesis. There is extensive death of small lymphocytes in the blood, thymus, lymph nodes and spleen, though the mechanism for this effect is not well understood, but is believed to be mediated through calcium influx. Much of the immunosuppressive action of steroids is, however, attributed to their anti-inflammatory properties. Cell-mediated immunity is depressed in most species.

The timing of steroid administration is probably not critical. It is often assumed that high-dose therapy must be started immediately rejection has been diagnosed if the graft is to be saved, and yet this may not be true. In the rat heart allograft model, a single bolus of methylprednisolone is more effective in prolonging graft survival when given late, rather than early, in the rejection process[37].

There are many different regimens for administering steroids to transplant patients. Our own regimen consists of 1 g methylprednisolone sodium succinate given intravenously during operation at the time of reperfusion of the donor heart, and further intravenous boluses of 125 mg 8-hourly for the first postoperative day. Thereafter, if the patient is absorbing oral fluids, an oral methylprednisolone dose of 0.3 mg/kg per day is given, divided into two doses. The dosage is slowly reduced (by 2–4 mg on each occasion) if endomyocardial biopsy confirms the absence of significant acute rejection.

Most centers use prednisone or prednisolone in similar dosage, 1 mg prednisone being the equivalent of 0.8 mg methylprednisolone. Prednisone is converted to methylprednisolone in the liver, and is a very much cheaper drug. Unless there are features of liver dysfunction, the patient should be switched to prednisone in the early post-transplant period. Some groups maintain prednisone therapy at 0.2 mg/kg per day thereafter, but in approximately 50% of patients it is possible to discontinue corticosteroids completely within 6 months (or earlier) in the absence of features of acute rejection[38]. Our own policy is for steroids to be withdrawn cautiously over several months; it is unusual at our center for the drug to be discontinued within the first 3 months.

When ATG is not part of the immunosuppressive regimen, rather higher initial doses of corticosteroids may be administered. The University of Minnesota group begins with an initial oral prednisone dosage of 1 mg/kg per day (given in four divided doses) (Table 12.1). If the progress of the patient is satisfactory, this dosage is reduced at 3-day intervals by approximately 0.125 mg/kg per day until a dosage of approximately 0.4 mg/kg per day is reached. This is administered for a month with further gradual reductions at monthly intervals to a dosage of 0.2–0.3 mg/kg per day at 3 months, and 0.125 mg/kg per day at 6 months. This dose is maintained indefinitely.

For an 80 kg patient, for example, the total daily dosage would be 80 mg initially, reducing by 10 mg every 3 days until a dosage of 30 mg/day was achieved. This would be maintained for 1 month. By 6 months, the daily dosage would have been reduced to 10 mg/day where it would remain indefinitely.

Antithymocyte (or antilymphocyte) globulin

The immunosuppressive effect of antilymphocyte globulin (ALG) was first demonstrated in the rat skin graft model[39]. The properties of ALG depend to a large extent on its method of preparation. It can be prepared against a wide variety of antigens, including those on thoracic duct or blood lymphocytes and thymocytes. ALG is prepared by immunizing, most commonly, horses, rabbits, or goats with human lymphocytes or thymocytes. A clear description of the steps involved in its preparation is given by Touraine et al.[40]. The dosage varies widely, depending on the preparation used. Several commercial preparations are currently available; there are variations in potency between them.

ALG has been shown to prolong renal allograft survival[41-43], and was first documented in cardiac transplantation by Cooley and his colleagues in 1968[44].

Until recently, our own policy with regard to ALG therapy was to administer an initial dose during operation, once the patient was on cardiopulmonary bypass; we adopted this policy following rapid circulatory deterioration from an anaphylactic-like reaction in two patients who were receiving ALG immediately before induction of anesthesia. The dose was estimated as that necessary to reduce the circulating T-lymphocytes to the therapeutic range of 50–150 cells/mm^3. We have always given this drug intravenously. The usual loading dose has been approximately 2 mg IgG/kg.

After operation, the T-11 lymphocytes were counted daily by flow cytometry using monoclonal antibodies (or by the sheep red cell rosetting test), and the dosage of ALG estimated accordingly. To maintain the T-lymphocytes at the desired level, we have given ALG in doses of up to 1000 mg/day (approximately 12 mg IgG/kg per day), though the daily dosage has varied widely from patient to patient. The drug is diluted in 100–200 ml normal saline, and is usually given as a single daily infusion over a period of 4 hours. When severe acute rejection is occurring, and the T-lymphocytes multiplying rapidly, we have on occasions counted the T-lymphocytes every 8 hours and administered ALG 8-hourly. The drug can be given intramuscularly, but repeated injections can cause local inflammation and pain[45].

ALG was administered daily until such time that the trough CsA level was considered adequate and consistent. This usually took only a few days, rarely requiring more than 1 week of ALG therapy; at this time, ALG was discontinued. It was introduced once again only when required in the management of an acute rejection episode.

In our experience, allergic reactions to ALG have been uncommon, but it has been our policy to give an antihistamine such as promethazine hydrochloride (12.5–25 mg) intravenously immediately before drug infusion.

Recently, concerned by the increasing incidence of cytomegalovirus (CMV) infection in our patients during the first few post-transplant months, we have discontinued the initial course of ATG, immunosuppressing the patient with only azathioprine and methylprednisolone until adequate cyclosporine levels can be obtained. We have no evidence that the administration of ATG results in a higher incidence of CMV infection, but we hope and believe that an overall reduction in the level of immunosuppressive therapy might lead to a reduction in this troublesome infectious complication. We therefore reserve ATG only for those patients in whom it is not possible to administer cyclosporine (e.g. due to neurotoxic or nephrotoxic effects) and those undergoing a severe rejection episode unresponsive to intravenous corticosteroid therapy alone.

The several potential complications of each of these immunosuppressive agents – cyclosporine, azathioprine, corticosteroids, and ALG – are discussed in Chapter 22.

Other immunosuppressive agents

Monoclonal antibody (OKT3)

OKT3, a murine monoclonal antibody of the IgG-2a series, is a pan-T-cell suppressor. It can only be given intravenously. OKT3 causes an immediate but temporary decline in circulating T-cells which persists while the antibody is being administered. OKT3 blocks all known T-cell functions. A rapid and concomitant decrease in the number of T3 (CD3), T4 (CD4), and T8 (CD8) cells occurs within minutes of administration of OKT3. There is some recovery in the numbers of T4 and T8 cells within the first week of administration, though the T3 cells remain undetectable in the peripheral blood. Recovery of T3 cells to pretreatment levels occurs within a week once administration is discontinued.

OKT3 monoclonal antibody has been used experimentally in heart transplantation for nearly 2 years[46]. Experience with it has rapidly accumulated, and most programs now use it to treat rejection unresponsive to conventional therapy (Chapter 16). A smaller number of centers is beginning to consider its use in the early postoperative period as a prophylaxis to prevent rejection. The various indications for its use are, therefore, (1) treatment of refractory rejection; (2) treatment of life-threatening rejection when it is elected not to wait to assess the full response of conventional therapy; and (3) rejection prophylaxis. Discussion of its value in the treatment of an established acute rejection episode can be found in Chapter 16.

It is recommended that 5 mg of OKT3 be administered daily for 10–14 days, each dose being given intravenously over 1 min. This dose may require adjustment to maintain the T-3 lymphocyte subset at about 20 cells/mm^3. To prevent excessive immunosuppression (and thus increase the risks of infection), most groups suggest that, during therapy, concomitant immunosuppressive therapy should be decreased to approximately half the maintenance level. Others advocate discontinuing concomitant immunosuppressive therapy entirely. Normal maintenance immunosuppressive doses (of CsA, etc.) should be resumed 3 days prior to completion of OKT3 therapy.

Serum levels of OKT3 can be measured by an ELISA (enzyme-linked immunosorbent serum assay). A mean trough level of 0.9 μg/ml (achieved with the recommended dose) has been shown to block T-cell effector functions *in vitro*.

Premedication with acetaminophen 650 mg orally, methylprednisolone 1 mg/kg i.v., and diphenhydramine 100 mg i.v. 30 min prior to administration of OKT3 is given to minimize allergic reactions. It is recommended that 100 mg of i.v. hydrocortisone be given intravenously 30 min after the injection of OKT3; further acetaminophen and antihistamines are optional.

One of the few cardiac transplant groups to have more than minimal experience with OKT3 is the Utah group[46–48]. When OKT3 was given during the first 2 weeks following transplantation as prophylaxis against rejection, there was improved patient and graft survival when compared with patients receiving ATG as prophylaxis during the same period of time. Because of excellent patient and graft survival in the conventionally-treated group, however, the sample size was not sufficient to demonstrate a reduction in mortality or graft loss in the OKT3-treated patients.

IgM anti-OKT3 appears in approximately 21% of patients receiving this agent, while IgG anti-OKT3 is seen in 86%, and IgE anti-OKT3 in 29%, occurring approximately 20 days after treatment is begun. The numbers of T-3 cells should be carefully monitored, and if they increase despite OKT3 therapy, the dosage of the monoclonal antibody should be increased at least 2–3 times. Patients who develop large quantities of IgG anti-OKT3 antibodies, and therefore fail to respond to OKT3 therapy, may not be candidates for another OKT3 treatment. However, in the Utah study, of six cardiac transplant patients with refractory rejection who had previously received OKT3 prophylaxis, only one showed evidence of the development of sensitization, as deduced from CD3 markers remaining above 1–2%. The other patients went on to receive a second course of 7–10 days' treatment of OKT3, and had favorable responses, with ultimate resolution of the rejection episode in three cases. It appears, therefore, that the majority of patients treated with OKT3 prophylaxis in a protocol that includes measures to inhibit antibody production may be re-treated for refractory rejection.

In patients with kidney transplants, however, reports of anti-idiotypic antibody development, which is a prominent feature of the immune response to OKT3, and probably other monoclonal antibodies, can lead to a block in their therapeutic effectiveness and can arise despite intense immunosuppression[49]. This response may require the use of different idiotypes for prolonged or repeated courses of therapy, and may be the major obstacle to the use of monoclonal antibodies.

The potential adverse reactions to OKT3 are discussed in Chapter 22.

Vincristine

The Utah group has evaluated adjunctive therapy using vincristine 0.025 mg/kg intravenously for eight doses over a 12-week period in combination with CsA and AZA[38]. Vincristine was shown to have an immunosuppressive effect, though there were numerous adverse factors which included muscle weakness, sensory neuropathy, constipation, arthralgia, and alopecia. Vincristine has also been shown to be immunosuppressive in animal models[50,51]. It would seem that vincristine would not be an ideal drug to use routinely, and that a combination of the other available immunosuppressive agents should generally suffice in preventing rejection.

Cyclophosphamide

In occasional patients who show refractory or repeated acute rejection despite triple or quadruple drug therapy, or in those in whom AZA is associated with hepatic dysfunction, we have found cyclophosphamide to be a useful agent. In view of its potential to cause severe bone marrow depression, however, it must be used cautiously. Its use is further discussed in Chapter 16.

COMMENT

With triple or quadruple drug therapy (CsA, AZA, steroids, and ALG), the development of severe acute rejection is rare, and has been seen in less than 2% of endomyocardial biopsies at our center during the past 2 years. This combination of drugs is, therefore, potent and efficient, and care has to be taken to avoid over-immunosuppression. Changes suggestive of mild or moderate acute rejection remain relatively common, but frequently do not warrant extra immunosuppressive therapy.

The efficacy of CsA has allowed steroid dosage to be significantly reduced, and in an increasing number of patients it can be discontinued entirely. This is a major advance that reduces the debilitating effects and complications associated with high-dose steroid therapy. Unfortunately, the use of triple or quadruple drug therapy has not yet been shown to reduce the incidence of graft arteriosclerosis (chronic rejection), which still occurs in a significant percentage of patients and is discussed in Chapter 19.

References

1. Greeley, W.J., Leslie, J.B., Reves, J.G. and Watkins, W.D. (1986). Eicosanoids (prostaglandins) and the cardiovascular system. *J. Cardiac Surg.*, **1**, 357
2. Fonger, J.D., Borkon, A.M., Baumgartner, W.A., Achuff, S.C., Augustine, S. and Reitz, B.A. (1986). Acute right heart failure following heart transplantation: improvement with prostaglandin E1 and right ventricular assist. *J. Heart Transplant.*, **5**, 317
3. Armitage, J.M., Hardesty, R.L. and Griffith, B.P. (1987). Prostaglandin E1: an effective treatment of right heart failure after orthotopic heart transplantation. *J. Heart Transplant.*, **6**, 348
4. Ferreira, S.H. and Vane, J.R. (1967). Prostaglandins: their disappearance from and release into the circulation. *Nature (London)*, **216**, 868
5. Gorman, R.R. (1980). Biochemical and pharmacological evaluation of thromboxane synthetase inhibitors. *Adv. Prostaglandin Thromboxane Leukotriene Res.*, **6**, 417
6. Mathe, A.A. (1977). Prostaglandins and the lung. In Ramwell, P.W. (ed.) *The Prostaglandins*. Vol. 3, p. 169 (New York: Plenum Press)
7. Bremner, W.F., Taylor, K.M., Baird, S., Thomson, J.E., Thomson, J.A., Ratcliffe, J.G., Lawrie, T.D.V. and Bain, W.H. (1978). Hypothalamo–pituitary–thyroid axis function during cardiopulmonary bypass. *J. Thorac. Cardiovasc. Surg.*, **75**, 392
8. Robuschi, G., Medici, D., Fesani, F., Barboso, G., Montermini, M., D'Amato, L., Gardini, E., Borciani, E., Dall'Aglio, E., Salvi, M., Gnudi, A. and Roti, E. (1986). Cardiopulmonary bypass: 'a low T4 and T3 syndrome' with blunted thyrotropin (TSH) response to thyrotropin-releasing hormone (TRH). *Hormone Res.*, **23**, 151
9. Novitzky, D., Human, P.A. and Cooper, D.K.C. (1988). Inotropic effect of triiodothyronine (T3) following myocardial ischemia and cardiopulmonary bypass. 1. An experimental study in pigs. *Ann. Thorac. Surg.*, **45**, 50
10. Norman, D.J., Illingworth, D.R., Munson, J. and Hosenpud, J. (1988). Myolysis and acute renal failure in a heart-transplant recipient receiving lovastatin. (Letter) *N. Engl. J. Med.*, **318**, 46
11. East, C., Alivizatos, P.A., Grundy, S.M., Jones, P.H. and Farmer, J.A. (1988). Rhabdomyolysis in patients receiving lovastatin after cardiac transplantation. (Letter) *N. Engl. J. Med.*, **318**, 47
12. Thompson, C.B., June, C.H., Sullivan, K.M. and Thomas, E.D. (1984). Association between cyclosporine neurotoxicity and hypomagnesaemia. *Lancet*, **2**, 1116
13. Schmitz, N., Eulen, H.H. and Loffler, H. (1985). Hypomagnesaemia and cyclosporine toxicity (Letter). *Lancet*, **1**, 103
14. Salaman, J.R. (ed.) (1981). *Immunosuppressive Therapy*. (Philadelphia; Lippincott)
15. Schwartz, R.S. (1968). Immunosuppressive drug therapy. In Rapaport, F.T. and Dausset, J. (eds.) *Human Transplantation*. p. 440 (New York: Grune and Stratton)
16. Santos, G.W. (1972). Chemical immunosuppression. In Najarian, J.S. and Simmons, R.L. (eds.) *Transplantation*. p. 206. (Philadephia; Lea and Febiger)
17. Bach, J.F. (1976). The pharmacological and immunological basis for the use of immunosuppressive drugs. *Drugs*, **11**, 1
18. Hurd, E.R. (1977). Drugs affecting the immune response. In Holborow, E.J. and Reeves, W.G. (eds.) *Immunology in Medicine*. p. 1067. (London: Academic Press)
19. Berenbaum, M.C. (1975). The clinical pharmacology of immunosuppressive agents. In Gell, P.G.H., Coombs, R.R.A. and Lachman, P.J. (eds.) *Clinical Aspects of Immunology*. p. 689. (Oxford: Blackwell Scientific)
20. Borel, J.F., Feurer, C., Gubler, H.U. and Stahelin, H. (1976). Biological effects of cyclosporin-A: a new antilymphocytic agent. *Agents Actions*, **6**, 468
21. Dreyfuss, M., Harri, E., Hofmann, H., Kobel, H., Pache, W. and Tscherter, H. (1976). Cyclosporin-A and C: new metabolites from *Trichoderma polysporum*. *Eur. J. Appl. Microbiol.*, **3**, 125
22. White, D.J.G. (ed.) (1982). *Cyclosporin-A*. (Amsterdam: Elsevier Biomedical)
23. Morris, P.J. (1981). Cyclosporin-A. *Transplantation*, **32**, 349
24. Borel, J.F. (1982). Immunological properties of cyclosporin-A. *Heart Transplant.*, **1**, 237
25. Andreone, P.A., Olivari, M.T., Elick, B., Arentzen, C.E., Sibley, R.K., Bolman, R.M., Simmons, R.L. and Ring, W.S. (1986). Reduction of infectious complications following heart transplantation with triple-drug immunotherapy. *J. Heart Transplant.*, **5**, 13
26. Donatsch, P., Abisch, E., Homberger, M., Traber, R., Trapp, M. and Voges, R. (1981). A radioimmunoassay to measure cyclosporin-A in plasma and serum samples. *J. Immunoassay*, **2**, 19
27. Sgoutas, D.S. and Hammarstrom, M. (1989). Comparison of specific radioimmunoassays for cyclosporine. *Transplantation*, **47**, 668
28. Schroeder, T.J., Brunson, M.E., Pesce, A.J., Hindenlang, L.L., Mauser, P.A., Ruckrigl, D.I., Weibel, M.L., Wadih, G. and First, M.R. (1989). A comparison of the clinical utility of the radioimmunoassay, high-performance liquid chromatography, and TDx cyclosporine assays in outpatient renal transplant recipients. *Transplantation.*, **47**, 262
29. Gmur, D.J. (1985). Modified column-switching high-performance liquid chromatographic method for measurement of cyclosporin in serum. *J. Chromatogr.*, **344**, 422
30. Speck, R.F., Frey, F.J. and Frey, B.M. (1989). Cyclosporine kinetics in renal transplant patients as assessed by high-performance liquid chromatography and radioimmunoassay using monoclonal and polyclonal antibodies. *Transplantation*, **47**, 802
31. Lake, K.D. (1988). Cyclosporine drug interactions: a review. *Cardiac Surgery: State of the Art Reviews*, **2**, 617
32. Calne, R.Y. (1961). Inhibition of the rejection of renal homografts in dogs by purine analogues. *Transplant. Bull.*, **28**, 65
33. Hersh, E.M., Carbone, P.P. and Freireich, E.J. (1966). Recovery of immune responsiveness after drug suppression in man. *J. Lab. Clin. Med.*, **67**, 566

34. Gleason, R.E. and Murray, J.E. (1967). Report from Kidney Transplant Registry: analysis of variables in the function of human kidney transplants. *Transplantation*, **5**, 360
35. Kries, H., Lacombe, M., Noel, L.H., Descamps, J.M., Chailley, J. and Crosnier, J. (1978). Kidney graft rejection: has the need for steroids to be re-evaluated? *Lancet*, **2**, 1169
36. Goodwin, W.E., Kaufman, J.J., Mims, M.M., Turner, R.D., Glassock, R., Goldman, R. and Maxwell, M.M. (1963). Human renal transplantation. I. Clinical experiences with six cases of renal homotransplantation. *J. Urol.*, **89**, 13
37. Salaman, J.R. and Couhig, E. (1980). Timing of anti-rejection therapy. *Transplantation*, **29**, 468
38. Gilbert, E.M., Renlund, D.G., O'Connell, J.B., Eiswirth, C.C., Rothstein, G., Gay, W.A., Bristow, M.R. and the Utah Cardiac Transplant Program (1987). Immunosuppressive efficacy of vincristine in heart transplantation: a preliminary report. *J. Heart Transplant.*, **6**, 369
39. Woodruff, M.F. and Anderson, N.F. (1963). Effects of lymphocyte depletion by thoracic duct fistula and administration of antilymphocytic serum on the survival of skin homografts in rats. *Nature (London)*, **200**, 702
40. Touraine, J.L., Malik, M.C. and Traeger, J. (1981). Antilymphocyte globulin and thoracic duct drainage in renal transplantation. In Salaman, J.R. (ed.) *Immunosuppressive Therapy*. p. 55. (Lancaster: MTP Press)
41. Nagaya, H. and Sieker, H.O. (1965). Allograft survival: effect of antiserums to thymus glands and lymphocytes. *Science*, **150**, 1181
42. Davis, R.C., Cooperband, S.R. and Mannick, J.A. (1969). Preparation and *in vitro* assay of effective and ineffective antilymphocyte sera. *Surgery*, **66**, 58
43. Levey, R.H. and Medawar, P.B. (1966). Some experiments on the action of antilymphoid antisera. *Ann. N.Y. Acad. Sci.*, **129**, 164
44. Cooley, D.A., Hallman, G.L., Bloodwell, R.D., Nora, J.J. and Leachman, R.D. (1968). Human heart transplantation: experience with 12 cases. *Am. J. Cardiol.*, **22**, 804
45. Baumgartner, W.A., Reitz, B.A., Oyer, P.E., Stinson, E.B. and Shumway, N.E. (1979). Cardiac homotransplantation. *Curr. Probl. Surg.*, **16**, 1
46. Gilbert, E.M., De Witt, C.W., Eiswirth, C.C., Renlund, D.G., Menlove, R.L., Freedman, L.A., Herrick, C.M., Gay, W.A. and Bristow, M.R. (1987). Treatment of refractory cardiac allograft rejection with OKT3 monoclonal antibody. *Am. J. Med.*, **82**, 203
47. Bristow, M.R., Gilbert, E.M., Renlund, D.G., De Witt, C.W., Burton, N.A. and O'Connell, J.B. (1988). Use of OKT3 monoclonal antibody in cardiac transplantation: review of the initial experience. *J. Heart Transplant.*, **7**, 1
48. Bristow, M.R., Gilbert, E.M., O'Connell, J.B., Renlund, D.G., Watson, F.S., Hammond, E., Lee, R.G. and Menlove, R. (1988). OKT3 monoclonal antibody in heart transplantation. *Am. J. Kidney Dis.*, **11**, 135
49. Jaffers, G.J., Fuller, T.C., Cosimi, A.B., Russell, P.S., Winn, H.J. and Colvin, R.B. (1986). Monoclonal antibody therapy: anti-idiotypic and non-anti-idiotypic antibodies to OKT3 arising despite intense immunosuppression. *Transplantation*, **41**, 572
50. Medleau, L., Dawe, D.L. and Calvert, C.A. (1983). Immunosuppressive effects of cyclophosphamide, vincristine and L-asparaginase in dogs. *Am. J. Vet. Res.*, **44**, 176
51. Sensenbrenner, L.L., Owens, A.H., Zawatzsky, L.S. and Elfenbein, G.J. (1972). The comparative effects of selected cytotoxic agents on transplanted hematopoietic cells. *Transplantation*, **14**, 347

13
Physiology and Pharmacology of the Transplanted Heart

A.R. HORAK

INTRODUCTION

The primary function of the heart is to deliver oxygenated blood to the tissues of the body in accordance with their metabolic requirements. When alterations in metabolic demands occur, the response of the heart and peripheral circulation is integrated by a number of intrinsic and extrinsic control mechanisms which ensure a controlled, appropriate response to the altered stress[1-3].

The major factors which determine the cardiac output, and its distribution are outlined in Figure 13.1[1]. Many of these factors are intricately regulated by the central nervous system (sympathetic and parasympathetic), humoral mechanisms (circulating catecholamines) and intrinsic metabolic and electrolyte alterations. Cardiac transplantation, by altering these control mechanisms, significantly affects the manner in which the heart and the peripheral circulation respond to alterations in demands.

PHYSIOLOGY OF THE TRANSPLANTED HEART

Cardiac transplantation results in complete denervation of the heart, which is permanent[4-10], thereby depriving the

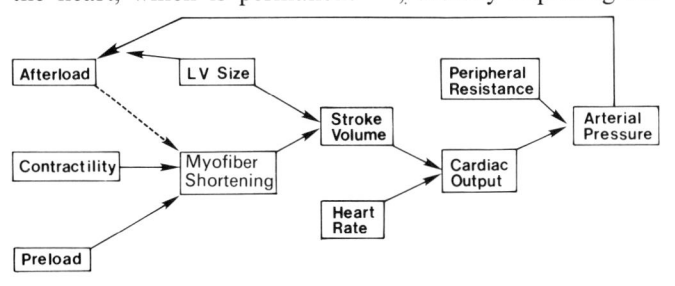

Figure 13.1 Diagram showing the interactions between the various components regulating cardiac activity (after Braunwald)[1]. Solid lines represent an increasing effect; the dotted line indicates a depressant effect. The numerous factors which affect these components themselves have not been included. Note, however, that left ventricular (LV) size is a determinant of both the afterload and the stroke volume. The preload, by altering LV size may therefore influence the afterload

heart of the important neural regulating mechanisms. Nevertheless, the actions of a number of other compensatory mechanisms allow the circulatory system to meet the increased demands placed upon it at times of stress, thus enabling a large proportion of transplant recipients to be rehabilitated successfully and returned to an active life[11,12].

THE RESTING STATE

Heart rate

Following the abolition of the usually dominant inhibitory vagal influences (by denervation), the resting rate of the transplanted heart is generally higher then normal[4-10,12-17], and does not reflexly alter in response to the Valsalva maneuver[4,5], carotid sinus massage[5], alterations in body position[4,5,18], or drugs such as phenylephrine, atropine or amyl nitrate[4-6].

Cardiac dynamics

Although the cardiac index of the transplanted heart is lower than that of normally innervated control hearts, it remains in the normal range; resting cardiac dynamics are essentially normal[6,7,10]. Immunosuppressive therapy with cyclosporine and prednisone appears to alter resting hemodynamics, causing systemic hypertension in almost all patients[17,19,20], while right atrial, pulmonary artery, pulmonary capillary wedge and left ventricular end-diastolic pressures, although in the normal range, tend to be higher than in control patients[17,19,20]. In the long term, resting hemodynamics may be altered by the onset of rejection or coronary artery disease.

Contractility and left ventricular performance

Left ventricular performance of transplanted hearts, as measured by hemodynamics (see above) or by ejection phase indices determined echocardiographically[21], by surgically implanted radio-opaque markers[8,9] or by radionuclide angiography[16,22] is normal. Left ventricular performance reflects a complex interaction between the contractile state and the loading conditions. When measured by load-independent echocardiographic indices, left ventricular contractility and contractile reserve are also normal[23].

Diastolic function

The echocardiographic isovolumic relaxation time and Doppler mitral valve pressure half-time (indices of diastolic function of the ventricle) are longer in cyclosporine-treated transplant recipients than in normal controls[24], indicating an abnormality of the diastolic compliance of the left ventricle. This may be a reflection of ischemic damage sustained at the time of transplantation, though one would generally expect associated poor systolic function in such cases, or a reflection of hypertrophy induced by the cyclosporine-related hypertension. Acute rejection alters these indices (shortening them) as well as increasing the peak early mitral inflow velocity, in keeping with an increased pulmonary capillary wedge pressure seen in rejection[24].

Humoral factors

Cardiac denervation after heart transplantation depletes the myocardium of norepinephrine and epinephrine because of interruption of postganglionic cardiac sympathetic nerves[25]. In contrast, myocardial dopamine levels are only modestly decreased. Increased sensitivity to circulatory catecholamines ensues[5,26,27], which appears to be mediated by a change in the state of the β-receptors ('up-regulation').

Atrial natriuretic peptide (ANP) levels in transplant recipients have recently been measured[28]. Levels of ANP are elevated above normal control levels. The origin of the ANP (donor atrium or residual recipient atrial remnant) was not determined. Further, levels are higher for a given right atrial pressure in transplant recipients than in patients with coronary artery disease, suggesting that factors other than atrial filling pressure may be important in determining ANP levels. The clinical significance of these findings is not yet clear.

RESPONSE TO EXERCISE

Isometric exercise

In normal healthy subjects

Isometric exercise causes an increase in systemic arterial blood pressure[29,30]. Sustained isometric contractions of more than 15% of the voluntary maximum (irrespective of the size of the muscle involved) result in the accumulation of muscle metabolites which stimulate reflex afferents, causing sympathetic activation and vagal inhibition. Thus, heart rate increases, peripheral vasoconstriction occurs and cardiac output increases slightly.

Following cardiac transplantation

Patients performing isometric exercise increase their systolic and diastolic blood pressures in a manner identical to that of control subjects[15,31,32]. The cardiac acceleration observed in control subjects does not occur, but cardiac output in both control subjects and transplant recipients rises slightly, though not significantly. The major alteration, accounting for the observed rise in blood pressure, is an increase in the peripheral vascular resistance. Peripheral resistance rises equally in both groups[31,32].

Dynamic exercise

Dynamic exercise differs from static isometric exercise in that cardiac output must also be increased and appropriately distributed in order to deliver nutrients to, and remove metabolites from, the periphery.

The fact that transplant recipients are able to perform significant amounts of dynamic exercise is well recognized[6,10,13,16,18]. The transplanted, denervated heart is able to increase its output significantly in response to exercise, but it does appear that maximal work capacity may be less than that achieved by age-matched control subjects[10,16,18]. There are some striking differences in the mechanisms whereby normal and transplanted hearts increase their cardiac output in response to an increase in demand.

Heart rate

In normal healthy subjects, the heart rate is determined not only by the intrinsic rate of spontaneous depolarization in the sinoatrial node, but also by extrinsic neural (sympathetic and parasympathetic) and humoral (circulating catecholamines) mechanisms. With the onset of exercise (and even occasionally preceding exercise) heart rate rises rapidly, remains elevated for the duration of exercise and subsides promptly after the cessation of exercise. These alterations are mediated predominantly by the neural mechanisms (sympathetic stimulation and parasympathetic inhibition).

The heart rate of the transplanted heart, which is generally higher at rest than that of controls, does rise with dynamic exercise, but the pattern of response is different from that of controls. The heart rate of transplant recipients rises much more gradually after the onset of exercise, never reaches the same peak heart rate, and subsides more slowly after cessation of exercise[4,5,8,9,14,16]. This change in heart rate is mediated predominantly by a rise in the levels of circulating catecholamines[8,33–35]. Changes in heart rate correlate with changes in the levels of circulating epinephrine[8], and can be inhibited by β-receptor blockers. If the effects of circulating catecholamines are blocked pharmacologically, a small rise of about 10 beats per minute still occurs in response to exercise[33,34]. This is probably related to the chronotropic effect of right atrial distension produced by increased venous return.

Cardiac output and work

In normally innervated hearts, changes in heart rate account for most of the increased cardiac output which occurs, while stroke volume remains virtually unchanged. Vasodilation of the blood vessels supplying the exercising muscles results in a decreased peripheral vascular resistance and an increased venous return. With more strenuous exercise, the increased preload (due to the increased venous return) results in an increase in the stroke volume (the Frank–Starling mechanism), thus further increasing the cardiac output[1–3,36–38].

The transplanted heart, despite the initial lack of cardioacceleration, is able to increase its output rapidly in response to dynamic exercise[5–10,13,14,16]. In contradistinction to the normally innervated heart, the Frank–Starling mechanism appears to play a major role early in this response, as the left ventricular end-diastolic pressure[5–8,10,13] and volume[8,16] rise early in exercise, and stroke volume[16] and cardiac output increase concomitantly (before any change in heart rate). Peripheral circulatory changes are similar to those which occur in the normal subject.

At higher work loads, the chronotropic and inotropic effects of circulating catecholamines, such as epinephrine, play a more prominent role[6,8,9], increasing the heart rate, circumferential fiber shortening[8], and ejection fraction[9] of the transplanted heart, causing a further increase in the cardiac output[6,8,9,16]. These effects may be enhanced by the known sensitivity of the denervated heart to catecholamines[5,26,27].

It is apparent, however, that despite these compensatory mechanisms, the cardiac output of the transplanted heart, both at rest and at peak exercise, may be lower than that of normally innervated control hearts[6,10,15], by as much as 25%[16]. Similarly, the duration of the period of exercise which can be maintained is less than in control subjects[10,18] (though this may, of course, be influenced by the development of conditions unrelated to the heart, such as corticosteroid-induced skeletal myopathy). Even if work load is increased gradually to allow the somewhat delayed compensatory mechanisms of the denervated, transplanted heart to take effect, transplant recipients produce more lactate and are able to utilize less oxygen than controls, suggesting that they are undergoing a greater degree of anaerobic metabolism[18]. Furthermore, transplant recipients performing exercise have a demonstrably increased arteriovenous oxygen difference compared with controls, indicating an increased extraction of oxygen from hemoglobin by the tissues, and suggesting that cardiac output is comparably lower than in controls[6,8].

It has been suggested that these findings, which imply suboptimal cardiac function, may be the result of subclinical rejection[18], as dogs with autotransplants are able to perform maximally[39].

Training effects

Adequate physical training does not cause a reduction in resting heart rate of the transplanted heart (though it does in control subjects), but the heart rate at submaximal work rates is significantly reduced when compared to pretraining levels. Work capacity is markedly improved. Thus, cardiac innervation is not required to produce increased work capacity following physical training[14,40].

TIME COURSE OF THE PHYSIOLOGIC EFFECTS OF HEART TRANSPLANTATION

Heart transplantation causes an almost immediate improvement in circulatory hemodynamics. Right and left heart filling pressure decline in parallel[41], reaching normal levels at 2 weeks after transplantation. There is rapid resolution of moderate pulmonary hypertension (within 2 weeks), while pulmonary vascular resistance decreases by 10–84% at 1 year post-transplant[41]. The greatest decrease occurs in patients with the highest preoperative values. Right ventricular dilation in response to the abnormal pulmonary circulatory dynamics occurs immediately after transplantation and persists despite resolution of the pulmonary hypertension[41]. Normalization of the sympathetic nervous system (as reflected by measurements of plasma norepinephrine levels) occurs within 2 weeks of transplantation[42].

PHYSIOLOGY FOLLOWING HETEROTOPIC HEART TRANSPLANTATION

When heterotopic heart transplantation is performed, the parallel linkage of the compliant donor transplanted heart with the failing non-compliant recipient heart leads to complex changes.

As there is no pressure difference between the anastomosed atria, filling of the transplanted and recipient ventricles is determined by their relative compliance (Figure 13.2). Filling of the more compliant donor left ventricle therefore accounts for most of the pulmonary venous return, and the contribution of this ventricle to the total cardiac output is consequently far greater. Not uncommonly, the

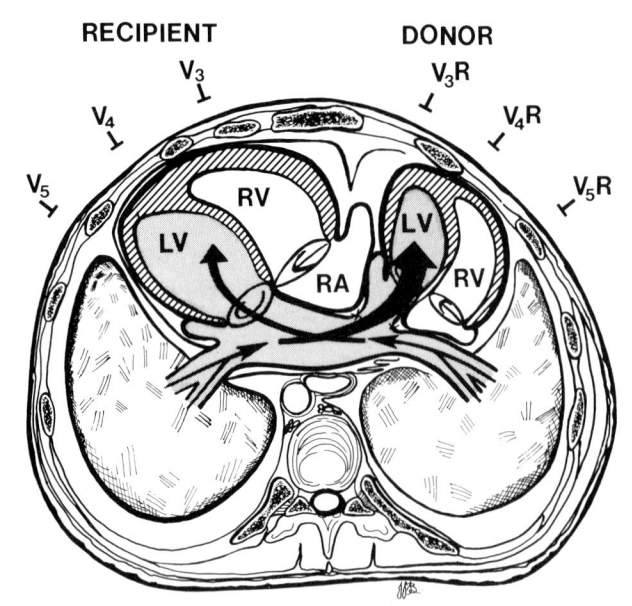

Figure 13.2 Diagram of a tranverse section through the thorax of a patient with a heterotopic heart transplant. The donor heart is situated in the right pleural cavity. (The sites of electrocardiographic electrode placement are also indicated.) Blood flow from the common left atrial chamber is governed by the relative compliances of the two left ventricles. Unless rejection of the donor heart is occurring, the compliance of the donor left ventricle will be greater than that of the diseased recipient left ventricle; blood in the common left atrial chamber will therefore drain predominantly to the donor left ventricle

donor left ventricle effectively assumes total left ventricular work and the native left ventricle fails to generate sufficient pressure or output to open the aortic valve[43-46]. Thus, diastolic compliance as well as systolic mechanical function determine preferential flow through the donor ventricle. This situation may be altered by the onset of rejection, which can markedly decrease the compliance of the donor ventricle, and would therefore tend to reverse the pattern of distribution of the pulmonary venous return.

The relative contribution of the two right ventricles to pulmonary blood flow is similarly determined by the diastolic compliance of the ventricles and by their systolic function. If there is no pulmonary hypertension and if pulmonary vascular resistance is initially normal, the total effective right heart output is shared by both right ventricles. However, if the pulmonary vascular resistance is significantly elevated pretransplant, the donor right ventricle is not able, initially, to contribute significantly to the pulmonary blood flow and the load is carried mostly by the native (recipient) right ventricle[43]. This situation may change with time as the pulmonary vascular resistance decreases post-transplant (see above) and as right ventricular hypertrophy of the donor heart develops.

In addition to these considerations, complex beat-to-beat alterations in preload occur, and these can also strikingly affect the performance of the recipient heart. If the hearts are allowed to beat spontaneously and happen to contract synchronously[44], or if they are paced synchronously[45], then the contribution of the recipient heart to the stroke volume of the synchronized beat falls dramatically. The recipient ventricle is frequently unable to raise its peak left ventricular pressure above aortic pressure and, therefore, ejection from this ventricle does not occur[44-46]. The bolus of blood in this ventricle may be shunted via an incompetent mitral valve through the common left atrium into the donor ventricle and ejected into the aorta[46].

Conversely, recipient heart function is optimized if the two hearts beat (or are paced) sequentially[44,45]. At least one patient has had a double atrial-triggered pacemaker implanted in order to assure sequential contraction of the hearts and optimize recipient heart function[47].

Subsequent work, however, has shown that, although the ejection fraction and output of the recipient heart are increased during sequential pacing, no real advantage is gained from this procedure as the donor heart is capable of maintaining a normal cardiac output in the absence of any recipient heart function[45,46]. Furthermore, the total output of the spontaneously beating recipient heart is not significantly different from the total output of the sequentially paced heart, as the spontaneously beating heart seldom beats synchronously with the donor heart for prolonged periods[45]. Sequential atrial pacing is, therefore, not used routinely when heterotopic heart transplants are performed at our institition[48].

A theoretical advantage of heterotopic heart transplantation is that it could allow time for recovery of native heart function. This does not seem to occur. Indeed, there is evidence to suggest that recipient heart function may deteriorate over a period of time following heterotopic transplantation[46,48]. Whether this is the result of the increased afterload on the recipient heart, or is simply a reflection of progression of the original disease process, is uncertain.

ELECTROPHYSIOLOGY OF THE TRANSPLANTED HEART

Minor electrophysiological abnormalities occur commonly in transplanted hearts. Following orthotopic transplantation, the residual recipient atrium and the donor atrium remain separated electrically, and independent activity (including arrhythmias) can be recorded electrophysiologically[49].

In the early postoperative period, sinus node dysfunction occurs in about half the patients studied[50]. If this dysfunction is persistent, it may indicate a poor prognosis[50]. Long-term survivors have a high incidence of abnormal sinus node function as measured by sinus node recovery time[51]. Conduction time through the atria is delayed in these patients with a resultant prolonged PR interval[51].

Denervation appears to have little influence on the resting electrophysiological characteristics of the atrioventricular conduction system[52]. However, on exercise, when heart rate is increased, the expected decrease in functional refractory period does not occur[53]. Some patients may have dual atrioventricular nodal pathways[51] but no episodes of sustained re-entrant tachycardia have been reported.

Extensive electrophysiological studies of the ventricles have not been reported[49].

Denervation does not protect the transplanted heart from arrhythmias[53,54]. In one study, atrial arrhythmias occurred in 72% of patients and ventricular arrhythmias in 57%. In other studies, ventricular premature activity was even more common[55]. Arrhythmias, especially atrial arrhythmias, appear to be related to periods of acute rejection[53,54] and respond to treatment of the rejection, or to antiarrhythmic drugs such as quinidine. Complex ventricular arrhythmias, usually related to underlying accelerated atherosclerosis, often herald sudden death[53,55]. The increased sensitivity of the transplanted heart to catecholamines[26,27], and the lack of suppressant vagal tone, may be significant factors in the pathogenesis of the arrhythmias[53,54].

PHARMACOLOGY OF THE TRANSPLANTED HEART

Data concerning the pharmacology of the transplanted heart are limited. A number of general principles may, however, be applied.

Firstly, drugs (such as atropine, edrophonium, digitalis, and pancuronium) whose effect is mediated via the autonomic nervous system (sympathetic and parasympathetic) will have no effect on the transplanted heart. Only drugs which act on the heart directly will have any effect. Secondly, denervation of the heart may result in an enhanced response to certain drugs (e.g. β-receptor stimulants). Thirdly, drugs which are negatively inotropic or which have an effect on the peripheral vasculature may have a profound effect on cardiac performance, as the transplanted heart relies mainly on the Frank–Starling mechanism and on changes in contractility for its stress response.

A few drugs should be considered in more detail.

Digoxin

The primary effect of digoxin in normally innervated hearts is mediated through the autonomic nervous system. Thus, digoxin has a significant vagally-mediated effect on atrioventricular (AV) nodal conduction, prolonging both the effective refractory period and the functional refractory period, irrespective of cycle length[56]. There is a lesser effect on sinus node function, with slight increases in cycle length, sinus node recovery time, and sinoatrial conduction time occurring in response to digoxin[57]. In the denervated, transplanted heart, digoxin has only a minimal[58] effect on the AV node[28,58] with mild depression of AV nodal conduction becoming evident after long-term administration. There is virtually no effect on sinus node function[57] (although sinoatrial exit block has been produced in one patient).

The therapeutic implications of these findings are that the effect of digoxin on AV conduction in the transplanted heart is blunted and the amount of slowing of the ventricular response in atrial fibrillation is less than occurs in innervated hearts.

In normally innervated hearts, digoxin in higher dosage has been shown to augment sympathetic nerve activity[59] and this may predispose to digoxin-induced ventricular arrhythmias. Whether arrhythmias caused by digoxin toxicity are less common in the transplanted heart is, however, unknown.

The direct inotropic effects of digoxin on the myocardium and the vasoconstrictive effects on the peripheral circulation remain unchanged[49].

Inotropic agents

Cardiac denervation results in depletion of myocardial catecholamines. Increased sensitivity to circulating catecholamines ensues, as can be evidenced by the enhanced inotropic and chronotropic response of the transplanted heart to agents such as epinephrine, norepinephrine and isoproteronol[5,26,27]. This sensitivity appears to be mediated by a change in the state ('up-regulation') of the β-receptors. Other inotropic agents (e.g. dopamine and dobutamine), whose actions are mediated via β-receptors, could be expected to have a similarly enhanced effect.

β-receptor blockers

The catecholamine-depleted transplanted heart is dependent on circulating catecholamines for chronotropic and inotropic alterations in response to exercise[27,34]. β-blocker administration, by inhibiting these responses to circulating catecholamines, dramatically reduces the exercise capability of transplant recipients[34].

β-blockers, nevertheless, appear to be reasonably well tolerated when used to treat cyclosporine-induced hypertension[49]. The resting heart rate of transplanted hearts, however, is not reduced by β-blockers[49], reflecting the lack of influence of circulating catecholamines on the transplanted resting heart rate.

Calcium antagonists

The calcium antagonists all have direct binding sites on the myocardium, and most of their cardiac effects are direct.

These direct cardiac effects may, however, be modified by reflex secondary effects mediated via the autonomic nervous system or by circulating catecholamines. The autonomic reflexes in response to vasodilation, however, are absent in transplant recipients.

Verapamil

The electrophysiological effects (negative chronotropic and negative dromotropic) of verapamil are accentuated in transplanted hearts[60] because of the absence of the indirect effect of verapamil (augmentation of sympathetic neural tone). The time course of action is also modified, the drug having a more rapid response.

Nifedipine

A mild tachycardia occurs in the transplanted heart 10–20 minutes after the administration of nifedipine[49], probably because of an increase in circulating catecholamines which result from the vasodilating effect of nifedipine. Nifedipine has no direct electrophysiological action on the sinus node or on the AV node[49].

Vasodilators

Vasodilators should be used cautiously as the abolition of reflex homeostatic mechanisms (e.g. reflex tachycardia) may exaggerate the hemodynamic effects of these agents.

Hydralazine has been used to control cyclosporin-induced hypertension with success.

Antiarrhythmic agents

Ventricular and supraventricular arrhythmias of the transplanted heart appear to be associated most commonly with acute rejection. Treatment of the rejection is normally sufficient to abolish these arrhythmias[53,54].

Quinidine gluconate has been used successfully as an antiarrhythmic agent in the transplanted heart, suggesting that innervation is not required for its antiarrhythmic actions[54]. In the denervated heart the vagolytic effect of quinidine is not seen and so both sinus rate and AV conduction are slowed (in contradistinction to its effect in the innervated heart)[61]. Intraventricular conduction is also slowed (as in the innervated heart).

Most antiarrhythmic agents are negatively inotropic and some may have effects on the peripheral circulation. They should thus be used with due caution.

References

1. Braunwald, E. (1974). Regulation of the circulation. *N. Engl. J. Med.*, **290**, 1124 (part 1), 1420 (part 2)
2. Braunwald, E. and Ross, J. (1979). Control of cardiac performance. In Berne, R.M. (ed.) *Handbook of Physiology*. Section 2, Vol. 1, p. 533. (Bethesda: American Physiological Society)
3. Braunwald, E. (1971). Structure and function of the normal myocardium. *Br. Heart J.*, **33** (Suppl.), 3
4. Beck, W., Barnard, C.N. and Schrire, V. (1969). Heart rate after cardiac transplantation. *Circulation*, **40**, 437
5. Carleton, R.A., Heller, S.J., Najafi, H. and Clark, J.G. (1969). Hemodynamic performance of a transplanted human heart. *Circulation*, **40**, 447
6. Stinson, E.B., Griepp, R.B., Schroeder, J.S., Dong, E. and Shumway, N.E. (1972). Hemodynamic observations one and two years after cardiac transplantation in man. *Circulation*, **45**, 1183
7. Beck, W., Barnard, C.N. and Schrire, V. (1971). Hemodynamic studies in two long-term survivors of heart transplantation. *J. Thorac. Cardiovasc. Surg.*, **62**, 315
8. Pope, S.E., Stinson, E.B., Daughters, G.T., Schroeder, J.S., Ingels, N.B. and Alderman, E.L. (1980). Exercise response of the denervated heart in long-term cardiac transplant recipients. *Am. J. Cardiol.*, **46**, 213
9. McLaughlin, P.R., Kleinman, J.H., Martin, R.P., Doherty, P.W., Reitz, B., Stinson, E.B., Daughters, G.T., Ingels, N.B. and Alderman, E.L. (1978). The effect of exercise and atrial pacing on left ventricular volume and contractility in patients with innervated and denervated hearts. *Circulation*, **58**, 476
10. Clark, D.A., Schroeder, J.S., Griepp, R.B., Stinson, E.B., Dong, E., Shumway, N.E. and Harrison, D.C. (1973). Cardiac transplantation in man: review of first three years experience. *Am. J. Med.*, **54**, 563
11. Christophersen, L.K., Griepp, R.B. and Stinson, E.B. (1976). Rehabilitation after cardiac transplantation. *J. Am. Med. Assoc.*, **236**, 2082
12. Hunt, S.A., Rider, A.K., Stinson, E.B., Griepp, R.B., Schroeder, J.S., Harrison, D.C. and Shumway, N.E. (1975). Does cardiac transplantation prolong life and improve its quality? An updated report. *Circulation*, **54** (Suppl.3), 56
13. Cory-Pearce, R., Wheeldon, D.R., Wallwork, J. and English, T.A.H. (1983). Late cardiac function after heart transplantation. *J. Am. Coll. Cardiol.*, **1**, 721
14. Savin, W.M., Gordon, E., Green, S., Haskell, W., Kantrowitz, N., Lundberg, M., Melvin, K., Sonnelson, R., Verschagin, K. and Schroeder, J.S. (1983). Comparison of exercise training effects in cardiac denervated and innervated humans. *J. Am. Coll. Cardiol.*, **1**, 722
15. Savin, W.M., Schroeder, J.S. and Haskell, W.L. (1982). Response of cardiac transplant recipients to static and dynamic exercise: review. *Heart Transplant.*, **1**, 72
16. Phlugfelder, P.W., Pulves, P.D., McKenzie, F.N. and Kostuk, W.J. (1987). Cardiac dynamics during supine exercise in cyclosporine-treated orthotopic heart transplant recipient: assessment by radionuclide angiography. *J. Am. Coll. Cardiol.*, **10**, 336
17. Corcos, T., Tamburino, C., Leger, P., Vaissier, E., Rossant, P., Mattei, M., Drudon, P., Gandjbakhch, I., Pavie, A., Cabrol, A. and Cabrol, C. (1988). Early and late hemodynamic evaluation after cardiac transplantation: a study of 28 cases. *J. Am. Coll. Cardiol.*, **11**, 264
18. Savin, W.M., Haskell, W.L., Schroeder, J.S. and Stinson, E.B. (1980). Cardio-respiratory responses in cardiac transplant patients to graded symptom-limited exercise. *Circulation*, **62**, 55
19. Greenberg, M.L., Uretsky, B.F., Reddy, P.S., Bernstein, R.L., Griffith, B.P., Hardesty, R.L., Thompson, M.E. and Bahnson, H.T. (1985). Long-term hemodynamic follow-up of cardiac transplant patients treated with cyclosporine and prednisone. *Circulation*, **71**, 487
20. Frist, W.H., Oyer, P.E. and Shumway, N.E. (1987). Long-term hemodynamic results after cardiac transplantation. *J. Thorac. Cardiovasc. Surg.*, **94**, 685

21. Deniveni, R., McKenzie, N., Kostuk, W.J., Heimbecker, R.O., Keown, P., Stiller, C. and Silver, M.D. (1983). Cyclosporine in cardiac transplantation: observations on immunologic monitoring, cardiac histology and cardiac function. *Heart Transplant.*, **2**, 219
22. Hastillo, A., Wolfgang, T.C., Tatum, J., Romhilt, S., Szentpetery, S., Lower, R. R. and Hess, M.L. (1983). Long-term prospective evaluation of cardiac allograft function utilizing exercise treadmill testing and gated pool scintigraphy. *Circulation*, **68** (Suppl.3), 183
23. Borow, K.M., Neumann, A., Arensman, F.W. and Yacoub, M.H. (1985). Left ventricular contractility and contractile reserve in humans after cardiac transplantation. *Circulation*, **71**, 866
24. Valentine, H.A., Fowler, M.B., Hunt, S.A., Naasz, C., Hatle, L.K., Billingham, M.E., Stinson, E.B. and Popp, R.L. (1987). Changes in Doppler echocardiographic indices of left ventricular function as potential markers of acute cardiac rejection. *Circulation*, **76** (Suppl.5), V86
25. Mohanty, P.K., Sowers, J.R., Thames, M.D., Beck, F.W.J., Kawaguchi, A. and Lower, R.R. (1986). Myocardial norepinephrine, epinephrine and dopamine concentrations after cardiac autotransplantation in dogs. *J. Am. Coll. Cardiol.*, **7**, 419
26. Donald, D.E. and Shepherd, J.T. (1965). Supersensitivity to L. norepinephrine of the denervated sinoatrial node. *Am. J. Physiol.*, **208**, 255
27. Ebert, P.A. (1968). The effects of norepinephrine infusion on the denervated heart. *J. Cardiovasc. Surg.*, **9**, 414
28. Magovern, J.A., Pennock, J.L., Oaks, T.G., Campbell, D.B., Burg, J.E. and Hersey, R.M. (1987). Atrial natriuretic peptide in recipients of human orthotopic heart transplants. *J. Heart Transplant.*, **6**, 193
29. Kivowitz, C., Parmely, W.W., Donoso, R., Marcus, H., Ganz, W. and Swan, H.J.C. (1971). Effects of isometric exercise on cardiac performance. The grip test. *Circulation*, **44**, 994
30. Helfant, R.H., DeVilla, M.A. and Meister, S.G. (1971). Effect of sustained isometric handgrip exercise on left ventricular performance. *Circulation*, **44**, 982
31. Savin, W.M., Alderman, E.L., Haskell, W.L., Schroeder, J.S., Ingels, N.B., Daughters, G.T. and Stinson, E.B. (1980). Left ventricular response to isometric exercise in patients with denervated and innervated hearts. *Circulation*, **61**, 897
32. Haskell, W.L., Savin, W.M., Schroeder, J.S., Alderman, E.A., Ingels, N.B., Daughters, G.T. and Stinson, E.B. (1981). Cardiovascular responses to handgrip isometric exercise in patients following cardiac transplantation. *Circ. Res.*, **48** (Suppl. 1), 156
33. Donald, D.E. and Samueloff, S.L. (1966). Exercise tachycardia not due to blood-borne agents in canine cardiac denervation. *Am. J. Physiol.*, **211**, 703
34. Bexton, R., Milne, J., Cory-Pearce, R., English, T.A.H. and Camm, A.J. (1983). Effect of β-blockade on the exercise response following cardiac transplantation. *J. Am. Coll. Cardiol.*, **1**, 722
35. Barnard, C.N. and Beck, W. (1972). The physiology of the transplanted heart. In Wells, C., Kyle, J. and Dunphy, J.E. (eds.) *Scientific Foundations of Surgery.*, 2nd ed. p. 185. (London: Heinemann Medical)
36. Starling, E.H. (1915). *The Linacre Lecture of the Law of the Heart.* (London: Heinemann Medical)
37. Frank, O. (1959). On the dynamics of cardiac muscle. (Translated by Chapman, C.B. and Wasserman, E.). *Am. Heart J.*, **58**, 282 and 467
38. Sarnoff, S.J. and Berglung, E. (1954). Ventricular function. I. Starling's law of the heart studied by means of simultaneous right and left ventricular function curves in the dog. *Circulation*, **9**, 706
39. Donald, D.E. and Shepherd, J.T. (1964). Initial cardiovascular adjustment to exercise in dogs with chronic cardiac denervation. *Am. J. Physiol.*, **207**, 1325
40. Niset, G., Poortmans, J.R., Leclerc, Q., Brasseur, M., Desmet, J.M., Degre, S. and Primo, G. (1985). Metabolic implications during a 20 km run after heart transplantation. *Int. J. Sports Med.*, **6**, 340
41. Bhatia, S.J.S., Kirshenbaum, J.M., Shemin, R.J., Cohn, L.H., Collins, J.J., Di Sesa, V., Young, P.J., Mudge, G.H. and Sutton, M.G. St. J. (1987). Time course of resolution of pulmonary hypertension of right ventricular remodelling after orthotopic cardiac transplantation. *Circulation*, **76**, 819
42. Olivari, M.T., Levine, T.B., Ring, W.S., Simon, A. and Cohn, J.N. (1987). Normalization of sympathetic nervous system function after orthotopic cardiac transplant in man. *Circulation*, **76** (Suppl.5), V62
43. Allen, M.D., Naasz, C.A., Popp, R.L., Hunt, S.A., Goris, M.L., Oyer, P.E. and Stinson, E.B. (1988). Non-invasive assessment of donor and native heart function after heterotopic heart transplantation. *J. Thorac. Cardiovasc. Surg.*, **95**, 75
44. Beck, W. and Gersh, B.J. (1976). Left ventricular bypass using a cardiac allograft: hemodynamic studies. *Am. J. Cardiol.*, **37**, 1007
45. Losman, J.G., Barnard, C.N. and Bartley, T.D. (1977). Hemodynamic evaluation of left ventricular bypass with a homologous cardiac graft. *J. Thorac. Cardiovasc. Surg.*, **74**, 6695
46. Melvin, K.R., Pollick, C., Hunt, S.A., McDougall, R., Goris, M.L., Oyer, P.E., Popp, R.L. and Stinson, E.B. (1982). Cardiovascular physiology in a case of heterotopic cardiac transplantation. *Am. J. Cardiol.*, **49**, 1301
47. Kennelly, B.M., Piller, L.W., Tarjan, P.P., Losman, J.G., Barnard, C.N. and Beck, W. (1978). Use of a double atrial triggered standby pacemaker system for a patient with a biventricular bypass heterotopic cardiac homograft. *Am. J. Cardiol.*, **41**, 341
48. Cooper, D.K.C. (1984). Orthotopic and heterotopic transplantation of the heart – the Cape Town experience. *Ann. Roy. Coll. Surg.*, **66**, 228
49. Thompson, M.E., Dummer, J.S., Griffith, B.P., Hardesty, R.L., Shapiro, A.P. and Rabin, B.S. (1985). Cardiac transplantation 1985; hope – promise – reality. *Prog. Cardiol.*, **14**, 191
50. Mackintosh, A.F., Carmichael, D.J., Wren, C., Cory-Pearce, R. and English, T.A.H. (1982). Sinus node function in the first three weeks after cardiac transplantation. *Br. Heart J.*, **48**, 584
51. Bexton, R.S., Nathan, A.W., Hellestrand, K.J., Cory-Pearce, R., Spurrell, R.A.J., English, T.A.H. and Camm, A.J. (1984). The electrophysiologic characteristics of the transplanted human heart. *Br. Heart J.*, **50**, 555
52. Bexton, R.S., Nathan, A.W., Hellestrand, K.J., Cory-Pearce, R., Spurrell, R.A.J., English, T.A.H. and Camm, A.J. (1984). The electrophysiologic characteristics of the transplanted human heart. *Am. Heart J.*, **107**, 1
53. Berke, D.K., Graham, A.F., Schroeder, J.S. and Harrison, D.C. (1973). Arrhythmias in the denervated transplanted human heart. *Circulation*, **48** (Cardiovascular Surg. Suppl. 3), 112
54. Schroeder, J.S., Berke, D.K., Graham, A.F., Rider, A.K. and Harrison, D.C. (1974). Arrhythmias after cardiac transplantation. *Am. J. Cardiol.*, **33**, 604
55. Romhilt, D.W., Doyle, M., Sagar, K.B., Hastillo, A., Wolfgang, T.C., Lower, R.R. and Hess, M.L. (1982). Prevalence and significance of ventricular arrhythmias in long-term survivors of cardiac transplantation. *Circulation*, **66** (Suppl.1), 219
56. Goodman, D.J., Rossen, R.M., Cannon, D.S., Rider, A.K. and Harrison, D.C. (1975). Effects of digoxin on atrioventricular conduction studies in patients with and without autonomic innervation. *Circulation*, **51**, 251
57. Goodman, D.J., Rossen, R.M., Ingham, R., Rider, A.K. and Harrison, D.C. (1975). Sinus node function in the denervated human heart. Effect of digitalis. *Br. Heart J.*, **37**, 612
58. Gillis, R.A., Raines, A., Sohn, Y. J., Levitt, B. and Standaert, F.G. (1972). Neuroexcitatory effects of digitalis and their role in the development of cardiac arrhythmias. *J. Pharmacol. Exp. Ther.*, **183**, 154
59. Goodman, D.J., Rossen, R.M., Cannom, D.S., Rider, A.K. and Harrison, D.C. (1975). Effect of digoxin on atrioventricular conduction; studies in patients with and without cardiac autonomic innervation. *Circulation*, **52**, 251
60. Qi, A., Tuna, I.C., Gornick, C., Barragry, T.P., Blatchford, J.N.,

Ring, W.S., Bolman, R.M., Walker, M.J. and Benditt, D.G. (1987). Potentiation of cardiac electrophysiologic effects of verapamil after autonomic blockade or cardiac transplantation. *Circulation*, **75**, 88

61. Mason, J.W., Winkle, R.A., Rider, A.K., Stinson, E.B. and Harrison, D.C. (1977). The electrophysiologic effects of quinidine in the transplanted human heart. *J. Clin. Invest.*, **59**, 481

14
Immunobiology of Allograft Destruction
D. NOVITZKY AND D.K.C. COOPER

INTRODUCTION

The processes involved in donor antigen presentation and recognition, in host cell activation and proliferation, ultimately leading to graft destruction, are complex, and, as more is known of them, are becoming increasingly so. No attempt will be made in this chapter to detail the many ramifications of what is known regarding the mechanisms of allograft destruction, but an effort will be made to outline and illustrate the major steps involved.

The mechanism by which the recipient's immune system attempts to destroy the allograft involves both cellular[1] and humoral[2] responses, which respectively take a few days and approximately 2 weeks to become effective in the non-sensitized subject. The cellular response is largely a function of the T-lymphocytes, though other cells are involved. The humoral response, the production of antibodies, is a function of B-lymphocytes.

The two major subpopulations of lymphocytes are T-lymphocytes, whose maturation depends on the thymus, and B-lymphocytes, which in mammals are derived from bone marrow cells. The T-lymphocytes are further subdivided into at least three main groups: (1) cytotoxic T-cells (CTC), which cause the lysis of allograft cells, (2) helper T-cells (TH), which are responsible for enhancing both the humoral and cell-mediated responses, and (3) suppressor T-cells (TS), which may inhibit these responses (for example, by suppressing antibody formation by B-cells).

A delicate balance exists between two key cells in the body – T-helper and T-suppressor – and is essential for immunological equilibrium in the normal subject. An imbalance in this equilibrium, e.g. towards the T-helper cells, may precipitate an autoimmune disease, such as lupus erythematosus or other collagen disease[3]. Similarly, any imbalance involving, for example, B-cells may alter this equilibrium.

THE MAJOR HISTOCOMPATIBLITY COMPLEX

The major histocompatibility complex (MHC) – in man, the human leukocyte antigen (HLA) system (Chapter 8) – regulates the immune response. Class I MHC antigens, determined by the HLA-A, B, and C loci, are found on the surface of virtually all nucleated cells and platelets[4], and are recognized by unprimed cytotoxic T-cells, which bear distinctive surface molecules known as CD8 (CD = cluster of differentiation). Several laboratories have reported low levels of MHC Class I antigens on myocytes[4,5], though these can be increased in certain pathological states.

The donor organ interstitium presents dendritic cells of mononuclear–macrophage lineage, as well as other mononuclear cells, such as lymphocytes; these can be grouped together under the name 'passenger leukocytes'[6]. (Following transplantation, these dendritic cells are replaced within a few weeks by those of recipient lineage.) This group of cells has a rich expression of MHC Class II antigens[7], which represent the HLA-D (DP, DQ, and DR) loci. These donor dendritic cells and macrophages are capable of presenting donor antigens directly to host lymphoid cells. Alloantigens on some parenchymal cells of the transplanted organ are taken up by recipient monocytes/macrophages, which, because they enable the antigens to be recognized by the T-helper cell (bearing CD4 molecules), are known as antigen-presenting cells (APC)[8]. Donor dendritic cells and macrophages that process and present their own antigens are thus able to act as their own antigen-presenting cells.

Vascular endothelial cells express low levels of both Class I and Class II antigens[9].

Following allografting, the introduction of one or more mismatch across the MHC Class I and/or Class II barrier (or across a minor histocompatibility complex) will be recognized by host cell surface receptors, resulting in the activation of an immunological cascade characterized by activation of various lymphocytes, macrophages, and monocytes, and the production of humoral factors such as antibodies and eicosanoids; other factors, such as complement, may also be involved[5] (Figure 14.1). The effect of this antigen recognition and cell proliferation is a cellular response within the graft, resulting in acute rejection (Figure 14.2). The inflammatory infiltrate in the transplanted cardiac graft is targeted to the antigens expressed on connective

THE TRANSPLANTATION AND REPLACEMENT OF THORACIC ORGANS

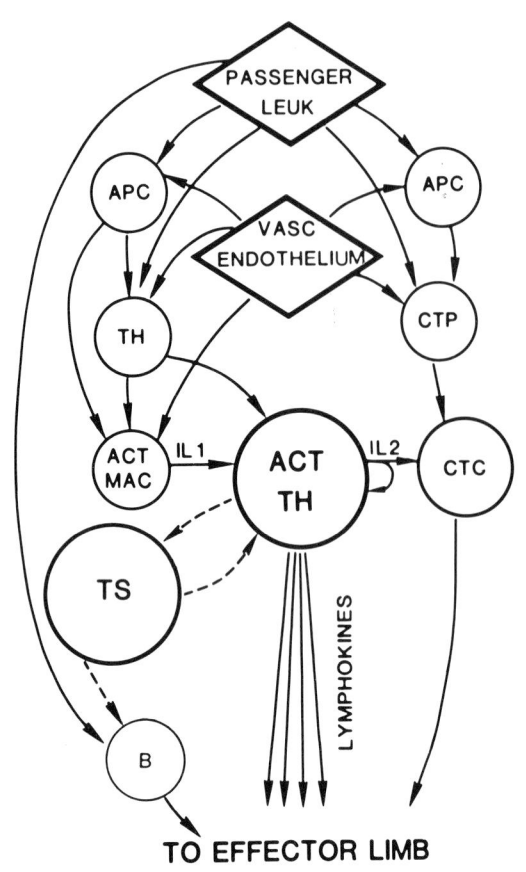

Figure 14.1 The first stages in the immune response to an allografted organ – antigen processing and presentation, cell differentiation and proliferation.

Alloantigen is expressed on (1) passenger leukocytes (dendritic cells, lymphocytes and plasma cells) in the grafted organ and (2) the vascular endothelium of the organ. This antigen may be taken up by antigen-presenting cells (APC) which expose it to T-helper cells (TH), unprimed cytotoxic T-cells (CTP), and macrophages (MAC). The influence of activated macrophages on T-helper cells, in part by the production of interleukin-1 (IL1), sometimes known as T-cell growth factor, is essential to enable the T-helper cells to become fully activated (ACT.TH). These, in turn, produce a variety of bioactive proteins known as lymphokines, including interleukin-2 (IL2) which plays a part in the maturation of cytotoxic T-cells (CTC).

B-cells, cytotoxic T-cells, and the lymphokines produced by T-helper cells play a major role in the so-called effector limb of allograft destruction (Figure 14.2). T-suppressor cells (TS) may play a significant role by modifying the activity of many other cells, particularly activated T-helper cells. The sequence of events that leads to T-helper cell activation is largely dependent on presentation and recognition of HLA Class II antigens, whereas those that result in cytotoxic T-cell maturation are largely dependent on presentation and recognition of HLA Class I antigens

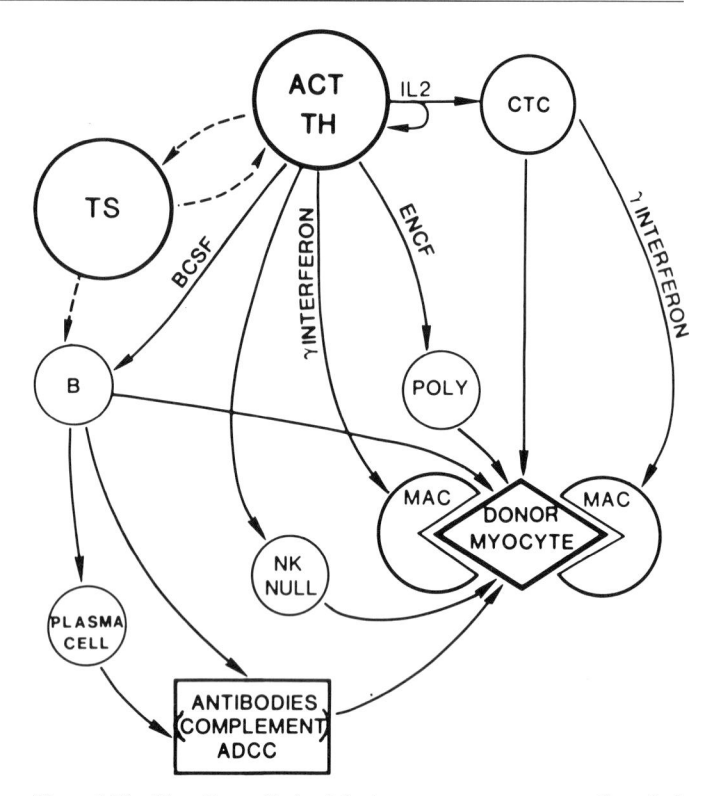

Figure 14.2 The efferent limb of the immune response to an allografted organ – destruction of the graft.

Cell-mediated rejection is effected by a diverse range of white blood cells, including T-helper cells (TH) (sometimes referred to as CD4-cells as they bear a distinctive surface protein molecule), cytotoxic T-cells (CTC) (CD8-cells), antibody-forming B-cells (B), and macrophages (MAC). The lymphokines produced by the activated T-helper cells (ACT.TH) recruit and influence several other cells (e.g. B-cells (B), natural killer (NK) and null cells, macrophages (MAC), and polymorphs (POLY) toward destruction of the graft (the donor myocyte). Examples of lymphokines shown in this figure are (1) B-cell stimulating factor (BCSF), (2) γ interferon or macrophage-activating factor (γ interferon), (3) eosinophil–neutrophil chemotactic factor (ENCF), and (4) interleukin-2 (IL2). B-cells and plasma cells produce antibodies that may destroy the graft alone (in the presence of complement) or may be essential for the destructive activity of certain cells – the so-called antibody-dependent cytotoxicity (ADCC).

T-suppressor cells (TS) may play a significant role in modifying the action of other cells

tissue cells (dendritic cells, monocytes, macrophages), blood vessels (vascular endothelium), and the surface of myocytes[5,6].

Myocyte and endothelial injury has been observed during brain death, and also during any ischemic period, such as ischemic transportation of the heart. This injury may 'up-regulate' Class I and Class II antigens on the cell surfaces, resulting in a more vivid expression of the antigens, and therefore a more rapid activation of host cells[7].

THE AFFERENT LIMB – ANTIGENIC RECOGNITION, CELL DIFFERENTIATION AND PROLIFERATION (Figure 14.1)

The induction of the immunological stimulus for graft rejection is currently based on the Lafferty–Bach–Bachelor concept[8–10]. The afferent limb of the rejection response is initially characterized by antigen presentation and processing. The first pathway results from the presence of donor histocompatibility antigens on graft passenger leukocytes (in particular, those expressed on dendritic cells) and vascular endothelial cells[5]. There is presentation of graft antigens by donor or recipient antigen-presenting cells to host lymphocytes and macrophages[11], resulting in 'activation' of macrophages and T-helper cells.

The antigen-presenting cells and activated macrophages also provide a second signal, interleukin-1 (IL-1), which helps to stimulate T-helper cell (CD4) activation. The response of the host is thought by some to be proportional to the extent of Class II MHC expression on the donor endothelial cells and passenger leukocytes[5]. Activated macrophages are essential in the process of activating the T-helper cells, partly by the production of IL-1. In turn, the activated T-helper cells up-regulate the expression of Class II antigens on the myocytes, thus enhancing graft antigen recognition further[8]. Interleukin-2 (T-cell growth factor), produced by the activated T-helper cells, contributes to proliferation of cytotoxic T-cells.

A strong blastogenesis and proliferation of recipient lymphoid cells is then observed in the graft[12]. The proliferative response spreads throughout the recipient's lymphoreticular system. Different activated cells will appear in the circulating blood, as will the by-products (e.g. alloantibodies) of differentiated lymphocytes[13].

THE EFFERENT LIMB – ANTIBODY PRODUCTION AND CELLULAR INFILTRATION OF THE GRAFT (Figure 14.2)

Once antigenic recognition has taken place, there is cell differentiation, resulting in a balance in favor of T-helper cells (over T-suppressor cells). Several different effector pathways have been identified. The T-helper cells synthesize a variety of bioactive proteins called lymphokines that recruit and activate other cells (e.g. natural killer cells, polymorphs, macrophages) against the allograft[3]. Important lymphokines include γ interferon (macrophage activating factor (MAF)), and B-cell stimulating growth factor (BCSF). Antibody-dependent cytotoxicity is also stimulated by the influence of T-helper cell-produced lymphokines on B-cells[2].

The effector limb is primarily characterized by cellular infiltration of the graft[5,6]. The first cells to appear in the allograft are lymphocytes and monocytes. There follows a blastogenic response in situ[14]. Lymphocytes are primarily confined to the perivascular regions of the graft. Mononuclear macrophages are distributed throughout the allograft parenchyma, making close contact with the myocytes. These features would suggest that the various inflammatory cell groups display different and specific functions to bring about destruction of the allograft[5,6]. The intense perivascular cuffing, seen mainly around small vessels and capillaries, would indicate that these structures stimulate a greater response of host cells.

In unmodified rejection, there is cell migration to and from the allograft, with an exponential increase of this exchange up to day 4. After this, the exchange declines. Lymphocytes continue to proliferate in their original compartment – either in the graft or the host lymphoreticular system – with exchange of cells between these compartments[5,6].

In acute cellular rejection, the T-cell response is dominant. The B-cell response is variable, being frequently small or imperceptible after allografting in non-sensitized individuals, but often playing an important role in patients sensitized by previous transplantation, blood transfusion, or pregnancy. The final differentiation of B-lymphocytes is into plasma cells, which mediate humoral mechanisms of acute rejection (the production of alloantibodies) and sensitization of the recipient, and play a role in both hyperacute and chronic rejection. When it is involved in the rejection process, the humoral mechanism is characterized by a strong B-cell proliferation in the graft. The proliferating B-blast produces immunoglobulins (IgM and IgG). On occasions, the humoral response can be particularly aggressive, and destruction of myocardial cells may be rapid[15].

Though so much is now known about the complex steps which occur during antigen recognition, cell differentiation and proliferation, and even of the effector mechanisms, less is certain about the exact mode by which these cells bring about destruction of the myocytes. There is evidence that direct cytolysis[16] and delayed-type hypersensitivity[17] play a role in graft destruction.

Cytotoxicity in the form of actual lysis of donor cells can be induced by (1) T-lymphocytes, (2) natural killer (NK) cells, (3) macrophages, and (4) complement. T-cell cytotoxicity is thought to be the most important mechanism by which allografts are destroyed. Cytotoxic T-cells kill donor cells rapidly in an antigen-specific fashion without requirement for antibody. Antibody-dependent cell-mediated cytotoxicity (ADCC) is another important pathway which can cause destruction of the allograft[18,19]. Various cell types require antibodies for killing; their effect will therefore be delayed until antibodies have been produced. The cell must attach itself to the exposed Fc fragment of antibody already bound to the target cell in order to produce damage. The role of NK cells remains unclear, although they can be found at the allograft site in large numbers. The activated macrophage also contributes to graft destruction by various mechanisms[20], including the production of proteases and eicosanoids. Antibodies produced by B-cells can also cause cell destruction, but only in the presence of complement; this occurs in episodes of hyperacute rejection[15,19].

Each of these types of cytotoxicity may act alone or in concert to destroy an allograft. Current and future improvements in immunosuppression depend on a knowledge of these mechanisms and on our ability to modify them.

MECHANISMS OF IMMUNOSUPPRESSIVE DRUGS IN MODIFYING THE IMMUNE RESPONSE

(Drug therapy in the prevention and treatment of acute rejection is also discussed in Chapters 12 and 16).

Corticosteroids

The beneficial effect of corticosteroids is mediated partly by inhibition of interleukin-1[21]. Since interleukin-2 release is dependent on interleukin-1, corticosteroids therefore also indirectly reduce interleukin-2 production[22,23]. Much of the efficiency of corticosteroid therapy is related to non-specific immunosuppressive and anti-inflammatory effects, and to the inhibition of migration of immune cells to the graft. There is also evidence they (1) impair antigen recognition, (2) interfere with macrophage function, and (3) at very high doses, interfere with some membrane functions of lymphocytes[24-26]. Corticosteroids may also have a cytotoxic effect on lymphocytes, probably by increasing cytoplasmic calcium.

Azathioprine

Azathioprine, a purine analogue, is useful in the prevention of acute rejection rather than the reversal of established rejection. Its effect is as an antimetabolite to DNA replication[27]. Azathioprine's effect is basically non-specific, affecting all rapidly dividing cells[28]. It reduces or prevents the rapid cell division that is an important part of the immune system response, thus blunting the ability of the host to generate cytotoxic T-cells[29]. Though it is active on B-cells, this activity is much less than on T-cells, which accounts for its suppression of cell-mediated rejection with less effect on antibody production.

Cyclophosphamide

Cyclophosphamide, an alkylating agent, has a more marked effect on B-cells than does azathioprine[27]. The alkyl groups attach to DNA, interfere with its integrity, and thereby produce significant cytotoxic effects.

Cyclosporine

The immunosuppressive effect of cyclosporine is much more specific than that of corticosteroids, azathioprine, or cyclophosphamide. The critical phase in the maturation of T-helper cells is the synthesis of lymphokines; cyclosporine blocks this synthesis. Its main mechanism of action is to inhibit interleukin-2 production and, to a lesser extent, interleukin-1[30,31]. This action effectively prevents the development of mature cytotoxic T-cells, and also prevents release of both γ interferon (macrophage-activating factor) and B-cell activating factors.

Cyclosporine has little or no effect on antigen-presenting cells, and does not result in bone marrow suppression. Its prime value is in the prevention of rejection by shutting down the effector limb (Figure 14.2). Cyclosporine decreases T-helper cell activity, though T-suppressor cell activity remains at a normal level. The drug has no direct effect on macrophage function[32].

T-cell antibodies (monoclonal and polyclonal)

Monoclonal T-cell antibodies are directed to, and block, the recognition of antigen by the recipient circulating T-cells. Receptors are found on all circulating human T-cells[33], and monoclonal antibodies can be raised against any T-cell subset. The modes of action of monoclonal antibodies include removal of T-cells from the circulation by complement-mediated lysis or by the reticuloendothelial system, and coating of cell surface antigens[34,35].

OKT-3 monoclonal antibody (which is directed against T-cells bearing the CD3 antigen, and is therefore virtually a pan-T-cell antibody) directly binds to the cell surface antigen, leading to loss of the cell's recognition apparatus[36]; these T-cells can therefore play no further part in the acute rejection process. The initial decline in the number of T-cells following institution of OKT-3 therapy is probably brought about by opsonization of the cell surface, and removal of the cells by the reticuloendothelial system of the host[37]. Many monoclonal antibodies (other then OKT3) have been, or are currently being developed, e.g. those directed toward other antigens present on T-cell surfaces, such as the T4 (CD4) antigen on T-helper cells, and those directed against interleukin-2 receptor sites.

Similar effects are observed after therapy with polyclonal antibodies, such as antithymocyte globulin (ATG) or anti-lymphocyte globulin (ALG), though the response is less specific. Theoretically, though this is not always so in practice, only T-cells are affected when ATG is administered, and both T- and B-cells are involved when ALG is administered. ATG has also been shown to decrease NK-cell cytotoxicity. The combined effect of this agent on both T- and NK-cell reactivity explains its potent antirejection activity relative to steroids and azathioprine. (A similar result can be obtained by thoracic duct drainage[38], though this method of immunosuppression has been replaced by drug therapy.)

Immunosuppression with monoclonal antibodies is clearly more specific than with ATG or ALG. Monoclonal antibodies have the advantages (over ATG and ALG) of better consistency in preparation, greater ease in monitoring serum levels, and administration of less foreign protein. As the immune response is so complex, however, at times there may be advantages of ATG or ALG in destroying or inhibiting a wider spectrum of lymphocytes.

Total lymphoid irradiation

Irradiation leads to DNA damage resulting in cell death during mitotic division[39]. The small lymphocytes, which are highly radiosensitive, are destroyed, resulting in loss of responsiveness to allogenic stimulation. There may also be a greater depletion of T-helper cells, creating an imbalance with T-suppressor cells[39].

COMMENT

Optimal combinations of immunosuppressive agents can only be arrived at rationally and effectively by a full understanding of the site and mode of action of each agent. As our knowledge of the various mechanisms that play a role in allograft destruction increases, so it should become possible to devise more sophisticated methods of blocking the sequence of events outlined in this chapter. For example, monoclonal antibodies are being developed against the various cellular components (e.g. macrophages) that play important roles in allograft destruction. The clinical employment of such agents may eventually enable graft destruction to be prevented, and yet allow the body to maintain all or most of its other host defense mechanisms.

References

1. Ascher, N.L., Hoffman, R.A., Hanto, T.W. and Simmons, R.L. (1984). Cellular basis of allograft rejection. *Immunol. Rev.*, **77**, 217
2. Milgrom, F. (1977). The role of humoral antibodies in transplantation. *Transplant Proc.*, **9**, 721
3. Neilson, E.G. and Zakheim, B. (1983). T-cell regulation, anti-idiotypic immunity, and the nephritogenic immune response. *Kidney Int.*, **24**, 289
4. Ahmed-Ansari, A., Tadros, T.S., Knopf, W.D., Murphy, D.A., Hertzler, G., Feighan, J., Leatherbury, A. and Sell, K.W. (1988). Major histocompatibility complex Class I and Class II expression by myocytes in cardiac biopsies post-transplantation. *Transplantation*, **45**, 972
5. Hayry, P., Willebrand, E., Parthenais, E., Nemlander, A., Soots, A., Lautenschlager, I., Alfoldy, P. and Renkonen, R. (1984). Inflammatory mechanisms of allograft rejection. *Immunol. Rev.*, **77**, 85
6. Mason, D.W. and Morris, P.J. (1986). Effector mechanisms in allograft rejection. *Annu. Rev. Immunol.*, **4**, 119
7. Milton, A.D. and Fabre, J.W. (1985). Massive induction of donor-type Class I and Class II major histocompatibility complex antigens in rejecting cardiac allografts in the rat. *J. Exp. Med.*, **161**, 98
8. Lafferty, K.J. (1980). Immunogenicity of foreign tissues. *Transplantation*, **29**, 179
9. Bach, F.H. (1980). Comment on Lafferty, K.J. Immunogenicity of foreign tissues. *Transplantation*, **29**, 182
10. Batchelor, J.R. (1978). The riddle of kidney graft enhancement. *Transplantation*, **26**, 139
11. Christmas, S.E. and Macpherson, G.G. (1982). The role of mononuclear phagocytes in cardiac allograft rejection in the rat. I. Ultrastructural and cytochemical features. *Cell. Immunol.*, **69**, 248
12. Hayry, P. (1984). Intragraft events in allograft destruction. *Transplantation*, **38**, 1
13. Renkonen, R., Soots, A., Von Willebrand, E. and Hayry, P. (1983). Lymphoid cell sub-classes in rejecting renal allograft in the rat. *Cell. Immunol.*, **77**, 187
14. Zeevi, A., Fung, J., Zerbe, T.R., Kaufman, C., Rabin, B.S., Griffith, B.P., Hardesty, R.L. and Duquesnoy, R.J. (1986). Allo-specificity of activated T-cells grown from endomyocardial biopsies from heart transplant patients. *Transplantation*, **41**, 620
15. Williams, G.M., Hume, D.M., Hudson, R.P., Morris, P.J., Kano, K. and Milgrom, F. (1968). 'Hyperacute' renal-homograft rejection in man. *N. Engl. J. Med.*, **279**, 611
16. Berke, G. and Amos, D.B. (1973). Mechanism of lymphocyte-mediated cytolysis. The LMC cycle and its role in transplantation immunity. *Transplant. Rev.*, **17**, 71
17. Ascher, N.L. and Simmons, R.L. (1988). Immunobiology of transplant rejection. In Cerilli, G.J. (ed.) *Organ Transplantation and Replacement.* p. 67. (Philadelphia: J.B. Lippincott)
18. Thomas, J.M., Thomas, F.T., Kaplan, A.M. and Lee, H.M. (1976). Antibody-dependent cellular cytotoxicity and chronic renal allograft rejection. *Transplantation*, **22**, 94
19. Descamps, B., Gagnon, R., Van der Gaag, R., Feuillet, M.N. and Crosnier, J. (1979). Antibody-dependent cell-mediated cytotoxicity (ADCC) and complement-dependent cytotoxicity (CDC) in 229 sera from human renal allograft recipients. *J. Clin. Lab. Immunol.*, **2**, 303
20. Hall, B.M., Dorsch, S. and Roser, B. (1978). The cellular basis of allograft rejection *in vivo*. I. The cellular requirements for first-set rejection of heart grafts. *J. Exp. Med.*, **148**, 878
21. Knudsen, P.J., Dinarello, C.A. and Strom, T.B. (1988). Unpublished. Quoted by Burdick, J.F., Strom, T.B., Belzer, F.O. *Immunosuppression in Transplantation: the Biology and Therapeutic Modalities.* Booklet sponsored by The American Society of Transplant Surgeons. Thomas G. Ferguson Associates, Inc.
22. Palacios, R. and Sugawara, I. (1982). Hydrocortisone abrogates proliferation of T-cells in autologous mixed lymphocyte reaction by rendering the interleukin-II producer T-cells to become unresponsive to interleukin-I and unable to synthesize the T-cell growth factor. *Scand. J. Immunol.*, **15**, 25
23. Kaplan, M.P., Lysz, K., Rosenberg, S.A. and Rosenberg, J.C. (1983). Suppression of interleukin-II production by methylprednisone. *Transplant. Proc.*, **15**, 407
24. Snyder, D.S. and Unanue, E.R. (1982). Corticosteroids inhibit murine macrophage Ia expression and interleukin I production. *J. Immunol.*, **129**, 1803
25. Du Pont, E., Wybran, J. and Toussaint, C. (1984). Glucocorticosteroids and organ transplantation. *Transplantation*, **37**, 331
26. Rinehart, J.J., Balcerzak, S.P., Sagone, A.L. and Lobuglio, A.F. (1974). Effects of corticosteroids on human monocyte function. *J. Clin. Invest.*, **54**, 1337
27. Bertino, J.R. (1973). Chemical action and pharmacology of methotrexate, azathioprine, and cyclophosphamide in man. *Arthritis Rheum.*, **16**, 79
28. Salaman, J.R. (1982). Non-specific immunosuppression. In Morris, P.J. (ed.) *Tissue Transplantation*, p. 60. (Edinburgh: Churchill Livingstone)
29. Bach, M.A. and Bach, J.F. (1972). Activities of immunosuppressive agents *in vitro*. II. Different timing of azathioprine and methotrexate in inhibition and stimulation of mixed lymphocyte reaction. *Clin. Exp. Immunol.*, **11**, 89
30. Borel, J.F. (1982). Immunological properties of cyclosporine-A. *Heart Transplant.*, **1**, 237
31. Green, C.J. (1986). Experimental transplantation. *Prog. Allergy*, **38**, 123
32. White, D.J.G. and Calne, R.Y. (1984). Chemical immunosuppression. In Calne, R.Y. (ed.) *Transplantation Immunology – Clinical and Experimental.* p. 254. (Oxford: Oxford University Press)
33. Meuer, S.C., Acuto, O., Hercend, T., Schlossman, S.F. and Reinherz, E.L. (1984). The human T-cell receptor. *Annu. Rev. Immunol.*, **2**, 23
34. Giorgi, J.V., Burton, R.C., Barrett, L.V., Delmonico, F.L., Goldstein, G. and Cosimi, A.B. (1983). Immunosuppressive effect and immunogenicity of OKT11A monoclonal antibody in monkey allograft recipients. *Transplant. Proc.*, **15**, 629
35. Estabrook, A., Berger, C.L., Mittler, R., Logerfo, P., Hardy, M. and Edelson, R.L. (1983). Antigenic modulation of human T-lymphocytes by monoclonal antibodies. *Transplant. Proc.*, **15**, 651
36. Chang, T.W., Kung, P.C., Gingras, S.P. and Goldstein, G. (1981). Does OKT3 monoclonal antibody react with an antigen-recognition structure on human T-cells? *Proc. Natl. Acad. Sci. USA*, **78**, 1805
37. Bristow, M.R., Gilbert, E.M., Renlund, E.G., De Witt, C.W., Burton, N.A. and O'Connell, J.B. (1988). Use of OKT3 monoclonal antibody in heart transplantation: review of the initial experience. *J. Heart*

Transplant., **7**, 1

38. Touraine, J.L., Archimbaud, J.P., Malik, M.C., Dubernard, J.M., Guey, A., Neyra, P., Mongin, D., Baurard, B. and Traeger, J. (1977). Improved results of human renal transplantation after thoracic duct drainage and antilymphocyte globulin treatment. In Touraine, J.L. *et al.* (eds.) *Transplantation and Clinical Immunology.* Vol. 10, p. 189. (Amsterdam; Excerpta Medica)

39. White, D.J.G. (1984). Total lymphoid irradiation. In Calne, R.Y. (ed.) *Transplantation Immunology – Clinical and Experimental.* p. 339. (Oxford: Oxford University Press)

15
Pathology of Acute Rejection

A.G. ROSE AND C.J. UYS

INTRODUCTION

Experimental cardiac transplantation using various animals preceded the first human-to-human cardiac transplant in 1967. Such experimental work provided a sound basis for understanding of the clinical and pathological features of cardiac rejection and their modification by immunosuppressive agents. Pioneering experimental work in animals was performed by Carrell and Guthrie[1], Mann et al.[2], Downie[3], Lower et al.[4], and Blumenstock et al.[5]. Cooper has reviewed the experimental development of cardiac transplantation[6] (Chapter 1), and Uys and Rose list key references to the pathology of experimental cardiac transplantation in dogs, rats, rabbits and baboons[7]. Thomson, in 1968, was the first to describe the pathology of a transplanted human heart[8], and this was followed shortly thereafter by the report of Lower et al.[9].

While irreversible severe acute rejection may sometimes lead to surgical removal of the donor heart and its examination by the pathologist, the usual problem facing the pathologist in centers where cardiac transplantation is performed is that of the histological recognition of acute rejection in endomyocardial biopsies taken from the right ventricle of the donor heart.

MACROSCOPIC APPEARANCES

Mild or moderate rejection may produce no naked-eye alterations in the transplanted heart. However, it has been shown that such rejecting allografts have an increased organ mass[10,11]. Heterotopically-placed hearts removed because of cessation of function following irreversible severe acute rejection (Figure 15.1) usually show extremely severe acute rejection changes, since immunosuppression is often greatly reduced in the period between cessation of graft function and surgical excision of the graft. Such hearts are commonly dilated and have a hemorrhagic-looking, swollen, mottled, myocardial cut-surface.

Focal pale areas of myocardial necrosis contrast sharply

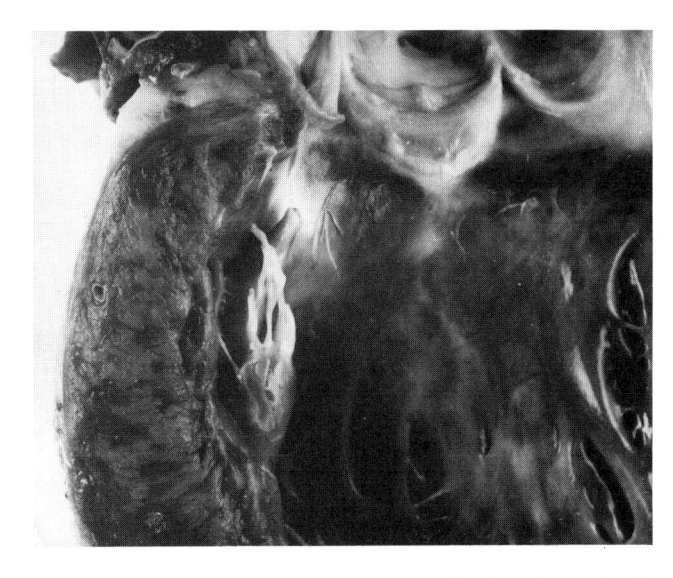

Figure 15.1 Close-up view of the left ventricle of a donor heart showing severe acute rejection. Subendocardial hemorrhage is widely distributed, and the myocardial cut surface shows pale areas of necrosis against a hemorrhagic background

with the plum-colored, viable myocardium. The ventricles may contain abundant apical stasis thrombi. Occasionally, stasis thrombus in the donor aortic valve pockets may extend upwards to occlude the donor coronary arteries, resulting in total or subtotal necrosis of the graft.

THE ROLE OF ENDOMYOCARDIAL BIOPSY IN THE DIAGNOSIS OF ACUTE REJECTION

The histopathology of acute rejection as seen in myocardial biopsies is similar to that seen in donor hearts removed surgically or at autopsy. The only difference is with regard to severity, which may differ from patient to patient and from biopsy to biopsy. Biopsy material is obviously limited in amount, and the pathologist has to detect rejection without having the multiple tissue sections which are available when the whole heart is examined.

Criticism of endomyocardial biopsy has focused primarily on the possibility of sampling error and the subtlety of the histologic changes in diagnosing rejection[12,13]. A study from our institution[14] attempted to validate the technique by examining 'biopsy' samples taken with a bioptome from formalin-fixed explanted human donor hearts, and comparing these in a blind fashion with standard histologic sections taken from the same hearts. Using a scoring system to grade severity of acute rejection, agreement of results between the bioptome samples and routine sections was found in 86% of cases. More important was the fact that in 285 biopsy samples, only two false-negative results were obtained. Rejection involved both ventricles equally.

Endomyocardial biopsy usually samples the septal wall of the right ventricle towards the apex. How many tissue samples should be taken at each biopsy procedure? From the pathologist's point of view, the more the better, and the larger each sample the better too. Four to eight samples is the optimum, but in practice we usually receive three or four endomyocardial samples per biopsy procedure. In our study referred to earlier, it was found that even as few as two endomyocardial samples revealed the presence of acute rejection[14]. Others consider that the myocardium is only adequately represented by a minimum of five endomyocardial samples per biopsy procedure[15]. Whilst the latter opinion was expressed regarding myocardial biopsy for suspected idiopathic cardiomyopathy, it is likely that the same principle should apply to rejection. If only one small endomyocardial sample is submitted, it is advisable for the examining pathologist to convey this information to the cardiac surgeon, since there is a possibility that significant rejection may be missed (false-negative biopsy). In the light of other clinical and laboratory parameters, the cardiac surgeon should decide whether an immediate or early repeat biopsy is indicated.

The size of the biopsy specimen varies according to the bioptome used. In our hospital, each endomyocardial sample is usually less than 3 mm in diameter. They are submitted to the laboratory in 5% buffered glutaraldehyde to facilitate subsequent ultrastructural examination of one of the fragments, if this is deemed necessary. The fragments for assessment of rejection are transferred into 5% buffered formaldehyde in the laboratory, and processed in a hypercenter tissue processor for expedited handling. Paraffin-embedded sections are stained by the hematoxylin–eosin, elastic van Gieson, and Unna-Pappenheim methods. One or two biopsies are also submitted fresh for immediate frozen section. This gives immediate information regarding the presence of rejection, and additional sections may be cut for the determination of lymphocyte subsets. Electron microscopy and immunofluorescence microscopy, however, play only a limited role in the recognition of rejection.

LIGHT MICROSCOPIC APPEARANCES

Classic features of acute rejection in patients receiving only azathioprine and corticosteroids

One of the earliest changes observed in acute rejection is the development of interstitial edema (Figure 15.2), which is most prominent perivascularly and less evident in the endocardium, which has a denser connective tissue component. The edema is probably a result of microvascular damage. Interstitial edema is less severe in patients receiving cyclosporine. The vascular endothelium is that portion of the graft which first encounters both humoral antibodies and the host cells which are attracted into the graft.

Since the host cells reach the graft via the bloodstream, in the early stages of acute rejection the small blood vessels within the graft may be observed to contain increased numbers of mononuclear cells (Figure 15.3). These cells may also be seen to be passing through the vessels' walls into the surrounding myocardium. The degree of interstitial edema does not always match the severity of the cellular infiltrate (Figure 15.4). The early infiltrating cells (Figure 15.5) consist mainly of non-activated lymphocytes and small unidentified mononuclear cells of lymphoid type, together with histiocytes and scanty neutrophils plus eosinophils. The cellular infiltration initially has a focal, mainly perivascular distribution. These cells soon develop a prominent cytoplasmic pyroninophilia, as do the endothelial cells of the small blood vessels. Focal infiltrations of similar cells are also noted in the endomyocardium. Cardiac histiocytes (Anitschkow myocytes), presumably of donor heart origin, also

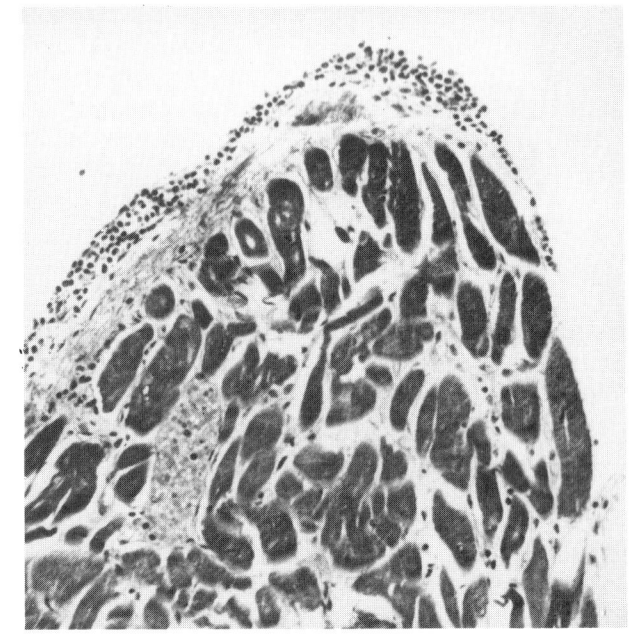

Figure 15.2 Early acute rejection. Mild interstitial edema spares the endocardium which contains an infiltrate of lymphoid cells (H&E × 135)

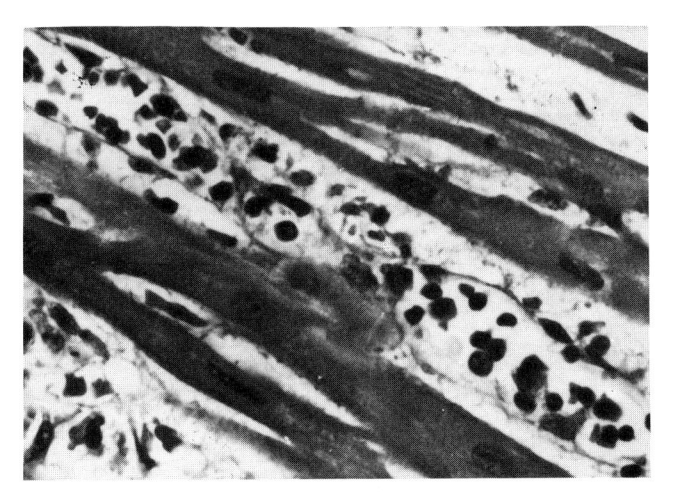

Figure 15.3 A capillary contains large numbers of mononuclear cells. Similar cells are present in the edematous interstitium of this rejecting graft (H&E × 420)

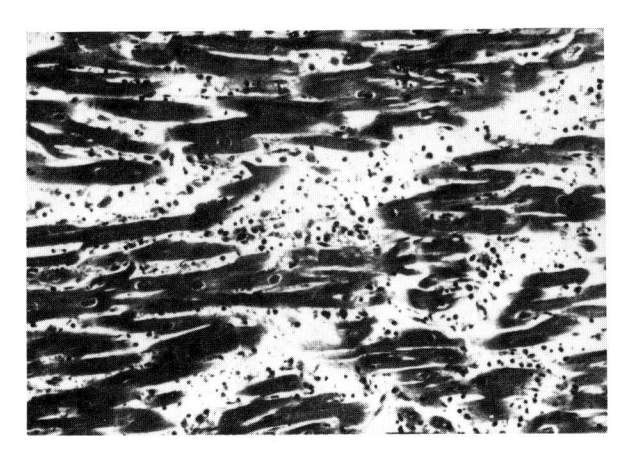

Figure 15.4 Prominent interstitial edema accompanies a moderate mononuclear cellular infiltrate of acute rejection (H&E × 120)

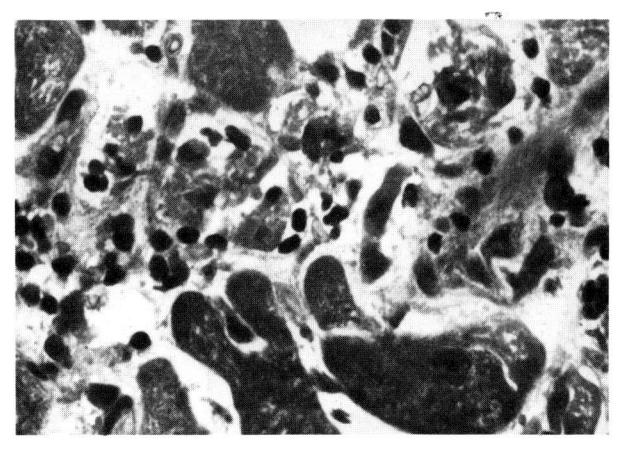

(a)

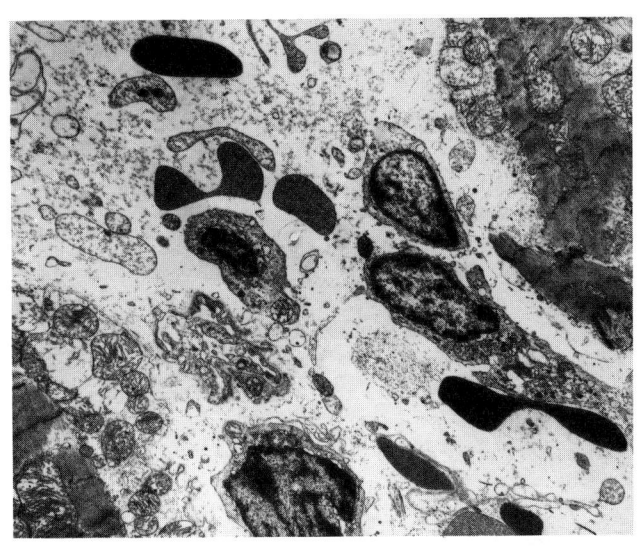

(b)

Figure 15.5 (a) Donor heart biopsy shows numbers of small lymphoid cells in relation to degenerating myocytes (H&E × 420). (b) The edematous interstitium between two myocytes (top right and bottom left) contains activated lymphocytes and some free-lying erythrocytes (lead citrate and uranyl acetate × 2400)

appear activated and prominent. Vascular changes in the graft are observed at an early stage; the endothelial lining cells become swollen and edema fluid accumulates in the intima (Figure 15.6). Sometimes this may lead to detachment of the endothelial cells.

If untreated, all of the above changes will progress and increase in intensity and be joined by other alterations associated with damage to the myocytes and blood vessels. Thus, interstitial edema becomes even more marked (Figure 15.4) and also separates bundles of myocytes, which previously had been in close apposition. Interstitial fibrin deposition also occurs, but fibrinolysis may render it inconspicuous microscopically[16]. With time, there is enlargement of the nuclei and cytoplasm of the lymphocytes, which now have the appearance of immunoblasts (Figure 15.7). Similar lymphoid-series cells within blood vessels are admixed with proliferating endothelial and intimal cells; the lymphoid cells may also be seen within the media and the adventitia (Figure 15.6). This cellular accumulation, together with the intimal edema and the sometimes-encountered microvascular thrombi, lead to lumenal narrowing.

Small vessel thrombi have been an inconspicuous feature of mild and moderate acute rejection in our human transplant material, but they have been encountered by others in canine cardiac allografts[17]. The occurrence of such thrombi in severe acute rejection in humans is not surprising, since there is evidence that rejection may activate the coagulation mechanism[18]. These microvascular changes, together with the cytotoxic effects of the infiltrating immunoblasts and humoral antibodies, combine to produce deleterious effects on the myocardium. Thus, the myocytes may show a range of appearances from normal through cytoplasmic swelling, lipid vacuolation, and colliquative myocyto-

(a)

(b)

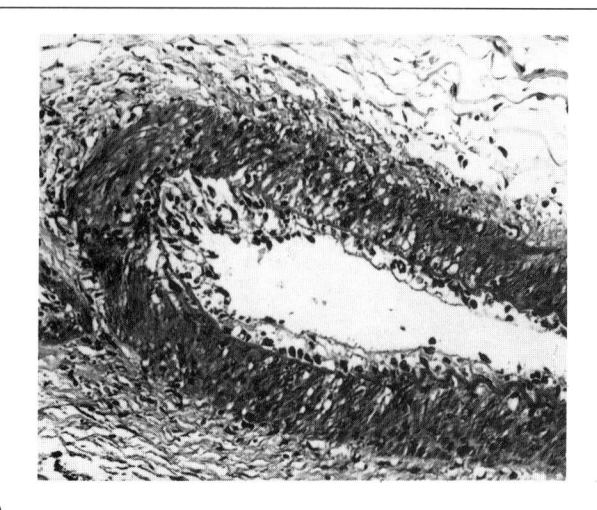

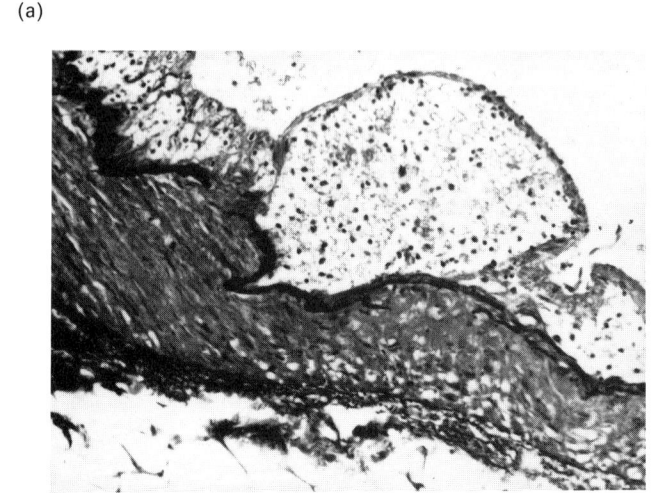

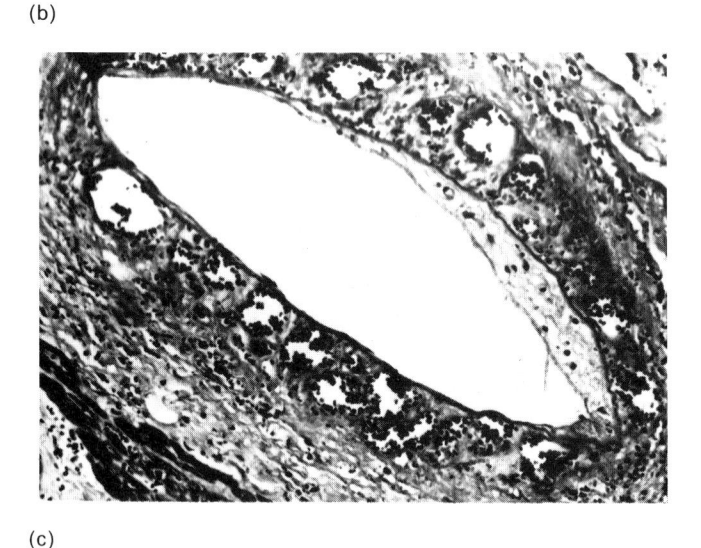

(c)

Figure 15.6 (a) Acute rejection has caused subendothelial intimal edema of this small coronary artery. Scanty mononuclear cells are present within the arterial wall. (b) At times the edema can be quite striking. (c) Small coronary artery shows outer medial defects of the kind associated with an immune-mediated arteritis (all H&E × 100)

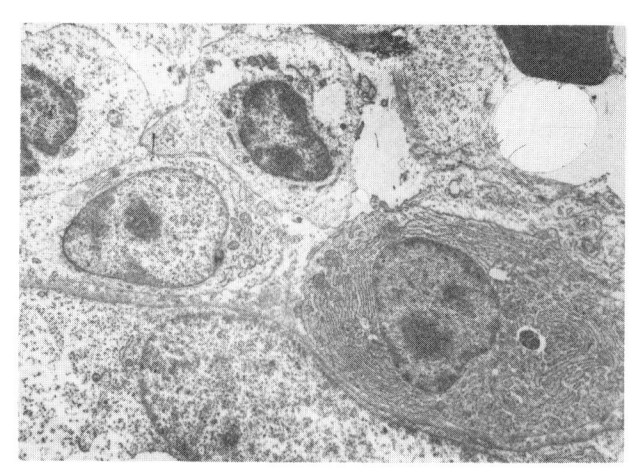

Figure 15.7 Acute rejection. A group of immunoblasts occupies the myocardial interstitium. A plasma cell is present (lower right) (lead citrate and uranyl acetate × 1350)

lysis, to coagulative necrosis (Figure 15.8). These changes may coexist in varying combinations. Myocytolysis is characterized by loss of cytoplasmic and nuclear detail, leaving an empty sarcolemmal sheath containing some lipofuscin granules as the tombstone of the vanished myofilaments. Hearts with such areas of necrosis also commonly show interstitial hemorrhages due to distintegration of capillaries.

In severe acute rejection the intramyocardial coronary arteries, as well as some of the smaller epicardial branches of the major coronary arteries, may show segmental fibrinoid necrosis (Figure 15.9) of a portion or of the entire circumference of the artery. Arteries of this size are seldom included in endomyocardial biopsies. Occlusive thrombosis is a frequent accompaniment of this lesion. For some unknown reason, the cardiac veins and the venules are seldom involved in the rejection changes described above[7]. (In Chapter 18

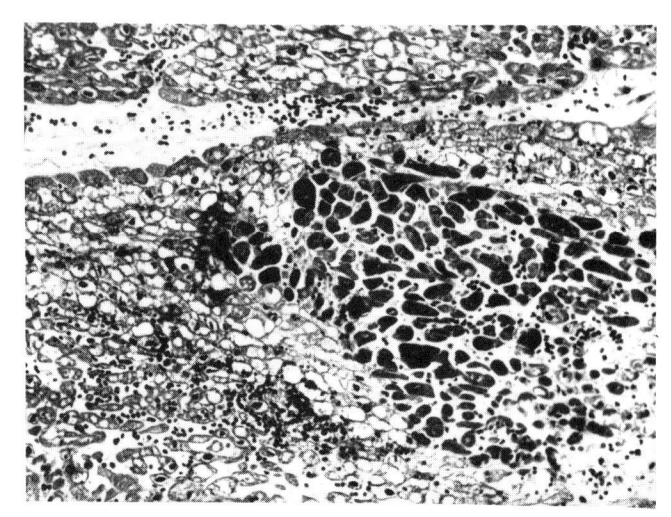

Figure 15.8 Severe acute rejection is associated with coagulative necrosis (dark-staining myocytes) and myocytolysis (empty sarcolemmal sheaths) (H&E × 110)

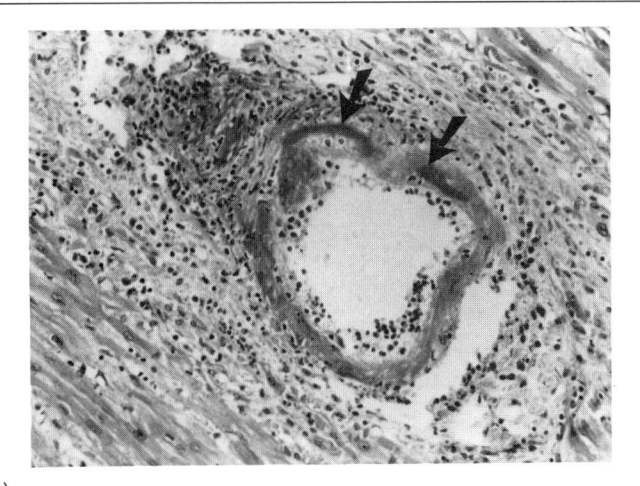

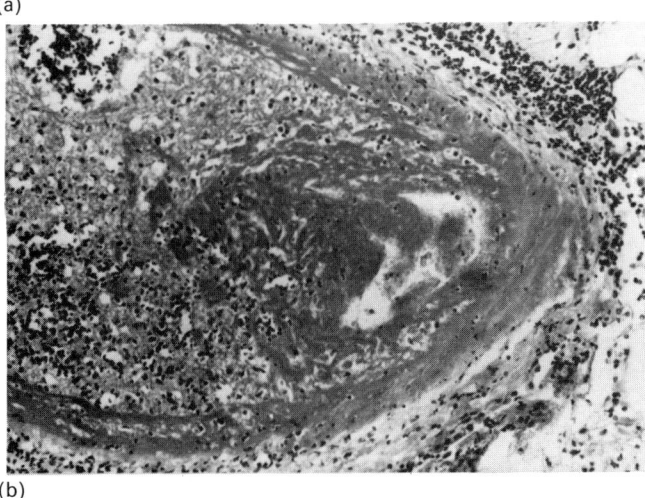

Figure 15.9 Severe acute rejection. (a) Early fibrinoid necrosis (arrows) of wall of an intramyocardial coronary artery. (b) Advanced fibrinoid necrosis of a small coronary artery with superimposed thrombosis (both H&E × 100)

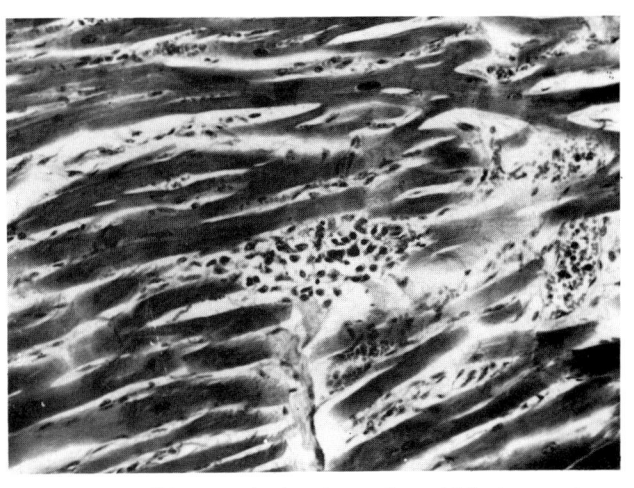

Figure 15.10 Mild acute rejection. Scanty interstitial edema and mononuclear cell infiltration (H&E × 110)

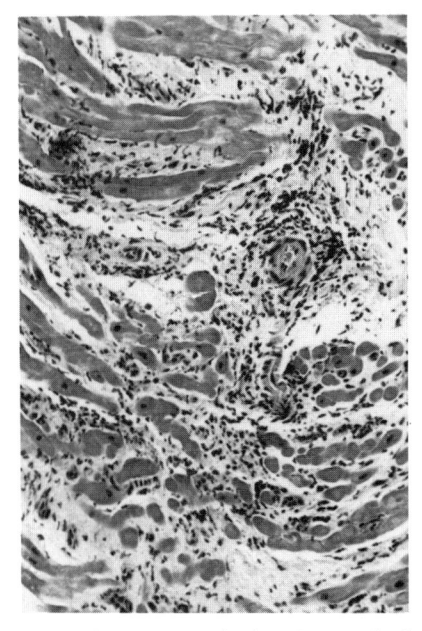

Figure 15.11 Moderate acute rejection. Increased edema and a more prominent cellular infiltrate are seen (H&E × 120)

we shall show how healing of acute rejection may lead to the constellation of myocardial and vascular changes in the donor heart which are referred to as chronic rejection.)

Examples of mild, moderate and severe rejection are given in Figures 15.10–15.12. Herskowitz et al.[19] have identified interstitial edema, perivascular karyorrhexis, and perivascular lymphocytic infiltration with intermyocyte extension as three histological abnormalities that help predict the future development of more severe acute rejection associated with myocyte necrosis.

Grading the degree of acute rejection

At Groote Schuur Hospital in Cape Town, we grade the severity of the rejection changes in the endomyocardial biopsies using a semiquantitative scoring system. This gives the clinician an easily-understood indication of the severity of the acute rejection changes present. The reproducibility of histological interpretation is enhanced since the same criteria are used each time to assess and score the biopsy specimens, rather than basing the diagnosis of rejection on an overall impression of the specimens. In serial biopsies, taken during an acute rejection episode, such a scoring system gives the clinician an easily interpretable guide as to the efficacy of increased immunosuppression. A lower histopathological score warrants less immunosuppressive therapy than a severe rejection episode, and reduces the risk of over-immunosuppression.

The histological scoring system we use[20] independently assesses five histological criteria: (1) interstitial edema, (2) interstitial mononuclear cellular infiltration, (3) cytoplasmic pyroninophilia of the mononuclear cells (the methyl-green pyronin stain identifies activated lymphocytes by staining

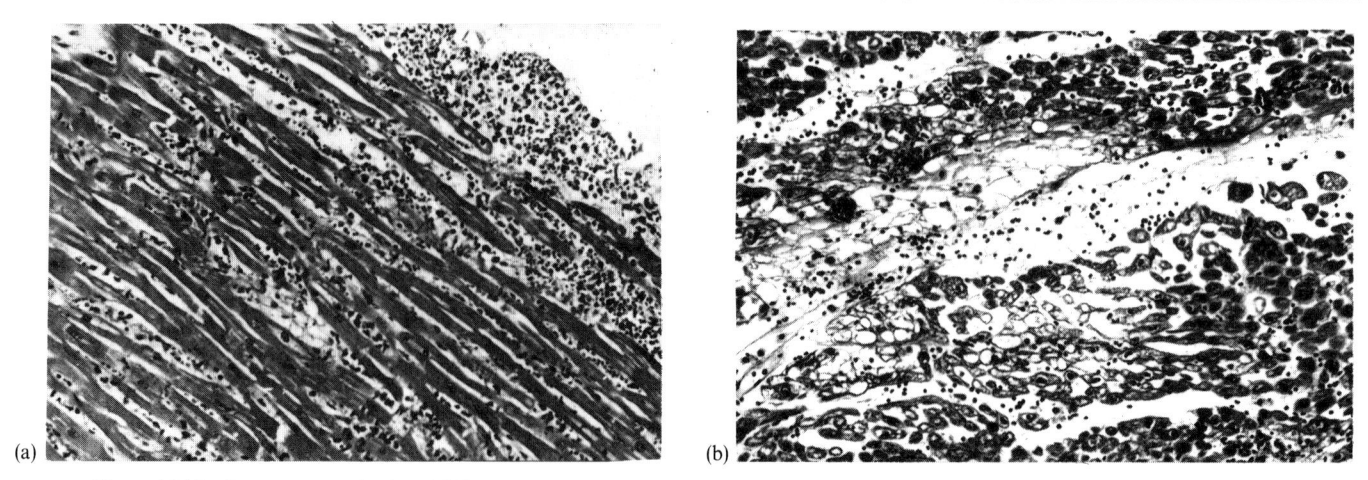

Figure 15.12 Severe acute rejection. (a) Very numerous mononuclear cells are present. (b) Myocytolysis is a prominent feature; this change is usually associated with occlusive arterial lesions (both H&E × 100)

the increased cytoplasmic RNA), (4) myocyte degeneration and/or necrosis, and (5) blood vessel alterations. Myocyte alterations include edema, vacuolation, loss of sharp contour, indistinct cross-striations, colliquative myocytolysis, fragmentation and coagulative necrosis. Contraction banding of the myocytes, which is present in most biopsies, is regarded as a biopsy-induced artefact and is not scored. Blood vessel alterations include intimal cell proliferation or necrosis, mononuclear cellular infiltration of the vessel wall, and medial cell loss.

The presence or absence of each of these five histological criteria is scored from 0 to 3 as follows: 0, absent or normal; 0.5, minimal change; 1, mild change; 2, moderate change; 3, severe change. The sum of these scores from the biopsy specimen is the final score. Theoretically, this may be as high as 15, though in clinical specimens scores above 6 are rarely encountered, and the latter score usually signifies irreversible damage to the graft. In the experimental animal, when acute rejection is allowed to progress unimpeded, an ultimate score of 15 is not uncommon. In our experience, a final score of 0 implies that no rejection is present; 0.5–2 denotes a mild rejection; 2.5–4 represents moderate acute rejection, and a score of greater than 4 indicates severe acute rejection.

Figure 15.13 compares four different grading systems for acute cardiac allograft rejection[20-23].

The choice of grading system used is less important than that there should be good communication between the

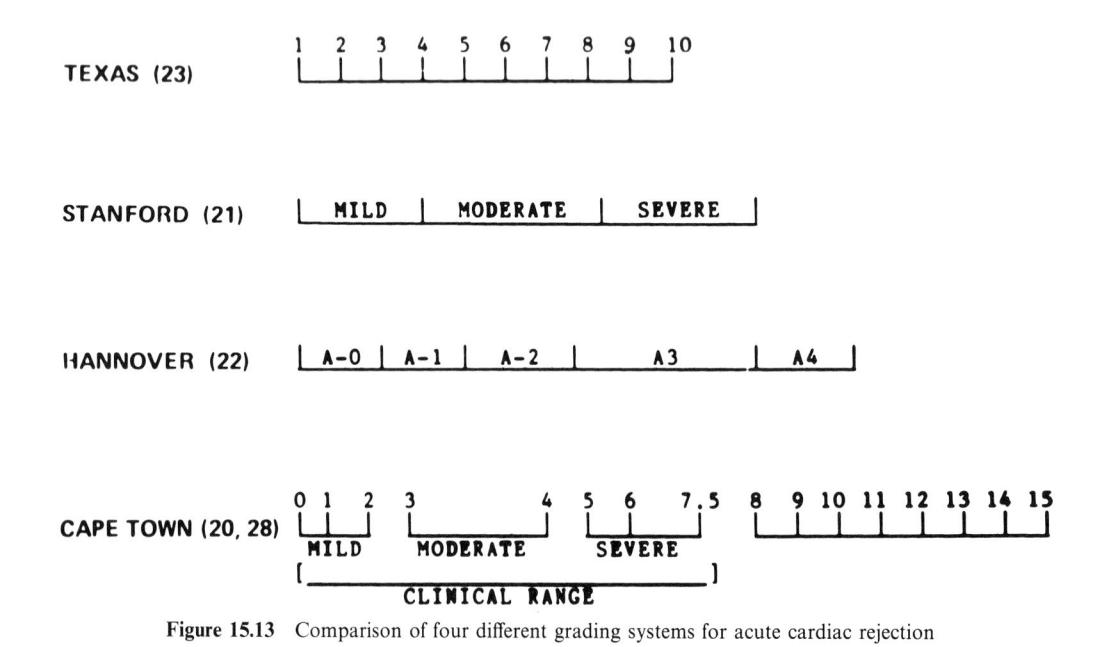

Figure 15.13 Comparison of four different grading systems for acute cardiac rejection

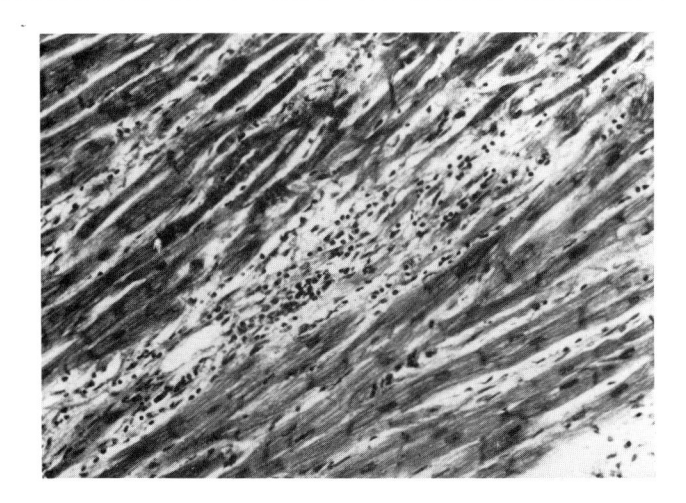

Figure 15.14 Resolving acute rejection shows few mononuclear cells and early stromal collapse fibrosis where some myofibers have been lost (H&E × 110)

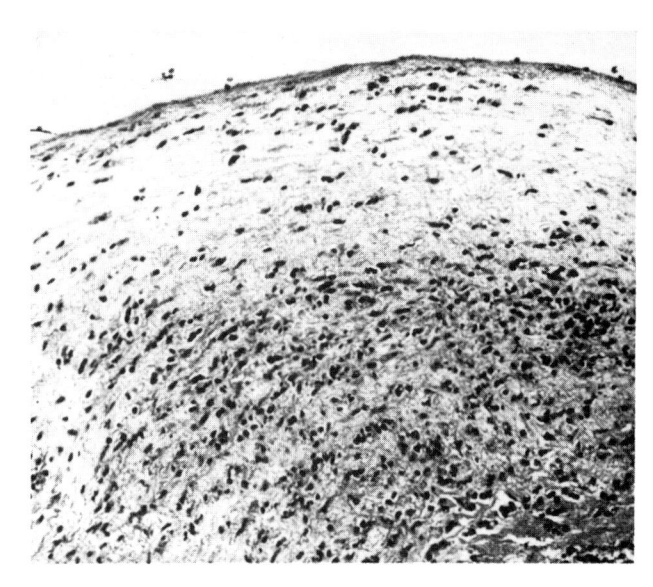

Figure 15.15 Mitral valve cusp of a patient with severe acute rejection contains numerous infiltrating lymphocytes (H&E × 135)

pathologist and the transplant surgeon. The pathologist must clearly transmit the degree of rejection present to the surgeon. The use of a scoring system has the advantage that the severity of rejection can be swiftly communicated without going into descriptive histological details which may confuse the clinician.

Resolving acute rejection

Resolving acute rejection (Figure 15.14) is encountered when augmented immunosuppression leads to the abolition of the acute rejection episode. However, it takes several days or even 1–2 weeks for all evidence of acute rejection to be resolved. Since the clinical concern is whether rejection has been controlled, this is a period in which further biopsies are commonly taken. Rapid dissolution of the mononuclear cellular infiltrate occurs within a day or two in patients receiving large doses of corticosteroids. However, in patients receiving cyclosporine-based immunosuppressive therapy, increased cyclosporine has a less dramatic immediate effect on the cellular infiltrate. With resolution of acute rejection, the remaining lymphoid cells show minimal pyroninophilia, and the removal of dead myocytes leads to early replacement fibrosis. The heart valves seldom show changes due to rejection, and such alterations are only occasionally seen with severe acute rejection (Figure 15.15).

Special features of acute rejection in patients receiving cyclosporine

The above-described histopathological changes of acute rejection are based upon our experience with cardiac transplants treated with an immunosuppressive regimen consisting of high-dose methylprednisolone, azathioprine and anti-thymocyte globulin. Since January 1983, our transplant patients have received the immunosuppressive agent cyclosporine[24], and the dose of steroids has been reduced.

When present, myocyte necrosis is a valuable indicator of acute rejection[21,25]. Such necrosis is rare in our experience, even in patients with prominent lymphocytic infiltrates. In patients receiving cyclosporine, myocyte necrosis may be associated with only a moderate degree of acute rejection. Ratliff et al.[26] have noted a unique form of reversible myocyte injury in cyclosporine-treated cardiac transplants associated with centralization of the myofilaments, which in turn are surrounded by a radially-oriented bundle of myofilaments. The myocyte injury of transplant rejection is generally reversible and is similar to apoptosis.

Endomyocardial biopsies from cyclosporine-treated cardiac recipients usually show a sparse, scattered, endocardiotropic infiltration of small mononuclear cells, which may not indicate significant acute rejection. Mild lymphocytic infiltration in the absence of evidence of myocyte necrosis has been considered to necessitate only frequent biopsy surveillance[27]. Antirejection treatment is withheld unless an increasingly severe infiltrate develops or active myocyte damage supervenes. Early acute rejection is heralded by an increase of plump, pyroninophilic, perivascular and interstitial mononuclear cells. Acute rejection develops more slowly (e.g. over a week) and takes longer to resolve. A fine, intermyocyte fibrosis has been observed in biopsies of some patients receiving cyclosporine, but this has thus far not been a notable feature in our patients. Similar changes may occur adjacent to a previous biopsy site[28]. A coarser form of focal stromal collapse fibrosis, following removal of necrotic myofibers, has been observed in a few of our biopsies showing resolving acute rejection.

Oyer et al.[27] suggest that the rejection process in cyclosporine-treated patients may be more focal than that seen in steroid–azathioprine-treated patients. They stress that at least three to five tissue samples from different areas of right ventricular endomyocardium should be obtained at each biopsy procedure in order to gain an accurate overall impression of the status of the rejection process. Our experience is that, even with steroid–azathioprine immunosuppression, the rejection changes are not uniformly distributed throughout the myocardium and the endocardium, but endomyocardial biopsy is representative of the overall situation[14].

Additional features categorizing cyclosporine-modified acute rejection are that, once established, acute rejection resolves slowly and myocyte damage may persist for about 2 weeks despite increased immunosuppression[24]. Severe acute rejection includes neutrophilic cells and hemorrhage, plus myocyte necrosis, as described for steroid–azathioprine-treated patients[29].

If repeated biopsies are totally negative for the presence of any lymphocytes, this should be discussed with the clinician, as there is the possibility of over-immunosuppression and the attendant danger of infection. This dictum is especially important in patients receiving cyclosporine, since endocardial lymphocytic infiltrations are commonly seen.

IMMUNOFLUORESCENT STUDIES

Immunofluorescent studies on autopsy and biopsy material from transplanted human and animal hearts in which the immunoglobulins IgG, IgM, and IgA, and complement (C3) were sought, yielded unhelpful results by both direct immunofluorescence and the immunoperoxidase methods. Moderate amounts of fibrinogen and C3 may be found within the walls of some intramyocardial blood vessels. A recent report, however, suggests a more positive role for immunofluorescence in the detection of rejection[30].

LYMPHOCYTE SUBPOPULATIONS IN ACUTE CARDIAC REJECTION

T-lymphocytes are the predominant cell type in acute cardiac rejection. The ratio of helper to suppressor T-lymphocytes in the cardiac biopsy does not correlate with rejection. However, the greater the number of cells in the biopsy, the greater is the likelihood of significant acute rejection. B-lymphocytes are seldom present in endomyocardial biopsies, and, if present, are seen in very scanty numbers only. Macrophages are more prominent in resolving acute rejection.

Cyclosporine suppresses the generation of inducer T-cells, but allows the generation of suppressor cells. Monoclonal antibodies, which destroy the T3 cell subset, are playing a small, but possibly increasing, role in the treatment of acute rejection.

ELECTRON MICROSCOPY

Ultrastructural examination of donor hearts and endomyocardial biopsies reveals a variable loss of myofilaments in the myocytes, leaving the Z-bands free within the sarcoplasm. Some Z-bands have a widened, smudgy, ill-defined appearance. Ratliff et al.[26] report an unusual, reversible form of myocyte damage, characterized by radially arranged myofilaments (see above). Severe acute rejection associated with vasculitis may cause complete myocyte destruction. Other features of note include swollen mitochondria, dilation of the T-tubules, cytoplasmic lipid vacuoles, and swelling or necrosis of capillary endothelial cells. The interstitial infiltration consists of ordinary lymphocytes, activated lymphocytes, histiocytes, and occasional neutrophils and eosinophils. In the early stages of acute rejection, there is a preponderance of mononuclear cells of undistinguished appearance.

Later, activated lymphocytes predominate. In resolving acute rejection one may observe mature-looking plasma cells, which are characterized by the presence of numerous polyribosomes and cisternae of rough-surfaced endoplasmic reticulum. Such cells stain weakly with the Unna–Pappenheim stain. In biopsies of cardiac allografts implanted in baboons, unidentified mononuclear cells comprised 53% of the interstitial cellular infiltrate overall in acute rejection[10].

SPECIAL PROBLEMS REGARDING THE LIGHT MICROSCOPIC DIAGNOSIS OF ACUTE REJECTION

There are certain special problems that may be encountered in the interpretation of biopsies from donor hearts[28,31,32].

Inadequate biopsy

Firstly, there is the adequacy of the endomyocardial sampling, which has been commented upon above. A not-infrequent situation which is encountered is that one or more of the endomyocardial biopsies submitted by the cardiologist is composed solely of fibrin thrombus. The source of the thrombus is not always clear, and possible sites of origin include the biopsy catheter itself, endocardial thrombus, or thrombus at the vein entry site. Since the biopsies are all taken from a limited area at the apical portion of the right side of the interventricular septum, there is a possibility that the thrombus may even be derived from a previous biopsy site if serial biopsies have been taken[31,32].

A localized lymphocytic response may also be evoked by the biopsy procedure, and this may lead the unwary to consider the presence of rejection[28,32]. The presence of organizing thrombus or hemosiderin deposits should provide a clue to the correct diagnosis.

Presence of fibrous tissue

Another problem which is encountered from time to time is the sample composed solely of fibrous tissue. While such a finding raises the possibility of chronic rejection, our experience is that chronic rejection commonly spares the myocytes that lie immediately subendocardial[20]. If the donor heart has a greatly reduced ejection fraction and endomyocardial biopsy shows no sign of acute rejection, the possibility of chronic rejection should be borne in mind. The larger the size of the bioptome sample, the better is the chance of detecting fibrosis due to chronic rejection. In several biopsies we have been able to identify fibrous tissue as being portions of tricuspid valve chordae tendineae (Figure 15.15). Such biopsies usually do not appear to result in significant valvular dysfunction. Occasionally, the bioptome may penetrate the ventricular wall and sample the fibrosed epicardium, with or without small epicardial blood vessels. A healed previous biopsy site may also show abundant fibrosis.

Donor heart infection

Fortunately, donor heart infection is rare; to detect infection by biopsy, therefore, the pathologist must be constantly on the alert for such a possibility. Infections include toxoplasmosis, coccidioidomycosis, cytomegalic inclusion disease, and Chaga's disease. Sarcocystis species, which may occasionally infect man, can produce a similar appearance to that of toxoplasmosis in the heart. These myocardial infections may elicit a mononuclear cellular infiltration that may be confused with acute rejection.

In one patient with a heterotopic transplant, we made the initial diagnosis of infection of both donor and recipient hearts by *Toxoplasma gondii* on endomyocardial biopsies (Figure 15.16). Electron microscopy and serology served to confirm the diagnosis[33]. We have since encountered a second such patient. Toxoplasmosis of the donor heart may interfere with the recognition of acute rejection in graft biopsy specimens. The interstitial mononuclear cell infiltration that follows release of the organisms from infected myocytes is very similar to that seen in acute rejection. This causes difficulty both in detecting cardiac rejection and in assessing its severity.

Pyroninophilia is not helpful in distinguishing the two conditions. The cellular infiltration in toxoplasmosis is said to be of a more mixed type and includes lymphocytes, plasma cells, histiocytes, and occasional eosinophils. In acute rejection, the cellular infiltrate consists almost entirely of activated lymphocytes[30]. Later, a few plasma cells may also be seen. Histiocytes may become active, but they usually do not comprise a prominent part of the cellular infiltrate in acute rejection.

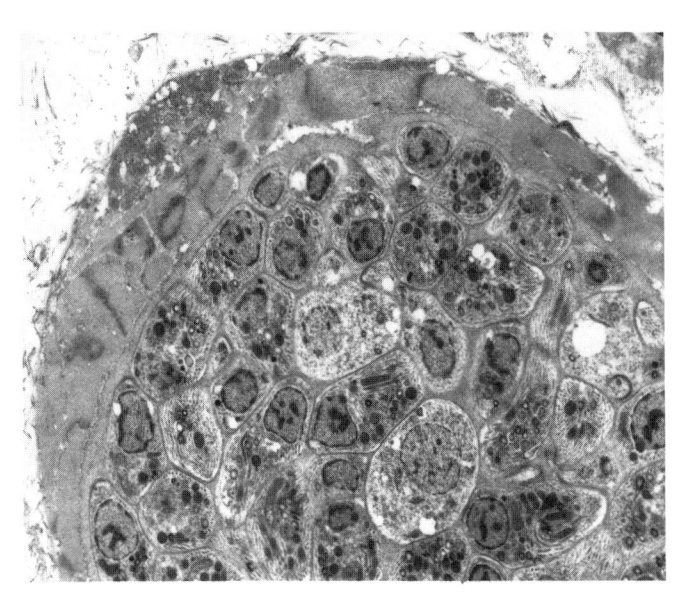

Figure 15.16 Donor heart biopsy shows numerous Toxoplasmas within a myocyte (lead citrate and uranyl acetate × 5180)

Despite these theoretical differences, there is no certain way of diagnosing acute rejection in the presence of an active cardiac infection by Toxoplasma. Since our first patient had a heterotopic transplant, the recipient heart served as a control for chemotherapy and for deciding whether a mononuclear cellular infiltration of the donor heart was likely to be due to rejection or toxoplasmosis.

Inadequate myocardial preservation

The paucity of human donor hearts available for transplantation has led to the concept of distant heart procurement, whereby the excised donor heart may be stored and transported in a cardioplegic solution in ice or by using a portable hypothermic perfusion system (Chapter 7). The major problem is the prevention of myocardial damage in the donor heart prior to implantation. Various forms of myocardial necrosis (coagulative, myocytolytic, and contraction band) may be observed. Widespread interstitial hemorrhage that is indicative of a reperfusion-type infarction may also be observed.

Effects of donor brain death

Donor heart biopsy is seldom performed in the first week after transplantation, and myocyte contraction banding is a frequent biopsy-induced artefact. The presence of abundant contraction bands has been taken as a sign of rejection by some[22]. More of a problem in the interpretation of early (first week) biopsies are possible myocardial alterations which represent persistence of donor brain death-related lesions (Chapter 6). Catecholamine overproduction associated with brain death produces myocyte injury which is recognized morphologically as showing heightened eosinophilia of myocytes, contraction banding, focal coagulative necrosis, and application of mononuclear cells to the surface of the damaged myocytes (Figure 15.17)[34-37]. The appearances can be similar to myocyte necrosis induced by acute rejection (Figure 15.18).

Lack of correlation with hemodynamic data

Hemodynamic function and inflammation or fibrosis detected on biopsy show a poor correlation. Greenberg *et al.*[37] found no significant difference in mean ejection fraction and left ventricular end-diastolic pressure between patients with and without fibrosis on biopsy, or between those with and without inflammation. In our institution, a good correlation has been noted between changes in left ventricular volumes and histological semi-quantitative scores for acute rejection[38] (Chapter 16).

COMMENT

Many non-invasive methods are being explored to find an acceptable substitute for endomyocardial biopsy in the diagnosis of acute rejection (Chapter 16). These include magnetic resonance imaging, assessment of peripheral blood lymphocytic activation, and soluble interleukin-2 receptor levels, but, for the near future, graft histology will remain the gold standard for the early diagnosis of acute rejection.

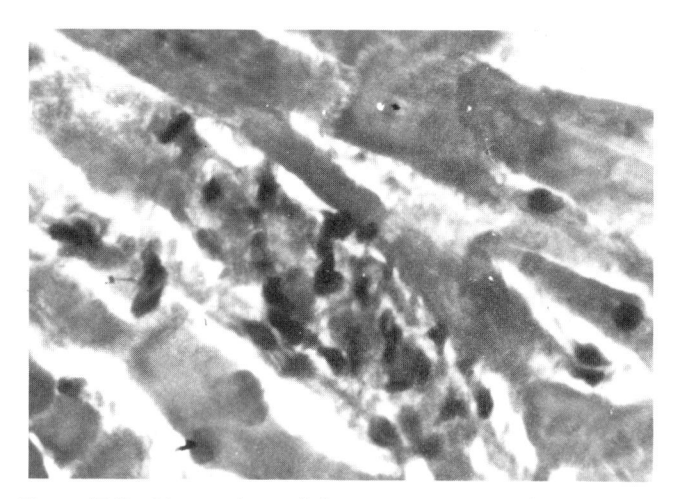

Figure 15.17 Mononuclear cellular response to necrotic myocyte in human donor heart damaged by brain death-induced catecholamine excess (H&E × 490)

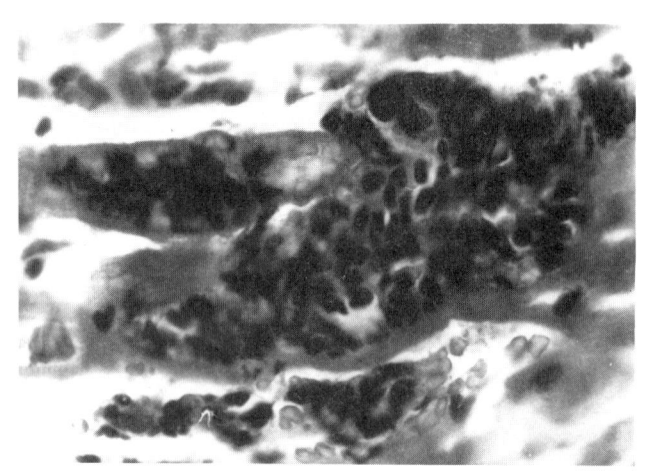

Figure 15.18 Myocytes damaged by severe acute rejection are covered by lymphocytes (H&E × 480)

References

1. Carrel, A. and Guthrie, C.C. (1905). The transplantation of veins and organs. *Am. Med.*, **10**, 1101
2. Mann, F.C., Priestly, J.T., Markowitz, J. and Yater, W.M. (1933). Transplant of the intact mammalian heart. *Arch. Surg.*, **26**, 219
3. Downie, H.G. (1953). Homotransplantation of the dog heart. *Arch. Surg.*, **66**, 624
4. Lower, R.R., Stofer, R.D. and Shumway, N.E. (1961). Homovital transplantation of the heart. *J. Thorac. Cardiovasc. Surg.*, **41**, 196
5. Blumenstock, D.A., Hechtman, H.B., Collins, J.A., Karetzki, A, Hosbein, J.D., Zing, W. and Powers, J.H. (1963). Prolonged survival of orthotopic homotransplants of the heart in animals treated with methotrexate. *J. Thorac. Cardiovasc. Surg.*, **46**, 616
6. Cooper, D.K.C. (1968). Experimental development of cardiac transplantation. *Br. Med. J.*, **4**, 174
7. Uys, C.J. and Rose, A.G. (1983). The pathology of cardiac transplantation. In Silver, M.D. (ed.) *Cardiovascular Pathology*. Vol. 2, p. 1329. (New York: Churchill Livingstone)
8. Thomson, J.G. (1968). Heart transplantation in man – necropsy findings. *Br. Med. J.*, **2**, 511
9. Lower, R.R., Lontos, H.A., Kosek, J.C., Sewell, D.H. and Graham, W.H. (1968). Experiences in heart transplantation. Technic, physiology and rejection. *Am. J. Cardiol.*, **22**, 766
10. Rose, A.G., Uys, C.J., Losman, J. and Barnard, C.N. (1979). Morphological changes in 49 Chacma baboon cardiac allografts. *S. Afr. Med. J.*, **56**, 880
11. Nowygrod, R., Spotnitz, H.M., Dubroff, J.M., Hardy, M.A. and Reemtsma, K. (1983). Organ mass: an indicator of heart transplant rejection. *Transplant Proc.*, **15**, 1225
12. Thomas, F.J. and Lower, R.R. (1978). Heart transplantation – 1978. *Surg. Clin. North Am.* **58**, 335
13. Copeland, J.G. and Stinson, E.B. (1979). Human heart transplantation. *Curr. Probl. Cardiol.*, **4**, 1
14. Rose, A.G., Uys, C.J., Losman, J.G. and Barnard, C.N. (1978). Evaluation of endomyocardial biopsy in the diagnosis of cardiac rejection. A study using bioptome samples of formalin-fixed tissue. *Transplantation*, **26**, 10
15. Baandrup, U., Florio, R.A., Roters, F. and Olsen, E.G. (1981). Electron microscopic investigation of endomyocardial biopsy samples in hypertrophy and cardiomyopathy. A semi-quantitative study in 48

patients. *Circulation*, **63**, 1289
16. Losman, J.G., Rose, A.G. and Barnard, C.N. (1977). Myocardial fibrinolytic activity in allogeneic cardiac rejection. *Transplantation*, **23**, 414
17. Kosek, J.C., Chartrand, C., Hurley, E.J. and Lower, R.R. (1969). Arteries in canine cardiac homografts. Ultrastructure during acute rejection. *Lab. Invest.*, **21**, 328
18. Lessof, M. (1978). Immunological reactions in heart disease. *Br. Heart J.*, **40**, 211
19. Herskowitz, A., Soule, L.M., Mellits, E.D., Traill, T.A., Achuff, S.C., Reitz, B.A., Borkon, A.M., Baumgartner, W.A. and Baughman, K.L. (1987). Histologic predictors of acute cardiac rejection in human endomyocardial biopsies: a multivariate analysis. *J. Am. Coll. Cardiol.*, **9**, 802
20. Cooper, D.K.C., Fraser, R.C., Rose, A.G., Ayzenberg, O., Oldfield, G.S., Hassoulas, J.N., Novitzky, D., Uys, C.J. and Barnard, C.N. (1982). Technique, complications, and clinical value of endomyocardial biopsy in patients with heterotopic heart transplants. *Thorax*, **37**, 727
21. Billingham, M.E. (1982). Diagnosis of cardiac rejection by endomyocardial biopsy. *Heart Transplant.*, **1**, 25
22. Kemnitz, J., Cohnert, T., Schafers, H.J., Helmke, M., Wahlers, T., Herrmann, G., Schmidt, R.M. and Haverich, A. (1987). A classification of cardiac rejection. A modification of the classification by Billingham. *Am. J. Surg. Pathol.*, **11**, 503
23. McAllister, H.A., Schnee, M.J., Radovancevic, B. and Frazier, O.H. (1986). A system for grading cardiac allograft rejection. *Tex. Heart Inst. J.*, **13**, 1
24. Lanza, R.P., Cooper, D.K.C., Novitzky, D. and Barnard, C.N. (1983). Survival after cardiac transplantation. (Letter) *S. Afr. Med. J.*, **64**, 1007
25. Griffith, B.P., Hardesty, R.L., Bahnson, H.T., Bernstein, R.L. and Starzl, T.E. (1983). Cardiac transplants with cyclosporin-A and low-dose prednisone: histologic graduation of rejection. *Transplant. Proc.*, **15**, 1241
26. Ratliff, N.B., Myles, J., McMahon, J., Golding, L., Hobbs, R., Rincon, G., Sterba, R. and Stewart, R. (1986). Reversible myocyte injury in cyclosporine treated cardiac transplants. (Abstract). *United States-Canadian Division International Academy of Pathology*, Annual Meeting, New Orleans
27. Oyer, P.E., Stinson, E.B., Reitz, B.A., Jamieson, S.W., Hunt, S., Schroeder, J.S., Billingham, M.E., Wallwork, J., Bieber, C.P., Baumgartner, W.A., Gamberg, P.L., Miller, J.L. and Shumway, N.E. (1982). Preliminary results with cyclosporin-A. In White, D.J.G. (ed.) *Cyclosporine A*. p. 461. (Amsterdam: Elsevier Biomedical)
28. Rose, A.G. (1986). Endomyocardial biopsy diagnosis of cardiac rejection. *Heart Failure*, **2**, 64
29. Uys, C.J., Rose, A.G. and Barnard, C.N. (1979). The pathology of human cardiac transplantation: an assessment after 11 years' experience at Groote Schuur Hospital. *S. Afr. Med. J.*, **56**, 887
30. Southern, J.F., Howard, C. and Fallon, J.T. (1987). Myocyte necrosis in cardiac transplant biopsies identified by immunofluorescence. (Abstract). *United States-Canadian Division International Academy of Pathology*, Annual Meeting, Chicago
31. Novitzky, D., Rose, A.G., Cooper, D.K.C. and Reichart, B.A. (1986). Histopathologic changes at the site of endomyocardial biopsy: potential for confusion with acute rejection. *J. Heart Transplant.*, **5**, 79
32. Rose, A.G., Novitzky, D. and Cooper, D.K.C. (1986). Endomyocardial biopsy site morphology. An experimental study in baboons. *Arch. Pathol. Lab. Med.*, **110**, 622
33. Rose, A.G., Uys, C.J., Novitzky, D., Cooper, D.K.C. and Barnard, C.N. (1983). Toxoplasmosis of donor and recipient hearts after heterotopic cardiac transplantation. *Arch. Pathol. Lab. Med.*, **107**, 368
34. Novitzky, D., Wicomb, W.N., Cooper, D.K.C., Rose, A.G., Fraser, R.C. and Barnard, C.N. (1984). Electrocardiographic and endocrine changes occurring during experimental brain death in the Chacma baboon. *J. Heart Transplant.*, **4**, 63
35. Novitzky, D., Wicomb, W.N., Rose, A.G., Cooper, D.K.C. and Reichart, B. (1986). Prevention of myocardial injury during brain death by total cardiac sympathectomy in the Chacma baboon. *Ann. Thorac. Surg.*, **41**, 520
36. Rose, A.G., Novitzky, D. and Factor, S.M. (1988). Catecholamine-associated smooth muscle contraction bands in the media of coronary arteries of brain-dead baboons. *Am. J. Cardiovasc. Pathol.*, **2**, 63
37. Greenberg, M.L., Uretsky, B.F., Reddy, P.S., Bernstein, R.L., Griffith, B.P., Hardesty, R.L., Thompson, M.E. and Bahnson, H.T. (1985). Long-term hemodynamic follow-up of cardiac transplant patients treated with cyclosporine and prednisone. *Circulation*, **71**, 487
38. Novitzky, D., Boniaszczuk, J., Cooper, D.K.C., Isaacs, S., Rose, A.G., Smith, J.A., Uys, C.J., Barnard, C.N. and Fraser, R. (1984). Prediction of acute cardiac rejection using radionuclide techniques. *S. Afr. Med. J.*, **65**, 5

16
Diagnosis and Management of Acute Rejection

D.K.C. COOPER

INTRODUCTION

Acute rejection is not a steady phenomenon, but occurs in sporadic waves, extending over a few days or a week or two. Since the introduction of cyclosporine (CsA) as an immunosuppressive agent, severe acute rejection episodes have become relatively rare (seen in less than 2% of endomyocardial biopsies at our center)[1]. Mild acute rejection (cellular infiltration) is seen fairly frequently, but many groups would not increase therapy in such cases. It is impossible to predict whether or not any individual patient will experience episodes of rejection and, when it occurs, it may be impossible to make the diagnosis on clinical evidence until it is extremely advanced.

These episodes of acute rejection diminish with time, the recipient's immune system appearing to adapt to the presence of the donor organ and its histocompatibility antigens. A state of unresponsiveness is achieved, and maintenance immunosuppressive therapy may be progressively reduced. No center involved in cardiac transplantation has yet, however, successfully weaned patients off immunosuppresive therapy altogether, even when several years have elapsed since the operation. It would appear that the possibility of an acute rejection episode is always present, even some years after transplantation, particularly if a patient fails to take his immunosuppressive medication regularly.

DIAGNOSIS OF ACUTE REJECTION

The patient may feel completely well until the rejection episode has progressed for some days and donor heart function has deteriorated (sometimes irreversibly) to the point that cardiac failure occurs. The clinical diagnosis of acute rejection may prove more difficult in a patient with a heterotopic heart transplant, in whom the recipient heart may assist the cardiac output for a considerable period of time, delaying the onset of symptoms and signs of cardiac failure. Irreversible damage of the myocardium may occur before clinical features become manifest. For successful therapy to be initiated at an early stage, the diagnosis must therefore be made before clinical features of cardiac failure occur.

Endomyocardial biopsy (EMB) remains the most reliable method - indeed, to date the only reliable method – of confirming rejection, and has a high sensitivity (97%) and specificity (100%)[2]; at most centers it is performed at least weekly during the first month after transplantation. The search for a simple, non-invasive method of detecting acute rejection in its early stages (or even predicting in advance) has continued for a number of years, but to date has eluded workers, though several potential methods are being investigated, some showing encouraging results. There are, however, some clinical features and simple investigations that may make the attending physician suspicious that a rejection episode is developing.

Clinical features

Acute rejection is frequently totally asymptomatic, particularly in its early stages. In a patient with an orthotopic allograft, the clinical diagnosis of rejection relies mainly on symptoms and signs indicating cardiac failure, particularly of right ventricular failure due to the decreased compliance associated with cellular infiltration and edema of the graft. In the early stages following cardiac transplantation, however, several other factors may affect the performance of the right ventricle, e.g. inadequate preservation of the heart during transportation and transplantation, an increased pulmonary vascular resistance, and fluid overload (secondary either to steroid therapy or impairment of renal function from CsA therapy). These factors may make a clinical diagnosis of rejection uncertain.

In the heterotopic transplant, however, due to the support given by the patient's own right ventricle, evidence of right ventricular failure may not occur during rejection and, therefore, such symptoms and signs cannot be relied upon in the diagnosis of this complication.

The onset of features of cardiac failure, however, should always be considered to be due to acute rejection until proved otherwise. If acute rejection is confirmed, the treatment is primarily increased immunosuppression rather than antifailure therapy, though this may be indicated also.

Any clinical features suggesting a reduction in cardiac output (e.g. cool periphery, diminished pulse volume, weight gain), muffled or reduced amplitude heart sounds, the development of a pericardial friction rub, tachycardia or gallop rhythm, or a dysrhythmia (in the absence of electrolyte or acid-base disturbance), should be viewed suspiciously until acute rejection has been excluded. Very occasionally, patients complain of vague chest discomfort or are feverish during an acute rejection episode.

Radiographic appearance

Radiographic evidence of rejection consists of progressive cardiomegaly, increasing pulmonary plethora, and, rarely, pulmonary edema. An increase in cardiac volume of more than 10% or 100 ml compared with the previous measurement, and a simultaneous increase of the cardiothoracic ratio of more than 2%, has been suggested as confirmation of acute rejection[3]. Using these criteria, sensitivity and specificity were 76% and 97%, respectively. Predictive values of a positive or negative test for the presence or absence of rejection were 82% and 96%, respectively. Such radiographic changes may well make the physician suspicious that rejection is occurring, but should not be relied upon exclusively.

Occasionally, the appearances are those of an exudate from the epicardium. Following orthotopic transplantation, fluid exuding from the epicardium may show up as a pericardial effusion (and may be associated with clinical features suggestive of subacute tamponade); after heterotopic transplantation, it may present as a right-sided pleural effusion.

In our experience, microscopic or biochemical examination of this fluid has not proved helpful in differentiating between an effusion resulting from underlying infection and one associated with acute rejection. The presence of a pericardial or pleural effusion should be considered suggestive of acute rejection until proved otherwise. A pleural effusion may, of course, suggest an underlying infective condition of the lung, which should also be aggressively sought. With satisfactory treatment of the acute rejection episode, these effusions will regress and disappear.

Effusions, however, may be absent in patients with severe acute rejection, or may appear very late in the episode. Their development cannot be awaited, therefore, as a reliable diagnostic aid in the recognition of early rejection.

Electrocardiography

For many years, mainly in the pre-CsA era, it was maintained that changes in the electrocardiogram (ECG) provided an indication that acute rejection was occurring[4-6]. Electrocardiographic evidence was based primarily on a decrease in QRS voltage of the donor heart, but was also said to include dysrhythmias[7], various degrees of heart block, occasional depression of ST segments, and a shift of axis[8,9].

There is now considerable evidence to suggest that the conventional 12-lead surface ECG is not helpful in monitoring rejection except in extremely advanced cases[10-14], and the amplitude of the QRS complex, in particular, is no longer measured in most centers. Other modalities of electrocardiographic monitoring, however, have shown some correlation with the presence of acute rejection.

In a study by Haberl et al.[15], two well-defined surface electrocardiographic recordings were analyzed by *fast Fourier transform* each day for 4 weeks after cardiac transplantation in 27 patients. Single-beat analysis of the QRS complex by this method revealed a progressive change of the spectral morphology on the days of rejection in 19 of 20 patients. After successful treatment, the frequency spectra returned to control within 1–2 weeks in most patients.

With a signal-averaged ECG, Keren et al.[16] were able to detect 92% of rejection episodes occurring in the late postoperative period in human transplant patients, but the technique was not sensitive enough to detect mild rejection nor rejection in the early post-transplant period.

Warnecke et al.[17] monitored rejection in nine patients by *intramyocardial electrogram* recordings transmitted by an implanted telemetric pacemaker. Of 33 rejection episodes, 29 were correctly predicted, with a voltage drop above 15% used as a criterion (sensitivity 88%). Eighty-three of 86 negative biopsy results corresponded to negative intramyocardial electrogram results, giving a specificity of 97%. Conversely, Wahlers et al.[18,19] concluded that measurements of intracardiac electrogram voltages by pacemaker telemetry, as well as single averaging of a single lead, failed to predict allograft rejection when compared with the endomyocardial biopsy. It seems unlikely that voltage changes obtained from the intramyocardial electrogram will be sensitive enough to allow reliable diagnosis of acute rejection as the voltage varies throughout a 24-hour period with significant diurnal changes, and is greatly influenced by exercise[18].

Unipolar peak-to-peak amplitude analysis has been shown to be a quantitative measure of ischemic myocardial injury. The technique requires placement of sutureless screw-in electrodes on the anterior and posterior aspect of each ventricle at the time of transplantation. In one clinical study, a unipolar peak-to-peak amplitude decline of 15% or greater occurred consistently 1–3 days before the biopsy detected rejection[20]. This gave the technique 100% sensitivity and 90% specificity in predicting and detecting cardiac allograft rejection.

Electrophysiologic monitoring using endocardial leads in transplanted hearts in dogs showed data that were inconclusive in predicting or detecting rejection[21]. In a detailed study in dogs with heterotopic heart transplants, Avitall and his colleagues[22], using epicardial electrodes, investigated changes in late diastolic thresholds, refractory periods of the left ventricle and right atrium, and conduction times from right atrium to left atrium, left ventricle to right ventricle, and right atrium to right ventricle. None of the measurements evaluated was shown to be a sensitive marker of mild rejection. In non-immunosuppressed pigs, however, ventricular voltage reduction from epicardial leads correlated with moderate to severe rejection but not with mild rejection[23].

Power spectrum analysis is a technique used to characterize beat-to-beat heart rate variability, which normally reflects ongoing autonomic modulation of cardiac function. Heart rate variability has been found to be greatly reduced in stable transplant recipients[24]. Increased broad-band heart rate variability became more marked during episodes of rejection in a small group of transplanted patients[24].

Some evidence has suggested that graft rejection in heart transplant recipients is accompanied by sinus node dysfunction[25]. ECG recordings of heart transplant patients who were in sinus rhythm were processed through patented digital routines that calculated the *power spectrum of the RR intervals*. A significant decrease in the peak spectral power of respiratory sinus arrhythmia was noted in patients who experienced rejection episodes. The sensitivity of this test was 100%, specificity 42%, positive predictive value 22%, and negative predictive value 100%.

Despite the relative accuracy of some of the above techniques, to my knowledge no major center involved in heart transplantation today is relying solely on any one or combination of them to detect rejection.

Hematological and immunological monitoring

A steady and progressive rise in the white blood cell (WBC) count, or in the total lymphocyte count, or, particularly, in the T-11 lymphocyte subset, may, on occasion, indicate that a rejection episode is occurring, but is unreliable[26]. A rise in the *T-cell fraction* has been considered helpful, and there is some evidence that fluctuations in the number of circulating T-cells may reflect an earlier phase of the host immune response to the cardiac allograft than that provided by endomyocardial biopsy[27,28]. This Stanford experience, however, was documented before the introduction of CsA, at a time when antithymocyte globulin (ATG) was administered regularly for several weeks post-transplantation. A rapid expansion of the circulating T-lymphocyte population, after discontinuation of ATG, was shown to correlate closely with the development of acute rejection.

In our experience, however, none of these parameters is reliable, though a persistent rise in the T-cell fraction in the early post-transplant period is suspicious in that it reflects that the host's immune system is responding to the presence of the foreign tissue. As CsA does not depress the number of circulating T-lymphocytes, monitoring of the T-cell fraction has not been put forward as such a valuable indicator of acute rejection in patients receiving this drug.

The development of *monoclonal antibody and fluorescent labelling of peripheral blood lymphocyte subsets* has refined standard T-cell monitoring[29], but changes in the ratio of the various subsets (e.g. T-helper (T4, CD4)/T-suppressor (T8, CD8) ratio) have not proved uniformly reliable in monitoring acute rejection[26,30–40]. *Transferrin receptors* (TRs) have been shown to be expressed on the surface of activated lymphocytes at an early stage in the cell cycle. An elevated percentage of TR-positive lymphocytes has been shown to be associated with rejection episodes[41,42], but also with infection. The T-helper/T-suppressor cytotoxic ratio was found to increase significantly during rejection (1.5 ± 1.0 to 1.96 ± 0.92), but remain low in infection (1.3 ± 1.5). The combined use of the percentage of TR-positive lymphocytes and the CD4/CD8 ratio may therefore be helpful in differentiating rejection from infection.

Cytoimmunological monitoring (CIM) is a combined morphological and T-cell subset analysis of peripheral blood lymphocytes that has been put forward as a predictor of acute rejection[43,44], but remains controversial[26,45]. An increase in the number of 'activated' (immunoblastic) lymphocytes in peripheral blood smears (Figures 16.1 and 16.2) is said to be a sensitive indicator that acute rejection is occurring or is about to occur; viral infection, an alternative and frequent cause of such activation, can be identified (and therefore excluded) by detecting a suppression of the CD4/CD8 ratio below 1.0. With CIM, cardiac rejection episodes were detected with a sensitivity of 94% and a specificity of 70%; a 6% false-negative rate was documented.

Other groups, however, have reported that neither CIM nor immunophenotyping is sensitive or specific enough to substitute for EMB in screening for tissue rejection[26,45]. In one detailed study, 83% of patients with biopsy-proven rejection and 81% without had increased levels of morphological activated lymphocytes[26]. Multiple other criteria for determining levels of activation were used without improving sensitivity or specificity. The use of CD4/CD8 ratios to discriminate between activation caused by rejection and that from viral infection and other inflammatory conditions yielded a sensitivity of 43% and specificity of 56%.

The group that introduced CIM (and others), however, continues to show good correlation with EMB, and it is

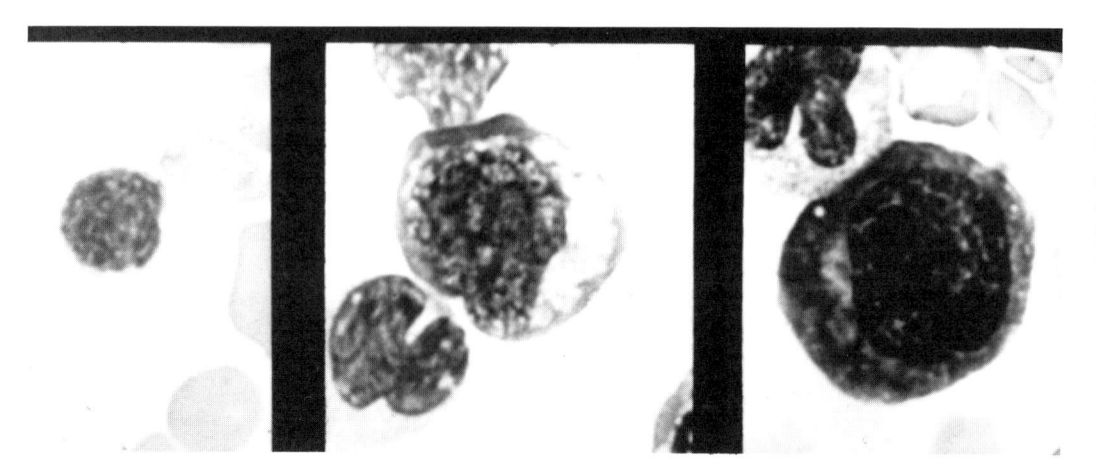

Figure 16.1 Circulating lymphocytes in different stages of 'activation'. *Left*: normal small lymphocyte; *Center*: activated lymphocyte; *Right*: T-lymphoblast. Note the difference in size, cytoplasm staining properties, and number of nucleoli (× 1100). (Courtesy of Dr C. Hammer, Munich)

possible that interpretation of the morphology is different at various centers. This, in itself, however, must be deemed a disadvantage of the method, and might restrict its widespread use. Its true value as a reliable predictor of rejection, therefore, remains questionable.

The *in vitro culture of activated lymphocytes* obtained by endomyocardial biopsy in media containing interleukin-2 (IL-2) showed correlation between positive cultures and acute rejection on EMB, and also appeared to have a predictive value in some cases with regard to the subsequent biopsy. The results, however, were not conclusive, and the test requires EMB as an initial step. It therefore remains invasive, and, furthermore, does not fulfil many of the other ideal criteria of a diagnostic test, e.g. the result cannot be obtained within minutes or hours[46].

Correlation has been found between the results of EMB and changes in the number of T-cells expressing *interleukin-2 receptors* (IL-2R)[47,48]. Interleukin-2 receptor is the protein that mediates the action of interleukin-2, an immune system growth hormone (Chapter 14). Normal resting T- and B-lymphocytes do not displace significant numbers of these receptors on their surface. When these cells are stimulated by a challenge to the immune system and begin to divide, the expression of IL-2R changes in 2 ways: (1) more molecules of IL-2R are expressed on the cell's plasma membrane, and (2) a form of the IL-2R protein is released by the activated cells into the fluid surrounding them. During a rejection episode (and during infection), therefore, interleukin-2 receptors are released from the T-cells into the plasma, where they can be measured. Initial high sensitivity and specificity, however, are lost after 5 weeks. The test is significantly influenced by the presence of a viral infection, making differentiation from rejection difficult or impossible. Elevation of soluble IL-2R beyond 2 weeks after transplantation would appear to be a poor prognostic sign regarding long-term survival[49-51]. This test appears promising, but requires further evaluation before its value can be fully assessed.

Serum levels of γ *interferon*, an important lymphokine produced by activated T-helper cells, and therefore a marker of T-lymphocyte activity, and *neopterin* were measured by Woloszczuk and his colleagues in both heart and kidney transplant patients[52]. Neopterin is a pteridine[53,54], which is produced by macrophages mediated by activated T-cells[55]; the mediator of this process is thought to be γ interferon. Rejection crises and infection were accompanied by distinct increases in serum neopterin. γ interferon levels were elevated for a short period 1 or 2 days earlier, both in infection and in rejection, though they were higher in infection. Each rise in γ interferon was followed by an increase of neopterin, but not every neopterin increase was preceded by a peak of γ interferon. It was concluded that both measurements allowed a simple, quick and reliable monitoring of the immune status of the transplant patient.

The role of neopterin in the immunologic defense mechan-

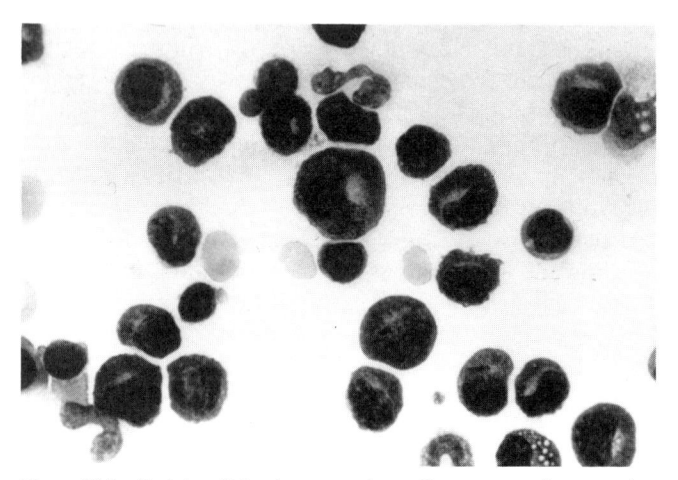

Figure 16.2 Peripheral blood mononuclear cell concentrate from a patient 7 days after heart transplantation. Lymphocytes in different stages of 'activation' can be seen, including small and activated lymphocytes and a lymphoblast (× 680). (Courtesy of Dr C. Hammer, Munich)

ism is still unknown. High levels of neopterin during graft rejection have been observed[53,55-57]. The highest increases have sometimes been noted almost 3 days before a positive endomyocardial biopsy, whereas on the day of the biopsy the neopterin changes were insignificant. There is also an increase in neopterin levels during the early postoperative period which can confuse the results[57]. Any event associated with increased activity of T-cells and macrophages (including infection) may cause an increased neopterin level[54,56,57]. Other factors, such as the immunosuppressive protocol used, also affect neopterin levels.

Havel and his colleagues[57] concluded that daily measurements of serum or urinary neopterin levels would be necessary to provide optimal sensitivity close to 100%. In practice, this would be possible only during hospitalization. In view of this limitation, these authors concluded that neopterin levels would not represent an alternative to EMB, but might be an indication for it during the early stages after transplantation.

There are some reports suggesting that *serum and urinary β-2-microglobulin* levels are useful for the diagnosis of acute kidney graft rejection[58,59] and may be a valuable adjunct in predicting and diagnosing acute cardiac rejection[60]. β-2-Microglobulin levels, however, may increase due to factors other than graft rejection (e.g. nephrotoxic antibodies and viral infections) and may vary if samples are not collected consistently or if the radioimmunoassay is not performed in a consistent fashion[60].

Urinary polyamine levels reflect cellular proliferation or degeneration in a variety of pathologic disorders, and have been proposed to be markers of lymphocyte proliferation on the basis of their synthesis in cultured human lymphocytes and their increasing intracellular concentration during lymphocyte transformation. Alterations in urinary polyamine levels may thus permit cellular proliferation in the immune system to be predicted before anatomic organ rejection. Carrier and colleagues[61] investigated urinary polyamines as non-invasive markers of unmodified heart allograft rejection in dogs, and noted that the urinary level rose during the first to third day after transplantation, which correlated with histopathological features of rejection. When the recipient dogs were immunosuppressed with CsA with or without steroids, each episode of rejection occurred from 1 to 4 days after a significant increase in urinary polyamine levels.

In heart transplant patients, the sensitivity of polyamine assays to predict rejection has been found to be 85%, the specificity 88%, and the positive predictive value 79%[62]. These results, though promising, would not appear good enough to warrant use of this method as the sole method of detecting rejection.

Prolactin has been shown to play a role in the modulation of the immune system, and there is some evidence to suggest that it might fluctuate as a function of immunologic events.

The Arizona group[63] followed prolactin blood levels in heart transplant patients. The sensitivity of prolactin to predict rejection was 79%, the specificity 92%, and the positive predictive value 61%. This accuracy was clearly inadequate for the test to be valuable in the clinical management of patients with heart transplants.

Immunologic events are accompanied by the release of arachidonic acid and its subsequent metabolism[64]. One such metabolic route gives rise to an unstable compound, thromboxane A2[65]. Increases in the urinary excretion of immunoreactive *thromboxane B2*, the stable breakdown product of thromboxane A2, have been documented in the rat during acute rejection of cardiac allografts[66], and in patients with kidney transplants[67]. This technique does not appear to have been evaluated thoroughly in patients with cardiac allografts.

Although a large number of hematological and immunological tests has been investigated as non-invasive markers of acute rejection, none has yet been found to be reliable enough to replace EMB. Several groups are, however, using one or more tests on a routine basis in the early post-transplant period as an adjunct to EMB, and have been able to reduce the frequency of biopsy during this period.

Arterial pulse wave monitoring

In patients with a heterotopic transplant, a comparison of the respective donor and recipient pulse waves, when measured on an external pulse trace (e.g. obtained by Doppler) taken over the femoral or carotid artery, has proved helpful in diagnosing acute rejection (Figure 16.3)[68,69]. The comparative heights of the two pulse waves demonstrate the relative contributions of the two hearts. In a severe acute rejection episode, when donor myocardial function is impaired, the donor wave diminishes relatively in height and the recipient increases.

Endomyocardial biopsy (EMB)

Percutaneous transvenous or transarterial EMB of right or left ventricle with a specially designed forceps, thus obtaining fragments of endocardium for histological examination, was first described by Sakakibara and Konno in 1962[70], and, 10 years later, was introduced as a clinical tool in heart transplantation by Caves and his colleagues[71]. At most centers, donor heart biopsy is performed at approximately weekly intervals during the first month after transplantation, with decreasing frequency during subsequent months. EMB is also performed whenever a rejection episode is suspected and to assess the efficacy of a course of antirejection therapy.

In patients with an orthotopic transplant, the percutaneous supraclavicular approach to either right or left jugular vein is our approach of choice (Figure 16.4), though the infraclavicular or femoral routes can be used. In those with

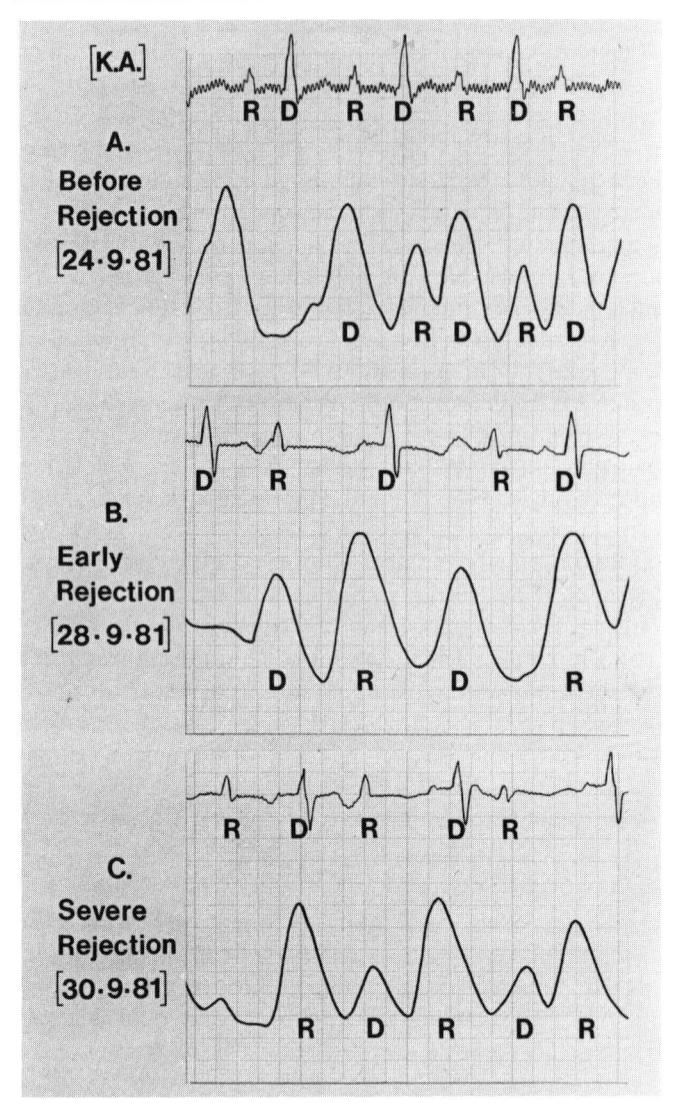

Figure 16.3 Recordings of electrocardiogram (ECG) (above) and arterial pulse waves (taken over femoral artery) (below) showing changes occurring during an acute rejection episode. R = recipient; D = donor

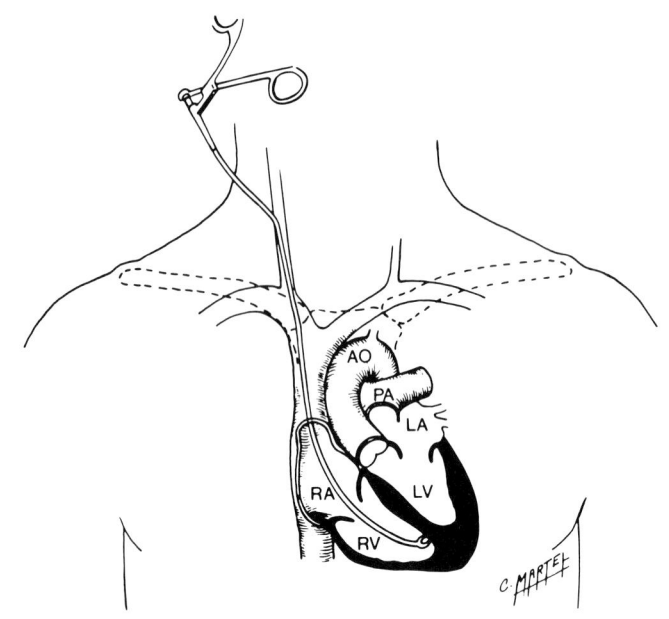

Figure 16.4 The technique of endomyocardial biopsy in a patient with an orthotopic heart transplant. The bioptome has been introduced into the right jugular vein, and passed via the superior vena cava and right atrium into the right ventricle

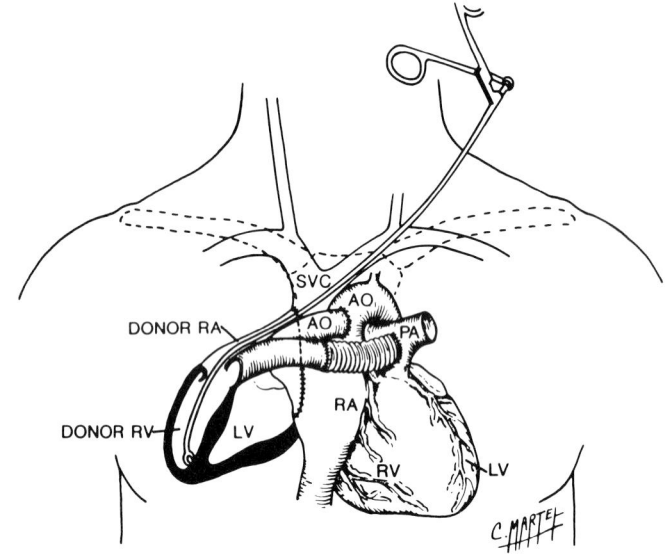

Figure 16.5 The technique of endomyocardial biopsy in a patient with a heterotopic heart transplant. The bioptome has been introduced into the junction of the left internal jugular and subclavian veins, and passed via the superior vena cava and donor right atrium into the donor right ventricle

a heterotopic transplant, the supraclavicular approach at the jugular–subclavian junction may be preferred (Figure 16.5). The techniques in both orthotopic[1,71,72] and heterotopic[2] transplant patients have been described fully elsewhere. In either case, the procedure takes 15–30 min and is performed in the cardiac catheterization laboratory. At least three (and preferably more) biopsies should be taken on each occasion to enable the histopathologist to make an adequate diagnosis. It is a relatively safe invasive procedure with few significant complications (0.3% at our institution[1]).

Cardiac perforation, with resulting hemorrhage (± tamponade) can occur, however, though the incidence is low (three of 10 000 biopsy procedures at Stanford, without mortality – M.E. Billingham, quoted by Locke et al.[73]). Coronary artery–right ventricular fistula has recently been described, and is more common than previously suspected[73–75] (Chapter 22). It was originally thought that repeated biopsy in any one patient could be undertaken without added complication[2], but the reported incidence of coronary artery fistula throws doubt on this conclusion.

The introduction of infection is also a potential hazard. Pulmonary embolism (or systemic embolism if a left ventricular biopsy has been taken) from dislodgement of mural thrombus, which may result from decreased myocardial contractions due to rejection, is also a potential complication. Other complications that have been reported include pneumothorax, the induction of arrhythmias, and temporary brachial or phrenic nerve paresis by the injection of local anesthetic[2].

Assessment of rejection is based on light microscopy (Chapter 15). Occasional or even repeated biopsies can be misleading, however, due to histopathological interpretations that are either incorrect or based on inadequate or unrepresentative tissue. The biopsy itself initiates an inflammatory response which results in a sequence of histological changes (cellular infiltration, interstitial edema and hemorrhage, and even myocyte necrosis) that may closely mimic acute rejection[76,77]. The pathophysiological changes that take place during the agonal period in the donor can also lead to myocardial changes (including mononuclear cell infiltration and myonecrosis) that can be erroneously interpreted as acute rejection in the early post-transplant period[78,79].

Echocardiography

During an acute rejection episode, because of a decreased compliance, altered diastolic ventricular function can be observed by Doppler echocardiography[80,81]. Isovolumetric relaxation times have been demonstrated to show considerable correlation with acute rejection, but the method is thought by some to be not sensitive enough to use as a substitute for cardiac biopsy[81-83]. A recent study from Paris confirmed that acute rejection was associated with a significant decrease of isovolumic relaxation time and especially of pressure half-time, with no change in heart rate and peak early mitral flow velocity[84]. With 20% decrease in pressure half-time as a criterion for acute rejection, sensitivity was 88%, specificity 87%, and positive predictive value 85%.

Some groups have been able to show some correlation between the measurements derived from the Doppler mitral flow velocity curve or the jugular venous flow velocity curve and acute rejection episodes[82,83,85], though others have been unable to demonstrate any such correlation[86]. The poor reproducibility of velocity half-time possibly makes this an unreliable measurement for clinical decision making.

Using two-dimensional (2D) echocardiography, left ventricular mass was shown to increase with reversible rejection episodes[87,88], without significant concurrent change in ejection fraction or end-diastolic volume. In another study (in dogs), however, changes in 2D echocardiography were found to be inconsistent[89]. Chandrasakaran et al. demonstrated that changes in echointensity estimated from serial 2D echocardiograms of the heterotopically transplanted dog heart were consistently associated with the early, reversible phase of rejection[90]. These authors, however, drew attention to the fact that the histologic changes of rejection observed in humans treated with various immunosuppressive drugs would not be as clear as they are in the experimental animal.

Changes in serial M-mode echocardiography have generally not been shown to correlate closely with rejection episodes[91,92]. Popp et al., however, demonstrated an increase in posterior wall thickness during rejection[93]. Estimating the left ventricular mass with M-mode has limitations; inherent variations in left ventricular mass are substantial, and the changes with rejection are believed by some to be too small to depend on this parameter[94].

The lack of agreement by the various investigators regarding the sensitivity of echocardiography in providing reliable information on which to base a diagnosis of acute rejection would suggest that this investigative procedure is not yet an acceptable alternative to EMB.

Scintigraphic techniques

Acute rejection leads to cellular infiltration and edema of the myocardium, together with damage of the myofibers, resulting in thickening of the ventricular walls, reduction in ventricular cavity volume (Figure 16.6), reduction of left ventricular compliance, and impairment of myocardial function. In patients whose therapy includes CsA, myocardial edema is less prominent, and therefore ventricular wall thickening is less obvious; cellular infiltration is present, however, resulting in a loss of compliance. Several of these features, e.g. lymphocyte infiltration, myocyte injury, or reduction in left ventricular cavity volume, can be demonstrated by scintigraphic techniques.

The infiltration of *indium-111-labelled lymphocytes or leukocytes* (or platelets) into allografts, indicative of rejection, is detectable non-invasively by γ scintigraphy, and has been investigated in monitoring for early detection of rejection[95,96]. Several groups have demonstrated the feasibility of detecting early rejection of heterotopic transplants in small laboratory animals with ^{111}In-labelled lymphocytes or leukocytes[95,97,98]; rejection could be detected 3-4 days before weakening of the heart beat[97]. Similarly, the results correlated well with endomyocardial biopsy findings after cardiac transplantation in dogs[99-101]. The technique appears to permit detection of rejection at an early enough stage to allow the process to be reversed by increased immunotherapy[102].

The uptake of labelled lymphocytes into the myocardium, however, cannot be construed to be an entirely specific phenomenon for detection of rejection[95,103]. Diseases associated with lymphocytic infiltration of the myocardium, such as toxoplasmosis and cytomegalovirus myocarditis, are likely to be detected as well. Ischemia-induced reperfusion injury may also be difficult to differentiate from rejection.

A similar technique using technetium 99m-labelled leukocytes has been investigated[104].

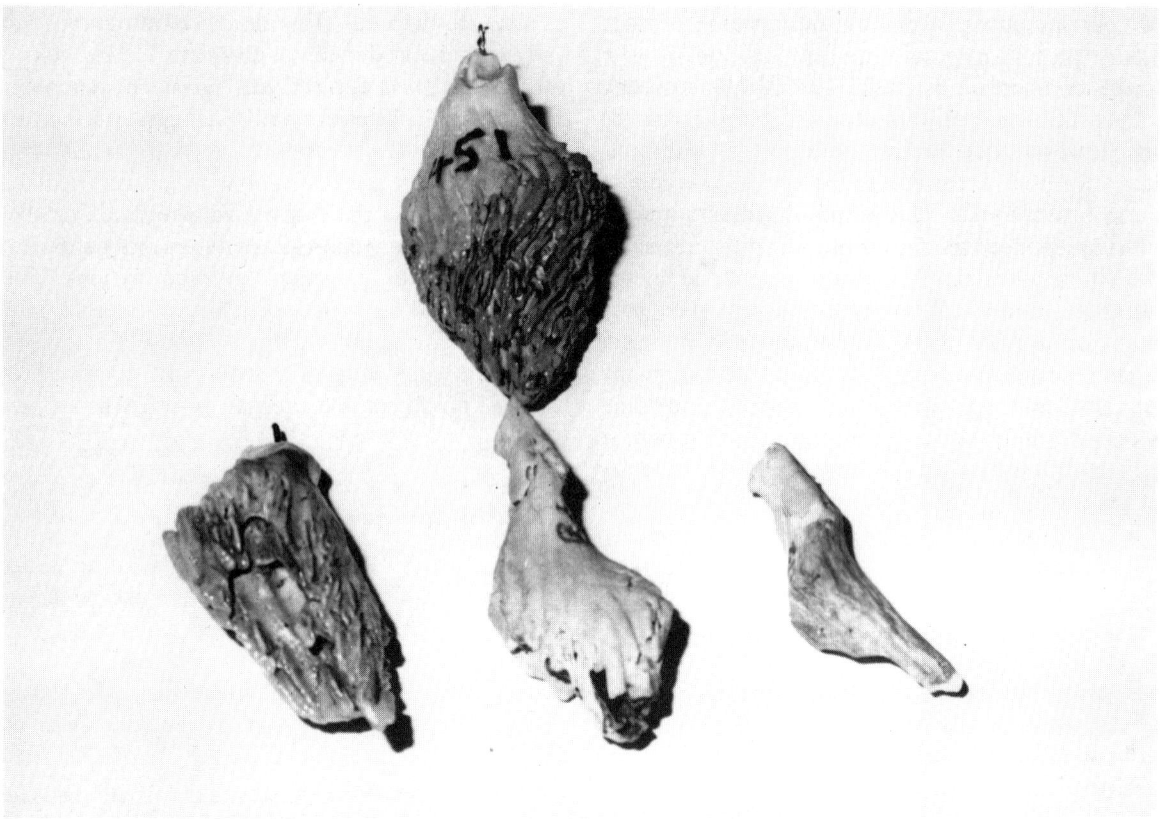

Figure 16.6 Casts of the left ventricular cavity after orthotopic heart transplantation in baboons of similar height and mass undergoing different degrees of acute rejection; A: no rejection (normal ventricular volume); B: mild acute rejection; C: moderate acute rejection; D: severe acute rejection. Note the decrease in left ventricular volume as rejection progresses. These changes in volume can be detected by radionuclide scanning techniques, such as technetium-99m labelling of red cells (Novitzky, D. et al[115])

The use of [111]In-*labelled antimyosin antibodies* to detect rejection after cardiac transplantation was first suggested by Khaw et al.[105]. As a result of disruption of the sarcolemma, myosin is exposed during an acute rejection episode. The loss of cell membrane integrity exposes myosin to extracellular fluid; antimyosin antibody, labelled with ^{111}In, can bind to the myosin, indicating evidence of myocardial damage[106,107]. Work in animal models suggests that antimyosin antibody uptake correlates with EMB scores, and can provide a non-invasive method to detect allograft rejection[88,108-110].

A recently completed study in cardiac transplant patients using ^{111}In antimyosin demonstrated both specificity and sensitivity of 80%[111]. Good correlation between EMB and antimyosin scintigraphy has also been demonstrated by Carrio et al.[107] and Schutz et al.[112]; in this latter study specificity was 100%.

A disadvantage of this technique is the requirement of a time interval of 48 hours between administration of the labelled antibody and the counts acquisition; the method, therefore, cannot provide immediate confirmation of rejection. Further disadvantages include: (1) the test becomes positive primarily in the presence of myocyte necrosis[113], and is less sensitive in early acute rejection; (2) the result is not easy to quantify; (3) false positives may occur[107] which may be related to an effect of cyclosporine[113]; and (4) human antimurine antibodies may develop in patients who undergo repeated study.

Radionuclide scanning of the volume and function of the donor left ventricle with *technetium-99m pyrophosphate-labelled red cells* has been used to monitor acute rejection after both heterotopic and orthotopic heart transplantation, and has been compared with histopathological evidence of rejection obtained from EMB. The technique of multigated blood pool scanning and calculation of left ventricular volumes has been detailed[114]. Ejection fraction, end-diastolic, end-systolic, and stroke volumes were calculated on each occasion. Changes in stroke volume, in particular, showed a high correlation with histopathological evidence of moderate and severe rejection ($p < 0.001$), whereas changes in ejection fraction showed no correlation[115,116]. This technique has proved a useful adjunct to EMB, but reproducibility can at times prove difficult, and it is not yet considered reliable enough to replace EMB.

Gallium-67 imaging is widely used to detect acute and chronic inflammatory lesions[117], including cardiac inflammatory processes such as myocarditis[118]. It is now clear that multiple factors contribute to the accumulation of ^{67}Ga in inflammatory lesions[119]. This technique has been investigated as a means of detecting acute rejection in cardiac allografts, both in rats[120] and man[119].

In a study comparing the results of ^{67}Ga scintigraphy with EMB in patients with cardiac transplants, the gallium scan showed an 83% sensitivity, with 17% false negatives and 9% false positives[118]. In its present form, therefore, this test is not reliable enough to warrant routine clinical use. Furthermore, the gallium has to be administered 48 hours before the scan is carried out, which would make it inappropriate for routine clinical application.

In vivo global *thallium kinetics* (distribution of thallium throughout the myocardium) were preserved during mild to severe acute transplant rejection in untreated rats[121]. The complex cellular and extracellular processes of acute rejection would appear, therefore, to limit the usefulness of thallium kinetics in the detection of rejection.

Of presently-available scintigraphic techniques, ^{111}In labelling of lymphocytes or leukocytes, or possibly radionuclide scanning to estimate changes in left ventricular volume, would seem to offer most prospect of providing a sensitive test for the detection of acute rejection in the immediate future.

Proton magnetic resonance imaging

Electrocardiographic-gated magnetic resonance imaging (MRI) is a non-invasive modality that provides high resolution images of the heart. Excellent morphological detail and tissue characterization have been obtained in various pathologic studies of the myocardium with this technique. MRI measurements, such as increased T1 and T2 relaxation times (associated with interstitial edema and infiltration of the myocardium by lymphocytes) and spin density, have been shown to be useful in detecting acute rejection in animal models[122,123]. MRI is also able to detect rejection by demonstrating progressively increasing myocardial wall thickness and decreasing ventricular chamber size[124,125].

Increases in T1 and T2 were seen in excised rejecting rat hearts[126]. In dogs, MRI demonstrated a potential for assessing the severity of cardiac rejection[127,128]. In one study, the linear relationship between the histological changes of rejection and MRI was 72%, while the correlation between T2 relaxation time and the water content was 92%[127].

In patients with heart transplants undergoing acute rejection, elevated T2 relaxation times have been recorded[129]. The accuracy of the technique is moderately high; MRI demonstrated a sensitivity of 78%, a specificity of 90%, and a negative predictive value of 93%. Similar changes may also be found, however, in any condition that results in edema of the myocardium[123], though this point remains debated[124].

Though these early results have been promising, further evaluation of MRI is required before its true value can be assessed.

^{31}P nuclear magnetic resonance spectroscopy

Several investigators have reported studies involving the use of ^{31}P nuclear magnetic resonance (NMR) spectroscopy to detect allograft rejection in experimental animals[130-132]. In a dog heterotopic heart transplant model, high energy phosphate metabolites, evaluated by this method, showed a progressive decrease in phosphocreatine during mild to moderate rejection, dropping to 30–40% of baseline levels with severe rejection[89]. In a similar rat model, there was a significant decrease in the phosphocreatine/inorganic phosphate ratio during rejection[132,133].

Though this technique looks promising, at present it is not applicable to orthotopic heart transplantation as the intervening bone and muscle would contribute to the spectrum, making the results difficult to interpret[134]. Other NMR techniques, including depth-resolved surface coil spectroscopy, are being developed which should allow for non-invasive detection of metabolic changes in an orthotopic heart[135]; such a technical advance is essential for any clinical application.

Comment

At the present time, there are some clinical, electrocardiographic and radiographic features that suggest that an acute rejection episode may be occurring, but EMB represents the only generally accepted reliable method of confirming the presence or absence of rejection. Even EMB can be misleading on occasions, however, and if biopsy proves negative and yet clinical suspicion of rejection is high, then EMB must be repeated as a matter of urgency. Most physicians involved in the care of heart transplant patients would agree that to-date there is no non-invasive technique that has equivalent sensitivity and specificity to EMB.

Technetium-99m scintigraphy, cytoimmunological monitoring, echocardiography, and magnetic resonance imaging have already proved helpful in some centers in suggesting that rejection may be occurring, but are not yet accepted at the majority of centers as negating the need for EMB. The measurement of IL-2R would seem potentially the most reliable *simple* test to indicate that a rejection episode is developing, though differentiation from infection is clearly difficult. Scintigraphy utilizing ^{111}In-labelled lymphocytes would appear particularly worthy of further study. Antimyosin scintigraphy may not prove ideal for day-to-day use. ^{31}P NMR spectroscopy requires further technical advances before its value can be fully assessed.

Many of the non-invasive tests being investigated require expensive, sophisticated equipment that may not be available at every center following heart transplant patients, and would certainly not be available to the average family practitioner. A simple blood test would clearly be the ideal form of monitoring for rejection. The measurement of soluble IL-2R in the peripheral blood would seem to offer most hope of fulfilling this role in the immediate future, although a rise related to the presence of infection would have to be excluded.

The procedure of EMB is unpopular with the majority of heart transplant recipients, and is not without risk (Chapter 22). The search for a non-invasive technique for diagnosing the presence of early rejection (or preferably for predicting the onset of rejection) should therefore continue. Further investigations and trials are required, however, before any non-invasive technique can be accepted as being totally reliable; only then will EMB prove unnecessary.

MANAGEMENT OF AN ACUTE REJECTION EPISODE

When is increased therapy indicated?

When acute rejection is confirmed, the first decision that has to be made is whether it is severe enough to warrant extra immunosuppressive therapy. In patients receiving maintenance triple drug therapy (CsA, azathioprine and a corticosteroid), evidence on EMB of mild acute rejection is relatively common (33% at our center), and our policy has been to give no extra therapy to such patients. *Severe acute rejection* has been infrequent (<2%), but clearly requires a course of increased therapy.

There is evidence that a significant proportion (± 30%) of *mild rejection* episodes progress to moderate rejection, and some groups would therefore advocate increasing the level of maintenance therapy, either by increasing the CsA[136] or corticosteroid dosage. Those who advocate increasing the blood level of CsA would raise the level by at least 50% (for 7–10 days), and have documented that this significantly reduces the number of cases where mild rejection progresses to moderate rejection[136]. No obvious side-effects were observed. Many groups, however, would offer no extra therapy in a patient with mild rejection, but would follow him closely until the episode either regressed or intensified.

The difficult decisions are frequently presented by the patient in whom *moderately severe acute rejection* is occurring. The decisions of whether to treat or not, and how much therapy to give, are based on several factors, in particular the patient's clinical course since transplantation. If previous biopsies or scans have confirmed no significant rejection, but there has been a sudden or progressive increase in rejection activity, then a course of extra therapy would seem to be indicated. Similarly, when there are any clinical features of impaired myocardial function, then a course of increased therapy would certainly seem justified.

In general, in patients with moderate acute rejection, our policy, and that of the majority of groups, is to augment therapy, though the form this augmentation should take remains uncertain and controversial. Whether extra therapy is given or not, careful monitoring of the patient is required, with a further biopsy within 4–7 days, to ensure that the rejection episode is subsiding. It is particularly in these cases where a non-invasive method of monitoring the heart would be so valuable.

Increased therapy – drugs and dosages

The standard treatment in patients with significant acute rejection has been the administration of 0.5–1 g 'pulses' of intravenous methylprednisolone sodium succinate on a daily basis. (Occasionally, the rejection episode may be so severe to warrant that the second dose be given only 12 hours after the first.) CsA and azathioprine dosages have not been altered. Some centers are reluctant to administer more than a total of 3 or 4 g of methylprednisolone during any one course of treatment. On rare occasions we have found it necessary to administer considerably more than this to obtain reversal of the rejection episode.

Whether increased *corticosteroid therapy* should be given intravenously or orally, and whether single doses of the magnitude of 1 g are essential, remain in question[137]. There is some evidence that much smaller daily doses would suffice in successfully reversing an acute rejection episode[138]. At Columbia University in New York, oral prednisone at 100 mg/day for 3 days, and then rapidly tapered over 1 week to the maintenance dose, was successful in reversing 90% of acute rejection episodes, with resolution of myocyte necrosis in every case[138]. A recent study from Hannover suggests that a 3-day course of methylprednisolone 250 mg/day i.v. is as effective in reversing acute rejection as courses of 500 mg or 1 g/day i.v.[139]. It would therefore seem that only in the severest cases are large doses of intravenous steroids warranted.

Our own policy in a moderately severe rejection episode (considered severe enough to warrant extra therapy) would be to give an attenuated dosage of methylprednisolone, possibly 1.5–3 mg/kg per day (or 200 mg/day) orally for 3 days, with half that dose (or 100 mg/day) for an additional 2 days. EMB would then be repeated, and, if the acute rejection were not resolving, a further course of corticosteroids (either oral or i.v.) would be administered. If rejection were worse, a short course of ATG would be added.

Certain groups are now administering intravenous corticosteroid pulses by nurses who attend the patient at home[140]. This arrangement has been found to be successful, with (1) no resulting infections, (2) marked financial savings, and (3) increased patient satisfaction. This approach will probably be used more extensively in the future.

In addition, in severe rejection, and certainly when the patient fails to respond to intravenous steroids alone, *ATG or ALG* should be administered intravenously on a daily basis to maintain the T-lymphocyte count in the therapeutic range (50–150 cells/mm^3)[141]. On occasions, when the T-cell count has been particularly high, we have reversed an acute rejection episode with ATG alone, though the immediate beneficial effects of corticosteroids make this the therapy of choice in the majority of cases.

Azathioprine dosage, if not already at the maximum tolerated dose as judged by features of bone marrow and hepatic toxicity, should probably be increased and maintained at that level; we would aim to maintain the total WBC count in the range of 4000–7000 cells/mm^3. Increased corticosteroid therapy, however, frequently greatly increases the total WBC count, which may subsequently fall fairly precipitously when corticosteroid therapy is reduced. This feature must be considered when decisions regarding azathioprine dosage are made.

If blood levels of *cyclosporine* remain in the therapeutic range, we have seen no reason to increase the CsA dosage, in view of the risk of inducing renal dysfunction or other drug-related complication. Other centers have shown, however, that a temporary increase in dosage can result in reversal of a rejection episode, without the need to give large doses of corticosteroids[136,142,143]. The Texas Heart Institute policy for the treatment of moderate rejection has been to administer a combination of intravenous (1–3 mg/kg per day) and oral (approximately 12 mg/kg per day) cyclosporine for 10–14 days[143]. The average CsA level was more than doubled, and moderate rejection was reversed in 80% of episodes. This adjustment of therapy would seem to be more suited to the treatment of a moderately severe (rather than a severe) rejection episode, where the need for rapid reversal of the histopathological changes, in order to prevent extensive permanent myocardial damage, is less urgent.

If severe rejection persists, and the total WBC count remains high despite high doses of azathioprine (3–5 mg/kg per day), we have on a number of occasions added a small daily oral dose of *cyclophosphamide* (0.5–1.5 mg/kg per day). (The therapeutic oral dose of cyclophosphamide is less than that of azathioprine.) This has been accompanied by a steady reduction in total WBC count and resolution of the rejection episode. Cyclophosphamide, however, has proved a difficult drug to manage, and is not without major complication, particularly in regard to bone marrow suppression. We have been forced to abandon its use in two patients as a result of this complication. It can, however, be valuable when administered as a short course in selected patients suffering severe acute rejection resistant to other therapy.

The effect of therapy is assessed by EMB within 4–7 days. If the acute rejection episode has regressed, then no additional treatment is necessary, but another biopsy is performed some 5–7 days later to confirm remission. If severe rejection continues, however, then the intravenous course of methylprednisolone (1 g/day) and ATG should be continued for a further 3 days. There is some indication, however, that a prolonged course of ATG together with CsA is associated with an increased risk of the development of lymphoma[144,145], and should be avoided. Similarly, the longer and more intense the course of antirejection therapy, then the higher the probable risk of infection, even though this infection may not present until some weeks or even months later.

The response to increased therapy is again monitored by repeating the EMB, again usually between 4–7 days later, depending on the severity of the episode. If two courses of methylprednisolone, each of 3 days, and ATG over the same period have resulted in a significant improvement in the histopathological features of rejection, then the dosage of corticosteroid may be reduced to maintenance levels, the rapidity of the reduction in dosage depending on the improvement in histopathological features on EMB. Many groups would reduce corticosteroid dosage to maintenance level slowly over a 7–14-day period; others would cut back more quickly. There do not appear to be hard data on which policy is preferable. It has been our policy to perform biopsy yet again within a further 7–14 days to ensure that the rejection episode continues in remission, and that relapse has not occurred following reduction of therapy.

If two courses of methylprednisolone and ATG for a severe acute rejection episode do not result in significant improvement, then our policy has been to consider the use of the monoclonal antibody *OKT3* though, in our experience, the need for this drug has been rare. All other immunosuppressive therapy is either discontinued or reduced by approximately 50%, and a 10–14-day course of OKT3 is administered as outlined in Chapter 12. OKT3 is said to reverse established rejection in more than 90% of cases, compared to only 70% responding to high-dose steroid therapy, and some groups would undoubtedly employ this drug at an earlier stage in the patient's care than we have done to date. The Utah group has found OKT3 to resolve refractory cardiac rejection completely in 57% of patients, and partially resolve it in 29%[146–148]. Life-threatening rejection responded completely in 50% of patients.

In a multicenter trial of OKT3 therapy for acute rejection of cadaveric renal transplantation, OKT3 reversed 94% of the rejection episodes, whereas conventional steroid treatment reversed only 75% ($p < 0.01$)[149]. This superior reversal rate with OKT3 was reflected in an improved 1-

year graft survival of 62% for the OKT3-treated group, as compared with 45% for the steroid-treated group ($p < 0.03$), in patients who were all selected by virtue of having had acute rejection.

Our own experience with the use of OKT3 is relatively small, mainly as the incidence of refractory acute rejection at our center has been negligible. The frequent side-effects of OKT3 therapy have also deterred us from using it unless all other therapies failed. It may be, however, that, although for several years we have been able to reverse all acute rejection episodes successfully using a combination of the other drugs available, this end-point might have been achieved more rapidly by a course of OKT3. The advantages and disadvantages of OKT3 therapy in patients with cardiac transplants require further clarification.

If all such therapy fails to reverse the rejection process, and graft failure is imminent, then urgent retransplantation is the only course of action that may result in patient survival (Chapter 20). Temporary mechanical support of the circulation by a ventricular assist device or artificial heart (Section IV) may be required until a suitable donor heart becomes available.

Acute or hyperacute vascular rejection

Rarely, extremely severe accelerated acute or hyperacute vascular rejection is associated with the development of anti-HLA lymphocytotoxic antibodies in the early post-transplant period. The histopathological features may show a mixture of cellular infiltration and vascular injury, with resulting hemorrhage and edema, as well as widespread myocyte injury. In our experience, this may occur in a patient who, though with a negative lymphocytotoxic screen pretransplant and a negative cross-match at the time of the transplant, has been subjected to previous blood transfusion, pregnancy, or organ transplantation. Though our experience is very limited, we have found plasmapheresis (to remove the anti-HLA antibodies) coupled with cyclophosphamide, cyclosporine, high-dose intravenous corticosteroids, and ATG therapy (to prevent antibody resynthesis and control the cellular elements) to be valuable in such a case. Similar experience has been reported by others[150,151]. When true immediate or early hyperacute rejection occurs, associated with either (1) a positive lymphocytotoxic cross-match, (2) ABO incompatibility[152], or (3) antibodies directed against vascular endothelium[153-156], the response to any combination of therapy is frequently poor, and the incidence of graft failure high. Myocyte destruction may be so rapid and so vigorous that no form of therapy has any significant effect.

Comment

Heavy immunosuppression is frequently associated with the appearance of herpes simplex lesions in the mouth and pharynx. Small ulcers appear, particularly on the tongue and buccal mucosa. In our experience, these rarely lead to systemic herpes viremia, but are an indicator that the patient is now heavily immunosuppressed. Their appearance acts as a warning that the limits of immunosuppression are being reached; any further increase in therapy may result in the development of serious infection. They can be uncomfortable or even painful for the patient, particularly when swallowing, and may limit dietary intake. Topical antiseptic and analgesic tablets or liquids provide symptomatic relief and will also help prevent secondary infection of these lesions, which spontaneously regress when the immunosuppression is reduced. When widespread, a course of acyclovir should be administered (Chapter 17).

Acute rejection no longer results in the high mortality it did before CsA was introduced, and today the greatest risk to the patient is over-zealous therapy. The antirejection drugs available provide an extremely powerful armamentarium, and, if life-threatening infection is to be minimized, must be used with caution.

References

1. Zuhdi, N., Shrago, S.S., Clark, R.M., Voda, J., Greer, A.G., Chaffin, J.S., Novitzky, D. and Cooper, D.K.C. (1989). Experience with myocardial biopsy in 23 patients with heart transplants. *J. Okla. State Med. Assoc.*, **82**, 109
2. Cooper, D.K.C., Fraser, R.C., Rose, A.G., Ayzenberg, O., Oldfield, G.S., Hassoulas, J., Novitzky, D., Uys, C.J. and Barnard, C.N. (1982). Technique, complications, and clinical value of endomyocardial biopsy in patients with heterotopic heart transplants. *Thorax*, **37**, 727
3. Laczkovics, A., Grabenwoger, F., Teufelsbauer, H., Dock, W., Wollenek, G. and Wolner, E. (1988). Noninvasive assessment of acute rejection after orthotopic heart transplantation: value of changes in cardiac volume and cardiothoracic ratio. *J. Cardiovasc. Surg.*, **29**, 582
4. Lower, R.R., Dong, E., Jr. and Shumway, N.E. (1965). Suppression of rejection crises in the cardiac homograft. *Ann. Thorac. Surg.*, **1**, 645
5. Lower, R.R., Dong, E., Jr. and Glazener, F.S. (1966). Electrocardiograms of dogs with heart homografts. *Circulation*, **33**, 455
6. Stinson, E.B., Dong, E., Jr., Bieber, C.P., Schroeder, J.S. and Shumway, N.E. (1969). Cardiac transplantation in man. I. Early rejection. *J. Am. Med. Assoc.*, **207**, 2233
7. Schroeder, J.S., Berke, D.K., Graham, A.F., Rider, A.K. and Harrison, D.C. (1974). Arrhythmias after cardiac transplantation. *Am. J. Cardiol.*, **33**, 604
8. Baumgartner, W.A., Reitz, B.A., Oyer, P.E., Stinson, E.B. and Shumway, N.E. (1979). Cardiac homotransplantation. *Curr. Probl. Surg.*, **16**, 1
9. Jamieson, S.W., Reitz, B.A., Oyer, P.E., Stinson, E.B. and Shumway, N.E. (1979). Current management of cardiac transplant recipients. *Br. Heart J.*, **42**, 703
10. Cooper, D.K.C., Charles, R.G., Rose, A.G., Fraser, R.C., Isaacs, S., Novitzky, D. and Barnard, C.N. (1985). Does the electrocardiogram detect early heart rejection? *J. Heart Transplant.*, **4**, 546
11. Semb, B.K.H., Abrahamson, A.M. and Barnard, C.N. (1971). Electrocardiographic changes during the unmodified rejection of heterotopic canine heart allografts. *Scand. J. Thorac. Cardiovasc. Surg.*, **5**, 120
12. Dear, M., Cooper, D.K.C. and Murtra, M. (1973). Electrocardiographic prediction of unmodified rejection in heterotopic canine cardiac allografts. *Cardiovasc. Res.*, **7**, 687

13. Losman, J.G., Rose, A.G. and Barnard, C.N. (1977). Myocardial fibrinolytic activity in allogenic cardiac rejection. *Transplantation*, **23**, 414
14. Losman, J.G., McDonald, J., Levine, H.D., Campbell, C.D. and Replogle, R.L. (1981). The variations of the electrocardiographic voltage during the day in normal adult subjects. *Heart Transplant.*, **1**, 39
15. Haberl, R., Weber, M., Reichenspurner, H., Kemkes, B.M., Osterholzer, G., Anthuber, M. and Steinbeck, G. (1987). Frequency analysis of the surface electrocardiogram for recognition of acute rejection after orthotopic cardiac transplantation in man. *Circulation*, **77**, 101
16. Keren, A., Billis, A.M., Freedman, R.A., Baldwin, J.C., Billingham, M.E., Stinson, E.B., Simson, M.B. and Mason, J.W. (1984). Heart transplant rejection monitored by signal-averaged electrocardiography in patients receiving cyclosporine. *Circulation*, **70**, (Suppl. I), 124
17. Warnecke, H., Schuler, S., Goetze, H.J., Matheis, G., Suthoff, U., Muller, J., Tietze, U. and Hetzer, R. (1986). Noninvasive monitoring of cardiac allograft rejection by intramyocardial electrogram recordings. *Circulation*, **74** (Suppl. III), 73
18. Wahlers, T.H., Haverich, A., Schafers, H.J., Frimpong-Boateng, K., Fieguth, H.G., Herrmann, G., Borst, H.G. and Arvanitidou, V. (1986). Changes of the intramyocardial electrogram after orthotopic heart transplantation. *J. Heart Transplant*, **5**, 450
19. Wahlers, T., Haverich, A., Busselberg, C., Schafers, H.J., Fieguth, H.G., Frimpong, K., Hermann, G., Zuvietz, C., Kemnitz, J. and Borst, H.G. (1987). Electrocardiographic parameters in allograft rejection after orthotopic cardiac transplantation. *Transplant. Proc.*, **19**, 3784
20. Rosenbloom, M., Laschinger, J.C., Saffitz, J.E., Cox, J.L. and Bolman, R.M. (1989). Noninvasive detection of cardiac allograft rejection by analysis of the unipolar peak-to-peak amplitude of intramyocardial electrograms. *Ann. Thorac. Surg.*, **47**, 407
21. Kitamura, M., Sakakibara, N., Kurosawa, H., Imamura, E., Kasanuki, H., Sekiguchi, M. and Koyanagi, H. (1988). Electrophysiologic assessment of the transplanted canine heart: correspondence to histopathologic findings in acute rejection. *J. Heart Transplant.*, **7** 213
22. Avitall, B., Payne, D.D., Connolly, R.J., Levine, H.J., Dawson, P.J., Isner, J.M., Salem, D.N. and Cleveland, R.J. (1988). Heterotopic heart transplantation: electrophysiologic changes during acute rejection. *J. Heart Transplant.*, **7**, 176
23. Koike, K., Hesslein, P.S., Dasmahapatra, H.K., Wilson, G.J., Finlay, C.D., David, S.L., Kielmanowicz, S. and Coles, J.G. (1988). Telemetric detection of cardiac allograft rejection. Correlation of electrophysiological, histological, and biochemical changes during unmodified rejection. *Circulation.*, **78** (Supp. I), 106
24. Sands, K.E.F., Lilly, L.S., Schoen, F.J., Mudge, G.H., Jr. and Cohen, R.J. (1986). Heart rate variability patterns in stable and rejecting cardiac transplant recipients (Abstract). *J. Am. Coll. Cardiol.*, **7**, 190A
25. Zbilut, J.P., Murdock, D.K., Lawson, L., Lawless, C.E., Von Dreele, M.M. and Porges, S.W. (1988). Use of power spectral analysis of respiratory sinus arrhythmia to detect graft rejection. *J. Heart Transplant.*, **7**, 280
26. Hanson, C.A., Bolling, S.F., Stoolman, L.M., Schlegelmilch, J.A., Abrams, G.D., Miska, P.T. and Deeb, G.M. (1988). Cytoimmunologic monitoring and heart transplantation. *J. Heart Transplant.*, **7**, 424
27. Bieber, C.P., Griepp, R.B., Oyer, P.E., David, L.A. and Stinson, E.B. (1977). Relationship of rabbit ATG serum clearance rate to circulating T cell level, rejection onset, and survival in cardiac transplantation. *Transplant. Proc.*, **9**, 1031
28. Oyer, P.E., Stinson, E.B., Bieber, C.P., Reitz, B.A., Raney, A.A., Baumgartner, W.A. and Shumway, N.E. (1979). Diagnosis and treatment of acute cardiac allograft rejection. *Transplant. Proc.*, **11**, 296
29. Kung, P.C., Goldstein, G., Reinharz, E.L. and Schlossman, S.F. (1979). Monoclonal antibodies defining distinctive human T cell surface antigens. *Science*, **206**, 347
30. Cosimi, A.B., Colvin, R.B., Burton, R.C., Rubin, R.H., Goldstein, G., Kung, P.C., Hansen, W.P., Delmonico, F.L. and Russell, P.S. (1981). Use of monoclonal antibodies to T cell subsets for immunological monitoring and treatment in recipients of renal allografts. *N. Engl. J. Med.*, **305**, 308
31. Ellis, T.M., Lee, H.M. and Mohanakumar, T. (1981). Alterations in human regulatory T lymphocyte subpopulations after renal allografting. *J. Immunol.*, **127**, 2199
32. Severyn, W., Flaa, C., Fuller, L., Kyriakides, G.K., Esquenazi, V. and Miller, J. (1982). The role of immunological monitoring in transplantation. *Heart Transplant.*, **1**, 222
33. Rabin, B.S. (1983). Immunologic aspects of human cardiac transplantation. *Heart Transplant.*, **2**, 188
34. Ellis, T.M., Lee, H.M. and Mohanakumar, T. (1981). Alterations in human regulatory T-lymphocyte subpopulations after renal allografting. *J. Immunol.*, **127**, 199
35. Kerman, R.H., Van Buren, C.T., Payne, W., Flechner, S. and Kahan, B.D. (1983). Monitoring T-cell subsets and immune events in renal allograft recipients. *Transplant. Proc.*, **15**, 1170
36. Binkley, W.F., Valenzuela, R., Braun, W.E., Deodhar, S.D., Novick, A.C. and Steinmuller, D.R. (1983). Flow cytometry quantitation of peripheral blood T-cell subsets in human allograft recipients. *Transplant. Proc.*, **15**, 1163
37. Carter, N.P., Cullen, P.R., Thompson, J.F., Bewick, A.L.T., Wood, R.F.M. and Morris, P.J. (1983). Monitoring lymphocyte subpopulations in renal allograft recipients. *Transplant. Proc.*, **15**, 1157
38. Guttman, R.D. and Poulsen, R.S. (1983). Fluorescence activated cell sorter analysis of lymphocyte subsets after renal transplantation. *Transplant. Proc.*, **15**, 1160
39. Liebert, M., Rosenthal, J.T. and Merall, E. (1983). Peripheral blood T-lymphocytes found in renal allograft recipients treated with cyclosporine. *Transplantation*, **36**, 200
40. Kirklin, J.K., Bourge, R.C., White-Williams, C., Naftel, D.C. and Phillips, M.G. (1989). Prophylactic anti-rejection therapy early after cardiac transplantation: RATG versus OKT3 (Abstract). *J. Am. Coll. Cardiol.*, **13**, 62A
41. Mohanakumar, T., Hoshinaga, K., Wood, N.L., Szentpetery, S. and Lower, R.R. (1986). Enumeration of transferrin receptor expressing lymphocytes as a potential marker for rejection in human cardiac transplant recipients. *Transplantation*, **42**, 691
42. Hoshinaga, K., Mohanakumar, T., Pascoe, E.A., Szentpetery, S., Lee, H.M. and Lower, R.R. (1988). Expression of transferrin receptors on lymphocytes: its correlation with T-helper/T-suppressor cytotoxic ratio and rejection in heart transplant recipients. *J. Heart Transplant.*, **7**, 198
43. Hammer, C., Reichenspurner, H., Ertel, W., Lersch, C., Plahl, M., Brendel, W., Reichart, B., Uberfuhr, P., Welz, A., Kemkes, B.M., Reble, B., Funccius, W. and Gokel, M. (1984). Cytological and immunologic monitoring of cyclosporine-treated human heart recipients. *Heart Transplant.*, **3** 228
44. Ertel, W., Reichenspurner, H., Lersch, C., Hammer, C., Plahl, M., Lehmann, M., Kemkes, B.M., Osterholzer, G., Reble, B., Reichart, B. and Brendel, W. (1985). Cyto-immunological monitoring in acute rejection and viral, bacterial or fungal infection following transplantation. *J. Heart Transplant.*, **4**, 390
45. Pelletier, L.C., Montplaisir, S., Pelletier, G., Castonguay, Y., Harvey, P., Dyrda, I. and Solymoss, C.B. (1988). Lymphocyte sub-population monitoring in cyclosporine-treated patients following heart transplantation. *Ann. Thorac. Surg.*, **45**, 11
46. Carlquist, J., Anderson, J., Hammond, E. and O'Connell, J. (1989). Diagnostic applications of lymphocyte cultures from heart allograft biopsies (Abstract). *J. Am. Coll. Cardiol.*, **13**, 62A
47. Roodman, S.T., Miller, L.W. and Tsai, C.C. (1988). Role of interleukin-2 receptors in immunologic monitoring following cardiac transplantation. *Transplantation*, **45**, 1050
48. Fieguth, H-G., Haverich, A., Hadam, M., Kemnitz, J. and Dammenhayn, L. (1989). Correlation of interleukin-2 receptor positive circulating lymphocytes and acute cardiac rejection. *Transplant. Proc.*, **21**, 2517
49. Southern, J.T., Fallon, J.T., Dec, G.W., Jacobs, M., Cosimi, A.B., Brown, M.C., Kung, P.C. and Colvin, R.B. (1986). A comparison of serum interleukin-2 receptor levels and endomyocardial biopsy grades in the monitoring of cardiac allograft rejection (Abstract). *J. Heart Transplant.*, **5**, 370
50. Holland, V.A., Brousseau, K.P., Berger, M.B., Young, J.B., Noon, G.P., Short, H.D., Whisenhand, H.H., Debakey, M.E., Nelson, D.L. and Lawrence, M.D. (1988). Soluble interleukin-2 receptor levels following transplantation. Presented at the *International Symposium on Inflammatory Heart Disease*, Snowmass, Colorado, July
51. Wisecarver, J.L., Kendall, T.J., Costanzo-Nordin, M.R., Winters, G.L.,

Switzer, B.L. and McManus, B.M. (1988). Soluble IL2 receptor proteins in human heart allograft recipients: relationship to frequency and intensity of rejection. Presented at the *International Symposium on Inflammatory Heart Disease*, Snowmass, Colorado, July

52. Woloszczuk, W., Schwarz, M., Havel, M., Laczkovics, A. and Muller, M.M. (1986). Neopterin and interferon gamma serum levels in patients with heart and kidney transplants. *J. Clin. Chem. Clin. Biochem.*, **24**, 729
53. Huber, C., Fuchs, D., Hausen, A., Margreiter, R., Reibnegger, G., Spielberger, M. and Wachter, H. (1983). Pteridines as a new marker to detect human T cells activated by allogenic or modified self major histocompatibility complex (MHC) determinants. *J. Immunol.*, **130**, 1047
54. Wachter, H., Hausen, A. and Grassmayr, K. (1979). Increased urinary excretion of neopterin in patients with malignant tumors and with virus diseases. *Hoppe-Seylers Z. Physiol. Chem.*, **360**, 1957
55. Niederweiser, D., Gratwohl, A., Huber, C. et al. (1983). Neopterin excretion during allogeneic and syngeneic autologous bone marrow transplantation. In Wachter, H., Cutrius, C. and Pfleider, W. (eds.) *Biochemical and Clinical Aspects of Pteridines*. Vol. 2. (Berlin: Walter de Gruyter)
56. Margreiter, R., Fuchs, D., Hausen, A., Huber, C., Reibnegger, G., Spielberger, M. and Wachter, H. (1983). Neopterin as a new biochemical marker for diagnosis of allograft rejection. *Transplantation*, **36**, 650
57. Havel, M., Laczkovics, A., Teufelbauer, H., Muller, M.M. and Wolner, E. (1989). Neopterin as a new marker to detect acute rejection after heart transplantation. *J. Heart Transplant.*, **8**, 167
58. Vincent, C. and Revillard, J.P. (1980). Serum levels and urinary excretion of beta 2 microglobulin in patients under hemodialysis or after renal transplantation. *Acta Clin. Belg.*, **35** (Suppl. 10), 31
59. Rosenbaum, R.W., Kately, J., Sanchez, T.V., Hirota, T.F. and Mayor, G.H. (1980). Beta-2 microglobulin: an early indicator of renal transplant survival and function. *Trans. Am. Soc. Artif. Intern. Organs*, **26**, 77
60. Goldman, M.H., Lippman, R., Landwehr, D., Szentpetery, S., Wolfgang, T., Lee, H.M., Hess, M., Mendez-Picon, G., Hastillo, A. and Lower, R.R. (1983). Beta 2 microglobulin and the diagnosis of cardiac transplant rejection. *Transplantation*, **36**, 209
61. Carrier, M., Copeland, J.G., Russell, D.H., Perrotta, N.J., Davis, T.P. and Emery, R.W. (1987). Urinary polyamines are noninvasive markers of heart allograft rejection. *J. Heart Transplant.*, **6**, 286
62. Carrier, M., Russell, D.H., Davis, T.P., Emery, R.W. and Copeland, J.G. (1988). Urinary polyamines as markers of cardiac allograft rejection. *J. Thorac. Cardiovasc. Surg.*, **96**, 806
63. Carrier, M., Russell, D.H., Wild, J.C., Emery, R.W. and Copeland, J.G. (1987). Prolactin as a marker of rejection in human heart transplantation. *J. Heart Transplant.*, **6**, 290
64. Stenson, W.F. and Parker, C.W. (1982). Prostaglandins and the immune response. In Lee, J.B. (ed.) *Prostaglandins*. p. 39, (New York: Elsevier)
65. Foegh, M.L. and Ramwell, P.W. (1983). Physiological implications of products in the arachidonic acid cascade. In Pace-Asciak, C. and Granstrom, E. (eds.) *Prostaglandins and Related Substances*. p. xiii (New York: Elsevier)
66. Khirabadi, B.S., Foegh, M.L. and Ramwell, P.W. (1985). Urine immunoreactive thromboxane B2 in rat cardiac allograft rejection. *Transplantation*, **39**, 6
67. Foegh, M.L., Alijani, M., Helfrich, G.B., Schreiner, G.E. and Ramwell, P.W. (1989). Urine thromboxane as an immunological monitor in kidney transplant patients. *Transplant. Proc.*, In press
68. Barnard, C.N., Barnard, M.S., Cooper, D.K.C., Curchio, C.A., Hassoulas, J., Novitzky, D. and Wolpowitz, A. (1981). The present status of heterotopic cardiac transplantation. *J. Thorac. Cardiovasc. Surg.*, **81**, 433
69. Cooper, D.K.C., Novitzky, D., Hassoulas, J. and Barnard, C.N. (1982). Transplantation of the heart. *Br. J. Clin. Pract.*, **36**, 337
70. Sakakibara, S. and Konno, S. (1962). Endomyocardial biopsy. *Jap. Heart J.*, **3**, 537
71. Caves, P.K., Stinson, E.B., Graham, A.F., Billingham, M.E., Grehl, T.M. and Shumway, N.E. (1973). Percutaneous transvenous endomyocardial biopsy. *J. Am. Med. Assoc.*, **225**, 288
72. Caves, P.K., Stinson, E.B., Billingham, M.E. and Shumway, N.E. (1974). Serial transvenous biopsy of the transplanted human heart. Improved management of acute rejection episodes. *Lancet*, **1**, 821
73. Locke, T.J., Furniss, S.S. and McGregor, C.G.A. (1988). Coronary artery-right ventricular fistula after endomyocardial biopsy. *Br. Heart J.*, **60**, 81
74. Sandhu, J.S., Uretsky, B.F., Zerbe, T.R., Goldsmith, A.S., Reddy, P.S., Kormos, R.L., Griffith, B.P. and Hardesty, R.L. (1989). Coronary artery fistula in the heart transplant patient. A potential complication of endomyocardial biopsy. *Circulation*, **79**, 350
75. Henzlova, M.J., Nath, H., Bucy, R.P., Kirklin, K. and Rogers, W.J. (1989). Coronary artery to right ventricle fistulae in heart transplant recipients: a complication of endomyocardial biopsy? (Abstract). *J. Am. Coll. Cardiol.*, **13**, 243A
76. Rose, A.G., Novitzky, D., Cooper, D.K.C. and Reichart, B. Endomyocardial biopsy site morphology: an experimental study in baboons. *Arch. Pathol. Lab. Med.*, **110**, 622
77. Novitzky, D., Rose, A.G., Cooper, D.K.C. and Reichart, B. (1986). Histopathologic changes at the site of endomyocardial biopsy: potential for confusion with acute rejection. *J. Heart Transplant.*, **5**, 79
78. Novitzky, D., Rose, A.G., Cooper, D.K.C. and Reichart, B. (1986). Interpretation of endomycardial biopsy after heart transplantation. Potentially confusing factors. *S. Afr. Med. J.*, **70**, 789
79. Novitzky, D., Cooper, D.K.C., Rose, A.G., Wicomb, W.N., Becerra, E. and Reichart, B. (1987). Early donor heart failure following transplantation from myocardial injury sustained during brain death. *Clin. Transplant.*, **1**, 108
80. Paulsen, W., Magid, N., Sagar, K.B., Hastillo, A., Wolfgang, T.C., Lower, R.R. and Hess, M.L. (1985). Left ventricular function of heart allografts during acute rejection: an echocardiographic assessment. *J. Heart Transplant.*, **4**, 525
81. Dawkins, K.D., Oldershaw, P.J., Billingham, M.E., Hunt, S.A., Oyer, P.E., Jamieson, S.W., Popp, R.L., Stinson, E.B. and Shumway, N.E. (1984). Changes in diastolic function as a noninvasive marker of cardiac allograft rejection. *J. Heart Transplant.*, **3**, 286
82. Valantine, H.A., Fowler, M.B., Appleton, C.P. et al. (1986). Assessment of changes in diastolic function resulting from acute cardiac allograft rejection using doppler echocardiography (Abstract). *X World Congress of Cardiology*, Washington, DC, September
83. Valantine, H.A., Fowler, M.B., Hunt, S.A., Naasz, C., Hatle, L.V., Stinson, E.B., Billingham, M.E. and Popp, R.L. (1986). Changes in doppler echocardiographic indices of left ventricular function as potential markers of acute rejection. (Abstract). *Circulation*, **74** (Suppl. II), 159
84. Desruennes, M., Corcos, T., Cabrol, A., Gandjbakhch, I., Pavie, A., Leger, P., Eugene, M., Bors, V. and Cabrol, C. (1988). Doppler echocardiography for the diagnosis of acute cardiac allograft rejection. *J. Am. Cardiol.*, **12**, 63
85. Appleton, C.P., Valantine, H.A., Hatle, L. and Popp, R.L. (1986). Assessment of right heart filling in cardiac transplants during venous doppler echocardiography (Abstract). *X World Congress of Cardiology*, Washington, DC, September
86. Forster, T., McGhie, J., Rijsterborgh, H., Van De Borden, S., Laird-Meeter, K., Balk, A., Essed, C. and Roelandt, J. (1988). Can we assess the changes of ventricular filling resulting from acute allograft rejection with doppler echocardiography? *J. Heart Transplant.*, **7**, 430
87. Nowygrod, R., Spotnitz, H.M., Du Broff, J.M., Hardy, M.A. and Reemtsma, K. (1983). Organ mass: an indicator of heart transplant rejection. *Transplant. Proc.*, **15**, 1225
88. Sagar, K.B., Hastillo, A., Wolfgang, T.C., Lower, R.R. and Hess, M.L. (1981). Left ventricular mass by M-mode echocardiography in cardiac transplant patients with acute rejection. *Circulation*, **64** (Suppl. II), 216
89. Hall, T.S., Baumgartner, W.A., Borkon, A.M., LaFrance, N.D., Traill, T.A., Norris, S., Hutchins, G.M., Braun, J. and Reitz, B.A. (1986). Diagnosis of acute cardiac rejection with antimyosin monoclonal antibody, phosphorus nuclear magnetic resonance imaging, two-dimensional echocardiography, and endocardial biopsy. *J. Heart Transplant.*, **5**, 419
90. Chandrasekaran, K., Bansal, R.C., Greenleaf, J.F., Hauck, A., Seward, J.B., Tajik, A.J. and Bailey, L.L. (1987). Early recognition of heart transplant rejection by backscatter analysis from serial 2D ECHOs in a heterotopic transplant model. *J. Heart Transplant.*, **6**, 1
91. Devereux, R.B. and Reichek, N. (1977). Echocardiographic determination of left ventricular mass in man. *Circulation*, **55**, 613
92. Schroeder, J.S., Popp, R.L., Stinson, E.B., Dong, E., Shumway, N.E.

and Harrison, D.C. (1969). Acute rejection following cardiac transplantation: phonocardiographic and ultrasound observations. *Circulation*, **40**, 155
93. Popp, R.L., Schroeder, J.S., Stinson, E.B., Shumway, N.E. and Harrison, D.C. (1971). Ultrasonic studies for the early detection of acute cardiac rejection. *Transplantation*, **11**, 543
94. Clark, M.B., Spotnitz, H.M., Dubroff, J.M., Wong, C.Y.H., Vayda, J.L., Costello, D., Drusin, R., Rose, E.A. and Reemtsma, K. (1983). Acute rejection after cardiac transplantation: detection by two-dimensional echocardiography. *Surg. Forum*, **34**, 248
95. Eisen, H.J., Eisenberg, S.B., Saffitz, J.E., Bolman, R.M., Sobel, B.E. and Bergmann, S.R. (1987). Noninvasive detection of rejection of transplanted hearts with indium-111-labeled lymphocytes. *Circulation*, **75**, 868
96. Alivizatos, P.A., Rose, M.L., Aikenhead, J., Pomerance, A., Chisholm, P.M. and Yacoub, M.H. (1985). Migration of In-111 labeled autologous leukocytes to the grafts of heart transplant patients. *Transplant. Proc.*, **17**, 614
97. Oluwole, S., Wang, T., Fawwaz, R., Satake, K., Nowygrod, R., Reemtsma, K. and Hardy, M.A. (1981). Use of indium-111-labelled cells in measurement of cellular dynamics of experimental cardiac allograft rejection. *Transplantation*, **31**, 51
98. Wang, T.S., Oluwole, S., Fawwaz, R.A., Wolff, M., Kuromoto, N., Satake, K., Hardy, M.A. and Alderson, P.O. (1982). Cellular basis for accummulation of In-111-labeled leukocytes and platelets in rejecting cardiac allografts: concise communication. *J. Nucl. Med.*, **23**, 993
99. McKillop, J.H., Wallwork, J., Reitz, B.A., Billingham, M.E., Miller, R. and McDougall, I.R. (1982). The use of ^{111}In-labeled lymphocyte imaging to evaluate graft rejection following cardiac transplantation in dogs. *Eur. J. Nucl. Med.*, **7**, 162
100. Eisenberg, S.B., Eisen, H.J., Sobel, B.E., Bergmann, S.R. and Bolman, R.M. (1988). Sensitivity of scintigraphy with ^{111}In-lymphocytes for detection of cardiac allograft rejection. *J. Surg. Res.*, **45**, 549
101. Eisen, H.J., Rosenbloom, M., Laschinger, J.C., Saffitz, J.E., Cox, J.L., Sobel, B.E., Bolman, R.M. and Bergmann, S.R. (1988). Detection of rejection of canine orthotopic cardiac allografts with indium-111 lymphocytes and gamma scintigraphy. *J. Nucl. Med.*, **29**, 1223
102. Rosenbloom, M., Eisen, H.J., Laschinger, J., Saffitz, J.E., Sobel, B.E., Bergmann, S.R. and Bolman, R.M. (1988). Noninvasive assessment of treatment of cardiac allograft rejection with indium-111-labeled lymphocytes. *Transplantation*, **46**, 341
103. Bergmann, S.R., Lerch, R.A., Carlson, E.M., Saffitz, J.E. and Sobel, B.E. (1982). Detection of cardiac transplant rejection with radiolabeled lymphocytes. *Circulation*, **65**, 591
104. Farid, N.A., White, S.M., Heck, L.L. and Van Hove, E.D. (1983). Tc-99m labeled leukocytes: preparation and use in identification of abscess and tissue rejection. *Radiology*, **148**, 827
105. Khaw, B.A., Fallon, J.T., Russell, P.S., Rosseel, J., Ferguson, P. and Haber, E. (1981). New approach to determination of heart transplant rejection by ^{125}I-antimyosin antibody and ^{99m}Tc-fibrinogen (Abstract). *Clin. Res.*, **29**, 496A
106. Ballester-Rodes, M., Carrio-Gasset I., Abadal-Berini, L., Obrador-Mayol, D., Berna-Roqueta, L. and Caralps-Riera, J.M. (1988). Patterns of evolution of myocyte damage after human heart transplantation detected by indium-111 monoclonal antimyosin. *Am. J. Cardiol.*, **62**, 623
107. Carrio, I., Berna, L., Ballester, M., Estorch, M., Obrador, D., Cladellas, M., Abadal, L. and Ginjaume, M. (1988). Indium-111 antimyosin scintigraphy to assess myocardial damage in patients with suspected myocarditis and cardiac rejection. *J. Nucl. Med.*, **29**, 1893
108. LaFrance, N.D., Hall, T., Dolher, W., Koller, J., Cole, P., Barkon, A., Traill, T., Jacobus, W., Norris, S., Hutchins, G., Braun, J., Baumgartner, W., Reitz, B. and Wagner, H.N. (1986). In-111 antimyosin monoclonal antibody in detecting rejection of heart transplants. *J. Nucl. Med.*, **27**, 910
109. Aldonizio, L.J., Seldin, D.W., Esser, P.D., Johnson, R.E., Michler, C., Marboe, E.A., Rose, E.A. and Anderson, P.J. (1986). SPECT imaging of cardiac transplant rejection using In-111 antimyosin antibody. *Nucl. Med.*, **27**, 910
110. Nishimura, T., Sada, M., Sasaki, H., Yutani, C., Fujita, T., Amemiya, H., Kozuka, T., Akutsu, T. and Manabe, H. (1988). Assessment of severity of cardiac rejection in heterotopic heart transplantation using indium-111 antimyosin and magnetic resonance imaging. *Cardiovasc. Res.*, **22**, 108
111. Frist, W., Yasuda, T., Segal, L.G., Khaw, B.A., Strauss, H.W., Gold, H., Stinson, E., Oyer, P., Baldwin, J., Billingham, M., McDougall, I.R. and Haber, L.E. (1987). Non-invasive detection of human cardiac transplant rejection with indium-111 antimyosin (Fab) imaging. *Circulation*, **76** (Suppl. v), 81
112. Schutz, A., Fritsch, S., Weiler, A., Kugler, C., Temisan, C., Spes, C., Angermann, C., Gokel, J.M. and Kemkes, B.M. (1989). Antimyosin monoclonal antibodies for early detection of mild cardiac rejection (Abstract). *J. Heart Transplant.*, **8**, 88
113. Ueda, K., Takeda, K., LaFrance, N.D., Solez, K., Baumgartner, W.A., Reitz, B.A. and Herskowitz, A. (1988). Is In-111 antimyosin antibody a useful diagnostic marker for evaluation of early cardiac allograft rejection? *Transplant. Proc.*, **20**, 778
114. Novitzky, D., Boniaszczuk, J., Cooper, D.K.C., Isaacs, S., Rose, A.G., Smith, J.A., Uys, C.J., Barnard, C.N. and Fraser, R.C. (1984). Prediction of acute cardiac rejection using radionuclide techniques. *S. Afr. Med. J.*, **65**, 5
115. Novitzky, D., Cooper, D.K.C., Boniaszczuk, J., Isaacs, S., Fraser, R.C., Commerford, P.J., Uys, C.J., Rose, A.G., Smith, J.A. and Barnard, C.N. (1985). The significance of left ventricular volume measurement after heart transplantation using radionuclide techniques. *J. Heart Transplant.*, **4**, 206
116. Iturralde, M., Novitzky, D., Cooper, D.K.C., Rose, A.G., Boniaszczuk, J., Smith, J.A., Reichart, B. and Isaacs, S. (1988). The role of nuclear cardiology procedures in the evaluation of cardiac function following heart transplantation. *Sem. Nucl. Med.*, **18**, 221
117. Tsan, M.F. (1985). Mechanism of gallium-67 accumulation in inflammatory lesions. *J. Nucl. Med.*, **26**, 88
118. O'Connell, J.B., Henkin, R.E., Robinson, J.A., Subramanian, R., Scanlon, P.J. and Gunnar, R.M. (1984). Gallium-67 imaging in patients with dilated cardiomyopathy and biopsy-proven myocarditis. *Circulation*, **70**, 58
119. Meneguetti, J.C., Camargo, E.E., Soares, J., Jr., Bellotti, G., Bocchi, E., Higuchi, M.L., Stolff, N., Hironaka, F.H., Buchpiguel, C.A., Pileggi, F. and Jatene, A. (1987), Gallium-67 imaging in human heart transplantation: correlation with endomyocardial biopsy. *J. Heart Transplant.*, **6**, 171
120. Bergsland, J., Carr, E.A., Carroll, M., Wright, J.W., Feldman, M.J., Massucci, J., Bhayani, J.N. and Gona, J.M. (1985). Uptake of myocardial imaging agents by rejected hearts. *J. Heart Transplant.*, **4**, 536
121. Barak, J.H., Laraia, P.J., Boucher, C.A., Fallon, J.T. and Buckley, M.J. (1988). Thallium kinetics in rat cardiac transplant rejection. *Transplantation*, **45**, 687
122. Tscholakof, D., Aherne, T., Yee, E.S., Derugin, N. and Higgins, C.B. (1985). Cardiac transplantations in dogs: evaluation with MR. *Radiology*, **157**, 697
123. Aherne, T., Tscholakof, D., Finkbeiner, W., Sechtem, U., Derugin, N., Yee, E. and Higgins, C.B. (1986). Magnetic resonance imaging of cardiac transplants: the evaluation of rejection of cardiac allografts with and without immunosuppression. *Circulation*, **74**, 145
124. Revel, D., Chapelon, C., Mathieu, D., Cochet, P., Ninet, J., Chuzel, M., Champsaur, G., Dureau, G., Amiel, M., Helenon, O., Vasile, N., Cachera, J.P. and Loisance, D. (1989). Magnetic resonance imaging of human orthotopic heart transplantation: correlation with endomyocardial biopsy. *J. Heart Transplant.*, **8**, 139
125. Wisenberg, G., Pflugfelder, P.W., Kostuk, W.J., McKenzie, F.N. and Prato, F.S. (1987). Diagnostic applicability of magnetic resonance imaging in assessing human cardiac allograft rejection. *Am. J. Cardiol.*, **60**, 130
126. Huber, D.J., Kirkman, R.L., Kupiec-Weglinski, J.W., Araujo, J.L., Tilney, N.L. and Adams, D.F. (1985). The detection of cardiac allograft rejection by alterations in proton NMR relaxation times. *Invest. Radiol.*, **20**, 796
127. Aherne, T., Yee, E.S., Tscholakof, D., Gollin, G., Higgins, C. and Ebert, P.A. (1988). Diagnosis of acute and chronic cardiac rejection by magnetic resonance imaging: a non-invasive *in-vivo* study. *J. Cardiovasc. Surg.*, **29**, 587
128. Nishimura, T., Sada, M., Sasaki, H., Amemiya, H., Kozuka, T., Fujita, T., Akutsu, T. and Manabe, H. (1987). Cardiac transplantation in

dogs: evaluation with gated MRI and Gd-DTPA contrast enhancement. *Heart Vessels*, **3**, 141
129. Lund, G., Morin, R.L., Olivari, M.T. and Ring, W.S. (1988). Serial myocardial T2 relaxation time measurements in normal subjects and heart transplant recipients. *J. Heart Transplant.*, **7**, 274
130. Walpoth, B.H., McGregor, C.G., Aziz, S., Billingham, M.E., Jardetzky, N.W., Jardetzky, O., Jamieson, S.W. and Shumway, N.E. (1984). Assessment of myocardial rejection by nuclear magnetic resonance (P-31NMR) (Abstract). *Circulation*, **70** (Suppl. 2), 165
131. Haug, E.G., Shapiro, J.I., Chan, L. and Weil, R. (1987). P-31 Nuclear magnetic resonance spectroscopic evaluation of heterotopic cardiac allograft rejection in the rat. *Transplantation*, **44** 175
132. Canby, R.C., Evanochko, W.T., Barrett, L.V., Kirklin, J.K., McGiffin, D.C., Sakai, T.T., Brown, M.E., Foster, R.E., Reeves, P.C. and Pohost, G.M. (1987). Monitoring the bioenergetics of cardiac allograft rejection using *in vivo* P-31 nuclear magnetic resonance spectroscopy. *J. Am. Coll. Cardiol.*, **9**, 1067
133. Haug, C.E., Shapiro, J.I., Cosby, R.L., Chan, L. and Weil, R., III (1988). ^{31}P nuclear magnetic resonance spectroscopy of heart, heart-lung, and kidney allograft rejection in the rat. *Transplant. Proc.*, **20**, 848
134. Fraser, C.D. Jr., Chacko, V.P., Jacobus, W.E., Soulen, R.L., Hutchins, G.M., Reitz, B.A. and Baumgartner, W.A. (1988). Metabolic changes preceding functional and morphologic indices of rejection in heterotopic cardiac allografts. *Transplantation*, **46**, 346
135. Bottomley, P.A. (1985). Non-invasive study of high-energy phosphate metabolism in human heart by depth-resolved ^{31}P NMR spectroscopy. *Science*, **229**, 769
136. Kobashigawa, J., Stevenson, L.W., Moriguchi, J., Westlake, C., Wilmarth, J., Kawata, N., Chuck, C., Lewis, W., Drinkwater, T. and Laks, H. (1989). A randomized study of high dose oral cyclosporine therapy for mild acute cardiac rejection. *J. Heart Transplant.*, **8**, 53
137. Salaman, J.R. (1983). Steroids in organ transplantation. *Heart Transplant.*, **2**, 118
138. Michler, R.E., Smith, C.R., Druisin, R.E., Reison, D.S., Hickey, T.J., Lamb, J., Reemtsma, K. and Rose, E.A. (1986). Reversal of cardiac transplant rejection without massive immunosuppression. *Circulation*, **74** (Suppl. III), III-68
139. Wahlers, T.H., Heublein, B., Lowes, D., Dammenhayn, L., Fieguth, H.G., Haverich, A. and Borst, H.G. (1989). Treatment of rejection following cardiac transplantation: what dosage of pulsed steroids is necessary? (Abstract). *J. Heart Transplant.*, **8**, 96
140. Miska, P.T., Bates, L.R., Collins, C.L., Bolling, S.F. and Deeb, G.M. (1988). Solu-medrol pulsing of heart transplant patients in the home. Presented to the *International Society for Heart Transplantation*, Los Angeles
141. Bieber, C.P., Griepp, R.B., Oyer, P.E., Wong, J. and Stinson, E.B. (1976). Use of rabbit antithymocyte globulin in cardiac transplantation. Relationship of serum clearance rates to clinical outcome. *Transplantation*, **22**, 478
142. Novitzky, D., Cooper, D.K.C. and Barnard, C.N. (1984). Reversal of acute rejection by cyclosporine in a heterotopic heart transplant. *Heart Transplant.*, **3**, 117
143. Radovancevic, B. and Frazier, O.H. (1986). Treatment of moderate heart allograft rejection with cyclosporine. *J. Heart Transplant*, **5**, 307
144. Hunt, S.A. (1983). Complications of heart transplantation. *Heart Transplant.*, **3**, 70
145. Pennock, J.L., Reitz, B.A., Bieber, C.P., Jamieson, S.W., Raney, A.A., Oyer, P.E. and Stinson, E.B. (1981). Cardiac allograft survival in cynomolgous monkeys treated with cyclosporin-A in combination with conventional immune suppression. *Transplant. Proc.*, **13**, 390
146. Gilbert, E.M., DeWitt, C.W., Eiswirth, C.C., Renlund, D.G., Menlove, R.L., Freedman, L.A., Herrick, C.M., Gay, W.A. and Bristow, M.R. (1987). Treatment of refractory cardiac allograft rejection with OKT3 monoclonal antibody. *Am. J. Med.*, **82**, 202
147. Bristow, M.R., Gilbert, E.M., Renlund, D.G., DeWitt, C.W., Burton, N.A. and O'Connell, J.B. (1988). Use of OKT3 monoclonal antibody in cardiac transplantation: review of the initial experience. *J. Heart Transplant.*, **7**, 1
148. Bristow, M.R., Gilbert, E.M., O'Connell, J.B., Renlund, D.G., Watson, F.S., Hammond, E., Lee, R.G. and Menlove, R.L. (1988). OKT3 monoclonal antibody in heart transplantation. *Am. J. Kidney Dis.*, **11**, 135
149. Ortho Multi-center Transplant Study Group (1985). A randomized clinical trial of OKT3 monoclonal antibody for acute rejection of cadaveric renal transplants. *N. Engl. J. Med.*, **313**, 337
150. Weil, R., Clarke, D.R., Iwaki, Y., Porter, K.A., Koep, L.J., Paton, B.C., Terasaki, P.I. and Starzl, T.E. (1981). Hyperacute rejection of a transplanted human heart. *Transplantation*, **32**, 72
151. Schuurman, H-J., Jambroes, G., Borleffs, J.C.C., Slootweg, P.J., Gamelig Meyling, F.H.J. and de Gast, G.C. (1988). Acute humoral rejection after heart transplantation. *Transplantation*, **46**, 603
152. Cooper, D.K.C. (1990). A clinical survey of cardiac transplantation between ABO blood group incompatible recipients and donors. *J. Heart Transplant.*, In press
153. Paul, L.C., Baldwin, W.M. and Van Es, L.A. (1985). Vascular endothelial alloantigens in renal transplantation. *Transplantation*, **40**, 117
154. Jordan, S.C., Yap, H.K., Sakai, R.S., Alfonso, P. and Fitchman, M. (1988). Hyperacute allograft rejection mediated by anti-vascular endothelial cell antibodies with a negative monocyte crossmatch. *Transplantation*, **46**, 585
155. Brasile, L., Zerbe, T., Rabin, B., Clarke, J., Abrams, A. and Cerilli, J. (1985). Identification of the antibody to vascular endothelial cells in patients undergoing cardiac transplantation. *Transplantation*, **40**, 672
156. Trento, A., Hardesty, R.L., Griffith, B.P., Zerbe, T., Kormos, R.L. and Bahnson, H.T. (1988). Role of the antibody to vascular endothelial cells in hyperacute rejection in patients undergoing cardiac transplantation. *J. Thorac. Cardiovasc. Surg.*, **95**, 37

17
Infectious Complications
E.D. BATEMAN AND A.A. FORDER

INTRODUCTION

Infection remains a major cause of death and morbidity in patients undergoing cardiac transplantation, especially in the first few months when immunosuppression is at its highest[1-9]. Study of these infections provides an alarming, though fascinating, insight into the delicate relationship between the transplant recipient and the wide variety of organisms, both pathogens and opportunists, in our environment. Although bacteria are the most common causative organisms (30–60%), other etiological agents such as viruses (20–50%), fungi (14–25%), and protozoa (up to 5%), account for a proportion of infectious episodes[3,4]. In our own and other centers, these complications have prompted a critical assessment of conditions favoring infection, of means for preventing them, and of diagnostic approaches to identification of causative organisms.

In this chapter we discuss several of the principles applied in the management of these patients. These principles include:

(1) The importance of maintaining immunosuppression at minimal effective levels, and the desirability of utilizing agents like cyclosporine, which may have less effect on host defence mechanisms;

(2) The importance of early mobilization of the patient;

(3) The maintenance of surgical sterility in the transplant ward;

(4) Careful surveillance for infection without waiting for the usual signs of disease;

(5) A more aggressive diagnostic approach;

(6) Isolation of possible pathogens before treatment is commenced; and

(7) The use of broad-spectrum therapeutic regimens because of the frequency with which infections are caused by multiple organisms.

INCIDENCE, TYPE AND SITE OF INFECTION

The incidence of infections has changed dramatically since the introduction of cyclosporine (CsA) into the immunosuppressive regimen in the early 1980s. Several reports, including a large comparative study from Stanford, have confirmed a reduction in overall infection rate, a decline in deaths attributable to infection, and a change in pattern of infections[4]. Major infection occurred in 22 of 40 heart transplant patients (55%) reported from our own institution between 1974 and 1981[3]. These episodes accounted for 39% of all deaths in this series, and for 59% of deaths occurring in the first year after transplantation.

The Stanford report compared infectious complications during the first year after transplantation amongst 72 patients treated with a CsA-based regimen between March 1982 and May 1984, with 38 historical controls treated with an azathioprine (AZA)-based regimen. Significantly fewer patients in the CsA group had an infection (71% versus 86%), infection contributed to death in fewer patients (11% versus 39%), and patient survival doubled (79% versus 53%)[4]. The University of Arizona experience showed a similar decline in infective episodes, from 2.8 ± 0.3 per patient on conventional treatment, to 1.2 ± 0.3 per patient on CsA, in the first post-transplant year[8].

The lower infection rate is partially attributable to fewer rejection episodes during CsA treatment (at the University of Arizona a reduction from 2.5 ± 0.4 to 1.5 ± 0.3 per patient)[6,8]. Short-term increases in immunosuppressive treatment for bouts of rejection are associated with a short-term increase in infection rate[7]. The converse is seen in older heart transplant recipients who, because of presumed declining immune functions, have fewer episodes of rejection, and require lower doses of immunosuppression. A lower frequency of serious infections has been observed in these patients[5].

Organisms gain access by several portals and, because of impaired host status, may present in a variety of ways. The relative frequency of these forms of presentation, and the systems involved, are listed in Table 17.1. Rubin *et al.* have

Table 17.1 Site of presentation of non-fatal infections after heterotopic cardiac transplantation at Groote Schuur Hospital (November 1974–October 1981)

Site	Presentation	Number of episodes (%)	Number of patients
Blood	septicemia	1 (4)	1
Lung	pneumonia, lung abscess, empyema	7 (27)	6
Skin, subcutaneous tissue	rash, cellulitis, abscesses	7 (27)	6
Bone	osteitis, arthritis	3 (12)	2
GI tract	diarrhea	3 (12)	3
Endocardium	septicemia, embolic brain abscess	2 (7)	2
Myocardium	cardiac failure, myocarditis	1 (4)	1
Brain meninges	encephalitis, meningitis	1 (4)	1
Cervix	vaginal discharge	1 (4)	1
Total		26 (100)	

Source: Cooper et al.[3]

described a pattern of infection occurring in renal transplant patients (Figure 17.1)[10].

In the first postoperative month, opportunistic (fungal, nocardial, and protozoal) infections are extremely rare. The major causes of infections are bacterial, and usually involve the wound, the lungs, mediastinum or, rarely, the urinary tract. These infections are readily treated with antibiotics. Non-bacterial infections provide a greater problem in diagnosis and treatment. The period 1–6 months after transplantation is the critical period for the recipient in terms of risk of life-threatening infection[10]. During this period immunosuppression reaches its peak, cytomegalovirus (CMV) and herpes simplex virus infections appear, and opportunistic infections become more common.

In the late post-transplantation period (more than 6 months after transplantation), chronic infection occurs, usually of viral etiology, in particular cytomegalovirus and hepatitis. Cryptococcal infections are also present during this period. Those diseases common in the community at the time must also be expected, e.g. tuberculosis or influenza.

A similar profile applies to cardiac transplant patients. At Stanford, the median onset for bacterial pneumonia and empyema was 17 days, 21 days for bacteremia; 25 days for legionella infections, mediastinal and sternal infections, and 98 days for urinary tract infections. Aspergillus infection occurred at 23 days and candidal infections at 44 days. Nocardial infections occurred at 150 and 260 days and two cases of pneumocystis pneumonia at 143 and 713 days[4].

Tables 17.2 and 17.3 summarize the fatal and non-fatal infections occurring in a sample of transplanted patients who received conventional immunosuppression (AZA, methylprednisolone, and rabbit antithymocyte globulin) in our own hospital between 1974 and 1983[3]. (CYA was introduced into our unit in March 1983.)

With the introduction of CsA, the pattern of infection has altered considerably. Viral infections are more numerous than bacterial, but are usually of only minor importance. In the Stanford series, none of the herpes simplex virus infections involved viscera; the incidence of CMV infection was reduced by half, and only 28% of these (compared with more than 50% in conventionally-treated patients) involved viscera[4]. The incidence of bacterial infection in the CsA group was also halved, much of this being attributable to fewer pulmonary infections (35% versus 63% in the control group). This reduction in the proportion of infectious respiratory complications has not been observed in all series[9]. The nature of respiratory infections has also been

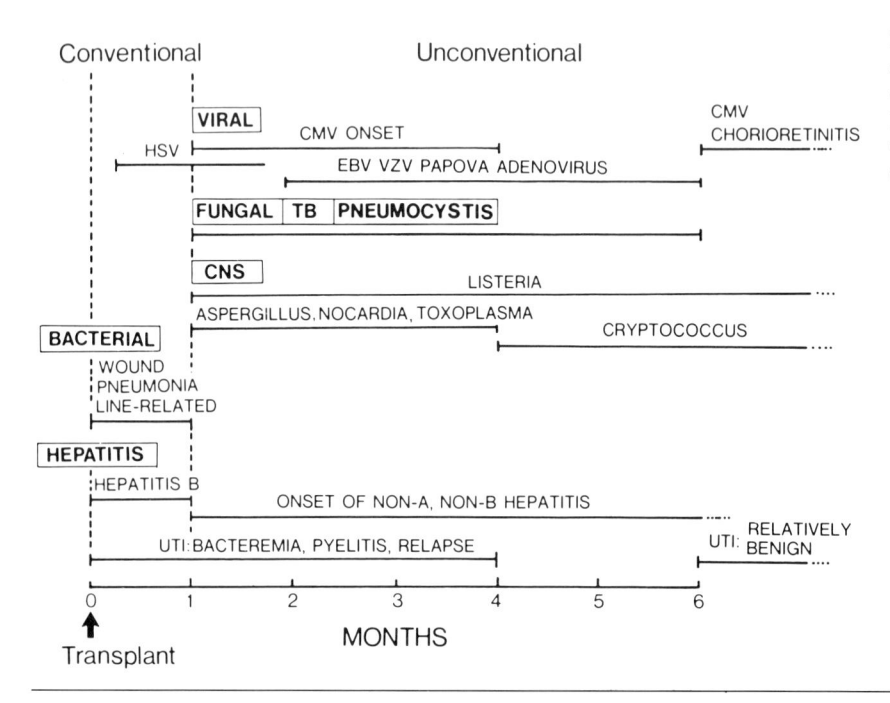

Figure 17.1 Common sequence of types of infection encountered in transplant patients (after Rubin et al.[10]). CMV = cytomegalovirus; HSV = herpes simplex virus; EBV = Epstein–Barr virus; VZV = varicella zoster virus; TB = tuberculosis; CNS = central nervous system; UTI = urinary tract infection

INFECTIOUS COMPLICATIONS

Table 17.2 Fatal infections after heterotopic cardiac transplantation at Groote Schuur Hospital (November 1974–October 1981)

	Site of origin	Organisms cultured or isolated	Clinical course	Time of death (days after transplantation)
Bacterial (4 patients)	?Leg	Leg: Clostridium perfringens	?Following endomyocardial biopsy performed through femoral vein; gas gangrene right leg; amputation	76
	Lungs	Sputum: Staphylococcus aureus Klebsiella pneumoniae Blood: Pseudomonas aeruginosa Escherichia coli	(Retransplant) Adult respiratory distress syndrome; tracheostomy; pneumonia; septicemia	24
	GI tract	Stools and blood: Salmonella group B Blood; (Serratia marcescens) (E. coli) (Enterobacter sp.)	Diarrhea; lung abscess; bronchopleural fistula; empyema	64
	Lungs	E. coli Enterobacter sp. Peptococcus	(Retransplant) Pneumonia	93
Fungal (4 patients)	Lungs	Aspergillus fumigatus	Pneumonia; dissemination	74
	Lungs	Aspergillus sp.	Pneumonia; dissemination	234
	Lungs	Petriellidium boydii	Pneumonia; dissemination	233
	Lungs	A. fumigatus	Pneumonia; dissemination	527
Viral (3 patients)	?Blood	Cytomegalovirus	Cytomegaloviremia	61
	?Blood	?Herpes simplex	Infection of esophagus, tongue and skin; encephalitis	220
	Lungs	Unidentified	Pneumonia	35

The significance of organisms in parentheses remains uncertain
Source: Cooper et al.[3]

reported to change. They are more diffuse, but with a lower incidence of respiratory failure[9]. Several centers report an increase in the proportion of legionella pneumonia, and possible decrease in the number of nocardial infections[4]. A reduction in bacteremic episodes, but paradoxically more local wound sepsis and mediastinitis, occurred in the CsA-treated group reported from Stanford, whereas urinary tract infections occurred with similar frequency with both treatment regimens (approximately 10%). Fungal (predominantly aspergillus) and pneumocystis infections are slightly less common in patients treated with CsA.

It is not clear whether the timing of these infections has altered with the introduction of CsA. No change was observed at Stanford, but Columbia University report a shift, two-thirds of pulmonary infections occurring after the third postoperative month[9].

FACTORS WHICH PREDISPOSE TO INFECTION

In the transplant patient, the basis for enhanced susceptibility to infection is exceedingly complex, and appears more so as new data become available. Nevertheless, it is important to attempt to identify individual elements of the weakened host defenses, as at least some of these may be strengthened by specific preventative or therapeutic measures, without disturbing the immunosuppression essential for graft survival. Aspects of host defenses and mechanisms which are disrupted are listed in Tables 17.4–17.6.

Immunosuppression following cardiac transplantation is generally more intense than with other organ transplants, and consequently is associated with a higher incidence of infection[11]. Immunosuppression may be specific or non-specific. The majority is *non-specific*, and readily achieved by one or more of a number of drugs and other agents. While non-specific immunosuppression is effective in preventing rejection, when profound it is associated with an unacceptably high incidence of infection, particularly in the first 3 months after transplantation, when drug therapy is heaviest. With time, however, adaptation permits reduction of therapy, with an associated lower risk of infection[12]. This accounts for the low incidence of fatal infections after the first year.

At all stages, a compromise has to be accepted between the possibility of rejection and suppression of resistance to infection. In practice, this is difficult to achieve because of individual susceptibilities to immunosuppressive drugs, the need to be guided by tests confirming rejection, and the lack of uniform virulence of different classes of organisms.

Table 17.3 Non-fatal infections after heterotopic cardiac transplantation at Groote Schuur Hospital (November 1974–October 1981)

	Site of origin	Organisms cultured or isolated	Months after transplantation	Clinical course
Bacterial (15 patients)	Blood	*Acinetobacter* sp.	3	Septicemia. Resolved with treatment (RWT)
	Endocardium	*Staphylococcus aureus*	18	Infection on prosthetic value; prosthesis removed; resolved
	Endocardium	*Salmonella dublin* *Bacillus cereus*	25	Septicemia; embolic brain abscess; infected saddle embolus (RWT)
	Lungs	*Haemophilus influenzae*	6	Pneumonia (RWT)
	Lungs	*H. influenzae*	12	Pneumonia (RWT)
	Lungs	*Streptococcus pneumoniae*	3	Pneumonia (RWT)
	Lungs	No organism identified	37	Pneumonia (RWT)
	Sternum	*Staph. aureus* (+7 other organisms)	1	Nine surgical drainage procedures; chronic discharging sinus for 36 months, resolved
	Sternum	Multiple organisms (10)	1	Three surgical drainage procedures; resolved
	GI tract	*Shigella dysenteriae*	1	(RWT)
	GI tract	*Salmonella* sp.	8	(RWT)
	GI tract	*Salmonella* sp.	1	(RWT)
	Subcutaneous tissue (leg)	*Citrobacter* sp.	5	Extensive abscesses of both legs; surgically drained; resolved
	Subcutaneous tissue (perineum)	*E. coli*	9	Perineal abscess following sigmoidoscopy and barium enema; surgically drained; resolved
	Subcutaneous tissue (perineum)	Non-hemolytic streptococcus	54	Perineal abscess; surgically drained; resolved
Mycobacterial (3 patients)	Lungs	*M. kansasii*	9	Chronic low grade pneumonia, treated but remained unresolved. Died at 14 months from disseminated Kaposi's sarcoma
	Lungs	*M. tuberculosis*	20	Chronic low grade pneumonia; refused treatment; died at 24 months from cerebral embolus
	Bone	*M. haemophilum*	48	Chronic discharging sinuses at left wrist, left thigh and left lower leg; low grade purulent infective arthritis left knee; not treated systemically; died at 54 months from chronic rejection
Fungal (1 patient)	Meninges	*Cryptococcus neoformans*	56	(RWT)
Viral (5 patients)	Face and scalp	Herpes zoster (clinical diagnosis)		Resolved
	Chest wall	Herpes zoster (clinical diagnosis)	36	Resolved
	Chest wall	Herpes zoster (clinical diagnosis)	9	Resolved
	Ear	Herpes simplex (identified in isolate)	35	Resolved
	Cervix	Herpes, unidentified (clinical diagnosis)	60	Resolved
Protozoal (2 patients)	Myocardium	*Toxoplasma gondii*	18	Seen on endomyocardial biopsy; ?transferred from donor; clinically asymptomatic (RWT)
	Lungs	*Pneumocystis carinii*	51	(RWT)

RWT = resolved with treatment
Source: Cooper et al.[3]

Even when severe infection occurs, prevention of graft rejection remains the priority (unlike the situation following renal transplantation, where immunosuppression may be reduced or even discontinued until the infection is controlled).

Ideally, antirejection therapy should leave host resistance intact. The highest degree of specificity likely to be achieved by drugs is one which interacts specifically and exclusively with the subpopulations of proliferating T-cells responsible for graft rejection (i.e. helper and killer T-lymphocytes). Even these drugs, however, would suppress the immunoproliferative response to pathogens. *Specific* immunosuppression, defined as treatment which directly or indirectly selectively suppresses the action of the lymphocyte clones responsible for rejection (i.e. antigen-specific, and directed at the histocompatibility antigens of the graft donor) will probably only be achieved by biological agents[13]. Until this is achieved, the threat of infection will remain.

A further consideration in the prevention of infections is the human factor. Patients who comply poorly with medical instructions and advice experience a higher incidence of infection[3,14]. In some instances, non-compliance is transient and associated with mild depressive disorders. These need to be recognized and treated, though it must be borne in mind that depression may be the first symptom of chronic illness, e.g. the development of tuberculous infection.

PREVENTION OF INFECTION

Literature relating to preventative and control measures in the transplant patient is often confusing and controversial, and it is difficult to distinguish those measures that are of proven efficacy from the many advocated on the basis of intuition or empiricism. Proof of efficacy is obtained only from properly designed clinical trials in homogenous groups

Table 17.4 Factors increasing the risk of infection in transplant patients

(1) Non-specific immunosuppression
   (a) *Iatrogenic*:
      Pharmacological agents
         glucocorticoids
         antimetabolites (e.g. azathioprine)
         cyclosporine A
         alkylating agents (e.g. cyclophosphamide)
      Biological agents
         antilymphocyte globulin
         (thoracic duct fistula)
         (plasmapheresis)
      Ionizing radiation
   (b) *Natural*:
      Debility from prolonged cardiac disease (poor nutrition and increased catabolism)
(2) Breach of surface barriers by:
   Central venous catheters/venous lines
   Chest drains
   Urinary catheter
   Endotracheal intubation and mechanical ventilation/tracheostomy
   Invasive procedures (e.g. endomyocardial biopsy)
(3) Increased exposure to micro-organisms
   Prolonged hospital stay
(4) Incorporation of prosthetic material (e.g. Dacron) (heterotopic transplantation)
(5) Neuropsychiatric disorders, non-compliance on the part of the patient

Table 17.5 Microbial infections associated with impaired T-lymphocyte function

Bacteria	Fungi
Brucella spp.	*Aspergillus* spp.
Listeria monocytogenes	*Candida* spp.
Mycobacteria spp.	*Cryptococcus neoformans*
Nocardia spp.	*Phycomycetes* spp.
Salmonella spp.	*Histoplasma capsulatum*
Viruses	Protozoa
Cytomegalovirus (CMV)	*Toxoplasma gondii*
Herpes simplex	*Pneumocystis carinii*
Vaccinia	
Varicella zoster	
Measles	

Table 17.6 Microbial infections associated with a shift in immunoglobulin type and poor opsonization

Streptococcus pneumoniae	*Streptococcus pyogenes* (group A)
Haemophilus influenzae	*Klebsiella pneumoniac*

of patients exposed to similar risk[15]. Furthermore, because infection in the transplant patient arises in a variety of circumstances, introduction of a single hygienic measure cannot be expected to bring about more than a modest reduction in the infection rate, worthwhile though this may be[15]. A large number of hygienic precautions has to be considered for inclusion in any infection control program. To submit more than a few of these to formal controlled trials is impractical. Because of the laborious nature of clinical trials and the numbers of patients needed, clinicians are at times forced to accept conclusions based on laboratory evidence alone, or derived from imperfectly controlled clinical studies and from situations not strictly comparable to the circumstances under consideration.

With these reservations in mind, the conditions which have prevailed, and policies which have been employed to control infections in heart transplant patients in our institution over the past two decades are presented below. More lenient policies employed in other centers will be presented later.

The transplant unit

All transplant patients are nursed in a specially designed unit, occupying a separate floor of the hospital. Separate nursing personnel care for the transplant patients; where possible, senior nursing staff are appointed on a permanent basis, and are specially trained in the care of such patients. The unit has three specialized single rooms equipped with intensive care facilities for the immediate postoperative care of the patients. There is air-conditioning (approximately 12 changes of air per hour) and terminal absolute filters in each room. Reliance is placed on ambient humidity in these areas, rather than upon artificial steam injection. The air is cooled by passage over refrigerated coils, and any condensate is drained away immediately. Spot checks are carried out on the plant by members of the Department of Medical Microbiology. The nursing station is equipped with gauges, indicating humidity, temperature, and the pressure gradient across the main air filter to each room, which are checked at regular intervals. All room finishes are designed to facilitate easy cleaning. Buckets are autoclaved between use; mops are disinfected in a freshly prepared solution of organic chlorine (500 ppm available chlorine).

Entry to the unit is by a change area only. All personnel entering the unit wear a gown, cap, mask, and overshoes, measures found to be very effective in keeping unwanted persons out of the area. Personnel and visitors with sore throats or septic and viral lesions (e.g. herpes) are excluded from the area. All bedpans, urinals, urine-measuring cylinders, and jugs are autoclaved on a regular basis in a sterilizing unit adjacent to the ward; all respiratory support equipment is delivered to the unit from a central pasteurizing/ethylene oxide gas sterilizing facility; and respiratory tubing and humidifiers are changed daily.

The patient

Strict attention is given to the location and elimination of all sources of infection prior to transplantation, though routine bacteriological screening of the patient is not undertaken. Preference is given to the careful daily monitoring of the patient for clinical signs and symptoms of infection, appropriate specimens being taken at the first indication of such infection.

As prophylaxis at the time of transplantation, the recipient is given 1 g of cephalosporin intravenously before operation, 6-hourly for 48 hours after surgery. Cephamandole 1 g 6-hourly was standard until recently, but cefotaxime 1 g 6-hourly is now recommended[7]. The duration of therapy is controversial, some recommending that the prophylaxis be continued until chest tubes are removed, and that it be reintroduced if further surgery or chest manipulation is performed[7]. At other times antimicrobial agents are not used unless indicated, and then only with laboratory guidance.

Infection introduced through an intravenous line, although reported in the literature, has not been a problem in our patients. This may relate to the strict aseptic care given to the infusion lines, but their relatively short stay in the patient is probably more important. The lines are inserted under sterile conditions, and the cutaneous sites of entry redressed and monitored daily for infection. In other series, bacteremia and candidemia have been encountered, and, in particular, *Escherichia coli*, *Serratia marcesens* and *Pseudomonas aeruginosa*, *Staphylococcus aureus*, candida and *Streptococcus milleri* have been a problem. The temperature often settles after removal of the infected catheter, and culture of the catheter tip enables one to identify the organism correctly and use specific antibiotic therapy. The duration of treatment is controversial, but should probably be for 10 days or until the temperature has settled for 5–7 days.

The following principles of management are employed routinely to reduce the incidence of pulmonary infections. The duration of postoperative intermittent positive pressure mechanical ventilation is kept to a minimum (usually less than 24 hours). To avoid necrosis of nasal mucosa and sinusitis, orotracheal intubation is preferred to nasotracheal. Tracheostomy is avoided unless absolutely necessary, since the stoma is a common site of colonization by organisms, and this often predisposes to pneumonia. Postoperative physiotherapy includes liberal use of intermittent positive pressure breathing with a pressure-cycled respirator for 15–20 minutes 4–6-hourly to prevent atelectasis. Early mobilization is encouraged to minimize the possibility of hypostatic pneumonia, an important cause of death in the early orthotopically-transplanted patients in the Cape Town series.

Additional prophylaxis is considered in two circumstances. Firstly, CMV-seronegative patients who received transplants from CMV-seropositive donors may be protected from developing overt infection by regular doses of intravenous CMV hyperimmune globulin[16]. Secondly, prophylaxis with pyrimethamine alone or combined with sulfisoxazole, given daily for 4–6 weeks, may prevent toxoplasma infections in recipients who are seronegative for this organism at transplantation and receive a heart from a seropositive donor[7,17,18].

Screening for hepatitis B virus infection is usual before transplantation and HBsAg positivity has generally been a contraindication to surgery. A recent study from Italy suggests that, provided pre-transplant liver biopsy shows only HBsAg and no HBcAg and HDBAg on immunoperoxidase staining, viral replication is very unlikely, and a flare-up of hepatitis with associated infectivity is unlikely[19].

Preoperative procedures, like long-term outpatient infusions of inotropic agents to control chronic heart failure, present new potential sources of infection[20]. Such infections must be controlled before transplantation is performed. Another determinant of infective complications after heart transplantation appears to be the closeness of match for HLA loci A and B between donor and recipient. Analysis of patients on a CsA-based regimen has confirmed that patients with three or four mismatches have significantly more infections than those with fewer, and a trend toward a higher number of deaths from rejection and infection[21].

Recently, in the light of the reduced incidence of infection since the introduction of CsA, debate regarding the necessity for complete reverse isolation has once more been called into question[22–25]. At Stanford, when simple handwashing, with cleaning of the ward by departmental staff rather than by a committed nurse, replaced sterile gown, cap and gloves, no change in survival was observed[25]. Other centers with more relaxed policies appear to have similar infection rates to those where stricter methods apply[23]. It is argued that fewer isolation restrictions lower unit costs, decrease staffing needs, and reduce anxiety for patients and family, without subjecting the patient to a significantly increased risk of infection.

None of these studies is conclusive, however, as they are small, and type 2 errors may be hidden in the analysis. It would seem prudent to apply a combination of the above measures as local hospital conditions, known surgical sepsis rates, and incidence of nosocomial infections dictate. Probably it is the skill and experience of the surgeon, and the dedication and care of the nursing staff who attend to details of management, that are most important, rather than details of a written protocol.

PRESENTING FEATURES OF INFECTION

The most alarming aspects of infections in the immunocompromised patient are their rapidity of onset and evolution, the paucity of physical signs, atypical presentation, and the wide variety of organisms to be considered. (One such example was a 31-year-old male recipient who on the fourth post-transplant day developed progressive breathlessness and pulmonary opacification on chest radiograph compatible with pulmonary edema, and who was found to have acid-fast bacilli in bronchial brushings obtained by fiberoptic bronchoscopy. There was no evidence of current or past tuberculosis at the time of surgery. Fever and leukocytosis were absent, as is frequently the case; patients may even by asymptomatic.) Herpetic or fungal mouth lesions and the presence of a cough, which is almost always dry in the initial phases of chest infection, are common, and sometimes herald the onset of more serious infection.

Urinary tract infections are less problematic than in renal transplant recipients, and are usually due to the presence of the indwelling catheter. The infecting organisms are usually sensitive to conventional antibiotics, and are treated in the usual way. Early removal of the urinary catheter is a desirable prophylactic measure. *Escherichia coli*, enterococcus, candida, and occasionally klebsiella and *Pseudomonas aeruginosa* are the usual pathogens.

PULMONARY INFECTIONS

The lung is by far the most common site of presentation of infection in the transplant patient, representing 27% of all infections in our early series, and between 40 and 51% of infections at Columbia University[9]. The distinction between primary and secondary involvement of the lung in septicemic dissemination of organisms is not always possible, since pleura, meninges, kidney, joints, and other sites may be involved early. Moreover, the pathogenic sequence of invasion, consolidation, and resolution by resorption or cavitation, that is usually seen in an infected lung, is variable in the immunocompromised patient.

Radiographic features of consolidation may be minor even with overwhelming pneumonia and septicemia, probably as a result of a poor leukocyte response. Cavitation often appears early, and rupture through to the pleural space, causing empyema, is not uncommon. This progression from tissue consolidation to cavitation with empyema formation has been observed in two patients in our own series. In one patient this followed diarrhea caused by Salmonella Group B, and in the other was caused by *Streptococcus milleri* septicemia.

Forms of bacterial pneumonia generally encountered in non-immunocompromised patients accounted for 24% of all infections in our series (Tables 17.2 and 17.3). This incidence is lower than that of the early Stanford series (45%)[11], but may reflect a different approach to the diagnosis of disseminating infection. These pneumonias may be divided along conventional lines into bacterial, mycobacterial, fungal, and viral. Cases of uncomplicated *Haemophilus influenzae* and *Streptococcus pneumoniae* pneumonia respond to conventional antibiotics. Bacterial pneumonias carry a worse prognosis when they occur in the presence of an endotracheal or tracheostomy tube, in association with adult respiratory distress syndrome, and/or respiratory failure requiring ventilatory support. Organisms such as *Staphylococcus aureus*, *Klebsiella pneumoniae*, *Pseudomonas aeruginosa*, *E. coli*, enterobacter species, and *Peptococci* have been encountered in this setting, with fatal consequences (Table 17.2).

Diagnostic approach to pulmonary infections

Investigations undertaken for suspected infection depend on the system involved. These have been reviewed by Armstrong[26] and Bartlett[27].

Blood cultures

These are performed in all cases since, when positive, they provide confirmation of the relevant organism. To avoid spurious positive results they are carried out according to a strict aseptic protocol involving full surgical preparation of the skin.

Chest radiography

Chest radiography is performed daily during the initial weeks after transplantation, and thereafter at each follow-up visit. Careful review of previous radiographs is essential to avoid missing subtle changes in the lung fields which give warning of developing infection. Any unexplained radiographic abnormality, especially in the presence of symptoms (dyspnea, cough, fever, malaise) or leukocytosis, is investigated. The approach to the patient with an abnormality on chest radiograph is aggressive and urgent, with emphasis on obtaining bacteriological confirmation *prior* to commencement of antibiotics, because of the poor yield from transbronchial procedures if performed after treatment is commenced.

Several methods for achieving *a bacteriological diagnosis* of lung infection are available, ranging in invasiveness from sputum examination to open lung biopsy. Each has its own sensitivity, specificity, and complication rate determined from series incorporating both non-immunocompromised and immunocompromised patients (reviewed by Matthay and Moritz)[28]. Series comprising heart transplant recipients alone have been too small to permit meaningful conclusions.

Sputum examination

Sputum, when available, is sent for Gram and Ziehl–Neelsen staining and culture, but its diagnostic usefulness is limited by frequent contamination by commensal organisms originating in the upper respiratory tract or mouth. The presence of pus cells in sputum increases the suspicion of an organism being relevant, but at most this finding serves as a guide. Identification of mycobacteria is almost always significant, but cryptococcus or aspergillus detected in this way are merely indications for further investigations. Candida and herpes simplex virus isolated from sputum usually reflect oral infections, and seldom require more than local treatment[26].

In order of invasiveness, alternative procedures are percutaneous transtracheal aspiration, percutaneous needle aspiration of the lung, fiberoptic bronchoscopy with brushing (with sheathed or unsheathed brushes), transbronchial biopsies and limited lavage of bronchial tree, and open lung biopsy. The advantages and disadvantages of these procedures are outlined in Table 17.7.

Transtracheal aspiration

Transtracheal aspiration specimens are more reliable than sputa, but negative results occur when infection is located peripherally and is not in communication with the bronchial tree[29]. In our experience it has a lower diagnostic yield, except in patients with extensive pneumonia. For smaller lesions, local sampling, as offered by needle aspiration and fiberoptic bronchoscopy, is preferred.

Ultrafine needle aspiration

Because of its comparative safety, ultrafine needle aspiration (with a 24 or 25 gauge needle) has replaced conventional needle aspiration of the lung, but is contraindicated in patients on anticoagulants or with overt bleeding disorders[30]. It is particularly useful for peripheral lesions, and when diagnostic pleural aspiration is also indicated. It carries the highest sensitivity and specificity of all procedures, but a marginally higher complication rate than fiberoptic bronchoscopy[30]. The procedure is, however, well tolerated, and preferred by patients, and has been used to good effect in several patients at our institution.

Fiberoptic bronchoscopy

The alternative procedures to ultrafine needle aspiration are performed through a flexible fiberoptic bronchoscope. These are favored when the process is extensive or diffuse and when transbronchial biopsy is indicated, e.g. for suspected *Pneumocystis carinii* infection.

Bronchoscopy is performed under local anesthetic through the nasopharynx, and for this reason, although it provides a higher bacterial yield than needle biopsy, approximately half the isolates obtained are upper respiratory tract flora. The use of brushes protected by double telescoping catheters (PTC brush), which are plugged distally to prevent contamination of the specimen with organisms from the bronchoscope, overcomes this disadvantage, and provides a smaller but more reliable yield[31]. Since each of these brushes can be used to sample in only one location,

Table 17.7 Advantages and disadvantages of methods used to diagnose pulmonary infections

Method	Advantages	Disadvantages/complications
(1) Sputum examination and culture	Easy	Irrelevant organisms obtained
(2) Transtracheal aspiration	Easy; performed in ward (false-negative 1%) (false-positive 21%)[28]	Subcutaneous emphysema 0.5% Hemorrhage 0.2% Paratracheal infection 0.2%
(3) Ultrafine (G 24–25) needle aspiration	Sensitivity 83% Specificity 100% (value of − ve result 70%) (value of + ve result 100%)[29]	Patient must be moved to fluoroscopy facility Pneumothorax 8% (requiring intercostal drainage 4%)[29]
(4) Needle aspiration (G 16–20)	As for 3 (above)[27]	Pneumothorax 30% Hemoptysis 10%[27]
(5) Fiberoptic bronchoscopy		
(a) Brush	High yield	Patient discomfort Hypoxia Irrelevant organisms obtained 52%
(b) PTC brush	Lower yield; specificity higher	Limited sample
(c) Biopsy	Useful for pneumocystis and tuberculous granulomata	Hemoptysis 1% Pneumothorax 1%[30]
(d) Limited lavage	Increases yield	None
(6) Open lung biopsy	Specificity	Risk of morbidity/mortality Not suitable for repeated examinations

an unsheathed brush should be routinely employed to sample from many other sites.

When brushes are removed, smears are made directly on to sterile glass slides, and the brush immersed in a sterile test tube containing 2 ml sterile saline. The specimens are halved, conveyed immediately to the bacteriology laboratory for staining, microscopy, and culture. Any organism detected on both brushes or the sheathed brush alone is considered potentially pathogenic. Results from unsheathed brushes alone are interpreted with caution.

A review of published results of fiberbronchoscopic procedures in immunocompromised patients indicates that transbronchial biopsy alone provides a specific diagnosis in 41% of cases, bronchial brushing alone in 27%, and combined brush in 52%[28]. Similar results were obtained in immunocompromised patients studied at Groote Schuur Hospital[32]. A notable difference between these two series was the lower incidence of complications in our own series. In the former series, the incidences of hemorrhage (of greater than 25 ml) and of pneumothorax were each 7%, whereas in our series the combined incidence of these complications in 809 bronchoscopies was less than 1%. The reason for this difference is not apparent, but the figures indicate the relative safety of the procedure. The problem of initiating a lower respiratory tract infection from nasopharyngeal organisms introduced during bronchoscopy[24,33] has not been recognized in our patients[32], possibly because the majority are placed on short-term broad-spectrum antibiotics after the procedure.

Ultrafine needle aspiration and fiberoptic bronchoscopy are used as complementary procedures to be employed when the other has failed to confirm the diagnosis. When necessary they may be performed repeatedly during resolution of the infective lesion.

The results of 15 consecutive fiberoptic bronchoscopies performed on heart transplant recipients at Groote Schuur Hospital between July 1979 and December 1983 for investigation of suspected infection are presented in Table 17.8. These results illustrate the improved yield when more than one form of specimen is taken (i.e. brush and biopsy specimens), and highlight the importance of withholding treatment until detailed bacteriological investigation has been attempted. Bronchoscopy failed to be diagnostic in all patients who had received or were receiving antibiotics at the time of the procedure (except in those with tuberculosis and pneumocystis, which broad-spectrum antibiotics would not be expected to clear). The diagnostic value of bronchoscopy in this group of cardiac transplant patients was significantly lower than that in a larger group of renal transplant recipients investigated concurrently, most of

Table 17.8 Results of fiberoptic bronchoscopy in heart transplant recipients at Groote Schuur Hospital (1979–1983)

Indication (on chest radiograph)	Brush	Transbronchial biopsy	Bronchial lavage	Outcome	Conclusion
(1) Segmental consolidation	–	ND	–	Resolved (on tetracycline)	Failed
(2) Small segmental consolidation	MSO	ND	ND	Resolved spontaneously	Failed
(3) Cavity L. midzone	MSO	ND	ND	Prior amoxycillin: resolved on cotrimoxazole	Failed
(4) Small segmental consolidation	–	ND	ND	Prior cephamandole; resolved without further treatment	Failed
(5) Bilateral basal consolidation	–	ND	ND	Prior cefoxitin; died E. coli (blood culture)	Failed
(6) Segmental consolidation	MSO	ND	ND	Prior clindamycin; resolved on clindamycin and cefoxitin	Failed
(7) Small segmental consolidation	–	ND	ND	Prior cotrimoxazole and cephamandole; resolved without further treatment	Failed
(8) Segmental consolidation	S. pneumoniae	+	ND	Resolved on erythromycin	Diagnostic
(9) Segmental consolidation	M. kansasii	ND	ND	UTNA also positive. Treated	Diagnostic
(10) Bilateral nodular infiltrate	M. tuberculosis	–	ND	Prior sulphatriad. Treated	Diagnostic
(11) Bilateral nodular infiltrate	–	M. tuberculosis	ND	Prior sulphatriad and daraprim. Treated	Diagnostic
(12) Bilateral nodular infiltrate	–	P. carinii	+	Prior ampicillin, tobramycin and metronidazole; resolved on treatment	Diagnostic
(13) Patchy lobar infiltrate	M. tuberculosis	+	–	Prior INH; resolved on treatment	Diagnostic
(14) Bilateral nodular infiltrate	M. tuberculosis	–	–	Four-drug TB therapy; resolved	Diagnostic
(15) Small segmental consolidation	–	ND	ND	Inactive scar, no treatment	Helpful

MSO = mixed salivary organisms; UTNA = ultra-thin needle aspiration; ND = not done; – = negative result; + = positive result

whom had not received antibiotics (50%)[35].

The spontaneous resolution of occasional pulmonary shadows seen on the chest radiograph in heart transplant patients raises the possibility that some are non-infective in origin. They may represent small pulmonary infarcts following endomyocardial biopsy, or regions of atelectasis.

Arising from these considerations, a sound policy is (1) to withhold all antibiotic treatment until bacterial investigations have been completed, (2) to routinely include with fiberoptic bronchoscopy use of a double sheathed brush, a standard brush, limited bronchial lavage for bacteriology and virology, and transbronchial biopsy for culture and histology, and (3) to utilize fluoroscopic screening with fiberoptic bronchoscopy to improve localization of small lesions.

Open lung biopsy

Open lung biopsy is reserved for patients in whom the above diagnostic procedures have failed to provide conclusive results. It is also performed rarely when there is failure of resolution despite what is considered appropriate treatment. (Open lung biopsy was indicated in one such patient at our center with active pulmonary tuberculosis (diagnosed bronchoscopically), who failed to improve after 4 weeks of supervised four-drug therapy. Biopsy confirmed pulmonary tuberculosis; organisms were identified in the tissue sections, but could not be cultured. The patient subsequently recovered fully.) We have not employed open lung biopsy as readily as has been advocated for bone marrow transplant recipients[36].

Computerized axial tomography

Computerized axial tomography (CAT) is a useful method for detecting localized pleural or extrapulmonary disease, and, following heterotopic heart transplantation, in demonstrating lesions of the right lower lobe whose presence on chest radiography may be obscured by the donor heart. In two of our patients, one with a tuberculous cavity and another with a lung abscess, lesions in this location were missed in the early stages. In the former, the CAT scan identified the site, and facilitated aspiration of the abscess.

SEPTICEMIA

Patients with septicemia may complain of symptoms similar to those with pulmonary infections. When no obvious pulmonary involvement is present, a detailed search for other primary sources should be made. This includes inspection of the wound, urine and throat swab cultures, mouth washings (obtained by gargling) for virological study, examination of the ears for middle ear infection, of the optic fundi for chorioretinitis and tubercles, and of the central nervous system to exclude meningitis and intracranial abscess. Any suspicion of the latter conditions is an indication for lumbar puncture, particular care being paid to identifying cryptococci; examination of 10 ml of cerebrospinal fluid is recommended for this purpose[37]. Urinary tract infections, although rare, are an important source of infection, and recurrent septicemia may originate from renal carbuncles. Examination and culture of aspiration and trephine biopsies of bone marrow are occasionally used, particularly when confirmation of disseminated tuberculosis is required; the yield, however, is fairly low[38].

Serology

Serological tests play only a minor role in the investigation of the pyrexial patient with suspected septicemia because of several shortcomings which seriously limit their usefulness[39].

(1) It is difficult to interpret a positive titer unless the previous antibody status is known. For this reason, serum levels of CMV antibodies are estimated before transplantation; changes in antibody titers can then be readily appreciated. For other organisms, a delay of up to 2 weeks in obtaining results is inevitable, and diagnoses can only be made with confidence retrospectively. In practice, therefore, if organisms like mycoplasma or legionella are suspected, the therapeutic regimen is adjusted to cover these organisms[7].

(2) Many immunocompromised patients fail to develop antibodies in response to infections. This has been observed in transplant recipients with fungal disease[39].

(3) Positive fungal antibody tests (e.g. immunodiffusion tests for aspergillus precipitins) do not distinguish between colonization and invasive forms of infection[39], and the diagnosis of new and possibly invasive infection can only be made if there has been recent seroconversion.

Organisms commonly tested for serologically prior to heart transplantation therefore include *Mycoplasma pneumoniae*, *Legionella pneumophila*, cytomegalovirus, herpes simplex virus, toxoplasma, influenza and adenoviruses, and hepatitis viruses. Occasionally, the Paul Bunnell, Weil-Felix, Widal, and Brucella serological tests are requested.

More promising techniques are being developed for demonstrating the presence of microbial antigens or other products of micro-organisms in tissue fluids and serum. These include immunofluorescent staining for antigens of *L. pneumophilia*[40], and demonstration of cryptococcal antigen in serum[41] or blood leukocytes[42] of patients with interstitial pulmonary disease.

Tests of limited usefulness for diagnosis of infection are the erythrocyte sedimentation rate (ESR) and the Limulus lysate test. This latter test is based on the ability of bacterial endotoxin (lipopolysaccharide) to cause extracts of the amoebocyte cell of Limulus polyphemus (the horseshoe crab) to coagulate. Although very sensitive *in vitro*, when applied to the diagnosis of human Gram-negative bacteremia, fewer than two-thirds have positive tests, and false-positive tests are not infrequent. False-negative results may arise from the presence in serum of antibodies to endotoxin or inhibitors[38].

CENTRAL NERVOUS SYSTEM INFECTIONS

Three patterns of infection of the central nervous system (CNS) have been described in renal transplant patients[43].

(1) Acute or subacute meningitis, almost invariably caused by *Listeria monocytogenes*.

(2) Subacute or chronic meningitis, caused by *Cryptococcus neoformans* or *Mycobacterium tuberculosis*.

(3) Focal brain infection giving rise to focal neurological signs, caused by listeria species, *Toxoplasma gondii*, candida species, *Nocardia asteroides*, and, most commonly, *Aspergillus fumigatus*[43].

Similar presentations have been seen in heart transplant recipients[3,37]. One patient in our series had viral encephalitis (probably herpetic)[3], and in the latter series[37] one had an abscess of bacterial origin (klebsiella). Occasionally rhinocerebritis caused by members of the class zygomycetes (rhizopus and mucor) are encountered[37].

Meningitis may occur at any time following transplantation, but frequently follows a temporary increase in treatment for rejection[37]. Headache, lethargy, and fever are common; examining the cerebrospinal fluid (CSF) is usually helpful in establishing the diagnosis. In cryptococcal meningitis, pleocytosis may be modest, and most cells are mononuclear; a mild elevation of protein is found. CSF glucose is low (compared with paired blood level), and the India-ink preparation and Gram stain show the large capsule and the budding yeasts respectively. By contrast, in listeria meningitis, pleocytosis is marked (both polymorphonuclear leukocytes and mononuclears), and although Gram stain may be negative, listeria colonies grow out on culture. CSF protein and glucose show the same abnormalities as in cryptococcal disease[37].

PRINCIPLES OF THERAPY OF BACTERIAL AND MYCOBACTERIAL INFECTIONS

Prospects for successfully treating infections in immunocompromised patients are improving with the introduction of newer antibiotics and antiviral agents. Nevertheless, the outcome of treatment is still largely dependent upon the patient's own antimicrobial defense mechanisms[36]. Other important factors are the nature of the invading organism, the stage at which the treatment is commenced, and the site of infection.

Bacterial infections

Since the first heart transplant was performed, important new antibiotics have been introduced into clinical practice which have influenced prescribing habits for transplant patients. Although it is impossible to provide statistical confirmation of the benefits of these newer agents, several of their advantages are self-evident.

The following is a summary of antibiotic prescribing policy for heart transplant patients.

(1) The preferred policy is to give specific, rather than 'blind', treatment for causative organisms. The difficulty is that delay in treating a rapidly progressing infection, while investigations are performed, may be disastrous. A compromise is often necessary, with 'presumptive' or 'best guess' antimicrobial therapy being introduced immediately after initiation of microbiological investigations, but before results of cultures are available. Adjustments to therapy, or its discontinuance, may be made subsequently as the results of laboratory tests become known.

(2) The choice of antimicrobials should be made in consultation with a microbiologist, particular attention being paid to *in vitro* sensitivity of organisms and the emergence of resistant hospital strains.

(3) Unless a specific antibiotic has already been indicated by the results of investigations, initial therapy should comprise two agents, and sometimes a third, depending on the clinical circumstances. The first two are an aminoglycoside paired with a B-lactam agent. The former may be tobramycin, gentamicin, or amikacin. Tobramycin is favored because of its greater antipseudomonal activity and its lesser nephrotoxicity[44]. The loading dose and maintenance dose are determined according to body surface area, and the therapy adjusted according to serum levels of aminoglycoside measured immediately before and 1 hour after each dose. There is a continuing debate as to whether the B-lactam agent should be a cephalosporin or an antipseudomonal penicillin, such as carbenicillin or piperacillin. In our patients, unlike recipients of bone marrow transplants, pseudomonal septicemia, with its associated high mortality, is relatively rare[36]. For this reason, penicillin or a cephalosporin is the preferred second agent.

Cefotaxime, a third-generation cephalosporin, has the advantage of broad-spectrum activity against both Gram-negative organisms and, to a lesser extent, staphylococci, and may be used alone, or occasionally in combination with metronidazole to cover anaerobes. This regimen avoids the risk of aminoglycoside-induced nephrotoxicity. When staphylococcal infection is proved or suspected, cloxacillin or fusidic acid are added to the regimen. Alternatively, clindamycin may replace the B-lactam agent. On occasions it may be necessary to introduce vancomycin where the staphylococcus isolated is resistant to all conventional antistaphylococcal agents.

(4) Treatment should be continued until the patient has been afebrile for 72 hours, provided there are no areas of infected tissue (pulmonary consolidation and abscesses must have cleared, urine cultures should be negative, etc.). A longer course of treatment is indicated if neutropenia or thrombocytopenia persist, and when patients are on high doses of corticosteroids and anti-inflammatory drugs which might be suppressing the pyrexia. Short courses of therapy (3–5 days) may be adequate for uncomplicated lower urinary tract infections and certain vascular and catheter-associated infections, provided the offending line is removed.

Mycobacterial infections

The incidence of mycobacterial infections in our series is high, reflecting a high prevalence of tuberculosis in the general population. For this reason, isoniazid (INH) prophylaxis (300 mg daily) for 6 months is now used in all transplant recipients who are noted to have evidence of healed primary tuberculous foci on chest radiographs before transplantation. Where previous postprimary or reactivation tuberculosis has occurred, the patient should be covered with INH and ethambutol or triple drug therapy for at least 1 year after transplantation.

Both *Myco. tuberculosis* and mycobacteria other than tuberculosis (MOTT) infections may follow an indolent course and be difficult to eradicate in spite of effective tuberculocidal drugs (rifampicin and INH) as part of four-drug combination therapy. In our experience they have rarely been responsible for the death of any patient. One recently described patient, however, died as a result of localized mycobacterial vasculitis of coronary arteries in association with disseminated disease[45]. Prolonged and intensive therapy is required for these infections[46].

CLINICAL FEATURES AND MANAGEMENT OF THE COMMONER OPPORTUNISTIC INFECTIONS

Viral infections

Members of the Herpesviridae are the viruses most frequently associated with serious disease in transplant patients. These include cytomegalovirus, varicella zoster, herpes simplex, and Epstein–Barr viruses.

Cytomegalovirus (CMV)

In common with other members of this family, the virus is widespread, is acquired during childhood, and lies latent in white blood cells and in the urogenital and other systems. The virus may be introduced into a non-immune recipient with the donor heart or, rarely, by blood transfusion[47]. In a series of heart transplant patients reported by Rand *et al.*[47], there was a higher incidence of death from pulmonary infection (pneumonia and lung abscess) in patients who, prior to transplantation, had no CMV antibodies, than in those with measurable antibody levels; the infections were caused by organisms other than fungi. CMV transmitted by blood transfusion was considered to be the cause of the increased mortality in this group. Blood transfusion has also been identified as a source of reinfection of patients who previously had antibodies to CMV[48].

Although most CMV infections in normal subjects are subclinical, amongst heart transplant patients receiving immunosuppression, they are a major cause of morbidity and mortality[4,15,49,50]. Approximately 20% of heart transplant subjects who become infective develop symptoms, and a quarter of these die as a result of the infection[4,49]. Considerable progress has been made recently in the early diagnosis and treatment of this condition. Viremia is a marker of active infection, and CMV immediate early antigens (CMV-IEA) may be detected by a 3-hour indirect immunoperoxidase staining method in blood leukocytes[42].

Prophylaxis against primary CMV infection may take three forms: (1) prevention of antibody-positive donor organs being implanted in antibody-negative recipients; (2) avoidance of antibody-positive blood transfusions; and (3) regular postoperative treatment with CMV hyperimmune globulin injections for CMV-negative recipients who receive an organ from a seropositive donor. The latter has proved successful in both renal[16] and heart transplant recipients[51]. The protocols in these two studies differed, the renal patients receiving intravenous injections at weekly intervals for 4 months, whereas heart recipients received only five doses. Furthermore, since reinfection may occur in previously seropositive subjects, and in view of the high incidence of subclinical CMV infection in many countries[51], it might arguably be administered to all heart recipients.

Common clinical features of CMV infection (in order of

frequency) are fever, leukopenia, thrombocytopenia, the presence of atypical mononuclear cells in the blood, abnormal liver function tests, lower respiratory tract infection, hepatic and splenic enlargement, and, rarely, pericarditis, arthritis, polyneuritis, pancreatitis, and encephalitis. Recently, hemorrhagic colitis, gastric ulceration[49], CMV-related coronary arterial thrombosis[50], and lobar lung consolidation[52] have been reported in heart transplant recipients. Primary infections occur 5–7 weeks after transplantation, and reactivation after approximately 5–12 weeks[53].

Until recently, no effective treatment has been available. A recent preliminary report suggests that 9-(1, 3-dihydroxy-2-proproxymethyl) guanine (DHPG) might be effective in infected heart and heart–lung transplant recipients[49,54]. Trisodium phosphonoformate is a new virustatic agent that selectively inhibits herpes virus DNA polymerase, and appears to have been effective in isolated patients with CMV pneumonitis after bone marrow, kidney, or heart transplantation[55]. Confirmation is required in larger studies.

Varicella zoster (VZ)

VZ infection occurs in transplant patients ten times more frequently than in normal adults, though the majority of cases follow a relatively benign course[53].

Herpes simplex virus (HSV)

HSV infections in the form of 'cold sores' of lips and oropharyngeal mucosa are common during the first post-transplant month[53]. Rarely, they spread to involve the face, eye, and alimentary tract, causing a fatal gastroenterocolitis. Clinical manifestations usually represent reactivation rather than primary infection. HSV infections, unless present in classical form, require laboratory confirmation by at least one or more of the following methods: (1) identification of the virus by immunological or other means, (2) isolation of the agent, and (3) serology.

HSV and VZ may be identified by electron microscopy (EM) or immunofluorescence, but culture is necessary for confirmation of EM results. CMV can be identified in urine, sputum, or respiratory tract washings by EM and culture; immunofluorescence is unreliable. Evidence of HSV and CMV infection has been found in lung tissue from approximately 40% of heart transplant patients dying of unrelated causes[56]. Complement fixation tests, although used routinely for HSV, VZ and CMV, are not as rapid or useful as immunofluorescence, radioimmunoassay, or enzyme-linked immunosorbent assay. The latter identify specific IgM antibodies, which are essential for diagnosis in immunosuppressed patients, particularly where primary infections are suspected[53]. The indirect immunoperoxidase staining method for detection of immediate early antigens of CMV in blood leukocytes may replace or supplement these tests for early diagnosis of primary infection.

Most viral infections cannot be successfully treated. Interferon holds some promise, but is not yet freely available for clinical trial. Acyclovir, an acyclic analogue of a natural nucleoside, is the most effective drug currently available for treatment of herpes simplex infections. Used intravenously, it is useful both prophylactically and therapeutically against HSV[57], and to a lesser degree in a VZ infection. It is of doubtful efficacy against CMV, and prior to the introduction of DHPG and trisodium phosphonoformate, the most effective measure for life-threatening CMV infections was to reduce immunosuppression, a difficult proposition in heart transplant patients[53].

Fungal infections

In our patients, as in other series[58], fungal infections are not uncommon (14%)[3], and, when disseminated, are associated with a high mortality. Fungal infections may be due to reactivation of latent infection acquired from the environment prior to transplantation, or to new opportunistic infection acquired following transplantation. Blastomycosis and coccidioidomycosis, which arise by the former route, seldom cause infection, but aspergillus, cryptococcus, and candida species are common opportunists.

Aspergillosis

Species of the aspergillus fungus are associated with several categories of lung disease in non-compromised hosts (allergic bronchopulmonary aspergillosis and mycetomas), but do not generally invade unless impairment of immunocompetence occurs. Invasive aspergillosis usually manifests as pneumonia, less often as brain abscess and meningoencephalitis, and rarely as gastrointestinal or skin lesions. In the lungs, almost any type of infiltrate, ranging from a diffuse interstitial one to focal cavitatory lesions may be seen. The tendency of the organisms to invade blood vessels may cause clotting and pulmonary infarction, and dispose to hematogenous dissemination. Sputum is positive (usually on culture only) in about one-third of patients with invasive pneumonia. Although false-positive results are common, the more often the sputum is positive, the greater is the likelihood that the result is relevant[58].

Aspergillus is also the commonest cause of meningoencephalitis and focal brain abscess in transplant patients. This frequently occurs early following transplantation[36], and patients present with disorientation and confusion, and progress to coma. Some have hemiparesis, hemianopia, and dysphagia. CSF examination is generally unhelpful, showing a modest degree of pleocytosis and raised protein, but not organisms. The diagnosis may be made by direct needle aspiration of the intracranial lesion, but should be strongly suspected when aspergillus is isolated from coexistent lung lesions[36]. Computed tomography of the brain has shown minimal non-specific, low-density lesions, which do not exhibit contrast enhancement[37].

Amphotericin B is the only proven effective treatment for invasive aspergillosis, but is of little use if given late or for CNS involvement. Intravenous therapy is given as indicated in Table 17.9.

Cryptococcosis

C. neoformans is an encapsulated yeast which gains access to the body via the respiratory tract. Isolation of cryptococcus from sputum or other specimens from the lungs of an immunocompromised patient is an indication for a careful search for pulmonary and extrapulmonary lesions caused by this organism[59,60]. Investigations for extrapulmonary disease involve aspiration or biopsy of any suspicious skin or bone lesions, examination and culture of CSF, of at least three specimens of urine, of blood, and possibly bone marrow. The presence of extrapulmonary lesions carries a poor prognosis[59]. Where no pulmonary or extrapulmonary lesions are found, vigilance with repeated cultures of sputum may be sufficient, since saprophytic occurrence of C. neoformans in sputum is known to occur[59-61].

Treatment of transplanted patients should comprise a combination of amphotericin B and 5-flucytosine (Table 17.9), even if the infection appears to be confined to the lung, since resistant organisms may emerge if flucytosine is used alone[61,62].

Surgical resection of pulmonary lesions adds little to the success of treatment, except perhaps when lesions are large and persist after several weeks of therapy; by reducing the mass of organisms, resection may shorten the course of the infection and diminish the potential for recurrence[60,61].

Candidiasis

Candidal infections of mucous membranes of mouth, pharynx, and esophagus are common problems in patients who are debilitated, immunosuppressed, and on broad-spectrum antibiotics. For this reason, transplant patients are given nystatin lozenges and suspension as prophylaxis from the time of operation until immunosuppression is reduced to low levels (usually during the second month) (Table 17.9). Several cases of fatal candidal infection have been reported in heart transplant patients[11].

The diagnosis of disseminated candidiasis, particularly in immunocompromised patients, and the associated problems of when to commence systemic therapy present several difficulties[63]. As with aspergillosis, definitive confirmation of the diagnosis is made only by histopathological demonstration of organisms invading visceral tissues – lungs, brain, meninges, myocardium, kidneys, skin, bone and eye. Blood cultures are frequently negative even in the presence of visceral involvement, nor is candidemia certain proof of dissemination. Indwelling venous catheters are a frequent source of candidemia; removal of the catheters may be all that is necessary to correct this situation. Isolation of candida from urine usually reflects local urinary tract infection, and, as an isolated finding, is an indication for

Table 17.9 Recommended therapeutic schedules of antifungal agents

Mode (site) of administration	Schedule	Toxicity
Intravenous		
Amphotericin B	Test dose: 1 mg in 250 ml 5% dextrose over 2–4 hours. Initial dose 5 mg in 500 ml 5% dextrose over 4 hours. Increase by 5 mg up to 1 mg/kg per day. Then administer 1 mg/kg every other day (limit 60 mg/day) in 500–1000 ml 5% dextrose. If creatinine rises, reduce dose by 10–20 mg and/or increase interval between doses (to up to 3 days)	Chills, fever, hypotension bronchospasm, phlebitis, nausea, vomiting, hypokalemia, hypomagnesemia, renal impairment, anemia, hepatic toxicity
Miconazole	400–600 mg 6-hourly i.v.	Phlebitis, nausea, hepatic toxicity
Intraventricular (cerebral)		
Amphotericin B	First dose 0.05 mg. Then increase by 0.05–0.1 mg increments daily or twice daily up to 0.5 mg/day. Thereafter, 0.5 mg/day or alternate days.	Headache, meningismus, seizures
Oral		
Nystatin	400 000–10 million units 4 times/day, mouth wash and swallow. Lozenge (suppository) 4 times day	Mouth soreness, nausea
5-Flucytosine	150 mg/kg per day in four divided doses.	Thrombocytopenia, pancytopenia (more common with renal failure); hepatitis
Bladder		
Amphotericin B	50 mg in 1000 ml of 5% dextrose; irrigate once or twice/day	Local irritation
Topical (skin)		
Nystatin	Apply 2–4 times/day	Local irritation and rash
Miconazole	Apply 2–4 times/day	Local irritation and rash

local treatment alone.

The following features have been suggested as indicative of dissemination requiring systemic therapy: (1) identification of candida in three or more of the following sites – oral or urogenital mucosa, venous catheter tip, blood, urine, or lung (via needle aspiration or sheathed brush); (2) the presence of peripheral embolic lesions, e.g. macronodular skin lesions (which can be biopsied for a rapid diagnosis) or endopthalmitis; (3) identification of candida in CSF or aspirates from bones or joints; and (4) histological confirmation in biopsy specimens, e.g. lung, liver, or kidney.

Petriellidosis

Infection by unusual organisms like *Petriellidium boydii* is occasionally encountered in cardiac transplant patients. This organism was found at necropsy in one patient in our series, the findings suggesting primary infection of the lungs with hematogenous dissemination to the brain, kidneys, and skin[3,56]. Disseminated petriellidosis has previously been described in patients on corticosteroids[64].

Trichosporon beigelii (cutaneum)

Trichosporon beigelii (*cutaneum*) infecting an artificial heart (the Penn State Heart) in a patient who subsequently underwent orthotopic cardiac transplantation resulted in later fatal disseminated infections. Treatment with amphotericin B and rifampicin did not appear to be effective and the patient died 1 month after admission[65].

Nocardiosis

Nocardia species, bacteria with branched filamentous morphology, are often misclassified as fungi. *N. asteroides* accounts for at least 85% of pulmonary or disseminated nocardiosis[46]. The importance of diagnosis lies in the satisfactory response of the infection to therapy, even in immunocompromised hosts. In specimens obtained from lung, identification is achieved by recognition of morphology, and positive staining in Gram, Ziehl–Neelsen, and methenamine-silver stained preparations. The diagnosis is confirmed by culture of nocardial colonies, which serves to distinguish them from actinomyces, with which they share morphological similarities. To confirm the diagnosis, invasive procedures are usually necessary, because sputum is positive in less than 30% of cases[46].

In most cases, infection enters via the lungs, and since nocardia are not part of the normal human flora, a positive sputum culture is highly suggestive of active infection[46]. Although some cases are mild, the majority of patients with nocardiosis have symptomatic lung disease features. Nocardial lung lesions may be solitary nodules, localized pneumonitis, or single or multiple lung abscesses. About 25% of patients develop CNS involvement (usually a brain abscess), on occasions after the pulmonary lesion has healed.

The treatment of choice is sulphonamides (high dose sulphadiazine 2–3 g 6-hourly), though cotrimoxazole, minocycline, and combinations of ampicillin and erythromycin have also proved effective in subjects allergic to sulphonamides[46]. A combination of amikacin and sulphonamide has given good results in some patients. Treatment should be continued for at least 6–8 weeks.

Protozoal infections

Pneumocystis

Pneumonia caused by *Pneumocystis carinii* is characterized by prominent dyspnea (91% of patients), fever (66%), and cough (50%), associated with cyanosis (39%), basal or widespread pulmonary crackles (33%), and hepatomegaly (35%). The pneumonia is generally not associated with sputum production and prominent signs of consolidation[66]. Diffuse bilateral infiltrates are seen on chest radiograph in almost all cases. Early diagnosis is important because of the profound disturbance of gas exchange and respiratory failure which ensues. The chances of recovery are greatly increased if ventilatory support can be avoided[67].

Fiberoptic bronchoscopy with transbronchial biopsies and/or bronchoalveolar lavage is usually necessary to establish the diagnosis, and should be done without delay if this condition is suspected. An alternative, which has been increasingly used in the investigation of patients with the acquired immunodeficiency syndrome (AIDS), is nebulized hypertonic saline, which induces a cough. In a significant percentage, the sputum induced contains pneumocystis organisms demonstrable by methenamine stain[68]. Bronchoalveolar lavage fluid needs to be pelleted by centrifugation, and the cell pellet stained for organisms. A relatively small volume of fluid (20 ml) may be sufficient to make this diagnosis, and larger volumes are usually not necessary[68].

Drug therapy consists of a combination of sulphamethoxazole (100 mg/kg per day) and trimethoprim (20 mg/kg per day)[67]. In most cases, a clinical response is observed within 4 days. Since approximately one-third of patients fail to respond to this therapy, progressive deterioration after 4 days is an indication for substituting pentamidine for the initial regimen[67]. Since pneumocystis infection is confined to the lung, and does not invade systemically, local treatment is a theoretical possibility. Recently, pentamidine delivered in the form of liposomes as an aerosol, has been shown to concentrate more than 30-fold in bronchial secretions (compared with systemic administration)[69]. This form of treatment is not yet in common use.

Prophylaxis with low-dose combined therapy (sulphamethoxazole 20 mg/kg per day and trimethoprim 5 mg/kg per day) given orally in two divided doses has been advocated, and has been proved effective in several categories of immunosuppressed patients[70]. This has not been given routinely in our patients as the incidence of infection with pneumocystis is low, and treatment is effective. Since pneumocystis infections frequently recur, however, prophylaxis is advisable for immunosuppressed patients who have previously been treated for pneumocystis infection[70].

Toxoplasmosis

The most serious consequences of infection with *Toxoplasma gondii* are encephalitis, pneumonitis, myocarditis, and chorioretinitis. The encephalitis is diffuse, but may occasionally be asymptomatic. Toxoplasma cysts and microglial nodules form, and abscess formation has also been described[37].

The most common route of infection is via the donor heart, when a seronegative patient receives a heart from a seropositive donor[6,71]. A primary infection follows, usually clinically evident within the first 6 weeks after transplantation[17]. Clinical signs of infection may follow reactivation in a previously infected host placed on immunosuppression[18]. The infection is usually fatal if prompt diagnosis and treatment are not achieved. Sero-conversion commonly precedes the appearance of symptoms, and may be detected by the latex agglutination test (as a screening test) and confirmed by dye, hemagglutination, and IgM tests, or by the protein blot method[72].

Several considerations are relevant to the use of these tests for early diagnosis of *Toxoplasma gondii* infection. Low titers of *T. gondii* antibodies may be acquired from blood transfusions at the time of surgery, but are usually at low titer, and disappear by 1 month. A four-fold or greater rise in the latex agglutination antibody titer is considered a positive result. This test frequently gives a false positive result during CMV infection (both primary and reactivation) due to the presence in sera of a non-CMV-specific IgM antibody. Seroconversion therefore needs to be confirmed by the dye or other serologic test[17].

In later stages of disease, aspirates from lesions (stained with Wright–Giemsa and hematoxylin and eosin stains) may show toxoplasma cysts and trophozoites, both extracellularly and inside inflammatory cells. Endomyocardial biopsies may also yield a positive result[17,71].

Sulphadiazine, pyrimethamine, and spiramycin treatment is successful in some patients. Prophylaxis with pyrimethamine administered as a single daily dose of 25 mg for 6 weeks postoperatively[18], or combined with sulfasoxazole 1 g intravenously 6-hourly for 1 month[7], appears to be effective prophylaxis for seronegative recipients who receive hearts from seropositive donors.

FUTURE DEVELOPMENTS IN THE CONTROL OF INFECTION IN THE IMMUNOCOMPROMISED PATIENT

Over the past 5 years significant progress has been made in the prevention and control of infections in the transplant patient. The single most important advance has been the introduction of cyclosporine in place of azathioprine, with an associated reduction in episodes of rejection with their attendant requirement for booster doses of corticosteroids. This progress illustrates the fact that the development of highly specific immunosuppression, that leaves the patient's antimicrobial defenses intact, is more important than other forms of microbial surveillance and treatment.

During the same period it has been shown that strict barrier nursing has little impact on the frequency of infections, providing that other nursing and medical practices for minimizing infection are strictly applied. Recently, renewed interest has been expressed in bowel sterilization as a means of reducing infections from endogenous sources. It is questionable whether this should be applied to patients undergoing heart transplantation.

Important progress has been made in the therapeutics of pneumocystis, toxoplasmosis, and CMV infections. Attention needs to be directed towards finding more effective antifungal measures for infections like aspergillosis. Initial promise that specific immunotherapy may be applied in these patients has not progressed to a point of clinical usefulness[73,74].

Infection no longer poses the same ominous threat to the heart transplant recipient that it did 5 years ago, and there are prospects that this source of morbidity and mortality will be reduced further during the next decades.

References

1. Baumgartner, W.A., Reitz, B.A., Oyer, P.E., Stinson, E.B. and Shumway, N.E. (1979). Cardiac homotransplantation. *Curr. Probl. Surg.*, **16**, 1
2. Barnard, C.N., Barnard, M.S., Cooper, D.K.C., Curchio, C.A., Hassoulas, J., Novitzky, D. and Wolpowitz, A. (1981). The present status of heterotopic cardiac transplantation. *J. Thorac. Cardiovasc. Surg.*, **81**, 433
3. Cooper, D.K.C., Lanza, R.P., Oliver, S.P., Forder, A.A., Rose, A.G., Uys, C.J., Novitzky, D. and Barnard, C.N. (1983). Infectious complications following heterotopic heart transplantation. *Thorax*, **38**, 822
4. Hofflin, J.M., Potasman, I., Baldwin, J.C., Oyer, P.E., Stinson, E.B. and Remington, J.S. (1987). Infectious complications in heart transplant recipients receiving cyclosporine and corticosteroids. *Ann. Intern. Med.*, **106**, 209
5. Renlund, D.G., Gilbert, E.M., O'Connell, J.B., Gay, W.A., Jones, K.W., Burton, N.A., Doty, D.B., Karawnde, S.V., DeWitt, C.W., Menlove, R.L., Herrick, C.M. and Bristow, M.R. (1987). Age-associated decline in cardiac allograft rejection. *Am. J. Med.*, **83**, 391
6. Baumgartner, W.A., Augustine, S., Borkon, M., Gardner, T.J. and Reitz, B.A. (1987). Present expectations in cardiac transplantation. *Ann. Thorac. Surg.*, **43**, 585
7. Gentry, L.O. and Zeluff, B.J. (1986). Diagnosis and treatment of infection in cardiac transplant patients. *Surg. Clin. North Am.*, **66**, 459
8. Emery, R.W., Cork, R., Christensen, R., Levinson, M.M., Icenogle, T.B., Riley, J., Ott, R.A. and Copeland, J.G. (1986). Cardiac transplant

patients at one year. Cyclosporine vs. conventional immunosuppression. *Chest*, **90**, 29
9. Schulman, L., Smith, C., Drusin, R., Rose, E., Enson, Y. and Reemtsma, K. (1986). Respiratory complications of heart transplantation. *J. Heart Transplant.*, **5**, 387
10. Rubin, R.H., Wolfson, J.S. and Cosimi, A.G. (1981). Infection in the renal transplant recipient. In Dixon, R.E. (ed.) *Nosocomial Infections*. p. 121. (New York: Yorke Medical Books)
11. Jamieson, S.W., Stinson, E.B. and Shumway, N.E. (1982). Cardiac transplantation. In Morris, P.J. (ed.) *Tissue Transplantation*. p. 147. (Edinburgh: Churchill Livingstone)
12. Baumgartner, W.A. (1983). Infection in cardiac transplantation. *Heart Transplant.*, **3**, 75
13. Fabre, J.W. (1982). Specific immunosuppression. In Morris, P.J. (ed.) *Tissue Transplantation*. p. 80. (Edinburgh: Churchill Livingstone)
14. Cooper, D.K.C., Lanza, R.P. and Barnard, C.N. (1984). Non-compliance in heart transplant recipients: the Cape Town experience. *Heart Transplant.* **3**, 248
15. Parker, M.T. (1978). Microbiological facilities for the surveillance and control of the spread of infection in hospitals. In Daschner, F. (ed.) *Proven and Unproven Methods in Hospital Infection Control*. p. 35. (Stuttgart: Fischer)
16. Snydman, D.R., Werner, B.G., Heinze-Lacey, B., Berardi, V.P., Tilney, N.L., Kirkman, R.L., Milford, E.L., Cho, S.I., Bush, H.L., Levey, A.S., Strom, T.B., Carpenter, C.B., Levey, R.H., Harmon, W.E., Zimmerman, C.E., Shapiro, M.E., Steinman, T., Logerfo, F., Idelson, B., Shroter, P.J., Levin, M.J., McIver, J., Leszczynski, J. and Grady, G.F. (1987). Use of cytomegalovirus immune globulin to prevent cytomegalovirus disease in renal-transplant recipients. *N. Engl. J. Med.*, **317**, 1049
17. Wreghitt, T.G., Gray, J.J. and Balfour, A.H. (1986). Problems with serological diagnosis of *Toxoplasma gondii* infections in heart transplant recipients. *J. Clin. Pathol.*, **39**, 1135
18. Hakim, M., Esmore, D., Wallwork, J., English, T.A.H. and Wreghitt, T. (1986). Toxoplasmosis in cardiac transplantation. *Br. Med. J.*, **202**, 1108
19. Minoli, L., Grossi, P., Marone, P., Maserati, R., Malfitano, A., Martinelli, L. and Sessa, F. (1986). Are HBsAg carriers suitable for heart transplantation? *J. Heart Transplant.*, **5**, 364
20. Applefeld, M.M., Newman, K.A., Sutton, F.J., Reed, W.P., Roffman, D.S., Talesnick, B.S. and Grove, W.R. (1987). Outpatient dobutamine and dopamine infusions in the management of chronic heart failure: clinical experience in 21 patients. *Am. Heart J.*, **114**, 589
21. Frist, W.H., Oyer, P.E., Baldwin, J.C., Stinson, E.B. and Shumway, N.E. (1987). HLA compatibility and cardiac transplant recipient survival. *Ann. Thorac. Surg.*, **44**, 242
22. Hess, N. (1986). Update on infection rates with only protective isolation. *J. Heart Transplant.*, **5**, 393
23. McKenzie, F.N., Menkis, A.H., Tadros, N., Stiller, C.R., Keown, P.A. and Kostuk, W.F. (1986). The limited role of protective isolation after heart transplantation. *J. Heart Transplant.*, **5**, 381
24. Gamberg, P., Miller, J. and Lough, M.E. (1986). Impact of protective isolation on the incidence of infection after heart transplantation. *J. Heart Transplant.*, **5**, 378
25. Preston, G.A., Larson, E.L. and Stamm, W.E. (1981). The effect of private isolation rooms on patient care practices, colonization and infection in an intensive care unit. In Dixon, R.E. (ed.) *Nosocomial Infections*. p. 285. (Atlanta: Yorke Medical Books)
26. Armstrong, D. (1981). The diagnostic microbiology laboratory in the care of the immunosuppressed patient. In Lorian, V. (ed.) *Significance of Medical Microbiology in Care of Patients*. p. 73. (Baltimore: Williams & Wilkins)
27. Bartlett, J.G. (1982). Making optimum use of the microbiology laboratory. *J. Am. Med. Assoc.*, **247**, 857 (Part 1), 1336 (Part 2), 1868 (Part 3)
28. Matthay, R.A. and Moritz, E.D. (1981). Invasive procedures for diagnosing pulmonary infection. A critical review. *Clin. Chest Med.*, **2**, 3
29. Bartlett, J.G. (1977). Diagnostic accuracy of transtracheal aspiration: bacteriologic studies. *Am. Rev. Respir. Dis.*, **115**, 777
30. Zavala, D.C. and Schoell, J.E. (1981). Ultra-thin needle aspiration of the lung in infectious and malignant disease. *Am. Rev. Respir. Dis.*, **123**, 125
31. Wimberley, N., Faling, L.J. and Bartlett, J.G. (1979). A fiberoptic bronchoscopy technique to obtain uncontaminated lower airway secretions for bacterial culture. *Am. Rev. Respir. Dis.*, **119**, 337
32. Willcox, P.A., Benatar, S.R., Potgieter, P.D., Ferguson, A.D. and Bateman, E.D. (1981). Fiberoptic bronchoscopy: experience at Groote Schuur Hospital. *S. Afr. Med. J.*, **60**, 651
33. Beyt, B.E., King, D.K. and Glew, R.H. (1977). Fatal pneumonitis and septicaemia after fiberoptic bronchoscopy. *Chest*, **72**, 105
34. Robbins, H. and Goldman, A.L. (1977). Failure of a 'prophylactic' antimicrobial drug to prevent sepsis after fiberoptic bronchoscopy. *Am. Rev. Respir. Dis.*, **116**, 325
35. Willcox, P.A., Bateman, E.D., Potgieter, P.D. and Benatar, S.R. (1987). Is fiberoptic bronchoscopy of value in the diagnosis of pulmonary shadows in renal transplant recipients? *Am. Rev. Respir. Dis.*, **135A**, 411
36. Meyers, J.D. and Thomas, E.D. (1981). Infection complicating bone marrow transplantation. In Rubin, R.H. and Young, L.S. (eds.) *Clinical Approach to Infection in the Compromised Host*. p. 507. (New York: Plenum)
37. Britt, R.H., Enzmann, D.R. and Remington, J.S. (1981). Intracranial infection in cardiac transplant recipients. *Ann. Neurol.*, **9**, 107
38. Young, L.S. (1981). Fever and septicaemia. In Rubin, R.H. and Young, L.S. (eds.) *Clinical Approach to Infection in the Compromised Host*. p. 75. (New York: Plenum)
39. Penn, R.L., Lambert, R.S. and George, R.B. (1983). Invasive fungal infections. The use of serologic tests in diagnosis and management. *Arch. Intern. Med.*, **143**, 1215
40. Rubin, R.H. and Greene, R. (1981). Etiology and management of the compromised patient with fever and pulmonary infiltrates. In Rubin, R.H. and Young, L.S. (eds.) *Clinical Approach to Infection in the Compromised Host*. p. 123. (New York: Plenum)
41. Fisher, B.D. and Armstrong, D. (1977). Cryptococcal interstitial pneumonia: value of antigen determination. *N. Engl. J. Med.*, **297**, 1440
42. Van der Bij, W., Van Dijk, R.B., Prenger, K.B., Prop, J., Torensma, R. and The, T.H. (1986). Antigen test for early diagnosis of active cytomegalovirus infection in heart transplant recipients. *J. Heart Transplant.*, **5**, 364
43. Rubin, R.H. (1981). Infection in the renal transplant patient. In Rubin, R.H. and Young, L.S. (eds.) *Clinical Approach to Infection in the Compromised Host*. p. 553. (New York: Plenum)
44. Smith, C.R., Lipsky, J.J., Laskin, O.L., Hellman, D.B., Mellits, E.D., Longstreth, S. and Lietman, P.S. (1980). Double-blind comparison of the nephrotoxicity of gentamicin and tobramycin. *N. Engl. J. Med.*, **302**, 1106
45. Tuder, R.M., Renya, G.S. and Bensch, K. (1986). Mycobacterial coronary arteritis in a heart transplant recipient. *Hum. Pathol.*, **17**, 1072
46. Simon, H.B. (1981). Mycobacterial and nocardial infections in the compromised host. In Rubin, R.H. and Young, L.S. (eds.) *Clinical Approach to Infection in the Compromised Host*. p. 229. (New York: Plenum)
47. Rand, K.H., Pollard, R.B. and Merigan, T.C. (1978). Increased pulmonary superinfections in cardiac transplant patients undergoing primary cytomegalovirus infection. *N. Engl. J. Med.*, **298**, 951
48. Chou, S. (1987). Cytomegalovirus infection and reinfection transmitted by heart transplantation. *J. Infect. Dis.*, **155**, 1054
49. Icenogle, T.B., Peterson, E., Ray, G., Minnich, L. and Copeland, J.G. (1987). DHPG effectively treats CMV infection in heart and heart–lung transplant patients: a preliminary report. *J. Heart Transplant.*, **6**, 199
50. Min, K.W., Wickemeyer, W.J., Chandran, P., Shadur, C., Gervich, D., Phillips, S.J., Zeff, R.H. and Song, J. (1986). Fatal cytomegalovirus infection and coronary arterial thromboses after heart transplantation: a case report. *J. Heart Transplant.*, **5**, 375
51. Havel, M., Laczkovics, A., Laufer, G., Spiss, C., Muller, M.M. and Wolner, E. (1986). Cytomegalovirus hyperimmunoglobulin prophylaxis after heart transplantation. *J. Heart Transplant.*, **5**, 398
52. Schulman, L.L. (1987). Cytomegalovirus pneumonitis and lobar consolidation. *Chest*, **91**, 558
53. Tobin, J.O.H. (1983). Virus infections in the immunocompromised. In Waterson, A.P. (ed.) *Recent Advance in Clinical Virology, No. 3*. p. 1.

(Edinburgh: Churchill Livingstone)
54. Watson, F.S., O'Connell, J.B., Amber, I.J., Renlund, D.G. and Bristow, M.R. (1986). Treatment of cytomegalovirus pneumonia in heart transplant recipients with DHPG. *J. Heart Transplant.*, **5**, 390
55. Locke, T.J., Odom, N.J., Tapson, J.S., Freeman, R. and McGregor, C.G.A. (1987). Successful treatment with trisodium phosphonoformate for primary cytomegalovirus infection after heart transplantation. *J. Heart Transplant.*, **6**, 120
56. Uys, C.J., Rose, A.G. and Barnard, C.N. (1979). The pathology of human cardiac transplantation. *S. Afr. Med. J.*, **56**, 887
57. Alford, C.A. (1982). Acyclovir treatment of herpes virus infections in immunocompromised humans. *Am. J. Med.*, **73** (Suppl.), 225
58. Armstrong, D. (1981). Fungal infections in the compromised host. In Rubin, R.H. and Young, L.S. (eds.) *Clinical Approach to Infection in the Compromised Host.* p. 195. (New York: Plenum)
59. Kerkering, T.M., Duma, R.J. and Shadomy, S. (1981). The evolution of pulmonary cryptococcosis. Clinical implications from a study of 41 patients with and without compromising host factors. *Ann. Intern. Med.*, **94**, 611
60. Butler, W.T., Alling, D.W., Spickard, A., and Utz, J.P. (1964). Diagnostic and prognostic value of clinical and laboratory findings in cryptococcal meningitis. A follow-up study of 40 patients. *N. Engl. J. Med.*, **59**, 270
61. Hammerman, K.J., Powell, K.E., Christianson, C.S., Huggin, P.M., Larsh, H.W., Vivas, J.R. and Tosh, F.E. (1973). Pulmonary cryptococcosis: clinical forms and treatment. A center for disease control cooperative mycoses study. *Am. Rev. Respir. Dis.*, **108**, 1116
62. Medoff, G. and Kobayashi, G.S. (1980). Strategies in the treatment of systemic fungal infections. *N. Engl. J. Med.*, **302**, 45
63. Edwards, J.E., Lehrer, R.I., Stiehm, E.R., Fischer, T.J. and Young, L.S. (1978). Severe candidal infections. Clinical perspective, immune defense mechanisms, and current concepts of therapy. *Ann. Intern. Med.*, **89**, 91
64. Walker, D.H., Adamec, T. and Krigman, M. (1978). Disseminated petriellidosis (Allescheriosis). *Arch. Pathol. Lab. Med.*, **102**, 158
65. Murray-Leisure, K.A., Aber, R.C., Rowley, L.J., Applebaum, P.C., Wisman, C.B., Pennock, J.L. and Pierce, W.S. (1986). Disseminated *Trichosporon beigelii* (cutaneum) infection in an artificial heart recipient. *J. Am. Med. Assoc.*, **256**, 2995
66. Walzer, P.D., Perl, D.P., Krogstad, D.J., Rawson, P.G. and Schultz, M.G. (1974). *Pneumocystis carinii* pneumonia in the United States: epidemiologic, diagnostic and clinical features. *Ann. Intern. Med.*, **80**, 83
67. Winston, D.J., Lau, W.K., Gale, R.P. and Young, L.S. (1980). Trimethoprimsulphamethoxazole for the treatment of *Pneumocystis carinii* pneumonia. *Ann. Intern. Med.*, **92**, 762
68. Luce, J.M. (1986). Sputum induction in the acquired immunodeficiency syndrome. *Am. Rev. Respir. Dis.*, **133**, 513
69. Debs, R.J., Straubinger, R.M., Brunette, E.N., Lin, J.M., Lin, E.J., Montgomery, A.B., Friend, D.S. and Papahadjopoulos, D.P. (1987). Selective enhancement of pentamidine uptake in the lung by aerosolization and delivery in liposomes. *Am. Rev. Respir. Dis.*, **135**, 731
70. Hughes, W.T., Kuhn, S., Chaudhary, S., Feldman, S., Verzosa, M., Aur, R.J.A., Pratt, C. and George, S.L. (1977). Successful chemoprophylaxis for *Pneumocystis carinii* pneumonitis. *N. Engl. J. Med.*, **297**, 1419
71. Rose, A.G., Uys, C.J., Novitzky, D., Cooper, D.K.C. and Barnard, C.N. (1983). Toxoplasmosis of donor and recipient heart after heterotopic cardiac transplantation. *Arch. Pathol. Lab. Med.*, **197**, 368
72. Potasman, I., Araujo, F.G., Desmonts, G. and Remington, J.S. (1986). Analysis of *Toxoplasma gondii* antigens recognized by human sera obtained before and after acute infection. *J. Infect. Dis.*, **154**, 650
73. Jones, R.J. (1981). Vaccines and antisera against Gram-negative bacilli. *J. Hosp. Infect.*, **2**, 105
74. Gaffin, S.L. (1982). Control of septic shock – present day concept. *S. Afr. J. Hosp. Med.*, **8**, 4

18
Pathology of Graft Atherosclerosis (Chronic Rejection)

A.G. ROSE AND C.J. UYS

INTRODUCTION

In the two decades since the first human heart transplant was performed by Barnard in 1967[1], this operation has become a well-established therapy for treating irremediable cardiac failure. Survival rates have progressively improved[2,3] (Chapter 31). In patients who die in the first few months after cardiac transplantation when immunosuppression is maximal, infection is a major cause of death[4,5] (Chapter 17). Rejection is also an important factor which, if not primarily responsible for the patient's death, contributes significantly to it, even when overwhelming infection is present[6,7]. The pattern of acute cardiac rejection, and the role of endomyocardial biopsy in its diagnosis, have been outlined in Chapter 15.

While the changes which characterize acute rejection may persist beyond the first few weeks post-transplantation, and indeed may occur in patients who die years after transplantation[7], they are progressively replaced by a chronic rejection response that is dominated by an obliterative lesion of the large coronary arteries. In 1968, Lower and his colleagues were the first to draw attention to the proliferative and obliterative intimal changes of chronic vascular rejection in the epicardial coronary arteries of long-surviving canine transplants[8]. The first description of a human heart with these obliterative vascular changes of chronic rejection was in 1969, when Thomson described the donor heart of a patient who had survived almost 20 months after transplantation[9]. Since then, with longer survival times, this lesion has been recorded with increasing frequency[6,7,10–17].

MACROSCOPIC APPEARANCES

The donor heart with chronic rejection shows a variable spectrum of macroscopic appearances (Figures 18.1 and 18.2). The anastomotic sites usually show signs of complete

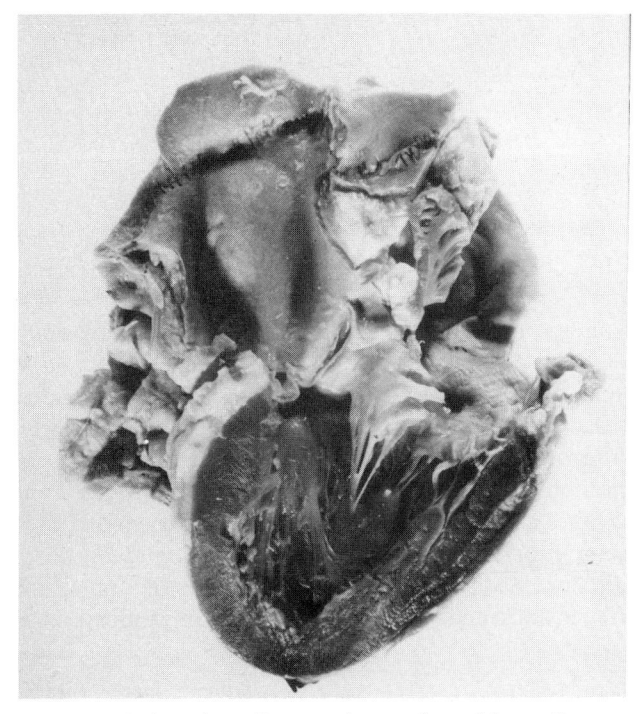

Figure 18.1 Orthotopic cardiac transplant, performed for cardiomyopathy, with postoperative survival 1.7 years, the patient dying of diffuse carcinomatosis. The coronary arteries showed no evidence of chronic rejection

healing. The sutures are often buried in connective tissue with smooth endocardial surfaces overlying the anastomoses; in none of our patients have these been the site of thrombus formation. Depending on the degree of chronic rejection, the ventricular myocardium in some appears near normal, while in others a varying extent of scarring, similar to healed infarction, is noted. In yet others there is evidence of superimposed acute infarction; this is particularly prominent in heterotopic transplants which have ceased to function for some time before the patient's death or before surgical extirpation of the heart.

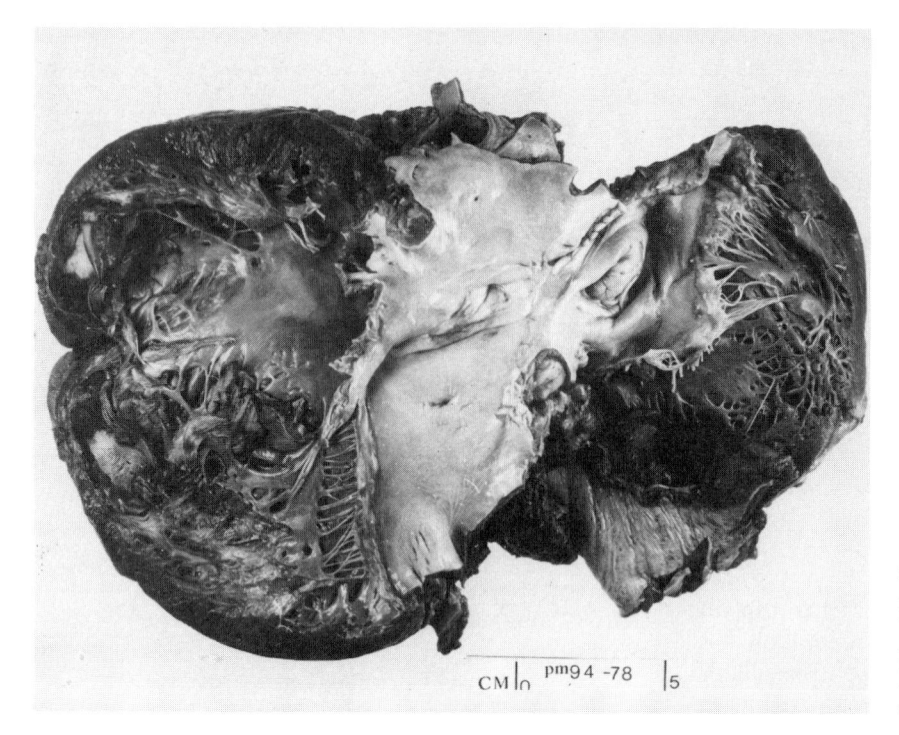

Figure 18.2 Heterotopic cardiac transplant, performed for chronic rheumatic valvular disease, with postoperative survival 0.64 years. Both hearts have been opened on the left side. The recipient ventricle is on the left and the donor ventricle on the right. Both contain antemortem mural thrombus. The donor heart showed acute-on-chronic rejection

In addition, in many such hearts, the coronary arteries appear strikingly abnormal. The epicardial branches of the main coronary arteries are thickened, have yellow-orange color due to lipid deposition in the vessel walls, and, on transverse section, show a marked reduction in lumenal cross-sectional area, sometimes with accompanying thrombotic occlusion. In heterotopic transplants with chronic rejection examined at autopsy, mural stasis thrombus often occupies a large portion of both ventricular cavities of the donor heart. The epicardial surface is bound by fibrous adhesions to adjacent structures, while the pulmonary arteries, aorta and valves are macroscopically unremarkable.

MICROSCOPIC APPEARANCES

Some microscopic changes of chronic rejection are usually detectable by 1 month postoperatively; in one of our cases the intimal thickening of early chronic vascular rejection was observed as early as 20 days after transplantation. It should be borne in mind that a donor heart, even from a young person, may occasionally exhibit significant focal coronary atherosclerosis before transplantation.

A gradual progression of the changes characterizing acute rejection to those of chronic rejection may be observed in the donor heart, depending upon the survival time of the recipient and whether death was primarily due to infection, late acute rejection, or chronic rejection. Even in patients who survive periods from 1 to 12 years, a proportion of the hearts at autopsy show evidence of coexistent acute rejection. These changes, similar to those already described (Chapter 15), take the form of infiltrates of lymphoid cells in the interstitium and subendocardial connective tissue (Figures 18.3 and 18.4). Many of these cells acquire abundant RNA-rich pyroninophilic cytoplasm. Features of myocyte damage, such as swelling and myocytolysis, are occasionally seen. Acute vascular rejection, presenting as fibrinoid necrosis of the media of large and medium-sized coronary artery radicles, associated with an infiltrate of lymphoid cells, infrequently co-exists (Figure 18.5). Where the signs of acute

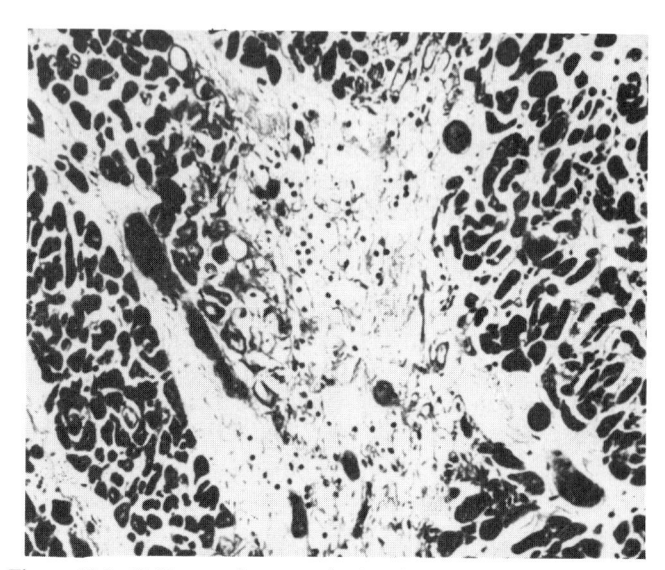

Figure 18.3 Evidence of acute rejection in a heart showing chronic rejection. Focal myocytolysis, interstitial edema, and a mild interstitial lymphocytic infiltrate are noted. Patient survived 2.7 years. Donor age 15 years (H & E x 150)

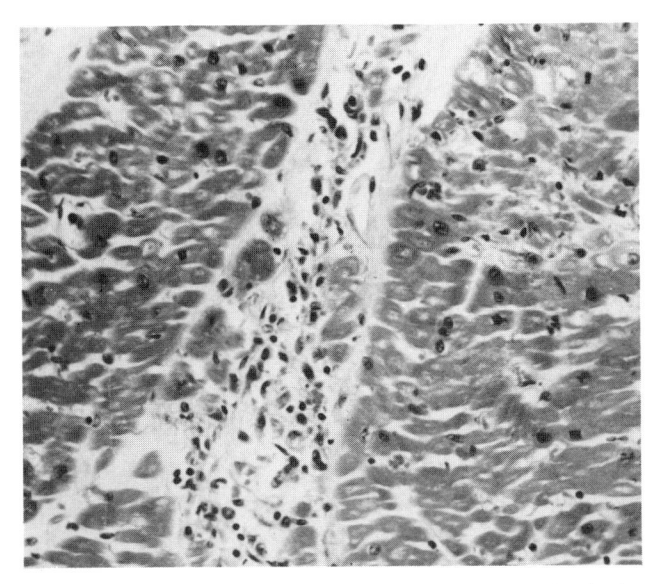

Figure 18.4 Persisting acute rejection in a patient with chronic rejection. Focal interstitial infiltration of lymphoid cells, some of which have acquired pyroninophilic cytoplasm. Patient survival 1.6 years. Donor age 25 years (H & E x 180)

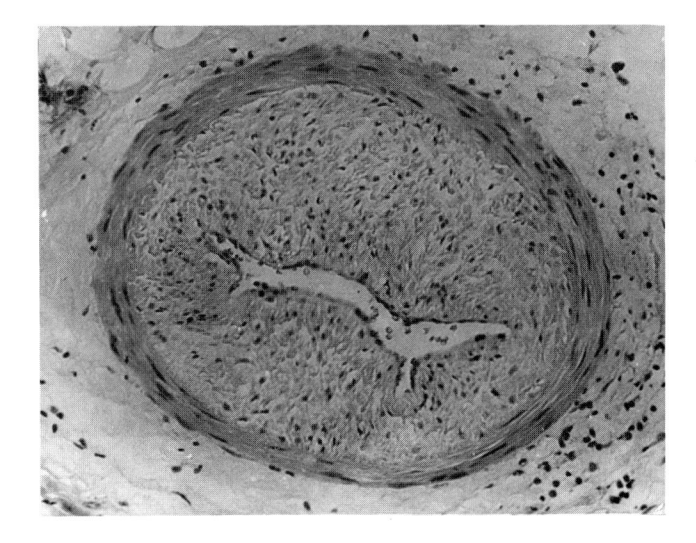

Figure 18.6 Chronic vascular rejection. Proliferation of intimal myofibroblasts has reduced the lumen of this small penetrating branch of the coronary artery to a mere slit. This is unassociated with lipid deposition, and no lymphocytes are present. Graft survival 1.6 years. Donor age 25 years (H & E x 150)

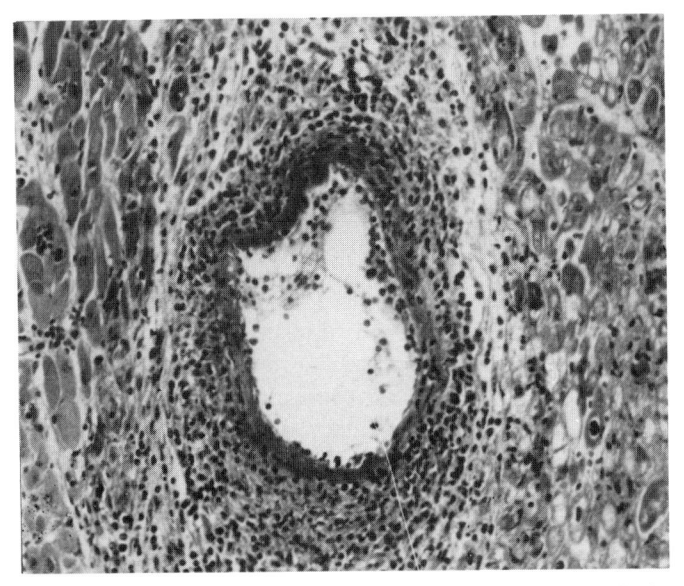

Figure 18.5 Persisting acute rejection. Fibrinoid necrosis of the wall of a small coronary artery radicle accompanied by an intense infiltration of lymphoid cells in the vessel wall and perivascular connective tissue. Graft survival 80 days (H & E x 150)

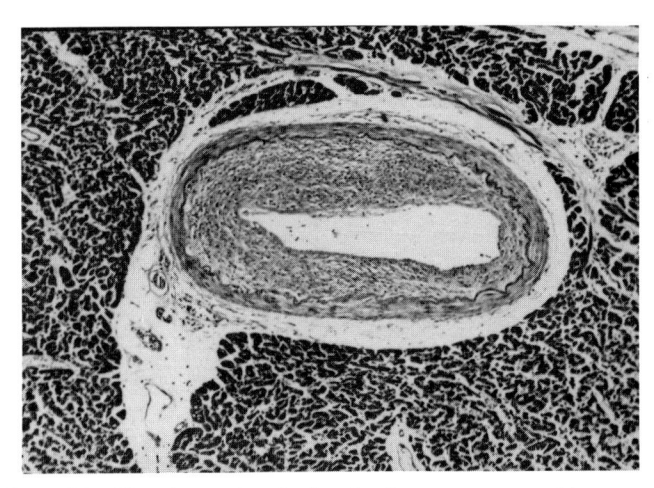

Figure 18.7 Chronic vascular rejection. Small coronary artery with severe intimal thickening due to myointimal cellular proliferation. Some fibrous replacement of media. Moderate lumen encroachment. Patient survival 12.5 years. Donor age 33 years (H & E x 60)

rejection are usually observed, they accompany those of chronic rejection, the latter being mostly of a severe degree.

The most striking and significant component of chronic rejection is the process of chronic vascular rejection which, due to continued proliferation of myointimal cells, leads to progressive obliteration of the lumena of the epicardial branches of the main coronary arteries and their penetrating branches (Figures 18.6 and 18.7). It should be noted that the latter (penetrating) arteries are usually unaffected by ordinary atherosclerosis. Lipid deposits are virtually never seen in the thickened intimas of these vessels in chronic rejection. Since the arterial changes in chronic rejection appear to be mainly those of accelerated atherosclerosis, understanding of the pathogenesis of atherosclerosis may be enhanced if the reason for this differential involvement of the penetrating branches of the epicardial coronary arteries could be elucidated.

Initially, the lipid deposits are observed in myofibroblasts and macrophages. With progressive accumulation, these cells disintegrate and release free-lying lipid. There is a variable lymphoid cellular infiltration of the walls of the affected vessels. The internal elastic lamina may be fragmented, and large gaps may result from healed arteritis. These lesions of chronic rejection in the large coronary artery branches, particularly when associated with abundant lipid deposition in the thickened intima, bear a close resemblance to advanced atherosclerosis (Figures 18.8–18.10). The smaller coronary artery branches more often show reparative fibrosis of previous medial necrosis, giving the lesion the appearance of a healed arteritis. These changes, in the more severely affected large arteries, predispose to superadded thrombosis, which appears as fresh thrombus in a few cases (Figure 18.11), but in the majority as old occlusive thrombus, which has undergone fibrous replacement and recanalization (Figure 18.12). Veins are very seldom affected by this process.

In addition to the vascular changes, scanty interstitial and subendocardial lymphoid infiltrates still persist. However, the lymphoid cells acquire more cytoplasm and have the appearance of activated lymphocytes. Plasma cells become progressively more numerous. Frequent scars are noted in the myocardium. In some, the remnants of degenerate myocytes occurring in collapsed stroma in the presence of a lymphoid infiltrate suggest previous foci of myocytolysis (Figures 18.13 and 18.14). In others, the appearance of large acellular scars are indicative of fibrous replacement of ischemic infarcts (Figure 18.15). Extensive acute infarcts are observed in heterotopic transplants with thrombotic occlusion of severely narrowed coronary arteries.

The obliterative vascular changes may lead to extensive loss of ventricular myocardium, and the resultant massive

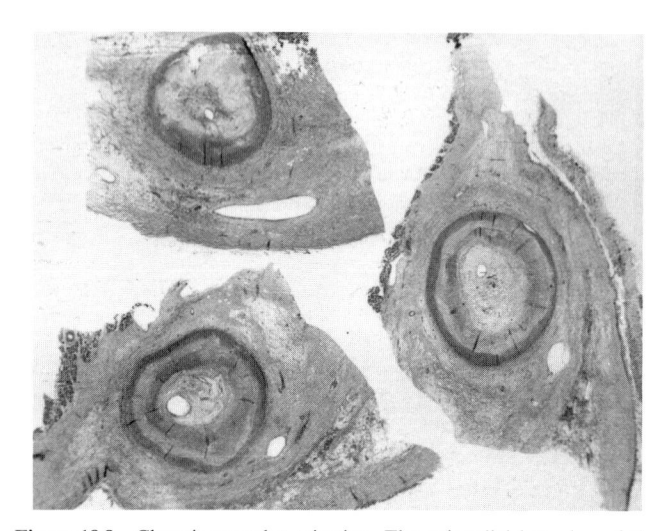

Figure 18.8 Chronic vascular rejection. The epicardial branches of the main coronary arteries are virtually obliterated by markedly thickened intima in which there is lipid deposition. Patient survival 12.5 years. Donor age 33 years (H & E x 4)

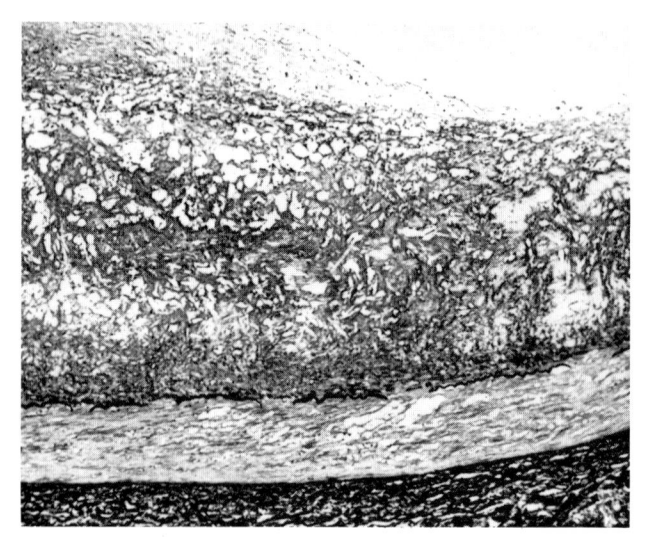

Figure 18.9 Chronic vascular rejection. A large coronary artery radicle shows intimal thickening with pronounced lipid deposition. There is a loss of smooth muscle from the media, and the internal elastic lamina is fragmented. Survival time 2.2 years. Donor age 30 years (H & E x 50)

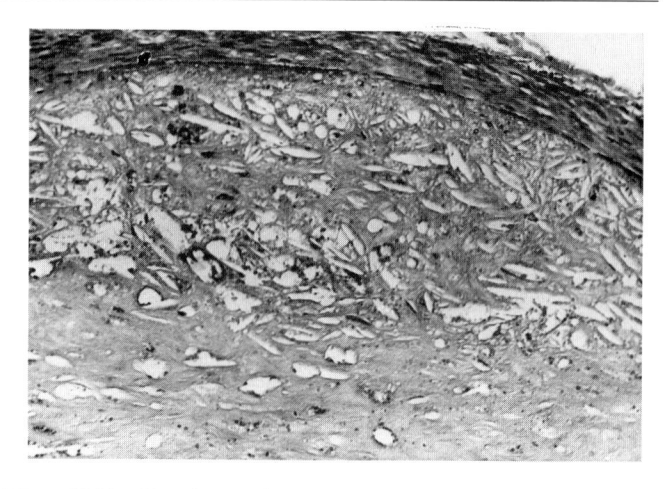

Figure 18.10 Chronic vascular rejection. Atherosclerotic-like appearance of advanced rejection. Patient survival 4.2 years (H & E x 110)

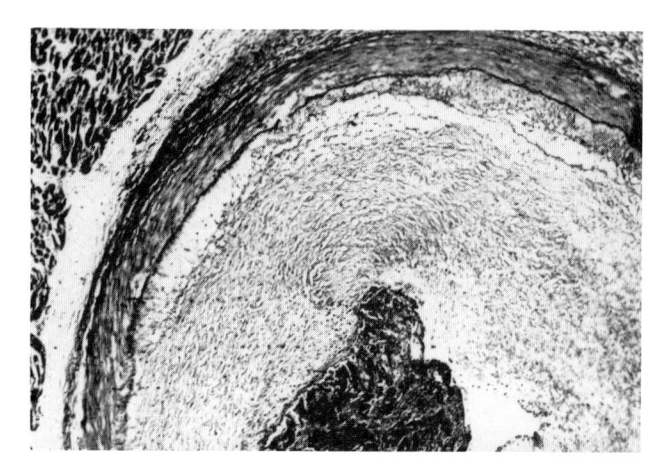

Figure 18.11 Advanced chronic vascular rejection. Pronounced lumen encroachment with superadded recent occlusive thrombus. Patient survival 2.7 years. Donor age 15 years (H & E x 40)

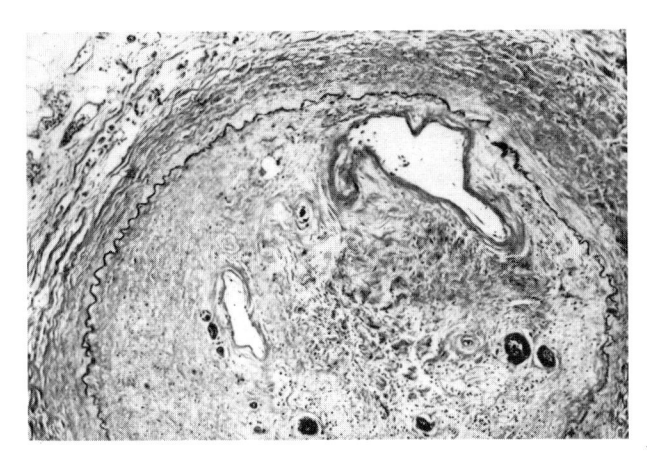

Figure 18.12 Advanced chronic vascular rejection. Lumen of altered artery obliterated by old organized and recanalized thrombus. Patient survival 2.2 years. Donor age 30 years (H & E x 40)

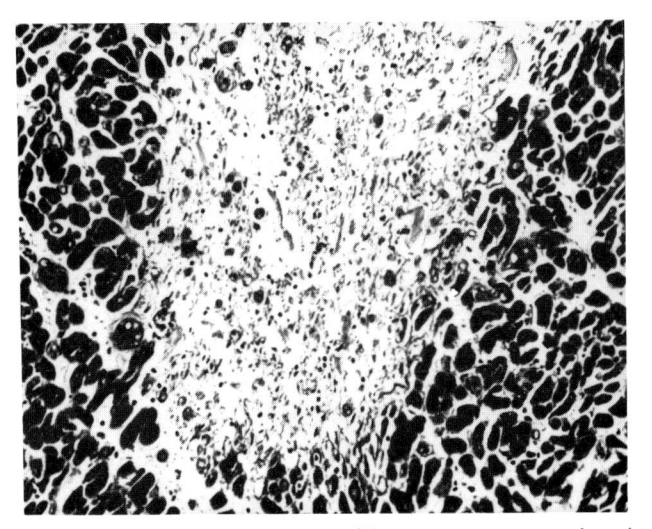

Figure 18.13 Scar showing remnants of degenerate myocytes and persisting lymphoid infiltrate suggestive of previous myocytolysis. Patient survival 2.7 years. Donor age 15 years (H & E x 130)

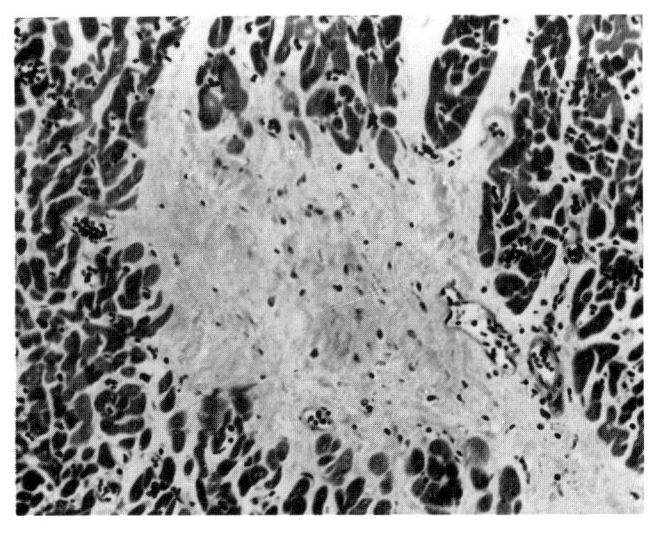

Figure 18.14 Small dense acellular scar, possibly due to previous myocytolysis with collapse fibrosis. No persistent cellular response. Patient survival 1.6 years. Donor age 25 years (H & E x 170)

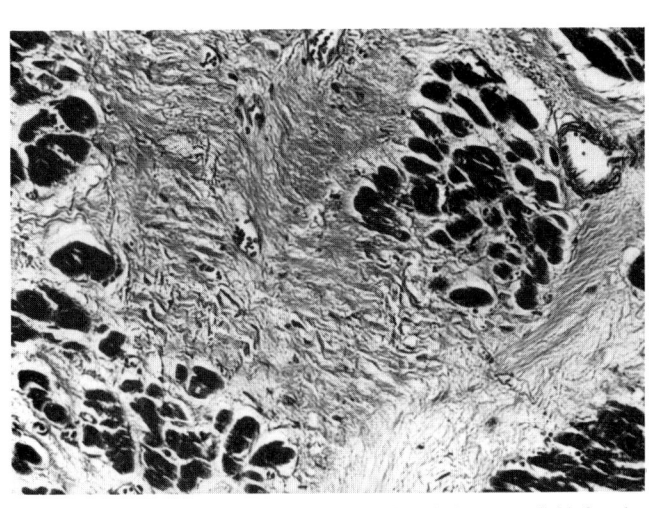

Figure 18.15 Large acellular fibrous scar of healed myocardial infarction. Patient survival 12.5 years. Donor age 33 years (H & E x 150)

fibrous replacement appears to be most marked in the right ventricle (Figure 18.16). Subendocardial myocytes (Figure 18.17) are kept alive by intra-cavity blood; this may be a cause of misleading results on endomyocardial biopsy.

Other cardiac structures are surprisingly little affected. Some loss of medial smooth muscle may be observed in the aorta and pulmonary arteries, with little accompanying cellular infiltration. Only in the presence of severe rejection are the valves affected by a focal lymphoid infiltration. Some valves thus affected show incipient platelet deposition along contact lines.

INCIDENCE OF CHRONIC REJECTION

The frequency with which chronic rejection changes occur in long-surviving cardiac transplants is illustrated in a personal study of 12 patients with 14 cardiac transplants, which had survival times longer than 1 year[18]. These consisted of three orthotopic and nine heterotopic transplants examined at autopsy, and two surgical specimens from patients who underwent heterotopic retransplantation. The grafts survived 1.1–12.5 years with a mean of 2.7 years.

Histologically, 29% of hearts showed evidence of persisting acute rejection, and 93% showed signs of significant chronic rejection. In the response of chronic vascular rejection, severe myointimal proliferation was present in most cases (86%), while a cellular infiltration of the vessel wall was generally absent (72%). The degree of vascular occlusion of chronic rejection bore no relationship to the severity of previous acute rejection episodes. Severe lumenal encroachment of between 51% and 100%, resulting from

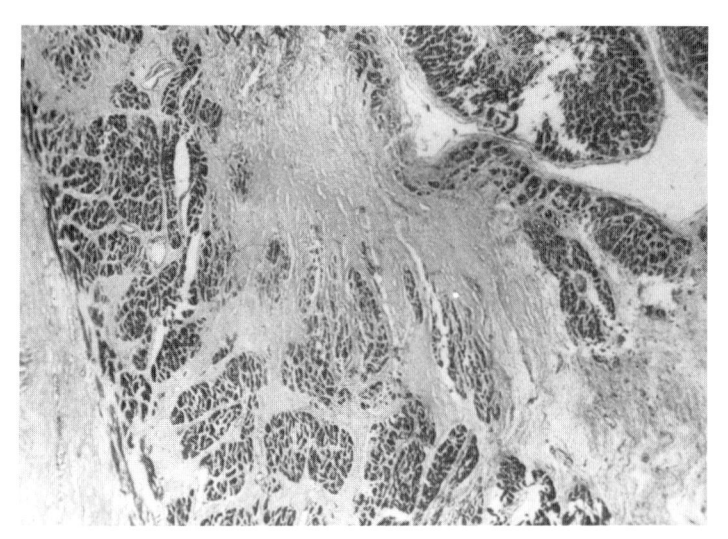

Figure 18.16 Massive fibrous replacement of the right ventricle due to chronic rejection. Note the subendocardial survival of myocytes. Patient survived 12.5 years with this allograft (H & E x 3.4)

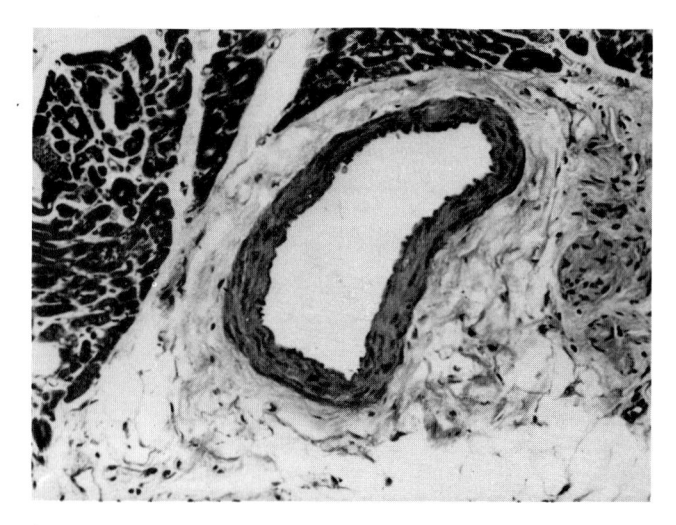

Figure 18.18 Normal-looking coronary artery in allograft which showed no chronic rejection at 1.7 years. Donor age 35 years (H & E x 150)

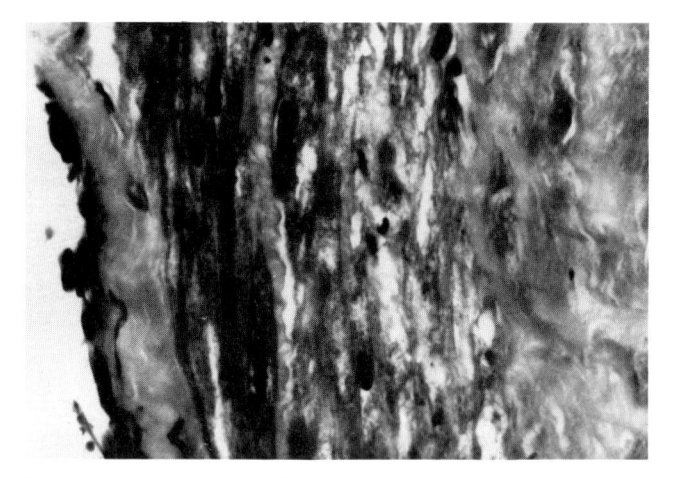

Figure 18.17 Degenerative changes in subendocardial myocytes in chronic rejection. Replacement fibrosis is seen deeper in myocardium (left). Patient survived 2 years (H & E x 115)

these changes, was frequently present (79%), while superadded thrombosis of the affected arteries was present in 72% of cases. Myocardial scars were present in 92% of hearts, while extensive acute infarction was present in 43% of heterotopic transplants. In only one case, with a survival time of 1.7 years, was there an almost complete absence of chronic rejection, the arteries being virtually normal (Figure 18.18). Further, it is striking that in all of the cases with chronic rejection there was an almost complete absence of infective lesions. A significant degree of rejection was responsible for the patient's death or graft failure in 79%.

COMMENT

The appearances of the vascular lesions described above are those of a reparative process following immune-mediated intimal and medial arterial damage. The entire length of the artery is affected by the immune insult. These changes probably represent the cumulative effect of multiple acute rejection episodes, whether these be overt or clinically silent. In severity, these lesions bear no constant relationship to the survival time of the graft or patient, and, in our patients, took from 1.1 to 12.5 years to evolve. Graft atherosclerosis differs from natural atherosclerosis by producing (1) consistently concentric intimal thickening, and (2) diffuse vessel involvement, (3) in affecting small arteries, (4) in its rapid development, and (5) by the rarity of associated calcification[19].

Not all vessels in the donor heart show accelerated atherosclerosis, which is surprising in view of the suspected immunological etiology. There is no correlation between the number and severity of clinically diagnosed acute rejection episodes and the subsequent development of chronic rejection. The determining factor for graft survival, in the presence of chronic rejection, is myocardial ischemia, manifesting as extensive recent or old infarction. The fact that donor hearts are generally procured from young people further underlines the significance of this event. This situation is ironic since ischemic heart disease is a frequent indication for cardiac transplantation.

While endomyocardial biopsy is an effective means of monitoring acute rejection episodes, it is of less use in chronic rejection. Experience has shown that extensive myocardial fibrosis may exist, which is not detected in the rather superficial endomyocardial biopsy, in which the subendocardial myofibers remain viable (Figures 18.16 and 18.17). Neither does the biopsy include medium-sized or large coronary arteries, which are the vessels affected by the process of chronic rejection.

Another feature in our series, which contains a significant number of heterotopic transplants, is the advanced nature of the chronic rejection reaction in the donor hearts, and of the ischemic lesions in the recipient hearts. These patients enjoy the benefit of two hearts, which jointly are able to maintain vital function in the presence of severely incapacitating lesions which have progressed far beyond that possible in a person supported only by a single heart. Consequently, the donor hearts generally show more advanced chronic rejection than orthotopic transplants, and the recipient hearts reveal a more severe degree of atherosclerosis, with accompanying ischemic manifestations, than would be possible in the natural state. Both lesions predispose to extensive mural thrombus formation (present in 50% of donor hearts with chronic rejection), which in turn results in an increased potential for peripheral embolization.

Chronic rejection has emerged as a major limiting factor to the success of cardiac transplantation.

References

1. Barnard, C.N. (1967). The operation. A human cardiac transplant; an interim report of a successful operation performed at Groote Schuur Hospital, Cape Town. *S. Afr. Med. J.*, **41**, 1271
2. Jamieson, S.W., Oyer, P.E., Reitz, B.A., Baumgartner, W.A., Bieber, C.P., Stinson, E.B. and Shumway, N.E. (1981). Cardiac transplantation at Stanford. *Heart Transplant.*, **1**, 86
3. Solis, E.K. and Kaye, M.P. (1986). The Registry of the International Society for Heart Transplantation: Third Official Report, June 1986. *J. Heart Transplant.*, **5**, 2
4. Baumgartner, W.A., Reitz, B.A., Oyer, P.E., Stinson, E.B. and Shumway, N.E. (1979). Cardiac homotransplantation. *Curr. Probl. Surg.*, **16**, 3
5. Cooper, D.K.C., Lanza, R.P., Oliver, S., Forder, A.A., Rose, A.G., Uys, C.J., Novitzky, D. and Barnard, C.N. (1983). Infectious complications after heart transplantation. *Thorax*, **38**, 822
6. Uys, C.J., Rose, A.G. and Barnard, C.N. (1979). The pathology of human heart transplantation. An assessment after 11 years' experience at Groote Schuur Hospital. *S. Afr. Med. J.*, **56**, 887
7. Uys, C.J. and Rose, A.G. (1983). Cardiac transplantation. Aspects of the pathology. In Sommers, S.C. and Rosen, P.P. (eds.) *Pathology Annual*. Vol. 17, pp. 147–178. (New York: Appleton-Century Crofts)
8. Lower, R.R., Kontos, H.A., Kosek, J.C., Sewell, D.H. and Graham W.H. (1968). Experiences in heart transplantation. *Am. J. Cardiol.*, **22**, 766
9. Thomson, J.G. (1969). Production of severe atheroma in a transplanted heart. *Lancet*, **2**, 1088
10. Bieber, C.P., Stinson, E.B., Shumway, N.E., Payne, R. and Kosek, J. (1970). Cardiac transplantation in man. VII. Cardiac allograft pathology. *Circulation*, **41**, 753.
11. Milam, J.D., Shipkey, F.H., Lind, C.J., Nora, J.J., Leachman, R.D., Rochelle, D.G., Bloodwell, R.D., Hallman, G.L. and Cooley, D.A. (1970). Morphologic findings in human allografts. *Circulation*, **41**, 519
12. Kosek, J.C., Bieber, C.P. and Lower, R.R. (1974). Heart graft arteriosclerosis. *Transplant. Proc.*, **3**, 512
13. Sinclair, R.A., Andres, G.A. and Hsu, K.C. (1972). Immunofluorescent studies of the arterial lesion in rat cardiac allografts. *Arch. Pathol.*, **94**, 331
14. Laden, A.M. (1972). Experimental atherosclerosis in rat and rabbit cardiac allografts. *Arch. Pathol.*, **93**, 240
15. Laden, A.M., Sinclair, R.A. and Ruskiewica, M. (1973). Vascular changes in experimental allografts. *Transplant. Proc.*, **5**, 737
16. Alonso, D.R., Storek, P.K. and Minick, C.R. (1977). Studies in the pathogenesis of atherosclerosis induced in rabbit cardiac allografts by the synergy of graft rejection and hypercholesterolemia. *Am. J. Pathol.*, **87**, 415
17. Rose, A.G., Uys, C.J., Cooper, D.K.C. and Barnard, C.N. (1982). Donor heart morphology twelve and a half years after orthotopic transplantation. *Heart Transplant.*, **1**, 329
18. Uys, C.J. and Rose, A.G. (1984). Pathologic findings in long-term cardiac transplants. *Arch. Pathol. Lab. Med.*, **108**, 112
19. Billingham, M.E. (1987). Cardiac transplant atherosclerosis. *Transplant. Proc.*, **19**, 19

19
Diagnosis and Management of Graft Atherosclerosis (Chronic Rejection)

D.M. EICH, R.J. QUIGG, A. HEROUX, A. HASTILLO, J. THOMPSON, G.R. BARNHART, R.R. LOWER AND M.L. HESS

INTRODUCTION

Cardiac transplantation has become an accepted therapeutic modality for end-stage heart failure. It is expected that each year approximately 2000 cardiac transplant procedures will be performed worldwide with a 1-year survival exceeding 80%[1]. These statistics reflect dramatic advances in cardiac transplantation over the past decade. Although rejection and infection are still primary concerns, they are no longer the nemesis of the allograft recipient who survives the immediate postoperative period. Instead, accelerated coronary artery disease (CAD) has become the leading cause of death among those transplant recipients who survive a year or longer after surgery.

HISTORICAL PERSPECTIVE

The rapid development of CAD in the cardiac allograft was a very early concern. The heightened awareness of accelerated CAD represents a resurgence of some early issues that were raised in the 1960s. In 1969, the report by Thomson detailing the pathologic findings of the first long-term cardiac transplant survivor revealed the presence of severe coronary disease[2]. These findings were viewed with some surprise as the donor heart had come from a previously healthy 20-year-old man. It was noted that the allograft recipient had been hyperlipidemic after operation, and it was postulated that immune endothelial injury secondary to chronic rejection was responsible. In 1967, Lower et al. had reported that virtually all long-term canine cardiac allografts developed vascular lesions that were felt to represent a form of chronic rejection[3]. However, this report was overshadowed by the excitement created by the first successful human cardiac transplant in South Africa.

The fervor over this new technique and its clinical applications was soon tempered as a myriad of problems became apparent involving donor availability, treatment of rejection, and infectious complications of immunosuppression. These problems resulted in grim short-term survival. Subsequently, many institutions abandoned the procedure. By the mid-1970s, there were only three major institutions performing cardiac transplantation. Gradually, advances were made in long distance procurement, immunosuppression, and the treatment of opportunistic infections. The development of cyclosporine led to improved treatment of rejection and a lower incidence of infectious complications[4]. These advances improved cardiac allograft survival and precipitated third-party reimbursement for cardiac transplantation in the United States. The improved survival and financial incentive for cardiac transplantation prompted a resurgence of interest in cardiac transplantation in the 1980s. By 1988, there were 125 centers performing cardiac transplantation in the United States alone.

As large numbers of patients were successfully transplanted and survived the immediate postoperative period, the problem of accelerated CAD became obvious. The incidence of accelerated CAD has been reported to vary between 1 and 4% at 1 year after transplantation to 44–50% by the fifth year after transplantation[5,6]. In 1982, the Stanford group reported that 11% of the deaths among their cardiac allograft recipients were attributable to the development of accelerated CAD[5]. At the Medical College of Virginia approximately 20% of the deaths in the cardiac transplant population have been attributed to CAD. Human autopsy reports confirm the previous pathologic findings of canine allografts in that virtually all long-term survivors have some degree of coronary artery pathology[7–9]. Coronary disease has been manifested over a broad range of time. At the Medical College of Virginia, this range has been observed to be between 1 and 15 years after surgery. Certainly, there are patients who, at 5 years after transplantation, have a well-preserved left ventricular ejection fraction and no clinical evidence of coronary disease. However, it appears that the severity of lumenal narrowing and subsequent complications such as thrombosis and infarction increase in parallel with the duration of graft survival[9]. It seems, therefore, that it is less a question of *whether* an allograft recipient will develop CAD, but rather, *when* will the patient develop CAD? What predisposes these individuals to such an aggressive form of coronary disease remains an unanswered question.

RISK FACTORS

Certain risk factors are known to be associated with the development of atherosclerotic cardiovascular disease in the general population. These include male sex, family history of early CAD, hypertension, diabetes mellitus, hyperlipidemia and smoking. It is believed that these risk factors, in conjunction with endothelial injury resulting from chronic rejection, may play a significant role in the pathogenesis of accelerated CAD. The exact roles of these risk factors in the transplant population have not been studied in detail and remain poorly understood. The assimilation of data pertaining to cardiac transplant patients with CAD has been limited to retrospective analysis of small sample sizes of patients on varied protocols.

Male sex

Although accelerated CAD is known to occur regardless of the etiology of the predisposing cardiomyopathy, many patients who require cardiac transplantation have end-stage ischemic heart disease. The majority of patients transplanted at the Medical College of Virginia have been males (86%). Therefore, there may be a baseline increase in risk factors in this population.

Hypertension

The appearance of hypertension has proven to be inevitable in transplant recipients as a result of cyclosporine immunosuppression. The etiology of cyclosporine-induced hypertension is not understood. Diastolic pressures of 110 mmHg or greater are often encountered. Left ventricular hypertrophy is a common echocardiographic finding after transplantation. Aggressive attempts to treat hypertension in these patients often result in the use of triple drug regimens.

Diabetes mellitus

Steroids are used as maintenance therapy at many institutions, and may contribute to the development of hypertension and/or steroid-induced diabetes mellitus. Patients on maintenance prednisone protocols frequently become hyperglycemic. Katz *et al.* reported a 10% incidence of steroid-induced diabetes in patients treated with cyclosporine and prednisone[10]. Although the presence of diabetes has been a relative contraindication to transplantation in the past, presently some centers are transplanting patients with well-controlled diabetes. Despite the known association of atherosclerotic vascular disease in the general diabetic population, no definitive association with accelerated allograft CAD has been demonstrated in small numbers of patients[11,12]. However, hyperglycemia has been associated with a significant increase in serum lipids[13].

Hyperlipidemia

The incidence of hyperlipidemia is quite high among the transplant population. This may be pre-existing or may be secondary to immunosuppressive therapy (Chapter 12). Although it is rare for the pretransplant patient to manifest increased serum cholesterol values, due to cardiac cachexia, the appearance of postoperative hyperlipidemia may be dramatic. Of our patients on a cyclosporine/prednisone protocol, 66% were hyperlipidemic (mean total cholesterol of 266 mg/dl) 1 year following transplantation[13].

In 1984, Hess *et al.* reported an association between hypercholesterolemia, humoral injury to the endothelium, and accelerated CAD[14]. Further clinical experience supports these observations. A review of serum lipid profiles of patients on conventional azathioprine/prednisone, and cyclosporine/prednisone immunosuppression, conducted at the Medical College of Virginia in 1986, revealed some interesting observations between those patients who developed CAD 2 years following surgery and those without clinical evidence of CAD at 5 years after surgery (Figures 19.1–19.4).

Figure 19.5 reveals cholesterol levels of two such patients. Patient T.C. was a 17-year-old male transplanted for an idiopathic cardiomyopathy. Patient M.S. was a 21-year-old female who underwent cardiac transplantation for a viral cardiomyopathy. M.S. is now 10 years post-surgery and is without clinical evidence of CAD. These data suggest a clear trend toward 'inferior' lipid profiles in those patients who develop CAD. Most recently, the Medical College of Virginia reported that high-risk total cholesterol levels, when indexed for age at 6 months after transplantation, are predictive of clinically significant CAD by the third year[11].

Smoking

Tobacco use is a risk factor that has also been associated with atherosclerosis in the general population. Although strongly discouraged, occasionally patients continue to smoke after transplantation. To date, however, no statisti-

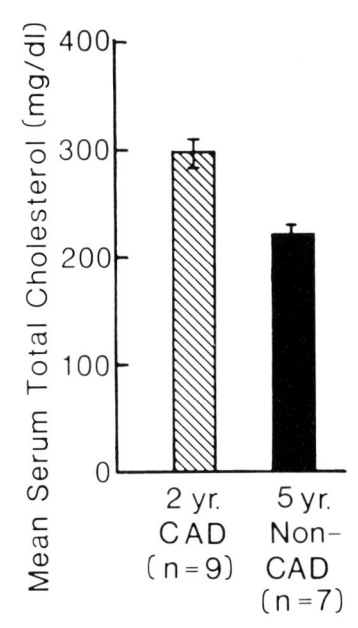

Figure 19.1 Mean total cholesterol values for patients *with* CAD at 2 years after surgery and for patients *without* CAD at 5 years after surgery. (The difference is significant at $p = 0.004$)

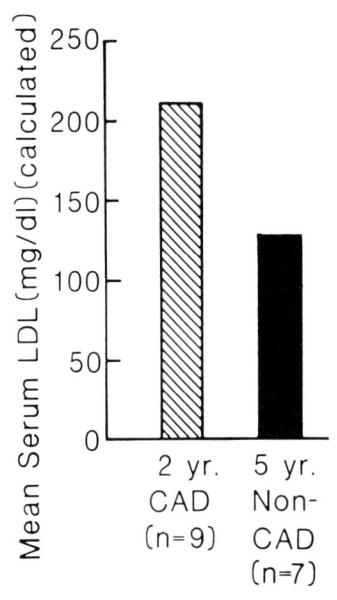

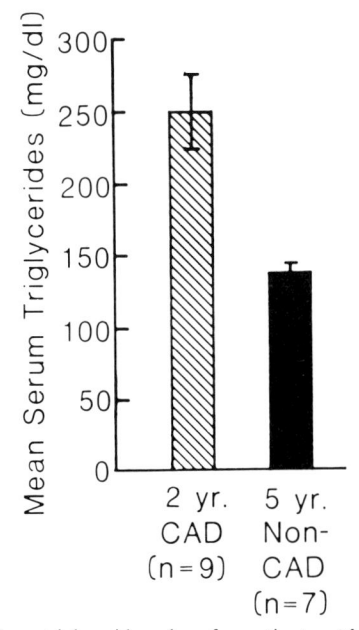

Figure 19.2 Mean triglyceride values for patients *with* CAD at 2 years after surgery and for patients *without* CAD at 5 years after surgery. (The difference is significant at $p = 0.0004$)

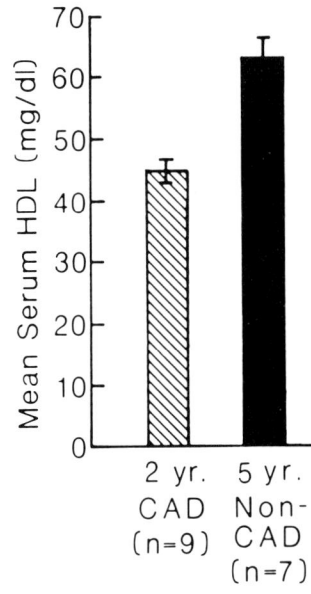

Figure 19.3 Mean LDL values for patients *with* CAD at 2 years after surgery and for patients *without* CAD at 5 years after surgery. (The difference is significant at $p < 0.05$ (Wilcoxon Rank Sum))

Figure 19.4 Mean HDL values for patients *with* CAD at 2 years after surgery and for patients *without* CAD at 5 years after surgery. (The difference is significant at $p = 0.0001$)

cally significant association has been drawn between tobacco use and allograft CAD; present experience remains anecdotal.

Acute and chronic rejection

Although there is a preponderance of risk factors in this population of cardiac transplant patients, it is obvious these factors alone cannot explain the accelerated nature of this disease. From the earliest days of transplantation, acute and chronic rejection have been felt to play a critical role in the genesis of these vascular lesions. The immune-mediated injury to the endothelium, with progression to the advanced intimal proliferative lesions of atherosclerosis, supports the revised response-to-injury hypothesis proposed by Ross[15]. Acute episodes of rejecton with associated endothelial injury by both humoral and cell-mediated mechanisms are well-

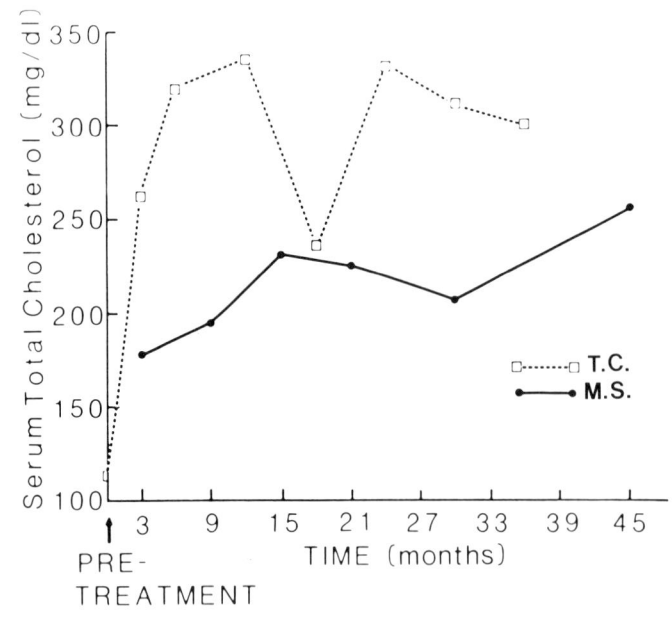

Figure 19.5 Total cholesterol values for two transplant patients. Patient T.C. was transplanted at 17 years of age for an idiopathic cardiomyopathy; he developed CAD 2 years after surgery. Patient M.S. was transplanted for a viral cardiomyopathy at 21 years of age: she is presently without clinical evidence of CAD 10 years after surgery

known to occur in cardiac transplant patients. Uretsky and colleagues reported an association between the number of episodes of acute rejection requiring treatment and the genesis of accelerated CAD[16], although no correlation was found by the Stanford group[12].

The concept of chronic rejection has been poorly understood. Pathologically, there is a continuum of rejection which we characterize as mild, moderate, or severe in accordance with the degree of cellular infiltration and myocyte injury. Severe rejection mandates immediate intervention with a host of immunosuppressants to avoid precipitous graft failure. Less is known about the long-standing consequences of 'mild' rejection. Certainly, there have been patients who have been without significant episodes of rejection but who eventually developed progressive graft atherosclerosis. In these patients the role of other associated risk factors may be critical. The work of Cathcart *et al.* revealed that when low-density lipoprotein is exposed to macrophages it is oxidized and becomes toxic to fibroblasts in culture[17]. This suggests a role for low-density lipoprotein cholesterol (LDL) in amplifying low-grade endothelial injury induced by ongoing cellular and humoral mechanisms.

Unfortunately, those risk factors that are known to predispose patients in the general population to CAD are exacerbated by our immunosuppressive protocols. In 1986, the Medical College of Virginia Transplant Program began treating patients with maintenance azathioprine/cyclosporine immunosuppression with the avoidance of prednisone. Prednisone is added to the regimen only if rejection episodes are particularly recalcitrant. Long-term follow-up in these patients reveals a significant decrease in total cholesterol and high-density lipoprotein cholesterol (HDL), a significant decrease in the incidence of hyperglycemia[10,13], but a small increase in the number of episodes of rejection. It remains to be clarified whether the elimination of prednisone will have an impact upon weight reduction, the development of steroid-induced diabetes and, therefore, the development of allograft CAD. Given ongoing endothelial injury associated with mild donor rejection, accelerated cardiac allograft CAD can be understood. The time course of the development of CAD would suggest a possible prolonged interaction between the cellular and humoral injury of rejection associated with known cardiovascular risk factors.

DIAGNOSIS

The pathologic picture of cardiac allograft atherosclerosis can be quite varied. Not only are there lesions closely resembling the discrete atheroma of the native CAD, but also one may find a diffuse process which involves the full extent of the coronary vasculature[7-9] (Figures 19.6 and 19.7). As a consequence of the spectrum of pathology, as well as the sympathetic denervation and absence of the typical warnings of anginal pain, the clinical presentation of this insidious disease can be either precipitous or indolent. Patients developing accelerated atherosclerosis can present with a variety of non-specific complaints, e.g. fatigue, persistent cough, or recurrent upper airway infection. Typical symptoms of congestive failure with dyspnea, orthopnea, and paroxysmal nocturnal dyspnea may herald progressive systolic dysfunction. Silent myocardial infarction may be noted on routine electrocardiograms. Sudden death may

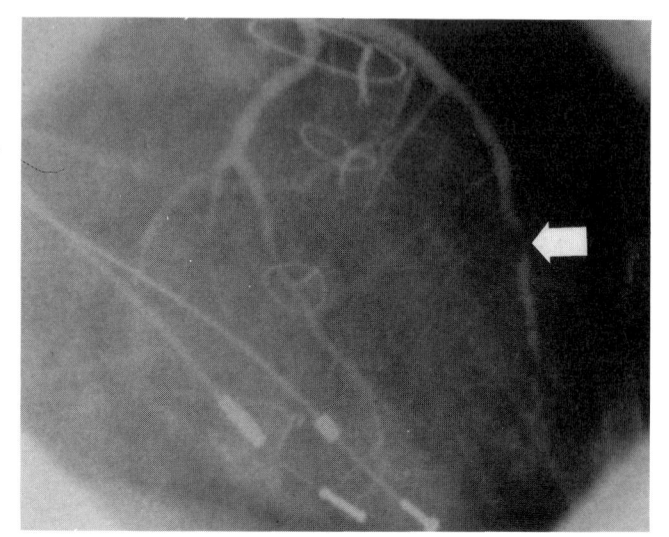

Figure 19.6 Right anterior oblique projection of a coronary angiogram taken of a cardiac transplant patient with accelerated CAD. Note the discrete stenosis of the mid-left anterior descending coronary artery (LAD) (arrow) and the pruning of the circumflex system

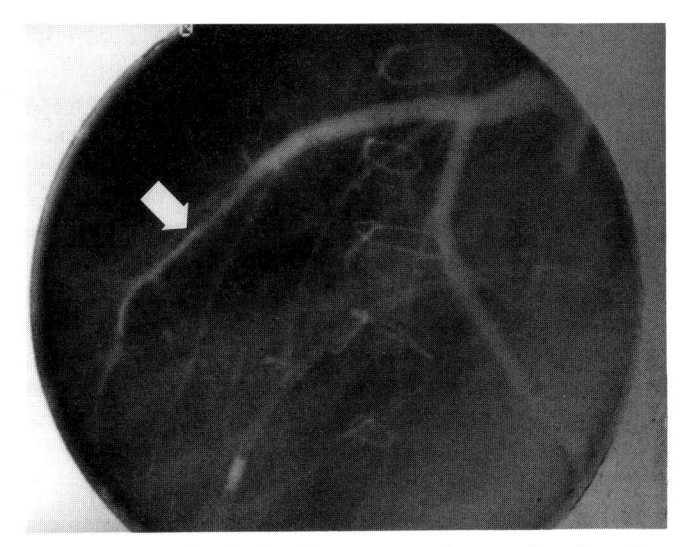

Figure 19.7 Lateral projection of a coronary angiogram taken of a cardiac transplant patient with accelerated CAD. Note the marked concentric narrowing of the LAD (arrow) with obliteration of diagonal and circumflex marginal branches. (Courtesy of Dr John Hodgson)

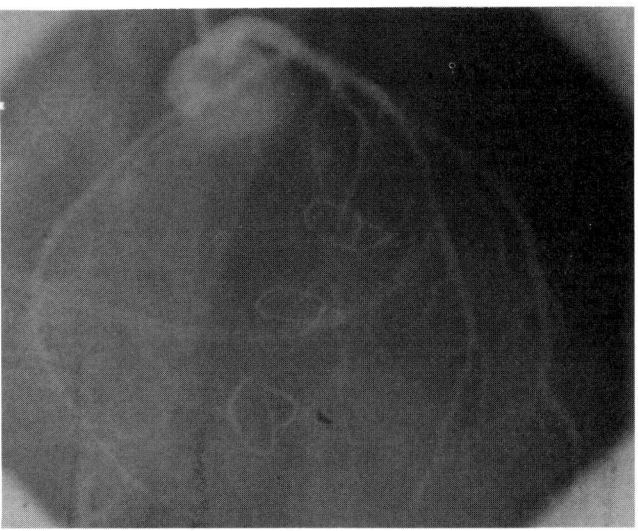

Figure 19.8 Angiogram taken of a cardiac transplant patient who had a precipitous drop in left ventricular ejection fraction and a stress thallium study which failed to demonstrate redistribution

also be the first clinical manifestation of this process.

At the Medical College of Virginia, a complement of invasive and non-invasive techniques is employed for the surveillance of accelerated atherosclerosis. Routine history and physical examination are supported by serial electrocardiograms to detect silent myocardial infarction. Nuclear ventriculography is employed to observe changes in both left and right ventricular systolic function and regional wall motion abnormalities. Two-dimensional echocardiography provides complementary data in assessing systolic and diastolic function. As the pathologic spectrum of cardiac allograft atherosclerosis often involves diffuse concentric disease involving the extent of the coronary vasculature, wall motion abnormalities seen on non-invasive examination may be global. A failure to observe discrete wall motion abnormalities therefore does not exclude coronary disease.

Exercise or dipyridamole thallium studies are utilized to screen for the presence of ischemic myocardium[18]. However, the sensitivity and specificity of this technique have not been proven in the cardiac transplant population, given the propensity to develop diffuse concentric disease (Figures 19.8 and 19.9). Abnormal thallium studies must be interpreted in the light of endomyocardial biopsy results since acute episodes of rejection have been found to result in false positive exercise thallium images. Holter monitoring has been shown by Romhilt et al. to be a useful diagnostic adjunct[19]. The detection of Lown Grade III ventricular dysrhythmias correlated with a poor prognosis and a high incidence of allograft CAD. Endomyocardial biopsy, although useful in the detection of allograft rejection, has not proven to be a reliable procedure in the diagnosis of allograft CAD.

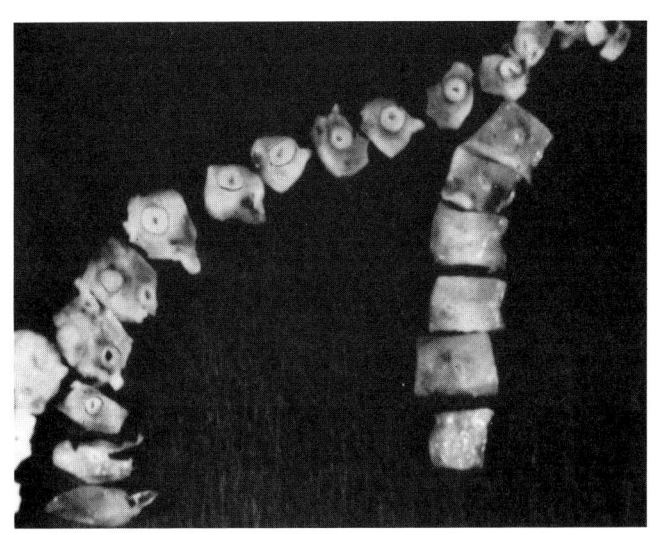

Figure 19.9 Pathologic specimen obtained at the time of retransplantation from the patient whose angiogram is shown in Figure 19.8. The specimen revealed marked concentric luminal narrowing of the epicardial vessels. (Courtesy of Dr Danna Johnson)

Coronary angiography has long been considered the gold standard for diagnosing CAD. At the Medical College of Virginia, angiography is performed only when non-invasive evidence suggests clinically significant CAD. Angiography is of particular value in circumstances where focal, discrete epicardial stenoses are present. The sensitivity of the angiogram is diminished, however, in cases where there is diffuse involvement of the coronaries with small vessel disease[20]. Diffuse concentric narrowing may be misinterpreted as 'small coronaries'. Therefore, adjunctive measures have been sought to increase the sensitivity of the angiogram. Paradoxic vasoconstriction has been observed by Ludmer in the normal population with CAD with intracoronary acetylcholine injection[21]. Fish and colleagues have demonstrated paradoxic vasoconstriction with intracoronary acetylcholine in allograft hearts[22]. Abnormal coronary flow reserve studies have been noted in human cardiac allografts with ongoing rejection[23]. Abnormal flow reserve studies are observed with non-specific endothelial injury as well as left ventricular hypertrophy and CAD. Normal coronary flow patterns virtually exclude significant disease.

TREATMENT

The only treatments available for cardiac allograft CAD are (1) percutaneous translumenal coronary angioplasty (PTCA) of discrete lesions, and (2) retransplantation. Neither approach is satisfactory in that lesions are rarely amenable to PTCA and the costs and risks of retransplantation are significant. We must therefore make every effort to prevent the development of this disease. Acute rejection must be treated aggressively in order to minimize the ongoing endothelial injury. Unfortunately, subclinical rejection cannot be completely eliminated given the limits of our present immunosuppressive protocols. Careful donor and recipient cross-matching, with aggressive management of individual episodes of rejection, can hopefully decrease the extent of endothelial injury.

Risk factors must be closely monitored in the cardiac transplant population. Dietary moderation of cholesterol consumption is encouraged, and diets with less than 300 mg cholesterol/day, with less than 30% total calories in fat, are recommended. Daily exercise is also encouraged, since these measures should have a beneficial effect on weight gain, and serum lipid levels.

Our immunosuppressive protocols are our greatest liability in the management of risk factors after cardiac transplantation. Patients maintained on cyclosporine and prednisone protocols have been reported to have the highest mean total cholesterol values[13,24]. Non-steroid protocols have been reported to have lower mean total cholesterol values, but also have been noted to have lower mean high-density lipoprotein cholesterol (HDL) values. The net effect of these alterations in lipid profiles on the genesis of accelerated CAD is unknown. Pharmacologic intervention with hyperlipidemia has been frustrating. The development of the HMG-CoA reductase inhibitor, lovastatin, is felt to be promising for this subset of patients. Although reports of rhabdomyolysis in patients treated with cyclosporine and lovastatin were very disappointing[25], anecdotal experience suggests that low doses of lovastatin may be used safely and effectively with close observation of serum creatine phosphokinase levels.

Cyclosporine-induced hypertension is a very difficult problem. Aggressive management often precipitates undesirable side-effects. The traditional first-line therapy of diuretics and β-blockers is minimally effective and often aggravates hyperglycemia and dyslipidemia. Angiotensin-converting enzyme inhibitors may be used effectively, but one must be cautious to avoid further exacerbation of cyclosporine-induced renal insufficiency. Calcium channel blockers may be employed as vasodilators. There have been recent reports demonstrating regression of atherosclerotic lesions using calcium channel antagonists[26,27]. Handley and colleagues observed a 44% decrease in atherosclerotic lesions induced in the rabbit carotid using isradipine[28].

Diuretic therapy may be a necessary adjunct to vasodilator therapy. Hydrochlorothiazide should be avoided as this agent is known to induce hyperglycemia and hyperlipidemia. Furosemide should be used in moderation to avoid inducing hypovolemia and further complicating renal insufficiency.

Obviously, tobacco abuse must be eliminated in this group of patients.

When the risk factor modification fails and there is angiographic evidence of a discrete lesion with significant myocardium in jeopardy, PTCA can be considered[29,30]. Given the nature of the process, with the likely presence of distal disease, PTCA must be considered as a palliative measure. The risk–benefit ratio of this procedure is further complicated by the absence of the usual safeguard to emergent coronary artery bypass in the event of procedural complications.

Progressive coronary atherosclerosis of the allograft frequently results in recurrent NYHA Class IV failure. For these patients retransplantation is a therapeutic option, but an option with considerable morbidity and mortality (Chapter 20). Although technically feasible, the long-term success of the second transplant has not been as favorable[31].

COMMENT

Accelerated CAD in the cardiac allograft is an old problem. Although first described in the 1960s, the magnitude of the problem did not become apparent until a sufficient number of patients survived the immediate postoperative period and lived long enough to develop the disease. At present, coronary disease appears to be an inevitable complication after transplantation. We must anticipate an ever-increasing number of patients coming to need retransplantation, and thereby further straining already limited donor resources. The diagnosis of accelerated CAD may be obvious in any given patient, but more often it requires the full complement of tests available to the cardiologist. Most importantly, the diagnosis requires a high index of suspicion. Once the diagnosis is made, treatment options are limited. We must therefore make every attempt to forestall the development of this disease by aggressive treatment of risk factors known to be associated with atherosclerosis. Finally, we must address our research endeavors towards this problem of accelerated coronary disease.

Acknowledgements

The authors of this chapter gratefully acknowledge Ms. Betsy Smithers for her assistance in the preparation of the manuscript, and Ms. Bettie Duke for her assistance with the computer database. Original work reviewed in this chapter was supported in part by grant RR00065 to the Clinical Research Center of the Medical College of Virginia.

References

1. Fragomeni, L.S. and Kaye, M.P. (1988). The Registry of the International Society for Heart Transplantation: fifth official report, June 1988. *J. Heart Transplant.*, **7**, 249
2. Thomson, J.G. (1969). Production of severe atheroma in a transplanted human heart. *Lancet*, **2**, 1088
3. Lower, R.R. and Cleveland, R.J. (1967). The current status of heart transplantation. *Proceedings of the First International Congress of the Transplantation Society*, **1**, 657
4. Fowler, M.B. and Schroeder, J.S. (1986). Current status of cardiac transplantation. *Mod. Concepts Cardiovasc. Dis.*, **55**, 37
5. Pennock, J.L., Oyer, P.E., Reitz, B.A., Jamieson, S.W., Bieber, C.B., Wallwork, J., Stinson, E.B. and Shumway, N.E. (1982). Cardiac transplantation in perspective for the future. *J. Thorac. Cardiovasc. Surg.*, **83**, 168
6. Barnhart, G.R. and Pascoe, E.A. (1988). Accelerated coronary atherosclerosis – cardiac transplant recipients. *Transplant. Rev.*, **1**, 31
7. Bieber, C.P., Stinson, E.B., Shumway, N.E., Payne, R. and Kosek, J. (1970). Cardiac transplantation in man. VII. Cardiac allograft pathology. *Circulation*, **41**, 753
8. Uys, C.J. and Rose, A.G. (1984). Pathologic findings in long-term cardiac transplants. *Arch. Pathol. Lab. Med.*, **108**, 112
9. Johnson, D.E., Gao, S.Z., Schroeder, J.S., Decampli, W.M. and Billingham, M.E. (1989). The spectrum of coronary artery pathology in human cardiac allografts. *J. Heart Transplant.*, **8**, 349
10. Katz, M.R., Barnhart, G.R., Szentpetery, S., Rider, S., Thompson, J.A., Hess, M., Hastillo, A. and Lower, R.R. (1987). Are steroids essential for successful maintenance of immunosuppression in heart transplantation? *J. Heart Transplant.*, **6**, 293
11. Thompson, J.A., Eich, D.M., Ko, D., Barnhart, G., Hastillo, A., Lower, R.R. and Hess, M. (1987). Hypercholesterolemia as a marker of early coronary artery disease post cardiac transplant. *Circulation*, **76** (Suppl. IV), 167
12. Gao, S.Z., Schroeder, J.S., Alderman, E.L., Hunt, S.A., Silverman, J.F., Wiederhold, Y. and Stinson, E.B. (1987). Clinical and laboratory correlates of accelerated coronary artery disease in the cardiac transplant patient. *Circulation*, **76** (Suppl. V), 56
13. Taylor, D.O., Thompson, J.A., Hastillo, A., Barnhart, G., Rider, S., Lower, R.R. and Hess, M.L. (1989). Hyperlipidemia after clinical cardiac transplantation. *J. Heart Transplant.*, **8**, 209
14. Hess, M.L., Hastillo, A., Mohanakumar, D.V.M., Cowley, M.J., Vetrovac, G., Szentpetery, S., Wolfgang, T.C. and Lower, R.R. (1983). Accelerated atherosclerosis in cardiac transplantation: role of cytotoxic B-cell antibodies and hyperlipidemia. *Circulation*, **68** (Suppl. II), 94
15. Ross, R. (1986). The pathogenesis of atherosclerosis: an update. *N. Engl. J. Med.*, **314**, 488
16. Uretsky, B.F., Muarli, S., Reddy, P.S., Rabin, B., Lee, A., Griffith, B.P., Hardesty, R.L., Trento, A. and Bahnson, H.T. (1987). Development of coronary artery disease in cardiac transplant patients receiving immunosuppressive therapy with cyclosporine and prednisone. *Circulation*, **76**, 827
17. Cathcart, M.K., Morel, D.W. and Chisholm, G.M. (1985). Monocytes and neutrophils oxidize low density lipoprotein making it cytotoxic. *J. Leukocyte Biol.*, **38**, 419
18. McKillop, J.H. and Goris, M.L. (1981). Thallium 201 myocardial imaging in patients with previous cardiac transplantation. *Clin. Radiol.*, **32**, 447
19. Romhilt, D.W., Doyle, M., Sagar, K.B., Hastillo, A., Wolfgang, T.C., Lower, R.R. and Hess, M.L. (1982). Prevalence and significance of arrhythmias in long-term survivors of cardiac transplantation. *Circulation*, **66** (Suppl. 1), 219
20. Mason, J.W. and Strefling, A. (1979). Small vessel disease of the heart resulting in myocardial necrosis and death despite angiographically normal coronary arteries. *Am. J. Cardiol.*, **44**, 171
21. Ludmer, P.L., Selwyn, A.D., Shook, T.L., Wayne, R.R., Mudge, G.H., Alexander, R.W. and Ganz, P. (1986). Paradoxical vasoconstriction induced by acetylcholine in atherosclerotic coronary arteries. *N. Engl. J. Med.*, **315**, 1046
22. Fish, R.D., Nabel, E.G., Selwyn, A.P., Ludmer, P.L., Mudge, G.H., Kirshenbaum, J.M., Schoen, F.J., Alexander, R.W. and Ganz, P. (1988). Responses of coronary arteries of cardiac transplant patients to acetylcholine. *J. Clin. Invest.*, **81**, 21
23. Hodgson, J.M., Cohen, M.D., Murphy, J.H., Szentpetery, S. and Thames, M.D. (1987). Reductions of ventricular function correlate with impairment of coronary flow reserve but not with endomyocardial biopsy following cardiac transplantation. *J. Am. Coll. Cardiol.*, **9**, 116A
24. Harris, K.P.G., Russel, G.I., Parviin, S.D., Veitch, P.S. and Walls, J. (1986). Alterations in lipid and carbohydrate metabolism attributable to cyclosporine A in renal transplant recipients. *Br. Med. J.*, **292**, 16
25. Norman, D.J., Illingworth, D.R., Munson, J. and Hosenpud, J. (1988). Myolysis and acute renal failure in a heart transplant recipient receiving lovastatin. (Letter). *N. Engl. J. Med.*, **318**, 46
26. Henry, P.D. (1985). Atherosclerosis, calcium and calcium antagonists. *Circulation*, **72**, 456
27. Weinstein, D.B. and Heider, J.G. (1987). Antiatherogenic properties of calcium antagonists. *Am. J. Cardiol.*, **59** (Suppl.), 163B
28. Handley, D.A., Van Valen, R.G., Melden, M.K. and Saunders, R.N. (1986). Suppression of rat carotid lesion development by the calcium channel blocker, PN 200-110. *Am. J. Pathol.*, **124**, 88
29. Hastillo, A., Cowley, M.J., Vetrovec, G.W., Wolfgang, T.C., Lower, R.R. and Hess, M.L. (1985). Serial coronary angioplasty for atherosclerosis following heart transplantation. *J. Heart Transplant.*, **4**, 192
30. Vetrovec, G.W. and Cowley, M.J. (1990). Application of percutaneous transluminal angioplasty in cardiac transplantation. *Circulation*, In press
31. Gao, S.Z., Schroeder, J.S., Hunt, S. and Stinson, E. (1988). Retransplantation for severe accelerated coronary vascular disease in heart transplant recipients. *Am. J. Cardiol.*, **62**, 876

20
Retransplantation

D.K.C. COOPER AND D. NOVITZKY

INTRODUCTION

When allograft failure or severe dysfunction of an orthotopically or heterotopically transplanted heart occurs from whatever cause, replacement of the heart may be indicated and can substantially extend patient survival. There are surprisingly few reported data on the indications for retransplantation, or on the complications and results of this procedure[1-9].

Cardiac retransplantation in a patient with a previous OHT was first performed at Stanford Medical Center as early as 1968[1]. The first such intervention after HHT took place in Cape Town in 1980[5]. Today, the number of patients undergoing retransplantation is steadily increasing and will undoubtedly continue to increase in the future. The introduction of cyclosporine (CsA), though undoubtedly reducing the incidence of severe acute rejection episodes, does not as yet appear to have prevented the development of graft arteriosclerosis, which today is the main indication for retransplantation. The demands made by the need for retransplantation may significantly reduce the number of donor hearts available to newly-selected potential recipients.

INDICATIONS FOR RETRANSPLANTATION

Retransplantation should be considered in any patient in whom the cardiac allograft undergoes failure or severe dysfunction from acute and/or chronic rejection. Retransplantation has also been performed on occasion for intractable arrhythmias of the donor heart, and for acute donor right ventricular failure due to an excessive pulmonary vascular resistance following orthotopic transplantation[1]; refinements of criteria for selection of both recipients and donors and the use of such agents as prostaglandins E_1 (PGE_1) to reduce pulmonary vascular resistance, have made these indications for retransplantation rare. Early donor heart failure from causes other than acute rejection accounts for 25% of the deaths of patients undergoing transplantation (Chapter 31); if a second donor heart can be obtained in time, or the patient can be maintained by prolonged pump-oxygenator support[7,9] or by an artificial heart or a mechanical assist device (Section IV), retransplantation may be lifesaving.

Intractable acute rejection of an orthotopic graft, though rare today, is clearly an urgent indication for retransplantation; when occurring in a heterotopic graft, the urgency is less acute, but nevertheless a second donor should be found as quickly as possible.

The decision to retransplant a patient undergoing chronic rejection (graft atherosclerosis) and, in particular, the timing of the procedure, may be difficult, as the patient's general condition may remain good, despite evidence of increasing coronary atherosclerotic changes. Both surgeon and patient may be reluctant to undertake retransplantation whilst the patient remains asymptomatic; delay, however, may result in sudden death from major myocardial infarction. Alternatively, the patient's general condition may have deteriorated from chronic infection or other complications of long-term immunosuppression, creating doubt as to his suitability for retransplantation.

SELECTION OF PATIENTS FOR RETRANSPLANTATION

All of the criteria for transplantation should be reassessed before retransplantation is performed (Chapter 2), since significant changes may have occurred since the patient was assessed initially. In particular, the increased immunosuppression that is necessary during acute rejection episodes, or the prolonged immunosuppression in patients who have survived long enough to develop graft atherosclerosis, may have resulted in foci of infection. If possible, these infections must be eradicated or suppressed before retransplantation is undertaken. If it is not possible to eradicate a significant focus of infection, then the patient may not be suitable for retransplantation.

The patient should also be carefully reassessed from a

psychological standpoint to ascertain whether he or she can cope with the stresses and strains of a further transplant procedure. Particular attention should be paid to the patient's compliance with medical guidance, and his or her adherence to therapy during the course of the first transplant. Retransplantation may be inadvisable if non-compliance had contributed toward failure of the initial allograft.

Meticulous testing of the recipient for the presence of lymphocytotoxic antibodies must be carried out, and antibodies against any new potential donor excluded. Antibody formation has occurred to a greater or lesser degree in many of the patients who have received cardiac allografts at our institution and may preclude retransplantation[10] (Chapter 8).

TIMING OF RETRANSPLANTATION

In intractable acute rejection

With the immunosuppressive agents currently available, intractable acute rejection is today a rare occurrence. When occurring in a patient with an orthotopic transplant, it is, of course, a surgical emergency, and either retransplantation must be carried out as an emergency, or the patient must be assisted by some form of mechanical device. Without such mechanical assistance, a second donor must be found within a day or two, or death of the patient will occur.

Heterotopic heart transplantation, however, may allow patient survival even when the donor heart has ceased functioning entirely[11] (Chapter 23). This is particularly likely in patients who undergo acute rejection of the graft within the first few weeks or months following transplantation, at which stage the patient's own heart is likely to remain sufficiently functional to allow patient survival until a second transplant procedure is performed.

In such patients, excision of the irreversibly acutely rejected heterotopic heart may be delayed, whenever possible, until the time of retransplantation. The patient is maintained on methylprednisolone 20 mg/kg per day orally in an effort to prevent symptoms from the toxic effects of tissue necrosis. At Groote Schuur Hospital in South Africa, this policy was successful in all cases except one, when the patient developed a high fever and was clearly unwell, necessitating immediate excision of the rejected donor heart[10].

In advanced chronic rejection

As with acute rejection, complete failure of an orthotopic allograft from chronic rejection results in the death of the patient; it is usually clear, however, that chronic rejection is occurring, and time is available to plan the retransplant procedure. Our experience with patients with heterotopic allografts has been that recipient heart function steadily deteriorates during the months following transplantation, irrespective of the underlying cardiac pathology. By the time graft atherosclerosis has occurred, recipient heart function has frequently ceased altogether or has become inadequate to sustain life. As with orthotopic transplants, complete graft failure, therefore, is frequently followed by the death of the patient.

The timing of retransplantation may prove difficult, therefore, in patients with either heterotopic or orthotopic grafts in whom chronic rejection is occurring. The decision to retransplant must not be delayed until graft function becomes totally inadequate, yet, on the other hand, retransplantation should not be undertaken until absolutely essential. The exact timing is influenced by many factors, notably the ease or difficulty with which a suitable donor will be obtained; for example, if the patient has a high level of circulating lymphocytotoxic antibodies, some delay may occur in obtaining a suitable donor, and the search should begin earlier rather than later.

The policy of the Stanford group has been to offer retransplantation to patients with evidence on coronary arteriography of life-threatening occlusive lesions in the major coronary arteries, irrespective of the patient's exercise tolerance[2]. This policy evolved following the sudden death of three long-term survivors with such lesions. Our own policy has been possibly rather less aggressive, as, until recently, we had not seen sudden death in an otherwise asymptomatic patient. We have generally waited until exercise tolerance has significantly deteriorated, and coronary arteriography and/or thallium scanning have confirmed advanced disease.

The recent sudden death of one patient, however, has forced us to reconsider this policy. This patient was demonstrated to have what was considered a minor stenosis of the proximal left anterior descending coronary artery 2 years after transplantation, but died suddenly 3 months later. Autopsy showed a very tight stenotic lesion. (It is of considerable interest that he suffered bouts of anginal pain for 2 to 3 months before his death. The pain was associated with ST segment changes on EKG suggestive of ischemia. To our knowledge, no other patient has suffered well-documented anginal pain after heart transplantation.)

The rate of development and progression of graft atherosclerosis is extremely variable. We have seen advanced disease as early as 3 months, yet no disease as late as 13 years, after transplantation. In our experience, the development of even moderately advanced disease may be compatible in many cases with an acceptable quality of life for several further months or even years. In one of our patients, a 50% stenosis of the right coronary artery was demonstrated 6 years before death; this progressed to complete occlusion of this vessel at its origin and widespread disease of the coronary system over the next 4 years. Some 2 years later the patient finally succumbed to the disease, retransplantation having been contraindicated on other grounds[12,13].

RETRANSPLANTATION – OPERATIVE CONSIDERATIONS

It is our present policy in all cases of retransplantation to prepare the femoral artery and vein and initiate pump-oxygenator support through this route before median sternotomy is performed. In all cases, inotropic agents should be available during induction of anesthesia. Some of these patients have particularly poor cardiac function, and are hemodynamically very unstable, and may require initiation of cardiopulmonary bypass by the femoral route (or at least, preparation of the femoral vessels) under local anesthesia before induction of general anesthesia.

In patients with orthotopic allografts

The operation of retransplantation in a patient with an existing orthotopic allograft presents the same technical problems and risks of reoperation as in any patient who has previously undergone cardiac surgery. Adhesions have invariably developed between pericardium and heart, frequently making the initial dissection time-consuming. As myocardial function in these patients is poor, particular care must be taken not to handle or disturb the heart more than is absolutely essential before pump-oxygenator support has been initiated; for this reason, frequently it may be necessary to resort to use of the femoral vessels to commence cardiopulmonary bypass.

After excision of the first donor heart, the second heart is inserted as described in Chapter 10.

In patients with heterotopic allografts

After the operation of heterotopic transplantation, the pericardium cannot be closed. Unless a sheet of prosthetic material, e.g. polytetrafluoroethylene, has been inserted between heart and anterior chest wall, adhesions are likely to develop between the right ventricle of the recipient's own heart and the posterior aspect of the sternum; the donor heart, lying in the right chest, adheres to the right lung and anterior chest wall. Retransplantation may, therefore, be a technically extremely difficult procedure. (We have used such a sheet to prevent both hearts from adhering to the anterior chest wall with considerable success on one occasion, greatly facilitating retransplantation.) Great care is required in opening the sternum and in dissecting out the structures of the chest. The recipient right ventricle may be inadvertently opened during sternotomy, necessitating emergency femoro–femoral cardiopulmonary bypass (if not already in progress) to maintain the circulation whilst the situation is controlled[5].

In patients with heterotopic heart transplants in Cape Town, the following operative procedures have been employed during retransplantation (Figure 20.1)[8]:

(1) Replacement of the heterotopic donor heart (in five cases).

(2) Replacement of the recipient heart, leaving the first heterotopic donor heart *in situ* (in three cases). Following excision of the recipient's heart, the stan-

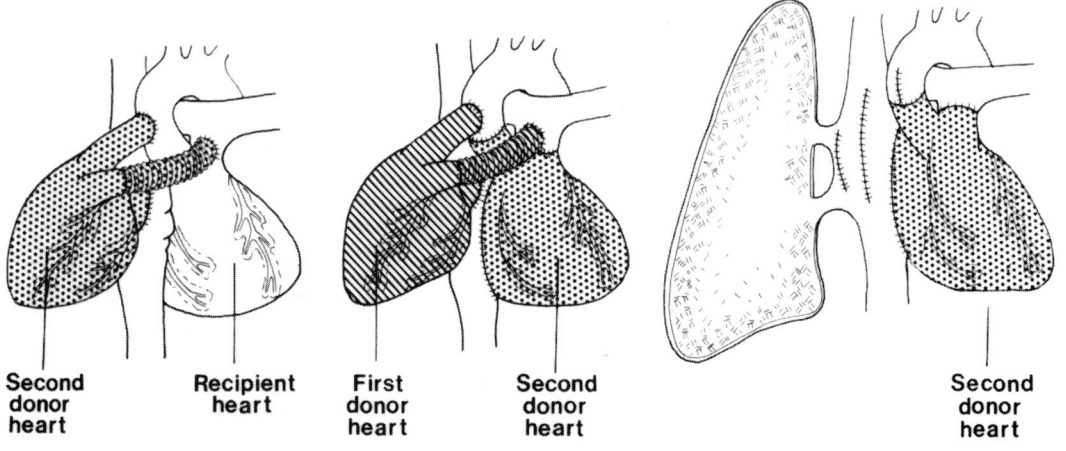

Figure 20.1 Different operative techniques used for retransplantation in patients with a heterotopic transplant. *Left*: technique 1 – replacement of the heterotopic donor heart; *center*: technique 2 – replacement of the recipient heart leaving the first heterotopic donor heart *in situ*; *right*: technique 3 – excision of both original donor and recipient hearts, and insertion of an orthotopic heart transplant; mobilization of the right lung is required to fill the space vacated by the heterotopic donor heart

THE TRANSPLANTATION AND REPLACEMENT OF THORACIC ORGANS

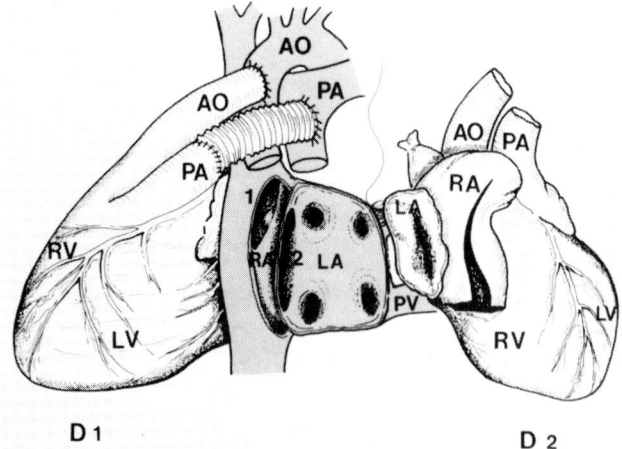

Figure 20.2 Replacement of the native heart in a recipient with a previous heterotopic transplant (D1) (technique 2). The native heart has been excised, and the second donor heart (D2) is about to be sutured into the orthotopic position (RA = right atrium; RV = right ventricle; PA = pulmonary artery PV = pulmonary vein; LA = left atrium; LV = left ventricle; AO = aorta)

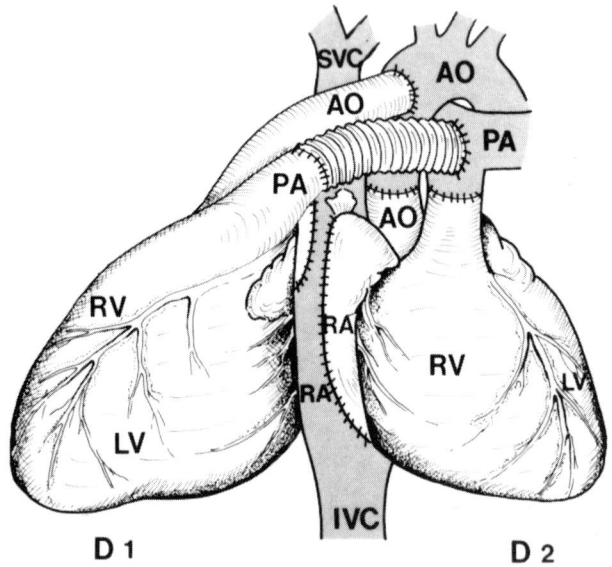

Figure 20.3 Replacement of the native heart in a recipient with a previous heterotopic transplant (D1) – the completed operation (technique 2). (SVC = superior vena cava; IVC = inferior vena cava. Other abbreviations as for Figure 20.2)

dard operation of orthotopic transplantation was performed (Figures 20.2 and 20.3).

(3) Excision of both original donor and recipient hearts and insertion of an orthotopic heart transplant; in these two cases, the right lower lobe required mobilization and re-expansion to fill the space vacated by the excised heterotopic heart.

Certain aspects of technique are worthy of note. Whenever it was decided to leave the heterotopic donor heart *in situ*, usually only its base and great vessels were mobilized. Similarly, whenever the recipient heart was to be left *in situ*, a full dissection was usually not carried out. If femoro-femoral bypass had already been initiated, a further single superior vena caval cannula was all that was required. If cardiopulmonary bypass was not already in progress, an arterial cannula was inserted into the aortic arch, and two venous cannulae placed, one in the superior vena cava, and one lower in the right atrium or inferior vena cava. While handling the superior vena cava, care was taken not to injure the azygos vein. Systemic cooling to 22°C was usually maintained.

Our approach to myocardial protection of the heart that was not to be replaced (i.e. either the heterotopic donor or the recipient heart) has varied over the years. Usually the aortic cross-clamp has been applied distal to the anastomosis of the donor aorta, thus rendering both hearts ischemic. On occasion, arrest of the retained heart by cardioplegia has been obtained, but on other occasions we have relied on topical cooling only. As, in every case, this heart (which was not to be removed) was badly diseased and therefore of little value to the patient, we have not always been meticulous in our efforts to protect the myocardium.

Decompression of the heart that was to be left *in situ* was readily achieved, as removal of the other heart rendered the left atrium open. At the end of the operative procedure, however, great care has to be taken to remove all air from both hearts. It has not been our policy to vent either heart, but a large air needle was placed in both aortic roots and in both left ventricles, either directly through the apex or, in the case of a heterotopic donor heart, through the anterior right ventricle and septum into the posteriorly placed left ventricle.

When the heterotopic donor heart required removal (techniques 1 and 3 above), this was performed once cardiopulmonary bypass had been initiated. On some occasions, air leaks and oozing of blood from the right lower lobe proved unavoidable. Excision of the first donor heart can be a difficult procedure in view of tight adhesions between this heart and the surrounding tissues, notably the lung. By leaving this heart *in situ*, the operating time is reduced and potential postoperative complications avoided.

Technique 3 is probably the least favorable, as removal of the original recipient heart together with the donor organ (and insertion of an orthotopic graft) also requires expansion of the right lower lobe, necessitating an extrapleural mobilization of much of the right lung, thereby increasing blood loss.

Excision of an acutely rejected heterotopic allograft in a patient with a functioning recipient heart

In patients with an irreversibly acutely rejected heterotopic allograft (and a functioning recipient heart), when the donor heart requires excision as a semi-emergency following the development of toxic symptoms from tissue necrosis, and when retransplantation cannot yet be performed due to the absence of a suitable donor or other contraindication, excision has been achieved without the need for cardiopulmonary bypass. The operation is performed through a median sternotomy. Vascular clamps are applied across the four sites of anastomosis (i.e. aorta, pulmonary artery, right atrium and left atrium), the donor tissue divided and excised, and the residual cuffs of tissue oversewn. There have been no complications associated with leaving cuffs of donor aorta or atria in the chest.

If a second heterotopic heart transplant is anticipated, the vacated cavity of the right chest has been maintained by filling it with a suitable foreign body, such as a silastic breast prosthesis. If this is not done, the space will fill with blood and other fluid and dense adhesions will form, making subsequent heterotopic transplantation exceedingly difficult, if not impossible.

POSTOPERATIVE CARE AND IMMUNOSUPPRESSION

The immediate postoperative care of patients who have undergone retransplantation does not differ significantly from that following the initial procedure (Chapter 12). If retransplantation is performed during or immediately following an irreversible acute rejection episode, care must be taken not to over-immunosuppress the patient, as he will almost certainly already have received a considerable amount of immunosuppressive therapy; preoperative 'loading' doses of the various drugs are probably unnecessary.

RESULTS OF RETRANSPLANTATION

In patients with orthotopic allografts

There are relatively few reports of series of patients undergoing retransplantation. Between January 1968 and March 1980, 202 hearts were transplanted in 185 patients at Stanford University Medical Center. Sixteen patients with orthotopic allografts received second transplants, eight for accelerated atherosclerotic coronary disease, six for unrelenting acute rejection, and two for dysrhythmia or right ventricular failure[4]. One patient required a third transplant because of donor left ventricular ischemia. All sequential transplants were managed similarly to the primary transplant.

Of the 16 initial transplant hearts at risk, 60% functioned for more than 1 year, and 57% for more than 2 years; these results were similar at that time to heart survival in patients not requiring retransplantation. Of the secondary transplant hearts at risk, however, only 31% survived for more than 1 year and 29% for more than 2 years, survival of approximately only 50% when compared with the primary group. The mortality was due largely to severe infection, and the development of malignant tumors.

Infection of the secondary transplant (retransplant) patient appeared to play a more dominant role in fatality. The patients in this group were suspected to be initially free of infection in spite of primary allograft immunotherapy. The number and type of infections, however, were not substantially different from those in the group receiving primary transplantation. Prolonged periods of immunosuppression during the perioperative period of the secondary transplant exposed these patients to this complication.

The Stanford group concluded that sequential orthotopic cardiac transplantation offers an acceptable alternative to patients with allograft failure, though survival was not as favorable because of the prolonged immunosuppression required.

In patients with heterotopic allografts

In the Cape Town series of nine sequential transplants[8], there were no operative deaths, though the procedures were difficult whenever the heterotopic donor heart required removal (techniques 1 and 3). Two patients died, however, after 24 days and 3 months, from bacterial pneumonias, and one hyperimmunized patient lost graft function after 5 days from accelerated acute rejection, but survived a further 17 months before dying from his underlying cardiomyopathy. Of the two patients who underwent a third transplant, one died after 1 month from aspergillus sepsis. At the time of this report, three of the four surviving patients remained well at 25, 33 and 64 months after their second operation, and one remained well some 4 months after his third transplant, having survived a total of 38 months following the second procedure.

In this small series, certain factors were considered which might influence survival.

Operative technique

Removal of the original donor heart, a technically difficult procedure with potential complications of bleeding and air leak, was followed by a higher morbidity and mortality than when this organ was left *in situ* and the second graft inserted in the orthotopic position.

Cause of failure of first transplant

Patients who were retransplanted for acute rejection did less well than those retransplanted for chronic rejection. This was possibly related to the immune status of the patient at the time of retransplantation, but in this small series was more readily explained on the basis of the immunosuppressive therapy available to the patient at the time of transplantation.

Immunosuppressive therapy

Of the four patients who continued to receive immunosuppression with only azathioprine and methylprednisolone after retransplantation, only one was a long-term survivor. Of the four patients in whom therapy was changed to include CsA at the time of the second intervention, three of four proved to be long-term survivors.

Two patients in this series survived with two donor hearts within their chest, the first (heterotopic) donor heart having been left *in situ*, and the patient's own heart having been replaced[5,8]. It was anticipated that the first donor heart, though severely affected by graft atherosclerosis, might lend support to the second donor organ should it be compromised by a severe acute rejection episode. In addition, in one of these two patients, the donor heart was taken from a 14-year-old girl weighing only 22 kg. Since the recipient weighed 56 kg it was felt that the small size of the donor heart might be insufficient to support the entire circulation alone during the initial few weeks or months, and the first donor heart might lend some support throughout this period, during which time the second donor heart would gradually hypertrophy. The first donor heart, affected as it was by severe graft atherosclerosis, eventually ceased to function. The retention of a chronically rejected, non-functioning heart did not cause problems.

From this experience, we would recommend that the first donor organ is left *in situ*, and that the recipient's own heart should be replaced at the second operation (Figures 20.2 and 20.3). This would also seem to be the operation of choice at third and subsequent procedures. The risk of major thromboembolism from a poorly or non-functioning heterotopic heart would seem small as long as anticoagulation is maintained (Chapter 23).

COMMENT

Though the technical problems faced in retransplantation, particularly in patients with an existing heterotopic heart transplant, are considerable, and, therefore, the risk of early postoperative complications probably increased, it would seem that retransplantation is certainly a worthwhile procedure, particularly since the introduction of CsA. The present indications for heterotopic heart transplantation are relatively few (Chapter 23) and, as reoperation in such patients is difficult, we believe that this procedure should only be performed when there is a definite contraindication to orthotopic transplantation.

References

1. Copeland, J.G., Griepp, R.B., Beiber, C.P., Billingham, M., Schroeder, J.S., Hunt, S., Mason, J., Stinson, E.B. and Shumway, N.E. (1977). Successful retransplantation of the human heart. *J. Thorac. Cardiovasc. Surg.*, **73**, 242
2. Baumgartner, W.A., Reitz, B.A., Oyer, P.E., Stinson, E.B. and Shumway, N.E. (1979). Cardiac homotransplantation. *Curr. Probl. Surg.*, **16**, 1
3. Copeland, J.G. and Stinson, E.B. (1979). Human heart transplantation. *Curr. Probl. Cardiol.*, **4**, 4
4. Watson, D.C., Reitz, B.A., Oyer, P.E., Stinson, E.B. and Shumway, N.E. (1980). Sequential orthotopic heart transplantation in man. *Transplantation*, **30**, 401
5. Novitzky, D., Cooper, D.K.C. and Barnard, C.N. (1984). Orthotopic heart transplantation in a patient with a heterotopic heart transplant. *Heart Transplant.*, **3**, 257
6. Novitzky, D., Cooper, D.K.C., Lanza, R.P. and Barnard, C.N. (1985). Further cardiac transplant procedures in patients with heterotopic heart transplants. *Ann. Thorac. Surg.*, **39**, 149
7. Wahlers, Th., Frimpong-Boateng, K., Haverich, A., Schafers, H.-J., Fieguth, H.G., Coppola, R., Jurmann, M. and Borst, H.G. (1986). Management of immediate graft failure after cardiac transplantation using cardiopulmonary bypass and intra-aortic balloon-pumping followed by cardiac retransplantation. *Thorac. Cardiovasc. Surg.*, **34**, 389
8. Novitzky, D., Cooper, D.K.C., Brink, J.G. and Reichart, B.A. (1987). Sequential – second and third – transplants in patients with heterotopic heart allografts. *Clin. Transplant.*, **1**, 57
9. Morris, J.S., Lower, R.R. and Szentpetery, S. (1987). Immediate graft failure treated with partial cardiopulmonary bypass and emergency cardiac retransplantation. *Transplant. Proc.*, **19**, 2497
10. Lanza, R.P., Campbell, E., Cooper, D.K.C., Du Toit, E. and Barnard, C.N. (1983). The problem of the presensitized heart transplant recipient. *Heart Transplant.*, **2**, 151
11. Novitzky, D., Cooper, D.K.C., Rose, A.G. and Barnard, C.N. (1984). The value of recipient heart assistance during severe acute rejection following heterotopic cardiac transplantation. *J. Cardiovasc. Surg.*, **25**, 287
12. Cooper, D.K.C., Charles, R.P., Fraser, R.C., Beck, W. and Barnard, C.N. (1980). Long-term survival after orthotopic and heterotopic cardiac transplantation. *Br. Med. J.*, **281**, 1093
13. Rose, A.G., Uys, C.J., Cooper, D.K.C. and Barnard, C.N. (1982). Donor heart morphology 12 1/2 years after orthotopic transplantation. *Heart Transplant.*, **1**, 329

21
Malignant Neoplasia in the Immunocompromised Patient
I. PENN

INTRODUCTION

With the proliferation of centers performing cardiac and cardiopulmonary transplantation, it is increasingly important that cardiologists and cardiac surgeons be familiar with the complications of such therapy. One of these is an increased risk for the development of certain types of cancer. Most of this chapter is based on experience obtained from renal transplantation, but, whenever possible, observations made in cardiac or cardiopulmonary graft recipients will be stressed. The report is based on data collected by the Cincinnati Transplant Tumor Registry (CTTR) until January, 1988.

We shall consider three categories of malignancies: (1) transplanted cancers; (2) pre-existing tumors that were present in the recipient before transplantation; and (3) *de novo* malignancies that developed in the recipient after transplantation.

TRANSPLANTED MALIGNANCIES

When assessing a potential cadaver donor for harvesting of the heart or heart and lungs, it is obligatory to determine whether or not he or she has cancer, or has been treated for it recently, as there is a danger of transmitting tumor cells with the transplanted organ(s)[1-4]. Under ordinary conditions, such foreign cells would be rejected promptly by the recipient. The immunosuppressive therapy used to prevent the graft(s) from being rejected, however, may also impair the host's immune defenses, and thus inhibit the destruction of the cancer cells, which may grow, invade adjacent structures, and even metastasize.

The CTTR has data on 113 recipients of organs from donors who had malignancies at the time of donation, or had been treated for them up to 5 years before transplantation, or who, in the case of several living donors, presented with neoplasms up to 2 years after donation. Donors with primary tumors confined to the brain were excluded from the study. After transplantation, 52 recipients (46%) developed malignancies identical to those in their original donors. These were confined to the allograft in 17 patients, while in another four there was invasion of adjacent structures. Thirty-one recipients had distant metastases, most of whom died of their neoplasms.

In the entire series, there were three cardiac transplant recipients. One patient is free of cancer, although three other recipients of organs from the same donor developed metastatic choriocarcinoma. The other two patients died of metastases from inadvertently-transplanted bronchial carcinoma and medulloblastoma respectively. In the latter case, the cerebellar tumor in the donor had been treated with a ventriculo–atrial shunt (see below).

Immunologic rejection of locally invasive or distantly metastatic cancer may occur if immunosuppressive therapy is discontinued and the tumor burden reduced by removing the neoplastic graft. While this has been successfully accomplished in five renal transplant recipients[1-4], it is not feasible in cardiac allograft patients unless an implantable artificial heart can be used, either as a permanent replacement, or for a period of several months until all evidence of malignancy has disappeared and a new cardiac allograft can be inserted.

It is, therefore, imperative to avoid using donors with tumors, except those with low-grade carcinomas of the skin or primary brain malignancies, which rarely spread outside the central nervous system. It is important, however, to have histologic proof that the cancers actually arose in the brain, as, in several instances, the cause of the donor's death was misdiagnosed as intracranial hemorrhage, cerebral angioma, or primary brain tumor, when, in fact, the donor died of metastases from choriocarcinoma, renal cell carcinoma, or bronchial carcinoma. We should also avoid using donors with primary brain tumors who have been treated with ventriculo–peritoneal or ventriculo–venous shunts, as these open pathways for dissemination[3,4].

PRE-EXISTING MALIGNANCIES

If a neoplasm were treated before transplantation, it is possible that the immunosuppressive therapy may impair the ability of the host's immune defenses to control any residual cancer cells. In a study of 427 patients who underwent renal transplantation and had been treated previously for tumors of the kidney or other organs, there was a 26% recurrence rate after transplantation[5]. In a few instances, recurrences occurred despite removal of the primary malignancy as long as 5–10 years beforehand. It was, therefore, recommended that, with the exception of patients with incidentally-discovered renal malignancies, non-melanoma skin cancers, or low-grade papillary thyroid carcinomas, transplantation should be delayed for at least 24 months after treatment of the tumors. During this time, renal transplant candidates can be kept alive by dialysis.

As regards potential cardiac transplant recipients, current experience with the artificial heart makes it extremely unlikely that they can be kept alive during this long waiting period. Because of the hopeless prognosis of potential cardiac allograft recipients who do not receive transplants, it is probably advisable to proceed expeditiously with transplantation as soon as a donor heart becomes available, except in individuals whose life expectancy is short because of the neoplastic disease.

Eighteen cardiac transplant recipients with pre-existing malignancies have been reported to the CTTR. Of 14 treated from 21.5 to 138.5 (average 93) months before transplantation, none has yet developed recurrence of the original neoplasm. In three other patients, the time of treatment of the neoplasm before transplantation is unknown. Of these three, one, with a basal cell carcinoma of the skin, developed multiple recurrences after transplantation. This is not surprising, as 53% of renal transplant recipients with pre-existing skin cancers developed recurrences after transplantation[5]. The final patient in the series of 18 had a lung cancer removed a few days after transplantation; apparently the tumor was not completely resected, and the patient died of the malignancy 11.5 months after transplantation.

Length of follow-up of the 18 patients ranged from 0.5 to 39 (average 14) months; in view of the short length of follow-up, it is possible that other patients may develop recurrences of their tumors in the future.

DE NOVO TUMORS

Incidence

The CTTR has data on 3398 patients who developed cancers *de novo* after transplantation[1,2,6]. Of these, 104 received heart (one also received a kidney) and three combined heart and lung allografts. There were also 3233 kidney transplant recipients and 58 recipients of other organs.

Data from several large renal transplant centers show an overall incidence of cancer ranging from 2 to 16%, with an average of 6%[1,2]. In a series of 182 cardiac transplant recipients who underwent 199 transplantations, the incidence was 10%[7]. Lanza et al.[8] compared the incidence of malignancies in cardiac and renal allograft recipients at the University of Cape Town. They found a two-fold greater increase of all neoplasms in the cardiac patients, with nearly a six-fold increase of visceral tumors ($p < 0.02$). They attributed the increased incidence to the more intensive immunosuppressive therapy used in the cardiac allograft recipients.

The number of patients who develop cancer increases with the length of follow-up after transplantation. A study of 3846 Australasian renal transplant recipients showed an incidence of 3% at 1 year, 14% at 5 years, and 49% at 14 years[9]. In 124 cardiac allograft patients, the actuarial risk of developing cancer was $2.7 \pm 1.9\%$ at 1 year, and $25.6 \pm 11.0\%$ at 5 years[10]. These figures underline the need to follow transplant patients indefinitely.

Age of recipients

Many of the patients were young at the time of transplantation. The average age was 40 years with a range from 5 months to 80 years. A total of 48% were aged 40 or younger.

Sex of recipients

Males made up two-thirds and females one-third of the patients with cancer, roughly the same proportions as those undergoing renal transplantation in general.

Time of appearance of the neoplasm

In the general population there is a latent period of 5–20 years, or even more, between exposure to many carcinogens and the development of malignancies. In transplant patients, however, tumors appear after a much shorter interval, at an average of 59 months[1,2].

Some cancers appear at fairly distinct intervals after transplantation[1,2]. Kaposi's sarcoma (KS) presents the earliest, at an average of 21 (range 2–225.5) months after transplantation. Lymphomas appear at an average of 36 (range 1–196.5) months, other neoplasms (excluding carcinomas of the vulva and perineum) 65 (range 1–253) months, and carcinomas of the vulva and perineum appear at the longest interval after transplantation at an average of 100 (9–241.5) months.

Types of tumors

Table 21.1 lists the neoplasms reported to the CTTR. The malignancies commonly seen in the general population, involving the bronchus, prostate, colon and rectum, female breast, and invasive carcinoma of the uterine cervix, are not increased in frequency in organ transplant recipients[1,2,6]. Instead, there is a disproportionately high incidence of certain neoplasms, particularly carcinomas of the skin and lips, lymphomas, Kaposi's sarcoma, *in situ* carcinomas of the uterine cervix, and carcinomas of the vulva and perineum[1,2,6,11,12].

These findings are confirmed by several epidemiological studies which show that, when transplant patients are compared with suitable age-matched controls, there is a 4–7-fold increase in skin cancer in people living in areas of low sunshine exposure, but a 21-fold increase in persons exposed to abundant sunshine[1,2]; a 29-fold increase in lip cancers[13]; a 28–49-fold increase in non-Hodgkin's lymphoma (NHLs)[14,15]; a 400–500-fold increase in Kaposi's sarcoma[16]; a 14-fold increase in carcinoma *in situ* of the uterine cervix[17]; and a 100-fold increase in carcinomas of the vulva and anus[13]. There are also small increases in incidence of carcinomas of the liver and biliary passages, leukemias, and carcinomas of the kidney[14,15].

Cancer of the skin and lips

Overall, these were the most common and comprised 1368 of the 3633 tumors (38%) (Table 21.1)[1,2]. An Australian study of 3846 renal transplant recipients showed that the incidence of skin cancer increased with the length of follow-up, with 11% having cancers at 5 years, 29% at 10 years, and 43% at 14 years[9]. Cardiac allograft recipients differ from the renal recipients in this series in that skin cancers were relatively uncommon, making up 23 of 109 (21%) of all tumors (Table 21.1). In part, this may be related to length of follow-up, which has been relatively short in many cardiac allograft recipients.

Several features distinguish the skin cancers of transplant patients from those in the general population[1,2,6,9]. Whereas basal cell carcinomas (BCCs) outnumber squamous cell carcinomas (SCCs) in the general population, the reverse occurs in CTTR patients in whom SCCs comprised 51% and BCCs 28%. (Another 14% had both types of malignancy.) Of the cardiac transplant recipients with skin cancers, 17 had SCCs, three had BCCs and three had SCCs and BCCs. In the population at large, non-melanoma skin cancers occur mostly in individuals in their sixties and seventies, whereas the average age of transplant patients is 30 years younger[1,2].

Multiple skin cancers occurred in 43% of patients in the CTTR. This incidence is remarkably high, and is comparable to that seen only in people in the general population who live in areas of abundant sunshine[1,2]. Several patients each had more than 100 skin cancers.

Malignant melanomas comprised 4.7% of skin cancers in the CTTR, in contrast with an incidence of 2.7% in the general population of the United States. This finding is consistent with an Australian study showing a five-fold higher incidence of malignant melanoma in transplant patients compared with age-matched controls[9]. Thus far, no melanomas have been reported in cardiac allograft recipients.

Most skin cancers in the CTTR were of low-grade malignancy, but a significant percentage of SCCs behaved much more aggressively than their counterparts in the general population[1,2,6,9]. Lymph node metastases occurred in 91 patients (7%), 75 of whom had SCCs, 12 of whom had malignant melanoma, and four of whom had other malignancies. Eighty patients (6%) died of their skin cancers, 52 with SCCs, 26 with malignant melanomas, one with BCC and one with Merkel's cell tumor. These findings are consistent with a more than 10-fold increase in mortality from SCCs of the skin observed in Australian renal transplant recipients[14]. The behavior of skin cancer in transplant patients is markedly different from that seen in the general population, in whom they cause only 1–2% of all cancer deaths, the great majority of which are from malignant melanoma.

Table 21.1 Most common types of *de novo* cancers in organ allograft recipients

Type of cancer	Non-cardiac recipients*	Cardiac recipients†
Cancers of skin and lips	1345	23
Lymphomas	441	56
Carcinomas of uterine cervix	182	0
Carcinomas of the lung	176	6
Kaposi's sarcomas	154	5
Carcinomas of colon and rectum	125	2
Carcinomas of breast	121	1
Carcinomas of the kidney	112	1
Carcinomas of vulva, perineum, penis or scrotum	98	1
Head and neck carcinomas (excluding thyroid, parathyroid and eye)	97	1
Leukemias	84	2
Metastatic carcinomas (primary site unknown)	81	1
Carcinomas of urinary bladder	81	1
Cancers of liver and bile ducts	58	0
Cancers of thyroid gland	50	0
Sarcomas (excluding Kaposi's)	44	1
Cancers of testis	43	0
Cancers of prostate	40	2
Cancers of stomach	39	1
Cancers of ovary	34	1
Cancers of pancreas	28	2
Miscellaneous cancers	91	2
Total	3524	109

*More than one type of tumor affecting different organs occurred in 219 patients, of whom 12 each had three separate types of cancer and one had four
†Two cardiac transplant recipients had two separate types of neoplasm

Most patients with SCCs who developed lymph node metastases, or who died of their cancers, had skin, rather than lip, lesions. In the overall series of patients with complications of their SCCs were three cardiac allograft recipients who developed lymph nodes metastases, two from lesions of the lip, and one from a lesion of the scalp. The two patients with lip cancers ultimately died of widely metastatic tumor.

Lymphomas

In the general population, lymphomas make up 3–4% of all cancers[1,2]. Their incidence is disproportionately increased in organ transplant recipients, in whom they comprised 497 of 3633 tumors (14%) (Table 21.1). If we exclude non-melanoma skin cancers and *in situ* carcinomas of the uterine cervix, which are omitted from most cancer statistics, the corrected incidence of lymphomas is 19%.

A remarkable feature of the cardiac transplant recipients in the CTTR is that lymphomas were the predominant tumor among them, comprising 56 of 109 neoplasms (51%) (Table 21.1). This is also a feature of recipients of other extrarenal organs (liver, pancreas, and bone marrow), in whom lymphomas comprised 45 of 58 neoplasms (78%). In contrast, lymphomas made up only 396 of 3466 tumors in renal transplant recipients (11%).

The most likely explanation for these striking differences is in the intensity of immunosuppression. When a renal transplant recipient has severe problems with rejection the physician can abandon efforts to save the transplant, discontinue the immunosuppression, and place the patient on dialysis. In contrast, when a cardiac or liver allograft is being rejected, every effort is made to reverse the process, as frequently it is not possible to obtain another cardiac or liver allograft to replace the one whose function is deteriorating. The consequence is that these patients tend to be heavily immunosuppressed during acute rejection episodes, usually in the first few months after transplantation, which is the time when most lymphomas occur.

This viewpoint is supported by a study of 75 survivors of heart and heart–lung transplantation who were treated with cyclosporine and prednisone, and in some instances antithymocyte globulin. Lymphomas occurred in six patients. Measured quantitative parameters of immunosuppression during the first 3 months after transplantation (mean cyclosporine level, total antithymocyte globulin dosage, number of days of T-cell suppression, and mean cyclosporine level during T-cell suppression) were higher in patients with lymphomas than in those who did not develop tumors[18].

In the overall series, the lymphomas were strikingly different from those seen in the general population[1,2]. The majority (92%) were non-Hodgkin's lymphomas (NHLs), whereas Hodgkin's disease is the most common lymphoma seen in the same age group in the general population.

Morphologically, most NHLs were reticulum cell sarcomas or large cell lymphomas. Of tumors studied by modern immunological techniques, 85% arose from B-lymphocytes, 14% were T-cell lymphomas, and 1% arose from null cells. Whereas extranodal involvement was reported in from 24% to 48% of NHL patients in the community at large, it occurred in 72% of NHLs in transplant patients. Furthermore, extranodal disease was confined to a single organ in 64% of the CTTR patients; most frequently the brain was involved.

In the general population, about 1% of NHLs involve the brain whereas in organ allograft recipients 32% affected the central nervous system (CNS), usually the brain. Spinal cord involvement was rare. Brain lesions frequently were multicentric in distribution. Another unusual feature was that in 67% of patients with CNS involvement the lesions were confined to the brain, whereas in the general population brain tumors are frequently associated with lymphomas in other viscera. A possible explanation for the highly unusual pattern of brain involvement is that this organ has poor immunologic reactions, so that lymphoma cells that arise in it, or are carried there from other sites, grow more readily in this relatively immunologically-privileged site than in other viscera[1,2].

A CNS lymphoma should be suspected whenever a transplant patient presents with neurologic symptoms[1,2]. A thorough work-up is necessary to exclude more common causes of these symptoms in these patients, including hypertensive encephalopathy, meningitis, brain abscess, or intracranial bleeding. Studies may include electroencephalography, brain scan, computerized axial tomography, examination of the cerebrospinal fluid, cerebral angiography, and magnetic resonance imaging.

Epstein–Barr virus (EBV) DNA has been isolated from some B-cell lesions in transplant recipients[19]. In immunosuppressed individuals it is believed to cause a spectrum of lesions, ranging from benign polyclonal B-cell hyperplasias on the one hand, to frank monoclonal B-cell lymphomas on the other[19]. We do not know the cause(s) of T-cell lymphomas in transplant patients.

Kaposi's sarcoma (KS)

KS comprise 159 of the 3633 cancers in the CTTR (4.3%) (Table 21.1). If we omit non-melanoma skin cancers and *in situ* carcinomas of the uterine cervix, then KS makes up 6.2% of neoplasms compared with its incidence in the general population of the United States of only 0.02–0.07% of all tumors (before the AIDS epidemic started)[1,2,11]. Among cardiac transplant recipients in the CTTR, KS composed 4.9% of all malignancies.

In the CTTR, patients with KS ($n = 159$) exceeded those with two common cancers, carcinomas of the colon/rectum ($n = 127$) and breast ($n = 122$), a remarkably high incidence[1,2,11]. Apart from individuals with AIDS, in which KS is enormously increased[11], there is probably no other series in which the numbers of KS patients exceed those with either of these two common cancers, except possibly in tropical Africa, where KS is common and colon cancer is infrequent.

KS was most common in organ transplant recipients who were Arabic, Jewish, black, or of Mediterranean ancestry[1,2,11]. Two-thirds had 'benign' KS, involving the skin, conjunctiva, or oropharyngolaryngeal mucosa, and one-third had the 'malignant' variety, with involvement of internal organs, most commonly the gastrointestinal tract and lungs[1,2,11].

After treatment, complete remissions occurred in 47 of the 96 patients (49%) with 'benign' disease. Whereas 32 remissions followed surgery, radiotherapy, or chemotherapy, 15 (32%) occurred when the *only* treatment was a drastic reduction of immunosuppressive therapy. In the malignant group, only six of the 63 patients (10%) had complete remissions after chemotherapy or radiotherapy, together with alteration of immunosuppressive therapy; only one patient had complete remission following cessation of immunosuppression only.

Of the five cardiac allograft recipients with KS, three had visceral disease and two non-visceral involvement. One patient in each category is currently alive.

Carcinomas of the uterine cervix

Carcinomas of the cervix occurred in 182 of the 1210 women in this series (15%) (Table 21.1). At least 78% were *in situ* lesions[1,2,17]. Thus far, none has affected cardiac allograft recipients. Nevertheless, it is advisable that all post-adolescent female patients have regular pelvic examinations and cervical smears to detect such lesions and also carcinomas of the vulva and perineum[1,2,12,17].

Carcinomas of the vulva and perineum

Carcinomas of the vulva, perineum, scrotum, penis, perianal skin, and anus occurred in 99 patients (68 women and 31 men) (Table 21.1)[1,2,12]. If non-melanoma skin cancers and *in situ* carcinomas of the uterine cervix are excluded, then carcinomas of the vulva and perineum constitute 4% of neoplasms in the CTTR, a much higher incidence than in the community at large. When compared with people with similar lesions in the general population, who are mostly in their sixties and seventies, the transplant patients were surprisingly young. The average age of the women at the time of transplantation was 29 (range 15–55) years, and of the men 37 (range 20–60 years).

In women there was sometimes a 'field effect', with involvement by cancer of the vulva, vagina, uterine cervix, and anus in varying combinations[1,2,12]. In some patients, a possible viral etiology of these malignancies is suggested by a preceding history of condyloma acuminatum and, less frequently, herpes genitalis[12]. Small neoplasms were treated by local excision. Large lesions required extensive operations, such as total vulvectomy and inguinal node dissection, or abdomino-perineal resection[12].

Multiple cancers

As can be seen from Table 21.1, only two cardiac transplant recipients had more than one different type of cancer involving different organs. Furthermore, none of the other non-renal transplant recipients had more than one type of malignancy. In contrast, multiple tumors were common in the 3233 renal allograft recipients, of whom 219 (6.8%) had more than one type of cancer, including 12 with three separate tumors, and one with four.

No doubt the much longer length of follow-up of the renal transplant patients permitted the development of additional malignancies. With prolonged follow-up of cardiac or cardiopulmonary transplant recipients, one should probably expect the same pattern to emerge.

Cyclosporine (CsA)-related malignancies

Since CsA has become the leading immunosuppressive agent in current use, concern has been expressed about its carcinogenic potential. With the limited experience gained thus far, it appears that the incidence of cancers following its use is no higher than with conventional immunosuppressive therapy (CIT), involving azathioprine and/or cyclophosphamide with prednisone or prednisolone, and, sometimes, antilymphocyte globulin[6,20].

The types of malignancies and their clinical behavior, however, show significant differences between the two forms of therapy[6]. We may compare 453 CsA-related tumors (in 444 patients – some patients had more than one type of neoplasm) with 3180 (in 2954 patients) that followed CIT[6]. The average time of appearance of all tumors after CIT was 65 (range 1–253) months, whereas the neoplasms that followed CsA administration occurred much earlier after transplantation, at an average of only 26 (range 1–234) months.

Of the CsA-related malignancies, a disproportionately high number occurred in recipients of extrarenal organs[6]. A total of 102 of the 444 patients (23%) received transplants of either the heart or heart–lung ($n = 61$), liver ($n = 28$), bone marrow ($n = 7$), or pancreas ($n = 6$). In contrast, only 63 of 2954 CIT patients (2%) were recipients of extrarenal organs. Most of the CsA-related cancers that occurred in extrarenal organ recipients (69 of 102 or 68%) were lymphomas. In fact, 69 of 131 CsA patients (53%) who developed lymphomas received extrarenal organs.

Skin cancers were the most common malignancies seen

after CIT, and comprised 40% (1272 of 3180) of tumors, whereas they comprised 96 of 453 CsA-related tumors (21%). In CIT patients SCCs outnumbered BCCs by 1.9 to 1. In CsA patients, the ratio of SCCs to BCCs was only 1.1 to 1. No CsA patient with skin cancer has yet developed lymph node metastases or died of the cancer, in contrast with the disturbing statistics (described in an earlier section) in CIT patients.

Lymphomas appeared a remarkably short time after transplantation in the CsA group, at an average of 12 (range 1–160) months compared with 45 (range 1–196.5) months after CIT. The CsA-related NHLs showed several important differences from those following CIT. In the CIT group, the great majority (78%) were extranodal and only 22% were nodal. The CsA group more closely resembled NHLs in the general population in that 44% were nodal and 56% extranodal. Small bowel involvement occurred in 10% in the CIT group, but in 24% of the CsA-related NHLs. The disease was localized to the small bowel in only 21% of the CIT group, but in 31% of the CsA group. A striking feature of NHLs in the CIT group was frequent involvement of the CNS, which occurred in 39%; of these, 70% were confined to the CNS. In contrast, only 13% of NHLs in the CsA group affected the CNS, and only 31% involved the CNS alone.

Epidemiologic studies have shown a 48-fold increase in mortality from lymphomas in CIT patients[14]. A gratifying feature of the NHLs in the CsA group is that the disease appeared to respond more readily to treatment than in the CIT group[6,21,22]. Complete regression of the lesions occurred in 35% of patients after various treatments, including reduction or cessation of immunosuppressive therapy, surgical excision, administration of acyclovir, radiation therapy, or chemotherapy. Eleven of the remissions occurred when the *only* treatment was reduction or cessation of immunosuppressive therapy. The great majority of the remissions occurred in patients whose disease was localized to a single organ.

There was a high incidence of KS in CsA patients (11% of all tumors). This figure became even more remarkable if non-melanoma skin cancers and *in situ* carcinomas of the uterine cervix were excluded, when the incidence rose to 14% in CsA patients versus 5% in CIT patients. The time of appearance of KS after transplantation was very short in CsA patients, averaging only 12 (range 2–21) months, compared with 24 (range 2–226) months in CIT patients.

There were 23 renal cancers among the 453 CsA-related neoplasms, twice the incidence seen in CIT patients, and much higher than their incidence in the general population[6]. In comparison with CIT patients, there was a relatively low incidence of *in situ* cervical carcinomas and cancers of the vulva and perineum in CsA patients. In part, this may be related to the relatively short length of follow-up of many CsA patients. Another possible explanation for their high incidence in CIT patients is that azathioprine has been shown to cause dysplastic changes in uterine cervical epithelium[17,23–25].

Why is there a heavy preponderance of NHLs and KS in CsA-treated patients as opposed to those receiving CIT? These are the tumors that appear in the early months of transplantation when immunosuppressive therapy is most intense. Probably their appearance signifies that many patients are being over-immunosuppressed[6,18,26,27]. Not only are we learning to use CsA, but we are learning to use it in combination with other potent immunosuppressive agents in triple, quadruple, and even quintuple treatment regimens. It is possible that with longer follow-up the other cancers mentioned above will manifest themselves; as already noted, skin cancers, in particular, show a progressive increase in incidence with the length of follow-up.

Treatment of *de novo* malignancies

In addition to standard therapy of the neoplasms, one must decide whether reduction or cessation of immunosuppressive therapy is necessary[1,2,11,12]. We know that cancers inadvertently transplanted with organ allografts, even when widely disseminated in the recipient, may regress completely when immunosuppressive therapy is discontinued and the cancerous allografts removed[1–4]. The immune system regains its ability to recognize and eliminate the foreign transplanted malignant cells.

Does such treatment help patients who have tumors arising from their own cells? As mentioned above, several cases of KS and several NHLs underwent complete regression after drastic reduction of immunosuppressive therapy. However, the CTTR has rarely received reports of remission of epithelial tumors following such treatment. Nevertheless, one may try to reduce immunosuppressive drug dosage in a patient with a highly malignant, or extensive, or advanced cancer, in the hope that the immune system may recover and help to eradicate the neoplasms. Before undertaking such therapy, however, the surgeon must weigh the risk of allograft rejection, which may mean return to dialysis therapy in renal allograft patients, but may be fatal in cardiac transplant recipients.

If patients need cytotoxic therapy for widespread cancers, it is advisable to stop or reduce azathioprine dosage during such treatment to prevent severe bone marrow toxicity[1,2]. As most cytotoxic agents have immunosuppressive side-effects, satisfactory allograft function may persist for long periods. Treatment with prednisone may be continued, as it is an important constituent of many cancer chemotherapy regimens.

Etiology of *de novo* malignancies

The causes of cancers in organ transplant recipients are not known, but a complex interplay of multiple factors is probably responsible[1,2]. A major role can be assumed for impaired immunity. Oncogenic viruses are also important, and may account for the short 'latent period' between transplantation and the development of many tumors.

Other factors that may play a role include: (1) possible carcinogenic effects of some immunosuppressive agents; (2) possible synergism of these agents with environmental carcinogens such as smoking, sunlight, radiation, food additives, etc.; (3) the administration of other potentially carcinogenic drugs to some renal transplant recipients (such as diphenylhydantoin or isoniazid); and (4) genetic susceptibility or resistance to certain types of neoplasia.

CONCLUSIONS

Although cancer is a complication of transplantation, it must be stressed that the great majority of organ transplant recipients do not develop this problem. Transplantation of malignancies nearly always can be avoided by careful selection of donors. Cardiac transplantation may be considered in patients who previously have been treated for cancers, except in those who have a short life-expectancy from their tumors.

Many patients who develop *de novo* cancers after transplantation have readily treatable *in situ* carcinomas of the cervix, low-grade skin cancers, and *in situ* cancers of the vulva and perineum (in one-third of this group of patients). With the limited experience gained thus far, however, cardiac transplant recipients appear to be more prone to develop potentially life-threatening malignancies, particularly lymphomas and cancers of various internal organs. Their occurrence may be related to the more intense immunosuppressive therapy that the physician is forced to give to some patients when compared that given to renal transplant recipients, in whom efforts to preserve a rejecting kidney may be abandoned in favor of a period of dialysis therapy, with no immunosuppressive therapy, until a second transplantation can be performed at a later date.

Acknowledgements

The author wishes to thank numerous colleagues, working in transplant centers throughout the world, who have generously contributed data concerning their patients to the Cincinnati Transplant Tumor Registry.

References

1. Penn, I. (1982). The occurrence of cancer in immune deficiencies. *Curr. Prob. Cancer*, **6**, 1
2. Penn, I. (1986). The occurrence of malignant tumors in immunosuppressed states. In Klein, E. (ed.) *Prog. Allergy*. Vol. 37, p. 259. (Basel: Karger)
3. Penn, I. (1986). Transmission of cancer with donor organs. *Transplant. Proc.*, **18**, 471
4. Penn, I. (1988). Transmission of cancer with donor organs. *Transplant Proc.*, **20**, 739
5. Penn, I. (1986). Kidney transplantation following treatment of tumors. *Transplant. Proc.*, **18** (Suppl. 3), 16
6. Penn, I. and Brunson, M.E. (1988). Cancers following cyclosporine therapy. *Transplant. Proc.*, **20** (Suppl. 3), 885
7. Weintraub, J. and Warnke, R.A. (1982). Lymphoma in cardiac allograft recipients. Clinical and histological features and immunological phenotype. *Transplantation*, **33**, 347
8. Lanza, R.P., Cooper, D.K.C., Cassidy, M.J.D. and Barnard, C.N. (1983). Malignant neoplasms occurring after cardiac transplantation. *J. Am. Med. Assoc.*, **249**, 1746
9. Sheil, A.G.R., Flavel, S., Disney, A.P.S. and Mathew, T.H. (1985). Cancer development in patients progressing to dialysis and renal transplantation. *Transplant. Proc.*, **17**, 1685
10. Krikorian, J.G., Anderson, J.L., Bieber, C.P., Penn, I. and Stinson, E.B. (1978). Malignant neoplasms following cardiac transplantation. *J. Am. Med. Assoc.*, **240**, 639
11. Penn, I. (1988). Kaposi's sarcoma – etiology: immunodeficiency. In Ziegler, J.L. and Dorfman, R.F. (eds.) *Kaposi's Sarcoma, Pathophysiology and Clinical Management*. p. 129. (New York: Marcel Dekker)
12. Penn, I. (1986). Cancers of the anogenital region in renal transplant recipients. Analysis of 65 cases. *Cancer*, **58**, 611
13. Blohme, I. and Brynger, H. (1985). Malignant disease in renal transplant patients. *Transplantation*, **39**, 23
14. Kinlen, L.J., Sheil, A.G.R., Peto, J. and Doll, R. (1979). Collaborative United Kingdom–Australasian study of cancer in patients treated with immunosuppressive drugs. *Br. Med. J.*, **2**, 1461
15. Kinlen, L. (1982). Immunosuppressive therapy and cancer. *Cancer Surveys*, **1**, 565
16. Harwood, A.R., Osaba, D., Hofstader, S.L., Goldstein, M.B., Cardella, C.J., Holecek, M.J., Kunynetz, R. and Giammarco, R.A. (1979). Kaposi's sarcoma in recipients of renal transplants. *Am. J. Med.*, **67**, 759
17. Porreco, R., Penn, I., Droegemueller, W., Greer, B. and Makowski, E. (1975). Gynecologic malignancies in immunosuppressed organ homograft recipients. *Obstet. Gynecol.*, **45**, 359
18. Brumbaugh, J., Baldwin, J.C., Stinson, E.B., Oyer, P.E., Jamieson, S.W., Bieber, C.P., Henle, W. and Shumway, N.E. (1985). Quantitative analysis of immunosuppression in cyclosporin-treated heart transplant patients with lymphoma. *Heart Transplant.*, **4**, 307
19. Hanto, D.W., Sakamoto, K., Purtilo, D.T., Simmons, R.L. and Najarian, J.S. (1981). The Epstein–Barr virus in the pathogenesis of post-transplant lymphoproliferative disorders. *Surgery*, **90**, 204
20. Cockburn, I. (1987). Assessment of the risks of malignancy and lymphomas developing in patients using Sandimmune. *Transplant. Proc.*, **19**, 1804
21. Makowka, L., Nalesnick, M., Streiber, A., Tzakis, A., Jaffe, R., Ho, M., Iwatsuki, S., Demetris, A.J., Griffith, B.P., Breinig, M.K. and Starzl, T.E. (1987). Control of post-transplant lymphoproliferative disorders and Kaposi's sarcoma by modulation of immunosuppression. In Good, R.A. and Lindenlaub, E. (eds.) *Symposia Medica Hoechst. The Nature, Cellular and Biochemical Basis and Management of Immunodeficiencies*. p. 567. (Stuttgart: F.K. Shattauer Verlag)
22. Starzl, T.E., Nalesnik, M.A., Porter, K.A., Ho, M., Iwatsuki, S., Griffith, B.P., Rosenthal, J.T., Hakala, T.R., Shaw, B.W. Jr., Hardesty, R.L., Atchison, R.W., Jaffe, R. and Bahnson, H.T. (1984). Reversibility of lymphomas and lymphoproliferative lesions developing under cyclosporine-steroid therapy. *Lancet*, **1**, 583
23. Gupta, P.K., Pinn, V.M. and Taft, D.D. (1969). Cervical dysplasia associated with azathioprine (Imuran) therapy. *Acta Cytol.*, **13**, 373

24. Kay, S., Frable, W.J. and Hume, D.M. (1970). Cervical dysplasia and cancer development in women on immunosuppressive therapy for renal homotransplantation. *Cancer*, **26**, 1048
25. Schramm, G. (1970). Development of severe cervical dysplasia under treatment with azathioprine (Imuran). *Acta Cytol.*, **14**, 507
26. Calne, R.Y., Rolles, K., White, D.J.G., Thiru, S., Evans, D.B., Henderson, R., Hamilton, D.L., Boone, N., McMaster, P., Gibby, O. and Williams, R. (1981). Cyclosporin-A in clinical organ grafting. *Transplant. Proc.*, **13**, 349
27. Editorial (1983). Cyclosporin and neoplasia. *Lancet*, **1**, 1083

22
Other Complications of Transplantation and Immunosuppressive Therapy

D.K.C. COOPER, J.S. MUCHMORE AND R.W. WELCH

INTRODUCTION

The fundamental problem associated with cardiac transplantation is undoubtedly the prevention and treatment of rejection, both acute and chronic. Anti-rejection therapy leads to complications, notably infection and, to a lesser extent, malignant tumor formation. There are many other potential complications, however, that are related to the transplantation operation or, particularly, to the immunocompromised status of the patient. These complications will be outlined and discussed below in the light of our own experience (at Oklahoma Transplantation Institute).

COMPLICATIONS OF THE OPERATION OF CARDIAC TRANSPLANTATION

Any of the complications of open heart surgery can, of course, occur following orthotopic or heterotopic transplantation. Technical complications are fortunately rare.

Hemorrhage

Hemorrhage is a potential early complication that may occur following the operation of either orthotopic or heterotopic transplantation. In both procedures there are long suture lines involving both low pressure venous systems and high pressure arterial systems. With care, however, postoperative bleeding should not be a major problem, though it may clearly be a major problem in patients undergoing transplantation of the heart and both lungs who have undergone previous operative procedures (Chapters 37 and 38).

Technical complications

In the preparation of the donor heart for both orthotopic and heterotopic transplantation, care must be taken to avoid the region of the sinoatrial node. In heterotopic heart transplantation, the recipient sinoatrial node must also be preserved.

Inadequate surgical technique may lead to narrowing at anastomotic suture lines, particularly following the rather more difficult operation of heterotopic heart transplantation; in this operation, faulty technique (or subsequent contraction from fibrosis) may result in narrowing of the superior vena cava–right atrial anastomosis, and may lead to difficulty in manipulating the endomyocardial bioptome into the donor right atrium. The avoidance of this problem is discussed in Chapter 11. Such narrowing may also result in hemodynamic derangement of the normal heterotopic heart transplant circulatory system. Blood returning from the systemic circulation will be directed almost entirely through the recipient right heart; after passage through the lungs, the blood will pass predominantly through the more compliant donor left ventricle. Though this circulation is unusual, the patient may remain asymptomatic.

Wound infection

Wound infection is fortunately relatively rare after major cardiac surgery, including transplantation, but can, of course, be potentially disastrous in the immunosuppressed patient.

Systemic and pulmonary emboli

Patients with poorly functioning orthotopic heart transplants (e.g. from acute or chronic rejection) are at risk of developing ventricular thrombi, which may be embolized into the pulmonary or systemic circulations. Pulmonary emboli have also been reported arising from a residual recipient right atrial appendage following orthotopic transplantation[1]; this appendage should be excised at operation.

A fatal paradoxical cerebral embolus (via an unnoticed patent foramen ovale in the donor atrial septum) resulted from a deep vein thrombosis in one of our patients; closure of any patent foramen ovale in either donor or recipient atrial septum should be carried out at operation in all cases.

The need to anticoagulate all patients with heterotopic heart transplants has been discussed in Chapter 23. Relatively few patients, however, have been seriously troubled by emboli; non-compliance of the patient with regard to meticulous attention to anticoagulant therapy has been a major contributing factor in almost all such cases. Again, poorly functioning ventricles are the sites of thrombus formation, though in these patients it is the native ventricles which are usually involved. (As the risk of thrombus formation (and infection) is clearly increased when a valve prosthesis is present, the presence of a prosthetic valve is now considered an absolute contraindication to heterotopic heart transplantation.)

COMPLICATIONS OF ENDOMYOCARDIAL BIOPSY

Endomyocardial biopsy is associated with an approximate 1–4% incidence of complication[2,3], though these have generally been minor complications such as pneumothorax and transient recurrent laryngeal nerve or brachial plexus paresis induced by local anesthesia.

A rare but potentially serious complication is perforation of the right ventricular myocardium at the time of taking the biopsy; acute cardiac tamponade may result. Thoracotomy may be required, though in patients with a heterotopic heart transplant intercostal tube drainage may be all that is required. Though it is fortunately a rare occurrence, occasionally the histopathologist will report that a biopsy shows epicardial fat or even normal lung; ventricular perforation has undoubtedly occurred and yet the patient has remained asymptomatic.

The development of a coronary artery–right ventricular fistula, thought to result from repeated biopsies in the same region[4-7], appears to be more common than hitherto suspected, being documented in 8% and 14% of patients, respectively in two reported series[4,5]. Though it rarely results in significant hemodynamic disturbance, it has on at least one occasion been associated with intractable failure necessitating retransplantation[7].

Pulmonary embolism (or systemic embolism in the case of left ventricular biopsy) from dislodgement of mural thrombus, which may result from decreased myocardial contractions due to rejection, is a potential hazard of endomyocardial biopsy following orthotopic or heterotopic transplantation. Ventricular ectopic activity induced by the catheter or bioptome frequently occurs, but is rarely more than transient.

The risk of introducing infection at the time of biopsy remains a potential hazard, but a sterile technique and the intravenous administration of a single dose of a suitable antibiotic (e.g. a cephalosporin) immediately before biopsy appears to minimize this risk.

COMPLICATIONS FROM IMMUNOSUPPRESSIVE DRUG THERAPY

The major potential complications of the various drugs presently used to immunosuppress patients with cardiac allografts are listed in Table 22.1.

Cyclosporine

Nephrotoxicity

Like many fungal antibiotics, cyclosporine (CsA) is nephrotoxic. The initial loading dose should be judged after considering the patient's general condition. In patients with already diminished renal function secondary to poor renal blood flow resulting from a low cardiac output, the initial dose of CsA should be withheld until the patient's renal function is clearly recovering after operation. A short period of hypotension during induction of anesthesia or during the operative procedure or early postoperative period, in the presence of a high blood level of CsA, can result in oliguria or anuria. Renal function usually recovers spontaneously as the CsA blood level falls, but even temporary dysfunction can be a major complicating factor in the early post-transplant period.

Impairment of renal function in cardiac transplant recipients often responds favorably to reducing the level of CsA and, when severe, to complete discontinuation of the drug for a short period[8]. Furosemide is also helpful in reversing the accompanying oliguria. Cyclosporine-induced nephrotoxicity appears to be relatively well tolerated, though short-term hemodialysis may be required on occasion. Close attention must be paid to monitoring both renal function and cyclosporine levels in the blood if the risk of renal failure is to be minimized.

Cyclosporine has also been reported to cause liver dysfunction, though it is doubtful whether this is a serious problem[9]. Liver dysfunction is usually dose-dependent and returns to normal levels when the dosage is reduced. More often, liver dysfunction in the early postoperative period reflects passive venous congestion.

Hypertension

Persistent hypertension has been noted as a complication of cyclosporine administration. Two years following cardiac transplantation fully 85% of patients may be expected to

Table 22.1 Major potential complications from immunosuppressive drug therapy

(1) *Cyclosporine*
    Nephrotoxicity
    Hypertension
    Neurotoxicity
    ? Hyperlipidemia
    Others (including hypertrichosis, gingival hyperplasia, tremor, hepatic dysfunction)

(2) *Azathioprine*
    Hematopoietic disorders (including leukopenia, thrombocytopenia, and anemia)
    Gastrointestinal disorders (including nausea and vomiting, hepatitis and biliary stasis)
    Others (including skin rashes, alopecia, fever, arthralgias, diarrhea, steatorrhea, and negative nitrogen balance)

(3) *Corticosteroids*
    Gastrointestinal disorders (including peptic ulcer, pancreatitis, and ulcerative esophagitis)
    Musculoskeletal disorders (including osteoporosis, vertebral compression fractures, pathological bone fractures, aseptic necrosis, muscle weakness, steroid myopathy, and loss of muscle mass)
    Endocrine disorders (including development of Cushingoid state, suppression of growth in children, menstrual irregularities, decreased carbohydrate tolerance and manifestations of latent diabetes mellitus, impotence)
    Metabolic disorders (including fluid and electrolyte disturbance and negative nitrogen balances, hyperlipidemia)
    Neurological disorders (including psychiatric complications and convulsions)
    Ophthalmic disorders (including cataracts, increased intraocular pressure, glaucoma and exophthalmos)
    Dermatological disorders (including acne, spontaneous hemorrhage, striae)

(4) *Antithymocyte globulin*
    Anaphylactic shock
    Others (including musculoskeletal pains, rash, fever, chills, and bronchospasm)

(5) *OKT3*
    Fevers, chills
    Aseptic meningitis
    Meningoencephalitis

(6) *Cyclophosphamide*
    Hematopoietic disorders (including leukopenia, thrombocytopenia, and anemia)
    Gastrointestinal disorders (including anorexia, nausea and vomiting)
    Genitourinary disorders (including sterile hemorrhagic cystitis)
    Gonadal suppression
    Pulmonary disorders (including interstitial pulmonary fibrosis)

have significant hypertension requiring treatment. Most are hypertensive in the first year, even if renal function appears normal. Its onset may be gradual over days or weeks, or at times, precipitous.

When rapid reduction in blood pressure is required, sublingual nifedipine (10 mg) is generally most effective. Nifedipine is often poorly tolerated, especially by older individuals, as long-term therapy.

Long-term therapy of hypertension in cardiac transplant patients is similar to standard antihypertensive treatment. Generally, blood pressure should be reduced below 155 mmHg systolic and 85 mmHg diastolic. Diuretics are used if needed for control of volume, but avoided if possible because of impairment of glucose tolerance, hypokalemia, hypomagnesemia, hyperuricemia, and adverse effects on cholesterol metabolism. The effects of agents that produce sedation (e.g. methyldopa) may also cause confusion when evaluating a patient who is experiencing weakness and fatigue.

We have found calcium channel antagonists (diltiazem, verapamil), central α-receptor stimulators (guanfacine, clonidine), and peripheral α-receptor blocking drugs (prazocin, terazocin) to be especially useful, alone or in any combination. Angiotensin converting enzyme (ACE) inhibiting medications (captopril, enalapril, lisinopril) may prove helpful additions to the antihypertensive regimen, though in some patients they have little effect. β-receptor blockers are less desirable, as it becomes more difficult to evaluate any changes in cardiac function. In many cases, hypertension is severe and requires the combination of three or more medications in full doses.

Occasionally, supine hypertension and orthostatic hypotension are encountered in patients with heterotopic cardiac transplants. Treatment is empirical. In our hands, diltiazem, starting with small (30 mg) doses, has been effective, perhaps because of the mild increase in circulating volume which accompanies this therapy. Treatment of the sitting/supine hypertension is not always possible without severe exacerbation of the orthostatic hypotension. Fortunately, the problem of orthostatic hypotension appears to diminish spontaneously with time.

Neuromuscular effects and neurotoxicity

Tremors, muscular weakness, and muscle cramps, particularly in the legs, are common and appear to occur more frequently in association with a low serum magnesium (Mg)[10,11]. Hypomagnesemia is common in cardiac transplant patients, possibly due to the renal effects of CsA. Hypomagnesemia may also lead to excessive cardiac irritability. We routinely monitor serum Mg and prescribe oral replacement therapy at a rate of 500–1500 mg Mg daily (in the form of magnesium oxide). The goal is to maintain the serum Mg at 0.8 mmol/l (1.5 mEq/l, 1.8 mg/dl) or greater. Tremor also improves when corticosteroid dosage is reduced, and muscle cramps improve when diuretic doses are reduced.

A neurotoxic effect of CsA, which occurs in patients with abnormally low serum levels of cholesterol, has been described following liver transplantation[12]. Clinical features consist of seizures, confusion, cortical blindness, quadriplegia, and coma. Computerized tomographic scanning and magnetic resonance imaging studies disclose a severe diffuse disorder of the white matter. All central nervous system effects and radiographic findings may be reversed by discontinuation or reduction of the dose of CsA.

We have recently seen severe neurological damage occur in a patient following transplantation of the heart and both lungs, who had a persistently low serum total cholesterol level[13]. It has since become our policy to reduce the dosage of CsA in patients with abnormally low serum levels of cholesterol. A substantial portion of the whole blood or serum content of CsA is carried in the low density lipoprotein (LDL) fraction of blood. It may be that when the LDL cholesterol is low, there is a higher proportion of CsA free in the serum.

Hypercholesterolemia

Some patients who have undergone heart transplantation will have underlying ischemic heart disease associated with persistent hypercholesterolemia. After transplantation, however, there is a significant increase in the serum cholesterol and triglycerides in the majority of patients[14-17]; this is believed to be related to cyclosporine and/or corticosteroid therapy. The average values for cholesterol and triglycerides, respectively in reported studies were 4.7 and 0.9 mmol/l (182 and 77 mg/dl) pretransplant and 6.2 and 2.3 mmol/l (240 and 200 mg/dl) post-transplant. Both post-transplant levels were moderately elevated, and might put the patients in a risk group for developing coronary artery disease at 2–3 times the normal rate. This risk, however, is further complicated by the possible influence of high cholesterol and/or triglyceride levels on the development of chronic rejection, so that the magnitude of accelerated risk is uncertain.

In one study, it was the LDL cholesterol level that was responsible for the main fraction of cholesterol[14]. The post-transplant cholesterol level was similar in those patients developing graft atherosclerosis (6.1 mmol/l, 236 mg/dl) and in those without graft atherosclerosis (5.8 mmol/l, 224 mg/dl). In contrast, the triglyceride level was 2.5 mmol/l (223 mg/dl) in those with coronary disease in the graft, but only 1.9 mmol/l (170 mg/dl) in the others, suggesting that the triglyceride component might be more reflective of the risk[14].

Our own policy in the management of patients who develop raised levels of cholesterol and triglycerides post-transplant is initially to encourage them to adhere strictly to an American Heart Association Phase II diet, which is low in cholesterol. If this fails to reduce cholesterol and triglyceride levels to within normal limits within 3 months, we prescribe a single cholesterol-lowering drug.

We originally chose probucol (500–1000 mg/day), but found that it was not uniformly successful. LDL levels were only moderately reduced, but so were HDL levels, increasing the LDL/HDL ratio, which was thought to be a less-than-ideal state for the patient. (Probucol was preferred to the bile acid sequestrant resins, such as cholestyramine and cholestipol, as it was believed that these might interfere with cyclosporine absorption. Preliminary observations, however, indicate that probucol administration may also be associated with a fall in the blood level of cyclosporine, necessitating increased dosages of the latter drug if therapeutic levels are to be maintained (Corder, C. et al., unpublished data).)

We were initially reluctant to use lovastatin in the treatment of hypercholesterolemia in our transplant patients because of the reported risk of rhabdomyolysis when this drug is administered to patients receiving cyclosporine[18,19]. Anecdotal reports from several centers, however, suggest that this drug can be safely prescribed in low doses (10–20 mg/day) and is effective in reducing total and LDL cholesterol levels in heart transplant patients. We have therefore recently begun to prescribe it at 20 mg/day, given late each evening, but it is too early yet for its effect to be accurately assessed. Should this dose of lovastatin prove inadequate to attain the desired result, it is our intention to add a bile acid sequestrant, taken in the morning.

Other side effects

A large number of other side effects of CsA has been described (Table 22.1).

Azathioprine

We have found azathioprine an easy and safe drug to use, and to be relatively free from serious complication, though its role in the occurrence of pancreatitis (see later) remains uncertain. It can be hepatotoxic. Whenever liver function abnormality is present, we have found it wise to use cyclophosphamide instead of azathioprine until function returns to normal.

Bone marrow suppression, involving both red and white cell precursors, has rarely proved a problem, as it develops slowly and recovers relatively quickly in the cardiac patient. Timely adjustment of dosage prevents severe suppression from occurring, though many patients remain mildly anemic.

Spontaneous hemorrhages into the skin (eccymoses) are commonly seen when azathioprine is used either alone or in combination with a corticosteroid; similar spontaneous bleeding can occur with corticosteroids alone.

Corticosteroids

The introduction of cyclosporine, by enabling greatly reduced steroid dosage, has reduced the incidence of complications of corticosteroid therapy, though they remain common.

Impotence/increased sexual appetite

There are few data available on the incidence of impotence following cardiac transplantation. In renal transplant series, however, impotence has been reported in 22–43% of male recipients[20]. Male potency is a complicated process, and the etiology of any impotency may be multifactorial.

Hypogonadotrophic hypogonadism occurs commonly immediately following cardiac transplantation or other open-heart surgery. We have documented reductions in serum testosterone from normal levels to levels at the lowest measurable limits in as few as 4 days following transplantation. The duration of this hypogonadism appears to vary with the clinical status of the patient. For those who suffer repeated illnesses, the hypogonadism will likely persist. Others who regain their vigor quickly may have a relatively few weeks of hypogonadism. Older patients have a more prolonged period of hypogonadism. Our patients who had cardiac transplantation prior to 1987 report impotence lasting from 2 weeks to several months following surgery.

Since 1987, we have routinely replaced testosterone following cardiac transplantation, mostly because low levels may be an important contributing factor in the rapid loss of trabecular bone which occurs in many patients. In this group, impotence is rarely reported. When it does occur, it is usually associated with prolonged illness, such as from cytomegalovirus infection, or psychological factors, which may include fear of immunological rejection or infection.

Erectile impotence, without loss of libido, may be reported by patients with extensive atherosclerotic vascular disease or peripheral neuropathy. Relative impotence may occur during the period of weaning from a prolonged course of testosterone replacement therapy. We normally wean replacement therapy by the third month post-transplant. Properly selected antihypertensive agents should rarely be a cause of impotence.

An increased sexual appetite is sometimes reported, and may equally lead to marital problems. Increased cardiac output will commonly restore lost potency, and an increased sexual appetite may follow the increased capability and improved feeling of well-being.

Diabetes mellitus

We have not considered uncomplicated diabetes to be a contraindication to transplantation, though we have not accepted the patient with significant diabetic complications, such as microvascular disease or neurotrophic foot ulcers. Some degree of impairment of glucose tolerance is seen in virtually all patients at some point in the transplantation process. Since the advent of convenient and rapid methods of estimating glucose in blood samples obtained by fingerstick, we have become more aware of the occurrence of hyperglycemia. In the post-transplant period, therefore, each patient must be willing to monitor his/her glycemia at home, keep records, and adjust therapy as prescribed. This has proved one more factor to complicate the daily life of the cardiac transplant patient.

It is easy to overlook the presence of diabetes or hyperglycemia in transplant patients since it is usually asymptomatic. We would emphasize the importance of routine monitoring of glycemia, particularly when corticosteroid therapy is instituted or increased. Certain patients will establish themselves as having a greater tendency towards hyperglycemia, and these patients should be monitored closely. Periodic monitoring of the glycosylated hemoglobin will help in identifying unacceptable hyperglycemia.

In its simplest form, hyperglycemia is seen in the first few days following transplantation during high-dose methylprednisolone therapy. It is seen again during the treatment of an acute rejection episode with methylprednisolone pulse therapy. In these circumstances, the hyperglycemia usually lasts only a few days. Without treatment, plasma glucose levels greater than 16.7 mmol/l (300 mg/dl) are commonly encountered. In the unproven belief that it is beneficial to maintain a near normal metabolic milieu, we routinely monitor and treat this hyperglycemia with the goal of maintaining glucose levels closer to 5.6 mmol/l (100 mg/dl), and certainly below 8.3 mmol/l (150 mg/dl). Granulocyte chemotaxis may be impaired at higher plasma glucose levels.

Some patients presenting for cardiac transplantation will have a pre-existing degree of impaired glucose tolerance

(IGT) or even frank diabetes. Those with long-standing congestive heart failure and its associated cachexia will have IGT. Typically, the pretransplant glycosylated hemoglobin ranges from 6.5 to 10% in this group. (Non-diabetics typically have a glycosylated hemoglobin of from 4.5 to 5.5%.) Following transplantation, the improved nutritional status of the patient, with restored vigor and muscular activity, is associated with resolution of the IGT. Usually, these patients require tapering doses of oral hypoglycemics in the first few post-transplant weeks only. Thereafter, they may display no sign of IGT or diabetes.

Many patients will present for transplantation with familial type II diabetes. The degree to which they display this diabetes will depend on several factors, which include (1) relative body masses of muscle and adipose, (2) diet, and (3) activity. Their diabetes can often be controlled with proper diet and activity. These persons are profoundly affected by pharmacological doses of corticosteroids. Until the corticosteroid dose is reduced to physiological levels, or eliminated entirely, treatment for diabetes will be required. In the long-term follow-up of such patients after reduction of corticosteroid dosage, those who follow the prescribed diet and activity instructions rarely require pharmacological treatment of their diabetes. Many patients, however, are unable or unwilling to follow such instructions, and require prolonged treatment, usually with oral agents.

At our own center, we have transplanted only one patient with uncomplicated type I diabetes. He has done well, but required large doses of insulin (< 300 Units daily) during the periods when he was taking corticosteroids in high or moderately high doses.

Rhenman et al.[21] described their experience with nine diabetic patients following cardiac transplantation. They found no statistically significant increase in infections, but encountered rejection episodes in all patients during the first month. Our experience regarding infection has been similar, but we have not encountered such a high incidence of rejection (Chapter 16).

Treatment of diabetes in the cardiac transplant patient is, as in other diabetics, largely empirical. In our own institution, we require home blood glucose monitoring, and prescribe a planned diet and exercise. Those patients with relatively normal fasting blood glucose levels, but with postprandial hyperglycemia, are given glipizide, which rarely produces fasting hypoglycemia. Those with fasting hyperglycemia are treated with glyburide. When these agents alone prove insufficient, regular (soluble) insulin is added before some or all meals. Some patients also require intermediate-acting insulin. As the patients' overall health improves, and corticosteroid dosages are lowered, the insulin may be phased out, and the diabetes treated with oral agents alone.

Good diabetic control is strongly encouraged. Our goal is to achieve pre-prandial glucose levels of 3.9–5.6 mmol/l (70–100 mg/dl) and 2 or 3 hours post-prandial glucose levels of less than 8.3 mmol/l (150 mg/dl). Not all patients are sufficiently disciplined to achieve these goals. In long-term follow-up, we monitor the glycosylated hemoglobin, the goal being to achieve levels of 7% or less. Levels of more than 8% are considered unacceptable. A glycosylated hemoglobin level of 9% would correspond approximately to an average glucose level of 8.3 mmol/l (150 mg/dl).

Osteoporosis and aseptic necrosis of bone

Aseptic necrosis of bone used to be a relatively common problem at many renal and cardiac transplantation centers, with an incidence varying from 4 to 41%[22-29], but since the introduction of CsA and reduction in corticosteroid dosage, it is fortunately now rare. The mechanism by which corticosteroids induce aseptic necrosis of bone is yet to be fully elucidated. There is considerable evidence from both experimental animals and man that steroids induce hyperlipidemia, fatty change of the liver, and consequent systemic fat embolization that leads to ischemic necrosis of bone[23]. Corticosteroids also induce loss of trabecular bone volume which may lead to trabecular collapse and subsequent bone necrosis[24,25].

The hip is the joint most commonly involved in aseptic necrosis, followed by the knee, shoulder, and elbow. Nonsurgical treatment includes reduction of the corticosteroid dosage to the lowest possible levels, and limitation of weight bearing by the affected joint for several months. Surgical treatment, in the form of joint replacement, may be necessary. At Stanford, approximately 2% of the early cardiac transplant patients developed aseptic necrosis of the head of the femur and required hip joint replacement[26,29].

Corticosteroid therapy is known to produce generalized osteoporosis. The effects are most evident in predominantly trabecular bone, such as the vertebral column, because this bone is metabolically the most active. The mechanism is not fully known. Factors believed to be causative include an increase in osteoclast-induced bone resorption, a decrease in bone matrix synthesis by osteoblasts, and a decrease in the intestinal absorption of calcium. At the Medical College of Virginia, 4% of the early cardiac transplant patients developed vertebral collapse[30], and at La Pitie Hospital in Paris 9% suffered from complications of osteoporosis[31].

At our own institution, we have seen two cases of severe and disabling multiple vertebral compression fracture syndrome (MVCF). Both patients responded gratifyingly to a regimen of reduced corticosteroid dosage, oral calcium therapy, and synthetic salmon calcitonin; pain and immobility resolved within 3 months, and no further compression fractures occurred. Since 1987, when we first noticed MVCF in our patients, we have monitored all cardiac transplant patients closely for evidence of trabecular bone osteoporosis. Our goals have been to learn more about the incidence and causes of osteoporosis and to prevent its more severe complications. This study has not yet been concluded, but some initial observations can be made.

Since 1987, all patients have been evaluated before and after transplantation (at intervals of 3-6 months) with single energy quantitated computed tomography of vertebral trabecular bone. All have received oral calcium therapy (800-1200 mg daily as calcium citrate). Hypogonadism, including the transient hypogonadism that may follow major surgery and illnesses, has been corrected using the appropriate sex steroid.

Pretransplant, many of the patients already demonstrated significant osteoporosis of trabecular bone. Densities of 60-110 mg of mineral per cubic centimeter of trabecular bone (versus a reference normal of 130-160 mg/cc) have been encountered commonly. The age of the patient and the duration and severity of congestive heart failure and other illnesses seem to be contributing factors; we also speculate that prior prolonged use of loop diuretics (which induce increased calcium excretion) may also contribute to the development of osteoporosis. A long history of smoking and heavy alcohol consumption may similarly be significant factors.

Following transplantation, some patients show only minimal (10-20%) further loss of trabecular bone, though others demonstrate severe loss to levels 50% or more below their pretransplant values. We have observed no patient who did not lose trabecular bone during the first 6 months following transplantation. Age, duration and severity of any posttransplant illnesses, and duration and severity of posttransplant hypogonadism all appear to be factors in the accelerated osteoporosis sometimes observed.

When a massive reduction in trabecular bone is documented (bone density falling to 70 mg/cc or less), we have instituted therapy with synthetic salmon calcitonin (50-100 IU subcutaneously daily). The response to this additional therapy has been variable; in some patients we have seen an improvement in bone density, in some stabilization of bone loss, and in others continued bone loss. Densities below 30 mg/cc have been observed in spite of calcitonin therapy, though in patients so treated we have not yet seen any instance of vertebral compression fracture. The side-effects of calcitonin therapy are minimal, consisting mostly of transient flushing and nausea, and can be reduced further by administering the medication subcutaneously; occasionally a reduction (or division) in dosage is required.

As greatly prolonged survival of transplant recipients is seen more frequently, osteoporosis may become an increasingly important development, if not complication. Much has yet to be learned of the treatment of osteoporosis in transplant patients as well as in the general population. Careful monitoring and treatment of this condition would seem important lest the development of MVCF complicates an otherwise successful cardiac rehabilitation program.

Growth retardation and delayed onset of puberty

Before the introduction of CsA, because of the complication of growth impairment, many renal, liver and cardiac transplantation units were reluctant to accept children as potential recipients. Growth retardation in children under the age of 12 or 13 could lead to such gross dwarfism that severe psychological problems ensued. The proportion of children who demonstrated normal growth following organ transplantation varied considerably from 13% to over 60% from one series to another[32,33].

Fortunately, it is now possible to immunosuppress some children without the need for steroid therapy (Chapter 24). In those that require steroids, there is some evidence that the growth retardation effect is minimized by administering a double dosage of steroids on alternate days with no therapy on intervening days[34,35].

Gastrointestinal tract complications

Several gastrointestinal diseases are not uncommon in the transplant patient. The severity and risks of these diseases are generally increased by corticosteroid therapy and, after heterotopic heart transplantation, by anticoagulation and anti-platelet therapy.

The first and most formidable of potential gastrointestinal tract complications is bleeding from the stomach or duodenum, which may result from the stress of surgery and/or prolonged high-dose steroid therapy. In general, endoscopic examination reveals the bleeding to be due to hemorrhagic gastritis or peptic ulceration.

Therapy for acute upper gastrointestinal tract bleeding is more complicated and hazardous in immunosuppressed patients, whether the treatment be by surgery or endoscopic thermal coagulation. We believe, therefore, that it is imperative to investigate and, where possible, treat all digestive diseases before transplantation. Peptic ulcer is the most important of these, and at our center all potential recipients are subjected to upper gastrointestinal tract evaluation if their cardiac condition allows such procedures. Upper or lower gastrointestinal endoscopy is today a benign procedure that can be tolerated by all except the most severely ill patients, and should not be postponed if indicated.

If the patient has no symptoms suspicious for acid peptic disease at the time of pretransplantation evaluation, an upper gastrointestinal tract radiological study is carried out. If acid peptic symptoms are present we prefer endoscopy because of its increased accuracy. When acid peptic disease is found, it is treated aggressively pretransplant; at our institution the H_2 blocker preference is ranitidine.

After transplantation, all patients receive H_2 blockers. If the patient had pretransplant acid peptic disease, ranitidine 150 mg twice daily is prescribed. If the pretransplant workup were negative, and the patient has no active ulcer symptoms post-transplant, ranitidine 150 mg daily (at night) is prescribed, the rationale for this being that the stress of the post-transplant period and steroid therapy may increase the patient's susceptibility to develop ulcer disease. Ranitidine therapy is continued at least until corticosteroids have been discontinued.

The wisdom of treating peptic ulcer disease prophylactically is well-supported by a review of the literature, since the complications of active severe ulceration, perforation, and gastrointestinal hemorrhage have been reported by a number of renal and cardiac transplant centers[36-39].

Gallbladder disease is a common entity in western civilization, and, in our experience, may become symptomatic early after transplantation. The pretransplant evaluation therefore always includes an upper abdominal ultrasound examination. If the ultrasound reveals gallstones, it is our feeling that further evaluation of the gallbladder using the hepatobiliary ^{99m}Tc-labeled aminodiacetic acid analog (HIDA) scan, coupled with calculation of gallbladder ejection fraction to cholecystokinin (CCK) stimulation, is indicated. If minimal or absent gallbladder function is identified, we consider the patient to be at high risk of developing cholecystitis in the post-transplant period. Good gallbladder function by this test reassures us that the likelihood of postoperative acute cholecystitis is low. A patient with severe active biliary tract symptoms prior to surgery is usually better managed by delaying cholecystectomy until after transplantation when his (or her) cardiac condition has stabilized. Active cholecystitis, however is a contraindication to proceeding with transplantation.

It is important to identify liver disease pretransplant because of the central role the liver plays in cyclosporine metabolism. In patients with a history of hepatitis or chronic alcohol ingestion, a nuclear scan of the liver and spleen is recommended. Splenomegaly and a shift of the isotope to the bone marrow help distinguish the cirrhotic patient from those with poor right heart function. Percutaneous liver biopsy is rarely needed pretransplant, but, if required, can be a safe procedure, even in the patient with a congested liver due to right heart failure.

Diverticulosis coli represents a major challenge to the managing clinician if it is active prior to transplantation. Immunosuppression often exacerbates the inflammatory and infectious component of this disease, and active diverticulitis in the pretransplant period is a relative contraindication to transplantation. At our institution, medical treatment pretransplant is instituted and, when the clinician feels the diverticulitis has become quiescent, the patient is placed on the transplantation waiting list.

Cytomegalovirus infection (Chapter 17) of the upper and lower gastrointestinal tracts has been a common and troublesome complication in the heart transplant patients at the Oklahoma Transplantation Institute; investigation should be aggressive and include endoscopy and biopsy for histological examination and viral culture. Therapy with DHPG (Syntex Ltd.) should be initiated as soon as possible.

Lenticular cataracts

Cataracts can be induced by prolonged high-dose steroid therapy and were fairly common in heart transplant patients before the introduction of CsA[30]. In renal transplant patients, the reported incidence of posterior subcapsular cataract varies from 12 to 60% (mean 37%)[40]. The typical lens opacity following long-term use of corticosteroid either systemically or topically is a posterior subcapsular opacity[41]. The high doses administered during rejection episodes produce subcortical crystalline opacities which usually affect the posterior pole of the lens. Low-dose corticosteroids sometimes provoke the development of cataracts, especially with prolonged use in excess of at least 12–18 months. In renal transplant patients there is a controversy as to whether cataract formation is dose-dependent[40,41]. Many patients who are started on steroid treatment have been chronically ill, and may already have cataracts when steroid therapy is begun. It is essential that they are informed, therefore, that there may be a progression of lenticular changes with long-term steroid treatment.

These cataracts may or may not progress and cause diminution of visual acuity. Surgical excision (possibly with intraocular lens implantation) is sometimes required.

There may be temporary fluctuations in vision related to steroid usage as well; these improve when steroid therapy is decreased.

Psychiatric complications

The incidence of psychiatric complications in patients receiving steroid therapy has been reported to be between 4 and 36%[42,43]. Symptoms vary in severity from insomnia, nervousness and mood changes, to manic or depressive symptoms, or agitation with paranoid ideation. Depression may or may not be related to the changes in physical appearance that may follow prolonged steroid therapy, e.g. Cushingoid features, hirsutism; fortunately, with the low dosage used today, extreme changes in physical appearance are rare. In patients with a pre-existing manic depressive, depressive, or schizophrenic disorder, or in those with a predisposition for these illnesses, the disorder can be exacerbated by the steroids.

Suicide has been successfully attempted by transplant patients. In the early experience of the University of Arizona, 12% of the cardiac transplant patients developed major psychiatric complications[35]. It is, however, difficult to determine whether such disorders are drug-related or occur as a result of the stress of the post-transplant period (Chapter 25). It seems likely that a combination of these factors exists in many cases.

Pancreatitis

The cause of post-transplant pancreatitis remains uncertain. Several etiologies have been implicated; these include drugs (corticosteroids, azathioprine, furosemide, epinephrine, and alcohol)[44-48], infections (cytomegalovirus, viral hepatitis, mumps, coxsackie and enteroviruses)[49-52], autoimmune disorders[53,54], ischemia[55] and biliary tract or peptic ulcer disease[56].

The University of Arizona reported a 6% incidence in cardiac transplant patients within the first 3 months[36]. Incidences of up to 7% with a mortality rate of more than 50% have been reported from several renal transplant centers. Though clinically severe acute pancreatitis is relatively uncommon after cardiac transplantation, a low-grade, asymptomatic pancreatitis has been noted in 49% of patients coming to necropsy[57]. Similarly, at Stanford, pancreatitis was found at necropsy in 70% of cardiac transplant patients[56].

Other complications

The list of other complications of corticosteroid therapy is long (Table 22.1). Fluid and salt retention can lead to hypertension and edema formation. Diuretic therapy can usually control these clinical features. Increased appetite and weight gain is common and may lead to obesity if not controlled by a strict diet (Chapter 27), and increased deposits of fat are seen particularly over the trunk. Changes in menstrual cycle, acne, night sweats, myopathy, joint pains, and spontaneous petechial hemorrhages in the skin are also common.

Antithymocyte or antilymphocyte globulin

We have observed circulatory collapse in two patients receiving antithymocyte globulin (ATG) whilst being prepared for heart transplantation, even though preliminary skin testing showed no sensitivity to the drug. As a result of this experience, we do not administer the first dose until the patient is supported by cardiopulmonary bypass.

There is a small risk of anaphylactic shock following its administration, whether this be intravenous or intramuscular. At Stanford, approximately 2% of patients exhibited frank anaphylaxis with the intramuscular use of ATG[29]. The risk of anaphylaxis may be reduced by administering a test dose subcutaneously and observing for a severe histamine skin reaction, and by administering steroids and an antihistamine before the ATG.

Patients who experience anaphylactic shock may require urgent steroid and epinephrine therapy, vasopressor support, and mechanically assisted respiration. They may, however, cautiously receive further ATG on subsequent occasions; in our experience, this reaction may be related to the batch of ATG used rather than to the ATG *per se*. Should the complication occur again, ATG produced in a second species of animal (e.g. rabbit or goat rather than horse) may be found not to provoke the reaction, and may be used safely.

A small proportion of patients receiving ATG develop a combination of symptoms which include rash, fever, chills, back and joint pain, and, less frequently, bronchospasm. During acute rejection episodes the chills and fever can be minimized by giving intravenous steroid therapy prior to the intravenous administration of ATG. Bronchospasm is treated as for anaphylaxis. Aspirin and antihistamines are useful in the treatment of joint pain and fever, and rash, respectively.

We have seen the clinical syndrome of serum sickness (fever, hepatomegaly splenomegaly and lymphadenopathy, associated with upper abdominal discomfort and pain) during intravenous ATG administration in two patients; it resolved after discontinuation of therapy.

Monoclonal antibody (OKT3)

The side-effects of OKT3 include fever (which occurs in 73% of patients), chills, dyspnea, chest pain, vomiting, wheezing, nausea, tremor, and diarrhea. Aseptic meningitis, exhibited by fever, headache, neck stiffness and photophobia, has been reported.

Because of the risk (less than 2%) of fatal pulmonary edema, OKT3 is contraindicated in patients with fluid overload, as determined by pulmonary congestion on a chest radiograph and by a weight gain of more than 3% within the week prior to the planned OKT3 therapy. It is recommended that a Swan–Ganz catheter should be inserted before treatment is begun, and that if the pulmonary capillary wedge pressure is seen to be unduly high, OKT3 therapy should be avoided.

The Utah group has shown, however, that OKT3 is generally well tolerated in the setting of cardiac transplantation[57]. In only one instance has therapy been interrupted for an adverse reaction thought to be related to OKT3, and that was due to the development of temporal arteritis. In addition, however, they have had one other serious effect. This was the development of meningoencephalitis that first presented 2 days after the last dose of a 10-day OKT3 prophylactic course. Headache was followed by confusion and fever 2 days later, necessitating hospital admission, a computer tomographic scan, and lumbar puncture. The cerebrospinal fluid contained 94 white blood cells per high-powered field, but remained sterile. This syndrome was self-limiting within 1 week, and was attributed to OKT3.

Cyclophosphamide

We have occasionally added small doses of cyclophosphamide to the immunosuppressive regimen in patients with unresponsive severe acute rejection when the total white blood count (WBC) remained high despite large doses of azathioprine (Chapter 16). A low dose (0.5–1.5 mg/kg per day) of this drug is generally sufficient to maintain a total white blood count within the desired range (5000–8000 cells/mm^3).

Though cyclophosphamide has undoubtedly been valuable on occasions, we have found it a difficult drug to use, and it must be administered with extreme caution. Unlike azathioprine, a fall in white blood count may be precipitous and result in a severe, life-threatening leukopenia (WBC < 1000/mm^3), which may persist for several days before recovery occurs.

Hemorrhagic aseptic cystitis may be a complication of cyclophosphamide therapy, necessitating its withdrawal.

BENIGN SKIN LESIONS

Patients on long-term immunosuppression not infrequently develop multiple benign skin lesions, which may require no treatment. Warts and keratoacanthomas are not uncommon. Several renal transplant groups have reported a greater than 40% incidence of warts, which are thought to result from reactivation of latent viruses rather than from primary infection[59,60]. It is important, however, to differentiate benign lesions from malignant tumors, such as squamous and basal cell carcinomata, which are the most common malignancies in immunocompromised patients (Chapter 21). All suspicious lesions should be biopsied or excised.

COMMENT

Long-term immunosuppressive therapy is clearly associated with a large number of side-effects and complications. Some of these can be avoided or minimized by careful selection of the patient or by pretransplant prophylactic treatment (e.g. for peptic ulcer), and others by post-transplant prophylactic medication. Avoidance of all such complications, however, cannot be ensured, and the potential risks must be considered when the potential recipient is initially assessed for cardiac transplantation.

COMPLICATIONS OF THE ORIGINAL DISEASE PROCESS

Progression of peripheral atheromatous vascular disease

Patients with widespread atheroma are, of course, at risk from progression of this disease in vessels other than the coronaries. Reconstructive surgery to peripheral vessels, especially in the legs, or even amputation for painful ischemic ulceration has been necessary in some patients with progressive peripheral arteriopathy.

Progression of cardiac disease (ischemic or myopathic) in patients with heterotopic heart transplants

A few of our heterotopic heart transplant patients with underlying ischemic heart disease have continued to show features of progressive atheroma of the coronary arteries of the native heart. One patient suffered a massive myocardial infarction of the recipient heart 3 months after transplantation. He experienced diaphoresis and severe typical ischemic chest pain radiating to the arms; an electrocardiogram confirmed the sudden onset of ventricular fibrillation. Throughout this episode, however, the donor heart maintained a steady rhythm and a systemic blood pressure of 110/70 mmHg. He did not demonstrate any other clinical features of shock. Analgesia was all that was necessary in the form of therapy.

Other patients with ischemic heart disease have subsequently lost coordinated electrical function of the native heart, but have suffered no adverse effects. Several of our patients with underlying cardiomyopathy have also lost function of the recipient heart. This has not led to problems, though we have been careful to continue anticoagulation. In one long-surviving patient, native heart ventricular fibrillation was demonstrated on one occasion, and coordinated contractions on subsequent occasions some months later, though it is unlikely that ventricular function was sufficient to open the aortic valve.

References

1. Ross, D. (1968). Report of a heart transplant operation. *Am. J. Cardiol.*, **22**, 838
2. Cooper, D.K.C., Fraser, R.C., Rose, A.G., Ayzenberg, T., Oldfield, G., Hassoulas, J., Novitzky, D., Uys, C.J. and Barnard, C.N. (1982). Technique, complications and clinical value of endomyocardial biopsy in patients with heterotopic heart transplants. *Thorax*, **37**, 727
3. Zuhdi, N., Shrago, S.S., Clark, R.N., Voda, J., Greer, A.E., Chaffin, J.S., Novitzky, D. and Cooper, D.K.C. (1989). Experience with endomyocardial biopsy in 23 patients with heart transplants. *J. Okla. Med. Assoc.*, **82**, 109
4. Fitchett, D.H., Forbes, C. and Guerraty, A.J. (1988). Repeated endomyocardial biopsy causing coronary arterial–right ventricular fistula after cardiac transplantation. *Am. J. Cardiol.*, **62**, 829
5. Sandhu, J.S., Uretsky, B.F., Zerbe, T.R., Goldsmith, A.S., Reddy, P.S., Kormos, R.L., Griffith, B.P. and Hardesty, R.L. (1989). Coronary artery fistula in the heart transplant patient. A potential complication of endomyocardial biopsy. *Circulation* **79**, 350
6. Henzlova, M.J., Nath, H., Bucy, R.P., Kirklin, J.K. and Rogers, W.J. (1989). Coronary artery to right ventricle fistulae in heart transplant recipients: a complication of endomyocardial biopsy? (Abstract). *J.*

Am. Coll. Cardiol. **13**, 243A
7. Locke, T.J., Furniss, S.S. and McGregor, C.G.A. (1988). Coronary artery–right ventricular fistula after endomyocardial biopsy. *Br. Heart J.*, **60**, 81
8. Griffith, B.P., Hardesty, R.L., Thompson, M.E., Dummer, J.S. and Bahnson, H.T. (1983). Cardiac transplantation with cyclosporine: the Pittsburgh experience. *Heart Transplant.*, **2**, 251
9. Green, C.F. (1981). Cyclosporin-A. In Salaman, J.R. (ed.) *Immunosuppressive Therapy.* p. 75. (Lancaster: MTP Press)
10. Thompson, C.B., June, C.H., Sullivan, K.M. and Thomas, E.D. (1984). Association between cyclosporin neurotoxicity and hypomagnesaemia. *Lancet*, **2**, 1116
11. Schmitz, N., Eulen, H.H. and Loffler, H. (1985). Hypomagnesaemia and cyclosporin toxicity (Letter). *Lancet*, **1**, 103
12. de Groen, F.C., Aksamit, A.J., Rakela, J., Forbes, G.S. and Krom, R.A.F. (1987). Central nervous system toxicity after liver transplantation: the role of cyclosporine and cholesterol. *N. Engl. J. Med.*, **317**, 861
13. Cooper, D.K.C., Novitzky, D., Davis, L., Huff, J.E., Parker, D., Schlesinger, R., Sholer, C. and Zuhdi, N. (1989). Does central nervous system toxicity occur in hypocholesterolemic transplant patients receiving cyclosporine? *J. Heart Transplant.*, **8**, 221
14. Billingham, M.I. (1987). Cardiac transplant atherosclerosis. *Transplant. Proc.*, **19**, 19
15. Ballantyne, C.M., Jones, P.H., Payton-Ross, C., Patsch, W., Short, H.D., Noon, G.P., Gotto, A.M., Jr., Debakey, M.E. and Young, B. (1987). Hyperlipidemia following heart transplantation: natural history and intervention with mebinolin (lovastatin). *Transplant. Proc.*, **19**, 60
16. Grady, K.L. and Herold, L.S. (1987). Comparison of nutritional status in patients before and after cardiac transplantation. *Circulation*, **76**, IV-145
17. Becker, D.M., Markakis, M., Sension, M., Vitalis, S., Baughman, K., Swank, R., Kwiterovich, P.O., Pearson, T.A., Achuff, S.C., Baumgartner, W.A., Borkon, A.M., Reitz, B.A. and Traill, T.A. (1987). Prevalence of hyperlipidemia in heart transplant recipients. *Transplantation*, **44**, 323
18. Norman, D.J., Illingworth, D.R., Munson, J. and Hosenpud, J. (1988). Myolysis and acute renal failure in a heart-transplant recipient receiving lovastatin (Letter). *N. Engl. J. Med.*, **318**, 46
19. East, C., Alivizatos, P.A., Grundy, S.M., Jones, P.H. and Farmer, J.A. (1988). Rhabdomyolysis in patients receiving lovastatin after cardiac transplantation (Letter). *N. Engl. J. Med.*, **318**, 47
20. Penn, I. and Makowski, E.L. (1981). Parenthood in kidney and liver transplant recipients. *Transplant. Proc.*, **13**, 36
21. Rhenman, M.J., Rhenman, B., Icenogle, T., Christensen, R. and Copeland, J. (1988). Diabetes and heart transplantation. *J. Heart Transplant.*, **7**, 356
22. Fisher, D.E. and Bickel, W.H. (1971). Corticosteroid-induced avascular necrosis – a clinical study of seventy-seven patients. *J. Bone J. Surg.*, **53A**, 859
23. Fisher, D.E., Bickel, W.H., Holley, K.E. and Ellefson, R.D. (1972). Corticosteroid-induced necrosis. II. Experimental study. *Clin. Orthop.*, **84**, 200
24. Briggs, W.A., Hampers, C.L., Merrill, J.P., Hagen, E.B., Wilson, R.E., Birtch, A.G. and Murray, J.E. (1972). Aseptic necrosis in the femur after renal transplantation. *Ann. Surg.*, **175**, 282
25. Solomon, L. (1973). Drug-induced arthropathy and necrosis of the femoral head. *J. Bone J. Surg.*, **55B**, 246
26. Burton, D.S., Mochizuki, R.M. and Helpern, A.A. (1978). Total hip arthroplasty in the cardiac transplant patient. *Clin. Orthop.*, **130**, 186
27. Morris, P.J., Oliver, D.O., Bishop, M., Cullen, P., Fellows, G., French, M., Ledingham, J.G., Smith, J.C., Ting, A. and Williams, K. (1978). Results from a new renal transplantation unit. *Lancet*, **2**, 1353
28. Merrill, J.P. (1978). Dialysis versus transplantation in the treatment of end-stage renal disease. *Annu. Rev. Med.*, **29**, 243
29. Jamieson, S.W., Bieber, C.P. and Oyer, P.E. (1981). Suppression of immunity for cardiac transplantation. In Salaman, J.R. (ed.) *Immunosuppressive Therapy.* pp. 177–179. (Lancaster: MTP Press)
30. Hess, M.L., Hastillo, A., Goldman, M., Rider, S., Mohanakumar, T., Ducey, K., Wolfgang, T., Szentpetery, S. and Lower, R.R. (1983). Cardiac transplantation at the Medical College of Virginia. *Heart Transplant.*, **2**, 246
31. Cabrol, C., Gandjbakhch, I., Pavie, A., Cabrol, A., Matter, M.F., Lienhart, A., Gluckman, J.C. and Rottembourg, J. (1983). Cardiac transplantation at La Pitie Hospital. *Heart Transplant.*, **2**, 244
32. Crosnier, J. and Broyer, M. (1979). Treatment of chronic renal failure in children. In Hamburger, J., Crosnier, J. and Grunfield, J.P. (eds.) *Nephrology.* p. 1361. (New York: Wiley)
33. Blodgett, F.M., Burgin, L., Tezzoni, D., Oribetz, D. and Talbot, N.B. (1956). Effects of prolonged cortisone therapy on the statural growth, skeletal maturation and metabolic status of children. *N. Engl. J. Med.*, **254**, 636
34. Soyka, L.F. and Saxena, K.M. (1965). Alternate-day steroid therapy for nephrotic children. *J. Am. Med. Assoc.*, **192**, 225
35. Potter, D.E., Holliday, M.A., Wilson, C.J., Salvatierra, O. and Belzer, F.O. (1975). Alternate-day steroids in children after renal transplantation. *Transplant. Proc.*, **7**, 79
36. Copeland, J., Fuller, J., Sailor, M.J. and McAleer, M.J. (1983). Heart transplantation at the Health Sciences Center of the University of Arizona. *Heart Transplant.*, **2**, 246
37. Kirkman, R.L., Strom, T.B., Weir, M.R. and Tilney, N.L. (1982). Late mortality and morbidity in recipients of long-term renal allografts. *Transplantation*, **34**, 347
38. Crosnier, J., Leski, M., Kreis, H. and Descamps, D. (1969). Non-renal complications of kidney allotransplantation. In Alwall, N. *et al.* (eds.) *Proceedings of the Fourth International Congress of Nephrology, Stockholm.* Vol. 3, p. 270. (Basel and New York: Karger)
39. Abele, R., Novick, A.C., Braun, W.E., Steinmuller, D., Buszta, C., Greenstreet, R. and Hinton, J. (1982). Long-term results of renal transplantation in recipients with a functioning graft for two years. *Transplantation*, **34**, 264
40. Debnath, S.C., Abomelha, M.S., Jawdat, M., Chang, R. and Al-Khader, A.A. (1987). Ocular side effects of systemic steroid therapy in renal transplant patients. *Ann. Ophthalmol.*, **19**, 435
41. Luntz, M.H. (1980). Clinical types of cataracts. In Duane, T.D. (ed.) *Duane's Series of Ophthalmology.* Volume 1, pp. 15 and 19. (Phildelphia: Lippincott)
42. Quarton, G.C., Clark, L.D., Cobb, S. and Bauer, W. (1955). Mental disturbance associated with ACTH and cortisone: a review of explanatory hypotheses. *Medicine*, **34**, 13
43. Ritchie, E.A. (1956). Toxic psychosis under cortisone and corticotrophin. *J. Ment. Sci.*, **102**, 830
44. Bourne, M.S. and Dawson, H. (1958). Acute pancreatitis complicating prednisolone therapy. *Lancet*, **2**, 1209
45. Mallory, A. and Kern, F. (1980). Drug-induced pancreatitis: a critical review. *Gastroenterology*, **78**, 813
46. Nakashima, Y. and Howard, J.M. (1977). Drug-induced acute pancreatitis. *Surg. Gynecol. Obstet.*, **145**, 105
47. Kawanishi, H., Rudolph, E. and Bull, F.E. (1973). Azathioprine-induced acute pancreatitis. *N. Engl. J. Med.*, **289**, 357
48. Jones, P.F. and Oelbaum, M.H. (1975). Furosemide-induced pancreatitis. *Br. Med. J.*, **1**, 133
49. Tilney, N.L., Collins, J.J. and Wilson, R.E. (1966). Hemorrhagic pancreatitis: a fatal complication of renal transplantation. *N. Engl. J. Med.*, **275**, 1051
50. Hume, D.M. (1968). Kidney transplantation. In Rapaport, F.T. and Dausset, J. (eds.) *Human Transplantation.* p. 110. (New York: Grune and Stratton)
51. Werbitt, W. and Mohsenifar, Z. (1980). Mononucleosis pancreatitis. *South. Med. J.*, **73**, 1094
52. Imrie, C.W., Ferguson, J.C. and Sommerville, R.G. (1977). Coxsackie and mumps virus infection in a prospective study of acute pancreatitis.

Gut, **18**, 53
53. Fujii, G. and Nelson, R.A. (1963). The cross-reactivity and transfer of antibody in transplantation immunity. *J. Exp. Med.*, **118**, 1037
54. Amos, D.B. and Stickel, D.L. (1968). Human transplantation antigens. *Adv. Intern. Med.*, **14**, 15
55. Feiner, H. (1976). Pancreatitis after cardiac surgery. *Am. J. Surg.*, **131**, 684
56. Karrer, F.M., Mammana, R.B. and Copeland, J.G. (1982). Survival following pancreatitis and surgical drainage of a pancreatic pseudocyst in a heart transplant recipient. *Heart Transplant.*, **1**, 325
57. Uys, C.J., Rose, A.G. and Barnard, C.N. (1979). The pathology of human cardiac transplantation. *S. Afr. Med. J.*, **56**, 887
58. Bristow, M.R., Gilbert, E.M., Renlund, D.G., De Witt, C.W., Burton, N.A. and O'Connell, J.B. (1988). Use of OKT3 monoclonal antibody in cardiac transplantation: review of the initial experience. *J. Heart Transplant.*, **7**, 1
59. Koranda, F.C., Dehmel, E.M., Kahn, G. and Penn, I. (1974). Cutaneous complications in immunosuppressed renal homograft recipients. *J. Am. Med. Assoc.*, **229**, 419
60. Spencer, E.S. and Anderson, H.K. (1970). Clinically evident, non-terminal infections with herpes viruses and the wart virus in immunosuppressed renal allograft recipients. *Br. Med. J.*, **3**, 251

23
Heterotopic Heart Transplantation – Indications and Special Considerations

D.K.C. COOPER

INTRODUCTION

The implantation of a natural auxiliary heart using the technique of heterotopic heart transplantation (HHT) may be on a permanent basis, or may occasionally be temporary as a means of support whilst recovery of the patient's own heart is awaited or a more definitive procedure is planned (as will be outlined later). Considerable clinical experience has now been amassed with auxiliary hearts implanted on a permanent basis[1]; all such hearts have to date been allografts. Clinical experience of temporary support by an auxiliary heart has been small, and it would seem that it is in this area of transplantation that xenografts may play a future role.

Early experimental work was mainly by the Russian surgeon, Demikhov[2] (Chapter 1), but it was not until Barnard and Losman developed their techniques of implanting an auxiliary heart in the chest in 1974[3-5] that a clinical program was initiated. The surgical technique of biventricular assist (Figure 23.1) has been described in Chapter 11. (The technique of left ventricular assist alone (Figure 23.2) is now very rarely performed.)

HHT has both advantages and disadvantages when compared with orthotopic heart transplantation (OHT) (Table 23.1)[1], which have been documented fully previously[6-8]. In particular, the heterotopic procedure may allow recipient survival despite temporary or permanent loss of donor heart function following acute or chronic rejection (Figure 23.3); the circulation may be maintained by the recipient's own heart for at least a period of time.

PERMANENT NATURAL AUXILIARY HEARTS

The introduction of the immunosuppressive agent, cyclosporine (CsA), which has significantly reduced the incidence of irreversible acute rejection (leading to permanent loss of donor heart function), has greatly reduced the indications for HHT. In the pre-CsA era, irreversible loss of the heterotopic donor heart did not necessarily lead to death of the patient, as the circulation might be maintained by the recipient native heart until retransplantation could

Table 23.1 Advantages and disadvantages of heterotopic over orthotopic heart transplantation

Advantages	*Disadvantages*

(1) Recipient heart acts as a built-in cardiac assist device and may maintain circulation.
(a) During reversible loss of donor heart function during:
  (i) period of recovery of donor heart from ischemia sustained during transplantation
  (ii) severe acute rejection episodes
(b) Following irreversible loss of donor heart function from:
  (i) acute, or
  (ii) chronic rejection (whilst patient awaits retransplantation)
(c) During adaptation of a very small donor heart to the demands of the circulation
(2) Allows for possible recovery of recipient heart, e.g. after viral myocarditis or rheumatic carditis
(3) Can be performed even in the presence of a high pulmonary vascular resistance if the hypertrophied recipient right ventricle can continue to support the pulmonary circulation
	(1) Risk of systemic emboli from thrombus in poorly contracting recipient left ventricle.
	(2) Requires long-term anticoagulation
	(3) Continuing angina related to ischemic recipient myocardium (rare)
	(4) Risk of infection and/or thrombus formation in relation to presence of valve prosthesis in recipient heart. This is a contraindication to heterotopic heart transplantation
	(5) Hemodynamically significant dysrhythmias of the recipient heart requiring high doses of antiarrhythmic agents may affect function of donor heart

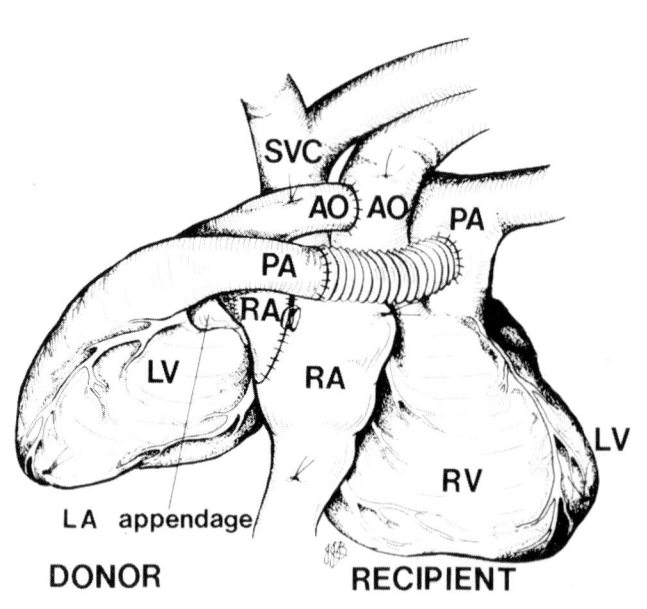

Figure 23.1 The completed operation of biventricular assist using a heterotopic heart transplant. The surgical technique is described in detail in Chapter 11. (SVC = superior vena cava; RA = right atrium; RV = right ventricle; PA = pulmonary artery; LA = left atrium; LV = left ventricle; AO = aorta)

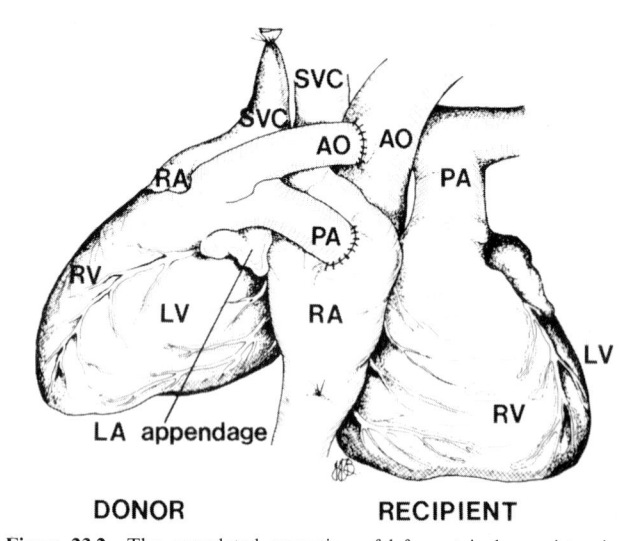

Figure 23.2 The completed operation of left ventricular assist using a heterotopic heart transplant. Anastomoses are performed between the donor and recipient left atria and aortae. Donor coronary venous return drains by the donor right atrium, right ventricle, and pulmonary artery into the recipient right atrium. (Abbreviations as for Figure 23.1)

be performed[6-8]. Today, however, irreversible rejection is relatively rare, and so this great avantage of HHT has become less important.

Indications

Nevertheless, HHT still has a role in certain specific conditions[1]:

(1) Whenever there is any possibility of recovery of the recipient's own myocardium, e.g. in acute myocarditis (of viral or rheumatic origin), then HHT should be preferred. Unfortunately, in patients with cardiomyopathy who undergo HHT, recipient heart function tends to deteriorate further over the next few months until the circulation is supported entirely by the donor heart.

(2) When there is any possibility that initial donor heart function will be less than adequate to maintain the circulation alone. This could be expected most commonly when there is a large discrepancy in body mass (greater than 25%) between recipient and donor. Although a small donor heart will eventually hypertrophy to adapt to the demands made upon it, it might fail in the early post-transplant period unless the recipient heart remains *in situ* to lend some support. In this respect, however, it should be remembered that a small child's heart may be technically impossible to insert heterotopically in an adult, as it may not be possible to join the two right atria (Chapter 11).

Similarly, when a donor heart has undergone a particularly long ischemic period during transportation and transplantation, or for some other reason is deemed less than ideal (and yet the recipient's cardiovascular status is deteriorating so rapidly that survival until the next donor becomes available is not expected), then again HHT would seem to be advisable; the support given by the recipient heart in the early transplant period may allow time for recovery of the donor heart.

Recovery of ischemic donor hearts was clearly demonstrated when two hearts in the Cape Town series were stored by hypothermic perfusion for periods of 7 and 13 hours respectively[9]. Diminished donor heart function was observed for 16–19 hours until full recovery occurred; the recipient heart was invaluable in supporting the patient during this period.

(3) When the patient is suffering severe anginal attacks unresponsive to full medical therapy and unrelieved (where possible) by myocardial revascularization procedures, and yet where left ventricular function continues to be good, it may on occasion be contra-indicated to excise the recipient heart and perform orthotopic transplantation (OHT). Following HHT, a well-functioning transplant would greatly diminish the demands on the ischemic recipient heart, thus reducing the oxygen requirement, and yet retain some support by the recipient left ventricle.

(4) A fixed pulmonary vascular resistance (PVR) greater than approximately 5 Wood units (400 dynes s^{-1} cm^{-5}) has long been considered a contraindication to OHT as it was anticipated that early failure of the donor right ventricle would occur. When the PVR is fixed greater than 8 Wood units (640 dynes s^{-1} cm^{-5}), it has generally been assumed that transplantation of the heart and both lungs should be

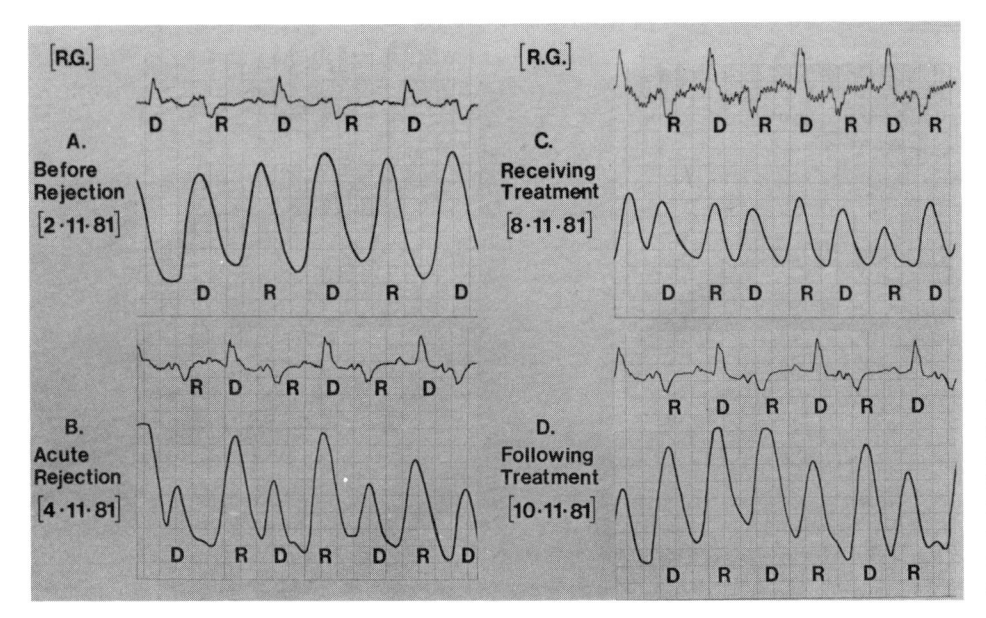

Figure 23.3 Diagram showing electrocardiogram (above) and femoral pulse trace (below) of donor (D) and recipient (R) hearts after heterotopic transplantation. Note the deterioration in the donor heart pulse in relation to the recipient heart pulse during an acute rejection episode, and the reversal of this trend following increased immunosuppressive therapy

carried out. When the PVR is fixed between 6 and 8 units, and where right ventricular failure is not severe, then HHT has been advocated. There have been few patients, however, where this theory has been put into practice, and the results clearly documented. Furthermore, the extent of reversibility of the PVR may be difficult to ascertain absolutely before transplantation.

A statistical study by Kirklin and his colleagues from Alabama confirms that elevated PVR is an incremental risk factor for premature death after heart transplantation[10]. The value of PVR used was that obtained closest to the time of transplantation without specific attempts to modify it by vasodilator or inotropic agents. The rate of rise in risk of death corresponded evenly to the progressive increase in PVR (particularly when expressed as Wood units × square meters), rather than abruptly increasing at a certain point. Although this study indicates that there is no precise level of PVR beyond which heart transplantation is contraindicated, there must come a point when the risk is so high that transplantation is no longer advisable, or, at least, an alternative surgical technique, e.g. heterotopic or heart–lung transplantation is indicated. Experience at many centers indicates that the arbitrary levels of 5 and 8 Wood units (suggested above) have been of value as guidelines. (The Alabama group stressed a preference for expressing PVR in Wood units × square meters (mean pulmonary artery pressure − pulmonary capillary wedge pressure/cardiac index (liters minute^{-1} square meters^{-1})); incorrect inferences may result from the use of simple Wood units.)

Many transplant groups believe that every attempt should be made at cardiac catheterization to demonstrate the degree of reversibility of the PVR − by the infusion of nitroprusside, nitroglycerin, prostaglandin E_1, or an inotropic agent, or by the administration of 100% oxygen. If the PVR cannot be reduced below 5 or 6 Wood units (400–480 dynes), and yet remains less than 8 units, then HHT may be indicated, but only if recipient right ventricular function remains demonstrably adequate and can clearly be predicted to support the pulmonary circulation (against the high PVR) after transplantation. If significant right ventricular failure is present, secondary to irreversible pulmonary vascular disease (as opposed to being secondary to left ventricular failure alone), then right ventricular function will not improve after HHT. In doubtful cases, we have found measurement of right ventricular ejection fraction by radionuclide scanning to be a valuable guide to the adequacy of right ventricular function. A right ventricular ejection fraction lower than 20% (i.e. approximately 50% of normal) would discourage us from performing HHT in the presence of a fixed PVR higher than 5 Wood units, and we would consider transplantation of the heart and both lungs.

A study from New York, however, indicated that, while in some cases an elevated PVR correlates with poor outcome from right ventricular failure, a high resistance is not an absolute contraindication even to OHT[11]. This study demonstrated that there is a very considerable reversible element in PVR in the majority of patients awaiting heart transplantation. OHT was successfully performed in such patients even if the PVR remained above 6 Wood units following nitroprusside infusion, though some such patients had significant though transient right ventricular failure after surgery. When the PVR had no demonstrable reversible element and remained significantly above 6 Wood units, then HHT could be performed successfully if there were no native right ventricular failure or significant tricuspid regurgitation; one patient underwent successful HHT with a fixed PVR of 15 Wood units.

Data from Stanford, however, suggest that the response of PVR to nitroprusside is of prognostic value in predicting the risk of early post-transplant mortality[12]. High-risk patients include those whose PVR cannot be reduced below 2.5 Wood units (in whom, in the Stanford series, there was a 42% mortality within the first 3 months post-transplant), as well as those whose PVR can be reduced below 2.5 only at the expense of systemic hypotension (in whom there was a 24% mortality). These data indicate that the detrimental effect of even a moderately high PVR on the outcome of heart transplantation may have been considerably underestimated in the past.

A further study, from Pittsburgh, has suggested that the transpulmonary gradient (TPG) (mean pulmonary artery pressure − pulmonary capillary wedge pressure), and not the calculated PVR, is a more accurate predictor of outcome following OHT[13]. In 187 patients undergoing OHT, neither the PVR (using 6 Wood units as the point of differentiation) nor the peak pulmonary artery systolic pressure (using 50 mmHg as the point of differentiation) significantly influenced early mortality as judged by 7- and 30-day actuarial survival. The TPG, however, seemed to affect survival in a significant fashion ($p < 0.05$). A TPG of more than 15 mmHg was associated with a higher mortality than when the TPG was between 10 and 15 mmHg; mortality was even lower when the TPG was less than 10 mmHg. This relationship persisted even when patients with known causes of death (infection, hyperacute rejection, technical, bleeding) were excluded from the analysis. There may, therefore, be a place for HHT in patients in whom the TPG is above 10 mmHg, though the level of TPG above which heart and lung transplantation should be performed remains uncertain.

The indication for HHT in relation to the PVR and/or TPG, therefore, still remains controversial, but it would seem reasonable to suggest that in patients with left ventricular failure from ischemic or cardiomyopathic disease, HHT should be preferred whenever there is serious doubt that the right ventricle of the transplanted heart will be able to support the pulmonary circulation successfully. This would certainly be suggested if the PVR were above 5 Wood units (and possibly above 2.5 Wood units) and showed no reversible element whatsoever, or if the TPG remained above 10 mmHg after an attempt to reduce it was made by infusion of nitroprusside and/or 100% oxygenation of the patient for a period of several minutes. In every case, however, it now seems clear that the higher the PVR, then the greater the early mortality associated with the operation[10,12], and this point must be carefully weighed in each individual patient.

If the PVR were fixed above 8 Wood units (or the TPG fixed above 15 mmHg, or actually increases) then heart–lung transplantation should be seriously considered.

In patients being considered for transplantation for congenital heart disease in whom there is a large left to right shunt which has resulted in a high PVR (and, of course, in patients with primary pulmonary hypertension), then transplantation of the heart and both lungs will almost certainly be indicated.

TEMPORARY NATURAL AUXILIARY HEARTS

The temporary insertion of a human auxiliary heart would seem to have little place in modern cardiac transplantation. It has been clearly demonstrated that temporary support of a failing circulation can be satisfactorily provided by one of the several ventricular assist devices or artificial hearts which are currently available (Section IV).

The use of an auxiliary non-human primate heart, however, as a bridge to transplantation would seem feasible, for it seems likely that chimpanzee hearts, in particular, will function satisfactorily for several days and possibly weeks or months. This would allow time for a suitable human heart to be located and inserted (with removal of both the chimpanzee organ and the recipient's native heart).

Indeed, this was one possibility in two patients in whom auxiliary cardiac xenografts (one baboon and one chimpanzee) were implanted by Barnard and his colleagues in 1977[14]. The baboon heart proved of insufficient size to support the circulation, and, in this pre-CsA era, the chimpanzee heart was rejected on the fourth postoperative day before a suitable human donor could be found.

Several aspects of the use of xenografts, even as heterotopically-placed natural auxiliary hearts or bridging devices, remain uncertain or controversial; these are discussed in Section IV.

References

1. Cooper, D.K.C., Novitzky, D., Becerra, E. and Reichart, B. (1986). Are there indications for heterotopic heart transplantation in 1986? A 2 to 11 year follow up of 49 consecutive patients undergoing heterotopic heart transplantation. *Thorac. Cardiovasc. Surg.*, **34**, 300
2. Demikhov, V.P. (1962). *Experimental Transplantation of Vital Organs.* Authorized translation from the Russian by Haigh, B. (New York: Consultants Bureau)
3. Barnard, C.N. and Losman, J.G. (1975). Left ventricular bypass. *S. Afr. Med. J.*, **49**, 303
4. Losman, J.G. and Barnard, C.N. (1977). Hemodynamic evaluation of left ventricular bypass with a homologous cardiac graft. *J. Thorac. Cardiovasc. Surg.*, **74**, 695
5. Novitzky, D., Cooper, D.K.C. and Barnard, C.N. (1983). The surgical technique of heterotopic heart transplantation. *Ann. Thorac. Surg.*, **36**, 476
6. Novitzky, D., Cooper, D.K.C. and Barnard, C.N. (1984). Reversal of acute rejection by cyclosporine in a heterotopic heart transplant. *Heart Transplant.*, **3**, 117
7. Novitzky, D., Cooper, D.K.C., Rose, A.G. and Barnard, C.N. (1984). The value of recipient heart assistance during severe acute rejection

following heterotopic cardiac transplantation. *J. Cardiovasc. Surg.*, **25**, 287

8. Cooper, D.K.C. (1984). Advantages and disadvantages of heterotopic transplantation. In Cooper, D.K.C. and Lanza, R.P. (eds.) *Heart Transplantation*. p. 305. (Lancaster: MTP Press)

9. Wicomb, W.N., Cooper, D.K.C., Novitzky, D. and Barnard, C.N. (1984). Cardiac transplantation following storage of the donor heart by a portable hypothermic perfusion system. *Ann. Thorac. Surg.*, **37**, 243

10. Kirklin, J.K., Naftel, D.C., Kirklin, J.W., Blackstone, E.H., White-Williams, C. and Bourge, R.C. (1988). Pulmonary vascular resistance and the risk of heart transplantation. *J. Heart Transplant.*, **7**, 331

11. Addonizio, L.J., Robbins, R.C., Reison, D.S., Drusin, R.E., Smith, C.R., Reemtsma, K. and Rose, E.A. (1986). Transplantation in patients with high pulmonary vascular resistance. *J. Heart Transplant.*, **5**, 394

12. Costard, A., Hill, I., Schroeder, J. and Fowler, M. (1989). Response to nitroprusside – predictor of early post-transplant mortality. (Abstract). *J. Am. Coll. Cardiol.*, **13**, 62A

13. Kormos, R.L., Thompson, M., Hardesty, R.L., Griffith, B.P., Trento, A., Uretsky, B.F. and Reddy, P.S. (1986). Utility of preoperative right heart catheterization data as a predictor of survival after heart transplantation. *J. Heart Transplant.*, **5**, 391

14. Barnard, C.N., Wolpowitz, A. and Losman, J.G. (1977). Heterotopic cardiac transplantation with a xenograft for assistance of the left heart in cardiogenic shock after cardiopulmonary bypass. *S. Afr. Med. J.*, **52**, 1035

24
Heart Transplantation in Infants and Children – Indications and Special Considerations

J.M. DUNN

INTRODUCTION

The first successful clinical cardiac transplant was performed by Barnard in 1967 in an adult[1]. In the same year Kantrowitz et al. reported a clinical transplant in a 16-day-old child with tricuspid atresia[2]. The following year Cooley et al. reported a transplant in a 2-month-old child with an atrioventricular canal defect[3]. Both of these pediatric transplants were ultimately unsuccessful.

In the 1980s, cardiac transplantation in the adult population has increased exponentially. Over 4000 cardiac transplants have been performed, most of them in the last few years[4] (Chapter 31). Despite this widespread increase in adult transplantation, and acceptance of it as an efficacious clinical tool for end-stage cardiac disease, pediatric cardiac transplantation remains controversial[5-8]. No doubt it is the palliative nature of transplantation, with as yet, insufficient long-term experience, that underlies our concerns. In the pediatric population, the problems and complications of transplantation are magnified. Transplant success, which is measured in years in the adult patient, must be measured in decades in the pediatric patient. Although there is no evidence that acute rejection is more severe in children, its detection is more difficult and cumbersome. The risk of infections is multiplied in the pediatric population because of their high incidence in childhood, lack of previous infectious exposure providing immunity in some cases, and frequently incomplete immunization record.

Nevertheless, there has been a steady increase in pediatric transplant experience over the last few years[8-14]. The Registry of the International Society for Heart Transplantation lists 258 children under the age of 19 years as having undergone cardiac transplantation[4].

The purpose of this chapter will be to delineate the similarities and, more specifically, the differences, in cardiac transplantation between children and adults.

INDICATIONS FOR CARDIAC TRANSPLANTATION IN CHILDHOOD

Very simply, cardiac transplantation is indicated in any child with end-stage heart disease when no further reasonable medical or surgical option is available.

The overwhelming majority of children undergoing cardiac transplantation have end-stage cardiomyopathy[15-17]. Ischemic cardiomyopathy is relatively uncommon, in contradistinction to the adult population; in children, myocardial ischemia is usually secondary to hypercholesterolemia or, in rare cases, an anomalous coronary artery arising from the pulmonary artery. The majority of pediatric cardiomyopathies are acquired, especially in older children, and are thought to be secondary to viral myocarditis, although the etiology is often uncertain. Dilated cardiomyopathy in the infant may be acquired, but may also be congenital, and may also be secondary to structural congenital abnormalities and previous surgery (Figure 24.1).

Hypertrophic cardiomyopathy may present with or without congestive heart failure[18]. This autosomally dominant trait with variable penetrance is usually managed medically or surgically without transplantation. Severe forms, with distorted and diminutive left ventricular chambers, severe outflow obstruction, and refractory ventricular arrhythmias may require transplantation (Figure 24.2).

A recent review of pediatric cardiomyopathies has demonstrated an extremely grave prognosis when (1) the myopathy develops after 2 years of age, (2) symptoms do not improve within a year, and (3) there are associated arrhythmias[19]. All such children should be considered urgently as transplant candidates.

Most congenital structural abnormalities of the heart can be corrected or palliated with good results, and should not be considered as indications for transplantation. Despite

THE TRANSPLANTATION AND REPLACEMENT OF THORACIC ORGANS

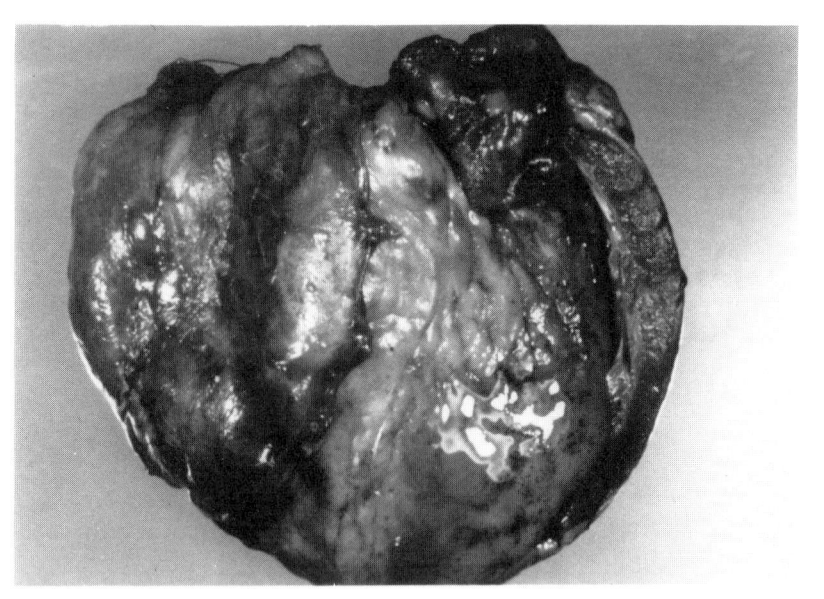

Figure 24.1 Dilated cardiomyopathy in a 12-year-old girl with Marfan's syndrome and severe mitral regurgitation. The patient was transplanted after mitral valve replacement resulted in no improvement of the cardiomyopathy

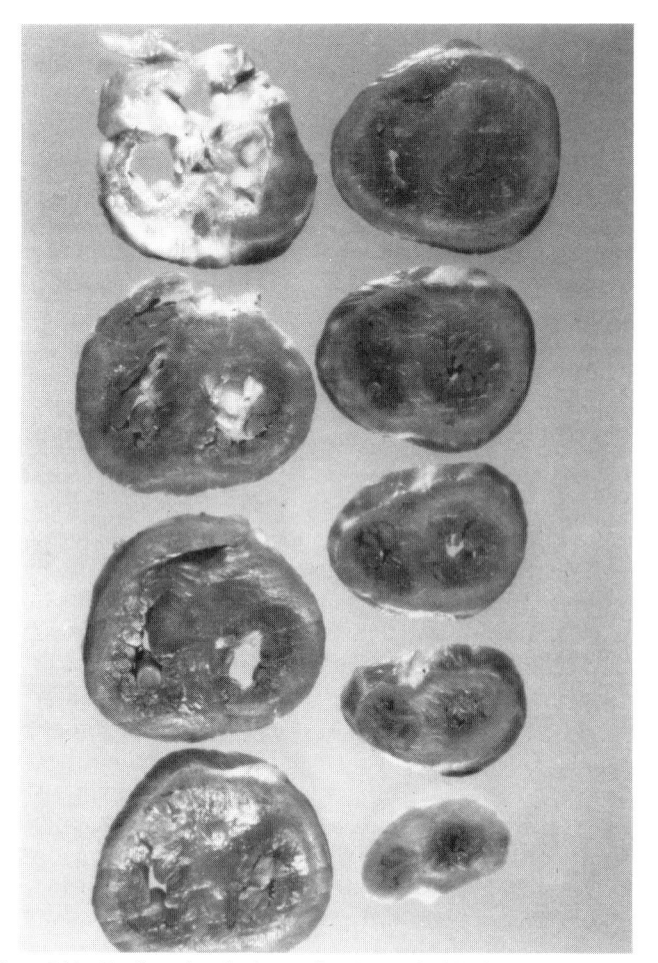

Figure 24.2 Explanted native heart of an 8-month-old infant transplanted for severe hypertrophic obstructive cardiomyopathy, with arrhythmias and congestive heart failure. Several sections demonstrated obliteration of the left ventricular chamber by hypertrophic muscle

appropriate surgical intervention, many children with correctable structural lesions go on to develop cardiomyopathy, which may make them transplant candidates[7]. This group includes those with ventricular failure secondary to mitral or aortic valve insufficiency, right ventricular dysfunction in transposition of the great vessels following atrial repair, and ventricular dysfunction following repair of tetralogy of Fallot.

Some structural congenital cardiac lesions defy complete surgical repair, and these infants may be candidates for transplantation. This group includes infants with single or univentricular hearts[20], and those with hypoplastic left heart syndrome[10-12]. As experience and the results of transplantation in children improve, it is anticipated that the criteria for transplantation will be widened to include other congenital lesions which are presently corrected or palliated but with less than perfect results[21].

Unresectable primary cardiac tumors represent another group requiring transplantation (Figure 24.3). Although primary cardiac tumors do not generally metastasize, concern about generalized and associated lesions exists. Patients with rhabdomyomas of the heart usually have central nervous system tuberous sclerosis, and may have mental retardation and seizure disorders. The symptomatic rhabdomyoma requiring transplantation in infancy remains an ethical dilemma, since the patient's neurologic status often cannot be completely evaluated.

CONTRAINDICATIONS

In general, contraindications to cardiac transplantation in children reflect those in the adult population (Chapter 2). Absolute contraindications include elevated irreversible

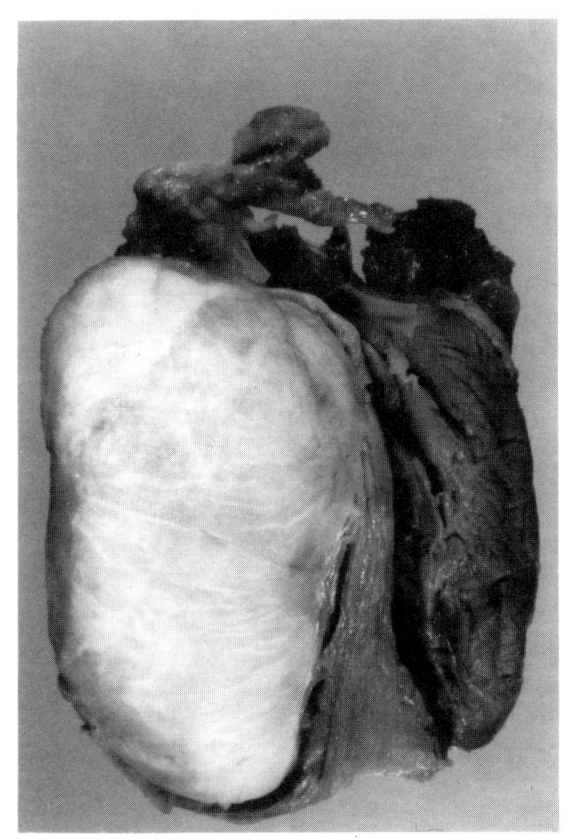

Figure 24.3 Heart of a 5-month-old infant with a large cardiac fibroma replacing the left ventricular free wall and obliterating the left ventricular cavity

pulmonary vascular disease, irreversible renal and hepatic disease, active infection, and malignancy. Relative contraindications include recent pulmonary infarction, reversible pulmonary vascular disease, psychosocial instability, drug or alcohol addiction, and an inadequate family support system.

PREOPERATIVE EVALUATION

Preoperative evaluation can usually be accomplished within a few days. Its purpose is to confirm the indications and contraindications for transplantation, demonstrate the feasibility of alternate medical or surgical management, and aid in the matching process once the patient has been accepted as a transplant candidate. Simultaneously, it offers the opportunity of pretransplant teaching of patient and/or family.

Evaluation is not unlike that in the adult. Cardiac catheterization is performed to confirm the cardiac lesion, and to measure the pulmonary vascular resistance (PVR) and its response to pharmacologic agents. Endomyocardial biopsy of the right ventricle is routinely performed. In most cases of cardiomyopathy, the biopsy will demonstrate characteristic muscle abnormalities, but rarely does it help diagnose the cause of the cardiomyopathy[22]. In the patient presenting acutely or subacutely, the presence of infiltrating cells may be helpful in confirming an active myocarditis. Diffuse muscle diseases may be diagnosed with peripheral skeletal muscle biopsies. As it is not known whether a diffuse muscle disorder will affect a transplanted heart, there is some concern whether transplantation should be performed in such patients.

Pulmonary vascular obstructive disease (PVOD) is a relative contraindication to transplantation when the PVOD is moderate, and an absolute contraindication when severe. It is our impression that elevation of PVR is more common in the pediatric cardiomyopathic patient than in our adult patients. When the PVR is raised, hemodynamic manipulations including oxygen therapy, infusion of pulmonary vasodilators, and 24-hour amrinone infusion, are employed to assess whether the elevation is reversible. A PVR of 6–8 Wood units is a relative contraindication to transplantation, and may foretell a prolonged post-transplant course with right ventricular failure. A PVR greater than 8 units is an absolute contraindication. Patients with end-stage cardiac disease secondary to congenital structural abnormalities have a greater likelihood of having PVOD than has the simple cardiomyopathic patient; this is a consequence of increased pulmonary blood flow and pressure, as well as of the cyanosis which is associated with congenital lesions.

Cardiac catheterization may also demonstrate structural abnormalities amenable to more traditional management, obviating the need for transplantation. For example, we recently evaluated a 2-year-old child who was found to have an anomalous left coronary artery arising from the pulmonary artery; surgical correction was performed. The problems of mitral, aortic, and/or tricuspid valve insufficiency, associated with cardiomyopathy, are more difficult to evaluate. When the valve lesions are major, and the cardiomyopathy minor, valve repair or replacement can be expected to be effective. All too often, however, severe cardiomyopathy associated with, or even secondary to, aortic or mitral valve insufficiency is not improved by valve repair or replacement (Figure 24.1). It remains difficult to determine when valve repair or replacement should be performed and when transplantation should be entertained initially.

The patient with a cardiac anomaly considered suitable for transplantation is screened for the presence of active infectious disease. Immunologic evaluation for donor match includes blood group and cross-matching, HLA tissue typing, and the presence and percentage of lymphocytotoxic reactive antibodies (Chapter 8). Blood group compatibility is essential, even in infants. HLA typing appears to be less important, as in the adult population (Chapter 8). The presence of reactive antibodies (greater than 10–15%) necessitates a lymphocytotoxic cross-match with the potential donor. In infants under 3 months of age, however, reactive antibodies are probably maternal, and their significance is thus questionable. In all infants, a maternal lymphocytotoxic screen is performed, as well as the infant's screen.

An interdisciplinary team approach is employed, utilizing members of the surgical, cardiological, infectious disease, psychiatric, and social services, and dietary, occupational/physical therapy, and nursing professionals. When a patient is found to be unacceptable for transplantation, the reasons and future management are discussed with the family and referring physician, and plans made for continued medical care.

PRETRANSPLANT CARE

Once accepted for transplantation, the pretransplant waiting period is utilized for patient and family teaching. Medical management is optimized to maintain the patient infection-free, with optimal renal and hepatic function. Care is on an outpatient basis unless the patient's cardiac status becomes inadequate.

Myocardial support

Cardiac support with digitalis, diuretics, and afterload reduction is the norm. When necessary, intravenous cardiotonic support is added; we have relied heavily on dopamine and amrinone. Experience with assisted circulation is limited in the pediatric population. Intra-aortic balloon counterpulsation can be effective in the smallest of children, but is limited by vascular access in the infant, the inability of the balloon to track at heart rates over 160 beats/minute, and poor augmentation in the relatively compliant pediatric aorta.

Pennington and his group have supported the circulation in 40 children with various support systems, including the ventricular assist device, intra-aortic balloon pump, and extracorporeal membrane oxygenation[23]. As in the adult population, assist devices as a bridge to transplantation may be an effective tool, especially when the bridge is needed for only a short period of time[24] (Section IV). Prolonged support, however, may be associated with severe complications, including bleeding, renal failure, infections, and neurologic deficit. No data are presently available on the ultimate success of transplantation in children following assisted circulation bridges.

Immunization program

One of the major concerns of transplantation in the infant and child is that of ultimate immunologic insufficiency in a subject who is already 'immunologically naive'. Every attempt should be made to complete a normal immunization program (Table 24.1) before the transplant procedure is

Table 24.1 Immunization schedule for children

Age	Vaccine
2 months	DTP, OPV
4 months	DTP, OPV
6 months	DTP (optional OPV)
15 months	MMR
18 months	DTP, OPV
2 years	HBPV
4–6 years	DTP, OPV
14–16 years	TD

DTP, diphtheria and tetanus toxoids with pertussis vaccine; OPV, oral poliovirus (live attenuated); MMR, measles, mumps, and rubella (live attenuated); HBPV, hemophilus 5 polysaccharide vaccine; TD, tetanus and adult diphtheria toxoid

performed. Once the child is receiving immunosuppressive therapy, the efficacy of immunization is questionable. In addition, immunosuppressed children may be at significant risk from common childhood illnesses. When the transplant procedure is urgent and imminent, full immunization must obviously be delayed. When elective, however, immunization should be completed, even if this necessitates delaying the transplant procedure for a short period of time.

When transplantation is urgent, or after transplant has been performed, the immunization protocol must be modified, utilizing only dead vaccines, and never live attenuated vaccines. Thus, oral polio virus vaccine (Sabin) should be avoided in the peritransplant period, and only dead vaccine (Salk) should be employed. Likewise, measles, mumps, and rubella vaccine (MMR) should be avoided in the peritransplant period.

SURGICAL TECHNIQUES

Technique of orthotopic heart transplantation for cardiomyopathy

Donor procurement

The donor operation is identical to that in the adult (Chapter 10). The donor is first evaluated by taking a medical (including trauma) history, and by assessment of hemodynamic and cardiac status, and by blood grouping. Hearts with severe congenital defects should clearly be avoided as donors.

The myocardium is protected with a suitable cardioplegic agent (e.g. St. Thomas's solution) and maintained in a cold crystalloid or saline solution for transportation. A total ischemic time of 3–4 hours appears to be acceptable. When infants and neonatal donors are available, it may be feasible to transport the entire donor in an isolette. This allows for donor and recipient procedures to be performed in adjacent operating rooms, and markedly limits ischemic time. We have done this in half of our infant transplants. In view of the paucity of pediatric donors, this method is valuable in allowing use of distant donors where transportation of the isolated heart would be time-prohibitive.

Simple defects, such as patent foramen ovale and patent ductus arteriosus, can be readily repaired in the explanted heart.

Recipient operation

The recipient procedure is similar to that in the adult (Chapter 10). Preoperative monitoring includes central venous and arterial pressures. A Swan–Ganz catheter is passed in the operative field through the new heart into the pulmonary artery, though in children under 10 kg we have avoided such a catheter as it is cumbersome and difficult to manage. After implantation of the donor heart, a 3 French catheter, with a thermistor tip, is placed directly through the right ventricle into the pulmonary artery, and secured with a pledgetted right ventricular mattress suture. This thermistor tip, in conjunction with a standard central venous catheter, allows reproducible thermal dilution cardiac output studies.

Technique of orthotopic heart transplantation for hypoplastic left heart syndrome

Bailey et al. have reported a technique for transplantation in patients with hypoplastic left heart syndrome (Figure 24.4)[1,2].

Donor operation

Bailey has recently reported the use of cardiopulmonary bypass to cool the donor, which has the advantage of cooling all organs for donation, and in addition obviates any possible detrimental effect of crystalloid cardioplegia in the neonate. Donor heart excision is performed, and any patent ductus arteriosus present is ligated and divided. The ascending aorta, complete aortic arch, and origins of the arteries to the head and upper limbs are dissected free and removed *in toto* so that the donor aortic arch and proximal descending aorta remain intact (Figure 24.5). The left and right pulmonary arteries are divided just distal to the bifurcation of the main pulmonary artery to afford a large pulmonary anastomosis. After heart excision, the patent foramen ovale is identified and closed with a figure-of-eight 4-0 suture.

Recipient operation

Until the recipient heart is removed, the patient is maintained on prostaglandin infusion to ensure patency of the ductus arteriosus. Surface cooling with ice may be used as a preliminary to sternotomy. Cardiopulmonary bypass is instituted, employing a single arterial perfusion catheter

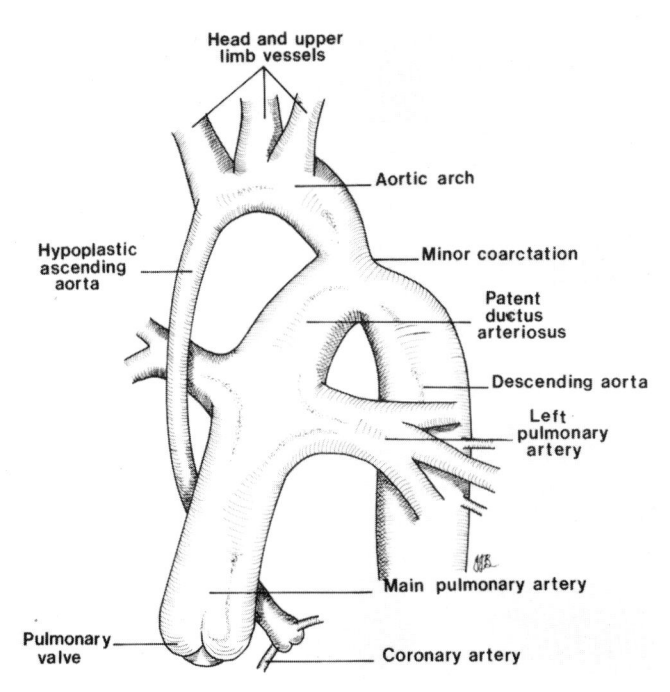

Figure 24.4 Anatomy of the great vessels in the hypoplastic left heart syndrome. The ascending aorta is hypoplastic and carries only blood (flowing retrograde) to the coronary arteries. Aortic perfusion is from the pulmonary artery via the very large patent ductus arteriosus. A severe coarctation of the aorta is most frequently present in a juxtaductal or preductal position

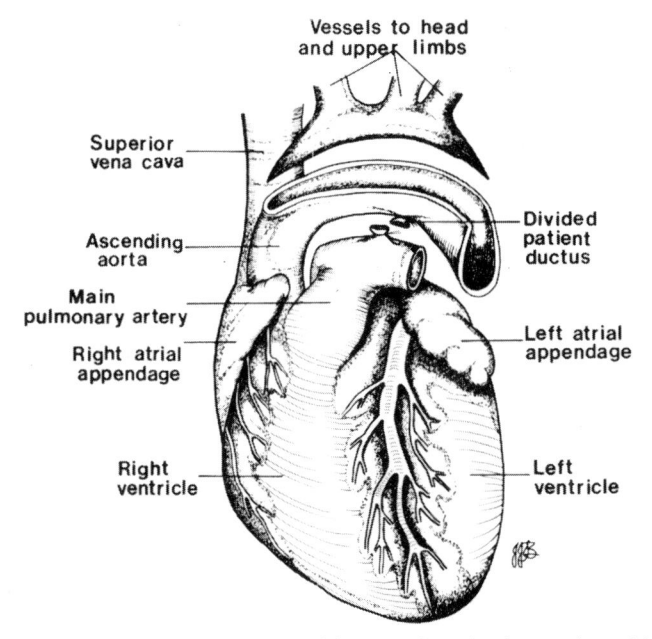

Figure 24.5 Donor heart prepared for transplantation in a patient with hypoplastic left heart syndrome. The patent ductus arteriosus has been divided between ligatures. The aortic arch and descending aorta are preserved after resecting the superior surface (or 'button') which includes the origins of the vessels to the head and upper limbs

placed in the aorta via the main pulmonary artery or ductus arteriosus, and a single venous cannula in the right atrium through the right atrial appendage. We prefer a 10 French Pacifico-type arterial perfusion catheter. A right-angled 18–21 Rygg venous cannula is appropriate for venous return. The patient is cooled on bypass with topical as well as core cooling. Regitine 0.1 mg/kg in the prime assures vasodilation and uniform blood distribution.

As soon as total bypass is instituted, the left and right pulmonary arteries are isolated at their origins from the main pulmonary trunk, and snared to prevent further pulmonary blood flow. Alternatively, a snare is tightened around the ductus containing the arterial perfusion cannula. The ascending aorta, aortic arch, and head and upper limb vessels are also isolated on snares. The ductus arteriosus, which represents the total systemic output, is dissected from pulmonary artery to descending aorta. The descending aorta is isolated at least 2 cm below the level of the ductus (and coarctation, when present).

When the rectal or nasopharyngeal temperature reaches 15–20°C, cardiopulmonary bypass is discontinued, and the blood drained from the patient into the pump-oxygenator. The aortic arch vessels are snared, and the distal thoracic aorta is cross-clamped. The arterial and venous perfusion cannulas are removed. The ascending aorta is ligated and divided (Figure 24.6). The ductus arteriosus is divided on the under surface of the aortic arch. Care is taken to remove all ductal tissue, which has the potential for both bleeding and contracting (with ultimate stenosis). The main pulmonary artery is divided at the pulmonary valve, and the heart removed at the atrioventricular groove. Any atrial septal defect is closed.

The cooled donor heart is brought into the pericardial cavity, and the left atrial anastomosis is performed first. In the hypoplastic left heart syndrome, the recipient left atrium is usually quite small, and plication of the donor atrium is usually necessary to complete this anastomosis. The majority of the donor atrial plication is performed along its septum to prevent external bleeding. Before completion of the left atrial anastomosis, a left atrial sump is passed through the mitral valve into the left ventricle. The right atrial anastomosis is next performed, as in the adult transplant.

The recipient pulmonary artery is usually 2–3 times larger than the donor pulmonary artery. This discrepancy can be overcome by spatulating the left and right pulmonary arteries of the donor (Figure 24.7). The origins of the vessels to the head and upper limbs arising from the donor aortic arch are discarded, and a long spatulated anastomosis performed between the two aortae, utilizing the donor aortic arch and descending aorta as an onlay patch to create continuity with the recipient aorta as well as to repair any coarctation (Figure 24.7). Cardiopulmonary bypass is reinstituted (with a venous cannula in the right atrium and an arterial cannula in the donor aorta) and the patient is warmed.

Figure 24.6 Excision of the native heart. Atrial excision is as in the adult. The ascending aorta is ligated and divided. The large ductus arteriosus is ligated and divided at the underside of the aorta. The aorta is incised longitudinally from the arch, beyond the coarctation, to the descending aorta. Care is taken to remove all ductal tissue from the aorta

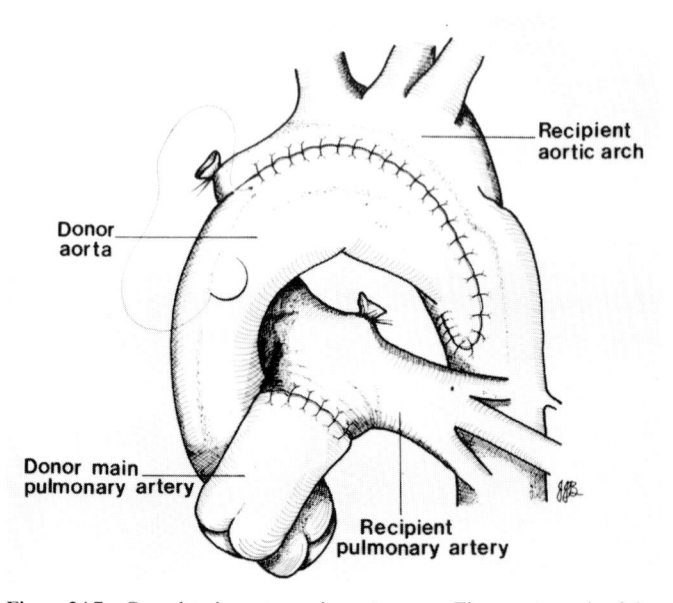

Figure 24.7 Completed great vessel anastomoses. The anastomosis of the pulmonary arteries is as in the adult. The donor aortic flap is anastomosed to the recipient aorta in such a way to recreate aortic continuity and to repair the coarctation

IMMUNOSUPPRESSION

Many different immunosuppressive protocols have been utilized in the pediatric population. There is much reticence to the long-term use of corticosteroids in children because of the fear of retardation of growth and development. Our own protocol is outlined below.

Maintenance therapy

Six hours pretransplantation, cyclosporine 5 mg/kg and azathioprine 2 mg/kg are given orally.

In the postoperative period, cyclosporine is titrated to maintain a whole blood radioimmunoassay (RIA) monoclonal level of 300–400 ng/ml. A daily dosage of between 1 and 10 mg/kg may be required. In older children cyclosporine is administered 12-hourly, but, because of an apparent increased metabolism of cyclosporine in young children and infants, we have found that 8-hourly administration provides appropriate blood levels without excessive dosage in these groups. Six to 8 months after transplantation, and if no rejection is evident, dosage is modified to maintain a whole blood RIA monoclonal level of 200–250 ng/ml.

Azathioprine is titrated with a daily dose[25] to maintain the white blood cell count at 5000–9000 cells/mm^3.

We utilize steroids preoperatively in all patients, and long-term in patients over 12 years of age. Methylprednisolone 10 mg/kg is given intravenously with initiation of reperfusion of the donor heart (when the aortic cross-clamp is removed). Daily maintenance is then begun with methylprednisolone (3 mg/kg intravenously) or prednisone orally, beginning with a dose of 3 mg/kg and tapering to 0.3 mg/kg per day in children over 12 years of age. In infants and growing children, steroids are discontinued after an initial three daily doses (each of methylprednisolone 10 mg/kg).

Antithymocyte globulin (ATG) 10 mg/kg is given intravenously over 6 hours at the completion of cardiopulmonary bypass, and once daily for 5 days. The ATG allows for maximum immunosuppression in the perioperative period when renal dysfunction may complicate full-dose cyclosporine[26].

Antirejection therapy

Early episodes of acute rejection are defined as rejection in the first 90 days after transplantation. Such an episode is managed with bolus intravenous methylprednisolone 10 mg/kg per day for 3 days. Persistence of rejection is an indication for a second such course. We have not experienced rejection refractory to such a protocol; in such an event, a course of ATG (or OKT3) would be administered.

Mild to moderate rejection occurring after 90 days post-transplant is treated with oral prednisone 1 mg/kg per day, and is tapered to maintenance level over a 3-week period. Severe rejection is managed with intravenous steroid bolus therapy.

The Loma Linda group has had excellent results utilizing single drug therapy, employing cyclosporine alone, initially intravenously and subsequently orally[11].

DIAGNOSIS OF REJECTION

Timely and accurate diagnosis of graft rejection is of primary importance to ensure prolonged survival of the transplant patient. In the adult patient, endomyocardial biopsy (EMB) serves as the standard against which all other diagnostic methods must be evaluated. At St. Christopher's Hospital for Children in Philadelphia, we have utilized EMB in all patients, including infants[27]. Our protocol includes EMB weekly for the first month, biweekly for the subsequent 2 months, monthly for the next 6 months, and at 3–6-month intervals after this time. In addition, EMB is freely performed for suspicion of rejection and in the presence of any unexplained symptoms.

In infants and small children, the EMB technique requires modification from that in the adult. Access is via the femoral vein, and a soft, flexible, disposable biopsy forceps (bioptome) (Cordis Corporation, Miami, Florida) is employed. A 7 French sheath is placed via the femoral vein. A balloon-tipped catheter is then floated into the right ventricle, after which the sheath is advanced over the catheter into the right ventricle. The balloon-tipped catheter is then removed. The bioptome is passed through the sheath into the right ventricle. A total of 3–6 biopsies are obtained. The technique of advancing the sheath into the ventricle is essential, since the small bioptome used has no preformed shape nor adequate 'memory', and cannot readily be passed into the ventricle without the support of the sheath. Added advantages of this technique include protection of the tricuspid valve, and the ease of passing the biopsy forceps repeatedly through the sheath without further significant manipulation. We have utilized this technique without complications. With the exception of biopsies performed during the initial period of hospitalization following transplantation, all biopsies are carried out on an outpatient basis.

The biopsy specimens procured by this technique are small, but adequate for evaluation of rejection. Histopathological interpretation is as in the adult (Chapter 15).

Bailey et al. have relied on clinical parameters and echocardiography in the diagnosis of acute rejection in infants, utilizing EMB only in older patients[11]. Diagnosis of rejection is entertained when there are symptoms or signs of fever, lethargy, poor feeding, tachycardia, tachypnea, and congestive heart failure. Clinical findings are supported by electrocardiographic, echocardiographic, and radiographic evidence of rejection, such as cardiomegaly, and by the presence of an elevated leukocyte count. These indicators have proved more than adequate, and this group has obtained excellent results.

COMMENT

Cardiac transplantation in children is now gaining widespread acceptance. Results, although not quite equal to those in adults, demonstrate that transplantation can be successful in treating end-stage heart disease and severe forms of congenital heart disease in children. There would appear to be no limitation regarding size or weight of the recipient, although it has proved difficult to procure an adequate number of suitable organs for our pediatric patients. Unless organs from other animal species (xenografts) are made available (Section VI), it would appear that the problem of organ shortage will become even more serious as transplantation is offered to an increasing number of infants and children.

References

1. Barnard, C.N. (1968). Human cardiac transplantation. An evaluation of the first two operations performed at the Groote Schuur Hospital, Cape Town. *Am. J. Cardiol.*, **22**, 584
2. Kantrowitz, A., Haller, J.D., Joos, H., Cerruti, M.M. and Carstensen, H.E. (1968). Transplantation of the heart in an infant and an adult. *Am. J. Cardiol.*, **22**, 782
3. Cooley, D.A., Bloodwell, R.D., Hallman, G.L., Nora, J.J., Harrison, G.M. and Leachman, R.D. (1969). Organ transplantation for advanced cardiopulmonary disease. *Ann. Thorac. Surg.*, **8**, 30
4. Kaye, M.P. (1987). The Registry of the International Society of Heart Transplantation: fourth official report – 1987. *J. Heart Transplant.*, **6**, 63
5. Baum, D., Stinson, E.B. and Shumway, N.E. (1981). The place for heart transplantation in children. *Pediatr. Cardiol.*, **4**, 743
6. English, T.A.H. (1983). Commentary. Is cardiac transplantation suitable in children? *Pediatr. Cardiol.*, **4**, 57
7. Penkoske, P.A., Freedom, R.M., Rowe, R.D. and Trusler, G.A. (1984). The future of heart and heart–lung transplantation in children. *Heart Transplant.*, **3**, 233
8. Pennington, D.G., Sarafian, J. and Swartz, M. (1985). Heart transplantation in children. *J. Heart Transplant.*, **4**, 441
9. Addonizio, L. and Rose, E.A. (1987). Cardiac transplantation in children and adolescents. *J. Pediatr.*, **3**, 1034
10. Bailey, L.L., Nehlson-Cannarella, S., Concepcion, W. and Jolley, W.B. (1985). Baboon-to-human cardiac xenotransplantation in a neonate. *J. Am. Med. Assoc.*, **254**, 3321
11. Bailey, L.L., Nehlsen-Cannarella, S.L., Doroshow, R.W., Jacobson, J.G., Martin, R.D., Allard, M.W., Hyde, M.R., Dang Bui, R.H. and Petry, E.L. (1986). Cardiac allotransplantation in newborns as therapy for hypoplastic left heart syndrome. *N. Engl. J. Med.*, **315**, 949
12. Bailey, L.L., Concepcion, W., Shattuck, H. and Huang, L. (1986). Method of heart transplantation for treatment of hypoplastic left heart syndrome. *J. Thorac. Cardiovasc. Surg.*, **92**, 1
13. Dunn, J.M., Cavarocchi, N.C., Balsara, R.K., Kolff, J., McClurken, J., Bordellino, M.M., Vieweg, C. and Donner, R.M. (1987). Pediatric heart transplantation at St. Christopher's Hospital for Children. *J. Heart Transplant.*, **6**, 334
14. Schmeltz-Lawrence, K. and Fricker, F.J. (1987). Pediatric heart transplantation: quality of life. *J. Heart Transplant.*, **6**, 329
15. Greenwood, R.D., Nadas, A.S. and Fyler, D.C. (1976). The clinical course of primary myocardial disease in infants and children. *Am. Heart J.*, **92**, 549
16. Keogh, A.H., Freund, J., Baron, D.W. and Hickie, J.B. (1988). Timing of cardiac transplantation in idiopathic dilated cardiomyopathy. *Am. J. Cardiol.*, **61**, 418
17. Michels, V.V., Driscoll, D.J. and Miller, F.A. (1985). Familial aggregation of idiopathic dilated cardiomyopathy. *Am. J. Cardiol.*, **55**, 1232
18. Schaffer, M.S., Freedom, R.M. and Rowe, R.D. (1983). Hypertrophic cardiomyopathy presenting before 2 years of age in 13 patients. *Pediatr. Cardiol.*, **4**, 113
19. Griffin, M.L., Hernandez, A., Martin, T.C., Goldring, D., Bolman, R.M., Spray, T.L. and Strauss, A.W. (1988). Dilated cardiomyopathy in infants and children. *J. Am. Coll. Cardiol.*, **11**, 139
20. Macoviak, J.A., Baldwin, J.C., Ginsburg, R., Fowler, M., Valentine, H., Oyer, P.E. and Stinson, E.B. (1988). Orthotopic cardiac transplantation for univentricular heart. *Ann. Thorac. Surg.*, **45**, 85
21. Reitz, B.A., Jamieson, S.W., Gaudiani, V.A., Oyer, P.E. and Stinson, E.B. (1982). Method for cardiac transplantation in corrected transposition of the great arteries. *J. Cardiovasc. Surg.*, **23**, 293
22. Edwards, W.S. (1983). Endomyocardial biopsy and cardiomyopathy. *Cardiovasc. Rev. Rep.*, **4**, 820
23. Pennington, D.G., Codd, J.E., Merjavy, J.P., Swartz, M.T., Kaiser, G.C., Barner, H.B. and Willman, V.L. (1983). The expanded use of ventricular bypass systems for severe cardiac failure and as a bridge to cardiac transplantation. *Heart Transplant.*, **3**, 38
24. Pae, W.E. and Pierce, W.S. (1987). Combined registry for the clinical use of mechanical ventricular assist pumps and the total artificial heart: first official report, 1986. *J. Heart Transplant.*, **6**, 68
25. Schneider, M., Cavarocchi, N.C., Jessup, M., McClurken, J.B., Dunn, J., Narins, B., Balsara, R., Vieweg, C. and Kolff, J. (1988). Azathioprine to reverse renal dysfunction after heart transplantation. *Transplant. Proc.*, **20**, 795
26. Deeb, G.M., Kolff, J., McClurken, J.B., Dunn, J., Balsara, R., Ochs, R., Badellino, M., Hollander, T., Eldridge, C., Clancey, M., Brownstein, L. and Coakley, J. (1987). Antithymocyte gamma globulin, low-dosage cyclosporine, and tapering steroids as an immunosuppressive regimen to avoid early kidney failure in heart transplantation. *J. Heart Transplant.*, **6**, 79
27. Bhargava, H., Donner, R.M., Sanchez, G., Dunn, J.M., Zaeri, N., Brickley, S. and Cavarocchi, N. (1987). Endomyocardial biopsy after heart transplantation in children. *J. Heart Transplant.*, **6**, 298

25
Psychiatric Aspects
E.S. NASH

INTRODUCTION

Cardiac transplantation emerged in 1967 as a dramatic new way of saving the life of a dying cardiac patient[1]. It was not so much the radical nature of the procedure that triggered the reactions, but the removal and replacement of an organ that is seen by some as a physiological pump and by others as the symbolic seat of love and loyalty.

Psychiatric experience in this field is indebted to contributions from two allied areas: firstly, the care of patients undergoing closed and open heart surgery, and secondly, the experience obtained from involvement in renal and liver transplantation programs. The psychiatric implications of closed and open heart surgery have been extensively documented[2-4]. Of particular relevance has been Kimball's identification of nuclear patterns of emotional reaction in patients who were assessed preoperatively; these patterns have been found to have predictive value. Out of the four groups that he identified, namely the adjusted, the symbiotic, the depressed, and those denying anxiety, it was the members of the latter two that caused concern. He reported that the depressed group had a high postoperative mortality rate, whilst those who denied anxiety had a high incidence of postoperative psychiatric complications[2].

The second area, i.e. psychiatric experience obtained from involvement in organ transplantation since the first kidney transplant was performed in 1950, has centered around the issues of selection criteria, organ incorporation versus rejection, postoperative psychosis, the complications of immunosuppressive medications, compliance and rehabilitation.

Psychiatric experience in heart transplantation over the past 20 years has been similar; recipients require psychosocial screening, develop early and late postoperative emotional or behavioral disturbances and have to incorporate a new life-giving organ. Heart transplant recipients have to face not only the physical challenges of organ rejection and systemic infections, but also the psychological challenges of re-organizing family relationships and of re-entering employment. It is in all these areas that psychiatric insights have helped transplant teams. Each of these aspects will be considered in greater detail.

The importance of the role of the psychiatrist is well illustrated by the observation at our own institute (Groote Schuur Hospital in Cape Town) that no fewer than 26% of deaths or loss of allograft function were related, in some part, to non-compliance on the part of the patient[5], thereby drawing attention to the psychological problems such patients display.

PATIENT SELECTION

'Patient selection is important because basic issues of social policy, the limits of medical responsibility, major ethical and legal considerations are encapsulated in the decision to choose or reject patients....'[6].

In the early years of cardiac transplantation, mental deficiency and overt psychosis were the only psychiatric grounds used to justify exclusion from a program[7]. With improved survival and the subsequent expansion of transplantation, the selection of suitable recipients has recently become an even more important issue[8]. Most centers now have a committee of medical personnel who take medical, psychological and social criteria into account (see also Chapter 26). A preliminary screening inevitably occurs prior to the actual referral, which reflects to some extent the responses of the referring physician to the patient's personality and to the character of his or her family. Self-referrals for cardiac transplantation must be viewed with some caution since this may be indicative of exhibitionistic traits in patients seeking publicity. (The self-referral of donors, however, requires immediate psychiatric intervention, since this suggests suicide intent.)

The psychiatric assessment of patients who have been referred for transplantation includes an in-depth interview that reviews the patient's personal development, family background and history of psychiatric illness, as well as his or her attitudes to the illness, disability, death and transplantation. During this interview it is of particular value to assess the patient's ego strengths such as his or her capacity to (1) understand the information offered, to think about problems in a rational way, to communicate needs and be motivated to regain health; (2) face reality, and not resort to excessive denial or fantasy; (3) maintain a stable mood, without wide emotional swings from elation to the depths of despair; (4) control basic impulses, such as anger, greed, sexuality and self-abuse; (5) use mature ego defenses in everyday life and under conditions of stress; (6) perform age-appropriate life tasks, e.g. education, employment and social responsibilities; (7) make mutually rewarding relationships and use social support; and finally (8) define his/her values, abide by these and use social resources that reinforce these. These ego strengths are based on those described by Beard[9] and Bellak[10].

Dreams are useful clues to reveal unspoken concerns. It is also important to examine current mental functioning using a standardized method[11], which should include inquiry about depression, suicidal ideas and memory impairment, as well as assessment of intelligence, insight and capacity to make sound judgments, with special relevance to the giving of informed consent. Formal psychological testing may be of assistance[12,13], but critically ill patients are frequently not able to carry out such tests.

Evidence of organic impairment may be found in patients with poor cerebral perfusion, but, if this is associated with neurological deficits, the impairment is likely to be permanent and due to brain damage. Where there are language barriers, competent and empathic interpreters, who are familiar with the transplant program, are invaluable.

Evidence of a disturbed personality, indicated by alcohol and drug dependence, an erratic work record, unstable interpersonal relations, and antisocial behavior, have been added in most programs to the original exclusion criteria of mental deficiency and overt psychosis[13]. The quality of the patient's psychosocial support is of great importance, and must also be taken into account[14,15]. This is particularly so in the occasional patient who has been fortunate in never before having had to make a major adjustment in his or her life; such patients may find the adjustments forced on them by the need for heart transplantation particularly difficult, thereby complicating their preparation for operation and their convalescence.

The nature of the heart disease in itself may be a clue to the patient's personality and his/her customary ways of adapting to stress. Since some candidates have a history of myocardial infarction (complicating coronary artery disease), they may well show features of the type A behavior pattern described by Friedman and Rosenman[16]. Such individuals characteristically show ambitiousness, striving, overcommitment to work, time urgency and impatience[17]. They strive to be 'good' patients postoperatively and are highly motivated to survive. Another identifiable group comprises those with cardiomyopathy, which has been associated with shorter survival when linked to significant alcohol abuse and unstable work and relationship patterns[5]. Careful thought has to be given before a transplant operation is performed on such unpredictable individuals.

Whilst patients with rheumatic or congenital heart disease, who have tolerated previous operative intervention, are likely to handle the stress of the transplantation procedure satisfactorily, they may have difficulty in relinquishing a well-established sick role; rehabilitation then becomes a major exercise.

Factors that are predictive of a favorable outcome include a patient's ability to discuss the possibility of his or her own death as well as having a clear use for the time gained by longer survival, reinforced by sound social support[18].

AWAITING A TRANSPLANT

Once a patient has been accepted for a program, he or she has to await a donor heart. Patients referred from distant places may have to live temporarily near the hospital and are often supported by only one family member. This alien environment can be stressful, especially if the patient has left a well-established support structure and has to wait many weeks. Initial optimism may give way to anxiety, despair and even depression. Individuals who use acting-out, impulsive behavior have difficulty tolerating this phase; exclusion from the program, even at this late stage, should be considered.

IMMEDIATE POSTOPERATIVE PERIOD

In the early days of cardiac transplantation many patients became psychologically disturbed during the initial postoperative period, just as they did in the early days of heart surgery[4]. These changes were attributed to the convergence of such factors as altered cerebral circulation, prolonged anesthesia, overstimulation by the monitoring system, the sensory deprivation of immobility, and the unfamiliar bland environment peopled by masked strangers.

The acute psychosis that can occur in this phase bears the features of both 'organic' and 'functional' disturbance; symptoms include reduced level of consciousness, hallucinations, paranoid delusions, disorientation for time and place, and mood disturbance such as depression or undue euphoria. Unconscious anxiety and fantasies about the transplanted heart may be voiced in this context[19].

More recent reports now indicate that there is little disturbance in the early postoperative period, which is possibly indicative of improved patient preparation prior to the procedure[12]. Although many patients are persistently euphoric at having survived the procedure, and are delighted with their increased vital capacity and physical strength, this state of well-being can be threatened by episodes of organ rejection or infection that may trigger depression and anxiety. If hospitalization is prolonged, boredom and social isolation may also take an emotional toll. The steroids required to combat organ rejection pose an additional hazard since they are known to produce depression and even psychosis[20].

Mild symptoms respond to a psychotherapeutic interview and program modification; more severe disturbances such as regressed behavior, irritability, paranoid fears, suicidal feelings and ideas may emerge and require treatment with neuroleptic medication such as chlorpromazine or thioridazine. Such drugs, however, have a relatively long half-life, and should be used with caution in debilitated patients; a butyrophenone, such as haloperidol, or a thioxanthine, may be preferable in such cases. Antidepressants such as the tri- or tetracyclic agents should also be administered with caution, again as they are long-acting, may share a metabolic pathway for degradation with cyclosporine, and may have an arrhythmogenic effect. Shorter acting non-tricyclics, such as trazodone and maprotiline, offer an alternative. In addition, it has been well-documented that emotional factors can influence the immunologic balance of the body, thereby affecting the organ acceptance or rejection[21].

Regressed behavior, which is often triggered by medical complications, responds to empathic and firm handling by staff. As dependency on the staff lessens, it becomes necessary for the patient to practice autonomy in taking control of some aspects of treatment. Many patients are anxious about leaving the security of the hospital and require gradual weaning from the intensive care unit and, later, the ward environment. The spouse also needs reassurance and instruction. The psychiatrist, clinical psychologist, or psychiatric social worker can help the surgical team understand the anxieties that inevitably occur during and after any hospitalization, particularly if the hospital stay has been for heart transplantation[22].

It is also very important to remember that disturbed behavior, confusion and headaches, may actually have a neurological cause, such as an intracranial viral, bacterial or fungal infection, which can occur more frequently in an immunologically compromised host. Epileptic fits, local pain, or paralysis are indications for immediate neurological investigation to rule out infarction or infection. Neoplasia may account for later neurological disturbance[23].

REHABILITATION

The successful transplant recipient has survived a unique life experience. Some survivors of cardiac arrest admit to thoughts of resurrection and fantasies of rebirth[24,25]. An effective donor heart pumps new life through the body and brain, bringing physical vigor, an enriched personality, improved memory and the promise of health. Cardiac resuscitation and cardiac surgery have introduced a new dimension of human experience; the patients both 'die' and are 'reborn' or 'resurrected'[26]. To quote Paul Coffey, a British heart transplant survivor, 'Following the transplant, and being given a second chance of life, one has time to think about what really matters'[27].

Integration of the new heart into the body image is effected in various ways. The organ has to be 'taken in' and become part of a healthy body representation. The heart is seen as a pump to the mechanically-minded patient, devoid of emotional significance, which can be replaced if worn out. At the other extreme, however, a few recipients unmistakably identify with the sex and personality of the donor. Reactions to the organ influence compliance with medication. Complete integration of the organ into the body image involves dealing at some level with feelings of guilt and indebtedness for having received an organ at the cost of another life[19,28]. Mai has observed that in 18 of the 20 heart transplant subjects that he studied, significant denial with respect to the graft, the donor or both, was present in the 30–90-day period following surgery[29].

Recipients of donor hearts have to deal with fantasies about the donor. At the present time most recipients are men; most donors are also men, frequently young men who have sustained head injuries in road traffic accidents[6]. Louis Washkansky, the first heart transplant patient, however, received a heart from a female donor. He enquired 'Do you think…that I might develop busts like a woman?…or become chicken-hearted?'[30]. Other male recipients receiving hearts from female donors have also had this type of reaction, though, with increasing frequency of the operation, such fantasies are becoming rare.

The early transplant patients' fame nourished the rehabilitation process and ensured a 'survivor mission' reaction which was frequently useful in gaining their co-operation in carrying out research, for example, on the physiology of the denervated heart[31]. For subsequent survivors the rehabilitation process has been a less dramatic affair, with mundane issues such as housing, employment and restored marital relationships to be faced (Chapter 26). As cardiac transplantation has become commonplace, however, the patient has had a greater exposure to the experiences of fellow recipients, and such interchange and sharing can be of great emotional support. Many centers have initiated support groups to enable patients to share their experiences and concerns.

While euphoria and improved self-esteem are found in many patients following operation, the steroid facies, which still occurs in a few, may make the recipient feel self-conscious, and unable to adapt to the new bloated appearance. In some patients there are difficulties in concentration, emotional lability, and irritability[20], while, in others, features of mild organic brain impairment can be found[32]. Recipients may show a morbid interest in their surgical 'twins' who have received organs from the same donor (e.g. kidneys), and identify closely with them.

Follow-up has to be carefully planned. On the one hand, transfer to physicians or surgeons remote from the transplant center, who have had little experience with transplantation programs, engenders insecurity and negative transference reactions, and this may jeopardize compliance with dietary instructions and medication – and hence survival. On the other hand, follow-up by the patient's own doctor lessens the overidentification with fellow transplant patients and grief at their death.

The return to the family means there has to be a reorganization of the family system[12]. Wives often feel insecure in adapting to a more active spouse, though marital relations may be jeopardized by drug-induced impotence[33]. Marital and family counselling may be required. The risk of rejecting the transplanted heart initially inhibits long-term planning. Nevertheless, favorable reports of the effective rehabilitation of 91% of the patients who had survived more than 6 months after transplantation at Stanford have spurred enthusiasm in transplant programs[34,35]. Improved survival has ensured official and community support for continuation and expansion of these programs.

TEAMWORK

Human organ transplantation is notable for its intensive interdisciplinary team work. It is a collaborative enterprise that requires the skills of surgeons, anesthesiologists, physicians (cardiac, renal, pulmonary), microbiologists, immunologists, hematologists, neurologists, psychiatrists, social workers, nurses, radiographers, physiotherapists and occupational therapists, as well as the technicians who assemble the heart–lung machine, and carry out the many necessary immunological and biochemical assays[6,8].

In a large center, a key individual is the liaison nurse, who mediates between the team that has to abandon the life-saving procedures on the donor, and the transplantation team, eager to receive organs in good condition. He/she has an important role in sustaining the donor's family in their grief and obtaining consent for organ usage, where this is legally required. Here too, psychiatric skills play a major role. Newcomers to the service, however, may find that the unique demands of the program tax their professional equilibrium, especially if they have unrealistic expectations of their roles. Psychiatric assistance may be necessary for such individuals if team support is not enough. Frequent team meetings are valuable to allow members to express their feelings and ensure good communication and support.

COMMENT

Heart transplantation raises the cosmic issues of death, resurrection and immortality that transcend the mundane daily concern of heart sounds, lymphocyte counts and blood cultures. A program of this kind demands the best that an academic or a research center has to offer, and stretches the imagination in seeking how to extend productive lives. 'Heart transplantation remains a major undertaking on the part of both patient and transplant team, but offers carefully selected patients with advanced myocardial disease the possibility of a good quality of life for a number of years'[5].

Psychiatrists and social workers have played a useful role in renal, liver and heart transplantation programs by assisting with selection and helping transplant teams handle the more complicated behavioral, emotional and family problems which regularly accompany major procedures that aim to prolong life. Donor families may also need support in coming to terms with their anger about delays in burial as well as with the finality of death that removal of the heart, in particular, confirms. These families often seek to find out the identity of the recipient, since the survival of the recipient gives their loss some meaning.

In addition, cardiac transplantation has opened up important ethical issues of selection, the finality of life, the definition of death, informed consent, and priorities in the allocation of scarce life-saving resources[32,36–38]. The giving and receiving of a body organ – a gift of enormous value – is the most significant aspect of human organ transplantation. It is not a private transaction between the donor and recipient, but rather takes place within a network of personal relationships that includes families, the medical team and society.

Mauss has described the gift relationship as a series of implied obligations – to give, to receive, and to repay[39]. In the context of cardiac transplantation, it is life that is given up, received, and renewed. Thus, donor, recipient, and kin can become bound to one another emotionally and morally in ways that can be fettering as well as self-transcending. Organ transplantation has brought issues of gift exchange and social solidarity to the fore, and has shown how technical advances tend to outstrip contemporary psychological and social organization. Heart transplantation highlights the value medical science places on individual human life, and the progress that is possible through the application of science with compassion.

References

1. Barnard, C.N. (1967). A human cardiac transplant: an interim report of a successful operation performed at Groote Schuur Hospital, Cape Town. *S. Afr. Med. J.*, **41**, 1271
2. Kimball, C.P. (1969). Psychological responses to the experience of open heart surgery. *Am. J. Psychiatr.*, **126**, 348
3. Abram, H.S. (1971). Psychotic reactions after cardiac surgery – a critical review. In Castelnuovo-Tedesco, P. (ed.) *Psychiatric Aspects of Organ Transplantation*. p. 70. (New York: Grune and Stratton)
4. Heller, S. and Kornfeld, D. (1986). Psychiatric aspects of cardiac surgery. *Adv. Psychosom. Med.*, **15**, 124

5. Cooper, D.K.C., Lanza, R.P. and Barnard, C.N. (1984). Non-compliance in heart transplant recipients: the Cape Town experience. *Heart Transplant.*, **3**, 248
6. Fox, R.C. and Swazey, J.P. (1974). *The Courage to Fail.* p. 242. (Chicago: University of Chicago Press)
7. Christopherson, L.K. and Lunde, D.T. (1971). The selection of cardiac transplant recipients and their subsequent psychosocial adjustment. In Castelnuovo-Tedesco, P. (ed.) *Psychiatric Aspects of Organ Transplantation.* p. 36. (New York: Grune and Stratton)
8. Freeman III, A.M., Watts, D. and Karp, R. (1984). Evaluation of cardiac transplant candidates: preliminary observations. *Psychosomatics*, **25**, 197
9. Beard, B.H. (1969). Fear of death and fear of life. *Arch. Gen. Psychiatr.*, **21**, 373
10. Bellak, L., Hurvich, M. and Gediman, H.K. (1973). *Ego Functions in Schizophrenics, Neurotics and Normals.* (New York: John Wiley)
11. Institute of Psychiatry, London (1987). *Notes on Eliciting and Recording Clinical Information.* 2nd ed. (London: Oxford University Press)
12. Allender, J., Shisslak, C., Kaszniak, A. and Copeland, J. (1983). Stages of psychological adjustment associated with heart transplant. *Heart Transplant.*, **2**, 228
13. Frierson, R.L. and Lippmann, S.B. (1987). Heart transplant candidates rejected on psychiatric indications. *Psychosomatics*, **28**, 347
14. Baumgartner, W.A., Reitz, B.A., Oyer, P.E., Stinson, E.B. and Shumway, N.E. (1979). Cardiac homotransplantation. *Curr. Probl. Surg.*, **16**, 1
15. Pennock, J.L., Oyer, P.E., Reitz, B.A., Jamieson, S.W., Bieber, C.P., Wallwork, J., Stinson, E.B. and Shumway, N.E. (1982). Cardiac transplantation in perspective for the future. *J. Thorac. Cardiovasc. Surg.*, **83**, 168
16. Friedman, M. and Rosenman, R.H. (1959). Association of specific overt behavior pattern with blood and cardiovascular findings: blood cholesterol level, blood clotting time, incidence of arcus senilis, and clinical coronary artery disease. *J. Am. Med. Assoc.*, **169**, 1286
17. Davies, M.H. (1981). Stress, personality and coronary artery disease. *Br. J. Hosp. Med.*, **26**, 350
18. Kaplan, H.I. and Sadock, B.J. (1985). *Comprehensive Textbook of Psychiatry*, IV. p. 1117. (Baltimore/London: Williams & Wilkins)
19. Castelnuovo-Tedesco, P. (1973). Organ transplant, body image, psychosis. *Psychoanal. Q.*, **42**, 349
20. Hall, R.C., Popkin, M.K., Stickney, S.K. and Gardner, E.R. (1979). Presentation of the steroid psychoses. *J. Ment. Nerv. Dis.*, **167**, 229
21. Freebury, D.R. (1974). The psychological implications of organ transplantation – a selective review. *Can. Psychiatr. Assoc. J.*, **19**, 593
22. Kraft, I.A. and Vick, J. (1971). The Transplantation Milieu, St. Luke's Episcopal Hospital, 1968–1969. In Castelnuovo-Tedesco, P. (ed.) *Psychiatric Aspects of Organ Transplantation.* p. 17. (New York: Grune and Stratton)
23. Hotson, J.R. and Pedley, T.A. (1976). The neurological complications of cardiac transplantation. *Brain*, **99**, 673
24. Blaiberg, P. (1969). *Looking At My Heart.* p. 120. (New York: Stein and Day)
25. Lunde, D.T. (1969). Psychiatric complications of heart transplants. *Am. J. Psychiatr.*, **126**, 369
26. Blacher, R.S. (1983). Death, resurrection, and re-birth: observations in cardiac surgery. *Psychoanal. Q.*, **52**, 56
27. Dopson, L. (1983). Every day is a bonus for us. *Nursing Times*, **79**, 8
28. Basch, S.H. (1973). The intrapsychic integration of a new organ. *Psychoanal. Q.*, **42**, 364
29. Mai, F.M. (1986). Graft and donor denial of heart transplant recipients. *Am. J. Psychiatr.*, **143**, 1159
30. Barnard, C.N. and Pepper, C.B. (1969). *One Life.* p. 322. (Cape Town: Howard Timmins)
31. Beck, W., Barnard, C.N. and Schrire, V. (1969). Heart rate after cardiac transplantation. *Circulation*, **40**, 437
32. Molish, H.B., Kraft, I.A. and Wiggins, P.Y. (1971). Psychodiagnostic evaluation of the heart transplant patient. In Castelnuovo-Tedesco, P. (ed.) *Psychiatric Aspects of Organ Transplantation.* p. 46. (New York: Grune and Stratton)
33. Wolpowitz, A. and Barnard, C.N. (1978). Impotence after heart transplantation. *S. Afr. Med. J.*, **53**, 693
34. Christopherson, L.K., Griepp, R.B. and Stinson, E.B. (1976). Rehabilitation after cardiac transplantation. *J. Am. Med. Assoc.*, **236**, 2082
35. Gaudiani, V.A., Stinson, E.B., Alderman, E., Hunt, S.A., Schroeder, J.S., Perlroth, M.G., Bieber, C.P., Oyer, P.E., Reitz, B.A., Jamieson, S.W., Christopherson, L.K. and Shumway, N.E. (1981). Long-term survival and function after cardiac transplantation. *Ann. Surg.*, **194**, 381
36. Paton, A. (1981). Life and death: moral and ethical aspects of transplantation. In Castelnuovo-Tedesco, P. (ed.) *Psychiatric Aspects of Organ Transplantation.* p. 161. (New York: Grune and Stratton)
37. Simmons, R.G., Klein, S.D. and Simmons, R.L. (1977). *Gift of Life: The Social and Psychological Impact of Organ Transplantation.* (New York: Wiley)
38. Oosthuizen, G.C. (ed.) (1972). *The Ethics of Tissue Transplantation.* (Cape Town: Howard Timmins)
39. Mauss, M. (1954). *The Gift: Forms and Functions of Exchange in Archaic Societies.* (Translated by Cunnison, I.). (London: Routledge and Kegan Paul)

26
Medico-social Aspects
W.D. PARIS

INTRODUCTION

Prior to 1967, patients with end-stage cardiac disease had little hope for the future. With the development of heart transplantation and the introduction of cyclosporine, patients who otherwise may not have survived have had an opportunity to extend and improve the quality of their lives. Survival statistics alone, however, do not reflect the challenges patients undergoing cardiac transplantation must face. Such patients must undergo what is ironically a life-threatening, but at the same time life-saving, procedure[1].

Medico-social work services have historically been available to patients and their families to help meet the challenges of transplantation. As a member of the heart transplant health care team, the social worker assists in the selection, follow-up and rehabilitation of transplant recipients. The patients and their families are assisted in their adjustment to the psychological, social, and financial impact of transplantation. As social workers, the challenge is to develop greater skill in assessing prospective candidates, and providing them with the appropriate follow-up.

Specifically, in this chapter, reference will be made to the selection process, the perioperative period, and the rehabilitation period.

ASSESSMENT AND SELECTION OF POTENTIAL RECIPIENTS

The selection phase tends to be the area of social work involvement that has received the most attention in the literature. Heart transplantation social workers initially relied on the expertise of dialysis social workers and their knowledge of patient selection and follow-up. As our professional expertise has burgeoned, there has been an increase in articles and publications specific to social work involvement with heart transplant patients and their families.

Preferably before admission or transfer to the transplant center, the social worker coordinates an assessment of the patient's personal and, in countries without socialized medicine, financial history. This preliminary work-up seeks to determine major psychiatric, social, and/or financial problems. When problems are identified, the social worker may provide counseling services or connect the family with appropriate community resources. Occasionally, these problems will be significant enough to preclude a patient's transfer to the transplant center.

Not infrequently, in countries such as the USA, with a health care system based largely on the patient's ability to pay, a major issue is one of finances. Hopefully, a prospective candidate will have medical insurance which will cover at least 80–100% of his expenses. If he does not have such insurance, he will have to rely on his own personal resources, local fund-raising activities, or, in the USA be fortunate enough to live in one of the few states that pays for this type of procedure and follow-up.

On admission, the psychosocial history is the next, and probably most important, contact that a social worker has with a prospective candidate and his family. The history should include an overall picture of the patient's personality, mental ability and level of functioning, and current social matrix. In particular, social data, medical compliance history, patient and family attitudes about transplantation, strengths and weaknesses of the family system, and motivation and potential for rehabilitation post-transplantation all need to be evaluated.

The importance of the psychosocial assessment in determining proper patient selection has been well documented. Historically, patients have been denied on the basis of poor medical compliance, history of mental illness, or evidence of alcoholism or drug abuse[2]. Some authors, however, are now questioning whether all candidates with such a history should be denied transplantation[3]. At the Oklahoma Transplantation Institute, our policy with regard to alcohol or drug abuse is to refuse patients with a current, continuing problem; however, we have accepted candidates who have maintained 2 years of sobriety and drug-free behavior prior to referral. Of these candidates, post-transplantation none has resumed alcohol or drug consumption to date. This outcome is consistent with that of heroin addicts who received renal transplants[4].

An important issue that must be addressed is the patient's compliance with medical instructions and advice. In heart transplant recipients, non-compliance has been found to be more common in younger patients (under 40), those single or divorced (and presumably lacking family support), those with a lower level of education (less than high school diploma), and those with no career skills[5]. Other authors believe that non-compliance may indicate ambivalence about surgery and/or survival, depression, intellectual deficit, or cognitive impairment[6]. Therefore, medication abuse or neglect, morbid obesity, smoking, or failure to make or keep appointments must be noted and explored. If there are social reasons for this behavior, attention and effort must be focused on identifying the underlying issues and helping the patient develop an effective plan of corrective action. When there is a psychological or intellectual basis for this behavior, its amenability to therapy must be assessed. Acceptance or denial of the candidate on to the transplant program will be based on the results of this evaluation.

The pretransplant psychosocial evaluation must also include an exploration of the probability of the candidate returning to work and the need for retraining or re-education post-transplantation. This should include an assessment of the patient's desire and potential to resume active employment once medical clearance has been received.

Potential recipients who have no future aspirations, and view the transplant as merely an advancement of the dying process, must be screened carefully and should receive psychiatric assessment. It is reasonable to expect that most recipients will be able to resume a fully functioning lifestyle post-transplant. The candidate's ability to identify meaningful tasks he would like to accomplish post-transplant and the presence of strong family support have been shown to be associated with a positive outcome after transplantation[2].

THE PERIOPERATIVE PHASE

The perioperative phase specifically refers to the time from selection through early convalescence. Others have identified individual phases which include: waiting period, immediate post-surgical period, recovery (first infection/rejection), hospital discharge, and early convalescence[7,8].

The waiting period has been reported to be a time of increased anxiety and depression for patient and family. Once accepted as a candidate the patient is encouraged to attend our transplant support group meetings. This is now a formalized component of our program, complete with educational sessions (see later). Communication with patients with transplants is encouraged, and has proven especially helpful to those awaiting donors. The immediate post-surgical period is, by comparison, a time of relatively little stress. The recovery phase can include at least one infection or rejection episode. It is at this time that a patient is confronted with the reality of having traded one set of symptoms for another. In general, the recovery phase is a time of increased frustration and depression for the patient, due to the slowness with which he progresses and to a feeling that he has little personal control over events taking place. Hospital discharge is a time of excitement and anxiety for both patient and family. A patient's physical and emotional care is shifted back to the family; role conflicts may begin to develop. Early convalescence is a furthering of this process, and intra-family conflict is likely to develop[7].

While the issues facing patients and their family members vary throughout these phases, the role of the social worker remains constant. The social worker functions as a support person who can provide educational or counseling services, and, when necessary, act as a referral source for additional community services.

A high level of involvement from the social worker is required at the time of discharge. While successful discharge means resolution of many of the medical factors that precipitated admission to hospital, what lies ahead may be uncertain. As a result, discharge is often an anxious time for both patient and family. Reactions can include confusion, shock, and denial[9]. Patient and family may be confronted by unrealistic expectations, and must learn to adapt to circumstances that may significantly affect their relationship.

The social worker will work with the patient and family to plan for the discharge by assessing the patient's post-hospital care needs. Whether the need is for referral to a community agency or purely for additional information, it is the social worker who, in consultation with the patient, family, and medical staff, will coordinate post-hospital care. All patients will require careful assessment at this time, and will require frequent review on an outpatient basis in the event problems arise.

REHABILITATION

The next phase of social work involvement is the rehabilitation process. Ideally, at this time, the patient is able to return to an independent emotional and physical functional status. A successful rehabilitated person can return to competitive employment or school, resume duties as a homemaker, or choose an active retirement[10].

Emotional support and stress management are equally important, and are issues which affect the patient's ability to attain his full rehabilitation potential. Our own experience has been that the patient may be faced by multiple family/support system problems within the first year post-surgery. In a group formed by our first ten patients who survived 3 months or longer, there were three divorces and two marital separations.

Denial is a common ingredient of the adaptation process in heart transplant patients[11]. It can be viewed as a way of coping with, or perhaps postponing, feelings until they can be better accommodated. At Oklahoma Transplantation Institute, in our first few patients adaptive use of this process was complicated by the local publicity associated with initiation of our program. Adjustment may be compounded further by the disparity between the identified needs of the patient and his spouse. Patients report the need for more open communication from their spouses, and also rely on them for physical care and transportation[12]. Spouses, meanwhile, feel the need for more informed local medical community support and advice; in particular, they request additional psychosocial support, with special attention on sexual counseling[13]. Major conflicts may arise due to the patient and family being unable to resolve minor problems.

In response to the needs of both patient and spouse, our support network and group meetings were established to promote the sharing of feelings and experiences of pre- and post-transplant patients and their families. The objectives of this group are to provide (1) an emotionally supportive environment, (2) the companionship of others with a similar medical condition, and (3) exposure to the coping skills needed to deal effectively with transplantation and its sequelae.

At our center, there has been a dramatic reduction in family/marital support system dysfunction in patients who have attended the group. In contrast to our first ten patients referred to above, in the following 18 long-term survivors there have been no divorces, marital separations, or complete breakdowns in the patient's support system. These observations support those of others, who have previously reported the benefits of heart transplant support groups[14].

However, not all patients benefit from such group meetings. In some cases, referral for private counseling is required. The staff social worker and psychiatrist should be available to provide this service.

How successful is rehabilitation after cardiac transplantation? There are limited data available. At our own relatively new center, of the first 33 patients who survived 6 months or longer, 33% resumed full-time employment, 19% are actively retired, while 48% are insurance disabled, and none was classified as medically disabled. This compares with data published from the University of Arizona, where 32% of their patients returned to work, 25% were retired, 35% were insurance disabled, and 7.5% were medically disabled[15].

Competitive employment may not always be possible, however, for heart transplant recipients. Nine of our 16 insurance disabled group have tried to find employment, but without success. The fact that they had undergone heart transplantation was undoubtedly a major factor in their lack of success. In general, however, these patients had been disabled for long periods prior to transplantation, had the lowest levels of academic achievement, and fewer work skills to offer; in addition, they tended to be in the older age range, making them less desirable as employees, and more ready to accept retirement as an alternative.

Of the seven who have not attempted to resume employment, all have some form of negative incentive to return to work; for example, if they resumed employment they would risk losing some form of income or medical insurance. Employment may, therefore, be possible in some cases, but may not be sufficiently desirable.

Vocational rehabilitation seems to be beneficial to patients undergoing other forms of heart surgery, but does not yet appear to have been so in those undergoing transplantation at our center. The reasons for this remain uncertain. Much work needs to be done – educationally, legally, and politically – before transplant patients can expect the same positive rehabilitation results as those undergoing other forms of heart surgery.

In summary, a review of our own patients' experiences would suggest that, if the patient's employment remains open to him after recovering from his heart transplant, then he will almost certainly return to full-time occupation. If, however, he was forced to give up work from physical disability before transplantation, and has no position to which to return, then he has almost no chance of obtaining employment even though he may be physically and mentally able to do so. In such cases, his best (and possibly only) hope is to retrain himself in a field where he can be self-employed.

COMMENT

Social work has been, and will continue to be, involved in all phases of transplantation, from evaluation through rehabilitation. A comprehensive knowledge of psychosocial issues and salient treatment modalities enables the social worker to be a vital link between the medical staff and the transplant patient. A professional commitment to respect self-determination has enabled the social worker to help patients and families explore the immediate and long-term impacts that cardiac transplantation may have upon them.

Embracing the holistic approach to health care puts the social worker in an excellent position to contribute positively toward the overall success of transplantation. It is incumbent, however, that social workers continue to expand their knowledge and expertise, and document their clinical and research experience through publication.

'Tis not enough to help the feeble up,
But to support him after.'
W. Shakespeare (Timon of Athens 1, i, 108)

Acknowledgements

The author wishes to thank Sharen Thompson LCSW and Mary Quisenberry ACSW for editorial assistance in the preparation of this chapter.

References

1. Brown, E.C. (1976). Casework with patients undergoing cardiac surgery. In Turner, F. (ed.) *Differential Diagnosis and Treatment in Social Work*. 2nd edn., p. 403. (New York: The Free Press)
2. Christopherson, L.K. (1979). Need for patient counseling. *Nursing Mirror*, **149**, 34
3. Mai, F.M., McKenzie, F.N. and Kostuk, W.J. (1986). Psychiatric aspects of heart transplantation: preoperative evaluation and postoperative sequelae. *Br. Med. J.*, **292**, 311
4. Gordon, M.J.V., White, R., Matas, A.J., Tellis, V.A., Glicklich, D., Quinn, T., Soberman, R. and Veith, F.J. (1986). Renal transplantation in patients with a history of heroin abuse. *Transplantation*, **42**, 556
5. Cooper, D.K.C., Lanza, R.P. and Barnard, C.N. (1984). Noncompliance in heart transplant recipients: the Cape Town experience. *Heart Transplant.*, **3**, 248
6. Lesko, L. and Hawkins, D. (1983). Psychological aspects of transplantation medicine. In Akhtar, S. (ed.) *New Psychiatric Syndromes*. (New York, London: Jason Aronson)
7. Allender, J., Shisslak, C., Kaszniak, A. and Copeland, J.G. (1983). Stages of psychological adjustment associated with heart transplantation. *Heart Transplant.*, **2**, 228
8. McAleer, M.J., Copeland, J., Fuller, J. and Copeland, J.G. (1985). Psychological aspects of heart transplantation. *Heart Transplant.*, **4**, 232
9. Blazyk, S. and Canavan, M.M. (1985). Therapeutic aspects of discharge planning. *Soc. Work*, **30**, 489
10. Christopherson, L.K., Griepp, R.B. and Stinson, E.B. (1976). Rehabilitation after cardiac transplantation. *J. Am. Med. Assoc.*, **236**, 2082
11. Mai, F.M. (1986). Graft and donor denial in heart transplant recipients. *Am. J. Psychiatry*, **143**, 1159
12. Rogers, K.R. (1987). Nature of spousal supportive behaviors that influence heart transplant patient compliance. *J. Heart Transplant.*, **6**, 90
13. Kennedy, J., Kavanagh, T. and Yacoub, M.H. (1987). Psychosocial problems of spouses of cardiac transplant patients. *Circulation*, **76**, 4
14. Suszycki, L.H. (1986). Social work groups on a heart transplant program. *J. Heart Transplant.*, **5**, 166
15. Meister, N.D., McAleer, M.J., Meister, J.S., Riley, J.E. and Copeland, J.G. (1986). Returning to work after heart transplantation. *J. Heart Transplant.*, **5**, 154

27
Nutrition and Diet
D. RAGSDALE

INTRODUCTION

The nutritional care of cardiac transplant candidates and recipients is a challenging and important part of overall patient care. Frequent reviews of the nutritional requirements of the patient are essential as they may differ markedly with changing clinical status. The nutritional status of cardiac transplant candidates and recipients significantly affects surgical outcome, length of hospitalization, quality of life, and mortality[1].

Over 50% of patients with a primary diagnosis of cardiac disease are likely to be significantly malnourished[2]. Advanced cardiac failure may result in cardiac cachexia, evidenced by multiple organ insufficiency (from hypoxia), muscle and adipose tissue loss, hypoalbuminemia, malabsorption, nausea, vomiting and anorexia. Risk of mortality and postoperative complications increases with each of these problems[3].

Literature regarding the specific nutritional needs of cardiac transplant recipients is limited, yet much information can be drawn from other patient populations and past experience. This chapter will discuss the primary areas of concern and recommendations for patient care.

NUTRITIONAL ASSESSMENT OF THE TRANSPLANT CANDIDATE

At a time when candidates for heart transplantation are more numerous than donors, long-term pretransplant nutritional care becomes increasingly difficult, especially for those who require support by a mechanical assist device or an artificial heart. Transplant candidates present in a wide variety of nutritional states, and nutritional status generally deteriorates while they await transplantation. Accurate initial and follow-up assessments will identify those patients at risk in each phase of transplant care.

The patient with slowly progressive disease (> 6 months) often has time to adjust metabolically. Although weight loss may appear minimal, it is usually masked by the presence of fluid overload[4]. Anthropometric measurements commonly detect a reduced lean muscle mass with varying degrees of adipose (caloric) reserves. Poor appetite, nausea and vomiting may reduce food intake at a time when all physical activities, including breathing, place greater nutritional demands on the patient. Abel et al. established that early malnutrition adversely affects cardiac function[5]. In turn, impaired cardiac function from nutritional deficit further interferes with food intake, creating a downward spiral of deterioration until parenteral nutritional support is initiated[4].

Pretransplant nutritional assessment includes recording of age, sex, height and weight, anthropometric measurements, and estimations of serum albumin, serum transferrin, and 24-hour urinary urea nitrogen and creatinine[6] (Table 27.1). A thorough diet history, with estimated nutrient and caloric intake levels, should be taken to detect potential deficiencies, and may suggest methods to improve oral intake. Dry weight should be estimated and used to determine the patient's percent weight change over a period of time; current weight should be compared with desirable weight standards. The estimated desirable weight is then used to determine basal energy expenditure (BEE)[7].

Caloric requirement

The total non-protein calorie requirements are calculated for maintenance and stress (e.g. surgery, sepsis) (Table 27.2). In the patient taking oral nutrition, requirements range from 20 to 50% above BEE values[1,8]. These additional requirements should be assessed on an individual basis. An extremely stressed patient receiving enteral or parenteral support may need up to 75% above BEE[8].

In advanced cardiac failure, tolerance of oral intake, enteral (tube feeding) or parenteral (intravenous) hyperalimentation support may be impaired. Ideally, support should be initiated before the patient is severely malnourished to allow gradual increases in caloric and fluid intake[4]. Supplying the optimal nutritional support requires constant reas-

Table 27.1 Nutritional assessment of the cardiac transplant patient

Height (cm): ____ Age: ____ Sex: ____
Weight (kg): ____ Usual wt: ____ wt.6 wks ago: ____ wt.6 months ago: ____
____ % change in ____ wks (based on Blackburn*)
Desirable wt. (based on Metropolitan ht/wt table): ____ ____ % of desirable

Triceps skin fold ____ mm ____ percentile (caloric reserves)
Arm circumference ____ cm ____ percentile (caloric reserves and muscle)
Arm muscle circumference ____ cm ____ percentile (lean body mass)

Albumin ____ Total protein ____ Transferrin ____ Lymphocytes ____ %
TLC ____ Hgb ____ Hct ____ WBC ____ BUN ____ Creatinine ____
24-hour BUN ____ 24-hour creatinine ____
Nitrogen balance study ____
Diet history:

*Blackburn's evaluation of weight change[7]

Time	Significant weight loss	Severe weight loss
1 week	1–2%	>2%
1 month	5%	>5%
3 months	7.5%	>7.5%
6 months	10%	>10%

*Values charted are for percentage weight change:

$$\text{Percentage weight change} = \frac{(\text{usual weight} - \text{actual weight})}{(\text{usual weight})} \times 100$$

Table 27.2 Estimation of nutritional needs

Basal energy expenditure at ____ wt. = ____ calories
Males = 66 + (13.7 × actual wt. in kg) + (5 × ht. in cm) − (6.8 × age) =
Females = 655 + (9.6 × actual wt. in kg) + (1.7 × ht. in cm) − (4.7 × age) =

Long's additional needs[8]

Activity factors		Stress factors	
Confined to bed	1.2	Minor operation	1.2
Out of bed	1.3	Skeletal trauma	1.35
		Major sepsis	1.6

sessment and monitoring. Overfeeding a patient can stress the heart, liver and kidneys, thus eliminating the benefits of such support[9].

Although BEE provides a reasonable estimate of average energy needs, the actual metabolic requirements of an individual patient are much more difficult to assess. For an individual patient, resting energy expenditure (REE), a form of indirect calorimetry, can be determined. It measures oxygen consumption and carbon dioxide production, and can be employed to determine the energy requirements of a non-ambulatory patient more precisely[9]. Maximum carbohydrate utilization is calculated to be 5 mg/kg per hour[8].

Protein requirement

The protein requirement of any individual patient is based on laboratory and anthropometric findings. Needs range from 1.2 to 1.5 g of protein per kilogram of appropriate dry body weight[1]. (It is not necessary to provide additional protein for adipose tissue maintenance in obese patients[3].) Protein requirements may increase to levels of 1.5–2.0 g/kg in the severely depleted patient, for example, the patient supported by an artificial heart. Renal failure should be treated by hemodialysis rather than by protein restriction.

NUTRITIONAL SUPPORT PRETRANSPLANT

The patient in the early stages of cardiac failure

The goal of nutritional support is to provide adequate calories, protein and other nutrients without overfeeding the patient. The New York Heart Association class II or III patient may show no problems with anorexia or weight loss (Table 27.3). Education regarding nutritional requirements, encouraging an intake of high protein, high calorie, moderate sodium foods, may be sufficient treatment at this stage.

The obese patient

The obese transplant candidate (> 20% above desirable body weight due to adipose tissue) is also at nutritional risk. Protein status, eating habits, and family eating patterns are often poor. Detailed histories of diet and eating patterns of both patient and family, of changes in weight, and of any

Table 27.3 Nutritional care in relation to New York Heart Association classification

NYHA class	Symptoms	Nutritional assessment	Nutritional intervention
I	Minimal or none	Diet history, food preferences, food preparation techniques	Basic nutrition counseling. Avoid high sodium foods
II	Dyspnea with unusual activity	As for I	Patient to record a diet diary for 3 days. Instruct on 2–4 g sodium diet if appropriate. Cholesterol and saturated fat restrictions as needed. Weight changes as needed
III	Dyspnea with usual activity	Complete assessment. Calorie count as needed. Nitrogen balance study	Ensure adequate protein, calories and nutrients. Restriction to 2 g sodium. Frequent small meals. Careful monitoring. Supplementation as needed
IV	Dyspnea at rest	As for III	Alternative support as needed. High calorie, protein diet. Close monitoring

significant family medical conditions or social situations that might influence the patient, are helpful. The extent of family support for modifications in the patient's diet are noted. If time allows, the patient should work with a dietitian and be guided toward gradual weight loss (1–4 lb/week) while maintaining adequate protein status. The patient should be instructed to seek professional guidance and monitoring in order to decrease weight, as, without guidance, severe protein and nutritional deficits can occur.

The patient in advanced cardiac failure

As cardiac function deteriorates, more intense support is necessary. Food intake may vary daily depending on gastrointestinal function and overall well-being. Cellular hypoxia, secondary to increasing cardiac failure, gradually leads to multi-system failure. Malabsorption occurs as the viscera become engorged with fluid, and the body is unable to utilize nutrients provided enterally[9]. Gastrointestinal motility often decreases, resulting in either constipation or diarrhea. A reduced renal blood supply results in conservation of nutrients and water by the kidneys[1]. Free water, from nutritional support and medications, is retained unless diuretics are provided. Diuretics deplete mineral and vitamin levels, which require careful monitoring and supplementation[10].

Sodium restriction is commonly advised, but should not compromise adequate nutritional intake, particularly of protein. A high protein diet can contain as little as 87–176 mEq (2–4 g) of sodium. Small frequent meals, snacks, and high protein shakes are recommended to enhance total protein intake.

Calorie and protein counts and nitrogen balance studies can determine daily intake. If oral intake is consistently at or below the calculated BEE, additional support will clearly become necessary. Alternative routes of nutritional support, such as enteral or parenteral hyperalimentation, are often required. While enteral support is preferred, tolerance is generally poor. Peripheral venous hyperalimentation can be beneficial in supplementing oral intake in hospitalized patients. Central venous hyperalimentation occasionally becomes necessary, and should not be postponed until serial laboratory studies reflect severe nutritional deficits.

The patient with cardiac cachexia

The patient with rapidly deteriorating cardiac function may develop cardiac cachexia while awaiting transplantation[2]. Nutritional treatment often includes a form of hyperalimentation. Although cachexia may be a compensatory mechanism to reduce oxygen consumption and decrease cardiac demands, at least minimal energy and nutrient needs should be supplied to maintain the patient's immune status and survival[9]. The absolute quantities and relative proportions of carbohydrate, protein and fat needed to maintain minimal nutritional support, yet reduce cardiac stress, remain highly debated and require further study.

The patient on a mechanical assist device or artificial heart

The artificial heart patient is under postoperative metabolic stress in addition to pre-existing malnutrition. Increased cardiac output and nutrient distribution to atrophied tissues stimulate the anabolic process. Energy and protein requirements will exceed those before operation. If the patient had been adequately nourished prior to implantation, his nutritional needs may not increase so significantly. A high protein, high calorie diet, with vitamin and mineral supplementation (and frequent 'snacks') is appropriate.

Oral intake may require supplementation in the form of tube feeding or intravenous hyperalimentation. The gastroenterologist, dietitian and nutrition support team should monitor intake and tolerance closely. Weekly calorie counts and nitrogen balance studies should be checked to assess adequacy of nutritional support.

NUTRITIONAL SUPPORT IMMEDIATELY POST-TRANSPLANT

Post-transplant patients require increased amounts of nutrients for wound healing at a time when renal and hepatic functions are frequently impaired, appetite may be poor, and the side effects of medications may result in gastrointestinal distress[3]. Postoperatively the patient's diet is advanced to solid foods as tolerated, the goal being to provide a high intake of calories (1.4–1.75 × BEE) and protein (1.4 g/kg body weight). Hyperalimentation may be continued to support a previously malnourished patient. To maximize intake, small frequent snacks between meals, including commercial liquid nutritional supplements, are continued, but may be modified to conform to new dietary restrictions. Intake is monitored by frequent calorie nutrient counts and nutritional assessments.

The patient's nutritional status and ability to consume food dictate the extent to which dietary restrictions can be implemented during the first week post-transplant. The restriction on sodium intake usually is relaxed to 176–220 mEq (4–5 g) per day, and sugar intake, especially in the form of concentrated sweets, is limited to minimize the effects of corticosteroids on glucose metabolism. Cholesterol and saturated fat restrictions are also implemented.

The protective isolation precautions used by some institutions may eliminate fresh fruits and vegetables from the patient's diet. Although aerobic Gram-negative bacilli are commonly found on such foods, they are no longer considered dangerous unless the patient is neutropenic[1,11]. Allowing fresh fruits and vegetables in the diet usually improves overall intake, and has not been associated with increased infection rates[12].

LONG-TERM NUTRITIONAL CARE

Long-term nutritional care is best provided in conjunction with follow-up appointments with the cardiologist or cardiac surgeon. The patient should be encouraged to record all food intake over a 3-day period at intervals, namely after discharge from hospital, after 6 weeks, and 6 months later. Careful review of these records will be helpful in determining compliance, and the necessity for further dietary education and guidance. Continuing patient monitoring and education are critical for long-term compliance with any special diet. Changes in the diet often cause confusion, and should be explained carefully.

Readmission or extended hospitalization is not uncommon in patients with heart transplants due to episodes of infection or rejection. Nutritional assessment, monitoring, and support are recommended upon readmission. In the case of sepsis and high metabolic needs, a high protein, high calorie diet with supplements may be necessary to maintain adequate nutrient intake. Antibiotic therapy and poor oral intake add to the nutritional risks.

Drug-related nutritional problems

The long-term nutritional care of the transplant patient must take into consideration drug-induced metabolic changes and the side effects of medications. Corticosteroids alter carbohydrate, protein and fat metabolism, and adipose distribution in the body. Altered carbohydrate metabolism can result in non-ketotic diabetes mellitus. Appetite and craving for sweets are also stimulated, contributing to obesity and elevated blood glucose. Protein catabolism results in muscle wasting, thinning of the skin, dissolution of vertical bone matrix, and poor wound healing[13]. The influence of steroids on fat tissue results in loss of subcutaneous fat from extremities and excessive deposition in the trunk areas[13]. Excessive fat in the trunk has been associated with increased risk of atherosclerotic disease[14].

Prednisone's antagonistic effects on vitamin D causes changes in the body's calcium balance, contributing to osteoporosis, and its mineralocorticoid effect may be associated with hypertension[13]. Zinc depletion, contributing to delayed wound healing, is another possible long-term effect[13]. These side effects are reduced when low-dose prednisone therapy is administered in conjunction with cyclosporine, though the incidence of hypertension may increase. Nutritional support aimed at reducing these effects of corticosteroids is a primary goal of post-cardiac transplant dietary care.

Cyclosporine therapy may be associated with hypertension, renal and hepatic dysfunction, an increased risk of viral infection, and the development of malignant tumors[15]. Intake of foods of high protein quality (e.g. meat and milk) and restricted sodium is recommended to counter these side effects.

Azathioprine therapy may be associated with hematologic changes, gastrointestinal problems, hepatitis or pancreatitis. Dietary modifications play an important part in the care of patients with such gastrointestinal problems, and should be based on individual symptoms.

Recommended diet for the cardiac transplant recipient

Total caloric intake, as well as the type of carbohydrate, protein and fat taken, are controlled to minimize the short- and long-term nutritional complications that may be associated with immunosuppressive therapy. Calorie intake should be adjusted to achieve and maintain ideal body weight. A low cholesterol, low saturated fat diet with limited sugar and no concentrated sweets, and a moderate restriction of sodium (approx. 132–220 mEq) (3–5 g) can be ordered for these patients. Cholesterol restriction is recommended on the basis that it may reduce the high incidence of atherosclerotic disease seen in patients with cardiac transplants (Chapter 19). Intake of polyunsaturated fat is increased to achieve at least a balance with saturated fat. Dietary sodium is primarily restricted to reduce the sodium and fluid-retaining effects of corticosteroids.

The pretransplant nutritional status of the patient will be an important factor in the strictness with which this diet can be applied in the early post-transplant period, though the long-term goal includes all of the restrictions listed. Specific recommendations for this special diet are listed in Table 27.4.

Vitamin and mineral supplementation may be necessary with such a diet. For example, if the patient avoids all red meats in order to reduce cholesterol and saturated fat, the intake of iron should be monitored carefully, and iron supplements given if necessary. Detailed adjustments for food preferences should be made for each patient. Adequate amounts of extra lean (> 95% fat free), high quality protein sources are encouraged to offset muscle wasting. A high intake of skim or 1% fat milk is beneficial as a source of protein, calcium, and vitamins A and D. However, milk intake should be limited if renal failure results in hyperkalemia.

If the patient is underweight, it is important to increase body weight so that there are adequate fat and protein reserves for periods of infection or rejection. On the other hand, once desirable body weight is attained, it is equally critical to prevent excessive weight gain since excessive weight places an added strain on the heart. Furthermore, obesity can lead to increases in blood cholesterol, triglyceride, and glucose levels, and in blood pressure, all of which are risk factors for coronary disease.

Table 27.4 Constituents of recommended diet*

The calorie level is calculated on an individual basis, to achieve and maintain desirable body weight.
The total number of calories should be made up of:
  carbohydrate 45–55%
    33% from simple sugars in fruits
    67% from complex carbohydrate high fiber (3–4 g/day)
  protein 25–30%
  fat 18–25%
    33% or less of calories from saturated
    33% monosaturated
    33% polyunsaturated
The daily diet should not contain more than approximately:
  200 mg cholesterol and
  176–220 mEq of sodium (4–5 g)

*Recommendations listed are modified American Dietetic Association and American Heart Association guidelines. The modifications listed were deemed necessary after experience with this specific patient population[1]

References

1. Ragsdale, D.A. (1987). Nutritional program for heart transplant. *J. Heart Transplant.*, **6**, 228
2. Blackburn, G.L., Gibbons, G.W., Bothe, A., Benotti, P.N., Harken, D.E. and McEnany, T.M. (1977). Nutritional support in cardiac cachexia. *J. Thorac. Cardiovasc. Surg.*, **73**, 489
3. Frazier, O.H., Van Buren, C.T., Poindexter, S.M. and Walenberger, F. (1985). Nutritional management of the heart transplant recipient. *J. Heart Transplant.*, **4**, 450
4. Alamini, M.A. (1987). The cardiac patient. In Lange, C.E. (ed.) *Nutritional Support in Critical Care*. (Rockville, MD: Aspen Publishers)
5. Abel, R.M., Grimes, J.B., Alonso, D., Alonso, M. and Gay, W.A. (1979). Adverse hemodynamic and ultrastructural changes in dog hearts subjected to protein-calorie malnutrition. *Am. Heart J.*, **97**, 733
6. Havel, R.J. (1982). Approach in the patient with hyperlipidemia. *Med. Clin. N. Am.*, **66**, 319
7. Blackburn, G.L., Bistrian, B.R., Maini, B.S., Schlamm, H.T. and Smith, M.F. (1977). Nutritional and metabolic assessment of the hospitalized patient. *JPEN*, **1**, 11
8. Long, C.L., Schaffel, N., Geiger, J.W., Schiller, W.R. and Blakemore, W.S. (1979). Metabolic response to injury and illness: estimation of energy and protein needs from indirect calorimetry and nitrogen balance. *JPEN*, **3**, 452
9. Heymsfield, S.B., Smith, J., Redd, S. and Whitworth, H.B. (1981). Nutritional support in cardiac failure. *Surg. Clin. N. Am.*, **61**, 635
10. Elwyn, D.H. (1987). Protein metabolism and requirements in the critically ill patient. *Crit. Care Clin.*, **3**, 57
11. Hess, N., Brooks-Brunn, J., Clark, D. and Joy, K. (1985). Complete isolation: is it necessary? *J. Heart Transplant.*, **4**, 458
12. Remington, J.S. and Schimpff, S.C. (1981). Please don't eat the salads. *N. Engl. J. Med.*, **304**, 433
13. Schneider, H.A., Anderson, C.E. and Coursin, D.B. (1983). *Nutritional Support of the Medical Practice*. (Hagerstown, MD: Harper and Row)
14. Rutten, P., Blackburn, G.L., Flatt, J.P., Hallowell, E. and Cochran, D. (1975). Determination of optimal hyperalimentation infusion rate. *J. Surg. Res.*, **18**, 477
15. Grady, K.L. and Herolf, L.S. (1988). Comparison of nutritional status in patients before and after heart transplantation. *J. Heart Transplant.*, **7**, 123

28
Exercise Rehabilitation
T.D. NOAKES AND G.L.G. KEMPENEERS

INTRODUCTION

There are a number of reasons why cardiac transplant recipients will have significantly impaired physical fitness both immediately before and after transplant surgery.

First, because of the incapacity caused by their progressively deteriorating cardiac status, cardiac transplant recipients have frequently participated in little or no meaningful physical exercise for many months or years prior to transplantation. Ultimately they may be bed-ridden. The deleterious effects of bed rest on cardiovascular and skeletal muscular function and on bone mineral content are well described[1-6].

Secondly, they will be on medication, particularly corticosteroids, which are known to influence skeletal muscle function adversely[7-9] (Chapter 22).

Thirdly, even after surgery, cardiac recipients can potentially have a residual central (cardiovascular) limitation for maximal exercise posed by the different pattern of response of the denervated heart to exercise as is discussed in Chapter 13. The heart rate of cardiac recipients rises more gradually after the onset of exercise, reaches a lower peak, and decreases more slowly after cessation of exercise than does the normally innervated heart[10-13]. In these patients, maintenance of an adequate cardiac output during submaximal exercise is achieved by augmentating preload and activation of the Frank–Starling mechanism[10]; at high workloads, cardiac output increases secondary to chronotropic and inotropic effects induced by steeply rising circulating norepinephrine levels[10,14]. Whether these adaptations can ensure that the maximal cardiac output of transplant recipients equals that of normal subjects is not clear[11,13,15], but seems unlikely[16]. In this context it should be noted that the prescription of β-receptor antagonist agents severely restricts the exercise tolerance of these patients in part because it prevents the essential chronotropic and inotropic actions of circulating catecholamines on the denervated myocardium[17].

Finally, a major long-term limitation is the process of chronic rejection, manifested by accelerated atherosclerosis of the donor coronary arteries and myocardial necrosis (Chapters 18 and 19). Savin *et al.* showed that work time during the maximal exercise test was inversely related to the history of rejection, and was least in those with the most frequent and severe episodes of rejection[11]. This relationship could be explained either by more frequent episodes of myocardial necrosis, or by the administration of higher doses of immunosuppressive agents in those undergoing frequent episodes of rejection.

The result of any and all of these four processes is that the exercise tolerance of cardiac transplant recipients is subnormal[11,16].

In this review, we present an approach to the evaluation of the cardiovascular and skeletal muscle function of cardiac transplant recipients, and describe how this information can be used to prescribe appropriate individualized exercise programs for such patients. It is likely that the benefits of such an exercise program for cardiac recipients are similar to those enjoyed by patients with coronary artery disease[16,18].

EXERCISE TESTING OF CARDIAC TRANSPLANT RECIPIENTS

The prescription of the appropriate individualized exercise training program hinges on a correct understanding of the physiological and pathological factors that limit the exercise tolerance of cardiac transplant recipients. These factors are identified during short-duration exercise of progressively increasing intensity, maintained by the patient until volitional exhaustion or until the onset of identifiable medical end-points, such as electrocardiographic changes compatible with myocardial ischemia, significant arrhythmias, hypotension, or angina pectoris.

Figure 28.1 shows, in diagrammatic form, the physiological variables that are usually measured and their response, during such a maximal exercise test, in persons without cardiovascular disease. The exercise test starts at a low workload, with progressive linear increases in oxygen consumption and heart rate with increased workload. Cardiac

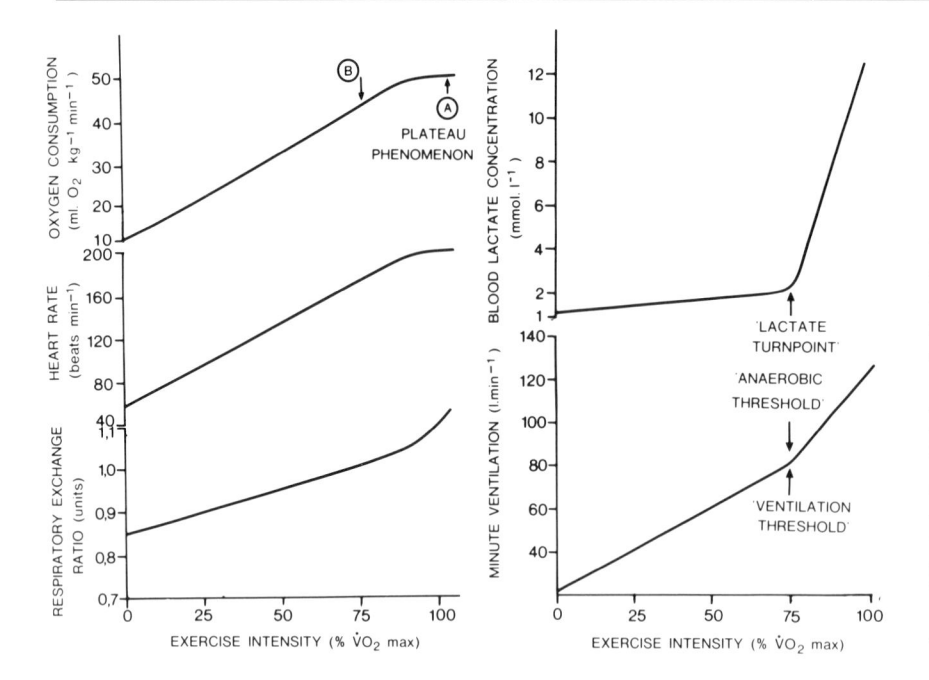

Figure 28.1 Diagrammatic representation of changes in oxygen consumption, heart rate, respiratory exchange ratio, blood lactate concentration, and minute ventilation, with progressive increases in exercise workload (exercise intensity).

The conventional belief is that maximal exercise always terminates after the development of an 'oxygen plateau' (point A: top left panel), indicating that tissue oxygen deficiency has developed, secondary to cardiorespiratory limitations in oxygen supply to the active muscles. When exercise terminates at point B, prior to the onset of the 'oxygen plateau', it would seem that this argument cannot be sustained. The 'lactate turnpoint' and the 'ventilation threshold', both of which are frequently referred to as the 'anaerobic threshold', are also indicated

output (not shown) also increases linearly with increasing workload due to increases in both heart rate and stroke volume[19]. Respiratory exchange ratio rises non-linearly with increasing exercise intensity.

A quite different response occurs in venous blood lactate levels, which are initially low and remain unchanged until an exercise intensity is reached above which blood lactate levels begin to rise steeply. The workload at which this phenomenon occurs is inappropriately (see later) called the 'anaerobic threshold' or 'lactate turnpoint'[20]. It is of interest that the increase in respiratory minute ventilation, which initially increases linearly with increased workload, deviates from linearity at workloads close to the 'lactate turnpoint' (Figure 28.1). This point has been called the 'ventilation threshold'.

The traditional view is that performance during maximal exercise of progressively increasing intensity is limited by a failure of the cardiovascular system to provide oxygen at a rate sufficiently fast to maintain oxidative adenosine triphosphate (ATP) production in the active skeletal muscles. Proponents of this belief argue that the rate of oxygen consumption always reaches a maximum or plateau (point A in Figure 28.1) prior to the termination of exercise. It is held that this plateau phenomenon indicates the onset of hypoxia in the active skeletal muscles due to a failure of the central (cardiovascular) mechanisms for oxygen delivery to the periphery. A corollary of this argument is that the 'lactate turnpoint' indicates the point at which this oxygen deficiency first becomes apparent so that 'anaerobic glycolysis' is activated, with increased production and release of lactate from the anaerobic muscles. This explains the interchangeable use of the two terms 'lactate turnpoint' and 'anaerobic threshold'.

Figure 28.2 indicates the traditional concept of how skeletal muscle anaerobiosis is believed to lead to the termination of maximal, short-duration exercise.

However, this view has been challenged on the basis that:

(1) The historical studies on which this assumption is based failed to show that oxygen consumption plateaued during maximal exercise[21].

(2) There is no evidence from modern studies that more than about 50% of subjects show this plateau phenomenon during maximal exercise[21]. In those subjects who terminate exercise prior to the development of a plateau in oxygen consumption (Figure 28.1, point B), the peak heart rates, respiratory exchange ratios and blood lactate levels may be relatively low. The low blood lactate levels, in par-

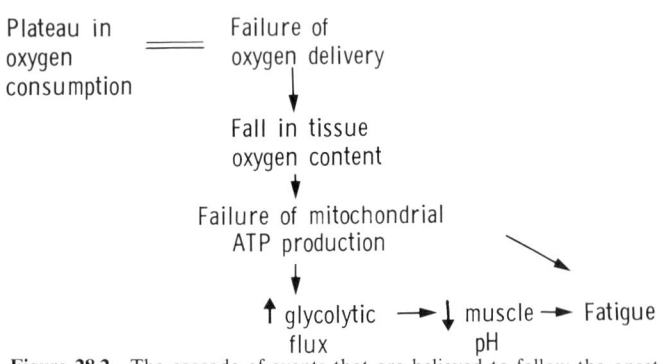

Figure 28.2 The cascade of events that are believed to follow the onset of tissue anaerobiosis that results from a central cardiorespiratory failure of oxygen delivery to the active muscle. The increased rate of glycolytic adenosine triphosphate (ATP) production leads to an increased skeletal muscle lactate and proton production, resulting in a fall in muscle pH, which causes fatigue. (Reproduced with permission from *Medicine and Science in Sports and Exercise*[21])

ticular, prove that tissue anaerobiosis could not have been the cause of the premature termination of exercise.

(3) There is no evidence that tissue anaerobiosis is present at the 'lactate turnpoint' or 'anaerobic threshold'.

(4) Blood lactate levels represent a balance between the rate of lactate production by the active muscles and its utilization by heart, liver, and other tissues, including skeletal muscle[20]. The findings that skeletal muscle produces lactate even at rest, proves that tissue anaerobiosis cannot be the most important explanation for the increased rates of lactate production by skeletal muscle during exercise[20]. It has been proposed that the rate of accumulation of lactate in blood depends on the balance between the rate of formation of pyruvate by glycolysis in skeletal muscle and its rate of oxidative disposal in the mitochondria[22], neither of which are determined solely by tissue oxygen content, at least during submaximal exercise in humans.

(5) There is no evidence that the non-linear increase in ventilation that occurs at the 'ventilation threshold' is causally related either to the onset of skeletal muscle anaerobiosis or the accumulation of lactate in the blood[22].

FACTORS LIMITING EXERCISE PERFORMANCE IN TRANSPLANT RECIPIENTS RECEIVING IMMUNOSUPPRESSIVE AGENTS

With this background, it is possible to interpret Figure 28.3, which compares our data for the physiological response of cardiac and renal transplant patients to exercise of progressively increasing intensity with that of control subjects. None of these patients terminated exercise prematurely because of the development of medical end-points, and most complained of leg fatigue.

The features of note are that both renal and cardiac transplant patients stopped exercising when their heart rates, blood lactate levels, rates of ventilation, and respiratory exchange ratios were lower than those of control subjects, and before there was evidence of a plateau in the rate of oxygen consumption. Even in the control subjects, there is no evidence for this oxygen plateau phenomenon. It should also be noted that far fewer of the transplant recipients were able to reach the higher exercise workloads.

Similar findings have recently been reported by Kavanagh et al. in 36 cardiac transplant recipients[16]. Similarly, none of the control or transplant subjects in the study of Savin et al. showed a plateau in oxygen consumption at the maximal workload[11].

The conclusion that must be drawn from these data is that the maximum exercise performance of none of the groups shown in Figure 28.3, but especially not that of the renal and cardiac transplant recipients, was limited by a central cardiorespiratory failure of oxygen delivery to the active skeletal muscles. The same would seem to apply to the subjects tested by Savin et al.[11] and Kavanagh et al.[16].

Thus, somewhat paradoxically, one must assume that the exercise performance of the majority of cardiac recipients is limited by peripheral, skeletal muscular factors, as also concluded by Kavanagh and his colleagues[16]. This skeletal muscular weakness could result either from prolonged inactivity or the use of certain drugs with myopathic effects. Studies in renal transplant recipients indicate that reversal of physical inactivity improves, but may fail to restore, normal skeletal muscle function[9]. This suggests that a drug-induced myopathy may limit the exercise tolerance of an indeterminate number, possibly the majority, of organ transplant recipients receiving immunosuppressive agents.

ASSESSMENT OF SKELETAL MUSCLE FUNCTION IN ORGAN TRANSPLANT RECIPIENTS

The presence of skeletal muscle weakness can be inferred from the results of the progressive maximal exercise test, as described above. Patients who terminate exercise at low rates of ventilation, low respiratory exchange ratios, and low venous blood lactate levels have a peripheral skeletal muscular, not central, limitation for their exercise tolerance. Currently there are two methods for quantifying *in vivo* skeletal muscle function in humans.

Isokinetic muscle strength and endurance can be measured using the Cybex isokinetic dynamometer (Lumex Inc., New York, USA). This system measures the dynamic muscular performance of different muscle groups during reciprocal contractions at different functional speeds. The training of renal transplant patients has been shown to increase dynamic muscle performance by between 20 and 40%[9].

The isokinetic cycle ergometer, developed by McCartney et al.[23,24], measures the *in vivo* power/velocity curve of skeletal muscle. A short (10s) maximal isokinetic cycling test measures peak torque and peak power produced at a range of pedaling cadences; a longer (30s) test measures the decline in power (fatigue index) during the test.

Whilst neither of these tests has yet been used for exercise prescription, they can be used (1) to quantify the peripheral component of the impaired exercise tolerance of transplant organ recipients; (2) to relate those changes to the dose of immunosuppressive agents prescribed to the patient, and (3) to follow the changes in muscle power that develop with training[9].

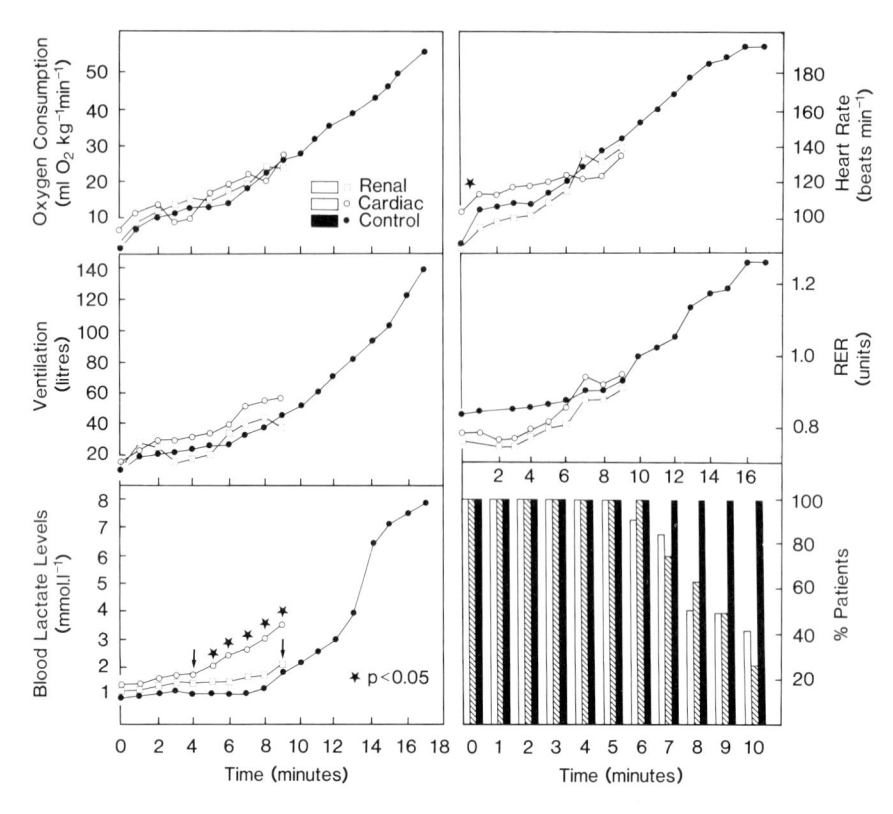

Figure 28.3 Progressive changes with increasing exercise intensity in oxygen consumption, heart rate, ventilation, respiratory exchange ratio, blood lactate levels, and the number of subjects completing each workload, in cardiac and renal transplant recipients and in matched controls. Note that the organ transplant recipients terminate exercise at lower rates of oxygen consumption and ventilation, and at lower heart rates, blood lactate levels, and respiratory exchange ratios. Fewer organ transplant recipients reach the higher exercise workloads. These findings are consistent with a non-oxygen-dependent, peripheral, skeletal muscle limitation for exercise performance in the organ transplant recipients

EXERCISE REHABILITATION PROGRAM FOR THE CARDIAC TRANSPLANT RECIPIENT

The exercise rehabilitation program provides the transplant recipient with a graduated exercise training program divided into three phases: (1) immediate postoperative, (2) inpatient, and (3) outpatient[25].

The intensive care unit and hospital inpatient phases

The intensive care unit phase of the rehabilitation program starts shortly after surgery, under the supervision of a physical therapist and the physician. When the patient's cardiac status is considered to be stable, he or she may start to perform a series of simple exercises. The aims of these exercises are to diminish the patient's risk of developing hypostatic pneumonia and thromboembolic phenomena, and to restrict the detrimental physical and psychological effects of deconditioning.

The formal exercise program will likely be conducted by a physiotherapist, and will usually be confined to exercises conducted in the bed or at the bedside[25,26]. Examples would be breathing exercises, upper limb exercises for the arms and shoulders, and leg raises and ankle exercises, all performed once a day. The energy cost of these activities is very low, increasing the heart rate of the order of 8 beats/min and the rate of oxygen consumption by about 2 ml/kg per min, or less than one metabolic equivalent (MET, which equals $3.5\,\text{ml}\,O_2/\text{kg}$ per minute)[27].

Depending on the length of stay in hospital and the patient's response to these exercises, additional exercises are added and the session increased to twice daily. 'Armchair mobilization' and standing at the side of the bed are encouraged, and walking is introduced. The intensity of all activities is carefully controlled by monitoring the patient's level of perceived exertion[28], and observing for the development of cardiac arrhythmias or the onset of inappropriate dyspnea[29].

Unresisted cycling, treadmill walking, and resisted cycling may be introduced subsequently. Progression at all levels is carefully monitored in accordance with the criteria that are well established for the exercise rehabilitation of patients with ischemic heart disease. An excellent in-hospital rehabilitation program for transplant recipients has been developed at Stanford University, and the details are available[25].

The outpatient phase

Our own experience has been with out-of-hospital rehabilitation, particularly of patients with ischemic heart disease, but also of renal[9] and cardiac transplant recipients. The requirements of all these patients are quite similar. The guidelines that we have evolved for the management of our patients with ischemic heart disease will be outlined. These guidelines have been adapted with minor modifications for our transplant recipients.

Experience with patients with ischemic heart disease has established the safety and value of early low-intensity exercise testing within 3–6 weeks after acute myocardial infarction, before hospital discharge[30]. It is more likely that because of their lesser risk of developing ventricular fibrillation during exercise, such criteria need not be applied with equal rigidity to all cardiac transplant recipients.

Early, low-intensity exercise testing may be performed prior to hospital discharge. In patients with ischemic heart disease, such testing usually stops at a heart rate of 120–130 beats/min, or at 30 beats/min above the resting heart rate in persons receiving β-receptor antagonist agents, or at 60% of the age-predicted maximum heart rate. Criteria for terminating the test in cardiac transplant recipients who lack the normal chronotropic response to exercise will, of necessity, be different. Probably the use of the Borg Scale would be most appropriate; the test should probably be terminated when the subject reaches a perceived exertion of 12–13 units, equivalent to a perceived exertion described as 'light to somewhat hard', or a workload equivalent to about 9 METs[29]. Patients with ischemic heart disease who develop electrocardiographic ST segment changes, either elevation or depression, arrhythmias or chest pain, or who achieve a low maximum workload, or who show evidence of poor myocardial function during such low-intensity testing, have a 1-year mortality rate of between 15 and 25% and require further cardiological investigation. Cardiac transplant recipients are unlikely to show any of these abnormalities during low-level exercise testing. Those who do would likely constitute poor candidates for an exercise rehabilitation program, and would require further, more invasive, cardiac evaluation prior to referral to a formal exercise program.

Patients who show none of these abnormalities during low-intensity exercise testing may undergo symptom- and sign-limited maximal exercise testing some time later, possibly within 2–6 months after transplantation[16,29]. It is very useful, specifically in cardiac recipients, to sample expired respiratory gases during such maximal exercise testing, in order to measure minute ventilation and oxygen consumption on-line, for the following reasons:

(1) A failure of oxygen consumption to rise with further increase in workload would indicate that the patient had reached his maximum aerobic workload and that no further information can be obtained by continuing the test further. As described, this is an unusual end-point in most cardiac transplant recipients.

(2) The workload corresponding to the ventilatory threshold can be identified (Figure 28.1). It serves little purpose to exercise the patient much beyond his ventilatory threshold as it is inappropriate to prescribe exercise at intensities that exceed this threshold, at least initially.

The medical criteria for terminating the exercise test are the same as those used in patients with ischemic heart disease, and have been detailed by Kavanagh and his colleagues[16]. These are:

(1) Adverse symptoms. It is important to recognize that a patient with a transplant heart does not sense anginal pain. Significant other symptoms include severe dyspnea, light-headedness, faintness, confusion, and severe fatigue.

(2) Adverse signs, including facial pallor; either a fall in heart rate or blood pressure, or the failure of either or both to rise with increasing effort; systolic blood pressure exceeding 280 mmHg, or diastolic blood pressure exceeding 140 mmHg.

(3) Adverse electrocardiographic changes, including frequent complex ventricular extrasystoles, ventricular tachycardia, sustained supraventricular tachycardia, atrial fibrillation, second- or third-degree heart block, or severe ST segment depression (horizontal or downsloping of greater than 4 mm).

Determining the appropriate exercise intensity

The symptom-limited maximal exercise test is used as the basis for determining the appropriate exercise intensity for the cardiac transplant recipient. A popular approach for patients with ischemic heart disease is to limit the patient to a maximum of 90% of the maximum symptom- or sign-limited heart rate achieved during the maximal exercise test, and to allow a 6 week training period before the patient is allowed to exercise regularly at that heart rate.

However, this is clearly inappropriate for the cardiac transplant recipient who has a blunted chronotropic response to exercise. Accordingly, it is more appropriate in these patients to prescribe exercise on the basis of the measured oxygen consumption, the ventilatory threshold, or the Borg Scale. The approach of Kavanagh et al.[16] has been to allow patients to exercise either at 60–70% of their peak oxygen consumption measured during the maximal exercise test, or at the exercise intensity corresponding to the ventilation threshold, or at an effort rating of 14 on the Borg Scale, equivalent to a perceived exertion described as 'somewhat hard'. A detailed walking/jogging program and the method of progression has been fully detailed[16].

Our own approach has been to devise a 24-week starter program that includes stretching, walking, jogging, and aerobics (Table 28.1), overseen by a sports medicine physician, physiotherapists and exercise physiologists. We have

Table 28.1 A 24-week initial physical training program for cardiac transplant recipients

Week	Stretching (min)	Walking (min)	Jogging (min)	Aerobics (min)	Perceived exertion rating (units)
1	30	10	0	20	10
2	30	10	0	20	10
3	25	15	0	20	11
4	25	15	0	20	11
5	20	13	2	25	12
6	20	13	2	25	12
7	20	11	4	25	12
8	20	11	4	25	12
9	15	14	6	25	13
10	15	14	6	25	13
11	15	12	8	25	13
12	15	12	8	25	13
13	10	15	10	25	13
14	10	15	10	25	13
15	10	13	12	25	13
16	10	13	12	25	13
17	10	16	14	20	14
18	10	14	16	20	14
19	10	12	18	20	14
20	10	10	20	20	14
21	10	13	22	15	15
22	10	11	24	15	15
23	10	8	27	15	15
24	10	5	30	15	15

found that these persons have special expertise for developing interesting and enjoyable exercise programs that are meaningful for all participants. They are also able to adapt the programs to new ideas that are fashionable amongst the popular exercise movement. For example, the inclusion of 'aerobics' in any exercise program would have been unthinkable 10 years ago; yet it is perfectly acceptable today.

The prescribed intensity is determined by the Borg Scale and increases gradually as the program progresses (Table 28.2). Table 28.2 lists equivalent values for the % maximum heart rate, the % VO_2 max., and the rating of perceived exertion according to the data of Ekblom and Goldbarg[31] and others[32]. It shows that, to a first approximation, the VO_2 max. is 10% lower than the % maximum heart rate at any exercise intensity, and that the rating of perceived exertion can be calculated as the % VO_2 max. multiplied by 0.2. Thus the training heart rate zone of between 60 and 80% maximum heart rate, within which the patient should maintain his heart rate during exercise, corresponds to 50–70% VO_2 max. and ratings of perceived exertion of 10–14, equivalent to subjective feelings of 'light to somewhat hard'.

Whilst this approach is not as exact as that of Kavanagh et al.[16], it accomodates a great diversity of sporting interests amongst the patients, who may be less committed to a program that includes only walking and jogging. Our belief is that there is no evidence that patients who exercise more vigorously necessarily derive greater benefit than those who exercise more conservatively. On the other hand, it would seem that the risk of cardiac complications arising during exercise, at least in patients with ischemic heart disease, increases with intensity of exercise[33,34]. Thus, our approach has been to encourage patients to exercise at a lower intensity for a longer time rather than at a higher intensity for a shorter time.

Monitoring during the exercise sessions

During each exercise session, careful attention should be paid to the following:

(1) Each patient's level of perceived exertion and heart rate is regularly checked. At first, these are measured every few minutes, but later, as the patient's ability to monitor his exercise intensity improves, only once every session. The heart rate checks are essential to identify abnormal heart rhythms. Patients are instructed to report any cardiac rhythm abnormalities to the attending exercise specialists. To reinforce these practices, all patients are required to fill out an activity card at the end of each exercise session. The card includes information on resting heart and blood pressure, on exercising heart rates, on time spent in each activity, on the presence of symptoms, and any medications that might have been taken.

(2) All symptoms must be immediately reported. Our experience in patients with ischemic heart disease is that the majority of patients at risk of sudden death will develop warning symptoms[33], and only if these symptoms are ignored will problems develop. Symptoms such as excessive dyspnea, unusual fatigue, general malaise and tiredness, and light-headedness must be taken extremely seriously. They are an immediate indication to reduce the training load, and for further cardiac evaluation. As angina does not occur in the denervated heart, the presence of myocardial ischemia must be detected by careful attention to these other symptoms.

(3) The patient is not allowed to exercise during or within 1 week of a pyrexial illness, due to the possible, albeit low, risk of fatal myocarditis.

Table 28.2 Comparative values for % maximum heart rate, % maximum oxygen consumption (VO_2 max.), and rating of perceived exertion

Maximum heart rate (%)	VO_2 max. (%)	Rating of perceived exertion (units)	Subjective description
50	36	7.2	very, very light
60	46	9.2	very light
70	58	11.6	light
80	70	14.0	somewhat hard
90	82	16.4	very hard
100	100	19.2	very, very hard

From data of Ekblom and Goldbarg[31]

(4) Episodes of rejection also call for a modification of the training program.

Patients are also instructed that they must train regularly without peaks of activity, must avoid competition, and must reduce their exercise training load should mental tension and depression develop. It is our feeling that work tension and business stress, particularly when travel is involved, are important causes of transient exacerbation of symptoms. Smoking is prohibited. Particular attention is paid to patients with type A personalities because they are notoriously difficult to control in any exercise rehabilitation program. They will frequently exceed their exercise prescription and fail to report symptoms. Thus they may be more likely to be at risk of complications, and require particular attention[34].

BENEFITS OF TRAINING

There are relatively few reports of the effects of exercise training in organ transplant recipients. Squires et al. trained two patients, beginning 6 weeks after each had undergone orthotopic cardiac transplantation[29]. After 8 weeks of low-intensity exercise training, the maximal exercise capacity of both patients had increased, and their heart rates and rating of perceived exertion were decreased at all submaximal workloads.

In the most comprehensive study yet reported, Kavanagh et al. followed 36 cardiac transplant recipients who participated in a more vigorous walking/jogging training program for up to 17 months[16]. The average peak power output of the transplant recipient was less than one-half that of the untrained normal controls in the pretraining maximal exercise test. After training, lean body mass was increased, heart rate and blood pressure at rest were reduced, as were heart rate, minute ventilation and perceived exertion, but not cardiac output, during submaximal exercise. At exhaustion, peak heart rate, peak power output, and peak rate of oxygen consumption ($\dot{V}O_2$ max.) were increased. They concluded that the exercise training program was justified as it increased the working capacity of the patients, and thus the quality of their lives. For reasons that have already been presented, they argued that the main effect of training appeared to be a 'strengthening of the peripheral muscles' rather than a direct effect on the transplanted heart.

Our related study with renal transplant recipients[9,35] confirms this assumption. We showed that the exercise capacity of these patients was subnormal before training, and was not completely restored with training. The patients adapted to training in the expected manner, as described by Kavanagh et al.[16]. In addition, we showed that the peak isokinetic torque produced by the quadriceps and hamstring muscles, and the total isokinetic work produced by those muscles during 25 maximal contractions, increased by between 20–70%. We have also concluded that the factor limiting the exercise performance of these patients was a peripheral myopathy, almost certainly resulting from the drugs used to control rejection, and that the major effect of training was to increase peripheral muscle strength. We have also considered whether a program designed specifically to increase the patients' muscle strength rather than their 'cardiorespiratory endurance' would not be an equally effective training method.

COMMENT

Certain physiological and pathological features of the cardiac transplant recipient demand that adaptations be made to the conventional principles underlying exercise prescription for patients with ischemic heart disease. In particular, the use of heart rate monitoring to control the exercise intensity is less applicable, and an alternate method using the Borg Scale of Perceived Exertion would appear to be more appropriate.

In addition, the cardiac transplant recipient is more likely to have a peripheral limitation to his exercise capacity, probably due to a myopathic effect of the drugs used to control rejection. This peripheral limitation to exercise, combined with the likelihood that such patients have, at least initially, less florid coronary atherosclerosis, probably places them at a lesser risk of sudden death during exercise than patients with ischemic heart disease.

It would seem that cardiac transplant recipients adapt in the normal way to exercise training with the exception that the peripheral skeletal muscular adaptations would appear to dominate. The use of additional or alternate training programs specifically to increase skeletal muscle strength would seem to be justified.

Whether continued exercise training can prevent progressive drug-induced myopathic changes and can reduce or delay the onset of rejection-related accelerated coronary atherosclerosis would seem worthy of further study.

Acknowledgements

The personal research included in this chapter was funded by Lennon Laboratories; additional funding was provided by the Medical Research Council of South Africa and the Nellie Atkinson and Harry Crossley Research Funds of the University of Cape Town.

References

1. Deitrick, J.E., Whedon, G.D. and Shorr, E. (1948). Effects of immobilization upon various metabolic and physiologic functions of normal men. *Am. J. Med.*, **4**, 3
2. Dock, W. (1944). The evil sequelae of complete bed rest. *J. Am. Med. Assoc.*, **125**, 1083

3. Harrison, T.R. (1944). Abuse of rest as a therapeutic measure for patients with cardiovascular disease. *J. Am. Med. Assoc.*, **125**, 1075
4. Trudel, J., Dewolfe, J., Young, J. and Lefevre, F. (1963) Disuse phenomena of lower extremity. *J. Am. Med. Assoc.*, **185**, 1129
5. Saltin, B., Blomqvist, G., Mitchell, J.H., Johnson, R.L., Wildenthal, K. and Chapman, C.B. (1968). Response to exercise after bedrest and after training. A longitudinal study of adaptive changes in oxygen transport and body composition. *Circulation*, **38** (Suppl. VII), 1
6. Issekutz, B., Blizzard, J.J., Birkhead, N.C. and Rodall, K. (1966). Effect of prolonged bedrest on urinary calcium output. *J. Appl. Physiol.*, **21**, 1013
7. Morris, P.J. (1979). *Kidney Transplantation, Principles and Practices.* (New York: Grune and Stratton)
8. Capaccio, J.A., Gallasi, T.M. and Hickson, R.C. (1985). Unaltered aerobic power and endurance following glucocorticoid-induced muscle atrophy. *Med. Sci. Sports Exerc.*, **17**, 380
9. Kempeneers, G.L.G., Myburgh, K.H., Wiggins, T., Adams, B., Van Zyl-Smit, R. and Noakes, T.D. (1988). The effect of an exercise training program on renal transplant recipients. *Transplant. Proc.*, **20** (Suppl. 1), 381
10. Pope, S.E., Stinson, E.B., Daughters, G.T., Schroeder, J.S., Ingels, N.B. and Alderman, E.L. (1980). Exercise response of the denervated heart in long-term cardiac transplant recipients. *Am. J. Cardiol.*, **46**, 213
11. Savin, W.M., Haskell, W.L., Schroeder, J.S. and Stinson, E.B. (1980). Cardiorespiratory responses of cardiac transplant patients to graded, symptom-limited exercise. *Circulation*, **62**, 55
12. Savin, W.M., Gordon, E., Green, S., Haskell, W.L., Kantrowitz, N., Lundberg, M., Melvin, K., Sammuelsson, R., Verschagin, K. and Schroeder, J.S. (1983). Comparison of exercise training in cardiac denervated and innervated humans. *J. Am. Coll. Cardiol.*, **1**, 722
13. Schroeder, J.S. (1979). Hemodynamic performance of the human transplanted heart. *Transplant. Proc.*, **11**, 304
14. Donald, D.E. (1968). Capacity for exercise after denervation of the heart. *Circulation*, **38**, 225
15. Stinson, E.B., Griepp, R.B., Schroeder, J.S., Dong, E. and Shumway, N.E. (1972). Hemodynamic observations one and two years after cardiac transplantation in man. *Circulation*, **45**, 1183
16. Kavanagh, T., Yacoub, M.H., Mertens, D.H., Kennedy, J., Campbell, R.S. and Sawyer, P. (1988). Cardiorespiratory responses to exercise training after orthotopic cardiac transplantation. *Circulation*, **77**, 162
17. Bexton, R.S., Milne, J.R., Cory-Pearce, R., English, T.A.H. and Camm, A.J. (1983). Effect of beta blockade on exercise response after cardiac transplantation. *Br. Heart J.*, **49**, 584
18. Roos, R. (1986). Exercise training for heart transplant patients. *Physcn. Sports. Med.*, **14**, (Sept.), 165
19. Rowell, L.B. (1986). *Human Circulation: Regulation During Physical Stress.* (New York: Oxford University Press)
20. Brooks, G.A. (1985). Anaerobic threshold: review of the concept and directions for future research. *Med. Sci. Sports Exerc.*, **17**, 22
21. Noakes, T.D. (1988). Implications of exercise testing for prediction of athletic performance: a contemporary perspective. *Med. Sci. Sports. Exerc.*, **20**, 319
22. Brooks, G.A. and Fahey, T.D. (1987). *Fundamentals of Human Performance.* (New York: Macmillan)
23. McCartney, N., Heigenhauser, G.J.F., Sargeant, A.J. and Jones, N.L. (1983). A constant-velocity cycle ergometer for the study of dynamic muscle function. *J. Appl. Physiol.*, **55**, 212
24. McCartney, N., Heigenhauser, G.J.F. and Jones, N.L. (1983). Power output and fatigue of human muscle in maximal cycling exercise. *J. Appl. Physiol.*, **55**, 218
25. Sadowsky, H.S., Rohrkemper, K.F. and Quon, S.Y.M. (1986). Rehabilitation of cardiac and cardiopulmonary recipients. An introduction for physical and occupational therapists. (Stanford University Hospital)
26. Levine, S.A. and Lown, B. (1952). 'Armchair' treatment of acute coronary thrombosis. *J. Am. Med. Assoc.*, **148**, 1365
27. Dehne, P.A. and Protas, E.J. (1986). Oxygen consumption and heart rate responses during five active exercises. *Physical Ther.*, **66**, 1215
28. Borg, G. (1970). Perceived exertion as an indicator of somatic stress. *Scand. J. Rehab. Med.*, **2**, 92
29. Squires, R.W., Arthur, P.R., Gan, G.T., Muri, A. and Lambert, W.B. (1983). Exercise after cardiac transplantation: a report of two cases. *J. Cardiac Rehab.*, **3**, 570
30. Constant, J. (1986). Prognostic information from early post-infarction exercise testing. *Am. J. Med.*, **81**, 655
31. Ekblom, B. and Goldbarg, A.N. (1971). The influence of physical training and other factors on the subjective rating of perceived exertion. *Acta Physiol. Scand.*, **83**, 399
32. Birk, T.J. and Birk, C.A. (1987). Use of ratings of perceived exertion for exercise prescription. *Sports Med.*, **4**, 1
33. Noakes, T.D. (1987). Heart disease in marathon runners. A review. *Med. Sci. Sport. Exerc.*, **19**, 187
34. Van Camp, S.P. and Peterson, R.A. (1986). Cardiovascular complications of outpatient cardiac rehabilitation programs. *J. Am. Med. Assoc.*, **256**, 1160
35. Kempeneers, G.L.G., Noakes, T.D., Van Zyl-Smit, R., Myburgh, K.H., Lambert, M., Adams, B. and Wiggins, T. (1989). Skeletal muscle limits the exercise tolerance of renal transplant recipients: effects of a graded exercise training programme. In press

29
Non-cardiac Surgery in Patients with Heart Transplants – Anesthetic and Operative Considerations

E. BECERRA AND D.K.C. COOPER

INTRODUCTION

As cardiac transplantation becomes increasingly successful, there is a growing possibility that patients with heart transplants may require surgery for conditions unrelated to the heart. Such patients clearly present special management problems, which include, in particular, atypical responses to both stress and certain pharmacological agents, and increased susceptibility to infection.

CONDITIONS FOR WHICH SURGERY MAY BE NECESSARY IN PATIENTS WITH HEART TRANSPLANTS

Between 12 and 30% of the patients who undergo heart transplantation may develop a pathological condition requiring one or more non-cardiac operations[1-3]. The need for such an operation has been documented from 2 hours to more than 10 years after transplantation[2]. In a study at Pittsburgh, the incidence of significant general surgical complications developing within 30 days after transplantation was 7%[1]. Patients with cardiac transplants may, of course, develop any unrelated disease requiring surgical intervention (e.g. carcinoma of the stomach, cholecystitis), as may any member of the population, but, in addition, they are at special risk of requiring surgery for several reasons (Table 29.1).

They may develop a complication of the transplant operation (e.g. incisional hernia, wound infection, gastric outlet obstruction secondary to vagus nerve injury occurring during heart–lung transplantation[1]), or of a subsequent diagnostic procedure (e.g. right ventricular perforation, pneumothorax or hemothorax following endomyocardial biopsy).

Systemic thromboembolism may occur in patients with a heterotopic heart transplant from a poorly functioning recipient (native) left ventricle, but may also occur rarely in patients with an orthotopic transplant when donor heart function is decreased either during an acute rejection episode or when chronic rejection is advanced. Anticoagulant therapy and antiplatelet agents may increase the risk of gastrointestinal bleeding and hematoma formation following trauma. When cardiac transplantation has been performed for ischemic heart disease, the atheromatous disease process may progress in peripheral vessels and lead to ischemic complications, particularly in the lower limbs or brain. Aortic dissection or aneurysm formation may also occur. All of these conditions may require surgery.

In addition, however, certain complications of long-term immunosuppresive therapy may require a surgical procedure, notably because immunosuppressed patients are more susceptible to infection (Chapter 17). The immunosuppressive agents themselves, particularly the corticosteroids, may lead to complications which require surgical treatment (Chapter 22). Corticosteroid therapy may result in musculoskeletal disorders (e.g. osteoporosis, vertebral compression fractures, pathological bone fractures, aseptic necrosis), gastrointestinal disorders (e.g. peptic ulceration and pancreatitis) and ophthalmic disorders (e.g. cataract, glaucoma,

Table 29.1 Conditions for which patients with heart transplants may require surgery

(1) Unrelated
(2) Complications of transplant operation
(3) Complications of diagnostic procedures (e.g. endomyocardial biopsy)
(4) Complications of immunosuppressive therapy, particularly corticosteroids
(5) Complications of other drug therapy (e.g. anticoagulation)
(6) Systemic thromboembolism (especially in patients with a heterotopic heart transplant)
(7) Continuing atheromatous disease (in patients with ischemic heart disease)

exophthalmos), all of which may require operative procedures.

The differential diagnosis of an acute abdominal complication in a patient with a heart transplant may prove difficult, but requires urgent assessment in order to avoid delay of treatment. Despite steroid therapy, the history and physical examination are generally reliable, though the white blood count may be misleading[1]. When perforation of the bowel is present, the patient almost always manifests with pain, tenderness and muscular rigidity[1]. Peptic ulcer disease and cytomegalovirus gastritis or duodenitis should be included in the differential diagnosis of abdominal pain[4]. Free intraperitoneal air on an abdominal radiograph suggests bowel or stomach perforation. In the early postoperative period, however, if no pain or muscular rigidity are present, free air may be associated with accidental opening of the abdominal cavity at the time of sternotomy. For the same reason, pneumothorax in the early post-transplant period (or even later[1]), possibly a complication of endomyocardial biopsy, may also progress and present as air in the abdomen. Assessment of the acute abdomen may include gastrointestinal endoscopy, computerized tomographic scanning, gastrografin contrast radiography, and ultrasound studies. Pancreatitis is a not unusual complication of immunosuppresive therapy, but it should be noted that the serum amylase is often increased after cardiopulmonary bypass[5]. In doubtful cases, early exploratory laparotomy is advocated[1].

PREOPERATIVE ASSESSMENT

If time permits, before any major surgical procedure is undertaken, the status of the patient with regard to both acute and chronic rejection should be checked. This may involve clinical examination for features of cardiac failure of dysrhythmias, blood cell counts and plasma chemistry, electrocardiographic studies, endomyocardial biopsy or other technique, such as radionuclide scanning, to detect acute rejection, and even coronary angiography or thallium scanning if significant chronic rejection is suspected. Elective surgical procedures should be postponed if the total white blood cell count is particularly low (less than 2000–3000 cells/m^3).

Patients receiving long-term anticoagulation therapy should have this therapy reduced to a safe level for the period of operation, but it should be instigated again 48 hours after operation unless there is a contraindication. Antiplatelet therapy should be discontinued for the day of operation only. In an emergency, fresh frozen plasma can be administered to normalize the coagulation state of the patient before surgery.

Unless the operative procedure is being undertaken for an infective complication, e.g. the drainage of an abscess, and a specific antibiotic is therefore indicated, our policy has been to prescribe an antistaphylococcal antibiotic as prophylaxis over the period of the operation; this should be administered initially approximately 1 hour before the surgical procedure begins so that high blood and tissue levels are present, and discontinued within 24–48 hours to minimize the risk of growth of resistant bacterial or fungal organisms.

SPECIAL PROBLEMS OF ANESTHESIA

The special problems faced in managing patients with cardiac transplants who require operative procedures include: (1) atypical responses to stress and to certain drugs, since the transplanted heart remains denervated; (2) increased susceptibility to infection; (3) increased tendency to arrhythmias, particularly during the first 3 months after transplantation or when acute or chronic rejection is occurring[6]; and (4) risk of complications related to drugs such as anticoagulants, corticosteroids, and cyclosporine.

With regard to drug-related complications, the increased risks of managing a patient who has been on long-term anticoagulation therapy are obvious, and the need for increased corticosteroid therapy in patients receiving these drugs over a long period of time, since their own adrenal cortical response to stress is suppressed, is also well known. Cyclosporine may result in impaired renal and/or hepatic function, which may complicate the perioperative period, and may also have resulted in systemic hypertension, for which the patient may be receiving additional antihypertensive therapy.

Maintenance azathioprine, cyclosporine and corticosteroid therapy is continued. In patients receiving long-term steroid therapy, hydrocortisone 100–200 mg should be given intravenously immediately before the induction of general anesthesia and may be required after operation for 24 or 48 hours[2,7]. Standard general anesthetic techniques may be used in these patients, care being taken to maintain good oxygenation. (Orotracheal intubation has been suggested as being preferable to nasotracheal to diminish the risk of lung infection[8,9].) Muscle relaxation, where necessary, may sometimes require larger doses than usual, since azathioprine antagonizes neuromuscular blocking agents by its phosphodiesterase-inhibiting properties[10]. Agents such as morphine may be used as necessary[2].

Particularly when a major surgical procedure is undertaken, adequate hemodynamic monitoring is essential. Arterial and central venous pressure lines are inserted, employing strict sterile technique. Continuous ECG monitoring is necessary. Percutaneous suprapubic rather than transurethral catheterization has been advocated in order to avoid urinary tract infections[11], though many groups, including our own, would feel this to be unnecessary.

Since transplantation results in complete and permanent

Table 29.2 Mortality of non-cardiac surgery in patients with heart transplants

Center	Authors (year)	Number of patients	Number of operations	Early mortality
Stanford, USA	Reitz et al. (1977)[11]	2	2	0
Stanford, USA	Kanter and Samuels (1977)[13]	16(?)	24	4
New York, USA	Eisenkraft et al. (1981)[7]	1	2	1
Pittsburgh, USA	Steed et al. (1985)[1]	17	17	4
Cape Town, South Africa	Cooper et al. (1986)[2]	15	39	1
Stanford, USA	Isono et al. (1987)[12]	10	10	0

denervation of the heart, it can no longer respond to neurally-mediated stimuli. During stress or exercise, the heart initially increases cardiac output by an increase in stroke volume rather than by cardioacceleration (Chapter 13). To avoid hypotension and maintain cardiac output during stress, therefore, an adequate preload must be available. In addition, steps may be required to increase heart rate rapidly and also enhance contractile force, namely by the administration of inotropic agents; the response of myocardial adrenergic receptors has been shown to be normal or increased.

POSTOPERATIVE MANAGEMENT

To reduce the risk of infection, the patient should be extubated and all drains and vascular and urinary catheters removed as soon as possible after operation. Since pulmonary infection is particularly common in immunosuppressed patients, they should receive respiratory therapy until fully mobilized; chest radiographs should be taken frequently during the early postoperative days to monitor pulmonary status. Since these patients are frequently receiving long-term corticosteroid therapy, this should be supplemented to cover the operative procedure; it is not necessary to continue this extra therapy for longer than 48 hours after operation unless there is some specific indication. As corticosteroids may impair wound healing, sutures should be left *in situ* for rather longer than usual. For a similar reason, when a gastrointestinal or biliary leak is present, it is advisable to maintain the drain for a longer period of time than usual to allow adequate healing.

After gastrointestinal surgery it may prove necessary to administer cyclosporine intravenously rather than orally, since absorption can be variable, though care must be exercised as, in our experience, the intravenous route is more commonly associated with nephrotoxicity. The intravenous dosage should initially be small (1–2 mg/kg infused over 24 hours) and adjusted when blood levels have been measured. Alternatively, most patients can be managed for several days, if necessary, without cyclosporine if ALG is administered on a daily basis to suppress the T-11 lymphocyte subset.

Early postoperative mobilization of the patient to minimize the risk of venous thrombosis and pulmonary embolism is as important as in other patients undergoing surgery; this complication has been documented in most of the published series[7,12].

RESULTS OF SURGERY IN PATIENTS WITH HEART TRANSPLANTS

A summary of published results of such surgery in patients with heart transplants is shown in Table 29.2. As some patients at Stanford may have been included in more than one study, it is not possible to estimate accurately the combined mortality in these series. It is clear, however, that the mortality was relatively low. Most of the deaths were related to the underlying pathology rather than any anesthetic or surgical complication. Almost one-half of the total deaths were from one series which included a number of extremely complex abdominal conditions[1]; this mortality would probably have been lower if some of the patients had presented for medical consultation earlier in the course of their illness. The authors of this paper stress the importance of early diagnosis. Pulmonary infections and embolism were the most frequent postoperative complications.

General anesthesia and surgical intervention in patients with heart transplants would, therefore, appear to be a relatively safe procedure if care is taken to monitor the patient and avoid the special complications which may be associated with immunosuppressive therapy.

References

1. Steed, D.L., Brown, B., Reilly, J.J., Peitzman, A.B., Griffith, B.P., Hardesty, R.L. and Webster, W.W. (1985). General surgical complications in heart and heart–lung transplantation. *Surgery*, **98**, 739
2. Cooper, D.K.C., Becerra, E.A., Novitzky, D., Ozinsky, J., Horak, A. and Reichart, B. (1986). Surgery in patients with heart transplants: anaesthetic and operative considerations. *S. Afr. Med. J.*, **70**, 137
3. Samuels, S.I. and Wyner, J. (1986). Anaesthesia for surgery in patients with a transplanted heart. *Br. J. Anaesth.*, **58**, 1119
4. Bramwell, N.H., Davies, R.A., Koshal, A., Tse, G.N.W., Keon, W.J. and Walley, V.M. (1987). Fatal gastrointestinal hemorrhage caused by cytomegalovirus duodenitis and ulceration after heart transplantation. *J. Heart Transplant.*, **6**, 303
5. Missavage, A., Weaver, D., Bouwman, D., Parnel, V. and Wilson, R. (1984). Hyperamylasemia after cardiopulmonary bypass. *Am. Surg.*, **50**, 297

6. Schroeder, J.S., Berke, D.K., Graham, A.F. and Harrison, D.C. (1974). Arrhythmias after cardiac transplantation. *Am. J. Cardiology*, **33**, 604
7. Eisenkraft, J.B., Dimich, I. and Sachdev, V.P. (1981). Anesthesia for major non-cardiac surgery in patients with a transplanted heart. *Mount Sinai J. Med. (NY)*, **48**, 116
8. Frater, R.W.M. and Santos, G.H. (1974). Sources of infection in open heart surgery. *N.Y. State J. Med.*, **74**, 2386
9. Kluge, R.M., Calia, F.M., McLaughlin, J.S. and Hornick, R.B. (1974). Sources of contamination in open heart surgery. *J. Am. Med. Assoc.*, **230**, 1415
10. Dretchen, K.L., Morgenroth, V.H., Standaert, F.G. and Walts, L.F. (1976). Azathioprine effects on neuromuscular transmission. *Anesthesiology*, **45**, 604
11. Reitz, B.A., Baumgartner, W.A., Oyer, P.E. and Stinson, E.B. (1977). Abdominal aortic aneurysmectomy in long-term cardiac transplant survivors. *Arch. Surg.*, **112**, 1057
12. Isono, S.S., Woolson, S.T. and Schurman, D.J. (1987). Total joint arthroplasty for steroid-induced osteonecrosis in cardiac transplant patients. *Clin. Orthop.*, **217**, 201
13. Kanter, S.F. and Samuels, S.I. (1977). Anesthesia for major operations on patients who have transplanted hearts: a review of 29 cases. *Anesthesiology*, **46**, 65

30
Non-cardiac Autopsy Findings in Patients with Heart (or Heart–Lung) Transplants

A.G. ROSE

INTRODUCTION

Patients who receive immunosuppressive therapy following organ transplantation have an iatrogenic, acquired (T-lymphocyte) immune deficiency. It is thus not surprising that they are prone to develop the same infective and neoplastic diseases that are commonly encountered in patients with the Acquired Immune Deficiency Syndrome (AIDS), which results from destruction of their T-lymphocytes by the human immunodeficiency virus. Patients with T-lymphocyte deficiency are prone to infection with *Pneumocystis carinii*, *Herpesvirus hominis*, Torula, and *Mycobacterium tuberculosis*, as well as malignant diseases, e.g. Kaposi's sarcoma. Fortunately, the immune deficit produced in the transplant recipient by the drug therapy is reversible and is proportional to the dosages used. Whilst cyclosporine-based therapy has a less depressive effect on the body's ability to deal with infective agents compared to the older steroid-based regimen, infection remains a potentially lethal problem.

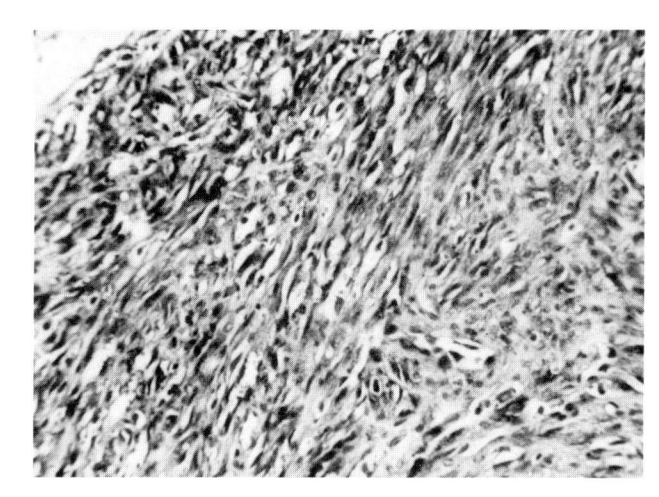

Figure 30.1 Kaposi's sarcoma in a heart transplant recipient is characterized by a proliferation of spindle-shaped, fibroblastic-looking cells enclosing numerous slit-like spaces (H & E × 120)

EXTERNAL APPEARANCE

On external examination the patient may show evidence of:

(1) A Cushingoid appearance due to steroid therapy (moon face, buffalo hump due to deposition of adipose tissue in the interscapular area, abdominal striae, truncal obesity).

(2) Peripheral edema which may be present if acute or chronic rejection has led to cardiac pump failure.

(3) Possible evidence of neoplasia in the skin, e.g. skin nodules due to Kaposi's sarcoma (Figure 30.1), squamous cell carcinoma, or general cachexia due to the anorexia associated with malignancy. Lymphadenopathy due to lymphoma may produce visible swellings.

(4) Skin infections by unusual organisms, e.g. mycobacteria other than *Mycobacterium tuberculosis*. Herpes zoster, varicella, and vaccina may also be detected on external examination. Hirsutism may be a side effect of cyclosporine therapy.

(5) Peripheral limb ischemia resulting from embolism, e.g. thromboembolism from thrombus within a recipient heart (ischemic or dilated cardiomyopathic) if heterotopic transplantation has been performed. Chronic rejection of the donor heart may lead to intracavity stasis thrombus that may be a potential source of thromboembolism.

(6) Finger clubbing which may persist in patients who have undergone heart–lung transplantation for long-standing chronic pulmonary infection.

LUNGS

Pulmonary infections are a major problem in transplant patients[1,2], and these include pneumonias due to a wide variety of organisms, including bacteria (e.g. *Staphylococci albus* and *aureus*, Klebsiella species, *Hemophilus influenzae*, and many others), fungi (e.g. *Aspergillus niger*, *Candida albicans*, *Cryptococcus neoformans*, Mucor), protozoal organisms (e.g. *Pneumocystis carinii*), and viruses (e.g. cytomegalovirus). Bacterial septicemia may cause diffuse pulmonary alveolar damage.

Cytomegalovirus (CMV), which is the commonest viral infection in immunosuppressed patients, may produce a pneumonitis with diffuse alveolar damage. The infection often co-exists with *Pneumocystis carinii* involvement of the lung. Cells infected with CMV are enlarged and show intranuclear inclusions that may be up to 17 μm in diameter, and are surrounded by a clear halo, giving an owl's eye appearance to the nucleus (Figure 30.2). CMV produced an overwhelming fatal infection in one of our early cardiac transplant patients, and the diffuse pulmonary involvement was associated with an area of intensive necrosis within one lung (Figure 30.3). Immune complexes were suspected of having played a role in the pathogenesis of the lesion, but none was demonstrated.

Lungs infected by *Pneumocystis carinii* are usually heavy and the cut surfaces appear yellow and consolidated with focal nodularity. The characteristic feature of the condition is the presence of foamy intra-alveolar exudate (Figure 30.4) containing a few macrophages that can lead one to strongly suspect the diagnosis before the confirmatory fungal silver stain is performed. The organisms are always confined to the intra-alveolar exudate, and, on hematoxylin–eosin sections, they are seen as tiny dots within the small cystic spaces occupying the intra-alveolar exudate. An interstitial pneumonitis is often present.

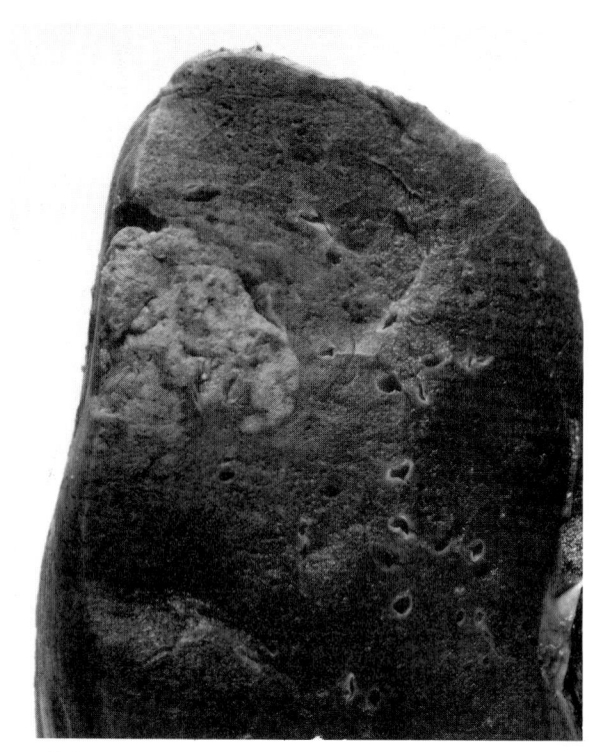

Figure 30.3 Area of necrosis in the right upper lobe of a recipient's lung that had a diffuse pneumonitis due to cytomegalovirus infection

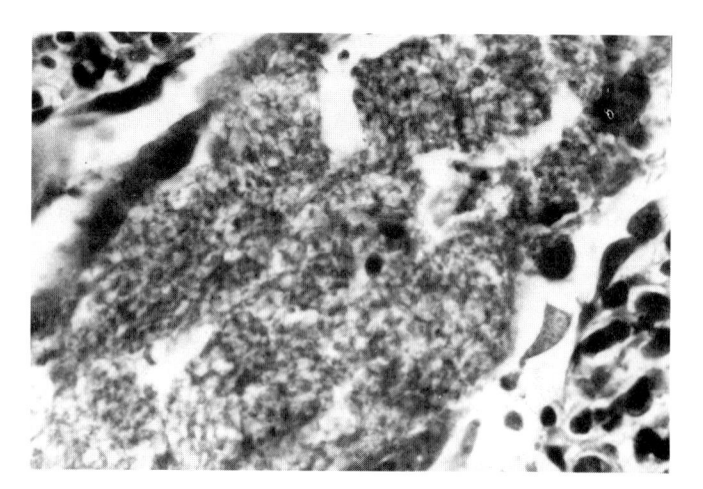

Figure 30.4 Foamy intra-alveolar exudate occupies an alveolar space in a transplant patient whose lungs are infected by *Pneumocystis carinii* (H & E × 480)

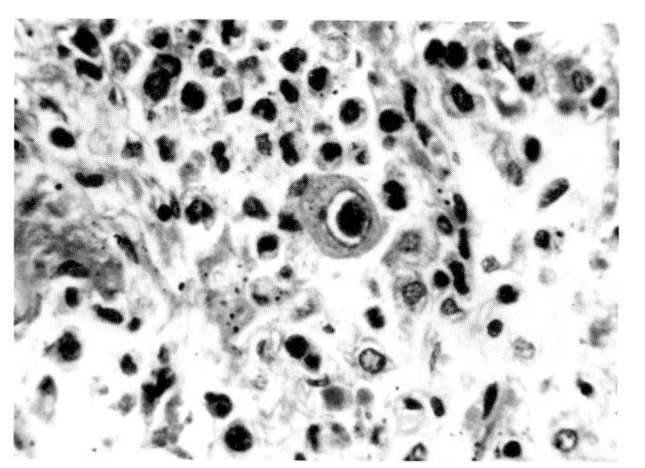

Figure 30.2 Pneumonitis due to cytomegalic inclusion body disease. An enlarged pneumocyte containing a typical intranuclear inclusion is present in the center of the field (H & E × 480)

In about 50% of cases, particularly in those with early infection, the characteristic intra-alveolar exudate may be absent and the microscopic features may simply be those of acute, diffuse alveolar damage. The Grocott (methenamine silver) stain will reveal the organisms as spherical, comma- or helmet-shaped structures, measuring up to 4 μm in diameter (Figure 30.5). Electron microscopy of the cystic form of the organism reveals an electron-dense, double-layered, membrane enclosing up to six dense sporozoites

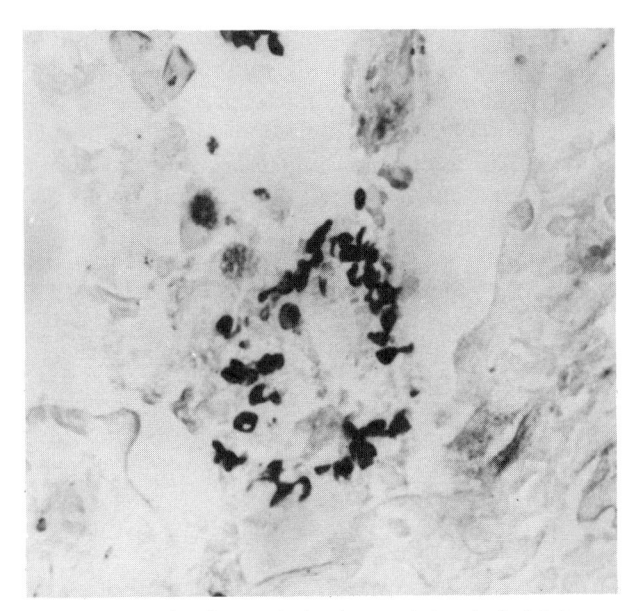

Figure 30.5 Fungal stain reveals the characteristic spherical, helmet- and comma-shaped forms of *Pneumocystis carinii* confined to the intra-alveolar exudate (Grocott methenamine silver × 600)

(daughter bodies), each surrounded by a membrane. The crescent-shaped forms contain no daughter bodies. Cell injury is thought to result from attachment of the organisms to the alveolar lining cells, which then undergo necrosis. This evokes reparative hyperplasia of the type II pneumocytes. Despite effective drug therapy, some patients may develop interstitial fibrosis and cor pulmonale.

In developing countries where tuberculosis is common, reactivation of dormant disease is prone to occur with immunosuppressive therapy. It is also a major problem in patients receiving immunosuppression after combined heart–lung transplantation since the donor lungs usually contain a 'healed' primary tuberculous complex which can be activated. Some patients may show subacute miliary tuberculosis.

Pulmonary abscesses may result from bacterial or fungal pneumonias.

In addition to the above possible changes, most patients will show residual evidence of pulmonary alterations due to the severe, long-standing left-sided heart failure that antedated the cardiac transplantation. Changes to look for include atherosclerosis of the major pulmonary arteries, as well as persistence of intimal fibrous thickening and medial hypertrophy of the smaller pulmonary arteries due to long-standing passive venous pulmonary hypertension. The lung parenchyma may show intra-alveolar hemosiderin-laden macrophages (so-called heart failure cells) as well as a degree of interstitial fibrosis with interstitial smooth muscle proliferation.

If death is due to graft rejection, then pulmonary edema related to left heart failure may be superimposed on the above changes. Pleural adhesions are related to the allografting operation.

MEDIASTINUM

Following cardiac or combined heart–lung transplantation, extensive adhesions usually develop between the donor organs and the surrounding mediastinal structures. If the pericardium has not been closed, adhesions develop between the heart and the back of the sternum. Dense pleural adhesions may develop around transplanted lungs.

RECIPIENT HEART (FOLLOWING HETEROTOPIC TRANSPLANTATION)

If heterotopic cardiac transplantation has been performed, with retention of the recipient's diseased heart, prolongation of the patient's life allows progression of cardiac pathology to an extent that would have been impossible if the patient had been dependent on his native heart alone. Native heart pathology may therefore progress to a severity usually unattainable.

In cases of ischemic heart disease, all three major coronary arteries may be totally occluded, and the left ventricle may consist almost entirely of fibrous tissue. Patients with idiopathic dilated cardiomyopathy may develop advanced dilation of the cardiac chambers with abundant stasis thrombi therein. Similarly, occlusive lesions of native (and prosthetic) valves may reach a very advanced state within the recipient's heart, without affecting the survival of the patient, who is kept alive by the donor heart.

LYMPH NODES

Lymph nodes may show caseous necrosis due to tuberculosis, or there may be viral inclusions, e.g. in cases of disseminated cytomegalic inclusion body disease. The latter has been associated with extensive necrosis of the lymph nodes in some instances. Due to the increased risk of neoplasia in transplant patients, either a primary tumor (malignant lymphoma) or metastatic tumor deposits (carcinoma or Kaposi's sarcoma) may be encountered.

SPLEEN

In patients dying of infection (e.g. bacterial pneumonia) the spleen commonly shows reactive features, and these tend to be especially prominent if a terminal septicemia has occurred. Disseminated tuberculosis may produce multifocal lesions in the spleen of miliary or subacute blood-spread tuberculosis. The spleen may also be infected by CMV infection or by *Toxoplasma gondii*.

LIVER

Patients who die shortly after cardiac transplantation may show residual evidence of previous chronic passive congestion of the liver, with atrophy or loss of centrilobular hepatocytes, and dilation of the adjacent sinusoids. Fatty change may also be noted. Similar changes may be seen in patients who demise late after transplantation from pump failure of the cardiac allograft from acute or chronic rejection. Disseminated CMV or Herpesvirus hominis infection may occasionally be encountered.

KIDNEYS

In therapeutic doses, cyclosporine may be nephrotoxic in some patients. There are currently no laboratory tests or histopathological findings that are specific for cyclosporine nephrotoxicity. Morphologic changes produced in the kidney by cyclosporine appear to be non-specific[3,4], and include an interstitial nephritis, tubular atrophy, diffuse interstitial fibrosis, peritubular capillary congestion, and an arteriolopathy, as well as fibrin thrombi within glomerular capillary loops.

The focal arteriolopathy in the kidney may take one of two forms: (1) massive protein deposits throughout the vascular wall, replacing necrotic smooth muscle cells, and (2) severe intimal mucoid thickening with lumenal narrowing sometimes associated with thrombosis. The nearest glomeruli may appear ischemic or may be segmentally sclerosed. Immunohistological analysis of the lymphocyte subsets in the kidney reveals a marked predominance of helper-inducer T-cells over cytotoxic-suppressor T-cells. (This may be helpful in patients with renal transplants receiving cyclosporine in whom a mononuclear infiltrate, due to cyclosporine toxicity, has to be distinguished from acute rejection).

Although the majority of patients receiving cyclosporine develop systemic hypertension, renal nephrosclerosis is not obtrusive, possibly due to the relatively short duration of the hypertension in the patients who come to autopsy.

ADRENAL GLANDS

Patients who have been receiving large doses of corticosteroid hormones for prolonged periods may show atrophy of the cortices of the adrenal glands.

BONES

Infarction of discrete areas within the long bones is more common in persons who have received large doses of corticosteroid hormones. The pathogenesis of the lesion is uncertain. The condition may be multifocal and can be quite disabling in some instances, e.g. resulting in aseptic necrosis of the femoral head with fracture formation, requiring major orthopedic surgery (metal pin) to correct. Histological sections of the affected bony region often show little else other than osteoporosis, but the precise relationship between steroid dose, duration of use, and risk of osteoporosis remains unclear. The axial skeleton is affected more than the limbs and may lead to vertebral compression fractures.

SKELETAL MUSCLE

The limbs may show a steroid-induced myopathy, which is characterized by wasting of the large proximal muscles of the limbs.

BRAIN

Cerebral lesions that may be encountered include brain abscesses, e.g. due to fungal infection (Figures 30.6 and 30.7)

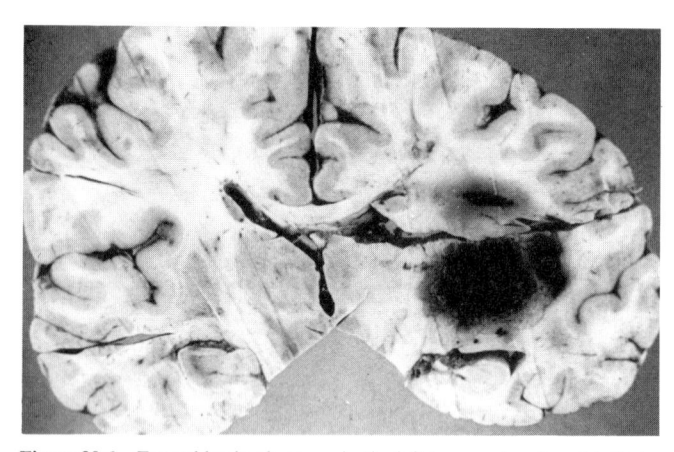

Figure 30.6 Fungal brain abscesses in the left temporal and parietal lobes

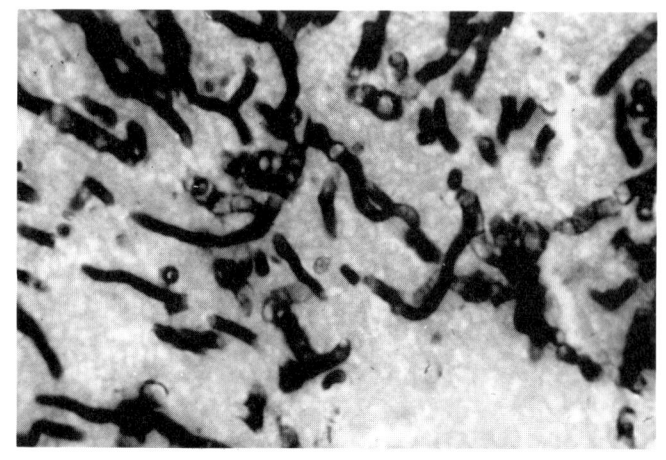

Figure 30.7 Fungal elements within the temporal lobe brain abscess shown in Figure 30.6 (Grocott methenamine silver × 480)

as well as primary lymphoma of the central nervous system. The brain is the commonest site of development of lymphoma in transplant patients[5] (Chapter 21). A total of 40% of lymphomas in cardiac transplant patients involve the central nervous system, compared with an incidence of only 28% in non-transplant patients. It has been claimed that patients with cardiomyopathy have a defect in mitogen-induced mononuclear suppressor cell activity, and that this renders such recipients more prone to develop lymphoma following organ transplantation and the institution of immunosuppressive therapy[6].

ARTERIES

Despite the presence of accelerated atherosclerosis in the epicardial and penetrating coronary arteries of the transplanted donor heart due to chronic rejection, the extracardiac arteries are unaffected by this process and show changes consistent with the age of the recipient. Heterotopic heart transplants are usually biopsied transvenously, but dissection of an artery may be a potential complication if cardiac catheterization has been performed transarterially, which has proved necessary in some such patients. In one of our patients, gangrene of the leg developed following femoral arterial catheterization. Thromboembolism has already been alluded to above.

VEINS

Organized or organizing thrombi within the deep calf veins or in the iliofemoral venous segment may be related to preoperative or postoperative cardiac failure.

OROPHARYNGEAL CAVITY

The mouth, tongue and throat may show herpetic ulceration (more common with steroids) or evidence of candidiasis ('thrush'). Fibrous hyperplasia of the gingiva may result from cyclosporine therapy. The clinical and histologic features are identical to the gingival hyperplasia induced by the anticonvulsant drug phenytoin (diphenylhydantoin).

ESOPHAGUS

Herpetic-induced ulceration of the esophagus is seldom seen with cyclosporine-based therapy, but used to be a frequent finding in patients who had received high doses of corticosteroid. Candidiasis may also occur.

STOMACH

The issue of whether peptic ulceration may complicate steroid therapy remains unresolved, but many believe that there is an increased risk of ulceration with prolonged steroid therapy. Kaposi's sarcoma may involve the stomach.

SMALL INTESTINE

The small intestine is said to be the commonest organ involved by Kaposi's sarcoma[7]. In one of two transplant patients in Cape Town who developed Kaposi's sarcoma, there was intestinal involvement, but in the second patient the tumor was confined to lymph nodes and skin. Whilst the first patient died of Kaposi's sarcoma, reduction of the second patient's immunosuppression led to regression of the sarcoma; this patient later died of chronic rejection and there was no evidence of tumor at autopsy. Kaposi's sarcoma is a multifocal malignant vascular neoplasm which usually presents with vascular-looking skin nodules on the extremities (Chapter 21). The precise histogenesis of the tumor remains uncertain since the tumor cells are negative for endothelial cell markers. If Kaposi's sarcoma complicates immunosuppression of the recipient, it usually occurs less than 2 years after the transplantation.

Histologically, the tumor is characterized by a proliferation of spindle-shaped, fibroblast-like cells arranged around numerous split-like spaces containing erythrocytes. Some of the tumor cells may contain characteristic eosinophilic inclusions within their cytoplasm. Iron-laden histiocytes are observed amongst the tumor cells. Electron microscopy shows necrotic endothelial cells, fragmentation of the basal lamina, as well as defects in capillary walls, which may account for extravasation of red blood cells. Reduction of immunosuppressive drug dosage may lead to significant control of this sarcoma.

PANCREAS

Steroid therapy often produces a mild pancreatitis, characterized by focal small zones of calcification of the interstitial fibroadipose tissue, due to the action of released pancreatic lipase.

EYES

Posterior subcapsular cataracts occur in 10–30% of patients receiving prolonged high-dose glucocorticosteroid therapy. This is not a major problem with cyclosporine-based regimens in which steroid dosages are much reduced.

References

1. Uys, C.J., Rose, A.G. and Barnard, C.N. (1979). The pathology of human cardiac transplantation: an assessment after 11 years' experience at Groote Schuur Hospital. *S. Afr. Med. J.*, **56**, 887

2. Cooper, D.K.C., Lanza, R.P., Oliver, S.P., Forder, A.A., Rose, A.G., Uys, C.J., Novitzky, D. and Barnard, C.N. (1983). Infectious complications following heterotopic heart transplantation. *Thorax*, **38**, 882

3. Banfi, G., Imbasciati, E., Fogazzi, G.B. and Tarantino, A. (1987). Renal lesions in cyclosporine-A treated kidney transplant patients. *Appl. Pathol.*, **5**, 95

4. Sacchi, G., Benetti, A., Falchetti, L., Grigolato, P., Cristinelli, L., Strada, A. and Maiorca, R. (1987). Ultrastructural renal findings in allografted kidneys of patients treated with cyclosporine-A. *Appl. Pathol.*, **5**, 101

5. Penn, I. (1979). Tumor incidence in human allograft recipients. *Transplant. Proc.*, **11**, 1047

6. Copeland, J.G. and Stinson, E.B. (1979). Human heart transplantation. *Curr. Probl. Cardiol.*, **4**, 1

7. Dorfman, R.F. (1984). Kaposi's sarcoma revisited. *Hum. Pathol.*, **15**, 1013

31
Results of Cardiac Transplantation and Factors Influencing Survival
1. International Society for Heart Transplantation Registry

C.F. HECK, L.S. FRAGOMENI, S.J. SHUMWAY AND M.P. KAYE

INTRODUCTION

After more than 20 years of experience with heart transplantation, significant changes have been witnessed regarding survival, the number of transplants performed annually, and the number of transplant centers performing this procedure. The operation has clearly been established as a successful form of treatment for end-stage heart disease.

Following the initial enthusiasm after the first transplant at Groote Schuur Hospital in South Africa, many centers around the world initiated clinical heart transplantation and obtained poor results. Further pioneering work, particularly at Stanford, and the introduction of cyclosporine as the major immunosuppressive agent at the beginning of this decade, stimulated many centers to restart or develop new programs. In 1988, the number of active centers totaled 173 (Figure 31.1)[1].

Figure 31.2 shows the increasing number of heart transplants performed annually since 1980, reflecting the current

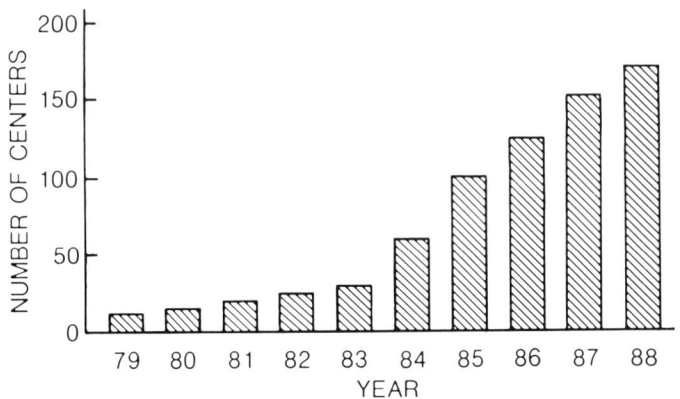

Figure 31.1 Number of active heart transplant centers worldwide during the period 1979-1988. (International Society for Heart Transplantation (ISHT) Registry, 1989)

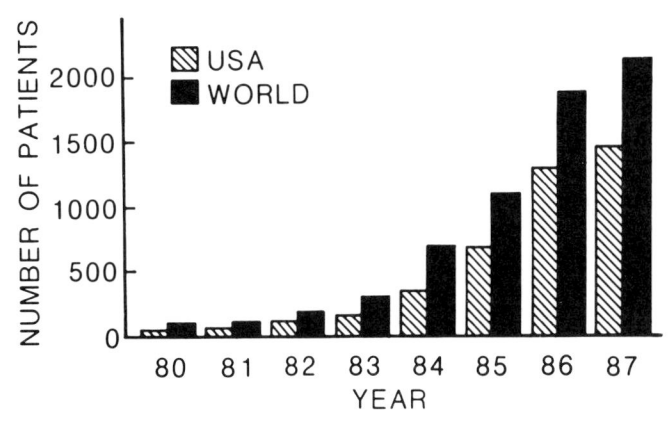

Figure 31.2 Number of heart transplants performed in the USA and worldwide during the period 1980-1987 (ISHT Registry, 1988). In 1988, 2450 transplants were performed worldwide

popularity of this therapy. The Registry of the International Society for Heart Transplantation has compiled data on 9417 patients operated on at 118 centers in the United States and at 84 centers in other countries[1,2]. In the years 1986-88 inclusive, over 6500 heart transplants were performed worldwide. The expansion in the number of transplant centers has led to a reduction in the number of transplants performed at each center. Less than 25% of the centers performed a total of more than 60 transplants during the 4-year period 1985-88. A total of 45% of the centers performed 20 or less transplants during this period.

The exponential increase in number of transplants and transplant centers is related to improved results. The number of transplants performed annually may now stabilize, mainly due to the lack of donors, although increasing numbers of patients are being assessed daily as possible candidates for cardiac transplantation.

The effects of various factors on survival (as seen through the Registry data)[1,2] will be discussed.

SELECTED FACTORS INFLUENCING GRAFT SURVIVAL

Recipient age

The mean age of patients undergoing heart transplantation is at present 44 years, with a population ranging from newborn to 70 years. Increasing numbers of both very young and older patients are being considered for transplantation. Of those under 10 years of age, 31% are infants (< 1 year)[1].

Although patient age does not significantly affect overall survival, the very young (patients aged 0–9 years) have a significantly higher 30-day mortality (25%) when compared with older recipients (approximately 10%).

The 5-year actuarial survivals of three different age groups are expressed in Figure 31.3[2]. Surprisingly, comparison among age groups shows that the most elderly group (55–68 years; $n = 710$) has the best 5-year survival, with 78% alive at the end of this period. In the middle age group (19–54 years; $n = 3023$), 5-year survival is 72%. In the younger age group (0–18 years; $n = 235$), the survival rate is slightly lower (70% at 5 years). Although the numbers in the younger and older groups are relatively small, the fact that the elderly group shows good (if not better) survival allows us to continue offering these patients the opportunity of cardiac transplantation. Careful selection of the potential recipient is clearly more important than the age factor alone.

Recipient sex

The majority of heart transplant recipients are male (83%). Women, although a minority group undergoing heart transplantation, appear to remain at increased risk of complications affecting survival.

Recipient's underlying cardiac pathology

Cardiomyopathy (52%) and coronary artery disease (30%) remain the most common indications for cardiac transplantation (Figure 31.4). Just under 10% of the patients reported to the Registry were reported as having unspecified congestive heart failure. Congenital heart disease, valvular disease, acute graft rejection, and myocarditis were less common indications. Prior to the use of cyclosporine, patients with cardiomyopathy seemed to show better survival following heart transplantation than patients with ischemic heart disease. Today, after the analysis of patients treated with triple immunosuppressive therapy (combination of cyclosporine, azathioprine, and corticosteroids) there is no significant difference in survival between these two groups.

Donor organ ischemic period

Donor organ ischemic time continues to be related to early mortality (Figure 31.5). Although many other variables, such as donor/recipient selection and donor management, may affect survival, the data suggest that we must continue to aim for the shortest possible ischemic time. A careful evaluation of all possible factors involved should positively influence these results in the future.

Operative procedure – orthotopic or heterotopic

Until 1988, only 180 hearts had been transplanted in a non-orthotopic position (Figure 31.6). Between the years 1983 and 1986, the number of heterotopic heart transplants

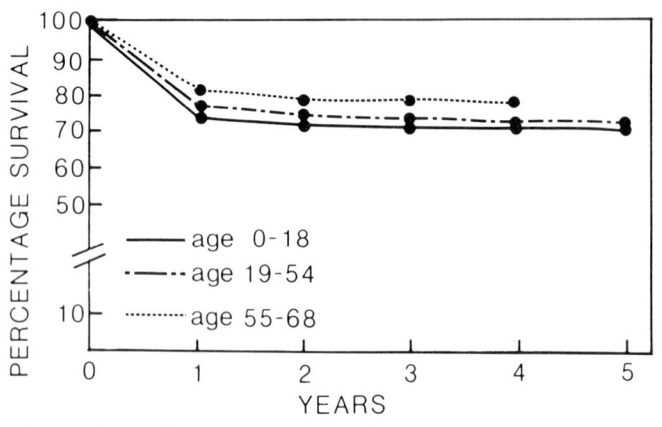

Figure 31.3 Influence of age on actuarial survival following heart transplantation (ISHT Registry, 1988)

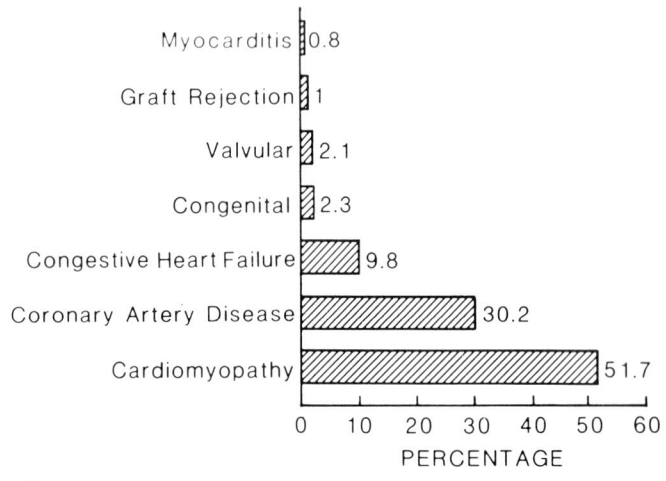

Figure 31.4 Underlying cardiac pathology in patients undergoing heart transplantation (ISHT Registry, 1988). In 1988, 52% of transplants were for cardiomyopathy, and 40% for ischemic heart disease[1])

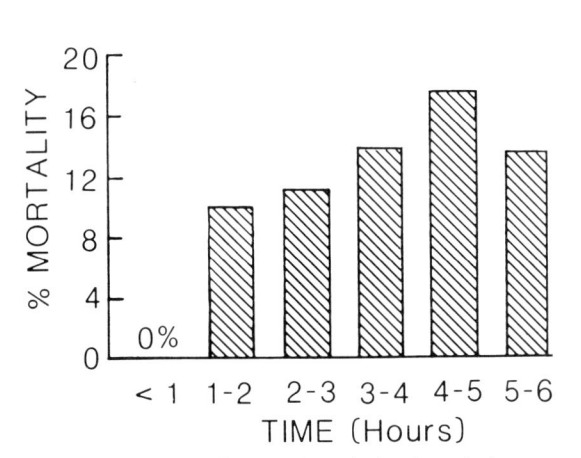

Figure 31.5 Relationship of donor heart ischemic period to mortality within 30 days following heart transplantation (ISHT Registry, 1988)

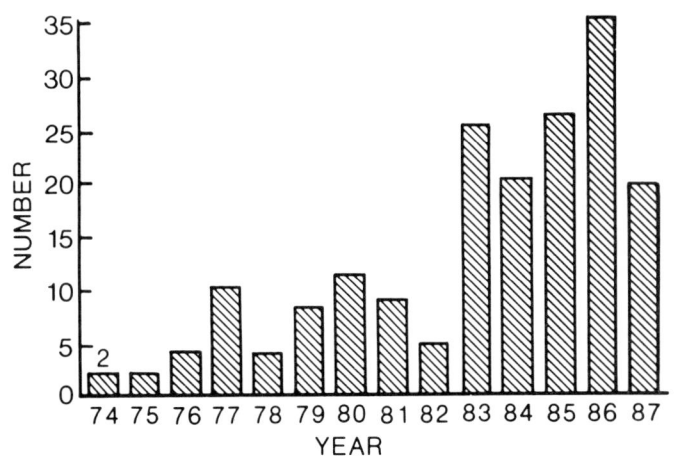

Figure 31.6 Number of heterotopic heart transplants performed annually: 1974–1987 (ISHT Registry, 1988). In 1988, 19 such transplants were reported in the Registry

remained relatively stable. With poorer results than after orthotopic heart transplantation, and 1- and 5-year actuarial survivals of 62% and 54%, respectively, the criteria for use of this modality of transplantation have become more specific. This attitude is reflected in the year 1987, when only 19 such transplants were performed. Heterotopic transplantation is frequently performed in patients unsuitable for orthotopic transplantation by virtue of a high pulmonary vascular resistance, and this factor alone is known to influence survival. The 74% 5-year survival associated with orthotopic heart transplantation is significantly better than the 54% 5-year survival following a heterotopic transplant.

Immunosuppressive therapy

Figure 31.7 compares 5-year actuarial survival between (1) all patients, (2) those receiving cyclosporine ± one other drug, and (3) those receiving triple therapy. The data suggest

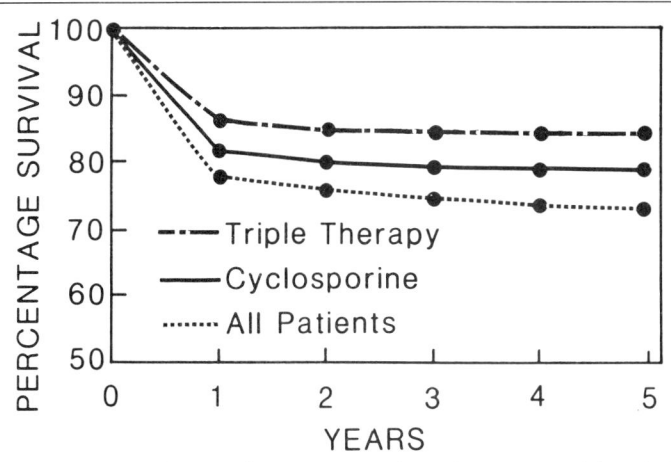

Figure 31.7 Influence of immunosuppressive regimen on actuarial survival following heart transplantation. Triple therapy = patients receiving combination therapy with cyclosporine, azathioprine, and a corticosteroid; cyclosporine = patients receiving cyclosporine ± one other drug; all patients = all patients irrespective of drug regimen (ISHT Registry, 1988)

that the combined use of cyclosporine, azathioprine, and corticosteroids is the most effective immunosuppressive regimen. The actuarial survival at 12 months for each of the 5 years (1982–86) is shown in Figure 31.8. With triple therapy, current (1988) 1-year survival is 86%. By comparison, in 1982, 12-month survival was 62%. The combination of improved immunosuppresive therapy and accumulation of expertise has clearly influenced the 1-year survival.

Increasing experience of transplant centers

Figure 31.9 shows 30-day mortality. As with 1-year survival, early survival has been steadily improving during recent years. The opening of many new centers performing cardiac transplantation, and the extension of the criteria for organ donation, may have contributed to the transient increase in mortality seen in 1987. The 9% mortality reported in 1988 is the lowest yet recorded by the Registry.

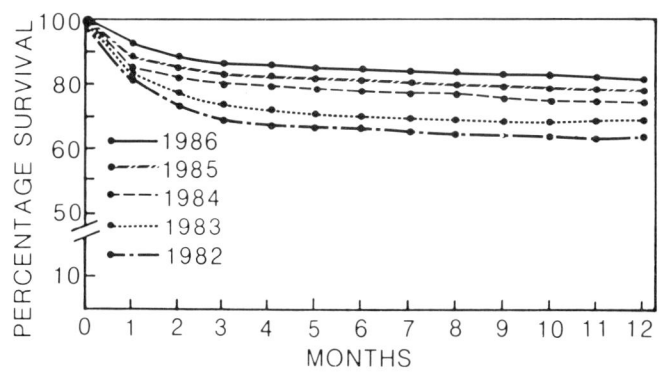

Figure 31.8 One-year actuarial survival of patients undergoing heart transplantation in the years 1982–1986 (ISHT Registry, 1988). One-year survival of patients operated on in 1987 was 86% (ISHT Registry, 1989)

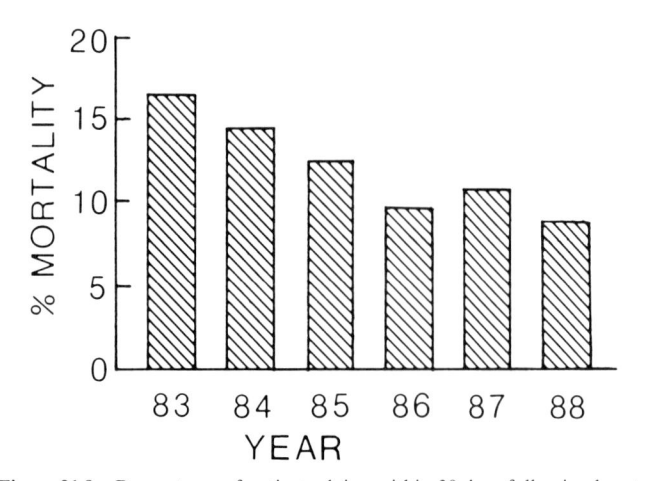

Figure 31.9 Percentages of patients dying within 30 days following heart transplantation in the years 1983–1988 (ISHT Registry, 1989)

The mean actuarial survival of patients receiving orthotopic heart transplants at centers performing 50 or more transplants between 1985 and 1988 is significantly better than that at centers doing fewer than 50 heart transplant procedures over the same period of time. One- and 3-year actuarial survivals were 83% and 80% at the busiest centers compared with 73% and 71% at the less active centers. This could signify that a certain minimum number of transplant procedures is necessary to maintain the skills of a proficient transplant team.

CAUSES OF DEATH FOLLOWING TRANSPLANTATION

Table 31.1 summarizes the causes of death following heart transplantation. Even the improved immunosuppression achieved with triple therapy has not diminished death from infection, with 37% of the transplanted patients dying from sepsis.

Deaths from cardiac causes (excluding rejection) continue to be high, with 21% of the patients in 1986 and 25% in 1987 dying from cardiac complications, such as a poorly functioning donor heart; in 1988, failure of the donor heart was the highest contributing factor to death of the patient within the first 30-day period. This high incidence may be related to the opening of new, less experienced, transplant centers and/or to less rigorous donor selection. Deaths from early donor heart failure provide an area for significant future improvement.

Acute rejection, although less common with triple therapy, is still responsible for 24% of deaths, usually in the early post-transplant period. Chronic rejection (graft atherosclerois) is being documented by yearly coronary angiography, and is the cause of 5% of deaths. Although longer follow-up is needed to assess the impact of chronic rejection on patient survival, accelerated graft atherosclerosis is seen in 15% of patients at 1 year and in 35% at 3 years. It seems that even the present antirejection therapy does not adequately control chronic rejection and subsequent graft atherosclerosis. It is hoped that progress will soon be made in this field, thus further improving the long-term results.

RETRANSPLANTATION

Until March 1988, retransplantation had been performed in 134 patients, mainly for chronic rejection and severe diffuse coronary atherosclerosis. Results following re-operation are poorer than after the first transplant, showing 1- and 5-year survivals of 57% and 53%, respectively. Until immunosuppressive therapy can be improved further, thus reducing the incidence of chronic graft atherosclerosis, it seems highly likely that the numbers of patients facing retransplantation will steadily increase, placing a greater strain on the limited number of donor hearts available.

RISK FACTORS

In order to evaluate the effect of such variables as age, sex, indications for transplantation, and immunosuppressive therapy on survival after heart transplantation, a Cox regression analysis was applied. Eighteen variables were examined. Table 31.2 shows that the presence of pulmonary hypertension more than doubles the risk associated with cardiac transplantation. In addition, for every 60 minutes of ischemic time, patient risk increases by a factor of 1.12. Treatment with cyclosporine and triple drug therapy significantly reduce the risk associated with heart transplantation. A logistic regression analysis of the significance of variables on 30-day survival after heart transplantation produced similar results.

The use of cyclosporine was the major beneficial factor influencing results. Further observations show that survival of patients who did not receive cyclosporine was poor; data from 538 patients operated on between 1978 and 1985 showed survival rates at 1 and 5 years of 66% and 55%, respectively. If the 30-day mortality is excluded, the survival rate at 4 years was even lower, with only 42% alive at the end of that period.

Table 31.1 Causes of death following heart transplantation: 1987

	< 30 days	> 30 days
Cardiac-related	24%	42%
Infection	48%	37%
Acute rejection	28%	12%
Chronic rejection	0%	5%
Pulmonary embolism	0%	2%
Malignant neoplasia	0%	2%
Total	100%	100%

Table 31.2 Influence of various factors on survival after heart transplantation (using Cox regression analysis)

Variable	Significance (p value)	Risk (hazard ratio) (normal = 1)
Pulmonary hypertension	> 0.001	2.21
Cyclosporine	< 0.001	0.46
Triple drug therapy	< 0.005	0.77
Donor ischemic period (60-min increments)	< 0.005	1.12

AVAILABILITY OF DONORS

The expansion of cardiac transplant programs is limited by the availability of donors, which at present is inadequate. Distant donor procurement continues to be a necessity. Present data show that only 20% of hearts were procured from donors located at the recipient hospital (Figure 31.10).

In an attempt to expand the donor population, older donors (> 40 years) are now accepted at many centers, although careful cardiac evaluation by echocardiography and coronary arteriography is mandatory in this group. Mean donor age at present is 26 years, with a range from 0 to 70 years. The majority of donors, however, is in the 10–40 years age group. The results of transplantation did not change when hearts from older donors were utilized.

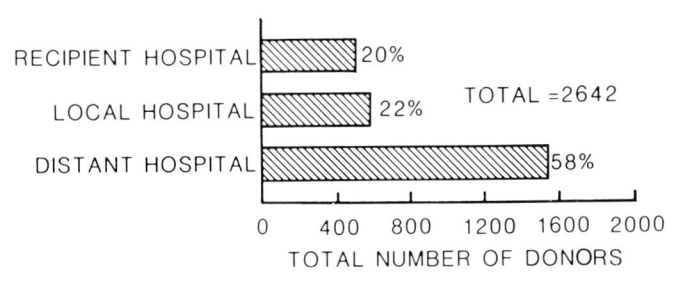

Figure 31.10 Percentages of donors retrieved (1) at the recipient hospital, (2) in the local community, and (3) at remote centers (ISHT Registry, 1988)

VENTRICULAR ASSIST DEVICES

Results of transplantation following the use of a ventricular assist device are discussed fully in Chapter 58. Ventricular assist devices are increasingly being used as a bridge to transplantation. It is still early to come to definite conclusions regarding the use of such devices. Such aspects as donor scarcity, financial cost, survival, and long-term outcome need to be considered carefully when the use of ventricular assist devices is evaluated.

COMMENT

Cardiac transplantation is today a highly effective form of therapy for end-stage cardiac disease. Although present techniques and immunosuppressive therapy have enhanced survival, there is still room for improvement. With future developments in the areas of patient selection, donor management, and immunosuppressive therapy, early and long-term results should improve further.

References

1. Heck, C.F., Shumway, S.J. and Kaye, M.P. (1989). The Registry of the International Society for Heart Transplantation: sixth official report, 1989. *J. Heart Transplant.*, **8**, 271
2. Fragomeni, L.S. and Kaye, M.P. (1988). The Registry of the International Society for Heart Transplantation: fifth official report, 1988. *J. Heart Transplant.*, **7**, 249

32
Results of Cardiac Transplantation and Factors Influencing Survival
2. Collaborative Heart Transplant Study
D.K.C. COOPER

INTRODUCTION

The Collaborative Heart Transplant Study was set up early in 1985 (by Dr Gerhard Opelz in Heidelberg, West Germany) to collect and collate data provided voluntarily by a large group of centers performing heart transplantation. At the present time, 68 centers participate in this project. The database now consists of almost 5000 heart transplants. It is clearly too early to look at factors that influence long-term survival following cardiac transplantation, but information on medium-term survival is already becoming available.

This chapter will present a brief summary of the effect of selected factors on 1-year survival[1-3]. All data relate to patients undergoing heart transplantation for the first time; retransplantation is not included. Graft removal or patient death was counted as graft failure.

OVERALL GRAFT SURVIVAL

During the past 4 years, overall 1-year graft survival in patients undergoing heart transplantation for the first time has been between 75 and 80%[1,2]. Current 2- and 3-year graft survival rates of transplants performed after 1984 (since when the yearly survival rates have remained stable) have been 73% and 68%, respectively[4].

SELECTED FACTORS INFLUENCING GRAFT SURVIVAL

Recipient age

Recipients aged less than 20 years fare less well than those above this age[1]. One-year graft survival in this younger group is approximately 60%, whereas in older patients it is approximately 80%. The poor results in the under 20-year-old group are partly accounted for by a higher mortality in infants and young children.

Recipient sex

Women make up less than 20% of the total of recipients of heart grafts. One-year graft survival in men (at approximately 80%) is noticeably better than that in women (less than 70%)[1].

Recipient's underlying cardiac pathology

One-year graft survival is no different whether the underlying disease is ischemic, cardiomyopathic, or valvular, being approximately 80% in each case[1]. Though the number of patients is small, those with congenital heart disease have a significantly worse prognosis, 1-year graft survival being less than 60%.

Clinical status of recipient at time of transplant

Based on clinical criteria available at the time of transplantation, each recipient was assessed as being a good, moderate, or poor risk. The difference in graft survival between good and poor risk patients is 25% at 1 year, with survival of those at moderate risk falling midway between these extremes[1].

Donor age

One-year graft survival in patients who received hearts from donors aged 40 years or older is 10% less than in those who received hearts from younger donors[1].

Donor organ ischemic period

A short ischemic period is associated with a trend toward improved graft survival at 1 year[1]. When the ischemic period was less than 1 hour, the 1-year graft survival rate is almost 10% better than when the ischemic period was greater than 3 hours[1].

ABO-compatibility

The recipient ABO blood group does not influence 1-year graft survival significantly[3]. An ABO blood group incompatibility between donor and recipient is associated with a high incidence of graft failure (G. Opelz, personal communication). ABO-compatible, but non-identical, donor–recipient pairing (e.g. O into A), as opposed to identical pairing (e.g. A into A), is not associated with any significant decrease in graft survival during the first year[3].

HLA matching

At the present time, the number of HLA-A and -B mismatched antigens between recipient and donor does not influence graft survival significantly, though grafts with no mismatch of either (1) HLA-A, B or (2) DR antigens fare better than mismatched grafts[2]. Although the numbers are small, graft survival is 10% higher (at almost 90%) in patients with no mismatch at the DR locus than in those with one or more mismatch[1]. One or no HLA-B and DR mismatch is associated with improved 1-year graft survival (approximately 90%) when compared with two or more mismatches ($< 80\%$) ($p < 0.05$, log rank)[2], though again the number of well-matched patients remains small[2].

Donor–recipient lymphocytotoxic cross-match

A positive lymphocytotoxic cross-match between donor and recipient is related to reduced 1-year graft survival ($< 65\%$) when compared with survival when the cross-match is negative (80%)[5].

COMMENT

The numbers of patients undergoing this procedure are still small when compared with those available for analysis of kidney transplants. Because of patient heterogeneity, center variation with respect to patient management, and variations in HLA typing techniques, some of the results summarized above must be considered preliminary.

The decline in overall graft survival seen during the first 3 post-transplant years, falling to 68% at this time interval, is virtually identical to that seen following kidney transplantation. (The 10-year renal graft survival is less than 40%, suggesting that this may also be the fate of heart grafts.)

In contrast, the International Society for Heart Transplantation Registry (Chapter 31) shows little decline in the survival curve after the first 3 months. No good explanation for the marked difference between these two computations has been put forward. Experience with the problem of accelerated graft atherosclerosis (chronic rejection) in patients with heart transplants would suggest that there is a small but definite annual decline in graft survival, and that the long-term results will be similar to those that have already been well-documented in the kidney transplant patient population.

References

1. Opelz, G., Mollner, H., Reichart, B. and Keppel, E. (1989). Preliminary results of the Collaborative Heart Transplant Study. In Reichart, B. (ed.) *Recent Advances in Cardiovascular Surgery*. p. 51. (Seehang: Schulz, R.S.)
2. Opelz, G. For the Collaborative Heart Transplant Study (1989). Effect of HLA matching in heart transplantation. *Transplant. Proc.*, **21**, 794
3. Opelz, G. (1989). Collaborative Heart Transplant Study Newsletter, 2
4. Opelz, G. (1989). Collaborative Heart Transplant Study Newsletter, 3
5. Opelz, G. (1989). Collaborative Heart Transplant Study Newsletter, 4

Section II

Transplantation of the heart and both lungs

33
Experimental Background and Early Clinical Experience

E. BECERRA, J. KAPLAN AND D.K.C. COOPER

INTRODUCTION

Transplantation of the heart and both lungs has only become a clinical reality in the 1980s, largely due to the introduction of cyclosporine, which has enabled the patient to be immunosuppressed adequately during the first 2–3 weeks without the need for a corticosteroid. The ability to immunosuppress the patient sufficiently without a corticosteroid has allowed time for healing of the tracheal suture line, which previously was a major source of early complication following this operation.

Research workers have been interested in heart–lung transplantation, however, for many years[1], and three clinical attempts at the procedure were carried out in the 1960s and 1970s.

EXPERIMENTAL BACKGROUND

Initial studies

The earliest attempt to transplant the heart and both lungs was by Carrel (Figure 1.1) at the beginning of this century, though this involved only transplantation into the neck of a recipient cat[2]; lung edema occurred with distention of the right side of the heart.

In 1946, Demikhov (Figure 33.1) transplanted the heart and lungs of a dog, and the recipient survived for 2 hours without its own organs, but it was not until 1949 that more prolonged survival was obtained[3]. The technique used was ingenious (Figure 33.2) as it enabled the blood supply to the brain to be maintained continuously throughout the operation, with the exception of 2–3 minutes at one critical stage. Demikhov took care to dissect out the phrenic and vagus nerves of the recipient with the intention of preserving the innervation of those structures, particularly the diaphragm, below the region of the heart and lungs. At this stage, the right lung was removed to facilitate later parts of the operation.

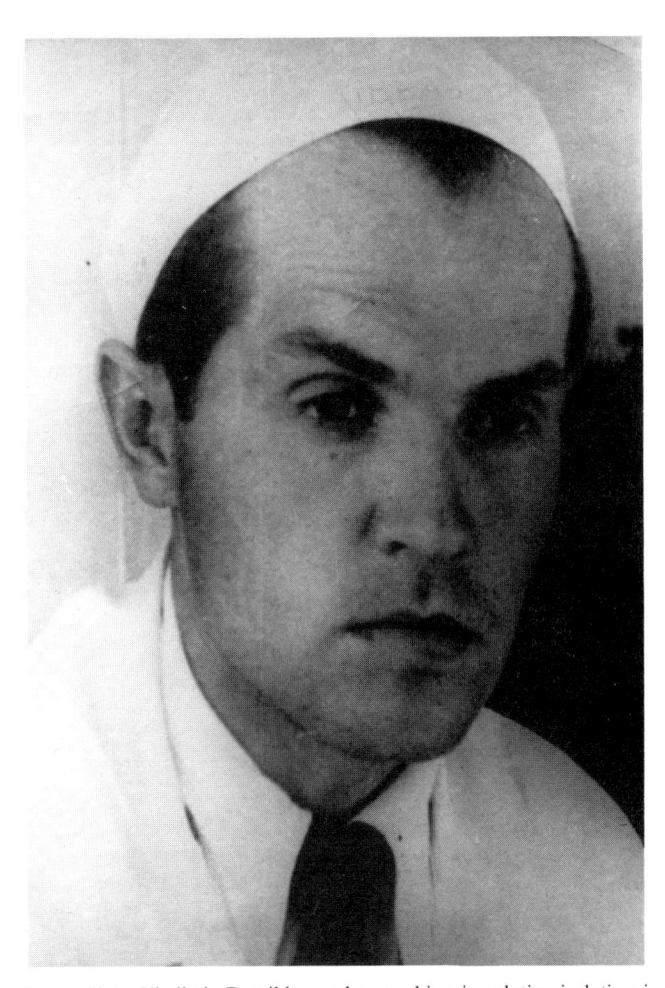

Figure 33.1 Vladimir Demikhov, who, working in relative isolation in the USSR, carried out extensive experimental work in the field of heart and heart–lung transplantation in the 1940s and 1950s

After preliminary mobilization, the donor heart–lung preparation was removed from the animal by clamping and dividing the thoracic aorta, the inferior cava, brachiocephalic

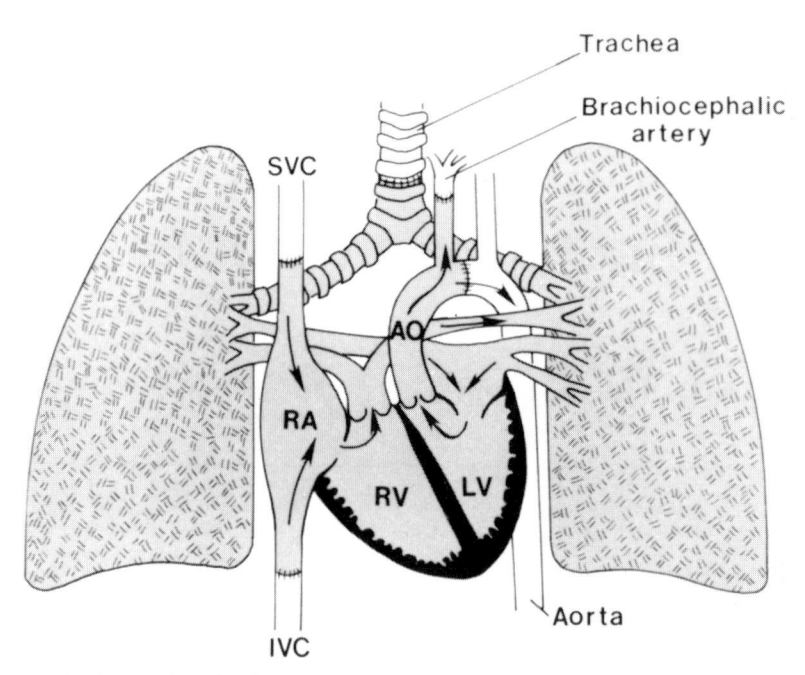

Figure 33.2 The completed operation of orthotopic heart–lung transplantation, using the technique described by Demikhov[3]

and subclavian arteries, and the superior vena cava. During transfer the donor heart–lung was kept viable by its own closed-circuit circulation, blood from the left ventricle being pumped into the arch of the aorta, from whence it passed through the coronary vessels supplying the myocardium and into the right atrium, the right ventricle, and the lungs; oxygenated blood was returned to the left atrium. This form of heart–lung preparation has subsequently been the basis of a means of transporting and temporarily preserving the heart and lungs[4-8] (Chapter 35).

The various vascular anastomoses were made either by suturing or by 'quick connects' over prosthetic tubes. During the inferior vena caval anatomosis the blood supply to the lower half of the body was temporarily interrupted for 15–20 minutes. The tracheas of the transplant and recipient were then connected, either by means of a special tube or by silk sutures, using a technique which avoided interference with respiration.

Of 67 attempts at this procedure, only six dogs survived for more than 48 hours with only two surviving for more than 4 days. Early deaths were from technical problems and thromboses at the various anastomoses, particularly of the brachiocephalic artery. Those dogs which did recover from the immediate effects of the operation appear to have been quite well for a few days until their demise. Respiration was generally slow, in the region of 12 per minute, and the pulse rate variable, though frequently fast. Certain dogs appeared to recover remarkably well, walking about their kennels, drinking water, eating meat, and reacting briskly to their surroundings. (One of them was even sent by train from Ryazan to Moscow on the fourth postoperative day and on arrival at its destination 'ran up the stairs by itself'.)

Several important observations and conclusions have resulted from Demikhov's pioneering studies. Most significant is the fact that following total replacement of the heart and both lungs many of these dogs did breathe spontaneously, and apparently adequately, until death, which did not appear to be the result of respiratory insufficiency unless caused by bronchopneumonia. This is a particularly important finding, but one that was not confirmed by all subsequent workers. Secondly, the respiratory rate was variable. On the day following operation one dog had a respiratory rate of 18 per minute. On the second postoperative day it was noted to have a pleural effusion; attempts to aspirate this led to vomiting for 5 minutes after which the dog was dyspnoeic 'and the respiratory rate rose to 135 per minute'. Four and a half hours later the rate returned to 12 per minute. Thirdly, the transplanted heart was able to maintain an adequate circulation for 6 days, and, despite the fact that it was totally denervated and neither atrium had been left *in situ*, it also showed considerable variation in rate.

During the period of Demikhov's studies, other workers, notably Marcus, Wong, and Luisada[9,10], were also studying heart–lung transplantation. Marcus *et al.* developed a technique for transplanting the heart and both lungs into the abdomen, thus giving the recipient two sets of heart and lungs (Figure 33.3). The purpose of this latter experiment was to determine whether the donor heart and lungs could be used as a pump-oxygenator unit to deliver oxygenated blood to a limited part of the host's body. Among their conclusions, these authors suggested the possibility of using

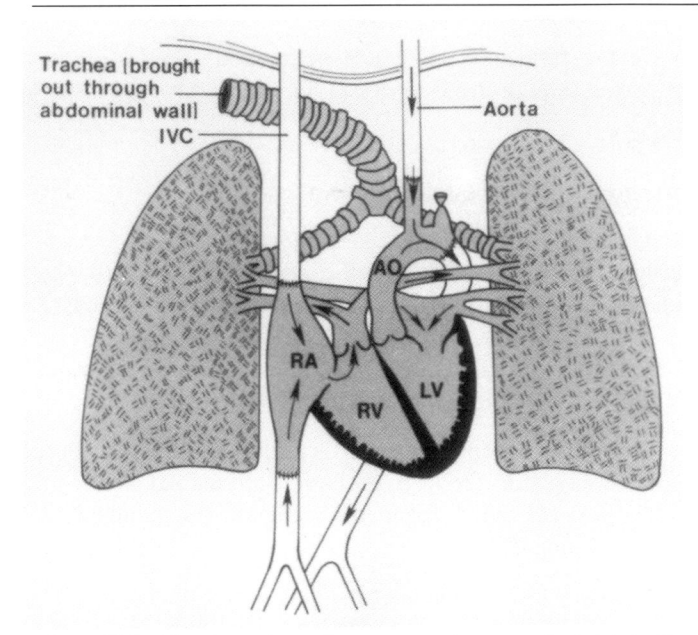

Figure 33.3 The donor heart–lung preparation transplanted into the recipient aorta–vena caval circulation in the abdomen, using the technique described by Marcus et al.[9,10]. The transplanted organs were able to function in accessory support of the host animal

a heterologous heart–lung preparation as an extracorporeal pump during intracardiac procedures. They also commented that the transplanted heart might act as an accessory pump to decrease the work load of the native heart, even if only temporarily.

Matejicek in 1956 briefly reported a study of the transplantation of the heart and right upper lobe of the lung into the chest, but no results were reported[11].

Advent of supportive techniques

With the advent of supportive techniques, total heart and lung excision and replacement became more feasible. In 1953, Neptune et al. reported the use of hypothermia to sustain life in the recipient while transplantation was proceeding[12]. The surgical technique, which became the basis for most of the subsequent experimental studies during the next 15 years, involved anastomosis or 'coupling' of the trachea, SVC, IVC, and aorta. The longest surviving animal recovered spontaneous respiration but died after 6 hours.

In 1957, Webb and his colleagues introduced cardiopulmonary bypass for the same purposes[13–15]. After a variety of experiments in dogs, Webb and his co-workers came to the conclusion that simultaneous bilateral pulmonary denervation of the heart and lungs, or even bilateral hilar stripping, resulted in respiratory dyfunction or even paralysis which made autotransplantation or allotransplantation of the heart and lungs impracticable.

They did suggest that while transplantation of the heart with one lung was technically more difficult, the technique might be feasible for use in patients with pulmonary hypertension. Such transplantation circumvented respiratory paralysis by leaving one innervated lung in the recipient. Continuing respiration appeared to be dependent on 'feedback' afferents from the respiratory system; they believed their studies indicated that respiratory paralysis was not due to phrenic nerve damage, excessive vagal or sympathetic dissection, or periods of shock accompanying the extensive dissection and trauma of the actual transplant. Accordingly, they concluded that transplantation of the heart combined with both lungs was probably a physiological impossibility.

Other investigators, however, reported the resumption of spontaneous respiration in dogs surviving after cardiopulmonary transplantation[16–19], and it was observed that oxygenation remained adequate despite the fact that the respiratory pattern was greatly altered; the tidal volume was increased and the respiratory rate diminished[17].

Lower (Figure 1.6) and his colleagues[17] carried out heart–lung transplantation in six dogs, two of whom survived until the fifth postoperative day. They were ambulatory, active, and eating until they became lethargic on the fourth day, at which time they began to die from respiratory insufficiency. These authors felt that their studies confirmed earlier work that the bronchial arterial supply to the lungs could be sacrificed without resulting necrosis, but the question of the possibility of prolonged survival after pulmonary denervation remained unanswered. It was evident that the sacrifice of peripheral innervation, which necessarily accompanies pulmonary transplantation, resulted, in the cases reported, not in respiratory paralysis but in an altered respiratory pattern which resembled that observed after bilateral cervical vagotomy. The operation appeared technically feasible, and spontaneous respirations with an altered pattern appeared to be sufficient to sustain life until allograft rejection supervened.

Both of the 5-day surviving dogs died from microscopic changes suggesting rejection of the lungs. The changes of acute rejection in the myocardium were less extensive than these authors had observed previously with cardiac allografts of longer duration. This observation has been confirmed by many subsequent workers in both the experimental animal[20,21] and in patients undergoing heart–lung transplantation[21,22]; the lung is generally more rapidly rejected than the heart, and, in fact, the heart may be protected in some way by the lungs (Chapter 39).

DeBono[19], using Neptune's technique, obtained six surviving dogs in whom spontaneous respiration of an apparently normal pattern occurred for periods from 2 to 10 hours, at which times the dogs were sacrificed. He pointed out that pulmonary edema, caused by a number of factors, diminished the ventilatory capacity and compliance of the lungs[19]. Similar observations of a changed respiratory pattern, which was often inadequate, were found by Longmore and his colleagues in 1969[6] and Grinnan et al. in

1970[23]. Longmore's group simplified the operation by anastomosing the two right atria rather than both the SVC and IVC. Only three anastomoses were now required – tracheae, right atria, and aortae (Figure 33.4). This technique forms the basis of that used currently in clinical practice (Chapter 37).

Further light was thrown on the effect of denervation of the lungs on subsequent respiratory function by studies on unilateral and bilateral lung transplantation. Bilateral lung denervation or bilateral lung transplantation resulted in a similar change in respiratory pattern. These studies are discussed further in Chapter 45, and clinical observations are summarized in Chapter 42.

Heart–lung transplantation in primates

In 1967, Nakae and his colleagues[24] carried out extensive pulmonary denervation in the dog, cat and monkey, and recognized the ability of primates to withstand total lung denervation. A normal pattern of spontaneous breathing was found in primates after lung denervation. These authors predicted that long-term survival could be achieved in this species. It was evident that primates tolerated total denervation of the lung, and did not require the Hering–Breuer reflex as did the dog, since spontaneous respiration, controlled by the mid-brain, was preserved. This observation was confirmed in 1972 by Castaneda and his colleagues[25] who reported long-term survival of 6–24 months after heart–lung autotransplantation in the baboon.

Both of these studies lent some degree of confirmation to the earlier work by Haglin and his colleagues in 1963[26] who showed that total denervation of both lungs did not prevent a return of adequate spontaneous respiration in primates, though it did in dogs.

Introduction of cyclosporine

Reitz and his colleagues[27], working with rhesus and cynomolgus monkeys, made significant contributions to the development of cardiopulmonary transplantation in the late 1970s and early 1980s, obtaining long-term survival through the introduction of immunosuppression with cyclosporine. Several contributions were made by this group.

(1) They demonstrated that cardiopulmonary bypass was preferable to hypothermic circulatory arrest to support the recipient during heart–lung transplantation;

(2) They established that median sternotomy provided the best approach to the chest cavity for this operation;

(3) They established that immunosuppression with cyclosporine and azathioprine, without a corticosteroid during the first 14 days to avoid its deleterious effect on tracheal healing, could be successful in preventing acute rejection;

(4) They described the successful management of post-transplant lung edema by fluid restriction and the administration of furosemide.

With regard to the technical aspects of their work, they utilized a low tracheal anastomosis, as used previously by many other workers, and a single right atrial anastomosis

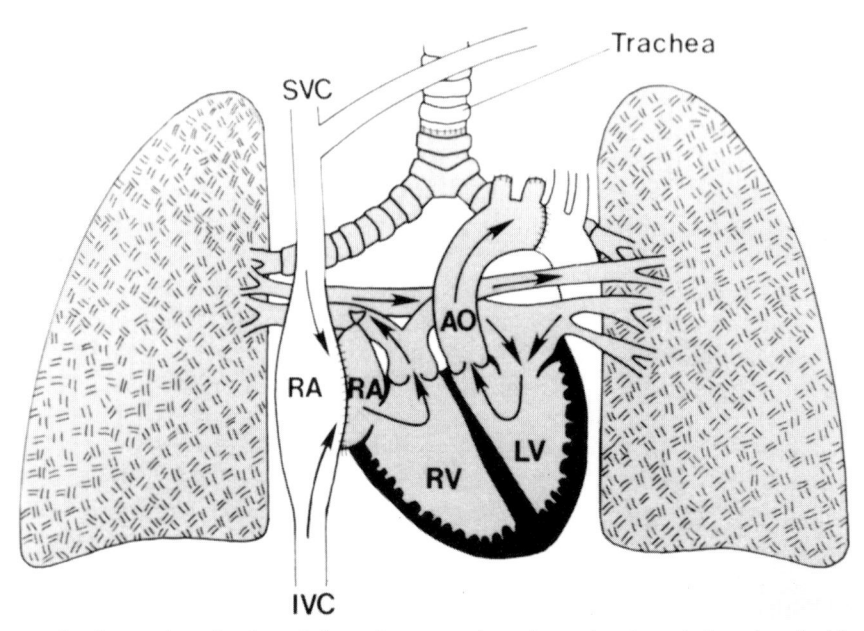

Figure 33.4 The completed operation of orthotopic heart–lung transplantation, using the technique described by Longmore et al.[6]

as proposed originally by Longmore et al.[6]. The relatively heavy immunosuppressive regimen used resulted in the development of histiocytic lymphoma in some of their experimental animals.

As a result of their studies, they proposed that endomyocardial biopsy could be used to diagnose both cardiac and pulmonary allograft rejection[27,28]. In retrospect, this proved to be an unreliable method of diagnosing lung rejection, as rejection rarely occurs simultaneously in both organs, pulmonary rejection being more frequent than cardiac rejection[20-22,29] (Chapters 38 and 39).

EARLY CLINICAL EXPERIENCE

The operation was first attempted clinically by Cooley on 31 August 1968[30]. The patient was a 2-month-old infant with a complete atrioventricular canal defect, pulmonary hypertension and pneumonia. The patient required reopening for bleeding, and died 14 hours after the initial transplant operation. In December 1969, Lillehei performed the second such operation on a 43-year-old patient with emphysema and pulmonary hypertension[31]; the patient survived 8 days, dying from pneumonia. The third operation was performed in Cape Town by Barnard (Figure 1.10) in July, 1971[32,33]. The bronchi, rather than the trachea, were chosen as the site of anastomosis of the air passages, as it was believed at that time that this would preserve both the blood supply to the recipient carina and the cough reflex in the carinal area more satisfactorily. The patient did well initially, but died on the 23rd day following the development of a right-sided bronchopleural fistula, which necessitated right pneumonectomy, and which was followed by septicemia.

All three of these early patients were immunosuppressed with only azathioprine and corticosteroids, as cyclosporine was not yet available.

It was not until another 10 years had elapsed that a fourth transplant of the heart and both lungs was reported, on this occasion (March 9, 1981) by Reitz (Figure 33.5) and his colleagues at Stanford University[28,34,35]. The availability of an improved immunosuppressive regimen, including cyclosporine, and a better understanding of both the reimplantation syndrome and the blood supply of the trachea and bronchi, resulted in the first long-term survival of such a patient. This first patient was a 45-year-old woman with primary pulmonary hypertension, who underwent heart and lung transplantation using the surgical technique and immunosuppression developed in this group's experimental program. She suffered two acute rejection episodes, both of which were reversed successfully, and, 10 months later, showed normal exercise tolerance.

Two other patients underwent the same operation during the following 4 months[36]. One of them was a 29-year-old woman with a complex transposition of the great vessels

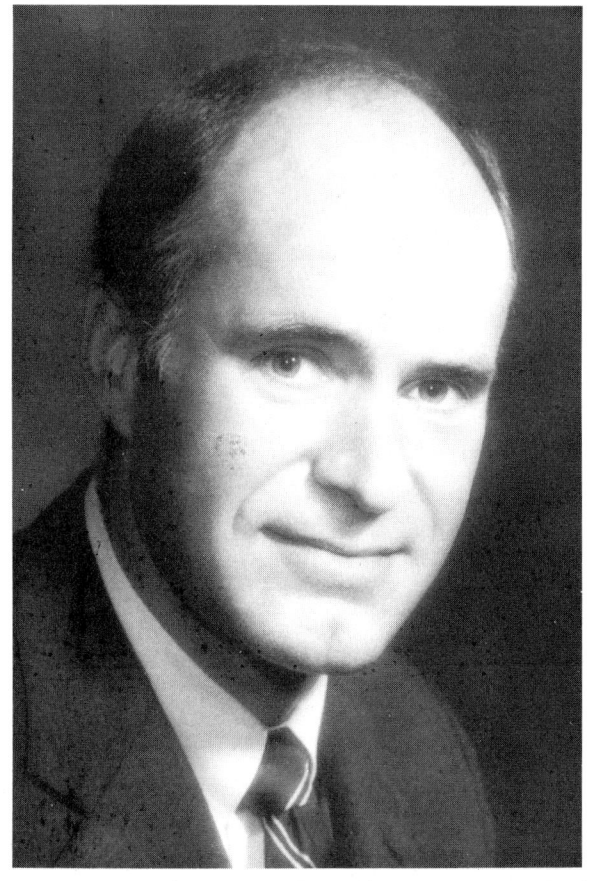

Figure 33.5 Bruce Reitz, who, working in Shumway's group at Stanford University in the USA, performed important experimental work on heart–lung transplantation. In 1981, he and Shumway (Figure 1.7) led a team that carried out heart–lung transplantation in a patient who became the first to survive long-term

who had undergone previous cardiac surgery. Dense adhesions led to technical problems and a coagulopathy associated with the long period of cardiopulmonary bypass. Renal, hepatic and pulmonary complications followed, the patient dying on the fourth postoperative day. Similar experiences at several centers have resulted in a reluctance of surgeons to attempt this procedure in patients who have undergone previous surgery of the chest[37]. Despite the hazards presented by adhesions from previous surgery, retransplantation of the heart and lungs has been successfully accomplished[37].

Although the results of transplantation of the heart and both lungs are still markedly inferior to those which can be expected after heart transplantation alone, the improved immunosuppressive regimen made available by the introduction of cyclosporine and increasing experience in the management of patients undergoing this procedure offer the possibility of long-term survival in well-selected patients[38].

References

1. Cooper, D.K.C. (1969). Transplantation of the heart and both lungs. I. Historical review. *Thorax*, **24**, 383

2. Carrel, A. (1907). The surgery of blood vessels. *Johns Hopkins Hosp. Bull.*, **18**, 18
3. Demikhov, V.P. (1962). *Experimental Transplantation of Vital Organs.* Authorized translation from Russian by Haigh, B. (New York: Consultants Bureau)
4. Robicsek, F., Pruitt, J.R., Sanger, P.W., Daugherty, H.K., Moore, M. and Bagby, E. (1968). The maintenance of function of the donor heart in the extracorporeal stage and during transplantation. *Ann. Thorac. Surg.*, **6**, 330
5. Robicsek, F., Tam, W., Daugherty, H.K. and Robicsek, L.V. (1969). The stabilized autoperfusing heart–lung preparation as a vehicle for extracorporeal preservation. *Transplant. Proc.*, **1**, 834
6. Longmore, D.B., Cooper, D.K.C., Hall, R.W., Sekabunga, J. and Welch, W. (1969). Transplantation of the heart and both lungs. II. Experimental cardiopulmonary transplantation. *Thorax*, **24**, 391
7. Cooper, D.K.C. (1975). A simple method of resuscitation and short-term preservation of the canine cadaver heart. *J. Thorac. Cardiovasc. Surg.*, **70**, 896
8. Hardesty, R.L. and Griffith, B.P. (1987). Autoperfusion of the heart and lungs for preservation during distant procurement. *J. Thorac. Cardiovasc. Surg.*, **93**, 11
9. Marcus, E., Wong, S.N.T. and Luisada, A.A. (1951). Homologous heart grafts: transplantation of the heart in dogs. *Surg. Forum*, **2**, 212
10. Marcus, E., Wong, S.N.T. and Luisada, A.A. (1953). Homologous heart grafts. I. Technique of interim parabiotic perfusion. II. Transplantation of the heart in dogs. *Arch. Surg.*, **66**, 179
11. Matejicek, E. (1956). Transplantation of organs. *Transplant. Bull.*, **3**, 167
12. Neptune, W.B., Cookson, B.A., Bailey, C.P., Appler, R. and Rajkowski, F. (1953). Complete homologous heart transplantation. *Arch. Surg.*, **66**, 174
13. Webb, W.R. and Howard, H.S. (1957). Cardiopulmonary transplantation. *Surg. Forum*, **8**, 313
14. Webb, W.R., Howard, H.S. and Neely, W.N. (1959). Practical methods of homologous cardiac transplantation. *J. Thorac. Surg.*, **37**, 361
15. Webb, W.R., Guzman, V. and Hoopes, J.E. (1961). Cardiopulmonary transplantation: experimental study of current problems. *Am. Surg.*, **27**, 236
16. Blanco, G., Adam, A., Rodriguez-Perez, D. and Fernandez, A. (1958). Complete homotransplantation of the canine heart and lungs. *Arch. Surg.*, **76**, 20
17. Lower, R.R., Stofer, R.C., Hurley, E.J. and Shumway, N.E. (1961). Complete homograft replacement of the heart and both lungs. *Surgery*, **50**, 842
18. Sen, P.K., Parulkar, G.B. and Kinare, S. (1965). Homologous canine heart transplantation: a preliminary report of 100 experiments. *Indian J. Med. Res.*, **53**, 674
19. De Bono, A.H. (1966). La transplantation cardiopulmonaire totale. *Ann. Chir. Thorac. Cardiovasc.*, **5**, 243
20. Prop, J., Kuijpers, K., Petersen, A.H., Bartels, H.L., Nieuwenhuis, P. and Wildevuur, C.H. (1985). Why are lung allografts more vigorously rejected than hearts? *J. Heart Transplant.*, **4**, 433
21. Novitzky, D., Cooper, D.K.C., Wicomb, W.N., Rose, A.G. and Reichart, B. (1985). Transplantation of the heart and both lungs: experimental and clinical experience and review of the literature. *S. Afr. Med. J.*, **67**, 575
22. McGregor, C.G.A., Baldwin, J.C., Jamieson, S.W., Billingham, M.E., Yousem, S.A., Burke, C.M., Oyer, P.E., Stinson, E.B. and Shumway, N.E. (1985). Isolated pulmonary rejection after combined heart–lung transplantation. *J. Thorac. Cardiovasc. Surg.*, **90**, 623
23. Grinnan, G.L.B., Graham, W.H., Childs, J.W. and Lower, R.R. (1970). Cardiopulmonary homotransplantation. *J. Thorac. Cardiovasc. Surg.*, **60**, 609
24. Nakae, S., Webb, W.R., Theodorides, T. and Sugg, W.L. (1967). Respiratory function following cardiopulmonary denervation in dog, cat, and monkey. *Surg. Gynec. Obstet.*, **125**, 1285
25. Castaneda, A.R., Zamora, R., Schmidt-Habelmann, P., Hornung, J., Murphy, W., Ponto, D. and Moller, J.H. (1972). Cardiopulmonary autotransplantation in primates (baboons). Late functional results. *Surgery*, **72**, 1064
26. Haglin, J., Telander, R.L., Muzzall, R.E., Kiser, J.C. and Strobel, C.J. (1963). Comparison of lung autotransplantation in the primate and dog. *Surg. Forum*, **14**, 196
27. Reitz, B., Burton, N.A., Jamieson, S., Bieber, C.T., Pennock, J.L., Stinson, E.B. and Shumway, N.E. (1980). Heart and lung transplantation. Autotransplantation and allotransplantation in primates with extended survival. *J. Thorac. Cardiovasc. Surg.*, **80**, 360
28. Reitz, B.A. (1981). Heart and lung transplantation. *J. Heart Transplant.*, **1**, 80
29. Cooper, D.K.C., Novitzky, D., Rose, A.G. and Reichart, B.A. (1986). Acute pulmonary rejection precedes cardiac rejection following heart–lung transplantation in a primate model. *J. Heart Transplant.*, **5**, 29
30. Cooley, D.A., Bloodwell, R.D., Hallman, G.L., Nora, J.J., Harrison, J.M. and Leachman, R.D. (1969). Organ transplantation for advanced cardiopulmonary disease. *Ann. Thorac. Surg.*, **8**, 30
31. Lillehei, C.W. Discussion of Wildevuur, C.R.H. and Benfield, J.R. (1970). A review of 23 human lung transplantations by 20 surgeons. *Ann. Thorac. Surg.*, **9**, 515
32. Barnard, C.N. and Cooper, D.K.C. (1981). Clinical transplantation of the heart: a review of 13 years personal experience. *J. Roy. Soc. Med.*, **74**, 670
33. Losman, J.G., Campbell, C.D., Replogle, R.L. and Barnard, C.N. (1982). Joint transplantation of the heart and lungs. Past experience and present potentials. *J. Cardiovasc. Surg.*, **23**, 440
34. Reitz, B.A., Pennock, J.L. and Shumway, N.E. (1981). Simplified operative method for heart and lung transplantation. *J. Surg. Res.*, **31**, 1
35. Reitz, B.A. (1982). Heart–lung transplantation: a review. *Heart Transplant.*, **1**, 292
36. Reitz, B.A., Wallwork, J., Hunt, S.A., Pennock, J.L., Billingham, M.E., Oyer, P.E., Stinson, E.B. and Shumway, N.E. (1982). Heart and lung transplantation: successful therapy for patients with pulmonary vascular disease. *N. Engl. J. Med.*, **306**, 557
37. Jamieson, S.W. and Ogunnaike, H.O. (1986). Cardiopulmonary transplantation. *Surg. Clin. North Am.*, **66**, 491
38. Jamieson, S.W., Reitz, B.A., Oyer, P.E., Billingham, M., Modry, D., Baldwin, J., Stinson, E.B., Hunt, S., Theodore, J., Bieber, C.P. and Shumway, E.B. (1983). Combined heart and lung transplantation. *Lancet*, **1**, 1130

34
Indications, Selection, and Management of the Recipient

A.G. MITCHELL

INTRODUCTION

Successful heart–lung transplantation can be dated to the beginning of the present decade, with the first reported case performed for primary pulmonary hypertension in 1981[1]. Since then there has been a steady increase in the number of operations performed[2], and a broadening of the indications for the procedure. The indications for transplantation of the heart and both lungs overlap to a certain extent on the one hand with those for cardiac transplantation, and, on the other hand, with those for single or double lung transplantation. This chapter will include our experience of transplantation at Harefield Hospital, where the first heart–lung procedure was performed in September, 1984. Since that time, 176 patients have received heart and lungs, and, of these, nine have required retransplantation for obliterative bronchiolitis.

INDICATIONS

Currently, patients who might be considered for heart–lung transplantation may have:

(1) Isolated pulmonary hypertension;
(2) Cardiac disease with severe pulmonary hypertension (Eisenmenger's syndrome) or underdeveloped pulmonary vasculature;
(3) Parenchymal lung disease irrespective of the cardiac state.

The indications for operation in the 176 patients undergoing heart–lung transplantation at Harefield Hospital are listed in Table 34.1. These are broadly similar to those in patients operated on at Papworth Hospital in England[3] and in Pittsburgh in the USA[4], though patients in the Stanford series, reported in 1986, were all pulmonary hypertensive[5]. As recently as 1986, some centers restricted the indications to pulmonary hypertension, and excluded patients with previous thoracic surgery[6].

Table 34.1 Indications for heart–lung transplantation in 176 patients at Harefield Hospital

Indications	Number of patients (%)
Congenital heart disease	72 (41)
Isolated pulmonary hypertension	48 (27)
Cystic fibrosis	23 (13)
Emphysema	14 (8)
Miscellaneous	19 (11)
Total	176 (100)

The largest group of patients at Harefield has had congenital heart disease, usually associated with pulmonary hypertension, either as part of the natural history of the disease or resulting from corrective or palliative surgery. The Eisenmenger response had developed following systemic–pulmonary arterial shunt procedures in a little over half of the patients, while the remainder had complex congenital defects. Those with congenital defects without pulmonary hypertension had pulmonary arteries unsuitable for any corrective procedure (e.g. inoperable pulmonary atresia).

In the Harefield series, isolated pulmonary hypertension was idiopathic (38 cases), thromboembolic (five cases), or veno-occlusive (two cases), and in two cases was associated with systemic lupus erythematosus. One patient had important kyphoscoliosis with pulmonary hypertension, but survived only a few days after transplantation. The principal parenchymal diseases have been associated with cystic fibrosis or extensive emphysema, of which five had α_1 antitrypsin deficiency. With a prevalence of approximately one in 2000 live births for cystic fibrosis, and half that for α_1 antitrypsin deficiency, these two conditions will continue to provide a substantial number of prospective young recipients[7].

Review of the early (1 month) and 1-year mortality of patients undergoing heart–lung transplantation at our center does not suggest that any major etiological group should be withdrawn from the program. Surprisingly perhaps, perioperative mortality was lowest (at 13%) for those with cystic fibrosis, with that of other groups between 20 and 30%; by 1 year, however, the difference was less marked.

Of the indications for heart–lung transplantation 11% are grouped as 'miscellaneous' with no more than three patients with any one diagnosis. Details are given in Table 34.2, together with the number dying within the first postoperative month. One additional case of lymphangioleiomyomatosis has been described[8], and the Papworth experience includes sarcoid (three cases) and histiocytosis X (one case)[3]. Fibrosing alveolitis and diffuse fibrosis would currently be considered indications for single lung transplantation in line with the experience of the Toronto group[9]; to date, eight such operations have been performed at Harefield. In general, malignant disease in the lungs should not be considered even though two patients have undergone transplantation, both having bronchoalveolar cell carcinoma without invasion of the pleura or mediastinum.

In adults with ischemic heart disease or cardiomyopathy it is unusual to find a pulmonary vascular resistance (PVR) fixed in excess of 8 Wood units (640 dynes^{-1} cm^{-5}). Measurement of the PVR needs to be carried out accurately and under optimal conditions – with adequate oxygenation and, if appropriate, the use of prostacycline. For many cases with a borderline PVR, it is appropriate to use a heterotopic cardiac transplant, or a donor heart taken from the recipient of a heart–lung transplant (and therefore conditioned to pulmonary hypertension).

This concept of the use of a 'conditioned' heart can be illustrated by a case example. Patient U.A., now aged 28 years, had evidence of cardiomyopathy at the age of 4 years; pulmonary artery pressures had been documented to increase from 52/21 mmHg at 4 years to 62/30 mmHg (PVR 4) at 16 years and 80/50 mmHg (PVR 12) at age 27. After intensive medical therapy for 3 months the pressures fell to 65/35 mmHg (PVR 7), but with no significant change on 100% oxygen. Cardiac transplantation from a pulmonary hypertensive donor was uncomplicated, and 1 year later the pulmonary artery pressure was 40/12 mmHg (PVR 3). The limits to which conditioned hearts may be used are not yet clear, but in children a PVR exceeding 4–5 Wood units currently requires heart–lung transplantation.

Table 34.2 Miscellaneous indications for heart–lung transplantation at Harefield Hospital

	Number of patients	Early (1 month) mortality
Fibrosing alveolitis	3	1
Pulmonary fibrosis	3	1
Cardiomyopathy + PHT*	3	0
Obliterative bronchiolitis	2	1
Acute respiratory distress syndrome	2	0
Carcinoma	2	1
Pulmonary lymphangioleiomyomatosis	1	0
Pulmonary hemangiomatosis	1	1
Pulmonary hemosiderosis	1	0
Ischemic heart disease + PHT*	1	1
Total	19	6

*PHT = pulmonary hypertension

CONTRAINDICATIONS

Table 34.3 lists the major and minor contraindications which should be considered. Major contraindications are likely to remain important for the foreseeable future, while minor ones are of less significance and can potentially be overcome in a majority of patients. In a developing program, few factors seem to be universally absolute prohibitions. Many of the contraindications are self-evident, and are based on the experience of cardiac transplantation. Our own policy has been to be relatively liberal and we have accepted patients who might have been unacceptable to some other programs.

Systemic infection precludes heart–lung transplantation, at least temporarily, but in cases of chronic lung disease, particularly cystic fibrosis and other cases of bronchiectasis, it may be impossible to keep the lungs consistently free of infection. Careful use of antibiotics is needed to supplement physiotherapy and postural drainage. Invasive fungal infections cannot be eradicated, and should be regarded as a very strong contraindication.

Severe chest deformity or muscular weakness prevent adequate ventilation of the transplanted lungs, but the degree to which either contraindicates transplantation remains a subjective assessment in conjunction with the measured lung volumes. In patients with severe venous congestion or marked tricuspid regurgitation, it is difficult to interpret standard liver function tests. Features of liver failure – spider nevi, encephalopathy, hypoalbuminemia, severe jaundice – are unlikely to improve, and preclude heart–lung transplantation. One case of heart, lung, and liver transplantation has already been described[10]. Mild jaundice and mild renal failure secondary to congestion do not absolutely preclude operation, though the postoperative course can be very difficult, and mortality and morbidity rise substantially. Intensive medical therapy, including hemofiltration, may significantly improve renal and hepatic function. Because of the risk of grand mal epileptic seizures during treatment for rejection, uncontrolled epilepsy must be included as a contraindication.

In contrast to our experience in orthotopic cardiac transplantation, where the outcome for suitably selected patients over 60 years of age is similar to that for younger patients[11], heart–lung transplantation seems better tolerated by younger patients. The perioperative and 1-year mortalities in relation to age are shown in Table 34.4, and indicate the increased risk in the 5th and 6th decades. It is unlikely that this effect is solely due to age, and well-motivated, otherwise suitable, candidates might still be considered up to their early fifties. At the lower age range,

Table 34.3 Contraindications to heart–lung transplantation

Major	Minor
Active systemic infection	Advanced age (>40 years)
Severe chest deformity	Previous thoracic surgery
Malignant disease	Presence of major or numerous bronchial collaterals
Severe renal/hepatic disease	Current corticosteroid therapy
Uncontrolled systemic disease	Diabetes mellitus
Severe central nervous system disability	Active peptic ulceration
Drug abuse/psychological instability	
Positive hepatitis or HIV serology	

Table 34.4 Mortality at 1 month and 1 year related to patient age (one infant of 2 months is excluded)

Patient age (years)	1 month Number of patients	Mortality (%)	1 year Number of patients	Mortality (%)
1–9	20	25	14	20
10–19	47	15	27	38
20–29	50	18	30	32
30–39	32	28	22	32
40–49	18	41	9	60
50–55	8	37	5	80
	Total 175	Mean 25%	Total 107	Mean 38%

prospects are more promising, with a 1-year survival of 80% for children between 1 and 10 years old.

The technical difficulties caused by bronchial collaterals and adhesions resulting from previous surgery have been well described[5]. The previous surgery may involve lateral thoracotomy or sternotomy, with particularly poor results of transplantation following the latter[4]. This is mainly a problem in patients with congenital heart disease who have undergone previous corrective surgery, systemic–pulmonary vascular shunts, or pulmonary artery banding. The importance of the presence of large bronchial collaterals cannot be overstressed. Many of our surviving patients, however, have undergone previous surgery for congenital lesions. Lobectomy for bronchiectasis had been performed in one patient with cystic fibrosis who remains alive and well following transplantation. Exploratory surgery should be avoided, if possible; there is rarely any need for open lung biopsy in patients with pulmonary hypertension. In individuals with cystic fibrosis, recurrent pneumothoraces may have led to the development of adhesions, or pleurectomy may have been performed; this may preclude transplantation by significantly increasing the operative risks.

Problems with healing of the tracheal anastomosis following heart–lung transplantation are well recognized[9]; preoperative steroid therapy should be greatly reduced or discontinued prior to surgery whenever possible.

PATIENT ASSESSMENT

To aid in the selection of patients referred for transplantation, an assessment protocol has been developed. This is aimed at determining the severity and nature of the presenting illness, the prognosis, and the importance of contraindications. Much of the screening can be performed by the patient's referring hospital so that the burden on the transplant center is reduced. The clinical history and examination cannot be overemphasized. Accepted patients are all severely restricted (New York Heart Association class III or IV) with a prognosis often under 1–2 years. Many of the patients with lung disease are dependent on oxygen, and cardiac patients may require intravenous inotropic support. The rate at which patients are deteriorating is a particularly important factor.

Social support may need to be arranged, particularly for patients traveling long distances to the transplant hospital, and it is helpful for the patient and family to discuss problems and prospects with staff – doctors, nurses, physiotherapists, etc. Dental hygiene should also be assessed. An opportunity to meet patients with successful transplants can put many of the worries of the prospective patient into perspective. Nevertheless, some potential candidates view transplantation with unreasonable euphoria, and this misconception should be corrected.

Screening includes blood count and tests of coagulation. Biochemical tests should cover renal and hepatic function, and, in patients with cystic fibrosis, malabsorption and abnormal glucose handling need to be defined. Patients with primary pulmonary hypertension should be checked for autoimmune disease. Although accelerated coronary atheroma has not been a problem in survivors without obliterative bronchiolitis, the fasting lipids are measured and dietary advice given. Bacteriological and fungal cultures need to be repeated frequently (from sputum and blood), particularly in patients with bronchiectasis. Serology for cytomegalovirus (CMV), hepatitis antigens, human immunodeficiency virus (HIV), and syphilis are checked.

The benefit of matching for CMV (i.e. use of a CMV-negative donor for a CMV-negative recipient) has been noted at several centers[12]. Preoperative serology titers against herpes simplex, Toxoplasma, pneumocystis, and Epstein–Barr virus form a useful baseline for postoperative comparisons. At our center, only ABO blood group compatibility is ensured between donor and recipient; we still perform, however, a full HLA typing of both donor and recipient, and document the presence of lymphocytotoxic antibodies in the recipient.

Pulmonary function tests include measurement of volumes, flow and ventilation rates, and diffusion capacity. Arterial blood gases are measured on air or oxygen. Most accepted patients are sufficiently restricted to make exercise testing unrewarding. If details of the lung structure are required they can be obtained by computerized tomography of the thorax, which is the preferred method of defining the extent of bronchiectasis in severely ill patients[13], and is essential if the presence of a malignant lesion is being considered. In order to match lung size between donor and recipient, the thoracic cage of the recipient is measured according to the scheme shown in Figure 34.1. This direct comparison of lung size is convenient for distant organ procurement; similar measurements can be made on the donor by the local hospital staff. Alternatively, comparisons can be made from chest radiographs taken to minimize magnification errors[14] (Chapter 35), and from lung volumes (measured in the recipient and estimated from the height and sex of the donor) (Chapters 36 and 38).

Although echocardiography with Doppler provides useful information of cardiac anatomy and pulmonary pressures, cardiac catheterization is routinely performed. In severe pulmonary hypertension, angiography carries a significant risk, even using isosmolar contrast agents, though a recent report suggests this risk may have been overstated[15]. If thromboembolic pulmonary hypertension is suspected, V/Q scanning is usually performed; the risk of embolism to the transplanted lungs requires a search for thrombus by venography and the exclusion of hypercoagulable states. Thromboembolic causes of pulmonary hypertension have been less common in our series than might be anticipated from the Mayo Clinic series[16]. In patients with complex congenital heart disease, definition of systemic collaterals is helpful; occasionally, abnormal systemic–venous connections can be demonstrated, knowledge of which might prove extremely helpful to the surgeon performing the transplant.

Use of the recipient's heart as a donor organ for cardiac transplantation

Unless there is a primary cardiac defect, at the time of heart–lung transplantation the recipient heart can be considered as a donor organ for cardiac transplantation in a second recipient. Heart–lung transplantation, with use of the recipient heart for subsequent heart transplantation in a second recipient, has been our policy following poor results obtained in a small number of patients in whom double lung transplantation was performed with the recipient retaining his own heart. The major problem in the cases where double lung transplantation was performed was poor healing or stricture formation at the tracheal anastomosis. Double lung transplantation is discussed in Chapter 50.

The successful use of the heart–lung recipient's own heart in a second recipient requires prior demonstration of normal left ventricular function, normal coronary arteries, adequate, though not necessarily normal, right ventricular function, and with no more than moderate tricuspid regurgitation. This latter is conveniently shown by echo–Doppler studies. The definition of pulmonary vascular resistance and estimation of right ventricular hypertrophy determines whether the heart can be used as an orthotopic cardiac transplant in a patient with elevated pulmonary arterial pressures.

Of 32 possible candidates, 25 live donor transplants were actually performed; 17 had underlying pulmonary disease (mainly cystic fibrosis) while eight had primary pulmonary hypertension. The 1-year survival of the recipients of these hearts, transplanted before July 1987, is 80%, which is similar to survival of patients receiving hearts from brain-

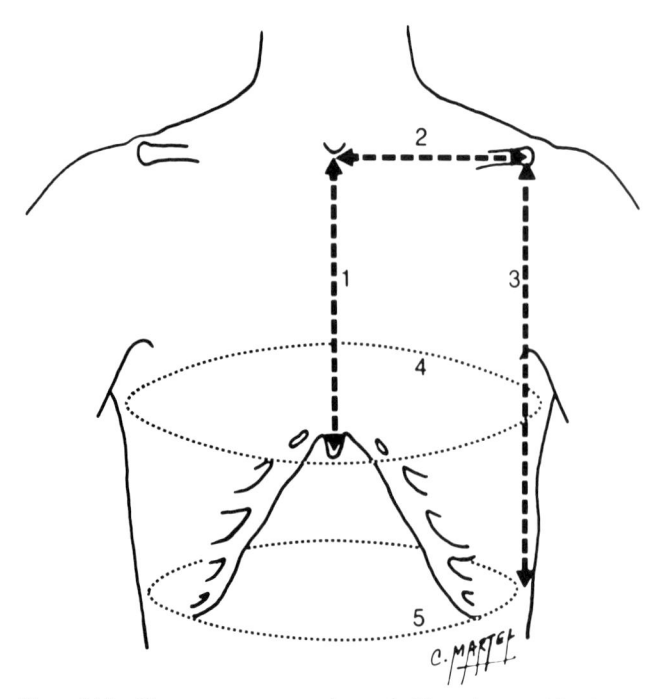

Figure 34.1 Chest measurements taken to facilitate size-matching between donor and recipient for heart–lung transplantation. (1) Suprasternal notch to xiphisternum; (2) suprasternal notch to acromium; (3) acromium to costal margin; (4) greatest circumference of chest; (5) circumference at lower costal margin. (See also Chapters 35, 36 and 38)

dead donors. The limits to which this practice is acceptable remain to be defined. Written consent for the use of the heart is requested from the patient when he or she has been accepted for heart–lung transplantation; to date, all have agreed willingly.

PATIENT SELECTION

In selecting individual patients for transplantation the high perioperative mortality and the unresolved problem of obliterative bronchiolitis provide notes of caution. Morbidity is higher than for cardiac transplantation, and the patients may remain in intensive care for long periods. These factors have important financial and logistic consequences, not only for the transplantation program but also for other cardiothoracic surgery performed at the transplant center.

The demand for heart–lung transplantation currently exceeds the availability of suitable donors. Of 177 adult patients referred and deemed suitable for transplantation over a 2-year period, only 40% received a donor; nearly 10% have already died on the waiting list, leaving approximtely 80 candidates currently awaiting a donor. This disproportion between the number of recipients and the supply of donors inevitably means some patients deteriorate markedly whilst on the waiting list. When a donor becomes available, it may be necessary to decide between a high-risk terminal patient and a healthier, better risk, alternative patient. In this climate, some patients may have to be removed temporarily or permanently from the list. Such decisions are unpalatable for the clinician to make, and difficult for the patient and relatives to accept. Moribund patients and those requiring prolonged ventilation are not suitable because of the high perioperative risks. Although two patients with acute adult respiratory distress syndrome have received transplants, the concept of such emergency procedures remains inappropriate at the present time.

It is now accepted that severe pulmonary hypertension can be managed only by transplantation of both heart and lungs. Terminal cystic fibrosis and emphysema are also definite indications. Final selection must make due allowance of significant contraindications and the patient's own attitude to transplantation. For the foreseeable future, there are going to be many disappointed deserving candidates.

PRE-OPERATIVE CARE

The period between acceptance for heart–lung transplantation and surgery can be protracted, with 30% of patients waiting longer than 1 year. These patients will have a lower priority, yet still are critically limited and often require periods of hospitalization for further deterioration. A period of intensive medical therapy may allow a few more months of relative stability.

For patients with isolated pulmonary hypertension, a poor prognosis has been related to a low cardiac output or a pulmonary artery saturation below 63%[16]. Right heart failure also carries a poor outlook, and syncope is particularly threatening[17]. Anticoagulants are essential, irrespective of evidence of thromboembolism[16]. By the time transplantation is recommended, vasodilators have usually been prescribed with varying degrees of success. The cardiac output is severely restricted, and changes in vasodilator regimens may be dangerous if the peripheral resistance is reduced unduly. Prostacycline, given intravenously, has been successful in reducing the PVR in a proportion of cases, and has been used as a 'bridging procedure' prior to transplantation, though a number of patients died whilst on therapy[18].

Diuretics are used widely, but require particularly careful manipulation, for even minor dehydration can produce a dangerous fall of blood pressure, increased cyanosis, and syncope. Volume replacement may be life-saving in some over-diuresed patients, and therapeutic challenges of a plasma expander should be used to obtain the optimum cardiac output. Adequate filling pressures may allow the reintroduction of vasodilators previously discontinued for hypotension. Intravenous inotropic agents can also be used to support the failing right ventricle. In congenital lesions with polycythemia, repeated venesections and fluid replacement may be required to maintain the hematocrit around 60%.

The prognosis for parenchymal pulmonary disease is less well defined. Patients have chronic respiratory failure with a low oxygen tension, and, although severe hypercapnia has been uncommon in our population, oxygen therapy must be used with all the usual care to avoid a marked rise in PCO_2. Mortality seems inversely related to arterial oxygen tension. Dependence on oxygen is usual, and there is little useful benefit from administration of bronchodilators which, if used in excess, may provoke arrhythmias. Because of the risks of infection and poor tracheal healing, steroids should be gradually withdrawn if possible. Infection in the lungs, particularly with pseudomonas, is a continuing threat and has a poor prognosis. If venous access becomes difficult, an implantable system may be used[19]. Many of the patients with cystic fibrosis and others in a chronically hypoxic state are in a poor nutritional state, and may benefit from parenteral nutrition or feeding via a gastrostomy during the period of assessment and whilst awaiting a donor. Factors associated with poor prognosis include forced expiratory volume in 1 second (FEV_1) and forced vital capacity (FVC) below 75% predicted and evidence of right heart failure[20].

For patients in respiratory failure, successful resuscitation from cardiopulmonary arrest may precipitate the need for prolonged ventilation. This adds to the risks of subsequent transplantation, and, if a donor is not readily available, the patient may have to be withdrawn from the program. Intensive regular physiotherapy, and occasionally aspiration of tracheobronchial secretions by bronchoscopy, are essential measures which may prevent respiratory arrest.

COMMENT

Heart–lung transplantation should be considered for patients with end-stage pulmonary and cardiopulmonary disease, particularly in younger patients. Near-moribund patients are not suitable. Transplantation will continue to be performed occasionally in relatively unsuitable patients on an experimental basis. Future analysis of late mortality and complications should help improve the selection process.

References

1. Reitz, B.A., Wallwork, J.L., Hunt, S.A., Pennock, J.L., Billingham, M.E., Oyer, P.E., Stinson, E.B. and Shumway, N.E. (1982). Heart–lung transplantation. *N. Engl. J. Med.*, **306**, 557
2. Kaye, M.P. (1987). The Registry of the International Society for Heart Transplantation: fourth official report – 1987. *J. Heart Transplant.*, **6**, 63
3. Scott, J.P., Hutter, J.A., Higenbottam, T.W. and Wallwork, J. (1988). Combined heart and lung transplantation. *Cardiol. Practice*, **6**, 21
4. Griffith, B.P., Hardesty, R.L., Trento, A., Paradis, I.L., Duquesnoy, R.J., Zeevi, A., Dauber, J.H., Dummer, J.S., Thompson, M.E., Gryzan, S. and Bahnson, H.T. (1987). Heart–lung transplantation: lessons learned and future hopes. *Ann. Thorac. Surg.*, **43**, 6
5. Burke, C.M., Theodore, J., Baldwin, J.C., Morris, A.J., McGregor, C., Shumway, N.E., Robin, E.D. and Jamieson, S.W. (1986). Twenty-eight cases of human heart–lung transplantation. *Lancet*, **1**, 517
6. Primo, G., Wellens, F., Leclerc, J.L. and De Smet, J.M. (1986). Current indications and experience with heart–lung transplantation. *Transplant. Proc.*, (Suppl. 3), 41
7. Hutchison, D.C.S. (1988). Natural history of α_1-protease inhibitor deficiency. *Am. J. Med.*, **84**, 3
8. Wellens, F., Estenne, M., De Francquen, P., Goldstein, J., Leclerc, J.L. and Primo, J. (1985). Combined heart–lung transplantation for terminal pulmonary lymphangioleiomyomatosis. *J. Thorac. Cardiovasc. Surg.*, **89**, 872
9. Cooper, J.D., Pearson, F.G., Patterson, G.A., Todd, T.R.J., Ginsberg, R.J., Goldberg, M. and Demajo, W.A.P. (1987). Technique of successful lung transplantation in humans. *J. Thorac. Cardiovasc. Surg.*, **93**, 173
10. Wallwork, J., Williams, R. and Calne, R.Y. (1987). Transplantation of liver, heart and lungs for primary biliary cirrhosis and primary pulmonary hypertension. *Lancet*, **2**, 182
11. Aravot, D.J., Banner, N.R., Khagani, A., Fitzgerald, M., Radley-Smith, R., Mitchell, A.G. and Yacoub, M.H. (1989). Cardiac transplantation in the seventh decade of life. *Am. J. Cardiol.*, **63**, 90
12. Hakim, M., Wreghitt, T., English, T.A.H., Stovin, P.G.I., Cory-Pearce, R. and Wallwork, J. (1985). Significance of donor transmitted disease in cardiac transplantation. *J. Heart Transplant.*, **4**, 302
13. Mootoosamy, I.M., Reznek, R.M., Osman, J., Rees, R.S. and Green, M. (1985). Assessment of bronchiectasis by computerized tomography. *Thorax*, **40**, 920
14. Hakim, M., Higenbottam, T., Bethune, D., Cory-Pearce, R., English, T.A.H., Kneeshaw, J., Wells, F.C. and Wallwork, J. (1988). Selection and procurement of combined heart and lung grafts for transplantation. *J. Thorac. Cardiovasc. Surg.*, **95**, 474
15. Perlmutt, L.M., Braun, S.D., Newman, G.E., Oke, E.J. and Dunnick, N.R. (1987). Pulmonary arteriography in the high-risk patient. *Radiology*, **162**, 187
16. Fuster, V., Steele, P.M., Edwards, W.D., Gersh, B.J., McGoon, M.D. and Frye, R.L. (1984). Primary pulmonary hypertension: natural history and the importance of thrombosis. *Circulation*, **70**, 580
17. Rozkovec, A., Montanes, P. and Oakley, C.M. (1986). Factors that influence the outcome of primary pulmonary hypertension. *Br. Heart J.*, **55**, 449
18. Jones, D.K., Higenbottam, T. and Wallwork, J. (1987). Treatment of primary pulmonary hypertension with intravenous epoprostenol (prostacycline). *Br. Heart J.*, **57**, 270
19. Stead, R.J., Davidson, T.I., Duncan, F.R., Hodson, M. and Batten, J.C. (1987). Use of a totally implantable system for venous access in cystic fibrosis. *Thorax*, **42**, 149
20. Hodson, M.E., Wise, A.E., Duncan, F. and Batten, J.C. (1985). Factors affecting survival of adult patients with cystic fibrosis. *Thorax*, **40**, 227

35
Selection of the Donor; Excision and Storage of Donor Organs

A. HAVERICH, D. NOVITZKY AND D.K.C. COOPER

INTRODUCTION

The first successful human heart–lung transplantation at Stanford in 1981[1] evolved as a logical consequence from what was, at that time, the most experienced heart transplant program. Extensive animal research had been performed prior to clinical application, and cyclosporine was available for immunosuppression[2]. These were probably the key reasons for the success of the clinical heart–lung transplant program that subsequently developed.

At Stanford, and in other centers, clinical activities have progressed slowly in this field when compared to the enormous increase in isolated cardiac transplants that has occurred in the ensuing years. The major obstacle to the expansion of heart–lung transplant programs has been the scarcity of donor organs suitable for combined heart–lung transplantation. It was not until methods of cardiopulmonary preservation allowing successful distant organ procurement were developed that the discrepancy between demand and supply of donor organs began to improve.

Such methods, where clinically applied, are described in this chapter. Donor selection and management, as well as the technique of excision, will also be detailed.

DONOR SELECTION

It has been estimated that less than 20% of potential heart donors are suitable for heart–lung transplantation[3]. Pneumonic changes may occur in brain-dead potential donors as a result of infection or aspiration and may preclude donation of lungs. Intubation, often performed as an emergency under less than optimal sterile conditions, and neurogenic pulmonary edema increase the risk of pulmonary dysfunction. Finally, a close size match between donor and recipient is required, because the donor lungs must fit within the fixed capacity of the recipient's thoracic cage.

In order to minimize the risk of pulmonary failure or infection after transplantation, a potential donor should meet the following criteria.

Age

Preferably, the donor should be less than 40 years (male) or 45 years (female) to reduce the risk of coronary artery disease. With the present severe shortage of suitable donors, this age limit might be extended if the donor appears suitable in other respects. Coronary angiography should, however, be performed (Chapter 6).

Medical history

Ideally, the donor should be a non-smoker with no history of significant lung or cardiac disease.

Cardiac function

Clearly, normal cardiac function is essential (Chapter 6).

Pulmonary function

Adequate gas exchange should be present. With positive end-expiratory pressure (PEEP) of 5 cm H_2O and an FiO_2 of 0.4 (40% O_2) or less, the PaO_2 should be greater than 100 mmHg. On an FiO_2 of 1 (100% O_2), the PaO_2 should be greater than 300 mmHg. Lung compliance should exceed 0.1 l/cmH_2O at a tidal volume of 10 ml/kg. In a patient with a non-obstructive endotracheal tube *in situ*, an inspiratory volume of 15 ml/kg should not result in a *static* pressure of more than 20 cmH_2O being measured. This will indicate a relatively normal lung compliance. The measurement should be repeated three times and an average taken. Possibly the simplest way of testing the lung compliance is by increasing the ventilatory tidal volume from a minimum of 500 ml in an adult by 100 ml increments to 1000 ml; *peak* inspiratory pressure should not rise above 30 mmHg. Airway resistance, though not a routine measurement, (on mechanical ventilation) should be less[3,4] than $1.6\,cmH_2O\,l^{-1}\,s^{-1}$.

In order to achieve or maintain such function, fluid restriction may be necessary, especially with respect to crystalloid solutions. Close monitoring of central venous pressure and cautious application of catecholamines are mandatory, as in cardiac donors. Prolonged artificial ventilation, an FiO_2 exceeding 0.5 (50%), and positive end-expiratory pressures greater than 10 mmHg should all be avoided.

Pulmonary infection

Due to nosocomial infections, mechanical ventilation in brain-dead subjects for more than 4–7 days will generally preclude use of the lungs for transplantation. The chest radiograph should be clear of major pulmonary infiltrates, including post-traumatic opacifications, suggesting contusion or infection, though some groups would not decline use of the lungs on these grounds alone if there were no confirmatory evidence of pulmonary damage or infection. Certainly, minor areas of infiltrate may not preclude donation. Before the donor operation, frequent aseptic and thorough endotracheal suction and toilet is mandatory, and a broad spectrum antibiotic should be administered.

The majority of heart–lung donors have bacterial and/or fungal colonization of the tracheobronchial tree despite normal radiographic appearances[3]. Therefore, specimens should be taken before (optimally via a bronchoscope) and during harvesting to allow immediate Gram stain and cultures. The presence of a purulent sputum with a large number of organisms on Gram stain, indicating the presence of an active infection, is usually considered to be a contraindication to donation. Many centers, however, might accept such a donor if the offending organism had been identified and specific antibiotic therapy initiated in both donor and recipient. The presence of some pus cells but no organisms detectable on a Gram stain generally will not preclude donation. Postoperative antibiotic treatment can be based on the results of culture.

Size match

In contrast to orthotopic heart transplantation, a close size match between donor and recipient thoracic cavities is required for cardiopulmonary transplantation. Undue compression of the donor lungs within the recipient's thoracic cage results in significant atelectasis and cardiac compression. Though fewer problems result from the use of smaller donor organs, the donor thoracic cavity dimensions should not deviate from those of the recipient by more than approximately 20%. Similarly, the donor heart may be too small to support the recipient circulation if the weight of the donor is less than approximately 75% that of the recipient.

To compare the relative sizes of the donor and recipient thoracic cavities, we believe that a comparison of the measurements taken on chest radiographs provides the most reliable information. Some surgeons, however, make external measurements of the donor chest to compare with those of the recipient chest (Chapter 34). Given the great variability in muscle and fat mass around the thoracic cage, we believe that a comparison of chest radiographs provides more reliable information. The chest radiographs to be compared should be taken at a standard distance from the subject (e.g. one meter) with both subjects in a supine position; if possible, both anteroposterior and lateral films should be available for comparison.

Measurements on the chest radiograph that have been found useful (at the Oklahoma Transplantation Institute) are illustrated in Figure 35.1. Alternative measurements that have been found useful (at the Medizinische Hochschule, Hannover) are (1) sternal notch to xiphoid, (2) sternal notch to lower rib margin, (3) sternal notch to acromion, (4) chest diameter halfway from sternal notch to lower rib margin, and (5) chest diameter at the level of the lower rib margin. All of these measurements can be readily obtained from the potential recipient during his or her initial evaluation, and from the donor at the time when brain death is established.

When the internal thoracic diameters of the donor are larger than those of the recipient, the donor will be excluded from donation. When the internal thoracic diameters of the donor are up to 20% less than those of the recipient, the donor will be acceptable.

Some centers no longer rely on comparison of chest and/or chest radiograph measurements, but prefer comparisons of height and weight or total lung capacity (measured or predicted) (Chapters 36 and 38).

DONOR MANAGEMENT

The donor will be maintained on a (physiological) PEEP of $5\,cmH_2O$ with the lowest possible FiO_2 required to maintain a PO_2 greater than 100 mmHg. The mean arterial pressure will be maintained at a minimum of 60 mmHg. As diabetes insipidus is present in most donors, urinary output is usually normal or excessive. Fluid replacement has to be kept at the minimum necessary to maintain normotension. Following blood volume correction, fluids will be administered to replace those lost by diuresis, but fluid overload must be prevented; it is important to ensure that the donor lungs do not become over-hydrated, and therefore every

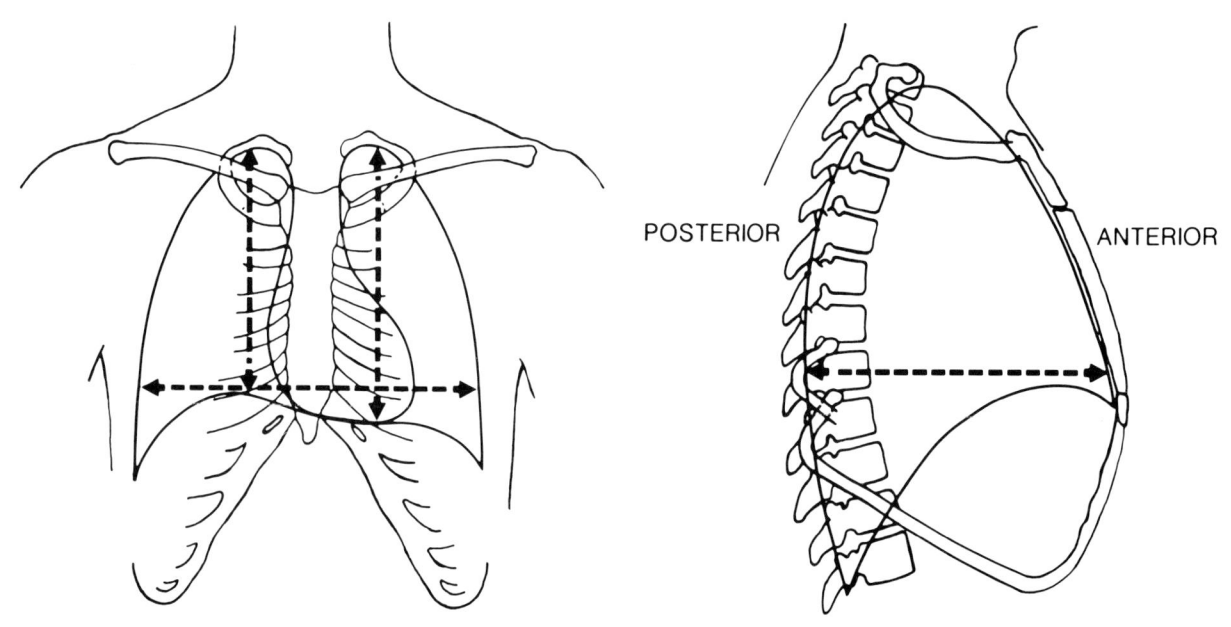

Figure 35.1 Measurements of anteroposterior and lateral chest radiographs found helpful in assessing relative sizes of donor organs and recipient thoracic cavity. All measurements are made on chest radiographs taken in the supine position with the camera at a set distance from the radiographic plate. Measurements include (1) vertical distance from the apex of the pleural cavity to the diaphragm on both right and left sides; (2) the transverse diameter at the widest point of the chest (this is usually near or at the costophrenic angle); (3) the anteroposterior diameters measured on the lateral chest radiograph from anterior surface of the vertebral column to the posterior surface of the sternum, and from the posterior curvature of the ribs to the back of the sternum, both of these measurements being made at the mid-sternal and diaphragmatic levels

effort should be made to maintain a relatively low CVP (approximately 5 cmH$_2$O) if this proves sufficient to sustain an acceptable arterial pressure.

EXCISION OF DONOR ORGANS – SURGICAL TECHNIQUE

The technique of excising the donor organs will be described irrespective of the mode of graft preservation used. In multi-organ donors, the chest is usually opened at the time the abdominal surgeons are beginning their procedures, as this enables the cardiothoracic surgeon to inspect the heart (and lungs, if necessary) and it also facilitates the dissection of the liver.

Irrespective of the preservation technique used for the heart and lungs, a median sternotomy is usually preferred. However, a bilateral anterior thoracotomy has also been suggested[6], purportedly allowing easier dissection of the posterior mediastinum and better control of bleeding. An anterior pericardiotomy is then performed, and the heart and aorta exposed up to the innominate and left carotid arteries (Figure 35.2). The pericardium, with adjacent pleura, is bilaterally excised. The presence of dense pleural adhesions will usually be a contraindication to use of the lungs for transplantation; the likelihood of causing multiple pulmonary lacerations and injury during the dissection of the donor lungs is high, and may lead to serious hemorrhage following implantation in the recipient. The superior vena cava (SVC), inferior vena cava (IVC), ascending aorta, and trachea (between the SVC and aorta) are all mobilized. The ascending aorta is dissected free from the main pulmonary artery. A tape is passed around the ascending aorta, and this structure is retracted to the left to expose the trachea. Minimal dissection is carried out around the trachea as it is important to disturb its blood supply from coronary collaterals as little as possible (Figure 35.3).

Two methods of preservation of the organs are commonly in vogue – simple hypothermic flush perfusion and cooling by pump-oxygenator (extracorporeal circulation (ECC)), both followed by storage in ice. Both methods will be elaborated later. For simple flush perfusion, a 14 French perfusion catheter is inserted into the main pulmonary artery and a cardioplegic infusion line placed in the ascending aorta. If donor cooling via ECC is preferred, aortic and right atrial (or SVC and IVC) cannulation is necessary. Both methods require prior full heparinization. For venting of the left heart, the tip of the left atrial appendage may be transected (flush perfusion), or a vent-catheter can be placed into the left atrium via the appendage or right superior pulmonary vein. The vent catheter can be placed in the apex of the left ventricle, though many feel it is best to avoid even this small degree of myocardial injury. If left ventricular venting is desired, the catheter can be passed from the atrium into the ventricle via the mitral valve.

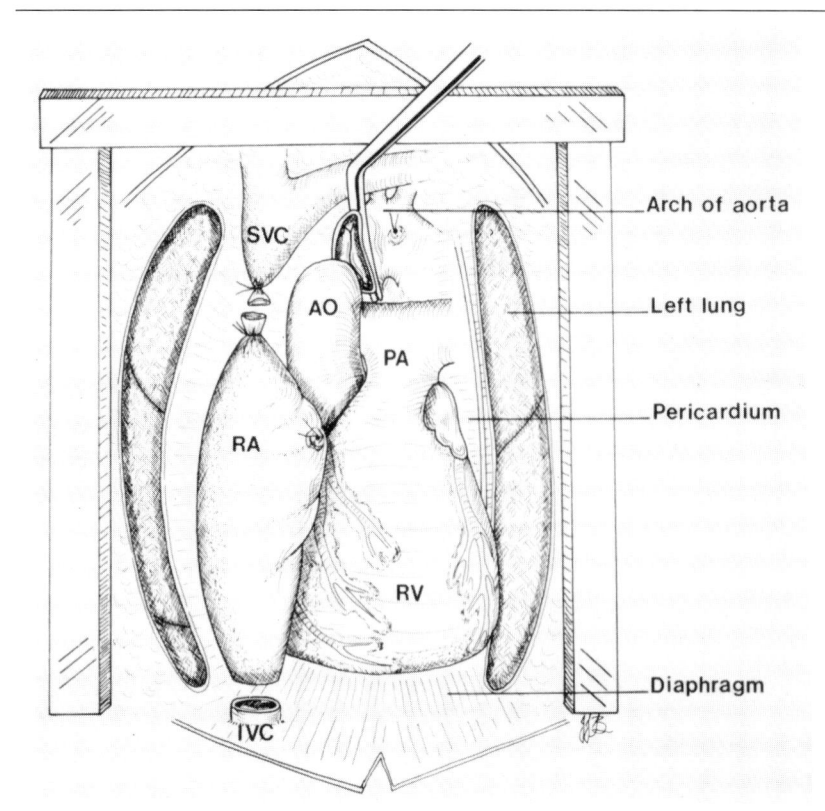

THE TRANSPLANTATION AND REPLACEMENT OF THORACIC ORGANS

Figure 35.2 Excision of donor organs. A median sternotomy has been performed, and pericardiectomy carried out. Both pleural cavities have been opened to allow inspection of the lungs. Cooling of the heart and lungs can be carried out by (1) a pump-oxygenator (bringing about total body cooling) and the infusion of a cardioplegic agent, or by (2) simultaneous infusion of a cardioplegic agent into the ascending aorta and a 'pulmoplegic' agent into the main pulmonary artery. In this figure cooling has been by pump-oxygenator. The aortic and right atrial cannulae have already been removed, but the sites of cannulation in the arch of the aorta and right atrial appendage are indicated. The cardioplegic infusion cannula is not shown. The superior vena cava has been doubly ligated and divided. The inferior cava has been divided. The ascending aorta has been cross-clamped as high as possible and divided. (Abbreviations used in this chapter: SVC = superior vena cava; RA = right atrium; IVC = inferior vena cava; RV = right ventricle; PA = pulmonary artery; PV = pulmonary vein; AO = aorta)

both caval veins are transected at the level of their pericardial reflections, the ascending aorta is divided as high as possible (Figure 35.2), and the trachea is divided as high as possible above the carina (Figure 35.4) after withdrawal of the endotracheal tube. The heart–lung graft is excised en bloc in a craniocaudal direction by dividing the posterior mediastinal tissues anterior to the esophagus and descending aorta (Figures 35.5–35.8). To avoid subsequent post-transplant bleeding in the recipient, electrocautery should be used wherever possible; the inferior pulmonary ligaments should be either stapled or suture-ligated. During explantation, the lungs should be handled with maximal care to prevent trauma.

Following excision (Figure 35.9), some surgeons prefer the lungs to remain partially inflated, though others advocate deflation. It is believed that partial inflation prevents prolonged post-transplant atelectasis. The heart and lung bloc is placed in a sterile container or bag filled with cold (4°C) fluid (blood or crystalloid solution), which in turn is placed in a box of approximate size filled with ice. The organs are then transported to the site of the recipient operation.

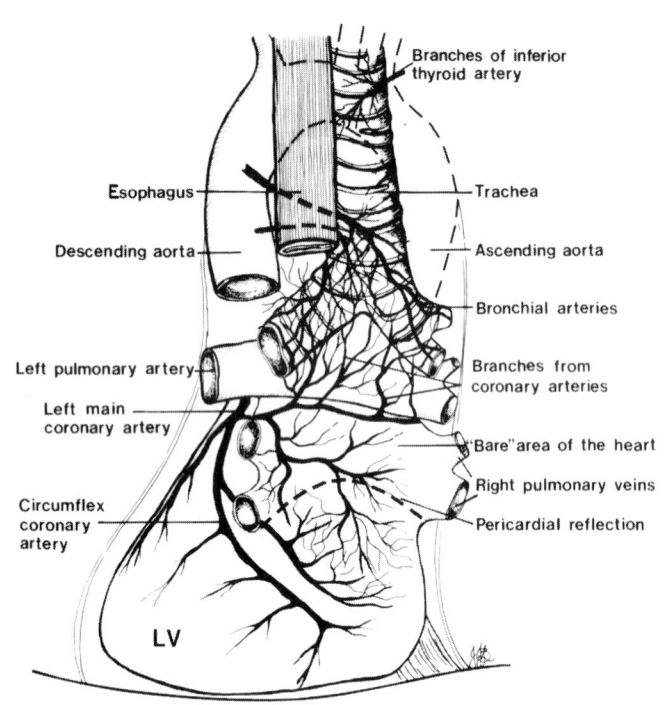

Figure 35.3 Posterior view of heart and trachea, showing blood supply to the trachea, carina and bronchi. (LV = left ventricle)

Cold saline is poured into both pleural (and pericardial) cavities to cool the lungs (and heart), which may or may not be maintained on mechanical ventilation (preferably using unheated room air) during this period.

Once satisfactory cooling of the organs has been achieved,

CARDIOPULMONARY PRESERVATION

With the first successful clinical heart–lung transplantation performed at the beginning of this decade[1], the question arose how to preserve morphological and functional pulmonary integrity during ischemia. At that time, no problems were apparent with respect to short-term myocardial pre-

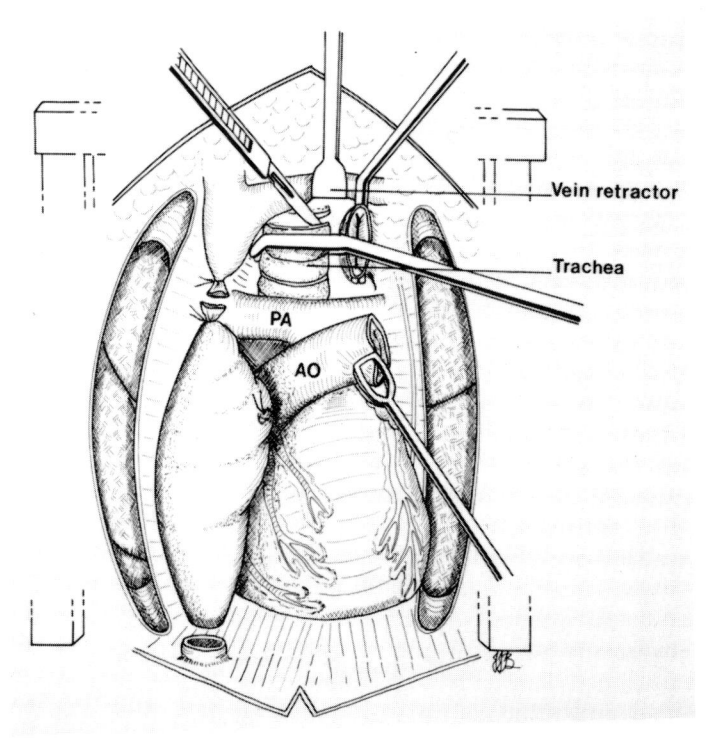

Figure 35.4 The ascending aorta has been retracted downwards and to the left, exposing the trachea, which has been clamped and divided as high as possible (after withdrawal of the endotracheal tube)

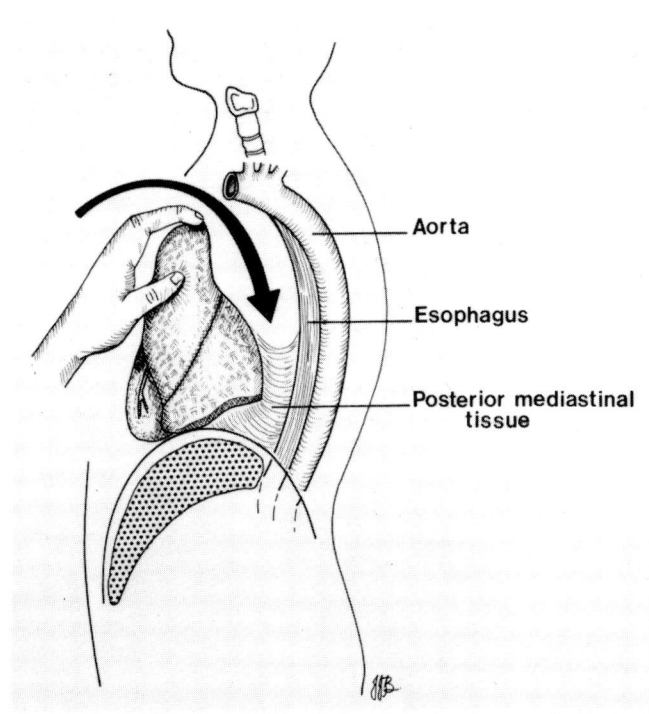

Figure 35.6 Indicates the plane of the dissection between heart (and lungs) and posterior mediastinal structures (esophagus and descending aorta)

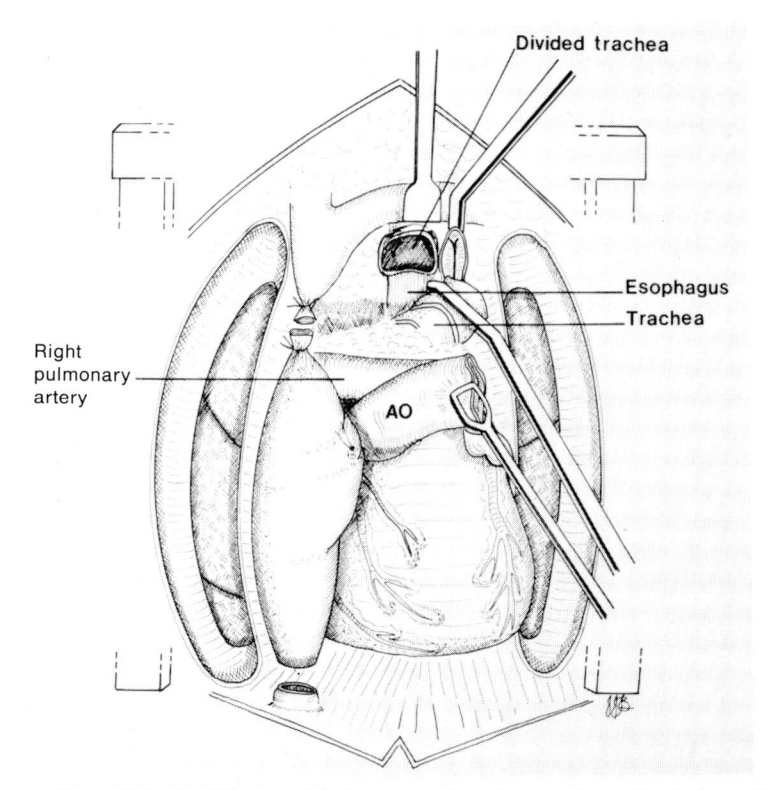

Figure 35.5 Mobilization of the heart away from the posterior mediastinal tissues is begun in a craniocaudal direction by retracting the distal trachea anteriorly and downwards, exposing the esophagus and descending aorta

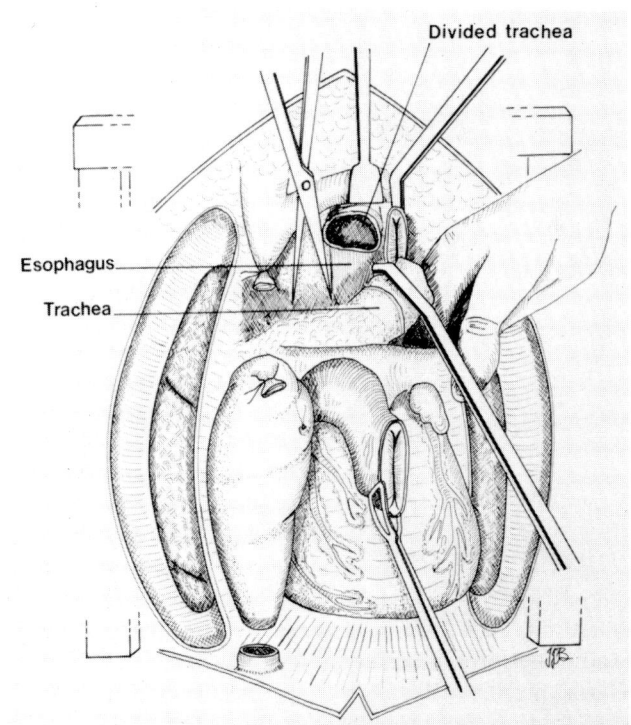

Figure 35.7 To facilitate the dissection, the surgeon's fingers are inserted posterior to the heart to retract this organ forwards and downwards

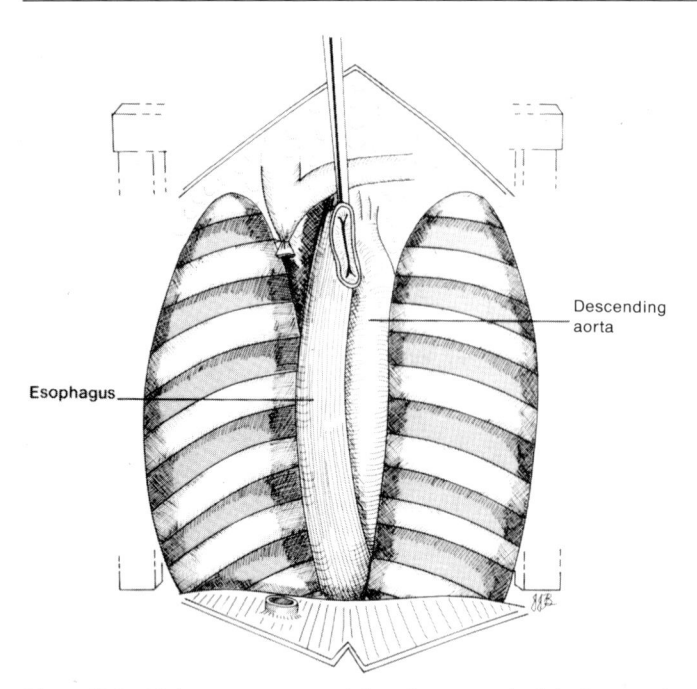

Figure 35.8 Major structures remaining after removal of the heart and lungs from the thoracic cavity

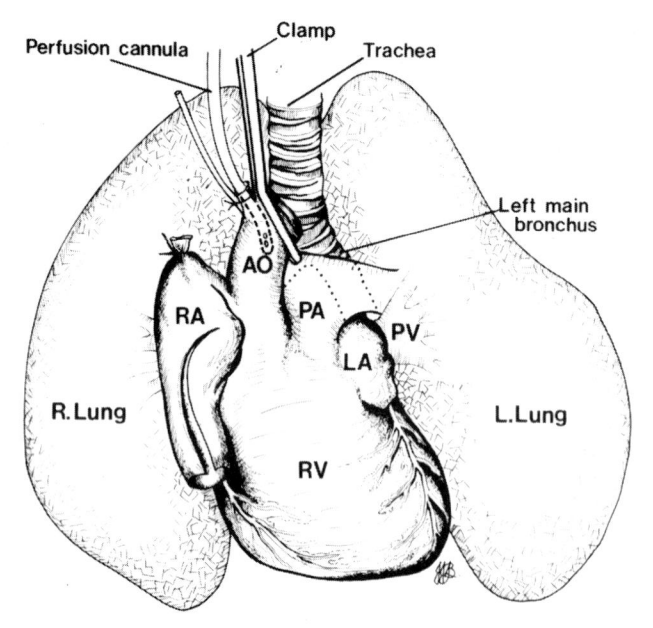

Figure 35.9 The excised organs. The cardioplegic perfusion catheter remains *in situ*. The right atrium has been incised in preparation for insertion into the recipient

servation. Based on the many experimental and clinical studies performed during the 1970s, which related to myocardial protection during open heart surgery, further studies, directly planned to facilitate transportation of donor hearts, have resulted in the introduction of distant organ procurement with extended periods of cold myocardial ischemia (Chapter 7).

The history of pulmonary preservation can also be traced back for more than 20 years. The majority of early experimental trials were performed following the first series of unilateral lung transplants in man (Chapter 45). These varied animal experiments have been reviewed previously[7], and will not be documented again here. In the 1970s, interest in pulmonary preservation studies decreased considerably following the dismal early results of unilateral clinical lung transplantation[8]. After the first successful combined replacement of heart and both lungs by Reitz and associates in 1981, however, interest was renewed. At Stanford, the first heart–lung transplants were carried out using a cold potassium cardioplegic agent for flush perfusion of both the coronary and pulmonary arteries[1]. Later, cold EuroCollins solution, modified by the addition of magnesium sulfate, was used to perfuse the lungs, with simultaneous protection of the myocardium[9].

This concept of crystalloid flush still represents one of three methods of pulmonary preservation used in clinical transplantation of the heart and both lungs. The other two modalities include (1) cooling of the lungs with cold blood by either the pump-oxygenator or flush perfusion (using cold donor blood), and (2) the use of an autoperfusing heart–lung preparation. The functional, biochemical and practical implications, as well as the results, of these methods of lung preservation will be detailed.

Hypothermic flush perfusion with crystalloid solution

Today, hypothermic flush perfusion is the basis of preservation of solid organs for purposes of transplantation. The vast majority of renal, hepatic, and cardiac allografts are harvested using simple perfusion with a crystalloid solution, followed by cold storage[10]. While numerous varied biochemical compositions have been created for this purpose, buffered solutions with an intracellular ionic composition and slightly increased osmolarity compared to serum, such as EuroCollins solution, are preferred by many centers. Ease of application and satisfactory graft function represent the chief advantages of this method. The topic of myocardial protection has been reviewed elsewhere (Chapter 7); it will not be discussed further here.

Unlike preservation studies in renal, cardiac, and hepatic transplantation, no controlled experimental studies on the efficacy of such storage solutions were performed prior to their clinical application for pulmonary preservation. In the initial clinical series, modified EuroCollins solution (at 4°C) (Table 35.1) was administered at a flow rate of 20 ml/kg body weight over a period of 5–7 minutes. This mode of application was revised following a study of unilateral lung transplantation in dogs which disclosed that a significant improvement in postoperative lung function could be obtained by increasing both flow rate and total volume of

SELECTION OF THE DONOR

Table 35.1 Composition of modified EuroCollins solution for lung preservation in clinical heart–lung transplantation

KH_2PO_4	2.05 g/l
K_2HPO_4	7.40 g/l
KCl	1.12 g/l
$NaHCO_3$	0.84 g/l
$MgSO_4$	1.00 g/l
Glucose	38.5 g/l
pH	7.3–7.4

the solution[11]. By infusing EuroCollins solution into the pulmonary artery at 60 ml/kg over 4 minutes (Figure 35.10), a more uniform distribution of EuroCollins solution within the lungs was obtained and a lower temperature was achieved (Figure 35.11). This modification allowed distant organ procurement in the clinical setting of heart–lung transplantation. While the infusion is taking place, the heart

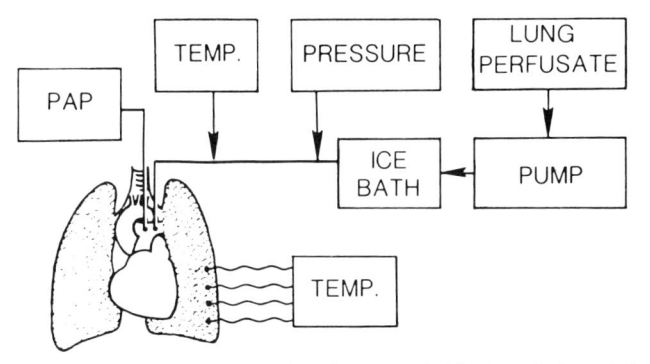

Figure 35.10 Experimental method for controlled flush perfusion of the lungs via the pulmonary artery. Note control of pulmonary temperature and pulmonary artery pressure (PAP)

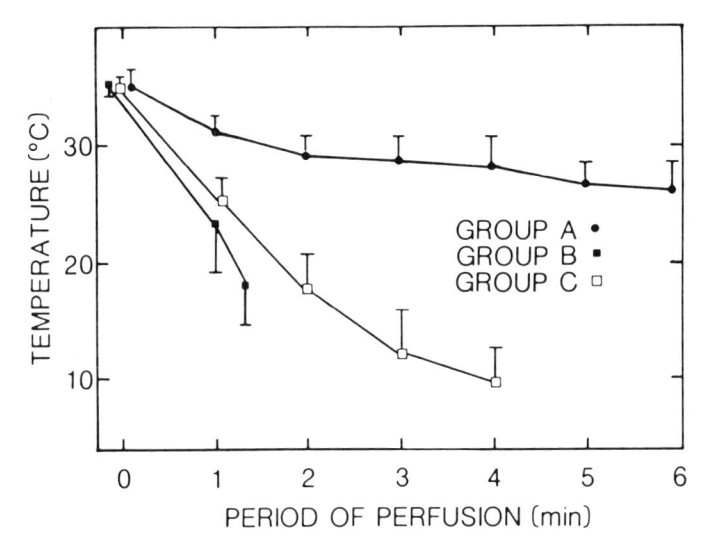

Figure 35.11 Changes in lung temperature during flush perfusion of the lung with EuroCollins solution at 4°C. Group A received 20 ml/kg of solution over 6 minutes; group B received 20 ml/kg over 1.3 minutes (at normal pulmonary arterial pressure during perfusion); group C received 60 ml/kg over 4 minutes (at normal pulmonary arterial pressure)[11]

and lungs are irrigated externally with cold (4°C) saline.

Further improvement of post-transplant pulmonary function was achieved by pretreatment of the donor using the prostaglandins analogue, PGE_1 (see below). PGE_1 is directly infused into the main pulmonary artery immediately prior to flush perfusion. The object is to obtain maximal vasodilation of the pulmonary vasculature and avoid spasm during pulmoplegic infusion. The infusion, containing 500–1000 µg of PGE_1, should be continued until the systemic systolic or mean arterial pressure falls by 30 mmHg. At this stage, flush perfusion should be begun.

Nevertheless, pulmonary function in a recipient of a cardiopulmonary allograft preserved by this simple method remains less than optimal. Additional concepts are being investigated at present to improve the preservation of pulmonary integrity. Recent studies have concentrated on aspects of reperfusion after the transplant has been performed (Chapter 7), since deleterious effects on both pulmonary vascular resistance and oxygenation have been identified. One possible mechanism of reperfusion damage is the generation of oxygen free radicals in the lung tissue during this period. Leukocytes may be responsible for this phenomenon since reperfusion by leukocyte-depleted blood reduces this effect[12]. Another observation supporting the hypothesis that oxygen free radical generation is injurious is that the addition of oxygen free radical scavengers is able to improve postoperative lung function after ischemic intervals of 6 hours[13].

Hypothermic flush perfusion with blood

The beneficial effect of perfusing a prostaglandins analogue through the donor lung before explantation has also been described when the lung has been preserved using cold blood. It is unclear whether this effect is achieved through the vasodilating or cytoprotective effect of the prostaglandins or through their ability to inhibit platelet aggregation. Nevertheless, the Cambridge group has achieved the goal of distant organ procurement for heart–lung transplantation by combining the administration of prostacycline with perfusion of the lungs by cold donor blood modified by the addition of buffers and protein solutions[14]. In terms of technical and instrument requirements, this approach is as simple to perform as flush perfusion using EuroCollins solution; cooling of the donor by means of extracorporeal circulation, however, is a more complicated procedure.

Cooling by extracorporeal circulation (ECC)

This latter mode of preservation for heart–lung transplantation was first described experimentally in 1984[15]. Later, the method was adopted for clinical distant organ procurement by the same center (Pittsburgh), and is now used for

279

the same purpose by the group in Harefield in the United Kingdom, currently the most active in this field[5] (Chapter 34). At the present time, the 'pumpers' – as opposed to the 'freezers' or 'flushers' – have performed a larger number of clinical transplants. The major drawback of this technique is the need to transport a relatively large amount of equipment to the donor center. Roller pump, perfusion circuits, heat exchanger, and oxygenator constitute the minimum requirements for this purpose.

There is good experimental evidence of a reduced post-transplant capacity for oxygenation by lungs preserved by ECC when compared to lungs preserved by flush perfusion with EuroCollins solution; pulmonary vasculature, in contrast, appears to be better preserved[16].

Autoperfusing heart–lung preparation

The final option for the preservation of cardiopulmonary function during medium-term ischemia of these organs is the autoperfusing heart–lung preparation (Figures 35.12 and 35.13). This method, as described by Robicsek and

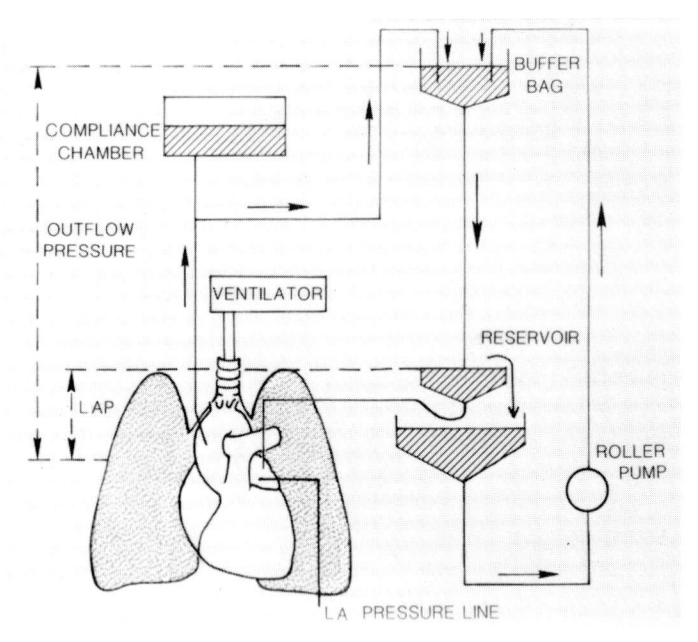

Figure 35.13 Schematic diagram of the autoperfusing heart–lung preparation as used for cardiopulmonary preservation

associates in the late 1950s, was developed primarily for the experimental storage of the heart alone, though it was used in experimental heart–lung transplantation by Longmore et al. in the late 1960s[22,23]. Following extensive animal investigations[17,18], it was utilized for clinical heart–lung transplantation by the Pittsburgh group[19]. Despite acceptable results, however, it was later abandoned and replaced by hypothermic flush techniques.

Application of the autoperfusing heart–lung preparation has been shown to be associated with two major disadvantages. First, the method results in hypostatic pulmonary edema and functional impairment[20,21]. Second, mechanical ventilation of the lungs via the donor trachea for prolonged periods (to allow transportation) possibly carries an added risk of introducing pulmonary infection. For these reasons, the autoperfusing heart–lung preparation has not been used recently in clinical cardiopulmonary preservation.

Reimplantation response

Though this is a postoperative complication of heart–lung transplantation, its development may be related to inadequate protection of the lungs during the ischemic period, and therefore a brief note on it would seem indicated here.

This complication, which is still poorly understood, has occurred in a number of the lung transplants performed to date, and may occur whether the transplant involves the heart and both lungs or a single lung[2,25]. Pulmonary function usually recovers promptly after operation, enabling the patient to be extubated within 24–48 hours. Chest

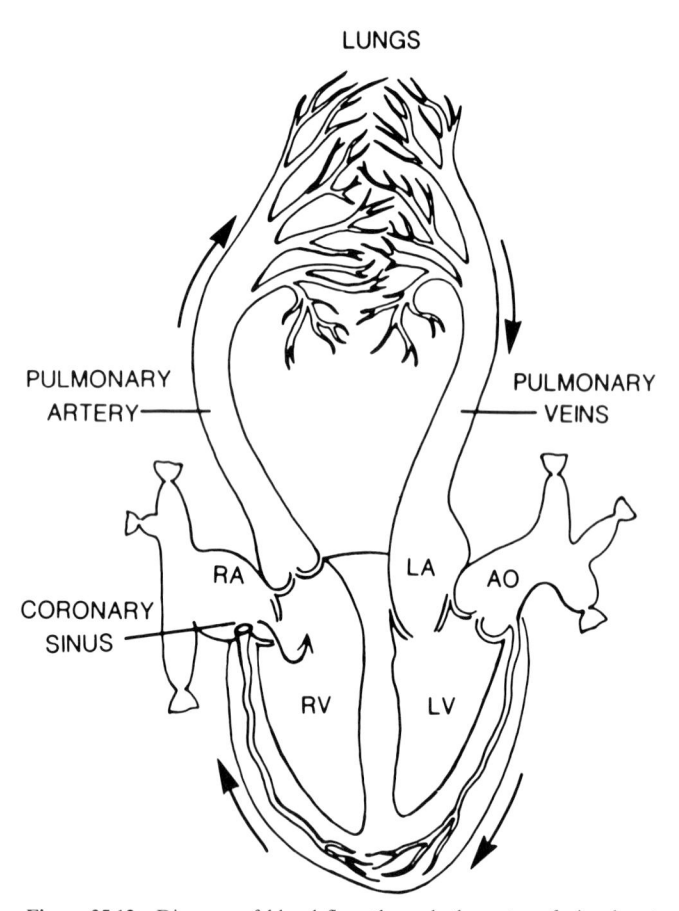

Figure 35.12 Diagram of blood flow through the autoperfusing heart–lung preparation (Demikhov[24]; Longmore et al.[22,23]). In the Robicsek modification, a buffer bag was inserted in the circuit to achieve a more constant aortic pressure (see Figure 35.13)

radiographs are normal. Within the first 24–48 hours, or during the next few days, however, the radiological appearances may change markedly, showing features of a diffuse pulmonary infiltrate. The patient may become febrile and tachypneic, and show signs of respiratory failure. These features are related to a loss of pulmonary compliance, elevation of the pulmonary vascular resistance, a marked fall in arterial PO_2 and an elevation of PCO_2, indicating pulmonary 'shunting' with ventilation–perfusion imbalance.

This clinical picture is difficult to differentiate from an acute rejection episode or from infection. The timing of this response may help in making a diagnosis. If it develops within the first 2–3 days, acute rejection is unlikely. Aggressive investigation for a possible pulmonary infection, however, must be carried out; this may involve fiberoptic bronchoscopy. Microscopic examination of fluid collected following bronchial lavage is of little value in differentiating the reimplantation response from acute rejection. It may be helpful, however, in differentiating infection, as microorganisms may be seen. Microscopic examination of lung biopsies may indicate acute rejection or infection. If both rejection and infection can be excluded, however, then a diagnosis of reimplantation response, as it has become known, can be made with some certainty.

The etiology of the reimplantation response is uncertain, but it appears likely that it is related to the ischemia which the lung has experienced during removal from the donor and reimplantation in the recipient. Though in several reported cases the ischemic time has been as short as 1 hour 30 minutes, this period is thought to be long enough for the lung to sustain damage. Several other factors, however, have been considered as possible etiologic factors, though these are probably of lesser importance than ischemia[26]. These include the effect of denervation of the lungs, disruption of the lymphatic circulation, and pulmonary trauma from manipulation during the operative procedure.

To a certain extent the reimplantation response can be prevented by maintaining a low venous pressure and inducing a diuresis during the early days following transplantation. Should the complication develop, then diuresis is essential, and oxygen should be administered by mask or nasal cannulae. If the pulmonary compliance continues to deteriorate and the arterial PO_2 cannot be maintained above 60 mmHg (8.0 kPa), then continuous positive airway pressure must be introduced. If this should prove inadequate, or if the patient becomes distressed by the respiratory effort, endotracheal intubation and ventilation may be necessary for several days until, hopefully, lung function recovers.

COMMENT

The lack of suitability of many brain-dead subjects as donors of heart and lungs has hindered the development of the combined transplantation of these organs. The technique of excision is now well-established. Advances are still required, however, in the field of preservation of the lungs. Both cooling the lungs by extracorporeal circulation and by cold flush perfusion, using either crystalloid or sanguineous fluids, each followed by cold static storage (in ice), offer simple and relatively efficient modes of graft preservation. Heart and lung ischemic intervals of up to 3–4 hours have been shown to be safe with either method, though the reimplantation response may still occur on occasions, and have allowed distant organ procurement for combined heart–lung transplantation in man.

References

1. Reitz, B.A., Bieber, C.P., Raney, A.A., Pennock, J.L., Jamieson, S.W., Oyer, P.E. and Stinson, E.B. (1981). Orthotopic heart and combined heart and lung transplantation with cyclosporin-A immune suppression. *Transplant. Proc.*, **13**, 393
2. Reitz, B.A., Burton, N.A., Jamieson, S.W., Bieber, C.P., Pennock, J.L., Stinson, E.B. and Shumway, N.E. (1980). Heart and lung transplantation. *J. Thorac. Cardiovasc. Surg.*, **80**, 360
3. Jamieson, S.W., Baldwin, J., Stinson, E.B., Reitz, B.A., Oyer, P.E., Hunt, S., Billingham, M., Theodore, T., Modry, D., Bieber, C.P. and Shumway, N.E. (1984). Clinical heart–lung transplantation. *Transplantation*, **37**, 81
4. Painvin, G.A., Reece, I.J., Cooley, D.A. and Frazier, O.H. (1983). Cardiopulmonary allotransplantation, a collective review: experimental progress and current clinical status. *Tex. Heart Inst. J.*, **10**, 371
5. Sale, J.P., Patel, D., Duncan, B. and Waters, J.H. (1987). Anaesthesia for combined heart and lung transplantation. *Anaesthesia*, **42**, 249
6. Hardesty, R.L. and Griffith, B.P. (1985). Procurement for combined heart–lung transplantation. *J. Thorac. Cardiovasc. Surg.*, **89**, 795
7. Haverich, A., Scott, W.C. and Jamieson, S.W. (1985). Twenty years of lung preservation - a review. *J. Heart Transplant.*, **4**, 234
8. Wildevuur, C.R. and Benfield, J.R. (1970). A review of 23 human lung transplantations by 20 surgeons. *Ann. Thorac. Surg.*, **9**, 489
9. Jamieson, S.W., Stinson, E.B., Oyer, P.E., Baldwin, J.C. and Shumway, N.E. (1984). Operative technique for heart–lung transplantation. *J. Thorac. Cardiovasc. Surg.*, **87**, 930
10. Karow, M. and Pegg, E. (1981). *Organ Preservation for Transplantation*. 2nd ed. (New York: Dekker)
11. Haverich, A., Aziz, S., Scott, W.C., Jamieson, S.W. and Shumway, N.E. (1986). Improved lung preservation using EuroCollins solution for flush-perfusion. *Thorac. Cardiovasc. Surg.*, **34**, 368
12. Till, G.O. and Ward, P.A. (1985). Oxygen radicals in complement and neutrophil-mediated acute lung injury. *J. Free Radic. Biol. Med.*, **1**, 163
13. Takayama, T., Auerswald, A., Schafers, H.-J., Dammenhayn, L. and Haverich, A. (1987). The protective effect of superoxide dismutase during reperfusion of the ischemic lung. *Transplant. Proc.*, **19**, 1332
14. Hakim, M., Higenbottam, T., Bethune, D., Cory-Pearce, R., English, T.A.H., Kneeshaw, J., Wells, F.C. and Wallwork, J. (1988). Selection and procurement of combined heart and lung grafts for transplantation. *J. Thorac. Cardiovasc. Surg.*, **95**, 474
15. Ladowski, J.S., Hardesty, R.L. and Griffith, B.P. (1984). Protection of the heart–lung allograft during procurement. Cooling of the lungs with extracorporeal circulation or pulmonary artery flush. *Heart Transplant.*, **3**, 351
16. Wahlers, T., Haverich, A., Fieguth, H.G., Schafers, H.-J., Takayama, T. and Borst, H.G. (1986). Flush perfusion using EuroCollins solution

vs cooling by means of extracorporeal circulation in heart–lung preservation. *J. Heart Transplant.*, **5**, 89

17. Robicsek, F., Masters, T.N., Duncan, G.D., Denyer, M.H., Rise, H.E. and Etchison, M. (1985). An autoperfused heart–lung preparation: metabolism and function. *J. Heart Transplant.*, **4**, 334
18. Ladowski, J.S., Kapelanski, D.P., Teodori, M.D., Stevenson, W.C., Hardesty, R.L. and Griffith, B.P. (1985). Use of autoperfusion for distant procurement of heart–lung allografts. *J. Heart Transplant.*, **4**, 330
19. Hardesty, R.L. and Griffith, B.P. (1987). Autoperfusion of the heart and lungs for preservation during distant procurement. *J. Thorac. Cardiovasc. Surg.*, **93**, 11
20. Taft, P.M., Collins, G.M., Grotke, G.T. and Halasz, N.A. (1976). Warm ischemic injury of the lung. *J. Thorac. Cardiovasc. Surg.*, **72**, 784
21. Otto, T.J., Trenkner, M., Stopczyk, A., Gawdzinski, M. and Chelstowska, B. (1968). Perfusion and ventilation of isolated canine lungs. *Thorax*, **23**, 645
22. Longmore, D.B., Cooper, D.K.C., Hall, R.W., Sekabunga, J. and Welch, W. (1969). Transplantation of the heart and both lungs. II. Experimental cardiopulmonary transplantation. *Thorax*, **24**, 391
23. Cooper, D.K.C. (1975). A simple method of resuscitation and short-term preservation of the canine cadaver heart. *J. Thorac. Cardiovasc. Surg.*, **70**, 896
24. Demikhov, V.P. (1962). *Experimental Transplantation of Vital Organs.* Authorized translation from the Russian by Haigh, B. (New York: Consultants Bureau)
25. Siegelman, S., Sinha, S.B.P. and Veith, F.J. (1973). Pulmonary reimplantation response. *Ann. Surg.*, **117**, 30
26. Reitz, B.A. (1982). Heart–lung transplantation: a review. *Heart Transplant.*, **1**, 291

36
Anesthetic Management

D.W. BETHUNE AND D.R. WHEELDON

INTRODUCTION

Following the introduction of cyclosporine into the immunosuppressive armamentarium in 1980, successful heart–lung transplantation has been reported[1]. The indications for the operation range from increased pulmonary vascular resistance, either primary idiopathic or as a consequence of cardiac disease, to the effects of disturbances in the lung parenchyma in emphysema and cystic fibrosis[2] (Chapter 34).

The anesthetic management of patients undergoing heart transplantation has been discussed in Chapter 9; only those aspects which differ significantly will be highlighted here.

Careful assessment of these patients is important in determining subsequent anesthetic management. Many patients with a primary disturbance of the lung parenchyma will have virtually normal cardiac function; in these patients, intravenous hypnotic agents will be of value in allowing high inspired oxygen levels to overcome the effects of intrapulmonary shunting. In patients with emphysema, difficulty in ventilation can be anticipated; in the period prior to initiation of cardiopulmonary bypass, PCO_2 levels of up to 10 kPa may have to be tolerated.

ASPECTS OF DONOR SELECTION AND MANAGEMENT

An anesthesiologist is always involved in selection and care of the donor, and travels with the donor team when heart and lungs are to be procured. Selection and assessment of the donor have been discussed in Chapter 35, but the subject of size match between donor organs and recipient thoracic cavity is worthy of further comment.

In our initial cases, measurements were taken from the chest radiographs of both recipient and donor. Two measurements of the transverse diameter (at the levels of T2 and T10) and two vertical measurements (1st rib to T10 and 1st rib to T12) were recorded. There proved to be difficulties, however, in identifying the lower vertebrae on some donor radiographs, and the relative magnification of the two radiographs was not always strictly comparable.

Currently, we use a formula (Chapter 38) based on the donor's height and sex to estimate a total lung capacity[3]. It is important to use the *actual* measured total lung volume of the recipient, as this may be increased in the emphysematous patient or restricted in a patient with pulmonary hypertension. The aim of the size matching is to select donor lungs that are smaller than the recipient's chest cavity by up to 10%.

In the case of the grossly emphysematous patient, the

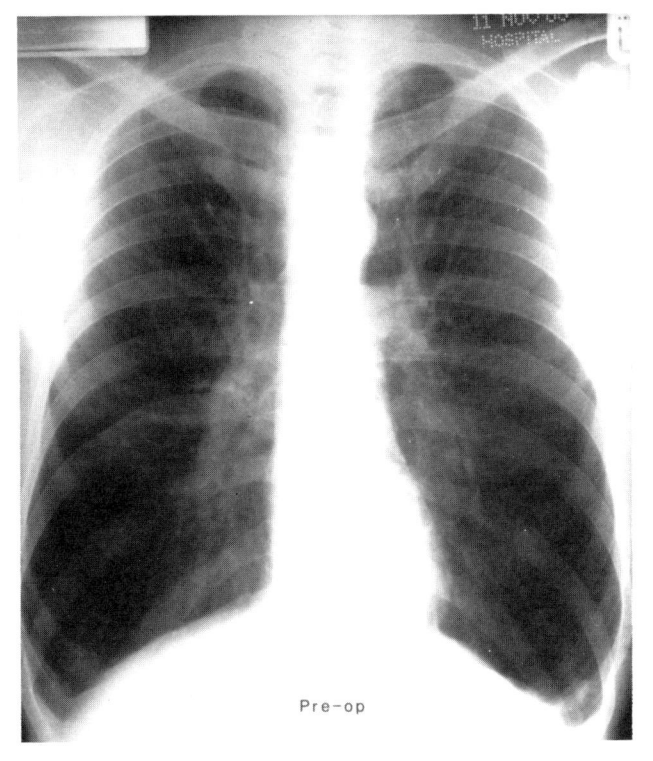

Figure 36.1 Chest radiograph of potential recipient showing marked emphysema; measured lung capacity > 10 liters

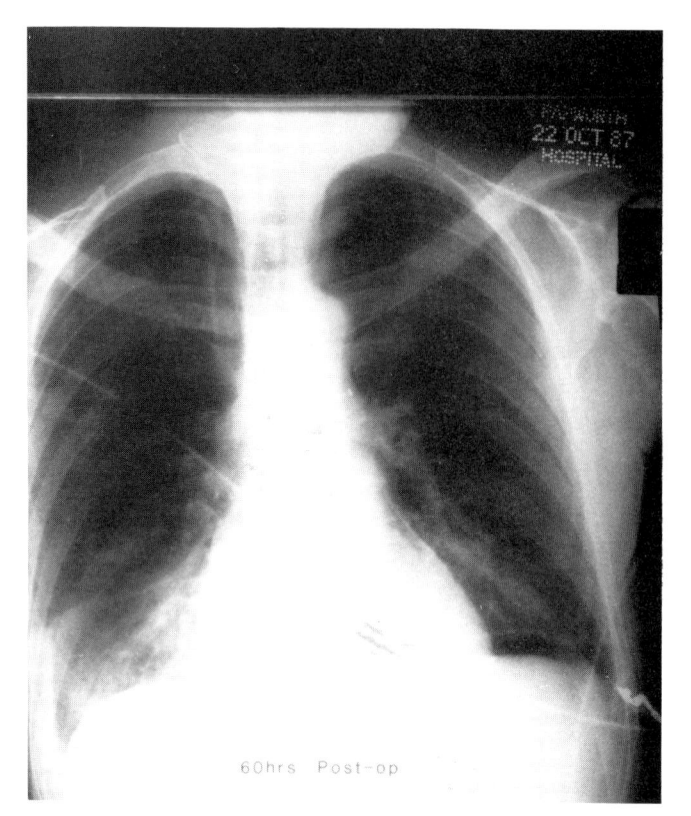

Figure 36.2 Chest radiograph of same patient (as in Figure 36.1) showing change in chest shape 60 hours after heart–lung transplantation

optimum size is difficult to determine. Figures 36.1 and 36.2 show the pre- and post- (60 hours) transplant chest radiographs of a recipient who underwent heart–lung transplantation for severe emphysema. The actual *measured* total lung capacity of the recipient was more than 10 liters, whereas the *estimated* lung volume was only 6 liters. The donor's *estimated* lung volume was also approximately 6 liters. These radiographs demonstrate the capacity of the emphysematous chest to assume a more normal configuration when the over-inflated lungs are replaced by smaller ones. In this particular patient, there were considerable problems with repeated pneumothoraces in the postoperative period, which was further complicated by an overwhelming infection, which led to the patient's death on the 29th day. It is almost certain that this patient's course would have been less problematic had larger donor organs been transplanted.

We now believe that, in the emphysematous patient, the *estimated* size of the donor lungs should be at least 80% of the recipient's *measured* total lung capacity. This will necessitate selecting lungs which have a greater volume than that *estimated* for the recipient by the height-based formula.

Until excision, the lungs are ventilated with an air–oxygen mixture (if air is available) or with nitrous oxide and oxygen, the intention being to maintain the lowest FiO_2 compatible with a PaO_2 of 15 kPa.

Our practice is to use cold cardioplegic solution (15 ml/kg) to arrest the heart, followed by the infusion of a flush perfusate (Tables 36.1 and 36.2) to cool and protect the lungs[4-6] (Figure 36.3). The pulmonary artery is cannulated with a 10–16 French gauge lighthouse tip venous cannula.

Table 36.2 Papworth pulmonary flush solution – final concentrations (per liter)

Sodium	126 mmol
Potassium	6.8 mmol
Calcium	1.8 mmol
Phosphate	251 mmol
Chloride	72 mmol
Mannitol	13 g
Glucose	1.7 g
Sodium citrate	1.7 g
Citric acid	216 mg
Adenine	18.2 mg
Hematocrit	8–15%
Osmolarity	330 mOsmol/kg
pH	6.5

Table 36.1 Preparation of Papworth flush solution

(1) Withdraw blood from donor into citrate–phosphate–dextrose (CPD) anticoagulant at an early stage of the operation.

(2) Make up the solution (as below) according to patient weight. Using a separate quill (port) for each ingredient, add each to a 3-liter parenteral nutrition (TPN) bag. Add the donor blood *last* to the TPN bag *via a transfusion filter*.

(3) Store in a cool box until ready for administration.

(4) Mix gently, to avoid foaming, before priming the infusion system.

(5) Infuse at 4°C at a pressure of 60 cmH$_2$O.

Patient weight (kg)	Donor blood (ml)	CPD (ml)	Ringers solution (ml)	20% albumin (ml)	20% mannitol (ml)	Heparin (units)	Total (ml)
70+	450	63	700	200	100	10 000	1 523
50–70	400	63–7 (56)	600	180	90	9 000	1 335
40–50	350	63–14 (49)	550	160	80	8 000	1 200
30–40	300	63–21 (42)	450	130	65	6 500	990
20–30	250	63–28 (35)	400	110	55	5 500	860
10–20	200	63–35 (28)	300	80	40	4 000	660

ANESTHETIC MANAGEMENT

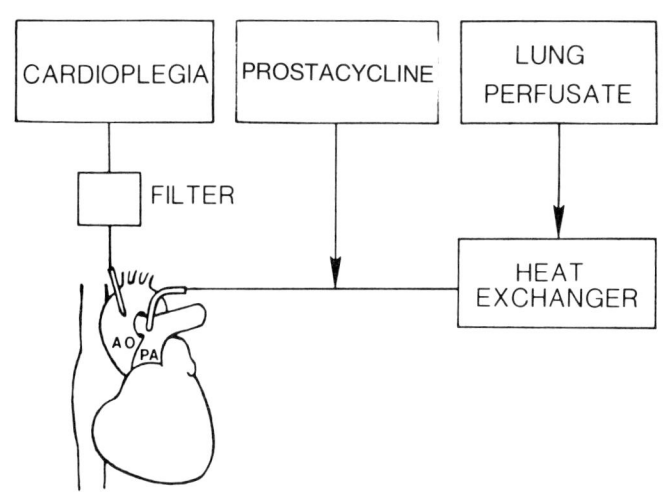

Figure 36.3 System for providing donor heart and lung cooling and protection (as used at Papworth Hospital)

A side-arm allows infusion of prostacycline (epoprostenol, Flolan, Wellcome, UK) at a rate of up to 20 ng/kg per minute to ensure vasodilation of the pulmonary vessels, which is commenced approximately 10 minutes prior to cardiac arrest (Table 36.3). The tip of the left atrial appendage is excised to decompress the left side of the heart. Cold saline (4°C) is poured over both heart and lungs to cool the organs externally.

When the heart has been arrested, the lungs are ventilated with air, either from the anesthetic machine or by using a

Table 36.3 Preparation of prostacycline infusate

(1) Add 10 ml of glycine buffer to the 0.5 mg ampoule of PGI_2.

(2) Mix well and, when totally dissolved, transfer this PGI_2/glycine mixture to the remaining 40 ml of glycine buffer.

(3) Remove 50 ml of normal saline from a 250 ml bag, and discard. Transfer the PGI_2/glycine mixture to the remaining 200 ml of saline via a 0.2 micron (Millipore) filter. This mixture contains 2 μg/ml.

(4) Store cold and protect from light.

(5) The table below gives a guide to infusion rates (when it is wished to administer the PGI_2 at 40 ng/kg per min). Begin the infusion at about 20% of the final planned dose, and increase over an approximate 10-minute period, depending on arterial blood pressure. Infuse 20% albumin to counter any increased venous capacitance. Increase infusion rate until the PGI_2 is being administered at 20–40 ng/kg per min.

Patient weight (kg)	Infusion rate (ml/h)	Graseby setting* (20 ml syringe)
80	96	32
70	84	28
60	72	24
50	60	20
40	48	16
30	36	12
20	24	8
10	12	4

*Graseby syringe driver type MS 16A (Graseby Medical, UK)

resuscitation bag; full expansion is confirmed by inspection. The trachea is clamped with the lungs held at 75% inflation. After excision, the trachea is stapled to allow removal of the clamp. The organs are transported in an insulated box which is maintained at 4°C by using a eutectic mixture[6].

MANAGEMENT OF THE RECIPIENT

Induction and maintenance of anesthesia

The recipient undergoes final assessment and is prepared for the operation. There is rarely time for premedication to be administered on the ward; once in the anesthetic room, incremental doses of midazolam and papaveretum are given to produce the desired level of sedation (Chapter 9). Once sedated, cannulae for monitoring and infusion are inserted (normally one in the left radial artery, two in the right internal jugular vein, and one peripheral venous). Antibiotics and immunosuppressive drugs are then administered. The relatives can then sit with the patient until it is time for the operation to commence, which is dependent on the progress of the donor team and the expected state of the recipient's chest; previous surgery and/or pleural infections can make dissection and hemostasis difficult and time-consuming.

Anesthesia can be induced with a variety of methods and agents. For those patients on the verge of cardiac decompensation, we prefer to use an inhalational technique with trichloroethylene, nitrous oxide, and oxygen. During induction it is important to monitor oxygen saturation continuously, and to adjust the inspired oxygen if necessary. In those patients with adequate cardiac reserve, intravenous hypnotics can be used with a high inspired oxygen. Relaxation is accomplished with either pancuronium or vecuronium, and the patient intubated with a cuffed orotracheal tube. Many of the patients will have suffered growth retardation, and it is desirable to have a selection of tubes available.

The patient is then connected to the ventilator, with a Pall BB50 filter as a heat and moisture exchanger[7]. We use a time-cycled flow generator (Nuffield 200) to ventilate the patient via a 'T' piece circuit prior to transplantation. By suitably adjusting the I:E ratio, it is possible to maintain oxygenation even in the very severely emphysematous patient, though a raised PCO_2 may have to be accepted as a consequence of air trapping. Post-transplantation, the ventilator is changed to a Servo 900C, either in the operating room or on return to the intensive care unit.

A urinary catheter is inserted, and the patient positioned for surgery. The heart–lung recipient may be in cardiac failure and may benefit from adjustment of pre- and/or afterload by venesection, head-up tilt, and/or the use of vasodilators in a similar manner to the heart transplant patient (Chapter 9). With the exception of the patient in whom air trapping is a problem, a patient with parenchymal lung disease rarely gives cause for concern as the inspired oxygen can be raised to counteract the effects of any V/Q mismatch.

Maintenance of anesthesia can be by a variety of agents. At Papworth we use a low concentration of a volatile agent (trichloroethylene) with nitrous oxide and oxygen. The FiO_2 is adjusted to maintain an oxygen saturation of at least 95%. An opiate supplement (papaveretum 0.3 mg/kg) is administered before sternotomy. The nitrous oxide is discontinued at least 10 minutes before cardiopulmonary bypass is initiated to minimize the effects of any gaseous microemboli arising from the pump-oxygenator[8].

Cardiopulmonary bypass

A standard cardiopulmonary bypass circuit is used with a membrane oxygenator[9] (Chapter 9). Facilities are available for hemofiltration and/or hemodialysis[10].

Post-cardiopulmonary bypass management

The hemodynamic behavior of the patient with transplanted heart and lungs is superior to that in the patient who has undergone heart transplantation alone. This is not surprising as the transplanted right ventricle of the heart–lung graft is not faced by a different, and possibly raised, pulmonary vascular resistance. Lung function has been universally good. (If the oxygen saturation is less than 99% on an FiO_2 of 30%, a discrete collapsed area of lung will invariably be found.) We have not been faced with the problem of lungs that were too big for the thoracic cavity, though in such a case there would inevitably be collapsed areas of lung.

The problem of very small lungs in relation to the size of the thoracic cavity is interesting; there are no obvious problems until the chest is closed. While the chest remains open, minimal positive end-expiratory pressure (5 cmH$_2$O) will ensure good expansion. Once the chest is closed it is our practice to apply suction at 10 kPa to maintain lung expansion and to encourage the drainage of any blood. On two occasions it proved impossible to ventilate such patients. Inflation pressures rose to 50–60 cmH$_2$O, and the cardiac output fell. The cause of such a problem is that the lungs are held fully expanded by the suction on the chest drains, but, as they do not fill the thoracic cavity, there is no inspiratory reserve to allow ventilation. The solution is to reduce chest suction to a level that will allow sufficient deflation of the lungs to give enough inspiratory reserve to allow normal ventilation. In these circumstances, positive end-expiratory pressure is not helpful. Some chest drain suction must be maintained; if the drains are merely connected to an underwater seal, there will be progressive collapse of the lungs once spontaneous respiration is established.

Weaning from the ventilator

In the patient who has become accustomed to a raised PCO_2, it is important to recognize that it will be some days before the respiratory center will return to normal function; when the patient is weaned from the ventilator, he will require a PCO_2 similar to the preoperative level. As with any immunosuppressed patient, it is desirable to extubate the patient as soon as possible.

Post-transplant bleeding

At our center, there is no question that the major problem immediately following heart–lung transplantation has been bleeding. This has occurred despite the liberal administration of platelets and fresh frozen plasma. The common cause is bleeding from adhesions that developed after previous surgery. Even in patients who had not undergone previous surgery, however, the extensive mediastinal dissection required can lead to difficulty in achieving complete hemostasis, particularly in areas that are no longer accessible through a median sternotomy once the heart and lungs are in position. The problem may be compounded in some patients by hepatic dysfunction consequent to chronic hypoxia or congestive cardiac failure. In two of our patients, a right thoracotomy was required to gain access to such bleeding points.

References

1. Reitz, B.A., Wallwork, J.L., Hunt, S.A., Pennock, J.L., Billingham, M.E., Oyer, P.E., Stinson, E.B. and Shumway, N.E. (1982). Heart–lung transplantation: successful therapy for patients with pulmonary vascular disease. *N. Engl. J. Med.*, **306**, 557
2. Hutter, J.A., Despins, P., Higenbottam, T., Stewart, S. and Wallwork, J. (1988). Heart–lung transplantation: better use of resources. *Am. J. Med.*, **85**, 4
3. Cotes, J.E. (1979). In *Lung Function – Assessment and Applications in Medicine*. 4th ed., p. 386. (London: Blackwell)
4. Wallwork, J., Jones, K., Cavarocchi, N., Hakim, M. and Higenbottam, T. (1987). Distant procurement of organs for clinical heart–lung transplantation using a single flush technique. *Transplantation*, **44**, 654
5. Hakim, M., Higenbottam, T., Bethune, D., Cory-Pearce, R., English, T.A.H., Kneeshaw, J., Wells, F.C. and Wallwork, J. (1988). Selection and procurement of combined heart and lung grafts for transplantation. *J. Thorac. Cardiovasc. Surg.*, **95**, 474
6. Wheeldon, D.R., Wallwork, J., Bethune, D.W. and English, T.A.H. (1988). Storage and transport of heart and heart–lung donor organs with inflatable cushions and eutectoid cooling. *J. Heart Transplant.*, **7**, 265
7. Shelley, M., Bethune, D.W. and Latimer, R.D. (1986). A comparison

of five heat and moisture exchangers. *Anesthesia*, **41**, 527
8. Bethune, D.W. (1976). Organ damage after open heart surgery. *Lancet*, **2**, 1410
9. Wheeldon, D.R., Bethune, D.W. and Gill, R. (1986). Perfusion for cardiac transplantation. *Perfusion*, **1**, 57
10. Hakim, M., Wheeldon, D., Bethune, D.W., Milstein, B.B., English, T.A.H. and Wallwork, J. (1985). Hemodialysis and hemofiltration on cardiopulmonary bypass. *Thorax*, **40**, 101

37
Surgical Technique of the Recipient Operation

D. NOVITZKY AND D.K.C. COOPER

INTRODUCTION

Careful selection of the donor organs (as outlined in Chapter 35) is essential for the success of the procedure. In particular, close matching of size between donor heart–lung bloc and the recipient thoracic cavity is important. We believe success of the operation is increased by ensuring as short an ischemic time as possible, as lung preservation techniques remain less than perfect. The technique of excision of the donor organs has been described in Chapter 35. The technique of the recipient operation was developed over many years in the laboratory (Chapter 33), and has been described by several authors, noticeably Jamieson et al.[1,2].

MOBILIZATION AND EXCISION OF RECIPIENT HEART AND LUNGS

A median sternotomy is performed. Dissection of the anterior mediastinal structures is carried out with electrocautery. The thymus is divided, and the left innominate vein is exposed. The pericardium is opened in the midline, the incision being extended from the diaphragmatic reflection to the reflection on to the aorta. Transverse incisions through the diaphragmatic reflections of the pericardium are extended laterally to expose the apex of the left ventricle and entire right atrium. Cranially, the pericardium is incised laterally in each direction to expose the arch of the aorta, and the origins of the brachiocephalic and left common carotid arteries.

The ascending aorta is mobilized from the pulmonary artery (Figure 37.1). The pericardium is dissected off the superior vena cava (SVC), exposing the vessel up to the origin of the azygos vein. Tapes are placed around the ascending aorta, SVC and inferior vena cava (IVC).

The sternal spreader is opened more widely, and the pleural cavities entered using electrocautery. On each side an incision is made in the pleura immediately posterior to the sternum, extending from the manubrium to the diaphragm. At each end the incision is continued posteriorly to within 3–4 cm of the phrenic nerve. Any pleural adhesions present between lung and chest wall are divided with cautery. Retraction on the thoracic organs is gentle, care being taken to avoid compromising hemodynamic stability.

Initiation of cardiopulmonary bypass

A single (or double) purse string suture of a suitable material is placed in the aorta as high as possible, the most convenient site being on the left anterolateral surface of the vessel between the origins of the brachiocephalic and left common carotid arteries (Figure 37.1). On the venous side, purse string sutures are placed anteriorly in the SVC just proximal to the azygos vein, and in the IVC close to the diaphragm. Following full heparinization, aorta, SVC and IVC cannulas are inserted (Figure 37.2).

Cardiopulmonary bypass is initiated, and body temperature is reduced to 24–26°C. While cooling is taking place, the SVC and IVC are snared (snugged) to bring about total cardiopulmonary bypass. An aortic cross-clamp is applied proximal to the aortic cannula (Figure 37.2).

Excision of recipient heart and lungs

The subsequent surgical procedures in the recipient consist of: (1) cardiectomy, (2) dissection and excision of the left atrial posterior wall, pulmonary veins and pulmonary arteries, (3) preparation of the pleuropericardial (phrenic, neurovascular) pedicles on each side, (4) bilateral pneumonectomy, (5) mobilization of the bronchi and carina in the posterior mediastinum, (6) division of the trachea above the carina, and excision of the tracheobronchial remnants.

THE TRANSPLANTATION AND REPLACEMENT OF THORACIC ORGANS

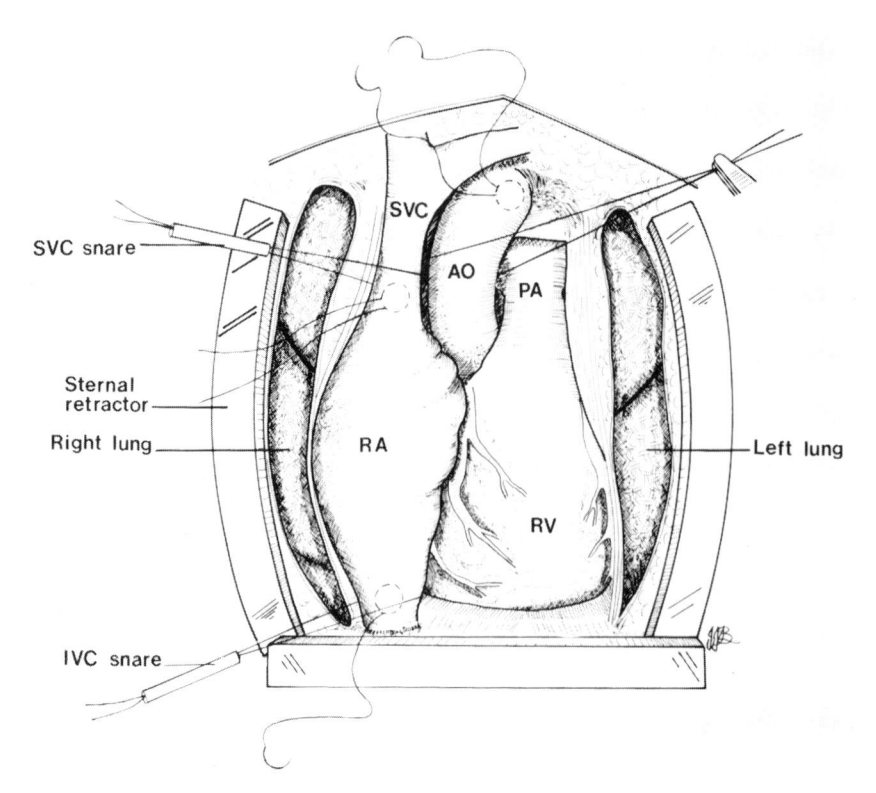

Figure 37.1 A median sternotomy has been performed. The ascending aorta has been mobilized from the pulmonary artery. Tapes have been passed around the ascending aorta, superior (SVC) and inferior (IVC) venae cavae. Purse-string sutures have been placed in the aorta, SVC and IVC. The pleura has been opened on each side anterior to the phrenic nerves, exposing the lungs. (Abbreviations used in this chapter. SVC = superior vena cava; RA = right atrium; IVC = inferior vena cava; RV = right ventricle; PA = pulmonary artery; LA = left atrium; LV = left ventricle; AO = aorta)

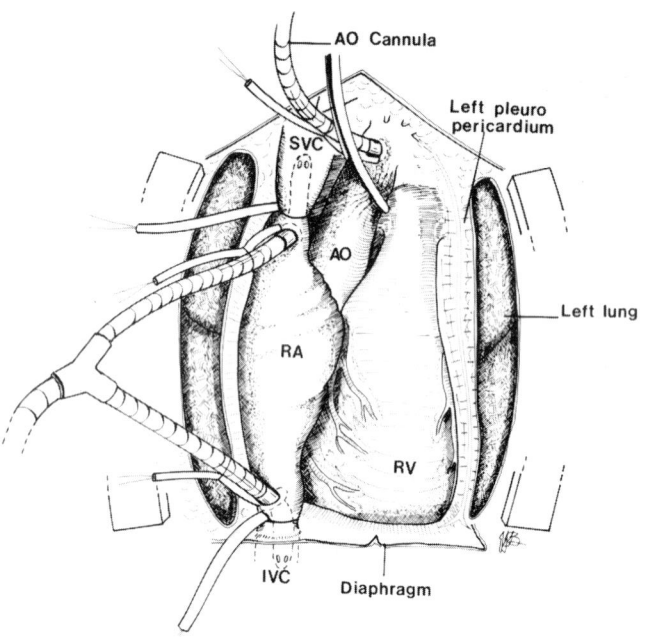

Figure 37.2 The aorta, SVC and IVC have been cannulated, and the ascending aorta cross-clamped

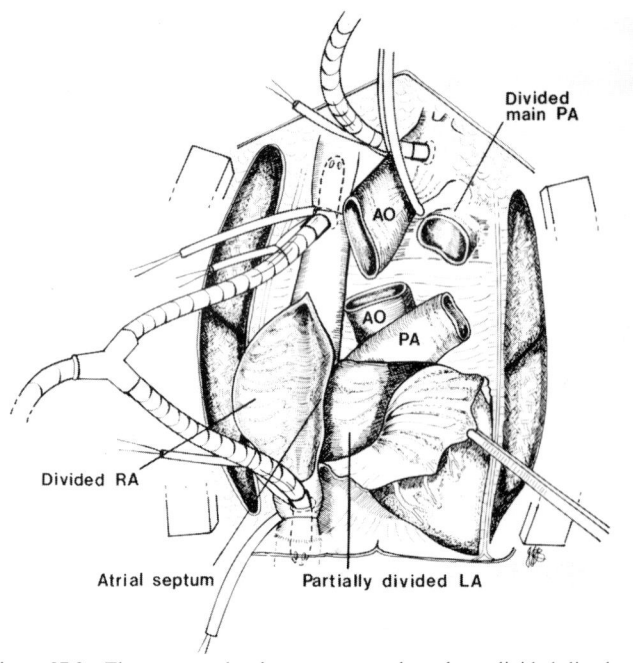

Figure 37.3 The aorta and pulmonary artery have been divided distal to their respective valves. The right atrium has been divided, and the left atrium is in the process of division

Cardiectomy

The aorta and pulmonary artery are divided immediately distal to their respective valves (Figure 37.3). The right atrium is transected (as for orthotopic heart transplantation (Chapter 10)), the incision being extended from the SVC–right atrial junction towards the IVC close to the atrioventricular groove; the right atrial appendage is included in the tissue removed. The interatrial septum is incised immediately proximal to the tricuspid valve. By lifting the heart anteriorly and to the right, the lateral wall of the left atrium is incised. Finally, the remaining (cranial) portion of the left atrial wall is transected. The heart has now been completely mobilized, and can be removed from the pericardial cavity.

Dissection and excision of left atrial posterior wall, pulmonary veins and pulmonary arteries

The posterior wall of the left atrium is divided in its midline (Figure 37.4); the transection involves those parts of the posterior wall that are both intra- and extrapericardial. Each half of the left atrium is then attached to its corresponding pulmonary veins. The left pulmonary veins (with attached posterior wall of left atrium) are mobilized towards the pulmonary hilum, at which point they are divided (Figure 37.5). The left half of the left atrium with its attached pulmonary veins can now be removed from the pericardial cavity.

The right side of the left atrium is attached to the interatrial septum, requiring careful dissection in that area. Injury to the posterior wall of the right atrium or SVC must be avoided. In the region close to the IVC, there is a fat pad providing a plane between the left atrium and interatrial septum, assisting in the dissection. In the mid-portion of the septum, however, dissection is difficult, and it is most convenient to leave the septum intact as a single unit.

Attention should now be turned towards the right pulmonary veins and that portion of the left atrium seen to the right side of the right atrium. The right-sided remnant of the left atrium is dissected from the interatrial septum, and the remaining posterior wall of the left atrium is mobilized. The pericardial reflections and the right pulmonary veins are incised, and the veins mobilized towards the pulmonary hilum, at which point they are divided and removed with the attached portion of left atrium.

Some surgeons feel that it is not essential to excise all of the posterior wall of the left atrium; if left *in situ*, mediastinal bleeding may be reduced.

The main pulmonary artery is excised, and the right and left pulmonary arteries divided in the midline at the bifurcation (Figure 37.6). Each artery is mobilized laterally as far as reasonably possible, and divided, allowing removal. A 'button' of the left pulmonary artery remains *in situ* attached to the left inferior wall of the arch of the aorta to ensure that the left recurrent laryngeal nerve is not damaged (Figures 37.6 and 37.7).

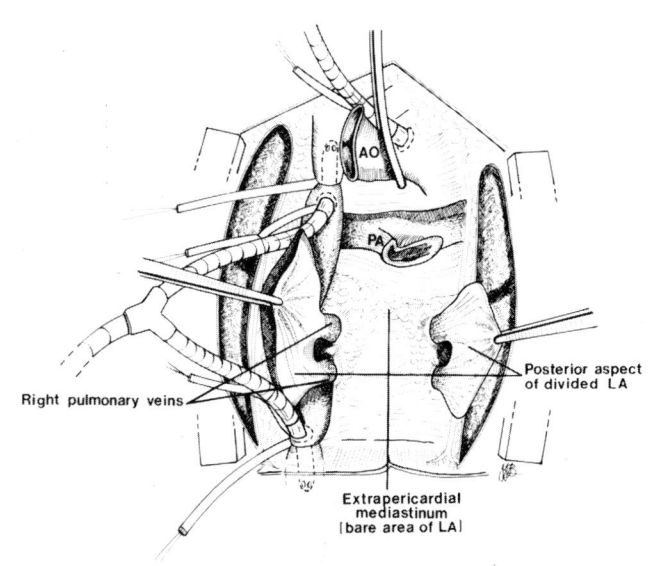

Figure 37.5 The pulmonary veins on both sides are being mobilized towards the pulmonary hila. The posterior walls of each half of the left atrium are being retracted anterolaterally by forceps

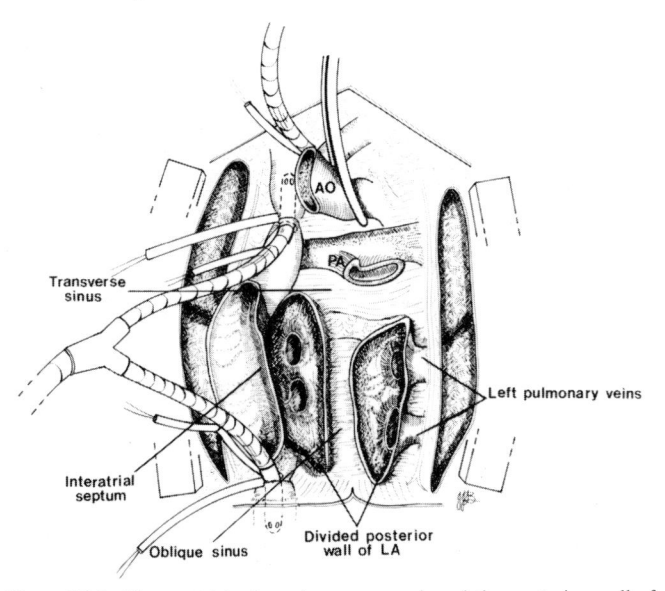

Figure 37.4 The ventricles have been removed, and the posterior wall of the left atrium has been divided in its midline

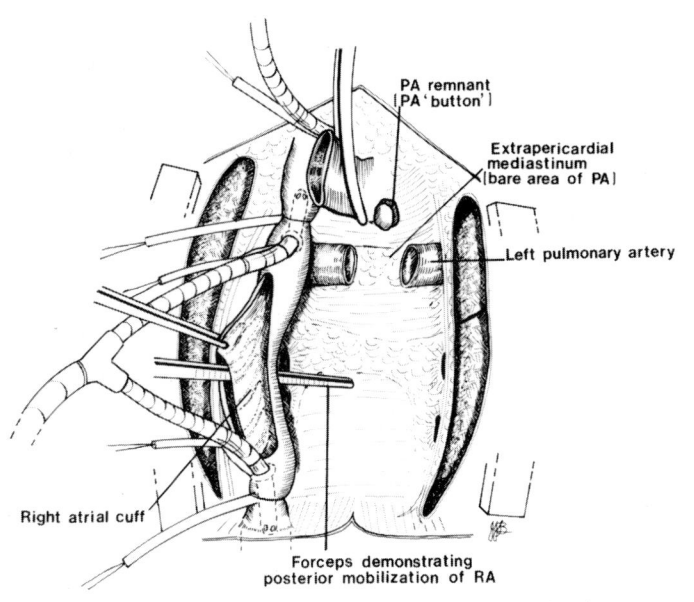

Figure 37.6 The posterior remnants of the left atrium and pulmonary veins have been excised. The right atrium has been mobilized posteriorly. The main pulmonary artery has been excised leaving a remnant ('button') attached to the aorta to protect the left recurrent laryngeal nerve

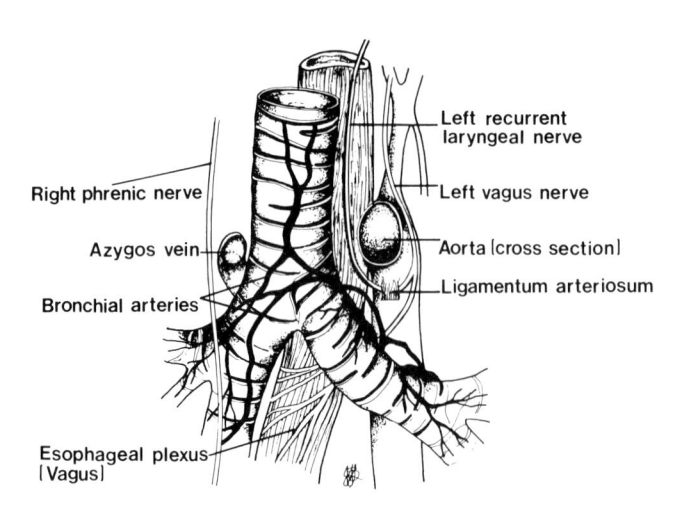

Figure 37.7 Drawing to illustrate the proximity of major thoracic nerves to the trachea, bronchi, and aorta. The potential sites of damage of these nerves during the operation of transplantation of the heart and lungs are obvious

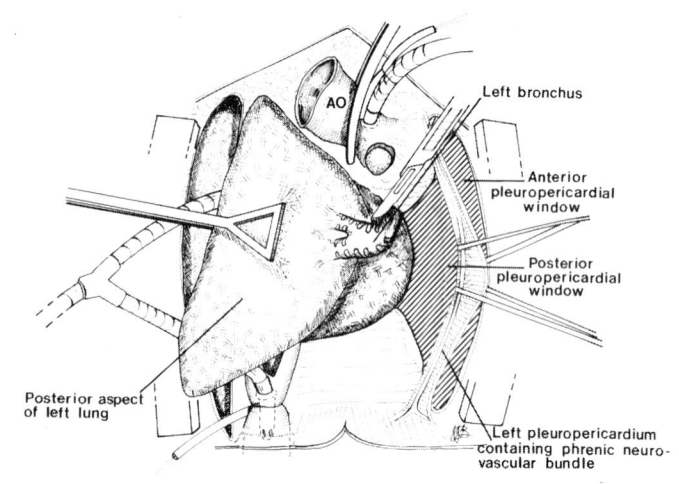

Figure 37.8 The left pleuropericardium has been incised posterior to the phrenic nerve. The left lung has been withdrawn from the left cavity into the pericardial cavity by passing it posterior to the phrenic neurovascular pedicle. The left bronchus has been dissected out and is about to be stapled and divided

Preparation of the pleuropericardial (phrenic, neurovascular) pedicles

Left side Following identification of the left phrenic nerve throughout the entire length of its course, the pleuropericardium is incised 2 cm anterior to the nerve at the level of the pulmonary hilum. The incision is extended caudally to the diaphragm, and cranially to the level of the aortic arch. The anterior excess of pleuropericardium is removed. Using a scalpel or scissors, the pleuropericardium is carefully incised posterior to the neurovascular pedicle immediately anterior to the hilum. There is usually a distance of only 1.5–2.0 cm between the hilar structures and the phrenic neurovascular bundle. The pleuropericardium is divided posteriorly parallel to the phrenic nerve, extending this incision for a similar distance to that made anterior to the nerve (Figure 37.8).

Right side The anterior incision in the right pleuropericardium is identical to that on the left side, with the exception that its cranial end will extend approximately to the level of the azygos vein. Usually the distance between the bundle and the right pulmonary hilum is less than that on the left, the phrenic nerve lying in close proximity to the right hilar structures. The distance between bundle and hilar structures is generally only 1 cm or less. The incision posterior to the neurovascular bundle must, therefore, be made with even more care than that on the left side.

Two silastic tapes are placed around each neurovascular pedicle to allow subsequent gentle retraction and help avoid traumatic manipulation.

Bilateral pneumonectomy

Left side The lungs are allowed to collapse completely. The left pulmonary ligament is divided with electrocautery.

The left lung is brought into the pericardial sac by passing it posterior to the phrenic neurovascular pedicle (Figure 37.8). The posterior pleural reflection to the left hilum is incised with cautery, care being taken not to injure the esophagus or descending aorta.

Using blunt dissection, the remnants of the left pulmonary veins are visualized within the pericardial sac. The remaining tissues are divided with extreme caution as many bronchial arteries, arising directly from the aorta, may be present, particularly in patients with congenital heart disease. Hemoclips are applied to bronchial arteries before their division. The vagus nerve is also close, its branches encompassing the esophagus, which lies immediately posterior to the point of dissection (Figure 37.7).

The dissection is extended cranially to mobilize the remnant of the left pulmonary artery. The left bronchus is palpated, and the surrounding tissue divided with cautery. At a convenient point, the left bronchus is stapled twice and divided between the rows of staples (Figure 37.8). The left lung is removed.

Right side The lung is mobilized cranially, and the pulmonary ligament exposed and divided, as on the left side. The right lung is introduced into the pericardial cavity by bringing it posterior to the right phrenic pedicle and right atrial cuff. The pleura posterior to the hilum is incised with cautery, and the same dissection carried out as on the left side to enable the right lung to be removed from the chest.

Mobilization of the bronchi, division of the trachea, and excision of the bronchial remnants

The posterior mediastinum can now be seen (Figure 37.9). The posterior pericardium remains intact anterior to the

SURGICAL TECHNIQUE OF THE RECIPIENT OPERATION

esophagus, and should be left in place, thus avoiding trauma to the vagus nerve and its branches. The aortic cross-clamp is rotated slightly to the left, thus retracting the aorta to the left and separating this vessel from the trachea, which is exposed posteriorly and to the right (Figure 37.9). The endotracheal tube can be readily palpated, confirming the position of the trachea. The bifurcation of the trachea into the two bronchi (the carina) is identified by palpation.

With electrocautery, the pericardium and areolar tissue anterior to the lower centimeter of the trachea are divided, exposing the lowest tracheal cartilages. The dissection is extended towards the left and right bronchi, which structures are completely mobilized. Division of the mediastinal tissue immediately lateral to the trachea should be avoided, as the right and left vagi lie in close proximity (Figure 37.7). The trachea is divided immediately proximal to the carina (Figure 37.9). The cranial trachea will immediately retract upwards. (Some surgeons prefer to insert one or two sutures into the trachea before final division to facilitate drawing it back into the surgical field when the tracheal anastomosis is to be performed.) A swab of any tracheal secretions is taken and sent for culture of micro-organisms. The right and left bronchial remnants can now be removed (Figure 37.10).

Further mediastinal tissue dissection should be avoided as the tissues surrounding the lower trachea carry small arteries essential for the blood supply of the retained trachea (Figure 37.11). The use of cautery should be avoided in this area as it may produce thermal necrosis of cartilage and may result in failure of healing of the tracheal anastomosis.

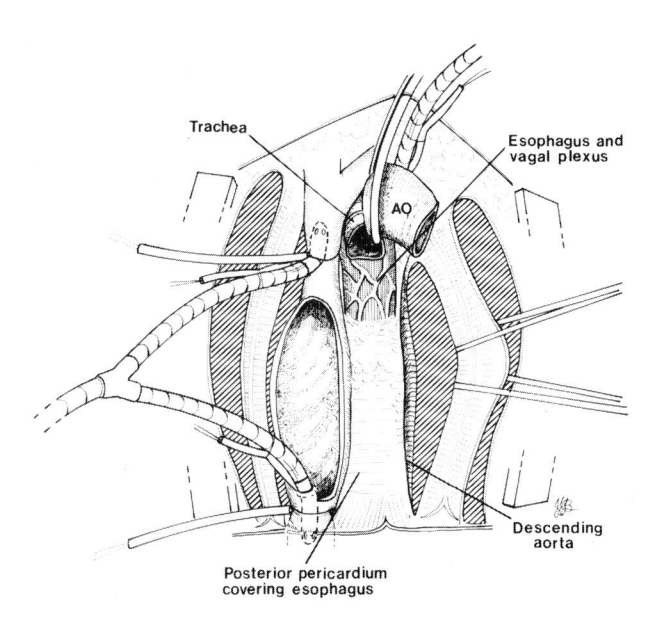

Figure 37.10 Excision of the lower trachea and two major bronchi has exposed the esophagus and vagal plexus. The recipient chest cavity is now prepared to receive the donor organs

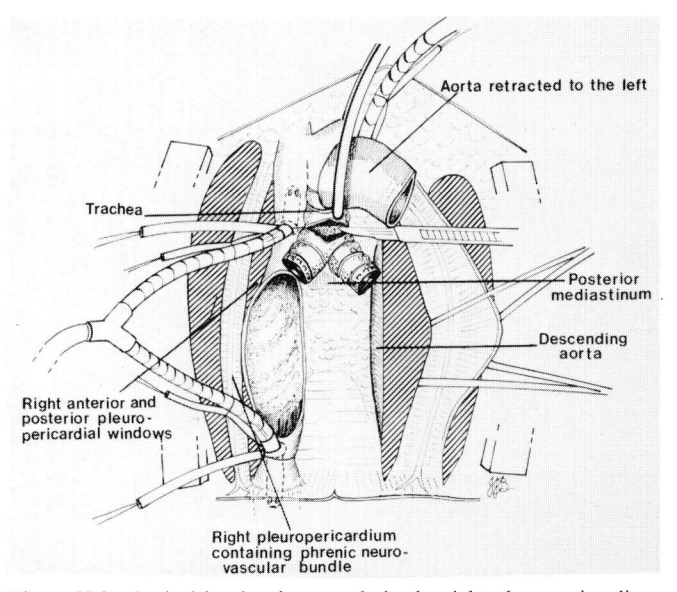

Figure 37.9 An incision has been made in the right pleuropericardium posterior to the right phrenic neurovascular bundle. The right lung has been withdrawn into the pericardial cavity, and has been excised (as was the left lung). The remnants of the two bronchi and lower trachea have been mobilized, and are being excised

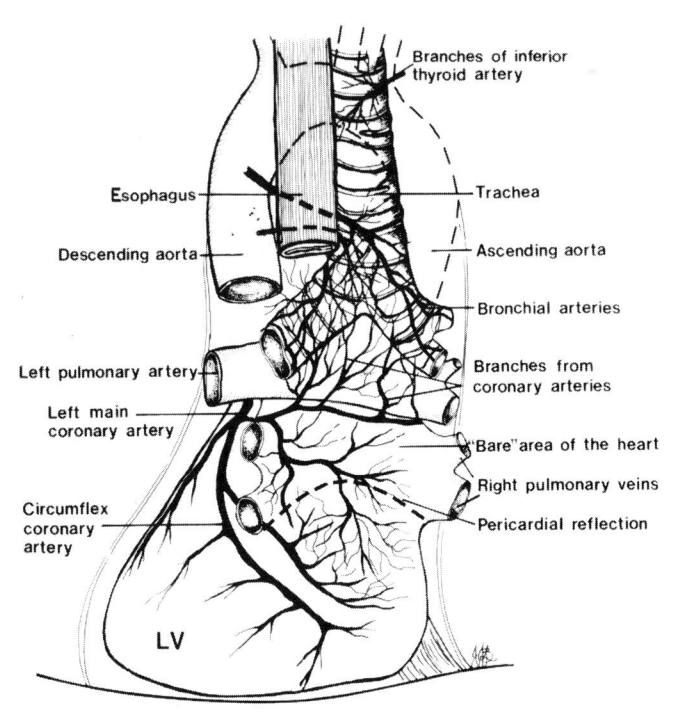

Figure 37.11 Posterior view of heart and trachea, showing sources of arterial blood supply to the trachea, carina, and bronchi

Hemostasis should be obtained by applying small hemoclips or sutures.

Hemostasis

It is essential to ensure that meticulous hemostasis is achieved in all of the dissected areas. In particular, careful examination should be carried out in the region of divided pleural adhesions, the pulmonary ligaments, and the 'bare area' of the mediastinum that lies anterior to the esophagus.

The recipient is now ready for implantation of the donor organs.

IMPLANTATION OF DONOR ORGANS

The donor organs are brought to the surgical field. Swabs for culture of micro-organisms are taken from both the bronchi, and mucus secretions are then aspirated from the bronchi; the suction device is discarded to prevent subsequent contamination of the surgical field.

Preparation of donor organs

The donor trachea is transected one or, at most, two cartilages superior to the origins of the bronchi (to minimize the risk of ischemic necrosis). Dissection of the areolar tissue around the lower trachea and bronchi, and of the tissue between the carina and left atrium, is avoided. It is believed valuable to preserve this tissue as a fine arterial network exists between the coronary arteries and the bronchial arteries (Figure 37.11); this network probably provides a small but important blood supply to the donor bronchi and trachea following transection and interruption of the blood flow from the bronchial arteries, thus helping to reduce the possibility of ischemic necrosis of these structures.

The donor right atrium is prepared by incising its anterolateral wall from the opening of the IVC into the base of the right atrial appendage (as in orthotopic heart transplantation), the length of the incision being judged primarily by the size of the recipient right atrial cuff (Figure 37.12). This incision in the donor right atrium can be lengthened, if necessary, immediately before or during performance of the right atrial anastomosis.

Positioning of donor organs in the chest

The heart–lung bloc is introduced into the recipient's chest (Figure 37.12). The heart is positioned in the pericardial cavity. The left lung is introduced into the left pleural cavity by passing it posterior to the left phrenic neurovascular pedicle. The right lung is introduced into the right pleural cavity by passing it posterior both to the right atrial cuff and to the right phrenic pedicle. It is convenient at this stage to identify each lobe, and position the lungs in such a way to ensure that rotation of the lung or lobe at the hilum is not present, as this will prevent proper air entry and/or blood flow subsequently when ventilation is commenced.

Three anastomoses are required – tracheal, right atrial,

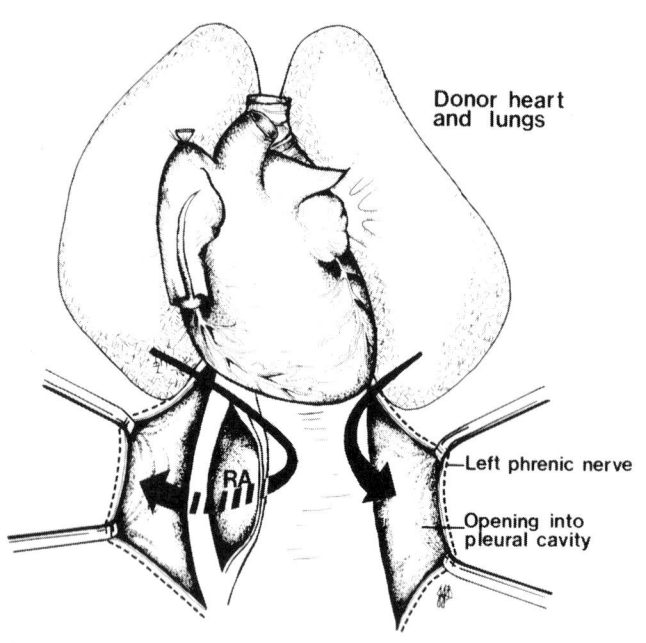

Figure 37.12 The donor heart and lungs will be inserted into the recipient chest by passing the donor right lung posterior to the recipient right atrium and right phrenic neurovascular bundle. The donor left lung will be passed posterior to the left phrenic neurovascular bundle. An incision has been made in the wall of the donor right atrium from the orifice of the IVC into the atrial appendage

and aortic. In between each anastomosis, copious amounts (1–2 liters) of cold saline (at 4°C) are applied over the heart and both lungs to prevent the tissues from warming rapidly. Ice or cold slush should not be used as thermal injury of the phrenic pedicles may result, leading to paralysis of the diaphragm.

Tracheal anastomosis

The anesthesiologist is asked to flex the head of the patient slightly to facilitate the tracheal anastomosis by making the recipient tracheal stump, which has retracted cranially, become more accessible to the surgeon. Two 'stay' sutures are placed, one on the right and one on the left, at the junction of the membranous–cartilaginous donor trachea, and then through similar points in the recipient trachea. These sutures are not tied, but are used both to hold the recipient trachea in the surgical field and as an aid to carrying out the anastomosis, especially if the two tracheas are of widely differing diameters. As the membranous portion is the most pliable part of the tracheal wall, any discrepancy in the two diameters should be corrected mainly in this area.

The performance of the tracheal suture line can be accomplished by several different techniques. Our own preference will be described. Using a double-ended 4.0 polypropylene suture, the tracheal anastomosis is begun in the membranous portion in the midline (Figure 37.13). This

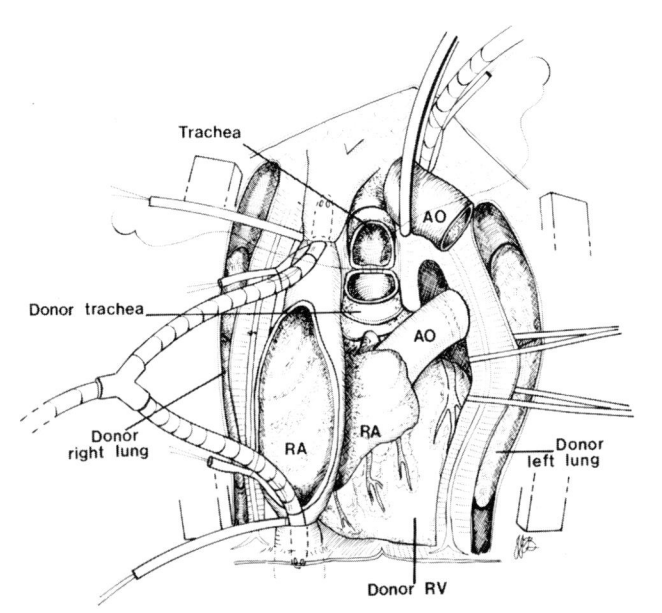

SURGICAL TECHNIQUE OF THE RECIPIENT OPERATION

Figure 37.13 The donor heart and lungs are now in position in the recipient's chest. The tracheal anastomosis is being carried out. (The stay sutures at the junction of the membranous–cartilaginous tracheas are not shown)

first suture is tied with the knot externally, anterior to the esophagus. The two membranous tracheas are anastomosed by continuous sutures carried in each direction (left and right). At this stage, the previously-placed 'stay' sutures at the membranous–cartilaginous junctions are tied down, and then further tied to the respective free end of the continuous suture. (It may be helpful to place a further 'stay' suture at the midpoints of the anterior walls of the trachea, again to help in adjusting for mismatch in tracheal size.)

From the junction of the membranous–cartilaginous portions of the trachea, each end of the 4.0 suture is brought anteriorly in a continuous running fashion, until they meet anteriorly in the midline, where they are tied. The sutures should preferably be introduced through the cartilaginous rings or immediately around the cartilage, avoiding the intercartilaginous membranes, as this may result in laceration and air leaks.

Once the tracheas have been anastomosed, the anesthesiologist is asked to ventilate the lungs at a pressure of not more than 30–40 cmH$_2$O. Saline is poured over the anastomosis and the suture line examined for any air leak. If an air leak is identified, it is closed with an interrupted suture of 4.0 polypropylene.

Some surgeons prefer to perform the anastomosis with interrupted sutures throughout, as they believe this technique is less likely to result in tissue ischemia, and therefore more likely to lead to satisfactory healing of the anastomosis. The best technique is as yet uncertain. If paratracheal dissection is kept to a minimum, and care taken not to denude either donor or recipient trachea of its surrounding areolar tissue with its microscopic vasculature, and if cautery is not used on the divided edges of the trachea, thus minimizing the risk of tissue (especially cartilage) necrosis, then we believe satisfactory healing of the tracheal anastomosis will take place with either suture technique. It would also seem to be important to divide the donor trachea as close as possible to the origins of the bronchi, thus minimizing the length of donor trachea that requires a blood supply.

Once the anastomosis has been completed and air leak excluded, the anterior and lateral surfaces of the suture line are covered with paratracheal mediastinal tissue (predominantly donor areolar tissue posterior to the left atrium), using interrupted sutures of 4.0 polypropylene (Figure 37.14). Each suture should endeavor to pick up, in order, (1) donor paratracheal tissue, (2) the tracheal anastomosis, and, finally, (3) recipient paratracheal tissue, including pericardium forming the posterior wall of the transverse sinus, before being tied. This results in the site of anastomosis being closely covered by mediastinal areolar and connective tissue, thus helping to seal the suture holes and anastomosis, and prevent any subsequent air leak, even if a minor degree of ischemic necrosis of one or other trachea occurs. The paratracheal tissue may also, in time, prove a source of blood supply to the region of the tracheal anastomosis, as microscopic vessels may grow from it across the adhesions which develop to the tracheal walls.

(Some surgeons believe it is advisable (or even essential)

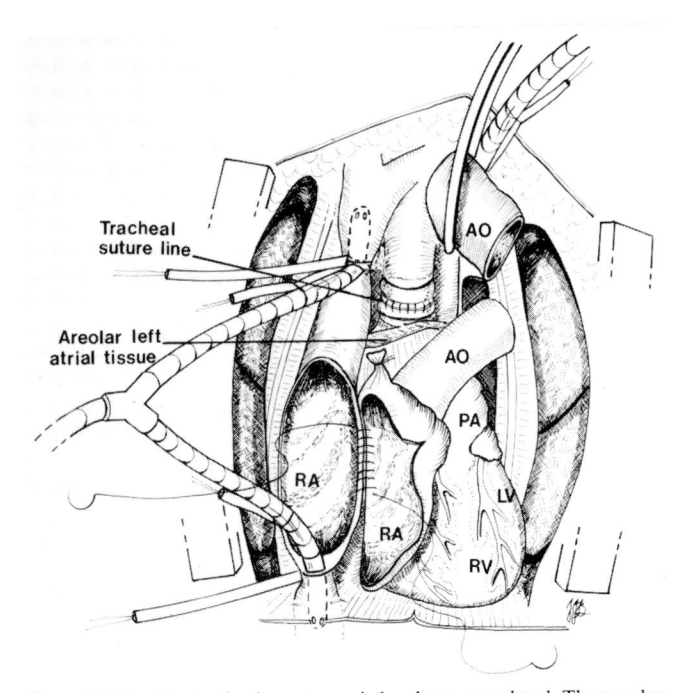

Figure 37.14 The tracheal anastomosis has been completed. The areolar tissue around the donor left atrium which is used to cover the site of the tracheal suture line is indicated, but in this drawing has not been sutured over the anastomosis. The two right atria are in process of being anastomosed

to bring up the omentum as a further protection against air leak, and as a further source of blood supply. If this is to be performed, mobilization of the omentum is done either at the beginning of the operation before heparin is given and cardiopulmonary bypass instituted, or after discontinuation of cardiopulmonary bypass and the administration of protamine sulfate; in this way, bleeding from the mobilization can be kept to a minimum. Though we do not believe this to be always essential, it should certainly be performed whenever there is any concern that the tracheal anastomosis is less than perfect. For example, when the tracheal anastomosis has been performed with some difficulty, or when there has been an air leak which proved difficult to control, or a lack of mediastinal tissue to cover the suture line, it is advisable to mobilize the omentum and wrap it circumferentially around the anastomosis both for extra protection and in an endeavor to provide a further vascular supply to this region (see below).)

Anastomosis of right atria

The donor right atrium is positioned anterior to the recipient right atrium (Figure 37.14). The oblique incision in the donor right atrial wall can be lengthened at this stage if necessary, to match the orifice of the recipient right atrium. Any patent foramen ovale in the recipient (or donor) septum can be closed at this stage. The right atrial anastomosis is accomplished with a continuous double-ended 4.0 polypropylene suture, starting at the midpoint of the medial (left) wall of the two right atria (the remnant of the atrial septum) and continuing first caudally around the IVC, and then cranially (Figure 37.14). Thereafter, the sutures are carried along the lateral (right) wall of the right atrium, and tied to each other at the midpoint of this wall.

Anastomosis of aortae

The lengths of the two aortae are assessed, and excess tissue trimmed from one or both ends. End-to-end anastomosis is performed with a continuous double-ended 4.0 polypropylene suture (Figure 37.15) (as in orthotopic heart transplantation (Chapter 10)).

(Before release of the aortic cross-clamp, it is our policy to administer 1 g of methylprednisolone. It is also our practice to give at this stage triiodothyronine (T3) 0.15 μg/kg patient weight i.v. via the pump-oxygenator (see Chapter 10).)

Removal of air from heart chambers

Air is removed from the heart and pulmonary vessels by inserting large-bore needles (e.g. a 14 gauge, the sheath of

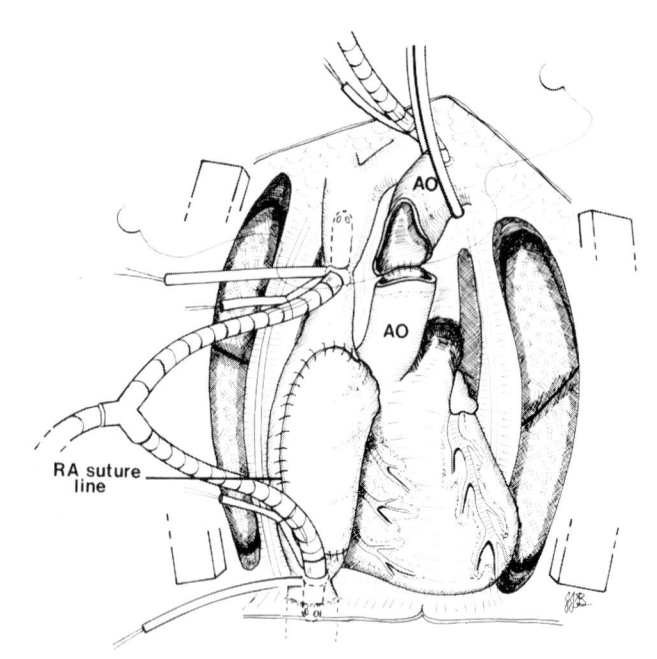

Figure 37.15 The right atrial anastomosis has been completed. The aortic anastomosis is in progress

which has been partially resected longitudinally ('slotted')), into the aorta, main pulmonary artery, and both left and right ventricles. In addition, an incision is made in the left atrial appendage (if this has not been performed during excision of the donor organs). The snares around the SVC and IVC are removed, thus increasing venous return to the right atrium, and full ventilation of the lung is initiated, thus increasing venous return to the left atrium, expelling any air from the pulmonary veins. The heart is gently massaged to expel air through the various needles, and the aortic cross-clamp is removed. At this stage, warming of the patient is begun.

Subsequent procedures and discontinuation of cardiopulmonary bypass

The aortic and right atrial suture lines are examined carefully, and further sutures inserted if necessary. If coordinated contractions do not develop spontaneously, but vigorous ventricular fibrillation occurs, the heart is electrically defibrillated. If this results in asystole or atrioventricular dissociation, the ventricles are paced, temporary pacing wires being inserted into the anterior wall of the right ventricle.

During rewarming, an oxymetric Swan–Ganz catheter can be introduced into the pulmonary artery by the anesthesiologist. When cardiac and pulmonary functions are considered adequate, with or without inotropic support (our own preference is for isoproterenol), then pump-oxygenator support can be discontinued. All cannulae can then be

SURGICAL TECHNIQUE OF THE RECIPIENT OPERATION

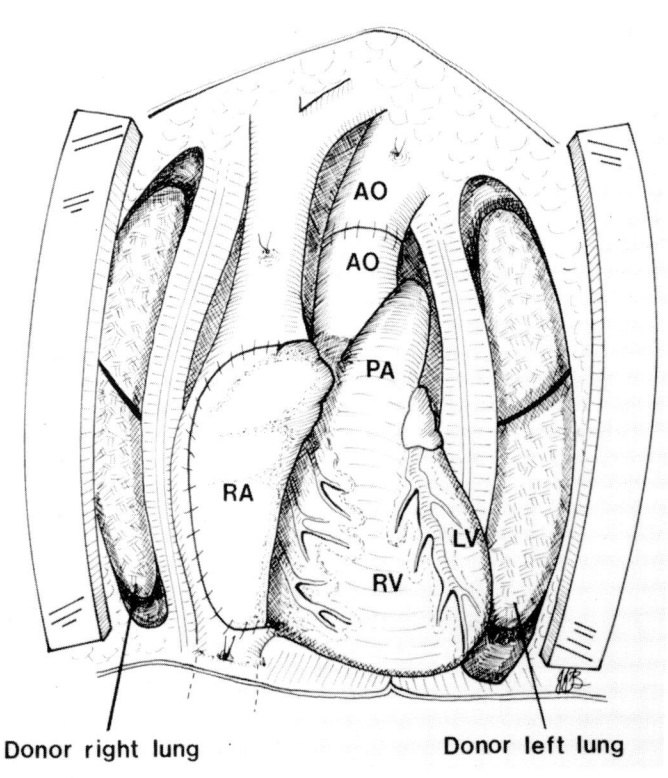

Figure 37.16 The aortic anastomosis has been completed, and all cannulae have been removed

removed (Figure 37.16) and protamine sulfate given. At this stage ventilation is with 100% oxygen (FiO_2 1.0). It is helpful to monitor the mixed venous oxygen as a reflection of both cardiac and pulmonary functions. If the oxygen saturation in the pulmonary artery remains satisfactory (60–70%), the FiO_2 can be progressively and rapidly reduced to 0.5 (50%). In the early post-bypass period, the cardiac preload (central venous pressure) should be maintained as low as possible; this may help reduce the development of pulmonary interstitial edema.

Mobilization of omentum

If a decision has been made to support the tracheal suture line with an omental wrap, the midline sternotomy incision is extended down into the anterior abdominal wall. The greater omentum is located, and brought through the abdominal incision. As its length is usually insufficient to reach to the area of the tracheal anastomosis, the omentum is dissected free from the transverse colon (Figure 37.17a). The omental vascular pedicles from the gastroepiploic arteries are preserved. Once enough length has been mobilized, the omentum is passed into the chest through an incision in the diaphragm, care being taken to avoid torsion of (or tension on) the greater curvature of the stomach (Figure 37.17b).

The omentum is probably best placed to the right side of the heart, between the right atrium and right lung, with its distal end lying between the aorta and trachea (Figure 37.18). The distal tip of omentum may be partially divided, forming a 'Y', allowing support of the tracheal anastomosis both anteriorly and posteriorly (Figure 37.18, inset). In this way, the entire tracheal suture line may be surrounded with viable tissue. A few interrupted sutures are placed through the trachea and omentum, to fix the omentum loosely in place. The omentum is also affixed to the diaphragm to prevent the possible subsequent development of a diaphragmatic hernia. The laparotomy incision is closed in a routine fashion.

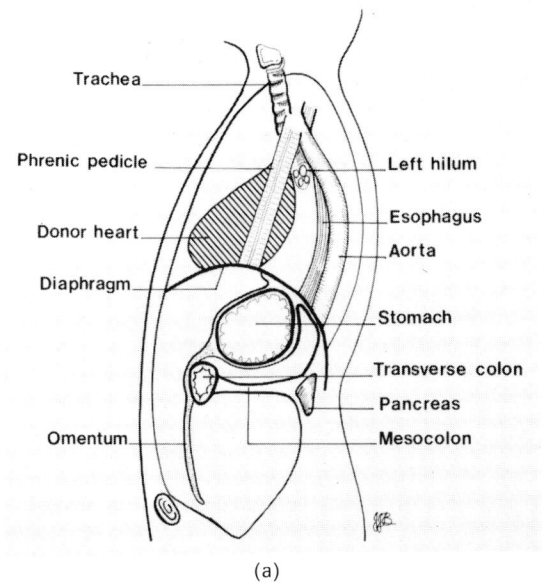

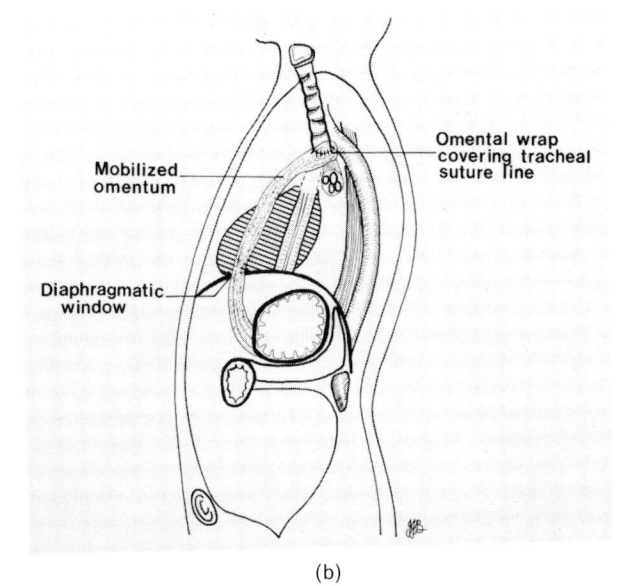

Figure 37.17 Diagrams to show basic anatomy of the omentum (a), which is mobilized and drawn into the thoracic cavity to allow it to be wrapped around the tracheal suture line (b).

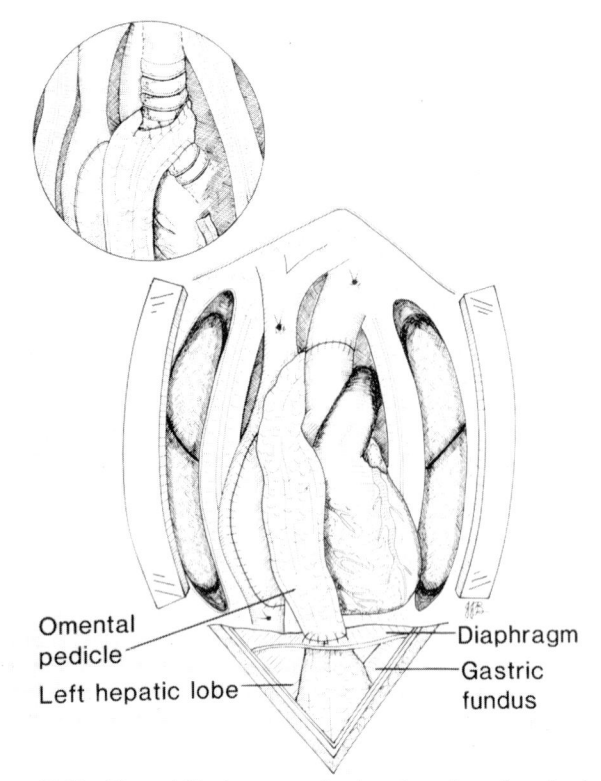

Figure 37.18 The mobilized omentum has been brought up into the chest, and in this drawing lies between the right atrium and right ventricle. It is passed posterior to the aorta and wrapped around the tracheal anastomosis (inset). The orifice in the diaphragm through which it was drawn up is closed by suturing the edges to the omentum

Chest drainage and closure

At least four drains are inserted, two in each pleural cavity, one of which is basal and one apical. With the pericardium so widely open, it is not essential to drain the pericardial sac, but it may be helpful to drain the most dependent part, inferior to the heart. The sternum is united with at least six wire or other strong sutures.

COMMENT

In patients with a previous laparotomy, or in those with an extremely short omentum, the creation of an intercostal muscle pedicle may be preferred. This can be performed on the right side (or bilaterally) at the level of the 4th or 5th intercostal space.

If bilateral injury to the vagus nerve is known to have occurred during the mediastinal dissection, it is probably advisable to perform a pyloroplasty.

If assessment of the relative sizes of the donor organs and recipient chest cavity has not been accurate, the insertion of an overly large bloc may lead to an inability to close the sternotomy. In extreme cases, lobectomy may help by reducing the pulmonary tissue volume, though this is not always successful. Occasionally only skin closure may be possible. Even this may prove impossible and the patient may have to be returned to the intensive care unit with the chest closed only by a sheet of silastic or other similar material. Usually a reduction in edema of the donor organs occurs during the next 24–48 hours, allowing sternal closure.

References

1. Jamieson, S.W., Baldwin, J., Reitz, B.A., Oyer, P.E., Billingham, M., Modry, D., Stinson, E.B., Hunt, S., Theodore, J., Bieber, C.P. and Shumway, N.E. (1983). Combined heart and lung transplantation. *Lancet*, **1**, 1130
2. Jamieson, S.W., Stinson, E.B., Oyer, P.E., Baldwin, J.C. and Shumway, N.E. (1984). Operative technique for heart–lung transplantation. *J. Thorac. Cardiovasc. Surg.*, **87**, 930

38
Postoperative Management, Surgical Complications, Diagnosis and Management of Acute Rejection

T.W. HIGENBOTTAM AND J. WALLWORK

INTRODUCTION

Combined heart–lung transplantation has advanced from an innovative surgical technique to a clinical treatment of severe pulmonary vascular disease[1], chronic end-stage lung disease[2], and cystic fibrosis[3]. Developments in organ preservation[4] (Chapters 7 and 35) and careful selection of recipients and donors, together with active investigation of lung rejection using transbronchial lung biopsy (TBB), have led to effective use of limited donor resources.

This review will concentrate upon the after-care of the patient following transplantation, and emphasize the effectiveness of shared medical and surgical care. Certain aspects of the pretransplant selection and preparation of both donor and recipient, however, require comment.

Selection of donor and recipient

Selection of donors, most of whom donate several organs, is based upon strict criteria (Table 38.1) (Chapter 35). Intracranial hemorrhage and head injury are the main causes of brain death.

Table 38.1 Selection criteria for heart–lung donors

Age below 40 years
No past history of pulmonary disease, including asthma
No major thoracic trauma
Short period of ventilation
No systemic or pulmonary infections
Normal findings on chest radiography
Normal lung compliance with a peak respiratory pressure < 20 mmHg, a tidal volume < 15 ml/kg, and a respiratory rate between 10 and 14 breaths/minute
Normal gas exchange (Pao_2 > 15 kPa on an Fio_2 of 30%)
Normal electrocardiographic findings
Inotropic requirement < 10 μg/kg per min of dopamine or dobutamine

The recipients we have selected are below 55 years of age, and can be classified into three major diagnostic groups; (1) Eisenmenger syndrome or pulmonary vascular disease, (2) chronic lung disease, including emphysema and cryptogenic fibrosing alveolitis, and (3) cystic fibrosis. No patient who continues to smoke is accepted, and those receiving an oral corticosteroid dose of more than 10 mg prednisolone/day are also excluded to minimize the problem of delayed wound healing.

Significant dysfunction of organs other than the heart and lung are exclusion criteria. The presence of liver cirrhosis can be treated with combined heart–lung and liver transplantation[5]. Insulin-requiring diabetes mellitus is a relative contraindication to heart–lung transplantation. Extrapulmonary sepsis, including mycetomas of *Aspergillus fumigatus*, where heart–lung transplantation may not eradicate the infection, remains an absolute exclusion criterion. Previous thoracotomy and/or corrective cardiac surgery are not contra-indications, but pleurectomy or pleurodesis is.

Compatibility and matching of donor and recipient

Donor and recipient must be of compatible ABO blood group. A direct cross-match for lymphocytotoxic antibodies is not performed unless prior testing of recipient serum against a random pool of lymphocytes had demonstrated cytolytic antibodies (Chapter 8).

It is often not possible to find donor lungs of similar size to those of the recipient, particularly if the patient has developed greatly enlarged lungs from, for example, emphysema, or conversely, small lungs from, for example, fibrosis. The size of the donor is assessed from his (or her) height, from which his predicted total lung capacity is estimated[6] (Figure 38.1). This is then matched with the recipient's

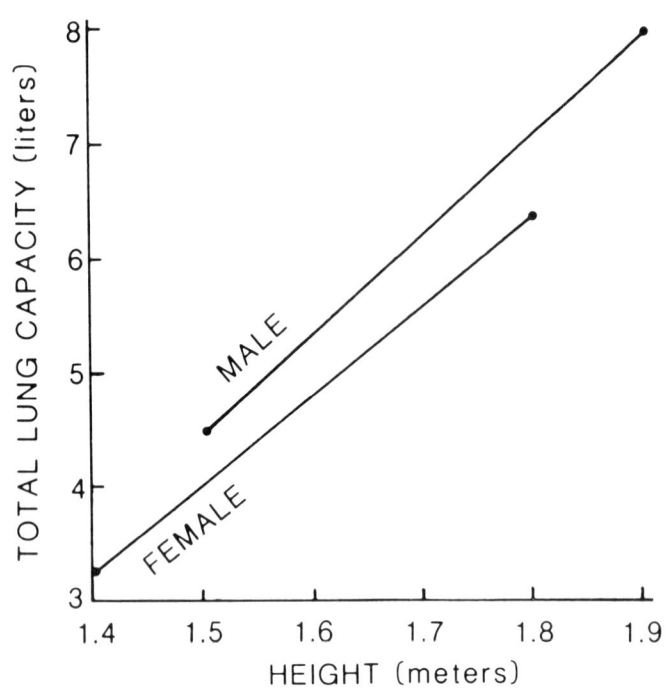

Figure 38.1 The total lung capacity of the donor can be calculated approximately from a knowledge of his/her height and sex (modified from Cotes, J.E.[6])

total lung capacity, which is already known, having been measured previously in the laboratory. A discrepancy of from 2 to 4 liters in pulmonary capacity between the donor and recipient lungs can be tolerated without the risk of complication such as atelectasis and intrapulmonary shunting, which have been reported in earlier series where donor lungs that were too large for that particular recipient were transplanted. We can therefore accept a considerable range of size of donors for each individual recipient (Figure 38.2).

Primary cytomegalovirus (CMV) pneumonitis has been the single most common cause of early postoperative death in our series[7]. It has occurred exclusively in those recipients who proved negative on serological testing for CMV, but who received organs from donors positive for CMV[8]. With the introduction of the rapid latex-agglutination test[9], it has proved possible to serotype the donor before excision of the organs; as a result, we now match CMV-positive donors with CMV-positive recipients. No deaths from CMV infection have occurred since the adoption of this policy (Table 38.2)[7]. Whilst it is possible to treat CMV pneumonitis successfully if diagnosed early enough, treatment requires hospitalization, is lengthy, and may be associated with an increased incidence of acute rejection. For these reasons, we have adhered strictly to our matching policy.

After transplantation, stored blood from each donor is tested for the presence of toxoplasma antigens, and, if positive and the recipient negative, prophylactic antibiotic therapy is administered (see below).

EARLY POSTOPERATIVE MANAGEMENT AND MAINTENANCE IMMUNOSUPPRESSION

General postoperative care

The principles of management consist of (1) early extubation (within 18–24 hours), (2) maintenance of a negative fluid balance by the judicious use of diuretics, and (3) early mobilization.

As soon as barrier nursing is withdrawn, the patient is usually returned from the intensive care unit to the ward, and is kept isolated from other patients for a further 4 days. Physiotherapy is individualized to the patient's needs. All are encouraged to mobilize as soon as possible; this includes standing, walking, and the use of pedal cycles. The special problems of the cystic fibrosis patient will be discussed later.

Antibiotics are given if the donor or recipient had infected sputum before surgery or if sputum volume increases after operation. The nature of the antibiotic is determined by the results of Gram stain and culture of the sputum. A patient previously serologically negative for toxoplasmosis, but who received organs from a donor who was seropositive, is given prophylactic pyrimethamine until seroconversion takes place.

Immunosuppressive therapy

At operation, the patient receives 1 g methylprednisolone i.v., followed by daily doses of methylprednisolone 125 mg i.v. for the first 3 days. Equine antithymocyte globulin (ATG) is also given daily for 3 days. Cyclosporine 4–6 mg/kg twice daily is given orally as soon as the patient can take an oral diet. During the 3 days of ATG therapy, the patient is 'barrier-nursed' under strict isolation conditions.

Oral maintenance immunosuppression consists of cyclosporine (approximately 6–10 mg/kg daily), ensuring a whole blood trough level of between 200 and 600 ng/ml, and azathioprine to keep the total white blood cell count below 5000 mm^3. Corticosteroid therapy is reserved only for those patients who experience repeated episodes of acute rejection (see later).

Postoperative monitoring

During the first 7 days after surgery, monitoring involves three main areas: (1) graft function, (2) the extent of immunosuppression, and (3) the presence or absence of infection.

Graft function is assessed by arterial gas samples and chest radiographs. The development of a pulmonary infiltrate, particularly with a hilar 'flare', together with pleural effusions occurring after the seventh postoperative day, can be associated with acute rejection.

Monitoring of the state of immunosuppression is basically

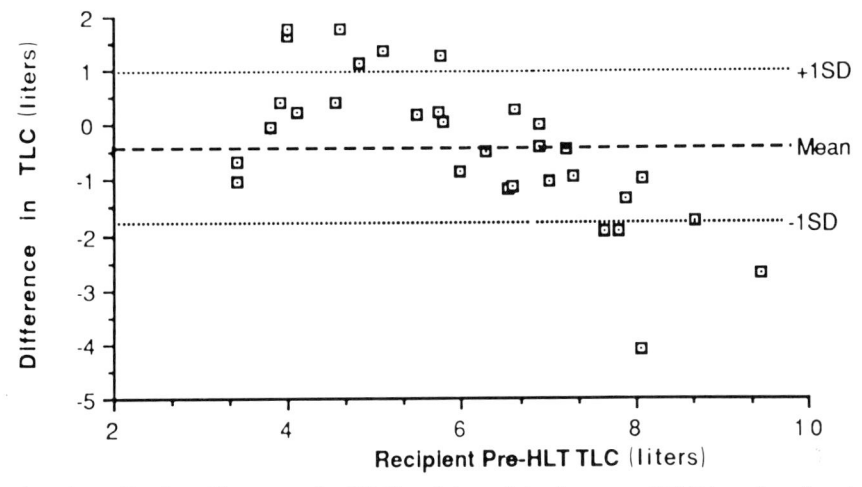

Figure 38.2 The donor's *predicted* total lung capacity (TLC) and the recipient's *measured* TLC have been found to be the best guides to size-match between donor and recipient. As a recipient may have a disease that greatly affects pretransplant TLC, matching by chest radiograph measurements alone is not considered satisfactory. In this graph, the difference between the *predicted* TLC of the donor and that of the recipient (*measured* before surgery) has been plotted against the recipient's presurgery TLC (for each of the patients in the Papworth series)

The TLC of the donor can be estimated approximately from the chart illustrated in Figure 38.1, or can be calculated accurately by one of the following two formulae, based on age, height, and sex:

Male TLC (in liters) = (7.8 × height in meters) − 7.3.
Female TLC (in liters) = (7.46 × height in meters) − (0.013 × age in years) − 6.42.

Lungs from a donor may prove to be up to 2 liters too large (e.g. when the recipient has pulmonary fibrosis) or 4 liters too small (e.g. when the recipient has emphysema) for the recipient's thoracic cavity (as measured on the chest radiograph), and yet show excellent function

Table 38.2 Influence of donor–recipient CMV serology matching policy on incidence of CMV infection

	Before introduction of policy (n)	After introduction of policy (n)
Total number of heart–lung transplants	17	16
CMV-positive recipients	10	7
CMV-negative recipients receiving CMV-positive organs	7	1
Recipients developing symptomatic CMV infection — non-fatal	3	0
Recipients developing symptomatic CMV infection — fatal	3	0

the same as in the cardiac transplant patient (Chapters 12 and 16).

Frequent samples for bacterial culture are taken of sputa, intercostal drainage sites, urine, and wounds.

Early complications

The two major early postoperative complications are persistent bleeding and persistent air leak.

Significant bleeding occurs in up to 30% of patients, principally those with Eisenmenger syndrome who have had previous cardiac surgery and those with cystic fibrosis[7]. Re-operation for such bleeding, if unilateral, is best performed by lateral thoracotomy, which enables large mediastinal collateral vessels to be identified and ligated; bilateral bleeding requires median sternotomy.

A persistent air leak and/or pneumothorax occurs in up to 20% of patients, and requires continued drainage by pleural drains maintained at a negative pressure sufficient to achieve a maximum degree of lung inflation. At our center, the longest period such air leaks have persisted has been 10 days.

MONITORING FOR ACUTE LUNG REJECTION AND PULMONARY INFECTION

Patients with heart–lung transplants remain acutely sensitive to changes in pulmonary function. Two to 3 days before a definite diagnosis of acute rejection is documented, the patient may complain of chest 'tightness' and breathlessness. Careful attention to such respiratory symptoms offers a simple means of detecting impending pulmonary rejection.

In both acute lung rejection and pulmonary infection, the principal histopathological abnormalities develop in the periphery of the lungs, with inflammatory infiltrates and edema of the alveolar septa and bronchiolar walls. These abnormalities are associated with physical signs on auscultation of the chest, namely late inspiratory crackles occasionally associated with wheezing. When acute rejection or infection occurs within the first month after operation each is often associated with fever.

Table 38.3 Mean values of parameters of lung function in patients with histological features of (1) normal lung, (2) acute rejection, and (3) infection on transbronchial lung biopsy. Figures in parentheses represent standard deviation of mean

	FEV_1 (liters/sec)	VC (liters)	TLC (liters)	DLCO (ml/min per mmHg)
Normal ($n = 19$)	101.5 (25)	89.5 (15)	101.4 (11)	67.1 (16)
Acute rejection ($n = 30$)	66.3 (20)	62.9 (17)	82.3 (20)	53.6 (16)
Infection ($n = 12$)	62.3 (20)	57.8 (17)	76.0 (15)	37.4 (13)

FEV_1 = forced expiratory volume in 1 second; VC = vital capacity; TLC = total lung capacity; DLCO = diffusing capacity for carbon monoxide

Pulmonary function testing on a daily basis is begun within 5 days of surgery using a hand-held battery-operated spirometer[10]. This device offers a means of measuring both the forced expired volume in one second (FEV_1) and the vital capacity (VC). At 1 week, formal testing in the laboratory is undertaken, including measurement of the FEV_1, VC, and total lung capacity (TLC), and the single breath carbon monoxide gas diffusion test (DLCO). Initially after median sternotomy, as a result of transient changes in chest wall configuration, the volumes FEV_1, VC and TLC are reduced, but increase progressively during the next 2–3 months as the chest wall movement recovers[11]. These changes are independent of the mechanical properties of the lung. Failure of the volumes to rise significantly during the first post-transplant month may be an early sign of lung rejection or infection[12].

From retrospective analysis of episodes of acute lung rejection or pulmonary infection diagnosed by histological examination, we have been able to confirm that a 5% reduction in FEV_1 or VC is associated with these complications (Table 38.3). The TLC and DLCO are more variably affected[12]. This has led us to institute a policy of monitoring the patient's spirometric function at home on a daily basis using the hand-held spirometer. All patients are discharged home with these measuring devices, and FEV_1 (and temperature) recorded daily. Full laboratory tests of pulmonary function are performed before discharge home, then at 3, 6 and 12 months, or when respiratory symptoms or a reduction in FEV_1 occur.

The chest radiograph is abnormal in almost 75% of episodes of acute lung rejection occurring during the first month after surgery (Table 38.4). The principal changes seen are diffuse alveolar infiltrates, often with pleural effusions (more on the right than the left)[13]. These changes cannot be distinguished, however, from those of CMV, pneumocystis, or staphylococcal pneumonia, all of which we have observed during this period[13]. Also, 26% of episodes of acute rejection occur with normal radiographic appearances. As a result, suspicion of the diagnosis must be placed more on the development of symptoms or abnormal physical signs, or failure of spirometric function to increase as expected[14].

After the first post-transplant month, less than 30% of the episodes of rejection are associated with radiological abnormalities (Table 38.4), and it is not possible to distinguish the changes from those of pneumocystis infection, which tends to occur later after surgery[13]. Again, the absence of radiological change must not prevent nor postpone aggressive investigation to confirm rejection or infection if either is suspected on other grounds.

Transbronchial lung biopsy (TBB)

To distinguish acute lung rejection from pulmonary infection, we perform TBB through a fiberoptic bronchoscope. Whilst invasive, the method can be performed easily and repeatedly, with the patient receiving intravenous diazepam as sedation and locally-applied anesthesia in the form of lidocaine (2% (w/v) gel to the nose and 2% (w/v) solution to the larynx).

Transbronchial biopsies are obtained from the periphery of the lung under fluoroscopic screening using the larger alligator forceps. Initially, our policy was to take four biopsies[14], but currently three biopsies are taken from each lobe of one lung (with the lingular being considered as a separate lobe on the left). Acute rejection can be demonstrated in up to 80% of biopsies from the lower lobes, but is found less commonly in biopsies from the upper lobes.

Each biopsy is fixed in neutral formaldehyde, and processed for 4 hours in a Shandon hypercenter. Standard stains and specific stains for trophozoites and fungi are undertaken on serial sections of each block of tissue[15].

Formal bronchoalveolar lavage (BAL) is also undertaken before TBB. At present, we do not undertake functional studies on T lymphocytes obtained from the BAL fluid. Although specific reactive cells can be demonstrated in the lavage fluid, the results from these studies are not obtained

Table 38.4 Correlation of abnormal features on chest radiograph with definitive diagnosis of acute rejection confirmed by lung biopsy

	Acute rejection episodes	
Chest radiograph	< 1 month after transplantation	> 1 month after transplantation
Normal	6	17
Abnormal	17	5
Total	23	22

for several days[16], and therefore are of no immediate therapeutic help. However, there is an increase in the absolute number of lymphocytes seen in the BAL fluid during a histologically-proven acute rejection episode, which is not seen in acute viral or bacterial infections or when rejection is not occurring[17]. At present, BAL offers supplementary information to TBB. Lavage material can be used to diagnose CMV pneumonitis and the presence of *Pneumocystis pneumoniae*; *Aspergillus fumigatus* and bacterial pathogens can be cultured from lavage specimens.

Complications from TBB and BAL are rare. In 187 TBBs only six specimens were inadequate for a diagnosis to be made. Three patients developed minimal pneumothoraces, and one suffered a severe hemoptysis requiring assisted ventilation for 1 hour. There have been no infectious complications in 30 studies of BAL.

Histological appearances of acute rejection and infection in transbronchial lung biopsy

From studies in primates it has been shown that acute lung rejection is associated with perivascular infiltrates of activated or immunoblastic lymphocytes, extending in the later stages to involve alveolar septa and bronchiolar mucosa. These changes are also seen in TBB specimens in acute rejection in patients[15] (see also Chapter 40). They are readily distinguished from the changes seen in CMV pneumonitis and pneumocystis pneumonia, where perivascular cuffing occurs, but with edema only; there are also more extensive abnormalities of the alveolar septa[15]. In CMV infection, 'owl's eye' inclusions are present, whilst in pneumocystis pneumonia foamy alveolar exudates are seen in which trophozoites can be demonstrated on silver staining[15].

The sensitivity of TBB to diagnose acute rejection (or infection) can be as high as 78%, with a specificity of 100% (Table 38.5)[14]. A biopsy may show the presence of both rejection and infection, in which case both should be treated.

The timing of transbronchial lung biopsy

Transbronchial lung biopsy is performed routinely 10 days after transplantation, at the time of discharge from hospital, at 3, 6 and 12 months, and thereafter annually. TBB is also performed when a patient develops pulmonary symptoms or signs, or when the FEV_1 or VC fall significantly. A normal chest radiograph does not preclude TBB. Currently, we are also undertaking TBB 2 weeks after treatment of an acute rejection episode.

Endomyocardial biopsy (EMB)

Initially, it was believed that EMB could be used to monitor acute rejection in heart–lung transplants[1]. However, both animal[18] and clinical[19] studies show that the heart undergoes rejection later than the lungs. In our first 17 patients, only one of 107 EMBs showed features of acute rejection, and this patient did not receive increased therapy. None of six concurrent EMBs has been positive when there was a biopsy-proven episode of acute lung rejection. As result of these observations, we have discontinued performing routine EMB[20], and our latest 30 patients have been managed without this investigation.

TREATMENT OF PULMONARY COMPLICATIONS (see also Chapters 41 and 43)

Acute rejection

An acute rejection episode is treated with intravenous methylprednisolone 0.5–1.0 g daily for 3 days, then oral prednisolone beginning with 1 mg/kg per day and steadily decreasing the dose over 10 days. If the patient experiences two or more episodes of acute rejection, confirmed by TBB, each severe enough to require treatment with methylprednisolone, then continuous triple therapy is initiated consisting of cyclosporine, azathioprine, and low-dose (10–15 mg/day) prednisolone.

CMV pneumonitis

When the recipient is serologically negative for CMV and receives organs from a CMV-seropositive donor, a course of intravenous DHPG (ganciclovir) is started. Hyperimmune globulin is also administered to the recipient from the time of surgery on a weekly basis. The course of hyperimmune globulin will lead to a rise in the titer of CMV IgG in the patient's blood. In the immunocompromised patient, without competent T or B-lymphocyte function, if the DHPG therapy is stopped before the infection has been satisfactorily controlled (i.e. before the patient has developed competent B-lymphocyte function) 'rebound' CMV infection can occur. At the present time, it is not possible to measure directly lymphocyte responsiveness to CMV. We have therefore used the appearance of seroconversion (i.e. the production of CMV IgM (and, later, a further rise in IgG) as an indication that the patient has become immunologically

Table 38.5 Correlation of histological features of acute rejection on transbronchial lung biopsy with a clinical diagnosis of acute lung rejection

	Clinical diagnosis	
Infiltrate	Rejection ($n = 36$)	No rejection ($n = 14$)
Perivascular	27	0
Mucosal	27	4
Interstitial	21	2

competent against CMV. When this occurs, we discontinue DHPG therapy.

Pneumocystis pneumonia

A combination of intravenous sulphadimidine and trimethoprim is used to treat pneumocystis pneumonia, when diagnosed on TBB. Intravenous sulphadimidine administration may be associated with a reduction in the whole blood cyclosporine level; close monitoring and adjustment of the cyclosporine dose is therefore necessary to avoid the development of acute rejection.

Aspergillus infection

Early diagnosis and treatment of this infection is essential if a fatal outcome is to be avoided. Intravenous amphotericin is used to treat invasive aspergillus. An initial dose of 15 mg is given; the daily dose is then steadily increased depending on renal function which is closely monitored. A total accumulative dose of 1.2 g must be given to eradicate the infection. Renal dysfunction, when it occurs, can be improved by administering the amphotericin on alternate days only.

Pyogenic pneumonia

The appropriate antibiotics are chosen from the sensitivities obtained from culture of TBB, BAL, and/or sputa. We emphasize intravenous therapy for at least 10 days.

Obliterative bronchiolitis

This is the name given to the disabling and fatal complication which occurred in up to 50% of long-term survivors in earlier series[21] (Chapters 40 and 43). There are experimental observations to suggest that it is the result of repeated untreated acute rejection episodes. In our own series, the incidence of obliterative bronchiolitis is lower, at less than 10%[7], probably as a result of using frequent TBB to detect acute rejection, which may have gone unobserved in earlier series.

Reviewing serial TBBs from the four patients in our series who have developed obliterative bronchiolitis (confirmed at autopsy or at retransplantation), the early biopsies showed intra-alveolar lymphocytic infiltrates. Later in the progress of the condition, these infiltrates organized into intra-alveolar fibrosis and alveolar septal fibrosis. We have assumed that the initial alveolar infiltrates represent a more aggressive acute rejection, and the subsequent fibrosis represents reparative changes which are associated with the characteristic bronchiolar fibrosis[22]. We now treat any patient with extensive infiltrates into the alveolar spaces with repeated courses of augmented triple drug immunosuppression until a normal biopsy is obtained.

SPECIAL PROBLEMS OF HEART–LUNG TRANSPLANTATION IN PATIENTS WITH CYSTIC FIBROSIS

After transplantation, these patients receive the H_2 antagonist ranitidine intravenously and n-acetyl cysteine by nasogastric tube to limit mucus impaction presenting in a form similar to meconium ileus. Pancreatic lipase supplements are begun when the patient begins an oral diet. Cyclosporine is taken orally with orange juice rather than with milk to minimize any reduction of small bowel absorption of this drug. In cystic fibrosis patients, we have found that 2–3 times the usual oral dose of cyclosporine is required to maintain adequate blood levels.

All patients receive colistin inhalations. Other antibiotics are given intravenously when indicated by the sensitivities of pathogens cultured from tracheal specimens obtained at the time of surgery. The presence of purulent sputum, infected with pseudomonas species, is commonly found after surgery in those with underlying cystic fibrosis, though these patients do not experience more episodes of pneumonia than other heart–lung transplant patients[3]. However, if the patient complains of increased sputum volume or other respiratory symptoms associated with infected sputum, then the appropriate antibiotics are administered.

COMMENT

This review sets out to offer a definitive guide to the medical care of patients after heart–lung transplantation. It represents our current approach, which has been associated with 1- and 2-year actuarial survivals of 78% and 68%, respectively. More than 75% of those surviving at 2 years have normal lung function.

References

1. Reitz, B.A., Wallwork, J., Hunt, S.A., Pennock, J.L., Billingham, M.E., Oyer, P.E., Stinson, E.B. and Shumway, N.E. (1982). Heart–lung transplantation: successful therapy for patients with pulmonary vascular disease. *N. Engl. J. Med.*, **306**, 557
2. Penketh, A., Higenbottam, T.W., Hakim, M. and Wallwork, J. (1987). Heart and lung transplantation in patients with end-stage lung disease. *Br. Med. J.*, **295**, 311
3. Scott, J., Higenbottam, T.W., Hutter, J., Hodson, M., Stewart, S., Penketh, A. and Wallwork, J. (1988). Heart–lung transplantation for cystic fibrosis. *Lancet*, **2**, 192
4. Hakim, M., Higenbottam, T.W., Bethune, D., Cory-Pearce, R., English, T.A.H., Kneeshaw, J.N., Wells, F.C. and Wallwork, J. (1988). Selection and procurement of combined heart and lung grafts for transplantation.

J. Thorac. Cardiovasc. Surg., **95**, 474
5. Wallwork, J., Williams, R.and Calne, R.Y. (1987). Transplantation of liver, heart and lungs for primary biliary cirrhosis and primary pulmonary hypertension. *Lancet*, **2**, 182
6. Cotes, J.E. (1979). In *Lung Function*. 4th edn., p. 386. (Oxford: Blackwell Scientific Publications)
7. Hutter, J.A., Despin, P., Higenbottam, T.W., Stewart, S. and Wallwork, J. (1988). Heart–lung transplantation: better use of resources. *Am. J. Med.*, **85**, 4
8. Hutter, J.A., Scott, J.P., Wreghitt, T., Stewart, S., Higenbottam, T.W. and Wallwork, J. (1989). The importance of cytomegalovirus in heart–lung transplantation recipients. *Chest*, **95**, 627
9. Gray, J.J., Alvey, B., Smith, D.J. and Wreghitt, T.G. (1987). Evaluation of a commercial latex agglutination test for detecting antibodies to cytomegalovirus in organ donors and transplant recipients. *J. Virol. Methods*, **16**, 13
10. Chowienczyk, P.J. and Lawson, C.P. (1982). Pocket-sized device for measuring forced expiratory volume in one second and forced vital capacity. *Br. Med. J.*, **285**, 15
11. Braun, S.R., Birnbaum, M.L. and Chopra, P.S. (1978). Pre and post-operation pulmonary function abnormalities in coronary artery revascularization surgery. *Chest*, **73**, 316
12. Otulana, B.A., Higenbottam, T.W., Hutter, J. and Wallwork, J. (1988). Close monitoring of lung function allows detection of pulmonary rejection and infection in heart–lung transplantation. (Abstract.) *Am. Rev. Respir. Dis.*, **137**, 245A
13. Millet, B., Higenbottam, T.W., Flower, C.R., Stewart, S. and Wallwork, J. (1989). The radiological appearances of infection and acute rejection of the lung following heart–lung transplantation. *Am. Rev. Respir. Dis.*, **140**, 62
14. Higenbottam, T.W., Stewart, S., Penketh, A.R.L. and Wallwork, J. (1988). Transbronchial lung biopsy for the diagnosis of rejection in heart–lung transplant patients. *Transplantation*, **46**, 532
15. Stewart, S., Higenbottam, T.W., Hutter, J.A., Penketh, A.R.L., Zebro, T.J. and Wallwork, J. (1988). Histopathology of transbronchial biopsies in heart–lung transplantation. *Transplant. Proc.*, **20**, 764
16. Rabinovich, H., Zeevi, A., Paradis, I. *et al.* (1990). Proliferative responses of bronchoalveolar lavage lymphocytes from heart–lung transplant patients. *Transplantation*, in press
17. Clelland, C., Higenbottam, T.W., Scott, J.A., Monk, J.A. and Wallwork, J. (1989). Lymphocyte counts and T-cell phenotypes in bronchoalveolar lavage (BAL) in relation to transbronchial lung biopsy (TBB) in patients with heart–lung transplants. *Thorax*, **44**, 873
18. Cooper, D.K.C., Novitzky, D., Rose, A.G. and Reichart, B.A. (1986). Acute pulmonary rejection precedes cardiac rejection following heart–lung transplantation in a primate model. *J. Heart Transplant.*, **5**, 29
19. McGregor, C.G.A., Baldwin, J.C., Jamieson, S.W., Billingham, M.E., Yousem, S.A., Burke, C.M., Oyer, P.E., Stinson, E.B. and Shumway, N.E. (1985). Isolated pulmonary rejection after combined heart–lung transplantation. *J. Thorac. Cardiovasc. Surg.*, **90**, 623
20. Hutter, J.A., Higenbottam, T.W., Stewart, S. and Wallwork, J. (1988). Transbronchial biopsy has eliminated the need for endomyocardial biopsy in heart–lung recipients. *J. Heart. Transplant.*, **7**, 435
21. Burke, C.M., Theodore, J., Dawkins, K.D., Yousem, S.A., Blank, N., Billingham, M.E., Van Kessel, A., Jamieson, S.W., Oyer, P.E., Baldwin, J.C., Stinson, E.B., Shumway, N.E. and Robin, E.D. (1984). Post-transplant obliterative bronchiolitis and other late lung sequelae in human heart–lung transplantation. *Chest*, **86**, 824
22. Scott, J.P., Higenbottam, T.W., Hutter, J.A., Stewart, S. and Wallwork, J. (1989). The natural history of obliterative bronchiolitis in heart–lung transplant recipients. *Transplant. Proc.*, **21** (1P + 3), 2592

39
Immunological Aspects
A.L. WESTRA AND J. PROP

INTRODUCTION

When in the early 1980s clinical heart–lung transplantation was reintroduced at Stanford University[1], it was assumed that the course of rejection of combined heart–lung transplants was similar to that of isolated cardiac transplants. Furthermore, it was assumed that rejection would occur simultaneously in heart and lungs. These assumptions were based on experimental findings in monkeys[2], and seemed to be confirmed by the first clinical observations[3,4]. In this perspective, there was no need for specific monitoring of rejection of the lung, because it would be mirrored by the concurrent rejection of the heart; for the detection of heart rejection, endomyocardial biopsy had been proven to be very reliable. With increasing experience, however, it has become evident that cardiac rejection is modulated by the concomitant transplantation of the lungs, and that rejection does not progress simultaneously in heart and lungs.

On the one hand, after combined heart–lung transplantation, cardiac rejection is significantly reduced (in fact, it occurs rarely) compared to cardiac rejection in recipients of isolated heart grafts[5-9]. This observation raised the idea of the 'combi-effect' – that the heart is protected in some way by the combined transplantation of the lungs. The possible mechanism of the 'combi-effect' will be discussed in the first part of this chapter.

On the other hand, in heart–lung transplanted patients the lungs are more prone to reject than the heart[10,11]. Observations of isolated pulmonary rejection were first made in monkeys[12]. At present, ample evidence is available from both clinical and experimental data[10-14] that rejection can affect the lungs while the heart is still normal. The consequence of this is that, from the immunological point of view, heart and lungs have to be regarded as separate organs instead of an 'en bloc' transplant. In the few instances in which it occurs, rejection of the heart causes little difficulty because its symptoms, and ways to monitor and treat it, are well-known from the experience with cardiac transplantation. In contrast, several uncertainties still exist with regard to the diagnosis and treatment of acute or chronic pulmonary rejection. The second part of this chapter will therefore focus on the rejection process in the lungs and methods of monitoring it.

THE 'COMBI-EFFECT' OF HEART–LUNG TRANSPLANTATION

The 'combi-effect' refers to the concept that survival of one graft is improved by combined transplantation of another graft. After combined heart–lung transplantation the combi-effect markedly reduces the incidence of rejection of the heart[15], which has important clinical significance[5-9]. For example, Wallwork and his colleagues in Cambridge decided that, because of the reduced incidence of cardiac rejection in heart–lung recipients, routine endomyocardial biopsy could be discontinued[9] (Chapter 38). Endomyocardial biopsies, taken at the times when transbronchial biopsies showed lung rejection, invariably demonstrated an absence of cardiac rejection.

The mechanism of the combi-effect is not well understood. In animal experiments, the surgical technique of transplantation has been documented to be unimportant as a major factor, although differences in technique influence graft survival to a small extent[15]. It was concluded that the combi-effect is caused by an immunological rather than a surgical-technical mechanism. Three immunological mechanisms can be considered:–

(1) It is possible that more immunosuppressive therapy is given after heart–lung (than after heart) transplantation. Immunosuppressive regimens for heart and heart–lung recipients differ largely in respect of the use of steroids, which are avoided during the first 2 weeks after heart–lung transplantation. Yet Baldwin *et al.*[6] were able to select groups of heart–lung and heart recipients who had received similar immunosuppressive treatment, and again demonstrated that the incidence of cardiac rejection was lower in the heart–lung recipients.

(2) The lungs may filter most of the anti-graft reactive cells out of the blood so that they do not reach the heart. Recipient cells have been found in large quantities in the bronchus-associated lymphoid tissue (BALT) of lung grafts as early as 24 hours after transplantation[16,17], and they also adhere to the endothelium of the extensive vascular bed in the lung. Baldwin et al.[6] called the lung a 'sink' for recipient lymphocytes; we prefer to compare it with a magnet.

(3) The third possible explanation of the combi-effect is that the lymphoid tissue in lung transplants stimulates the induction of donor-specific tolerance during cyclosporine (CsA) immunosuppression. In dogs, it has been found that lungs were not rejected after withdrawal of CsA therapy[18]. In rats, tolerance was induced by a single CsA injection on day 2 after transplantation of a lung graft[19] or combined heart–lung graft[15]. A similar tolerance can be induced by injection of donor lymphocytes during heart transplantation[20], although this is less effective than transplantation of a lung (Figure 39.1); we therefore postulate that it is the lymphoid tissue of the transplanted lung in combination with CsA that favors tolerance induction.

A better insight into the mechanism of the combi-effect may not only help improve the treatment of recipients of combined heart–lung transplants, but may also indicate ways for improved therapy for recipients of isolated heart and other organs.

ACUTE PULMONARY REJECTION

The various manifestations of pulmonary rejection have not yet been fully clarified. Acute pulmonary rejection has been diagnosed in some recipients of combined heart–lung transplants[10,21], but has probably been overlooked in many more cases because there was no accurate non-invasive method to monitor it[22]. Before discussing possible monitoring techniques, the pathology and immunology of rejection in heart–lung grafts in the rat will be briefly described; a more detailed description of the pathology in the human subject appears in Chapter 40.

Pathology of (heart–)lung rejection

The pathologic manifestations of rejection identified in combined heart–lung allografts are not different from those described for isolated heart or lung transplants by Billingham[23] and Prop et al.[16,24], respectively.

In the heart, there are essentially four grades of rejection: (1) *no evidence* of acute rejection, (2) *mild*, (3) *moderate*, and (4) *severe* acute rejection. This system of Billingham is widely used for grading of rejection after heart transplantation. Key parameters are the extent of perivascular lymphocytic infiltrates, interstitial infiltrates, and myocyte necrosis. Similar changes have been observed in the heart when the lungs have been transplanted concomitantly[14].

For isolated rat lung allografts, we initially described four phases of unmodified acute rejection[16,24], the sequence and rate of which proved the same as those observed later in the lungs of combined heart–lung allografts[14]. Observations in the latter studies, and additional experience gained clinically, led to minor alterations in defining these phases[14,25].

An overview of the most important features of the four rejection phases is given in Table 39.1. Consecutively, in the *latent* phase there is no evidence of acute pulmonary rejection; shortly after transplantation pathologic changes attributable to the reimplantation response[26] may be seen. The *vascular* phase is characterized by the early appearance of perivenous infiltrates of lymphocytes, followed by additional peribronchial and periarterial infiltrates while the immunological activity in the BALT is markedly increased. The early (cellular) *alveolar* phase is defined by the accumulation of lymphocytes and macrophages in the alveolar walls and spaces. In the late (edematous) alveolar

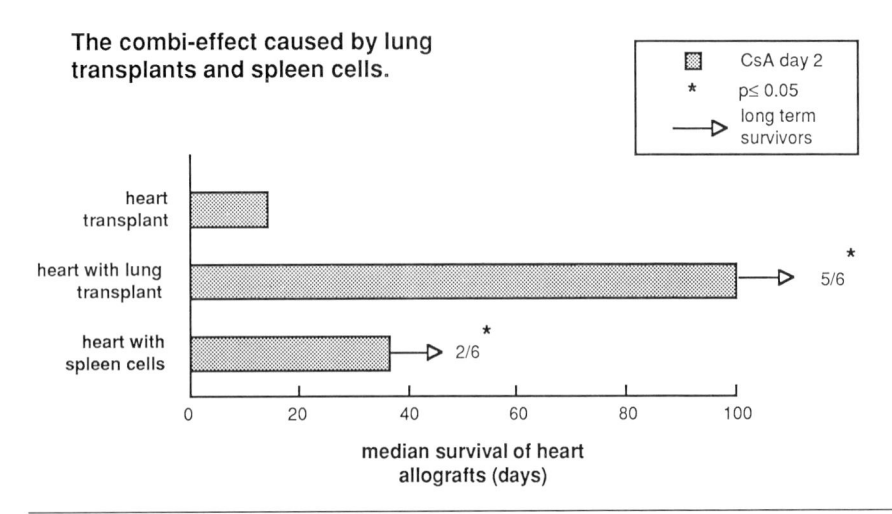

Figure 39.1 The combi-effect. The combi-effect prolongs survival of a heart allograft as a result of (1) combined transplantation with the lung, or (2) injection of donor lymphocytes in CsA-treated recipients. Three groups of rats are shown, receiving, respectively, a heart transplant, a heart and lung transplant, and a heart transplant with injection of 10^8 spleen cells at the time of transplantation. The combi-effect is most obvious in the group with lung transplants, where five of the six hearts survived indefinitely

Table 39.1 Features of the four pulmonary rejection phases

Features	Latent	Vascular Early	Vascular Late	Alveolar Early	Alveolar Late	Destructive
Infiltrates of						
perivenous lymphocytes		++	+++	+++	+++	+++
periarterial lymphocytes		+	+	+++	+++	+++
peribronchial lymphocytes		+	++	+++	+++	+++
interstitial lymphocytes				++	+++	+++
alveolar lymphocytes				+	+++	+++
alveolar PMNs				+	+++	+++
Increased immune activity in						
BALT	+	+++	**			
infiltrates		+	++	+++	+++	+++
Bronchiolar epithelium						
class II MHC antigens		+	++	+++	+++	+++
intra-epithelial lymphocytes				+	++	**
ulceration				+	++	+++
Edema						
perivascular	*				+	
peribronchial	*				+	
alveolar	*			(+)	++	
Necrosis						
of parenchyma						++
with hemorrhage						+
Fibrosis						+

+ some structures affected; ++ many structures affected: +++ all structures affected
* present during reimplantation response; should disappear completely before the end of the first postoperative week: ** cannot be recognized any more because of the extensive infiltration

phase intra-alveolar edema develops that is still reversible but quickly progresses into the destructive phase. The term *destructive* phase is reserved for that histologic picture associated with actual alveolar wall (parenchymal) necrosis. Sometimes intra-alveolar hemorrhage is seen in this phase. The four phases occur irrespective of the donor–recipient MHC barrier, only the pace of it varies (Figure 39.2).

Immunosuppression does not necessarily prevent all lymphocytic infiltration of the lung graft. In CsA-treated rats, the extent of the infiltrates corresponded with the vascular rejection phase. The changes were usually restricted to scattered perivenous and peribronchiolar infiltrates, leaving many of these structures throughout the lung unaffected. After cessation of CsA therapy, the infiltrates remained stable and did not cause obvious impairment of lung function.

Very little clinical pathologic experience had been obtained at the time that we described these four rejection

Rejection phases in lung allografts of five rat strain combinations.

rats strains

BN → LEW
LxB → LEW
LEW → BN
F 344 → LEW
LxF → LEW

— latent phase
▢ vascular phase
■ alveolar phase
▨ destruction phase

days after transplantation

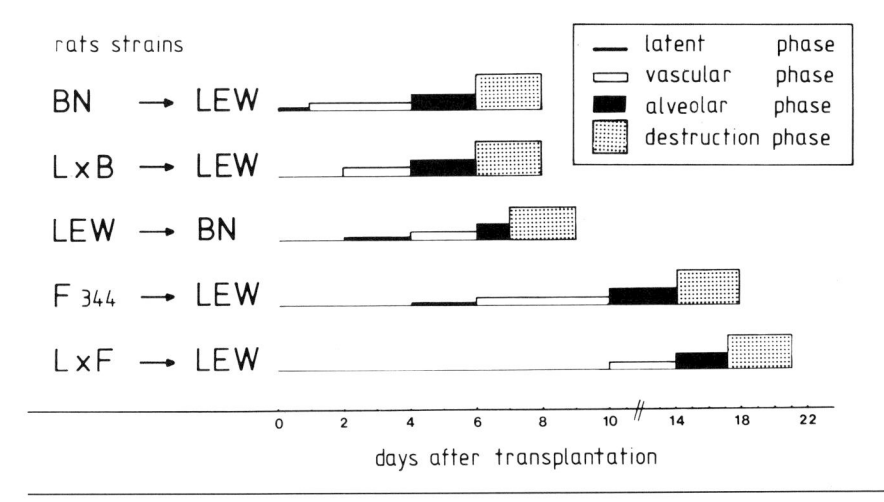

Figure 39.2 Relationship of pulmonary rejection phases and MHC mismatch. The four rejection phases occurred in all investigated combinations of rat strains. LxB and LxF are the F1 hybrids of LEW with BN and LEW with F344 respectively. In three combinations, BN to LEW, LxB to LEW, and LEW to BN, the full sequence of the rejection phases was completed in a week; donor and recipient rats of these combinations are mismatched for the major histocompatibility complex (MHC). In two combinations, F344 to LEW, and LxF to LEW, it took 3 weeks to complete the rejection sequence; these donor and recipient rats are only incompatible for minor (non-MHC) transplantation antigens. No animal received any immunosuppressive therapy

phases in rat lung transplants[16,24]. Now that the use of transbronchial biopsy has provided more lung tissue for pathologic analysis, it appears that the same rejection phenomena occur in human recipients. Whether these phenomena form the same sequence of phases is still difficult to determine because biopsies are taken less frequently in patients than in the animals. At least we can conclude, however, that clinical observations conform with the four described pulmonary rejection phases seen in the rat.

Immunology of acute (heart–)lung rejection

Acute rejection affects the lung more vigorously than the heart. This has been attributed to the 'lymphoid function' of the lung graft[17,27]. The lung contains a complete lymphoid system (BALT and less well-defined collections of lymphocytes and macrophages), whereas the heart lacks any significant lymphoid tissue. This pulmonary lymphoid system accelerates the early induction of the rejection process[16,27]. Donor lymphocytes disseminate from the lung graft into the recipient's lymphoid tissues where they induce a systemic rejection response[16,17]. Yet, the fact that lymphocytes potentiate the systemic rejection response seems to be of minor importance, since in untreated animals the disseminated lymphocytes do not accelerate rejection of the heart of heart–lung grafts, and in CsA-treated animals the lymphocytes even improve heart survival by the combi-effect[20].

More important than the systemic effect is the local effect of the pulmonary lymphoid system upon rejection of the lung. In the transplanted lung, the BALT is the first site of infiltration by recipient lymphocytes. Here, donor and recipient lymphocytes interact *in situ* in a two-way mixed lymphocyte response (MLR)[16]. Simultaneously, donor alveolar macrophages and recipient lymphocytes react in an *in situ* MLR, as was shown by the Pittsburgh group with cells recovered by bronchoalveolar lavage from heart–lung recipients[28].

In long-term surviving lung grafts the role of the pulmonary lymphoid system in rejection is probably negligible. The effect of the lymphoid system gradually weakens, because many of the donor lymphoid cells recirculate and are replaced by recipient cells. While the donor macrophages are being replaced over a period of some months, the alveolar MLR gradually disappears[28,29]. The BALT of the graft seems to degenerate, possibly because of injury caused by rejection; in long-term surviving lung allografts in rats, the BALT can be seen to be largely replaced by fibrinous tissue (Uyama and Prop, unpublished observations). The evidence is, therefore, that the lung's lymphoid system is not an important factor in the etiology of late rejection.

BRONCHIOLITIS OBLITERANS (see also Chapters 40 and 43)

The emergence of airway disease as a late complication in human heart–lung transplant recipients[30-32] has focused attention on a possible rejection process directed against the bronchi and bronchioles. That the airways are significantly involved in the rejection process has been clearly demonstrated in investigations in rats[25]; the sequential changes in the airways seen during the various phases of rejection ultimately lead to the development of a histologic picture of bronchiolitis obliterans, similar to that seen in biopsies from human heart–lung transplant recipients. Yet, in patients acute pulmonary rejection episodes were diagnosed in only a few cases before the development of bronchiolitis obliterans. We postulate, therefore, that undetected episodes of weak acute rejection or a chronic form of rejection lead to the development of bronchiolitis obliterans.

Etiology of bronchiolitis obliterans

Bronchiolitis obliterans is a non-specific response of the airways to injury[33]. Clinically, it occurs following toxic fume inhalation and various infections, in association with connective tissue disease as a localized lesion probably related to a focus of organizing pneumonia, and as a diffuse idiopathic process associated with a patchy organizing pneumonia.

Pathologically, it is characterized by a scarring inflammatory process involving the terminal and respiratory bronchioles (Chapter 40). In the presumed sequence of events the initial insult causes respiratory epithelial cell necrosis with sloughing of cell debris into the lumen and subsequent ulceration. This is accompanied by a fibrinous inflammatory exudate which gradually begins to reorganize. It eventually results in either of two forms of bronchiolitis obliterans[34].

In the form with primarily intra-airway organization, the characteristic appearance is that of intralumenal mucopolysaccharide-rich granulating tissue plugging the lumen (Masson bodies). This may eventually go on to obstruct the lumen completely. The second form results in a constrictive bronchiolitis obliterans in which there is external constriction of the lumen caused by the development of peribronchial or intramural fibrosis. In the end-stage of either process, however, the progressive scarring may result in a bronchiole which, without the aid of elastic tissue stains, is unrecognizable on microscopic sections[35].

Bronchiolitis obliterans in lung transplants

In the transplanted lungs of long-term human heart–lung recipients, Yousem *et al.*[36] observed developing bronchiolitis obliterans in various stages of pulmonary rejection; Tazelaar *et al.*[25] observed similar changes in rejecting rat lung grafts. In humans, the etiology of the process is unclear, because in the uncontrolled clinical situation it is impossible to be certain of the relative contributions of various factors. Rejection, together with other factors, is suspected of having an etiologic role (Chapter 43). This hypothesis has received recent support by the observation from Pittsburgh that bronchiolitis obliterans occurs in patients in whom lymphocytes lavaged from the lung grafts show positive antigraft responses[37].

In our own animal studies, a correlation of bronchiolitis obliterans with rejection is reasonably clear (Figure 39.3). The surgical procedure of transplantation itself is not responsible; no airway pathology, other than the early changes attributable to the reimplantation response; were seen in syngeneic transplant controls. Neither was there any evidence of mucus stasis in the bronchial tree as an etiologic factor. Furthermore, although the bronchial circulation and lymphatics are severed at the time of transplantation, this did not seem to affect the bronchi.

Although in animals the only obvious cause of bronchiolitis obliterans in lung allografts is the rejection process, it is still possible that, in the clinical situation, the progress of bronchiolitis obliterans is accentuated by one or more other postulated etiologies.

For example, pulmonary infection or inhaled agents in lungs undergoing rejection may conceivably lead to further insults to the airways: e.g. the epithelium is injured directly by rejection, while the rejection response is aggravated by infectious stimulation[38], and repair responses are inadequate as a result of immunosuppression and impaired mucociliary clearance. Cytomegalovirus (CMV) has been particularly suspect in the etiology of bronchiolitis obliterans[39], especially since the Pittsburgh group has documented successive viral infection, positive anti-graft lymphocytic reactions, and bronchiolitis obliterans in heart–lung transplanted patients[40].

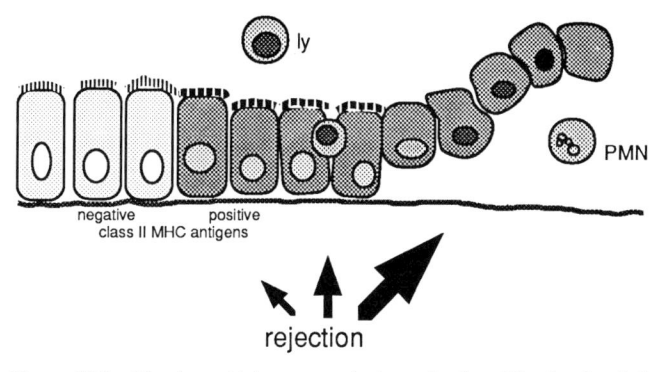

Figure 39.3 The bronchial mucosa during rejection. The insult of the bronchial mucosa by the pulmonary rejection process is depicted. The rejection process progresses from left to right. The mucosa first starts to express class II MHC antigens: lymphocytes (ly) infiltrate into the epithelium and the airways; damaged epithelium sloughs and fills the airways together with polymorphonuclear leukocytes (PMN)

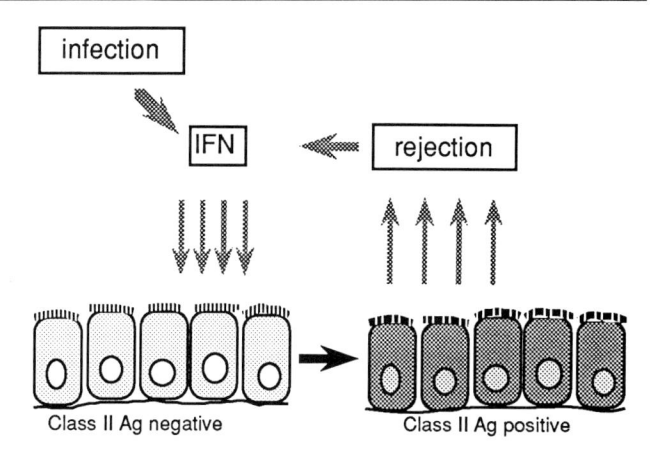

Figure 39.4 Class II MHC antigens on bronchial epithelium of lung allografts. A vicious circle is generated by class II MHC antigens on the bronchial mucosa. γ-Interferon (IFN), which is produced by activated T cells, stimulates normal epithelial cells to express class II antigens. The class II-positive epithelium is a stimulus for the rejection process, so that alloreactive T cells produce more IFN. This circle can be initiated by (viral) infections, which also cause IFN production

It is not surprising that the airways are involved in the pulmonary rejection process. In rat lung allografts, it has been shown that the bronchial epithelium starts to express class II MHC antigens during acute rejection and after insufficient CsA treatment[41]. It has been hypothesized that such *de novo* expression of class II antigens by non-lymphoid tissues is induced by locally activated, alloreactive T cells. Once induced, these antigens on epithelial cells may stimulate the activation of the rejection process (Figure 39.4), and are themselves targets of the rejection response[42].

The finding that, during corresponding rejection phases, the airway changes are more severe in MHC-mismatched allografts than in closely matched allografts[25] supports the hypothesis that class II MHC-antigens on epithelial cells may be a target for rejection. If this is true, then striving for close matching of donor and recipient for MHC antigens may reduce the incidence of bronchiolitis obliterans in the clinical setting.

MONITORING OF PULMONARY REJECTION

The lack of an accurate technique for monitoring pulmonary rejection has been a major obstacle that has prevented optimal treatment of heart–lung recipients. Although the concept that lung rejection is not difficult to diagnose still persists[43], most transplantation centers acknowledge the need for better monitoring techniques. This has become particularly important since endomyocardial biopsy was shown not to reflect pulmonary rejection, and since bronchiolitis obliterans was assumed to be a rejection phenomenon. Endomyocardial biopsy remains, however, the best method of detecting cardiac rejection in a patient with a combined heart–lung graft.

In general, monitoring techniques can be divided into (1) those detecting changes caused by the local rejection process in the graft itself, and (2) those showing manifestations of a systemic process. Local changes can be monitored by imaging and functional techniques, or by immunopathologic techniques. The systemic process is usually monitored by analysis of cells and other factors in the peripheral blood.

Monitoring of the local rejection process

The monitoring technique that is most commonly used for detection of pulmonary rejection is the chest radiograph. Low cost is its main advantage, but it is neither sensitive nor specific. Infiltrates appear on chest radiographs fairly late during rejection, i.e. in the alveolar phase, as changes in the vascular phase are too subtle for this technique to detect. Detected changes are not specific for rejection; they can have other causes such as infection and the reimplantation response[21].

More advanced imaging techniques, such as nuclear magnetic resonance and positron emission tomography, may in the future become helpful in rejection detection, but data on these techniques are not available at the present time.

Of the functional tests, only the measurement of the FEV_1 is used for monitoring of (chronic) rejection in lung allografts. A reduction in FEV_1 has been shown to indicate the development of bronchiolitis obliterans at a stage that can, to some extent, be reversed by corticosteroid therapy[44,45]. In cases of acute rejection, lung function is not affected until the alveolar phase, when gas exchange is impaired by cells infiltrating the alveolar walls (Figure 39.5). The rejection can still be treated in this phase, but it may have inflicted structural damage to the lung graft.

In investigating techniques for the immunopathologic detection of rejection in lung grafts, the main obstacle was how to obtain adequate graft material. Open lung biopsies have been used, but only occasionally, because this method is too invasive for use as a routine procedure. The Cambridge group has shown that transbronchial biopsies provide sufficient graft tissue to assess the progress of rejection[9,46] (Chapter 38). Transbronchial biopsies have revealed manifestations that correlate with the various phases of pulmonary rejection that have been described above[14,16,24,25]. Many transplantation centers have now accepted transbronchial biopsy as a reliable and safe technique for monitoring lung rejection.

Instead of tissue, cells for monitoring can be retrieved from lung grafts by bronchoalveolar lavage. Although in animals acute pulmonary rejection has been detected as early as the vascular phase by an increase in the number of alveolar lymphocytes[47], in patients analysis of lavaged cells has not been found to be sufficiently specific to detect

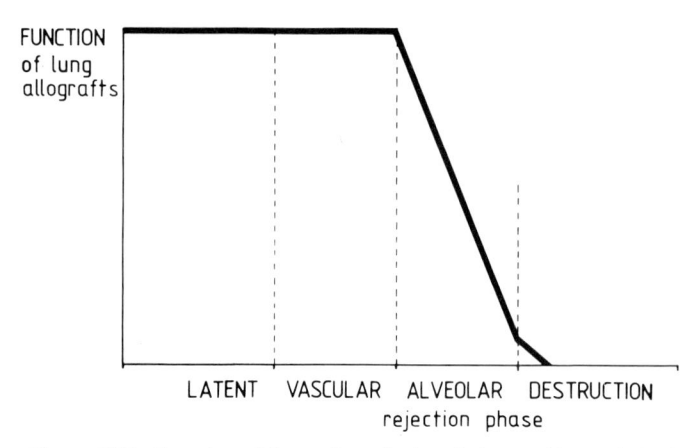

Figure 39.5 Function of lung allografts in relation to histopathologic rejection phase. Function and imaging tests which are commonly used (FEV_1, chest radiography, perfusion scintigraphy) demonstrate deterioration of lung function from the alveolar rejection phase onwards. More sensitive tests are needed to detect impaired function of lung allografts in an earlier phase

rejection[22,48]. Its clinical use has therefore been limited to the diagnosis of *Pneumocystis carinii* infection, though recently, Zeevi and colleagues[37] from Pittsburgh have suggested that bronchoalveolar lavage can predict the development of bronchiolitis obliterans. This group demonstrated that lavaged lymphocytes begin to respond strongly against donor antigens long before clinical symptoms of bronchiolitis obliterans emerge. In many cases positive responses were provoked by a preceding infection. It is possible, therefore, that the lymphocytic responses of lavaged cells can be used to detect chronic rejection well before the graft is irreversibly damaged.

Monitoring of the systemic rejection process

Monitoring of systemic rejection does not accurately reflect the rejection occurring in the lung graft, although there is a definite correlation. Many systemic monitoring techniques analyze peripheral blood leukocytes, because these are easy to obtain. They are analyzed in immunological assays for their functional and morphological properties. For many years, the inversion of the T4/T8 ratio was used as an indication of rejection[49,50].

A method combining morphological and antigen profiles is cytoimmunological monitoring (CIM), which was developed in Munich[51,52]. CIM evaluates the degree of lymphocyte activation in the blood by morphological criteria (size, cytoplasmic basophilia, and nucleus structure) (Figure 39.6). In addition, lymphocyte subsets are identified with monoclonal antibodies. CIM is used in Munich for rejection detection of heart transplant recipients. Some other centers

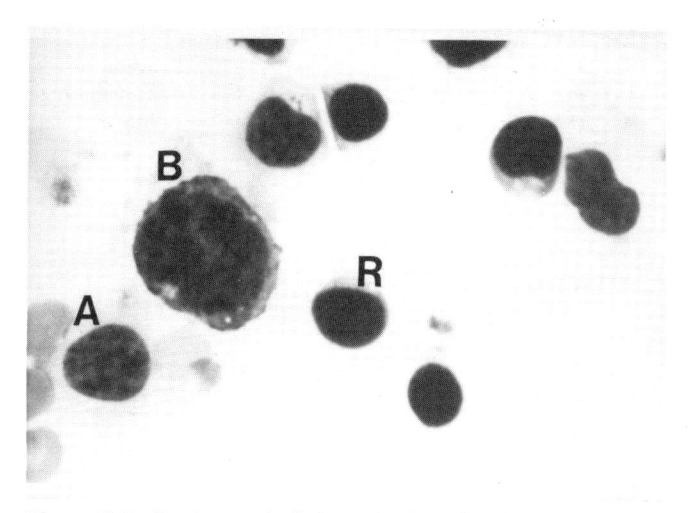

Figure 39.6 Cytoimmunological monitoring of activated lymphocytes during rejection. Activated lymphocytes can be distinguished from resting lymphocytes according to their size, basophilia of the cytoplasm, and structure of the nucleus. (R = small resting lymphocyte with a compact nucleus; A = activated lymphocyte with a larger and less dense nucleus; B = blast cell with a very large, open nucleus)

have also introduced CIM, but there are conflicting views about the applicability of the method for the detection of early cardiac rejection.

The value of CIM for monitoring pulmonary rejection after combined heart–lung transplantation has yet to be determined. Activation has been seen in a few patients, but whether this was a sign of rejection remained unclear. In dogs and rats we have found that CIM does show activation in cases of histologically confirmed pulmonary rejection, and in some experiments the method was more sensitive than bronchoalveolar lavage.

COMMENT

In conclusion, the heart and the lungs behave differently with regard to rejection after combined transplantation. The heart benefits from the simultaneously-transplanted lung so that it is rarely rejected; we have called this the 'combi-effect'. Difficulties in treatment of heart–lung recipients arise from the lung. Rejection affects the lung graft more frequently than the heart, a chronic or subclinical form of pulmonary rejection causes bronchiolitis obliterans, and pulmonary rejection is difficult to monitor.

For grading of acute rejection in human lung biopsies, a histopathologic system based on studies in the rat describing four rejection phases has been proposed.

A major step forward would be made by the development of better monitoring techniques of pulmonary rejection. At present, these include the histopathologic examination of tissue obtained by transbronchial biopsy for the diagnosis of acute rejection, and alloreactive assays of lavaged lymphocytes for the detection of the chronic form of rejection.

Acknowledgements

The original work presented in this chapter was supported by the Netherlands Heart Foundation (Grant 85113), the Netherlands Asthma Foundation, and J.K. de Cock-Stichting.

References

1. Reitz, B.A., Wallwork, J.L., Hunt, S.A., Pennock, J.L., Billingham, M.E., Oyer, P.E., Stinson, E.B. and Shumway, N.E. (1982). Heart–lung transplantation. Successful therapy for patients with pulmonary vascular disease. *N. Engl. J. Med.*, **306**, 557
2. Reitz, B.A., Burton, N.A., Jamieson, S.W., Bieber, C.P., Pennock, J.L., Stinson, E.B. and Shumway, N.E. (1980). Heart and lung transplantation. Autotransplantation and allotransplantation in primates with extended survival. *J. Thorac. Cardiovasc. Surg.*, **80**, 360
3. Reitz, B.A., Gaudiani, V.A., Hunt, S.A., Wallwork, J., Billingham, M.E., Oyer, P.E., Baumgartner, W.A., Jamieson, S.W., Stinson, E.B. and Shumway, N.E. (1983). Diagnosis and treatment of allograft rejection in heart–lung transplant recipients. *J. Thorac. Cardiovasc. Surg.*, **85**, 354
4. Jamieson, S.W., Baldwin, J.C., Reitz, B.A., Stinson, E.B., Oyer, P.E., Hunt, S., Billingham, M.E., Theodore, J., Modry, D., Bieber, C.P. and Shumway, N.E. (1983). Combined heart and lung transplantation. *Lancet*, **1**, 1130
5. Imakita, M., Tazelaar, H.D. and Billingham, M.E. (1986). Heart allograft rejection under varying immunosuppressive protocols as evaluated by endomyocardial biopsy. *J. Heart Transplant.*, **5**, 279
6. Baldwin, J.C., Oyer, P.E., Stinson, E.B., Starnes, V.A., Billingham, M.E. and Shumway, N.E. (1987). Comparison of cardiac rejection in heart and heart–lung transplantation. *J. Heart Transplant.*, **6**, 352
7. Glanville, A.R., Imoto, E., Baldwin, J.C., Billingham, M.E., Theodore, J. and Robin, E.D. (1987). The role of right ventricular endomyocardial biopsy in the long-term management of heart–lung transplant recipients. *J. Heart Transplant.*, **6**, 357
8. Wahlers, T., Khaghani, A., Martin, M., Banner, N. and Yacoub, M. (1987). Frequency of acute heart and lung rejection after heart–lung transplantation. *Transplant. Proc.*, **19**, 3537
9. Higenbottam, T., Stewart, S. and Wallwork, J. (1988). Transbronchial lung biopsy to diagnose lung rejection and infection of heart–lung transplants. *Transplant. Proc.*, **20**, 767
10. McGregor, C.G.A., Baldwin, J.C., Jamieson, S.W., Billingham, M.E., Yousem, S.A., Burke, C.M., Oyer, P.E., Stinson, E.B. and Shumway, N.E. (1985). Isolated pulmonary rejection after combined heart–lung transplantation. *J. Thorac. Cardiovasc. Surg.*, **90**, 623
11. Novitzky, D., Cooper, D.K.C., Rose, A.G. and Reichart, B. (1986). Acute isolated pulmonary rejection following transplantation of the heart and both lungs: experimental and clinical observations. *Ann. Thorac. Surg.*, **42**, 180
12. Scott, W.C., Haverich, A., Billingham, M.E., Dawkins, K.D. and Jamieson, S.W. (1984). Lethal rejection of the lung without significant cardiac rejection in primate heart–lung allotransplants. *Heart Transplant.*, **4**, 33
13. Cooper, D.K.C., Novitzky, D., Rose, A.G. and Reichart, B.A. (1986). Acute pulmonary rejection precedes cardiac rejection following heart–lung transplantation in a primate model. *J. Heart Transplant.*, **5**, 29
14. Prop, J., Tazelaar, H.D. and Billingham, M.E. (1987). Rejection of combined heart–lung transplants in rats. Function and pathology. *Am. J. Pathol.*, **127**, 97
15. Westra, A.L., Caravati, F., Petersen, A.H., Wildevuur, Ch.R.H. and Prop, J. (1989). Reduced heart rejection in combined heart–lung transplants. *Transplant. Proc.*, **21**, 455

16. Prop, J., Wildevuur, C. R. and Nieuwenhuis, P. (1985). Lung allograft rejection in the rat. II. Specific immunological properties of lung grafts. *Transplantation*, **40**, 126
17. Prop, J., Kuijpers, K., Petersen, A.H., Bartels, H.L., Nieuwenhuis, P. and Wildevuur, Ch.R.H. (1985). Why are lung allografts more vigorously rejected than hearts? *J. Heart Transplant.*, **4**, 433
18. Norin, A.J., Emeson, E.E., Kamholz, S.L., Pinsker, K.L., Montefusco, C.M., Matas, H.J. and Veith, F.J. (1982). Cyclosporin A as the initial immunosuppressive agent for canine lung transplantation. Short- and long-term assessment of rejection phenomena. *Transplantation*, **34**, 372
19. Prop, J., Bartels, H.L., Petersen, A.H., Wildevuur, Ch.R.H. and Nieuwenhuis, P. (1983). A single injection of cyclosporine-A reverses lung allograft rejection in the rat. *Transplant. Proc.*, **15**, 511
20. Westra, A.L., Petersen, A.H., Prop, J., Nieuwenhuis, P. and Wildevuur, C.R. (1988). Prolongation of rat heart allograft survival by perioperative injection of donor cells followed by cyclosporine treatment. *J. Heart Transplant.*, **7**, 18
21. Chiles, C., Guthaner, D.F., Jamieson, S.W., Stinson, E.B., Oyer, P.E. and Silverman, J.F. (1985). Heart–lung transplantation. The postoperative chest radiograph. *Radiology*, **154**, 299
22. Zeevi, A., Fung, J.J., Paradis, I.L., Dauber, J.H., Griffith, B.P., Hardesty, R.L. and Duquesnoy, R.J. (1985). Lymphocytes of bronchoalveolar lavages from heart–lung transplant recipients. *J. Heart Transplant.*, **4**, 417
23. Billingham, M.E. (1985). Endomyocardial biopsy detection of acute rejection in cardiac allograft recipients. *Heart Vessels*, **1** (Suppl.), 86
24. Prop, J., Wildevuur, C.R. and Nieuwenhuis, P. (1985). Lung allograft rejection in the rat. III. Corresponding morphological rejection phases in various rat strain combinations. *Transplantation*, **40**, 132
25. Tazelaar, H.D., Prop, J., Nieuwenhuis, P., Billingham, M.E. and Wildevuur, Ch.R.H. (1988). Airway pathology in the transplanted rat lung. *Transplantation*, **45**, 864
26. Prop, J., Ehrie, M.G., Crapo, J.D., Nieuwenhuis, P. and Wildevuur, Ch.R.H. (1984). Reimplantation response in isografted rat lungs. Analysis of causal factors. *J. Thorac. Cardiovasc. Surg.*, **87**, 702
27. Prop, J., Nieuwenhuis, P. and Wildevuur, C.R. (1985). Lung allograft rejection in the rat. I. Accelerated rejection caused by graft lymphocytes. *Transplantation*, **40**, 25
28. Fung, J.J., Zeevi, A., Kaufman, C., Paradis, I.L., Dauber, J.H., Hardesty, R.L., Griffith, B. and Duquesnoy, R.J. (1985). Interactions between bronchoalveolar lymphocytes and macrophages in heart–lung transplant recipients. *Human Immunol.*, **14**, 287
29. Paradis, I.L., Marrari, M., Zeevi, A., Duquesnoy, R.J., Griffith, B.P., Hardesty, R.L. and Dauber, J.H. (1985). HLA phenotype of lung lavage cells following heart–lung transplantation. *J. Heart Transplant.*, **4**, 422
30. Burke, C.M., Theodore, J., Dawkins, K.D., Yousem, S.A., Blank, N., Billingham, M.E., Van Kessel, A., Jamieson, S.W., Oyer, P.E., Baldwin, J.C., Stinson, E.B., Shumway, N.E. and Robin, E.D. (1984). Post-transplant obliterative bronchiolitis and other late lung sequelae in human heart–lung transplantation. *Chest*, **86**, 824
31. Burke, C.M., Theodore, J., Baldwin, J.C., Tazelaar, H.D., Morris, A.J., McGregor, C., Shumway, N.E., Robin, E.D. and Jamieson, S.W. (1986). Twenty-eight cases of human heart–lung transplantation. *Lancet*, **1**, 517
32. Jamieson, S.W. (1985). Recent developments in heart and heart–lung transplantation. *Transplant. Proc.*, **17**, 199
33. Epler, G.R. and Colby, T.V. (1983). The spectrum of bronchiolitis obliterans. *Chest*, **83**, 161
34. Gosink, B.B., Friedman, P.J. and Liebow, A.A. (1973). Bronchiolitis obliterans. Roetgenologic–pathologic correlation. *Am. J. Roentgenol.*, **117**, 816
35. Katzenstein, A.L.A. and Askin, F.B. (1982). *Surgical Pathology of Non-Neoplastic Lung Disease*. (Philadelphia: W.B. Saunders Co.)
36. Yousem, S.A., Burke, C.M. and Billingham, M.E. (1985). Pathologic pulmonary alterations in long-term human heart–lung transplantation. *Hum. Pathol.*, **16**, 911
37. Griffith, B.P., Paradis, I.L., Zeevi, A., Rabinowich, H., Yousem, S.A., Duquesnoy, R.J., Dauber, J.H. and Hardesty, R.L. (1988). Immunologically mediated disease of the airways after pulmonary transplantation. *Ann. Surg.*, **208**, 371
38. Prop, J., Jansen, H.M., Wildevuur, C.R. and Nieuwenhuis, P. (1985). Lung allograft rejection in the rat. V. Inhaled stimuli aggravate the rejection response. *Am. Rev. Respir. Dis.*, **132**, 168
39. Burke, C.M., Glanville, A.R., Macoviak, J.A., O'Connell, B.M., Tazelaar, H.D., Baldwin, J.C., Jamieson, S.W. and Theodore, J. (1986). The spectrum of cytomegalovirus infection following humam heart–lung transplantation. *J. Heart Transplant.*, **5**, 267
40. Paradis, I., Zeevi, A., Duquesnoy, R., Hardesty, R., Kormos, R., Nalesnik, M., Dummer, J.S., Dauber, J. and Griffith, B.P. (1988). Immunologic aspects of chronic lung rejection in humans. *Transplant. Proc.*, **20**, 812
41. Romaniuk, A., Prop, J., Petersen, A.H., Wildevuur, C.R. and Nieuwenhuis, P. (1987). Expression of class II major histocompatibility complex antigen by bronchial epithelium in rat lung allografts. *Transplantation*, **44**, 209
42. Burke, C.M., Glanville, A.R., Theodore, J. and Robin, E.D. (1987). Lung immunogenicity, rejection, and obliterative bronchiolitis. *Chest*, **92**, 547
43. Reitz, B.A. (1988). Heart–lung transplantation. In Fishman, A.P. (ed.) *Pulmonary Diseases and Disorders*. 2nd ed., p. 2459. (New York: McGraw-Hill)
44. Allen, M.D., Burke, C.M., McGregor, C.G.A., Baldwin, J.C., Jamieson, S.W. and Theodore, J. (1986). Steroid-responsive bronchiolitis after human heart–lung transplantation. *J. Thorac. Cardiovasc. Surg.*, **92**, 449
45. Glanville, A.R., Baldwin, J.C., Burke, C.M., Theodore, J. and Robin, E.D. (1987). Obliterative bronchiolitis after heart–lung transplantation: apparent arrest by augmented immunosuppression. *Ann. Intern. Med.*, **107**, 300
46. Stewart, S., Higenbottam, T.W., Hutter, J.A., Penketh, A.R.L., Zebro, T.J. and Wallwork, J. (1988). Histopathology of transbronchial biopsies in heart–lung transplantation. *Transplant. Proc.*, **20**, 764
47. Prop, J., Wagenaar-Hilbers, J.P.A., Petersen, A.H. and Wildevuur, Ch.R.H. (1988). Characteristics of cells lavaged from rejecting lung allografts in rats. *Transplant. Proc.*, **20**, 217
48. Gryzan, S., Paradis, I.L., Hardesty, R.L., Griffith, B.P. and Dauber, J.H. (1985). Bronchoalveolar lavage in heart–lung transplantation. *J. Heart Transplant.*, **4**, 414
49. O'Toole, C.M., Maher, P., Spiegelhalter, D.J., Walker, J.R., Stovin, P., Wallwork, J. and English, T.A.H. (1985). 'Rejection or infection' predictive value of T-cell subset ratio, before and after heart transplantation. *J. Heart Transplant.*, **4**, 518
50. Yacoub, M.H., Rose, M.L., Cox, J.H. et al. (1985). Immunological monitoring of heart transplant patients: clinical and experimental studies. In Thiede, A. et al. (eds.) *Microsurgical Models in Rats for Transplantation Research*. p. 327. (Berlin and Heidelberg: Springer-Verlag)
51. Hammer, C., Reichenspurner, H., Ertel, W., Lersch, C., Plahl, M., Brendel, W., Reichart, B., Uberfuhr, P., Welz, A., Kemkes, B.M., Reble, B., Funccius, W. and Gokel, M. (1984). Cytological and immunologic monitoring of cyclosporine-treated human heart recipients. *Heart Transplant.*, **3**, 228
52. Ertel, W., Reichenspurner, H., Lersch, C., Hammer, C., Plahl, M., Lehmann, M., Kemkes, B.M., Osterholzer, G., Reble, B., Reichart, B. and Brendel, W. (1985). Cytoimmunological monitoring in acute rejection and viral, bacterial or fungal infection following transplantation. *J. Heart Transplant.*, **4**, 390

40
Pathology of Heart–Lung Transplantation
S.A. YOUSEM

INTRODUCTION

With over 250 heart–lung transplantations performed worldwide, a clinical management scheme for these patients has emerged[1]. Clinicians specializing in heart–lung allografting have established consistent, reproducible data utilizing radiographic, immunologic, and pulmonary function information, which allow the identification of lung rejection or interposed infectious processes. Coinciding with this clinical progression, a reproducible, consistent pattern of histopathologic changes has been identified, which allows the diagnosis of both acute and chronic lung rejection[2-9].

This brief chapter represents a general approach to the histopathologic diagnosis of lung rejection. It is based on a review of pathologic material of over 100 patients transplanted at the University of Pittsburgh School of Medicine and Stanford University Medical Center.

The seminal work of Veith and his colleagues on experimental animals provided germinal information on the histopathologic changes in the immediate post-transplant period[4-11]. These alterations, which have been modified somewhat because of the use of cyclosporine[12], are now recognized as representing *acute* lung rejection. With clinical control and suppression of acute rejection, patients have survived longer and the increased survival (average 23 months) has led to the identification of unique pathologic alterations in long-term recipients, which differ from those occurring within the first 3 months after transplantation; these changes are currently believed to be a manifestation of chronic lung rejection[2,3,13-15].

This chapter will thus begin with a description of the earliest changes in the pulmonary parenchyma after transplantation, and proceed to a discussion of acute and chronic lung rejection.

IMMEDIATE POSTOPERATIVE COMPLICATIONS
'Reimplantation response'

Within the first week after transplantation, several alterations in the pulmonary parenchyma have been identified. First, occurring in all patients, is the so-called 'reimplantation response', which may be related to interruption of lymphatic routes, ischemia during transportation and transplantation, or division of nerves and bronchial arteries[16-18]. The consequence is pulmonary edema, which can clinically mimic acute lung rejection. Histologically, this is reflected in expansion of the interlobular septa and peribronchial and perivascular regions by pale eosinophilic edema fluid (Figure 40.1). This proteinaceous material is also found focally within air spaces. Occasionally scattered neutrophils are identified. This pathologic picture is identical

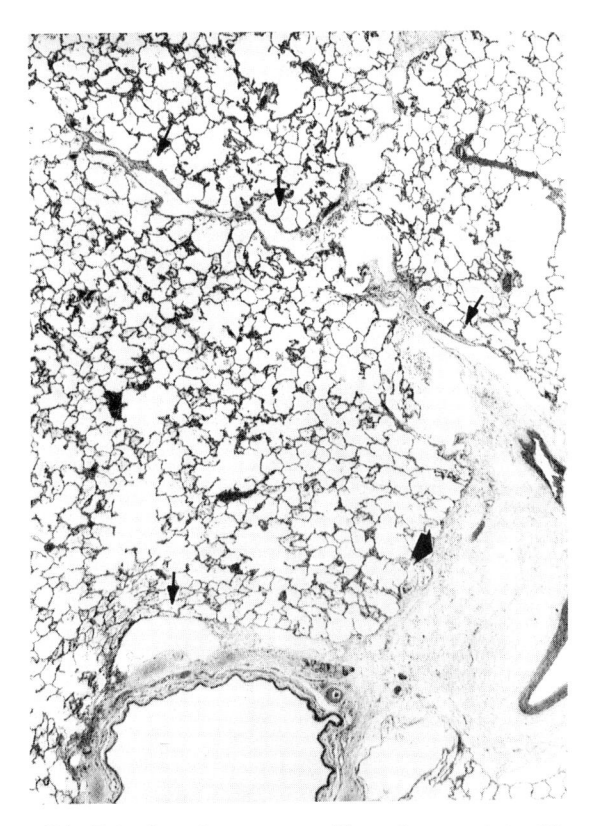

Figure 40.1 Reimplantation response. The pulmonary interstitium is edematous as reflected in perivascular pallor (large arrow) and marked dilation of lymphatic channels (small arrows)

to that of early congestive heart failure, and it slowly resolves with regrowth of lymphatics.

Tracheal dehiscence

Tracheal dehiscence was an early problem which has resolved with the use of lower steroid doses and the wrapping of the anastomotic site with an omental pedicle[4,14,17]. Histologically, the site reveals acute ulceration with necrosis of epithelium and submucosal connective tissue, and an acute inflammatory exudate. At the margins, acute ischemic changes are common and are presumably a result of bronchial artery ligation. A complication of this ischemic injury is infection. In one third of cases, colonization by candida has been identified; this is related to tracheal colonization in the donor and contamination of the operative field. In four cases at Pittsburgh and three at Stanford, aortic anastomotic infections were also seen which suggests candida fungemia may occur and lead to secondary sites of infection[3]. Other agents infecting anastomotic sites include herpes, adenovirus, mucormycosis, and cytomegalovirus.

Adult respiratory distress syndrome

In lungs with prolonged ischemia or inadequate preservation, diffuse alveolar damage and the adult respiratory distress syndrome may occur. Morphologically this is similar to diffuse alveolar damage (DAD) in non-transplanted patients. The interstitium (interlobular septa, bronchovascular bundles, and alveolar septa) is edematous, and hyaline membranes coat the surfaces of the respiratory bronchioles and alveoli. The alveoli contain an admixture of red blood cells, histiocytes, and necrotic alveolar lining cells. A mild neutrophilic infiltrate is commonly seen. With respiratory support in cases of mild injury, the hyaline membranes are resorbed into the interstitium and the type II alveolar pneumocytes proliferate over the denuded septa and then undergo metaplasia to type I cells. Inadequate response to ventilatory therapy or severe graft ischemia may lead to progression of the DAD into a proliferative phase, with young plugs of granulation tissue filling air spaces and the interstitium, and, with time, progression to end-stage pulmonary fibrosis and honeycomb lung.

ACUTE LUNG REJECTION

Within the first 3 months after transplantation, the major pulmonary abnormalities relate to infection and acute lung rejection[14,17,18]. Acute rejection of the lungs shows a similar distribution and cellular component to that commonly observed in other organ systems, e.g. heart and kidney. A predominantly mononuclear infiltrate is initially identified around small pulmonary venules in the interlobular septa, and progresses to cuff pulmonary arterioles (Figure 40.2)[2,4,5,9,19-21]. As the number of mononuclear cells increases, spillage into the periseptal alveolar walls is noted. The mononuclear cells are composed of small round lymphocytes and immunoblasts (large lymphoid cells with prominent nucleoli and pyroninophilic cytoplasm), which infiltrate the subendothelial zone, traverse the muscular wall, and form a perivascular concentric ring around the adventitia of the vessels. Endothelial cells become plump, mitotically active and hypertrophic and undergo epithelioid change. Individual cell necrosis is also observed as the lymphoid cells permeate and undermine the subendothelial regions (Figures 40.3 and 40.4).

Simultaneously, the peribronchial lymphoid tissue becomes hyperplastic, and is infiltrated by large numbers of transformed large lymphoid cells and immunoblasts. Presumably this relates to an *in situ* mixed lymphocyte reaction. This reaction is usually noted in the walls of bronchioles, between bronchioles and arteries, and in peribronchial and hilar lymph nodes.

As the severity of acute rejection increases, perivascular changes worsen and bronchiolar damage begins to occur

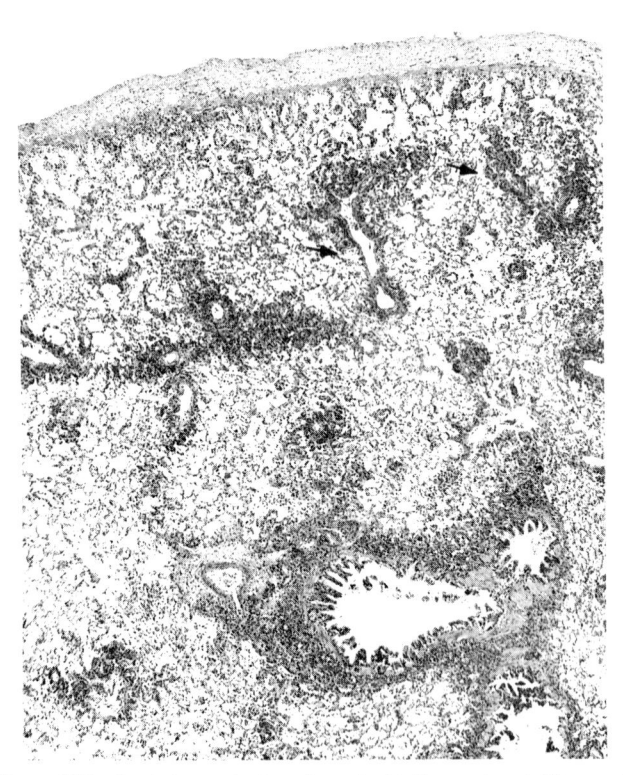

Figure 40.2 Acute lung rejection. A marked inflammatory infiltrate cuffs the pulmonary veins running in the pleura and interlobular septa (arrows). Concentric cuffing of bronchioles and arterioles is seen at lower right

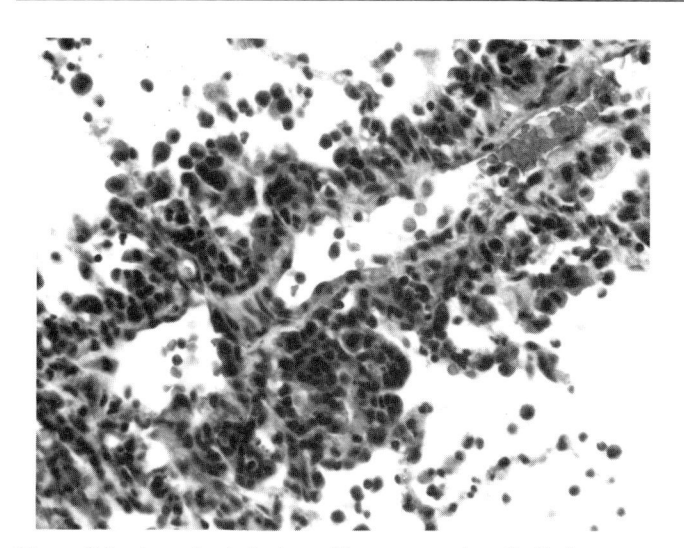

Figure 40.3 A small vein is rimmed by a concentric cuff of inflammatory cells. This represents the earliest manifestation of acute lung rejection

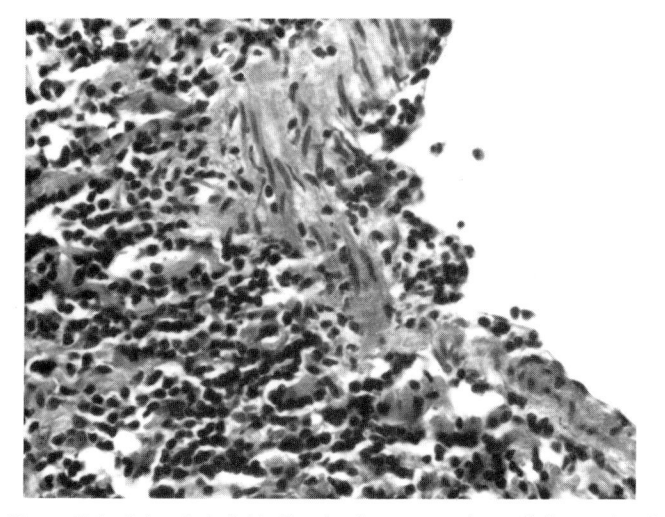

Figure 40.4 Subendothelial infiltration by mononuclear cells is associated with necrosis and reactive hyperplasia with epithelioid change in the endothelial cells. Mononuclear cells are small round lymphocytes and transformed large lymphoid cells. Phenotypically they represent T cells for the most part

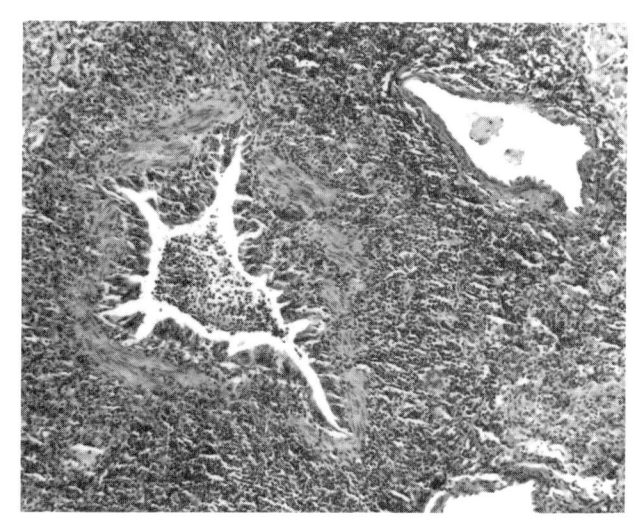

Figure 40.5 Late in acute lung rejection, an intense infiltrate envelops bronchioles and arteries, and spills into the alveolar septa. The latter reaction results in diffuse alveolar damage with necrosis of pneumocytes, and their shedding, along with macrophages, into air spaces

(Figure 40.5). Both arterial and venous walls become permeated with mononuclear cells, neutrophils and eosinophils, and the vessels undergo fibrinoid necrosis. Alveolar hemorrhage ensues. At the same time, inflammatory cells begin to permeate alveolar septa diffusely, and alveolar pneumocytes undergo necrosis, and slough into the air spaces as proteinaceous hyaline membranes form (diffuse alveolar damage). Infarct-like necrosis of parenchyma is a late consequence. As this perivascular and alveolar process occurs, bronchioles become rimmed by a similar cellular infiltrate. Individual lymphocytes insinuate themselves between the respiratory epithelial cells (emperipolesis), and individual cell necrosis is observed. With time, the mucosa becomes necrotic and sheds into the lumen where it becomes mixed with fibrin, acute and chronic inflammatory cells, and cellular debris. The final result is massive lung infarction and necrosis.

Acute lung rejection appears to be a *diffuse* process with a predisposition for the lower lobes[14]. Lung rejection may develop independently of cardiac rejection, and consequently right ventricular endomyocardial biopsy is not an adequate method of monitoring rejection[22,23]. It also appears to be significantly modified in its intensity by the use of cyclosporine[12]. Veith reported this phenomenon as a separate form of acute lung rejection[9]; it is likely, however, that this reaction represents only a muted or less severe form. The process of alveolar or 'atypical' acute lung rejection is not a distinct entity[11], but instead represents the phase of diffuse alveolar damage resulting from ischemic graft damage.

HYPERACUTE LUNG REJECTION

The author has experience with two cases which are unique and potentially represent hyperacute rejection of the lung, presumably as a result of previous antigen sensitization. In the first case, the patient developed a disseminated intravascular coagulation-like picture with diffuse oozing of blood from suture lines and pulmonary vessels immediately after discontinuation of cardiopulmonary bypass. At autopsy there was uniform filling of capillaries by fibrin thrombi and neutrophilic infiltration of the intima of vessels (Figures 40.6 and 40.7). Alveolar hemorrhage was also remarkable. IgG, IgM, and complement were found in the microthrombi and focally within vessel walls.

The second case was a solitary right upper lobe transplant of a father's lung to his son which, immediately after

Figure 40.6 Hyperacute lung rejection. Fibrin microthrombi fill small capillaries (arrows). This pattern may also be seen with sepsis and disseminated intravascular coagulation

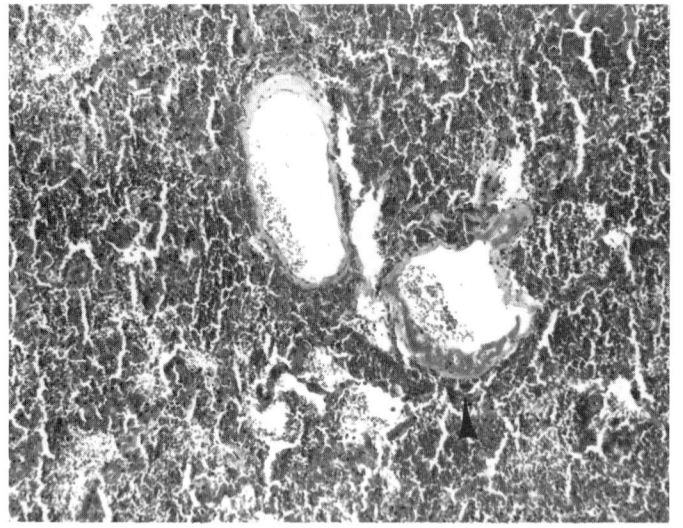

Figure 40.7 Hyperacute lung rejection. Fibrinoid necrosis of vessels (arrow) and marked alveolar hemorrhage is similar to hyperacute rejection in other organ systems

anastomosis, became suffused and violaceous. Autopsy 1 day later revealed fibrinoid necrosis of arteries, veins, and bronchial walls, with a leukocytoclastic vasculitis. Massive alveolar hemorrhage was present. No blood group mismatch occurred although a complete histocompatibility work-up was not performed. These two cases are currently being investigated further.

CHRONIC LUNG REJECTION

In approximately 50% of allograft recipients, a clinical syndrome of progressive respiratory dysfunction occurs[2,3,13,14]. These patients develop a dry or mucus-producing cough associated with mucopurulent sputum. Chest radiographs may show dilation of bronchi or peribronchial thickening. Pulmonary function studies reveal an obstructive defect with progressive reduction of air flow, resulting in a mixed obstructuve and restrictive pattern[24]. The histopathologic correlate of this is bronchiolitis obliterans, associated with a paradoxical dilation and ectasia of the proximal bronchial tree.

Understanding this change requires conceptual isolation of the large and small airway components. The large bronchi, with specimen radiography, display a pattern of cylindrical bronchiectasis[2,3]. There is usually mucostasis with focal areas of acute bronchitis, and the epithelium displays squamous metaplasia (Figures 40.8 and 40.9). The basement membrane is thickened, and the submucosa expanded by dense hyalinized collagen. A mononuclear inflammatory infiltrate is common. Smooth muscle appears atrophic and replaced by collagen, the cartilaginous plates are irregular, and the perichondrium thickened. Peribronchial fibrosis is also remarkable, and minor salivary gland tissue is atrophic (rather than hyperplastic). Bronchial arteries are atretic and show marked arteriosclerosis.

In contrast to the bronchi, the small terminal and respiratory bronchioles show the histologic spectrum of bronchiolitis obliterans (OB)[2,3]. The OB is panlobar, extensive, and patchy, and has been associated with changes of *acute* lung rejection in 30% of cases.

In any case of OB, one can find a temporally heterogeneous pattern of respiratory epithelial injury. In early lesions, the bronchioles are cuffed by a mononuclear infiltrate consisting of small round and plasmacytoid lymphocytes. Lymphocyte emperipolesis is noted with foci of diffuse

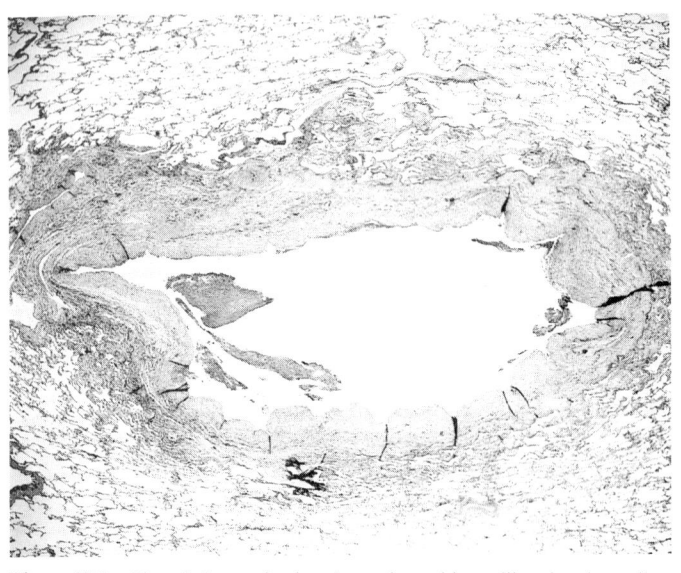

Figure 40.8 Chronic lung rejection. Large bronchi are dilated and usually contain a mucopurulent exudate. Note that adjacent air spaces are unremarkable. This histologic finding corresponds to cylindrical bronchiectasis on specimen bronchography

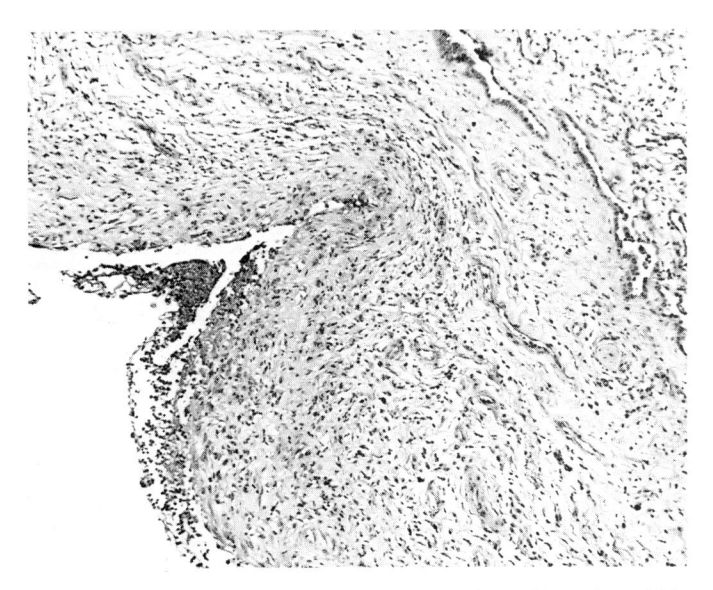

Figure 40.9 Chronic lung rejection. The epithelium of large bronchi is frequently ulcerated and inflamed and shows squamous metaplasia. The submucosa contains a granulation tissue-like reaction with extensive fibrosis, with loss of the bronchial smooth muscle wall. Bronchial arteries, which were ligated at surgery, often appear atretic and thrombosed

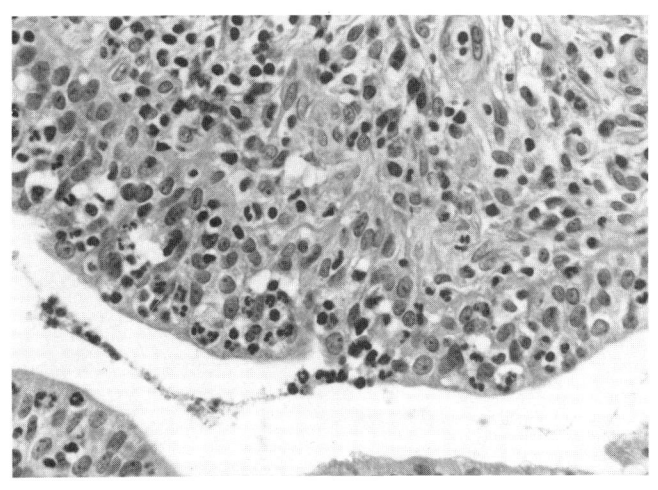

Figure 40.11 Chronic lung rejection. As injury to small bronchioles progresses with necrosis of cells, a mixed acute and chronic inflammatory infiltrate forms with the creation of an intralumenal plug of fibrin, acute inflammatory cells, and mucus

epithelial cell necrosis (apoptosis) (Figures 40.10 and 40.11). As the epithelial cells slough, they are enveloped in mucus, fibrin, and acute and chronic inflammatory cells. In the organizing phases, fibroblasts and endothelial cells from the submucosa infiltrate the inflammatory plug, filling the lumen of the bronchiole. This results in a sessile polyp of young myxoid granulation tissue protruding into the lumen of the bronchiole (Masson body) (Figures 40.12 and 40.13).

The subsequent healing of this myxoid polyp may proceed

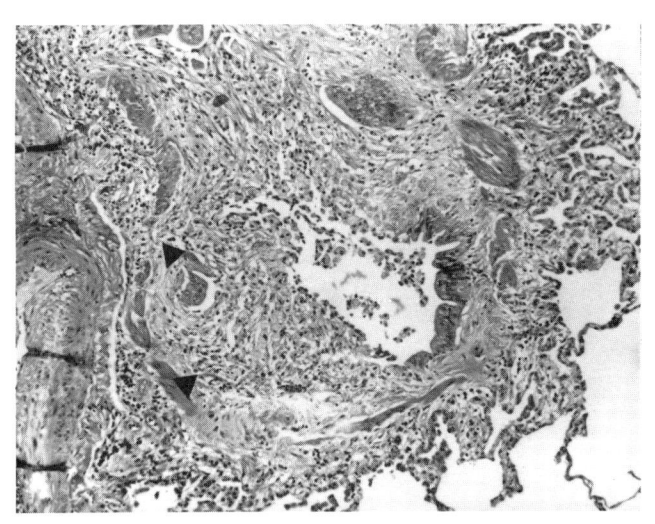

Figure 40.12 Chronic lung rejection. After the necrosis of epithelium, fibroblasts, histiocytes and endothelial cells infiltrate the lumenal debris and form an intralumenal plug of granulation tissue (arrows) which may entrap metaplastic epithelium (bronchiolitis obliterans). The epithelium is interrupted and shows squamous or basal cell metaplasia. Small terminal bronchioles are located adjacent to muscular arterioles and have a similar diameter

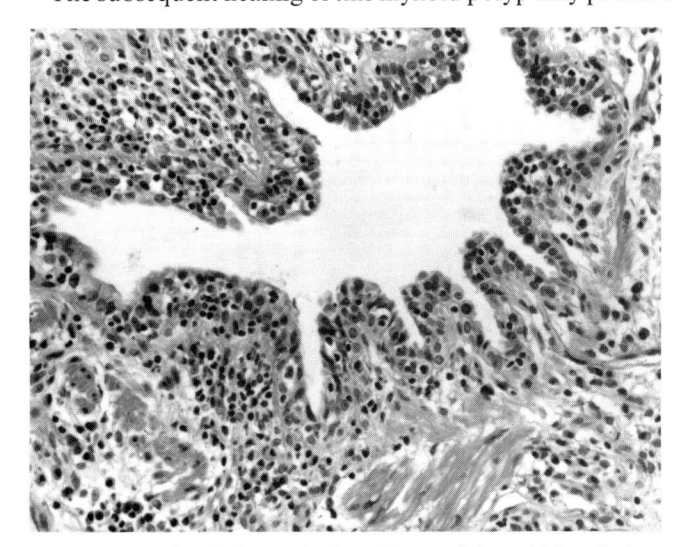

Figure 40.10 Chronic lung rejection. The small bronchioles display a submucosal mononuclear infiltrate, which extends into the overlying epithelium, resulting in necrosis of epithelium and basal-cell (cuboidal) metaplasia. Small lymphocytes percolate between epithelial cells (emperipolesis), probably initiating epithelial cell necrosis

along three pathways. First, if the injury is not severe, the granulation tissue may be re-epithelialized by metaplastic bronchiolar epithelium and the entire collagenous plug resorbed with only intermittent interruptions of the bronchiolar elastica as the residue of previous inflammation. To demonstrate this may require elastic tissue stains which, along with a trichrome stain, are essential in evaluating OB. Second, if only a segment of the bronchiole is injured, an eccentric hyaline scar of dense eosinophilic collagen may form (Figures 40.14 and 40.15). This is usually associated with breaks in the elastic lamina of the bronchiole and focal

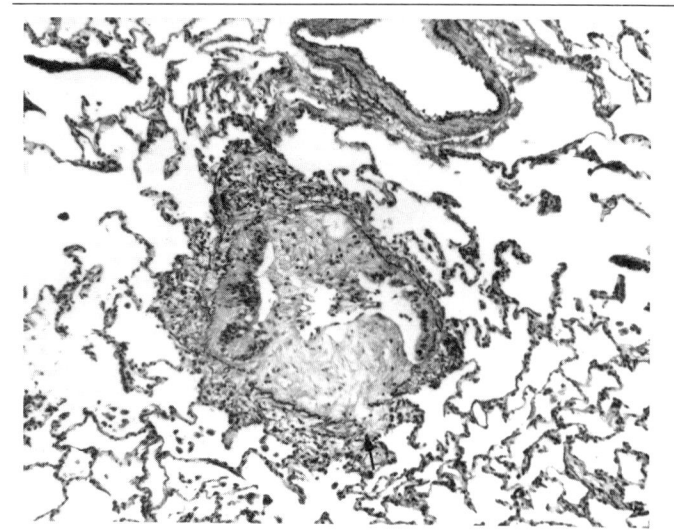

Figure 40.13 Chronic lung rejection. Elastic tissue stains show the polypoid plug of granulation tissue projecting into the lumen with a thin layer of metaplastic epithelial cells covering its surface. Note the interruptions of the bronchiolar elastica (arrow). A small muscular arteriole is seen in the superior portion of the field

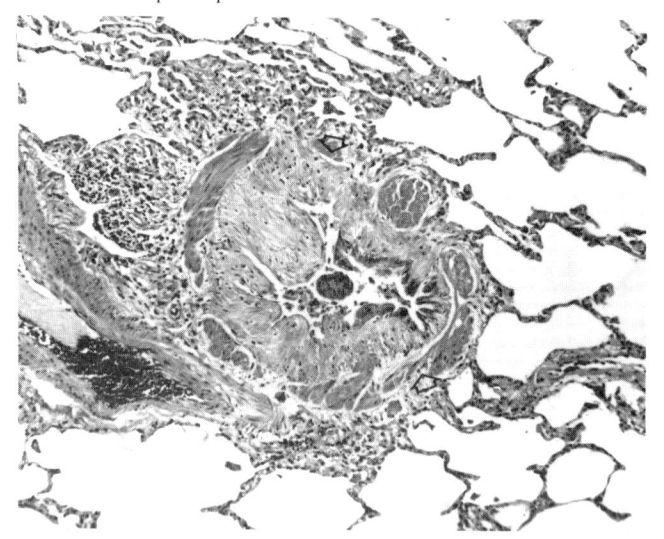

Figure 40.14 Chronic lung rejection. One consequence of bronchiolar injury is eccentric scarring of the submucosa which reduces the lumenal diameter of the bronchiole. Old scar tissue (arrows) forms an eccentric fibrous plaque

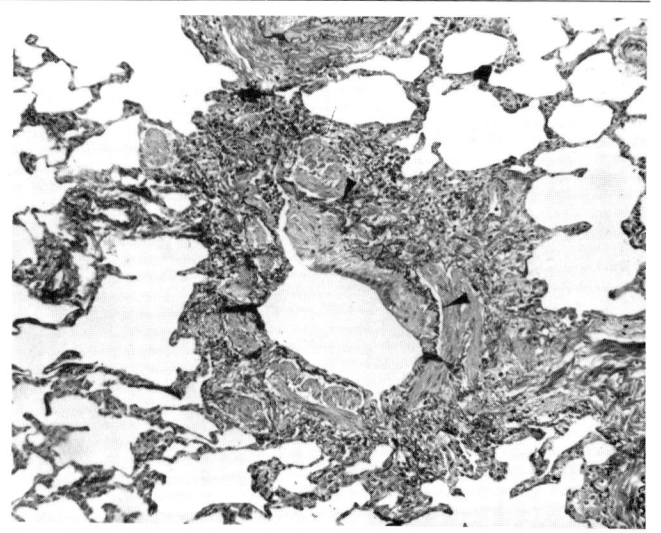

Figure 40.15 Chronic lung rejection. Elastic tissue stains show the subtle focal fibrous scarring of this small terminal bronchiole (arrows)

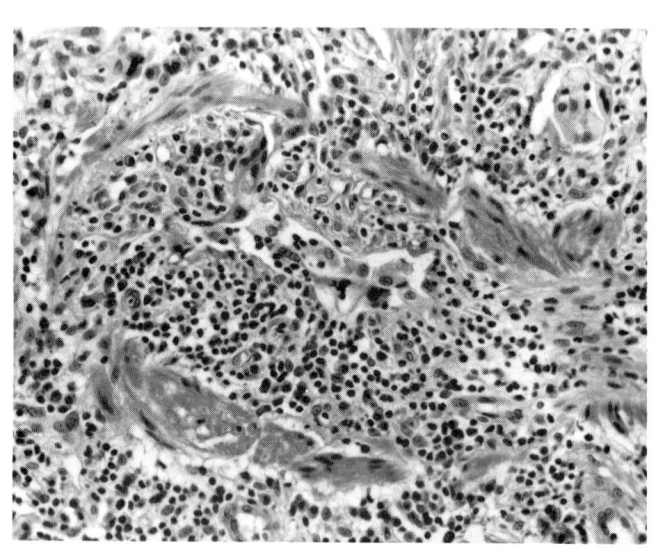

Figure 40.16 Chronic lung rejection. Concentric submucosal bands of fibrous tissue reduce the lumen of some bronchioles to a slit or fishmouth shape. The lumen contains foamy histiocytes, a consequence of the obstructive effect of bronchiolitis obliterans. A mononuclear infiltrate is common within the scar tissue of the lumen and submucosa

loss of the smooth muscle wall. If the entire bronchiolar epithelium is injured, a circumferential constricting cuff of collagen may also form and be coated with metaplastic cuboidal epithelium (Figure 40.16). Eccentric and concentric fibrosis results in significant lumenal compromise akin to small airways disease. Third, if epithelial injury is significant, the entire lumen of the bronchiole may be permanently occluded by dense scar tissue (Figure 40.17).

At each of these healing phases, a moderate submucosal chronic inflammatory infiltrate is present. Because of the lumenal compromise, bronchioles and alveolar ducts distant to the obstruction may contain inspissated mucus or foamy lipid-laden macrophages. Alveolar septa and air spaces lack an inflammatory infiltrate.

The effect of OB relates to the extent of disease in both lung (diffuse versus localized process) and severity of injury. In all cases studied at autopsy, OB is extensive, panlobar, and severe[3].

In addition to the airway damage, the second anatomic compartment showing abnormalities is the pulmonary vasculature. All long-term survivors show accelerated arteriosclerosis characterized by intimal fibroelastosis[2,3]. Myofibroblasts and fibroblasts form a concentric layer of myxoid collagen on the inner aspect of an intact internal elastica (Figures 40.18 and 40.19). This change is rarely associated with an infiltrate of mononuclear inflammatory

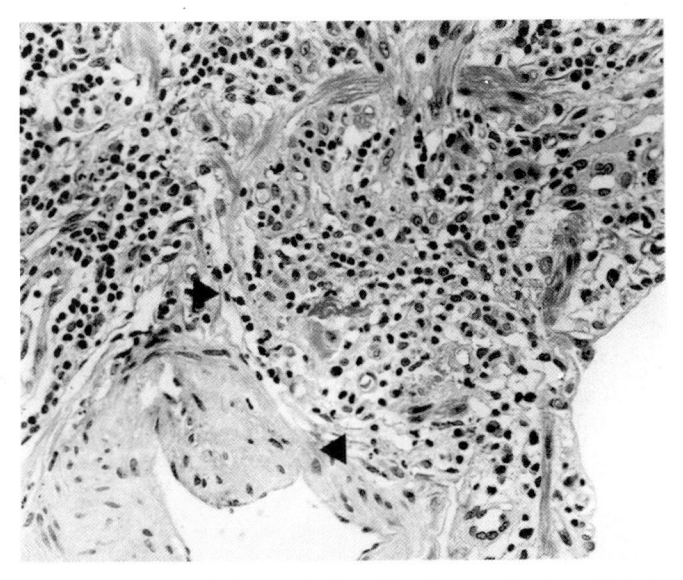

Figure 40.17 Chronic lung rejection. The lumen of a bronchiole is completely occluded by the old fibrous tissue and mononuclear inflammatory cells. Small capillaries supply this fibrous scar. Bronchioles may only be identified at this stage by their location adjacent to arterioles (lower left) or by elastic tissue stains. The smooth muscle wall of the bronchiole is destroyed focally (arrows)

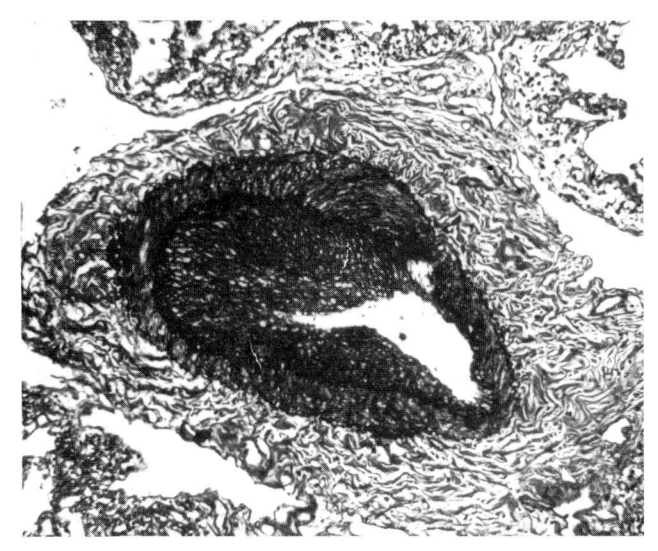

Figure 40.19 Chronic lung rejection. Elastic tissue stains show the intimal fibroelastosis occurring on the inner aspect of an intact internal elastic lamina, in the small muscular arteries

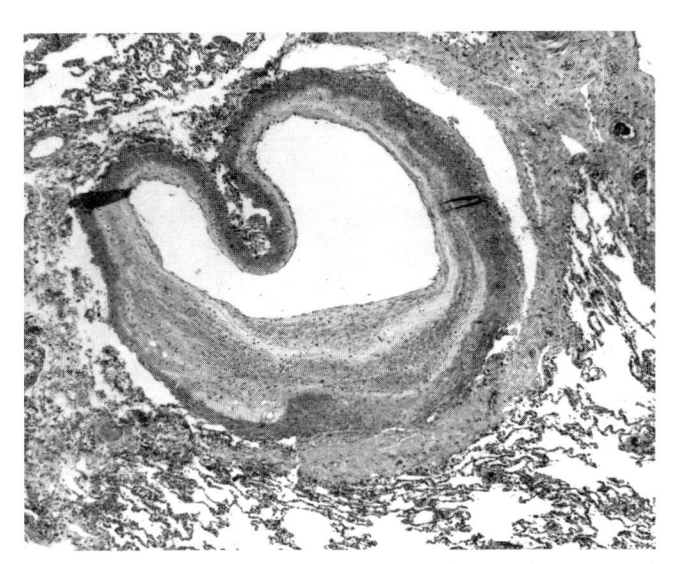

Figure 40.18 Chronic lung rejection. Large arteries may show concentric or eccentric plaques of myxoid fibrous tissue. A mild mononuclear cell infiltrate (endovasculitis) is occasionally seen as well

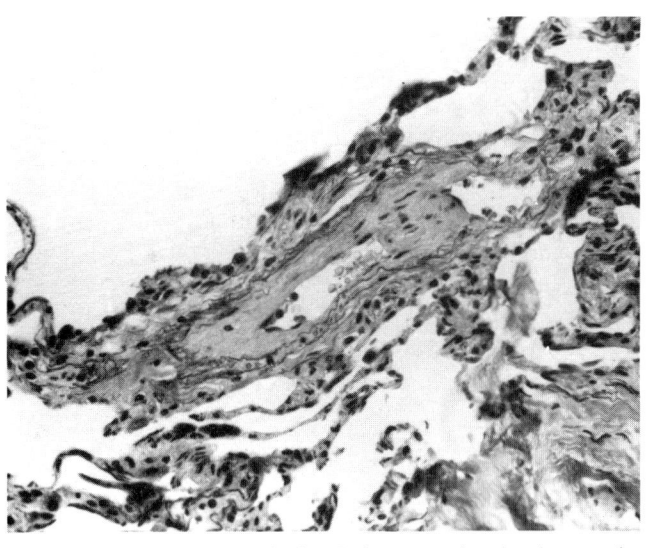

Figure 40.20 Chronic lung rejection. Pulmonary veins also show accelerated phlebosclerosis in this 22-year-old donor lung, 39 months after transplantation

cells (endovasculitis). For the most part, the intimal proliferation corresponds to Grade II of the Heath–Edwards classification of pulmonary hypertension[25], though these patients almost never show elevated pulmonary pressures. There is an association with accelerated coronary arteriosclerosis, where the coronary disease is more severe in OB patients and occasionally associated with myocardial infarcts[17,26].

The pulmonary venous system also shows a peculiar phlebosclerosis with waxy sclerotic eosinophilic thickening of veins (Figure 40.20). Again, the elastica of veins appears intact beneath the eosinophilic collagen plaques.

Subsidiary pulmonary findings include focal pleural adhesions and rare irregular parenchymal scars. Both tracheal and vascular anastomotic sites are usually intact. The trachea, however, shows squamous metaplasia and marked fibrous thickening of its wall with minor salivary gland atrophy. It is commonly dilated and histologically resembles a dense fibrous tube with scant smooth muscle. No epithelial or mesenchymal differences are observed above and below the anastomotic sites.

Associated pathology in other organs

Cardiac changes include hypertrophy of the heart and marked coronary arteriosclerosis (Figure 40.21). In 14% of patients, acute myocardial infarction has accounted for the death of long-term survivors of heart–lung transplantation[3,14].

Extrathoracic organ changes are not striking. Hilar lymph nodes show lymphoid depletion, fibrous scarring and hemosiderin deposits, presumably a result of the immunologic reaction between donor and recipient lymphoid cells. Mediastinal nodes are grossly and histologically unremarkable with the exception of mild paracortical hyperplasia. The kidneys usually show vascular and endothelial damage due to cyclosporine toxicity.

In patients *without* OB, the lung parenchyma is identical to that of age-matched controls with a mild increase in pulmonary arterial fibroelastosis (personal observations). Those patients who have expired have done so as a result of myocardial infarcts, infections, adult respiratory distress syndrome of uncertain etiology, and iatrogenic causes. Two patients have developed a post-transplant lymphoproliferation similar to those described in other organ systems.

IMMUNOHISTOCHEMISTRY

Although no systematic studies have been performed, the inflammatory infiltrate in acute rejection is composed of T cells, predominantly helper/inducer T cells. An admixture of T suppressor and cytotoxic cells is usually present in the submucosa of bronchioles involved by OB. Leu 7 cells appear to be more commonly seen in bronchioles with chronic rejection. Bronchoalveolar lavage data suggest larger amounts and different classes of type II MHC antigens on the bronchiolar epithelium in patients with OB[28,34].

PATHOGENESIS OF OBLITERATIVE BRONCHIOLITIS

The etiology of the long-term bronchial and bronchiolar changes has been the subject of many reports[2,3,13–15]. The current and favored hypothesis is that OB results from immunologic damage to bronchiolar epithelium, and therefore is a manifestation of chronic lung rejection. Supportive evidence includes reports from bone marrow transplant recipients who developed 'lymphocytic bronchiolitis' or OB as a result of graft-versus-host disease[35–41]. This is associated with functional obstruction and other sites of epithelial injury including skin, bursa, gastrointestinal tract, and sinuses.

We also suspect that OB is a host-versus-graft immunologic reaction. Supporting this would be four points: (1) the association of OB with histologic changes of acute lung rejection[2,3]; (2) the analogous development of OB in non-transplant patients with collagen vascular diseases due to autoimmune reactions[42–45]; (3) the fact that, in animal studies, the extent of bronchiolar damage is related to the degree of histocompatibility mismatch[21,46–49]; and (4) the response of patients with OB to increased immunosuppression[13,50]. It should be noted, however, that OB is not related to either the number of acute rejection episodes or clinical infections in human recipients[13,14].

A second possibility, however, is that infection is the cause of OB. Well-documented OB has been reported as a consequence of respiratory syncytial virus, adenovirus, parainfluenza virus, mycoplasma, legionella, hemophilus, cytomegalovirus, and chlamydia infections[51–54]. Certainly, these patients experience repeated upper and lower respiratory tract infections; the repeated injury may impair defense mechanisms in these immunocompromised hosts by inducing squamous metaplasia, mucus stasis with inadequate clearance, and therefore a propensity for bacterial superinfection. Some evidence has emerged that OB may be preceded by viral or pneumocystis infection, which activates cell surface antigens not normally seen, and/or up-regulates and stimulates the immunologic reactivity of host lymphocytes to the foreign epithelium[31,33,57].

Infection may also be responsible for the bronchiectasis by irreversibly scarring the major airways, and destroying smooth muscle. The loss of tone and resiliency may also be caused or made worse by a lack of neurogenic stimulation of the bronchial tree, and the impaired healing resulting from the loss of bronchial arteries, the major blood supplier of the proximal airways.

Other potential causes of OB include repeated aspiration, drug reactions, impaired mucociliary clearance and local defense mechanisms, e.g. macrophage function, and cyclosporine[13,14,51,53].

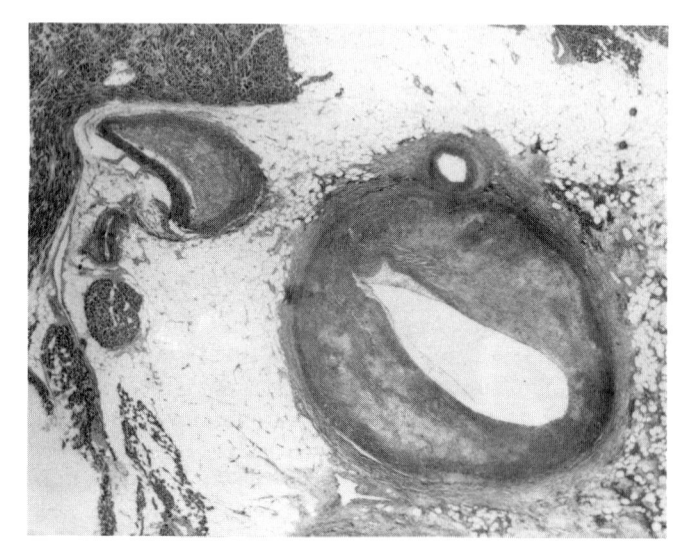

Figure 40.21 Marked coronary arteriosclerosis is seen in association with the pulmonary vascular changes, and may lead to silent myocardial infarcts. Scarred myocardium is seen at upper left

ROLE OF TRANSBRONCHIAL AND OPEN LUNG BIOPSIES

Recent reports have promoted the usefulness of transbronchial biopsy in the diagnosis of OB and chronic lung rejection[58], though the current author retains some skepticism in the value of this investigation. As indicated previously, OB can be a consequence of a finding in any pneumonic process. It may also be extremely subtle and not easily recognized in small biopsies. Because of this, and because of the extremely poor prognosis OB implies, we recommend an open-lung biopsy for the diagnosis if transbronchial biopsy is equivocal, at a time when the patient is not suffering from any superimposed acute pneumonia. This more frequently allows a confident, unequivocal diagnosis, and also eliminates false positive diagnoses.

Transbronchial biopsy and bronchoalveolar lavage, however, have been demonstrated to be of considerable value in the exclusion of infectious causes of pulmonary infiltrates.

References

1. Kaye, M.P. (1987). The Registry of the International Society for Heart Transplantation: fourth official report – 1987. *J. Heart Transplant.*, **6**, 191
2. Yousem, S., Burke, C. and Billingham, M. (1985). Pathologic pulmonary alterations in long-term human heart-lung transplantation. *Hum. Pathol.*, **16**, 911
3. Tazelaar, H.D. and Yousem, S. (1989). Heart–lung transplantation: an autopsy study. *Hum. Pathol.*, **19**, 1403
4. Veith, F., Sinha, S., Blumcke, S., Dougherty, J.C., Becker, N.H., Siegelman, S.S. and Hagstrom, J.W. (1972). Nature and evolution of lung allograft rejection with and without immunosuppression. *J. Thorac. Cardiovasc. Surg.*, **63**, 509
5. Halasz, N., Cantanzaro, A., Trummer, M., Tisi, G.M., Saltzstein, S.L., Moser, K.M. and Hutchin, P. (1973). Transplantation of the lung: correlation of physiologic, immunologic and histologic findings. *J. Thorac. Cardiovasc. Surg.*, **66**, 581
6. Byers, J., Sabanayagam, P., Zarins, C., Baker, R.R. and Hutchins, G.M. (1973). Pathologic changes in baboon lung allografts. *Ann. Surg.*, **178**, 754
7. Baker, R., Sabanayagam, P., Zarins, C., James, A.E., Hutchins, G.M., Byers, J.M., Katarajan, T.K. and Lee, J.M. (1973). Functional and morphologic changes after lung allografting in baboons. *Surg. Gynecol. Obstet.*, **137**, 650
8. Joseph, W. and Morton, D. (1971). Morphologic alterations in the transplanted primate lung. *Surg. Gynecol. Obstet.*, **133**, 821
9. Veith, F., Kamholz, S., Mollenkoph, F. and Montefusco, C. (1983). Lung transplantation, 1983. *Transplantation*, **35**, 271
10. Veith, F., Koerner, S., Siegelman, S., Kawakami, M., Kaufman, S., Attai, L.A., Hagstrom, J.W. and Gliedman, M.L. (1973). Diagnosis and reversal of rejection in experimental and clinical lung allografts. *Ann. Thorac. Surg.*, **16**, 172
11. Veith, F. and Hagstrom, J. (1972). Alveolar manifestations of rejection: an important cause of the poor results with human lung transplantation. *Ann. Surg.*, **175**, 336
12. Veith, F.J., Norin, A.J., Montefusco, C.M., Pinsker, K.L., Kamholz, S.L., Sliedman, M.L. and Emeson, E. (1981). Cyclosporin-A in experimental lung transplantation. *Transplantation*, **32**, 474
13. Burke, C.M., Theodore, J., Baldwin, J.C., Tazelaar, H.D., Morris, A.J., McGregor, C., Shumway, N.E., Robin, E.D. and Jamieson, S.W. (1986). Twenty-eight cases of human heart–lung transplantation. *Lancet*, **1**, 517
14. Griffith, B.P., Hardesty, R.L., Trento, A., Paradis, I., Duquesnoy, R.J., Zeevi, A., Dauber, J.H., Dummer, J.S., Thompson, M.E., Gryzan, S. and Bahnson, H.T. (1987). Heart-lung transplantation: lessons learned and future hopes. *Ann. Thorac. Surg.*, **43**, 6
15. Burke, C., Theodore, J., Dawkins, K., Yousem, S.A., Blank, N., Billingham, M.E., van Kessel, A., Jamieson, S.W., Oyer, P.E., Baldwin, J.C., Stinson, E.B., Shumway, N.E. and Robin, E.D. (1984). Post-transplant obliterative bronchiolitis and other late lung sequelae in human heart–lung transplantation. *Chest*, **86**, 824
16. Prop, J.M., Ehrie, M.G., Crapo, J.D., Nieuwenhuis, N.C.P. and Wildevuur, C.R.H. (1984). Reimplantation response in isografted rat lungs. *J. Thorac. Cardiovasc. Surg.*, **87**, 702
17. Reitz, B. (1982). Heart–lung transplantation: a review. *Heart Transplant.*, **1**, 291
18. Jamieson, S., Baldwin, J., Stinson, E., Reitz, B.A., Oyer, P.E., Hunt, S., Billingham, M., Theodore, J., Modry, D. and Bieber, C.P. (1984). Clinical heart–lung transplantation. *Transplantation*, **37**, 81
19. Prop, J.M., Wildevuur, C.R.H. and Nieuwenhuis, P. (1985). Lung allograft rejection in the rat. III. Corresponding morphological rejection phases in various rat strain combinations. *Transplantation*, **40**, 132
20. Prop, J., Nieuwenhuis, P. and Wildevuur, C.R.H. (1985). Lung allograft rejection in the rat. I. Accelerated rejection caused by graft lymphocytes. *Transplantation*, **40**, 25
21. Prop, J.M., Wildevuur, C.R.H. and Nieuwenhuis, P. (1985). Lung allograft rejection in the rat. II. Specific immunological properties of lung grafts. *Transplantation*, **40**, 126
22. Novitzky, D., Cooper, D.K.C., Rose, A.G. and Reichart, B. (1986). Acute isolated pulmonary rejection following transplantation of the heart and both lungs: experimental and clinical observations. *Ann. Thorac. Surg.*, **42**, 180.
23. McGregor, C.G., Baldwin, J.G., Jamieson, S.W., Yousem, S.A., Burke, C.M., Oyer, P.E., Stinson, E.B. and Shumway, N.E. (1985). Isolated pulmonary rejection after combined heart–lung transplantation. *J. Thorac. Cardiovasc. Surg.*, **90**, 623
24. Theodore, J., Jamieson, S.W., Burke, C.M., Reitz, B.A., Stinson, E.B., van Kessel, A., Dawkins, K.D., Herran, J.J., Oyer, P.E., Hunt, S.A., Shumway, N.E. and Robin, E.D. (1984). Physiologic aspects of human heart–lung transplantation. *Chest*, **86**, 349
25. Heath, D. and Edwards, J.E. (1958). The pathology of hypertensive pulmonary vascular disease. A description of six grades of structural changes in the pulmonary arteries with special reference to congenital septal defects. *Circulation*, **18**, 533
26. Billingham, M.E. (1979). Some recent advances in cardiac pathology. *Hum. Pathol.*, **10**, 367
27. Griepp, R., Stinson, E., Bieber, C., Reitz, R.B., Copeland, J.G., Oyer, P.E. and Shumway, N.E. (1977). Control of graft arteriosclerosis in human heart transplant recipients. *Surgery*, **81**, 262
28. Paradis, I.L., Marrari, M., Zeevi, A., Duquesnoy, R.J., Griffith, B.P., Hardesty, R.L. and Dauber, J.H. (1985). HLA phenotype of lung lavage cells following heart–lung transplantation. *J. Heart Transplant.*, **4**, 422
29. Zeevi, A., Fung, J.J., Paradis, I.L., Dauber, J.H., Griffith, B.P., Hardesty, R.L. and Duquesnoy, R.J. (1985). Lymphocytes of bronchoalveolar lavages from heart–lung transplant recipients. *J. Heart Transplant.*, **4**, 417
30. Gryzan, S., Paradis, I.L., Hardesty, R.L., Griffith, B.P. and Dauber, J.H. Bronchoalveolar lavage in heart–lung transplantation. *J. Heart Transplant.*, **4**, 414
31. Burke, C.M., Glanville, A.R., Theodore, J. and Robin, E.D. (1987). Lung immunogenicity, rejection and obliterative bronchiolitis. *Chest*, **92**, 547
32. Harjula, A., Baldwin, J.C., Glanville, A.R., Tazelaar, H., Oyer, P.E.,

Stinson, E.B. and Shumway, N.E. (1987). Human leucocyte antigen compatibility in heart–lung transplantation. *J. Heart Transplant.*, **6**, 162

33. Romaniuk, A., Prop, J., Petersen, A.G., Wildevuur, C.R. and Nieuwenhuis, P. (1987). Expression of class II major histocompatibility complex antigens by bronchial epithelium in rat lung allografts. *Transplantation*, **44**, 209

34. Romaniuk, A., Prop, J., Petersen, A.H. *et al.* (1987). Increased expression of class II MHC-antigens in rejecting and cyclosporine-treated rat lung allografts. *Transplantation*, **44**, 209

35. Dummer, J.S., Bahnson, H.T., Griffith, B.P., Hardesty, R.L., Thompson, M.E. and Ho, M. (1983). Infections in patients on cyclosporine and prednisone following cardiac transplantation. *Transplant. Proc.*, **15**, 2779

36. Wyatt, S., Nunn, J., Hows, J., Yin, J., Hayes, M.C., Cattovsky, G., Gordon-Smith, E.C., Hughes, J.M., Goldman, J.M. and Galton, D. (1984). Airways obstruction associated with graft-versus-host disease after bone marrow transplantation. *Thorax*, **29**, 887

37. Ralph, D., Springmeyer, S., Sullivan, K., Hackman, R.C., Storb, R. and Thomas, E.D. (1984). Rapid progressive airflow obstruction in marrow transplant recipients. *Am. Rev. Respir. Dis.*, **129**, 641

38. Beschorner, W., Saral, R., Hutchins, G., Tutschka, P.J. and Santos, G.W. (1978). Lymphocytic bronchitis associated with graft-versus-host disease in recipients of bone marrow transplants. *N. Engl. J. Med.*, **299**, 1030

39. Stein-Streilein, J., Lipscomb, M., Hart, D. and Darden, A. (1981). Graft-versus-host reaction in the lung. *Transplantation*, **32**, 38

40. Grebe, S. and Streilein, J. (1976). Graft-versus-host reactions: a review. *Adv. Immunol.*, **22**, 119

41. Urbanski, S.J., Kossakowska, A.E., Curtis, J., Chan, C.K., Hutcheon, M.A., Hyland, R.H., Messner, M. and Sculier, J.P. (1987). Idiopathic small airways pathology in patients with graft versus host disease following allogeneic bone marrow transplantation. *Am. J. Surg. Pathol.*, **11**, 965

42. Geddes, D.H., Corrin, B., Brewerton, D.A., Davies, R.J. and Turner-Warwick, M. (1977). Progressive airway obliteration in adults and its association with rheumatoid disease. *Quart. J. Med.*, **46**, 427

43. Epler, G., Snider, G., Gaensler, E., Cathcart, E.S., Fitzgerald, M.X. and Carrington, C.B. (1979). Bronchiolitis and bronchitis in connective tissue disease. *J. Am. Med. Assoc.*, **242**, 528

44. Murphy, K., Atkins, C., Offer, R., Hogg, J.C. and Stein, H.B. (1981). Obliterative bronchiolitis in two rheumatoid arthritis patients treated with penicillamine. *Arth. Rheum.*, **24**, 557

45. Herzog, C., Miller, R. and Hoidal, J. (1981). Bronchiolitis and rheumatoid arthritis. *Am. Rev. Respir. Dis.*, **124**, 636

46. Marck, K.W., Prop, J.M., Wildevuur, C.R.H. and Nieuwenhuis, P. (1985). Lung transplantation in the rat: histopathology of left lung isolated allografts. *J. Heart Transplant.*, **4**, 263

47. Prop, J., Kuijpers, K., Peterson, A.H., Bartels, H.L., Nieuwenhuis, P. and Wildevuur, C.R. (1985). Why are lung allografts more vigorously rejected than hearts? *J. Heart Transplant.*, **4**, 433

48. Tazelaar, H.D., Prop, J., Nieuwenhuis, P., Billingham, M.E. and Wildevuur, C.R.H. (1986). Airway pathology in the transplanted rat lung. *Am. J. Clin. Pathol.*, **86**, 394 (abstract)

49. Prop, J., Tazelaar, H.D. and Billingham, M.E. (1987). Rejection of combined heart–lung transplants in rats: function and pathology. *Am. J. Pathol.*, **127**, 97

50. Allen, M.D., Burke, C.M., McGregor, C.G.A., Baldwin, J.C., Jamieson, S.W. and Theodore, J. (1986). Steroid responsive bronchiolitis after human heart–lung transplantation. *J. Thorac. Cardiovasc. Surg.*, **92**, 449

51. Gosink, B., Friedman, P. and Liebow, A. (1973). Bronchiolitis obliterans. *Am. J. Roentgenol.*, **117**, 816

52. Becroft, D. (1971). Bronchiolitis obliterans, bronchiectasis and other sequelae of adenovirus type 21 infection in younger children. *J. Clin. Pathol.*, **24**, 72

53. Epler, G. and Colby, T. (1983). The spectrum of bronchiolitis obliterans. *Chest*, **83**, 161

54. Moran, T. and Hellstrom, H. (1958). Bronchiolitis obliterans. *Arch. Pathol.*, **66**, 691

55. Wohl, M. and Chernick, V. (1978). Bronchiolitis. *Am. Rev. Respir. Dis.*, **118**, 759

56. Brooks, R.G., Hofflin, J.M., Jamieson, S.W., Stinson, E.B. and Remington, J.S. (1985). Infectious complications in heart–lung transplant recipients. *Am. J. Med.*, **79**, 412

57. Prop, J., Jansen, H.M., Wildevuur, C.R.H. and Nieuwenhuis, P. (1985). Lung allograft rejection in the rat. V. Inhaled stimuli aggravate the rejection response. *Am. Rev. Respir. Dis.*, **132**, 168

58. Higenbottam, T., Stewart, S., Penketh, A. and Wallwork, J. (1987). The diagnosis of lung rejection and opportunistic infection by transbronchial lung biopsy. *Transplant. Proc.*, **19**, 3777

41
Infectious Complications
J.S. DUMMER

INTRODUCTION

In 1981 Reitz and his co-workers at Stanford University successfully introduced heart–lung transplantation into clinical practice[1,2]. Although the new form of transplantation was rapidly taken up by other centers, the pace of further development has been significantly slowed by the scarcity of suitable heart–lung donors. It was also soon appreciated that heart–lung recipients are at risk for a number of serious complications in the postoperative period, the most important of which are intrathoracic infections, particularly pneumonias[3]. These complications account for the fact that the healthy survival of heart–lung recipients is worse than other major organ transplant recipients[3-5].

This review will present what is known about infections after heart–lung transplantation, relying heavily on the local experience in Pittsburgh, discuss relevant problems of diagnosis and treatment, and outline the major infectious problems toward which further investigative efforts should be aimed.

FACTORS INCREASING SUSCEPTIBILITY TO INTRATHORACIC INFECTION

Even in the normal host the lung is relatively vulnerable to infection. In the lung transplant recipient a number of factors unique to this procedure may greatly enhance the susceptibility to intrathoracic infection. These can be broadly discussed under the headings of donor factors, intraoperative factors and postoperative factors.

Donor factors

Most lung donors are intubated, and their airways frequently colonized by bacteria and occasionally by yeasts. Even in the absence of clinical pneumonia there may be bronchial injury. Foreign material may be aspirated into the lung during a closed head injury or gunshot wound to the head, and cause no clinical signs in the donor lung until after transplantation. We have seen one such case, which was associated with a severe focal pneumonia in the postoperative period. In addition, subclinical edema, atelectasis, or even ischemia may produce injury to the donor lung before, during or after procurement, and subsequently impair its ability to handle micro-organisms. Finally, it is well-known that heart allografts may at times transmit latent infections with organisms such as cytomegalovirus and *Toxoplasma gondii*[6-8]. It is possible that lung allografts could additionally transmit infections, which are latent in the lung, such as tuberculosis or histoplasmosis.

Operative factors

Operative factors unique to heart–lung transplantation may predispose to infection. The transected trachea is a potential portal of entry of micro-organisms at the time of surgery, either from the recipient or the donor side, and even with avoidance of steroid therapy during the early weeks after surgery, breakdown of the tracheal anastomosis may occasionally occur[3]. Injury to the vagus or recurrent laryngeal nerves may predispose to pulmonary aspiration, and injury in the phrenic nerve may cause poor diaphragmatic dynamics and lead to poor cough and atelectasis. The extensive dissection required may be associated with severe surface hemorrhage in the mediastinum or along pleural surfaces. Retained blood clots in the chest may then be a nidus for infectious agents.

Postoperative factors

The lymphatic drainage of the transplanted lung is interrupted by the act of transplantation. This interruption may be responsible for the phenomenon of postimplantation edema (reimplantation response) in the first few days after surgery[9-11]. The transplanted lung is a denervated organ, and the distal trachea and bronchial tree are anesthetic. In practice, this means that the cough reflex may be suboptimal for clearing secretions during pulmonary infections[12]. Even the clearance provided by the mucociliary blanket may be impaired in some patients[13].

Finally, in these patients the lung is not only an organ of gas exchange, but also the target of the allograft reaction. During the first few months after transplantation immune cells from the allograft accomplish a slow transition from donor to recipient HLA phenotypes[14]. Zeevi has demonstrated that lymphocytes recovered from the lung during this period proliferate in response to resident macrophages, and has termed this reaction allogenic bronchoalveolar lymphocyte macrophage reaction[15-17]. It is not known to what extent this reaction affects macrophages, but it is conceivable that this reaction may impair key functions of the macrophage such as phagocytosis, killing or presentation of antigen[12,18]. More research needs to be done to better define the nature of local immune deficits in the allografted lung, but it now appears that this is an important factor in the transplant recipient's susceptibility to infection.

CLINICAL INFECTIONS

Published data

There are only two detailed reports of infections in heart–lung recipients, and each describes a series of only 14 patients[19,20]. After a brief discussion of these two reports I shall provide updated information on infections in the first 31 operative survivors at Pittsburgh.

Brooks reported on the infectious complications of heart–lung transplantation at Stanford[19]. Although only three patients died during the follow-up period, which averaged 1 year, there were 29 documented infections, the majority of which were bacterial pneumonias. Some patients developed recurrent bacterial lung infections which produced considerable morbidity. Two patients (14%) had disseminated candidiasis at postmortem. The series was remarkable for the absence of pneumonia due to *Pneumocystis carinii*, and the low incidence of serious cytomegalovirus infections; the latter was probably due to Stanford's exclusive use of blood products from donors with no cytomegalovirus antibodies. Other infections were two cases of legionella pneumonia, both cured by antibiotic therapy, and a disseminated herpes simplex virus infection.

On the basis of their experience, the authors commented that the diagnosis of lung infection in heart–lung transplant recipients was difficult, both because infection could not always be easily differentiated from rejection on the basis of a chest radiograph, and because samples of bronchial secretions, obtained from the patients by transtracheal aspiration or bronchoscopy, often yielded multiple species of bacteria.

Somewhat later, the Pittsburgh group reported on the infectious complications, also in 14 patients, and made comparisons between infections in recipients of heart–lung and heart transplants[20]. It was noted that infection rates in heart–lung recipients were twice that in heart recipients, and that two-thirds of the infections in heart–lung recipients were in the lung or chest cavity. Infectious complications were a contributing factor in all seven deaths in the Pittsburgh series. Some patients also had a pattern of recurrent bacterial bronchopulmonary infections that required hospital admission for treatment.

Although a direct comparison between the early Stanford and Pittsburgh experiences is difficult because of possible differences in the patient populations and case definitions, both suggested a high vulnerability of the lung allograft to serious infection. There were a few notable differences, particularly in the incidence of *Pneumocystis carinii* infection, which was seen in none of the Stanford patients but was diagnosed in six of 14 Pittsburgh patients. Pittsburgh also reported a high incidence of severe viral infections such as cytomegalovirus pneumonia and lymphoproliferative disease related to primary Epstein–Barr virus infection. The combined experience seemed to issue a caveat to any program embarking on heart–lung transplantation, that these patients would require intense follow-up and a search for innovative solutions to their infectious problems.

Pittsburgh update

Data are presented on the first 31 patients who survived more than 3 days after surgery. The mean follow-up in these patients was 492 days (range 6–1743) after transplantation, and the 1-year survival was 55%. The mean age of the patients was 32 years; 13 were men and 18 were women. Underlying diagnoses included primary pulmonary hypertension (11 patients), pulmonary hypertension secondary to congenital heart disease (12 patients), and other diagnoses (eight patients), which included a broad array of conditions including emphysema, interstitial fibrotic lung disease, veno-occlusive disease, cystic fibrosis, and eosinophilic granuloma.

Because most of the infections in our earlier series were severe, defined as those which required hospitalization for diagnosis or treatment, this review will report only on severe infections. Table 41.1 lists the severe infections seen in these patients during the follow-up period, and the number of deaths associated with each type of infection. Infections were considered to be associated with death, either if the infection was found at postmortem, or if the patient was being treated for the infection at the time of death.

Ninety-one severe infections were detected. Of these, 57% were bacterial, 19% viral, 12% protozoal, 10% fungal, and 2% were sternal wound infections due to *Mycoplasma hominis*.

Table 41.1 Severe infections complicating heart–lung transplantation in Pittsburgh*

Type	Cases	Deaths†
Bacterial ($n = 52$)		
lung	39	12
mediastinum	4	2
blood‡	4	1
pleural	3	0
abdominal	2	2
Viral ($n = 17$)		
cytomegalovirus	12	6
Epstein–Barr	3	1
herpes simplex	1	1
non-A, non-B hepatitis	1	1
Protozoal ($n = 11$)		
pneumocystosis	9	3
toxoplasmosis	2	1
Fungal ($n = 9$)		
candidiasis	6	5
aspergillosis	2	2
cryptococcosis	1	1
Mycoplasma ($n = 2$)		
M. hominis	2	1

*31 consecutive operative survivors, mean follow-up 492 days
†Indicates that the infection was being treated at time of death or was discovered at autopsy
‡Includes only bloodstream infections without a definite site of tissue infection

Bacterial infection

The majority of the bacterial infections were pneumonias or severe bronchitis. The organisms involved were most often enteric Gram negative rods, pseudomonas species and staphylococci, although in eight instances the bacterial flora were so mixed that a predominant species could not be identified. The specimens were most often obtained by bronchoscopy, and the quality of the cultured specimens was always confirmed by inspection of a Gram stain. No infections due to pneumococcus were seen, and only one due to Hemophilus influenzae was diagnosed. Also, no infections due to legionella, mycobacteria, or nocardia were identified.

Four patients in the series developed a syndrome of recurrent bacterial pulmonary infections more than 1 year after transplantation. In three cases this was associated with persistent colonization with Pseudomonas aeruginosa. In the fourth, multiple bacteria, including pseudomonas, were found. Two of these patients have died, one with septic complications, and the other after an attempt at retransplantation; the third is now undergoing recurrent hospitalization every few months for intravenous antibiotics, and the fourth has improved with a regimen of daily postural drainage and occasional hospitalization for antibiotic treatment. Two also had evidence of chronic lung rejection at postmortem; a component of chronic rejection is suspected but not proved in the other two.

Bacterial mediastinitis was diagnosed in four patients and was due to staphylococcal species in three. Bacteroides species were the only bacteria isolated from the fourth case, but the patient was on multiple antibiotics at the time of exploration for repair of a partial tracheal dehiscence. A tracheal leak was also the probable source in one of the other cases. These cases and those due to candida and Mycoplasma hominis (see below) combine to make a 22% rate of mediastinitis in this series, which is much higher than the rate of 1.5% for routine cardiac transplant cases in Pittsburgh[21].

Bacterial pleural space infections were due to Escherichia coli (two patients) and Staphylococcus aureus (one patient). Two occurred in the early postoperative period and appeared to be due to superinfections of pleural space hematomas, and one occurred more than 2 years after transplantation and had no clear source, although a radiographically-inapparent pneumonia was suspected. Other bacterial infections included bloodstream infections, three of which were line-related staphylococcal infections, and intra-abdominal infections, one of which was related to perforation of the small bowel at the site of a regressing lymphoproliferative lesion.

Cytomegalovirus infection

As in other transplant populations, cytomegalovirus (CMV) infections were the most important viral pathogen in this series. Table 41.2 shows data on the number of primary and reactivation CMV infections in the population. Overall, 21 patients (68% of the total group) were infected, defined by isolation of the virus in the post-transplant period. Twelve patients (57% of the infected patients) had symptoms due to CMV. Infection only occurred in about half of seronegative patients, but when it occurred it was symptomatic in all but one instance. By contrast, infection occurred in almost all seropositive patients, but was symptomatic in only 20%.

These rates of infection and disease, and the increased risk of symptomatic infection with primary infection, are similar to those noted in recipients of other types of transplants[22]. We previously noted a higher rate of CMV pneumonia in heart–lung recipients than in recipients of heart allografts[23]. This observation was upheld by the present series as ten patients (32% of the total group) had

Table 41.2 Primary and reactivated cytomegalovirus (CMV) infections in heart–lung transplant recipients

CMV antibody status before transplantation	Number of patients	Number with infection	Number of symptomatic patients	CMV pneumonia	CMV seropositive donors/number tested
Negative	20	11	10	8	3/14
Positive	11	10	2	2	1/7
Total	31	21	12	10	4/21

CMV pneumonia diagnosed by open lung biopsy or at autopsy. This is more than three times the rate of CMV pneumonia diagnosed in heart transplant recipients at our institution.

It strongly suggests that the lung allograft is more susceptible to CMV infection than native lungs. One explanation for this might be that the infection is transmitted by the donor lung and arises *in situ*. The information collected to date would tend to discount this explanation as most of the CMV pneumonias occurred in lungs harvested from seronegative donors (see Table 41.2). At present, we think it is likely that the allograft reaction in the donor lung promotes CMV infection, in some way analogous to the enhancement of CMV pneumonia in bone marrow transplant recipients with graft versus host reaction[24].

Given the serious nature of CMV disease in heart–lung transplant recipients, and the inadequacy of current treatment regimens, it seems best to try to avoid CMV infection. We now administer only CMV-negative blood products to our CMV-negative heart–lung recipients. If serious tissue infections with CMV occur, our current practice is to offer treatment with ganciclovir. This is a promising experimental agent with *in vitro* and *in vivo* activity against CMV, but insufficient data are currently available to define its role in treating transplant recipients[25,26]. The use of prophylactic immunoglobulins to attenuate the manifestations of CMV infection is another interesting approach, but requires further study[27].

Epstein–Barr virus

Lymphoproliferative disease related to Epstein–Barr virus (EBV) infection was seen in two young men in the series. Two more recent heart–lung recipients also developed this post-transplant complication. All four patients had primary EBV infection. Three had regression of their tumors with reduction of immunosuppression, and one died from abdominal sepsis after perforation of the small bowel at the site of an ileal tumor.

Heart and heart–lung transplant recipients have been reported to develop these tumors more frequently than other transplant recipients[28,29]. Their proper treatment is controversial. Hanto has advocated acyclovir therapy, especially for patients who present with symptoms of infectious mononucleosis and have polyclonal tumors[30]. Starzl, however, has noted that the tumors frequently regress with reduction of immunosuppression without acyclovir therapy[31]. Since the tumors appear to be much more common after primary EBV infection, it is important to study candidates before transplantation for EBV antibodies so that EBV-seronegative candidates at risk for primary infection can be detected.

Other viral infections

Other severe viral infections included a case of non-A non-B hepatitis and a case of herpes simplex esophagitis discovered at autopsy. In addition, we have diagnosed respiratory syncytial virus pneumonia in a pediatric heart–lung recipient. (The Stanford group has reported an adult patient with recurrent viral infections due to parainfluenzae virus and respiratory syncytial virus[32].) At present, the importance of community acquired respiratory viruses as pathogens in heart–lung recipients is not clear, but it is an intriguing area for further investigation.

Protozoal infection

Protozoal infections have been a common complication of heart–lung transplantation in Pittsburgh. In the series there were nine cases of *Pneumocystis carinii* infection that required hospitalization. Not listed in Table 41.1 are seven additional patients who had *P. carinii* discovered during routine outpatient bronchoscopy. These patients were asymptomatic and were treated with oral sulfamethoxazole/trimethoprim (SMX/TMP) as outpatients. By comparison, the incidence of pneumocystis infection in heart transplant recipients at our institution is 5% or less[33,34]. Fatal disease and relapses of pneumocystis infection have also been seen in heart–lung, but not in heart, recipients at our institution.

It is apparent from these high rates of pneumocystis infection that prophylaxis against pneumocystis infection would be desirable in heart–lung recipients. Unfortunately, we have been unable to maintain patients consistently on daily SMX/TMP prophylaxis because of gastrointestinal intolerance and rises of serum creatinine, which created confusion with cyclosporine toxicity. We have opted for a low-dose intermittent regimen (SMX/TMP 1–2 double strength tablets daily for 7 days out of each month). So far, no clinical pneumocystis infections have been diagnosed in patients on this regimen, but it requires further follow-up and study.

Two patients had toxoplasmosis. In one the infection was discovered in lung and brain at autopsy, but had been clinically obscured by multiple other infections. The other patient's only symptom was fever; the diagnosis was made serologically, and later confirmed by isolation of the organism from the bloodstream in tissue culture.

Pretransplant testing for toxoplasma antibodies is essential as serology is the most accessible approach to making or ruling out the diagnosis of toxoplasmosis. Donor antibody testing is probably also warranted, as many of these infections are transmitted by donor organs[7].

Fungal infection

Seven (23%) of the patients in the series developed nine invasive fungal infections. Candida was the most common pathogen and was either confined to the mediastinum and pleural spaces (three patients) or was disseminated (three patients). All of the candida infections occurred in the first 6 weeks after transplantation in patients in the intensive care unit. Disruption of the tracheal anastomosis was a likely conduit for infection in the three patients with infection isolated to the chest cavity.

Two patients with candidiasis also had invasive aspergillosis involving the lung. In one instance there was a secondary brain abscess. One patient had disseminated cryptococcal disease, which spared the central nervous system, 4 months after transplantation. Since these are very high rates of fungal infection, consideration could be given to some form of systemic prophylaxis for fungal infection in these patients. It is likely that only further experience and research, combined with better antifungal drugs will enable us to find the best approach to this problem.

Sternal wound infection with M. hominis

We recently reported on the occurrence of sternal wound infections due to *Mycoplasma hominis* in patients undergoing sternotomies[35]. This series included two heart–lung recipients, and we are currently treating a third for *M. hominis* infection in the mediastinum and both pleural spaces. All occurred 2–4 weeks after transplantation. Two presented with fever and mild erythema, tenderness and instability of the sternal wound. The third case was diagnosed when mycoplasma were isolated from pleural fluid, but sternal signs developed later.

The key to making the diagnosis is recognizing it as a possibility when there is purulent drainage combined with a negative Gram stain for bacteria and initially negative cultures. This should be followed by careful examination of anaerobic culture plates (Columbia nalidixic agar and blood agar) for the typical pinpoint, translucent colonies. Transfer of these to mycoplasma A7 agar (Remel Regional Media Laboratories, Lenexa, Kansas, USA) produces colonies with the fried-egg appearance typical of mycoplasma.

Unlike *Mycoplasma pneumoniae*, these mycoplasma are uniformly resistant to erythromycin. They are usually, but not always, sensitive to clindamycin and tetracycline[36]. Recently it has been found that they are also sensitive *in vitro* to some of the newer quinolone antibiotics, such as ciprofloxacin[37].

Mycoplasma mediastinitis is clinically milder than staphylococcal mediastinitis, and the organisms cannot usually be isolated after a few days of antimicrobial therapy; the infection, however, appears to compromise readily the integrity of sternal bone, and several patients have required reoperation for placement of a muscle flap to fill a large sternal defect. Because of the relatively poor structural results achieved so far with immediate drainage and debridement, we now consider delaying operative intervention (if no abscess is seen on a computerized tomographic scan of the chest) until antimicrobials have been administered for a number of days. The best operative management remains to be determined.

DIAGNOSIS OF INFECTION

Heart–lung recipients need to be evaluated before transplantation, and followed in a systematic fashion after transplantation in order to facilitate the prompt diagnosis of rejection and infection. The pretransplant evaluation for infection is similar to that for other transplant candidates, but should include, at a minimum, a brief history focusing on the candidate's past experience with infections, geographic aspects of their residence and travel, and possible exposure to tuberculosis. The most useful laboratory tests are antibody tests for herpesviruses, for the human immunodeficiency virus type 1, and for toxoplasmosis. The evaluation should include a tuberculin skin test, as the immunosuppressive medications used after transplantation will usually ablate positive reactions.

Following transplantation, we have tried to keep routine surveillance to a minimum. We have generally ordered cultures for CMV and herpes simplex virus (urine, throat wash, and buffy coat) every 2–4 weeks for the first 2 or 3 months after transplantation. This degree of screening is usually adequate to detect virtually all infections with CMV and most infections with herpes simplex virus. We do not perform repeat post-transplant antibody tests for viruses or toxoplasma unless this is dictated by the clinical situation. Transplant centers without an in-house virology laboratory, however, should probably obtain antibody tests for CMV every 2–3 weeks for 3 months after transplantation to screen for infection with this agent.

We have not found routine surveillance cultures for bacteria or fungi to be useful when following recipients of most solid organ transplants; a possible exception is the surveillance of sputum by Gram stain and culture in heart–lung recipients while they are intubated in the intensive care unit. Gram stains of sputum from patients in this setting often show bacteria and neutrophils, even in the absence of lung infection. But comparison of serial sputum Gram stains will frequently show a detectable increase in the number of bacteria and neutrophils, or a shift in the predominant flora, when pneumonia develops. An additional benefit of this practice is that the antibiotic sensitivities of colonizing bacteria may help to guide therapy when pneumonia develops.

A key element in our long-term follow-up of these patients has been the involvement of our pulmonary physicians (particularly Drs Irvin Paradis and James Dauber). They have introduced a program of serial bronchoscopy with bronchoalveolar lavage (BAL) on the patients after transplantation. These BALs are done routinely every 2–3 weeks during the postoperative hospitalization, every 3 months for the first 2 years, and at a reduced frequency of every 6–12 months thereafter. In practice the patients usually undergo BALs more frequently because they are also used as a diagnostic tool to investigate suspected infection or rejection in the lung. All BALs are submitted to a broad array of stains and cultures to diagnose infection. The cells in the BAL are enumerated, classified, and also submitted for *in vitro*, immunologic testing, which is a research arm of the project. A review of the experience with this investigative technique in heart–lung transplant recipients has recently been published[12].

In a patient with pneumonia, a decision about treatment is usually made shortly after the lavage, and is based on the clinical picture, Gram stain, cell counts and differential from the lavage. In addition to bacterial studies, fungal cultures, viral cultures, M-toluidine and silver stains for pneumocystis, and cytologies (to detect inclusion bodies), and stains and smears to detect mycobacteria, are usually processed on the BAL specimens. Although these tests detect a wide variety of infectious agents, they are not completely sensitive in diagnosing infection. In difficult cases we have not hesitated to perform open lung biopsy as the ultimate investigation to diagnose infection and distinguish it from rejection.

This simple schema is somewhat more complicated in practice, and depends on communication between the various physicians caring for the patient and meticulous evaluation of the clinical situation. From 2–3 months after transplantation, the patients usually do not reside near the transplant center and are seen relatively infrequently for clinical follow-up. This makes their evaluation for infection more difficult. However, the number of likely infectious agents also decreases with time, since fungal disease is seen mostly in the very early post-transplant period, CMV disease is predominantly a problem in the first 6 months, and pneumocystis infection can generally be prevented by antibiotic prophylaxis.

RELATIONSHIP OF REJECTION AND INFECTION

Some understanding of the clinical aspects of rejection in heart–lung recipients is critical for an approach to infectious problems, as rejection may mimic infection in a number of ways. There appear to be two major clinical forms of rejection. The first is acute rejection of the lung, which usually occurs 1–6 weeks after transplantation, and most often presents with the rapid appearance of lung infiltrates, often of a diffuse distribution, together with arterial oxygen desaturation. Fever may also be present, and a heart biopsy usually will not show rejection. In general, the rejection responds quickly to a few intravenous doses of corticosteroids[12,38–40].

Chronic rejection presents from a few months to greater than 1 year after transplantation, and has a more indolent course with breathlessness and cough, which may be productive or non-productive. There is measurable deterioration of pulmonary function with obstructive and occasionally restrictive findings. The patients do not usually have fever. Chest radiographs may be normal or show a generalized patchy increase in lung markings. Histologically, the lung shows obliterative bronchiolitis, interstitial and pleural fibrosis and arteriosclerosis. The response to increased immunosuppression is not as reliable as in acute rejection[4,41–43]. (It should be noted that these are paradigmatic illustrations based on relatively small numbers of cases; as experience increases, a broader spectrum of rejection phenomena may be characterized.)

It is apparent that either of these presentations might mimic infection or cause diagnostic confusion by coexisting with infection. One of the major challenges in caring for heart–lung recipients is to develop diagnostic tools powerful enough not only to distinguish these two entities, but to detect each in the presence of the other. Recently the concept has emerged that chronic immune damage to the airways may lead to bronchiectasis, and then to recurring episodes of bronchitis and pneumonia[12]. Two of the four patients in this series with recurring bacterial lung infections more than 1 year after transplantation had definite histological evidence of chronic rejection. In the other patients, chronic rejection was suspected, but no definite tissue evidence was obtained.

More intriguing is the possibility that infectious episodes might trigger chronic rejection. Gryzan *et al.* have noted an association between pneumocystis infection and the subsequent emergence in BAL fluid of lymphocytes reactive against donor spleen cells[44]. Two of three patients in whom these alloreactive lymphocytes were found later developed chronic rejection. A similar pattern of alloreactivity has been noted after CMV infection[12]. These findings are provocative, but it should be noted that infections such as CMV and pneumocystis are so common in this population that associations by chance alone could explain these findings.

It is likely that the chronic respiratory dysfunction seen in some patients after heart–lung transplantation may have elements of both rejection and infection, but there is a spectrum of clinical presentation ranging from predominantly infectious to predominantly non-infectious.

COMMENT

Current data suggest that the rate of infections in heart–lung recipients is significantly higher than that in heart recipients. Most of the increased risk is probably due to technical aspects of the surgery and unique aspects of infection arising in the allograft.

Future progress will likely arise from further technical improvements in surgery, from intense investigation of infection and rejection in the lung allograft, and from the development of safe prophylactic regimens to prevent viral and fungal disease after transplantation. In the meantime, meticulous attention to clinical management by physicians experienced in the care of such patients offers the best hope for a favorable outcome.

References

1. Reitz, B.A., Wallwork, J.L., Hunt, S.A., Pennock, J.L., Billingham, M.E., Oyer, P.E., Stinson, E.B. and Shumway, N.E. (1982). Heart–lung transplantation. Successful therapy for patients with pulmonary vascular disease. *N. Engl. J. Med.*, **306**, 557
2. Jamieson, S.W., Reitz, B.A., Oyer, P.E. et al. (1983). Combined heart and lung transplantation. *Lancet*, **1**, 1130
3. Griffith, B.P. (1987). Cardiopulmonary transplantation – growing pains. *Int. J. Cardiol.*, **17**, 119
4. Morris, A.J.R. and Jamieson, S.W. (1987). Combined heart–lung transplantation for end-stage right ventricular failure. *Cardiol. Clin.*, **17**, 251
5. Thompson, M.E., Dummer, J.S., Paradis, I., Zeevi, A., Griffith, B.P. and Hardesty, R.L. (1987). Heart–lung transplantation – the courage to succeed. In Yu, P. (ed.) *Progress in Cardiology*. Vol. 16 (3). (Philadelphia: Lea and Febiger)
6. Pollard, R.B., Rand, K.H., Gamberg, P., Gallagher, J.G. and Merigan, T.C. (1982). Specific cell mediated immunity and infections with herpesvirus in cardiac transplant recipients. *Am. J. Med.*, **73**, 679
7. Luft, B.J., Naot, Y., Araujo, F.G., Stinson, E.B. and Remington, J.S. (1983). Primary and reactivated toxoplasma infection in patients with cardiac transplants. *Ann. Intern. Med.*, **99**, 27
8. Wreghitt, T.G., Hakim, M., Cory-Pearce, R., English, T.A.H. and Wallwork, J. (1986). The impact of donor-transmitted CMV and *Toxomplasma gondii* disease in cardiac transplantation. *Transplant. Proc.*, **18**, 1375
9. Siegelman, S.S., Sinha, S.B.P. and Veith, F.J. (1973). Pulmonary reimplantation response. *Ann. Surg.*, **177**, 30
10. Jamieson, S.W., Stinson, E.B., Oyer, P.E., Reitz, B.A., Baldwin, J., Modry, D., Dawkins, K., Theodore, J., Hunt, S. and Shumway, N.E (1984). Heart–lung transplantation for irreversible pulmonary hypertension. *Ann. Thorac. Surg.*, **38**, 554
11. Mancini, M.C., Borovetz, H.S., Griffith, B.P. and Hardesty, R.L. (1985). Changes in lung vascular permeability after heart–lung transplantation. *J. Surg. Res.*, **39**, 305
12. Dauber, J.H. and Zeevi, A. (1988). Lung transplantation: lessons learned about local immune function and pulmonary defense mechanisms. In Daniele, R.P. (ed.) *Pulmonary Immunology*. p. 625. (New York: McGraw Hill)
13. Mancini, M.C. and Tauxe, W.N. (1986). Assessment of pulmonary clearance in heart–lung transplant recipients using technetium99 minimicronized albumin colloid (MMAC). *Am. Rev. Respir. Dis.*, **133**, A11
14. Paradis, I.L., Marrari, M., Zeevi, A., Duquesnoy, R.J., Griffith, B.P., Hardesty, R.L. and Dauber, J.H. (1985). HLA phenotype of lung lavage cells following heart–lung transplantation. *J. Heart Transplant.*, **4**, 422
15. Fung, J.J., Zeevi, A., Kaufman, C., Paradis, I.L., Dauber, J.H., Hardesty, R.L., Griffith, B. and Duquesnoy, R.J. (1985). Interactions between lymphocytes and macrophages in heart–lung transplant recipients. *Human Immunol.*, **14**, 287
16. Zeevi, A., Fung, J.J., Paradis, I.L., Dauber, J.H., Griffith, B.P., Hardesty, R.L. and Duquesnoy, R.J. (1985). Lymphocytes of bronchoalveolar lavage from heart–lung transplant recipients. *J. Heart Transplant.*, **4**, 417
17. Zeevi, A., Fung, J.J., Paradis, I.L., Gryzan, S., Dauber, J.H., Hardesty, R.L., Griffith, B., Trento, A., Saidman, S. and Duquesnoy, R.J. (1987). Bronchoalveolar macrophage–lymphocyte reactivity in heart–lung transplant recipients. *Transplant. Proc.*, **19**, 2537
18. Muggenburg, B.A., Bice, D.E., Haley, P.J., Mauderly, J.L., Dauber, J.J., Heron, K. and Griffith, B.P. (1987). Immune response in the transplanted canine lung. *Am. Rev. Respir. Dis.*, **135**, A103
19. Brooks, R.G., Hofflin, J.M., Jamieson, S.W., Stinson, E.B. and Remington, J.S. (1985). Infectious complications in heart–lung transplant recipients. *Am. J. Med.*, **79**, 412
20. Dummer, J.S., Montero, C.G., Griffith, B.P., Hardesty, R.L., Paradis, I.L. and Ho, M. (1986). Infections in heart–lung transplant recipients. *Transplantation*, **41**, 725
21. Griffith, B.P., Kormos, R.L., Hardesty, R.L., Armitage, J.M. and Dummer, J.S. (1988). The artificial heart: infection-related morbidity and its effect on transplantation. *Ann. Thorac. Surg.*, **45**, 409
22. Ho, M. (1982). *Cytomegalovirus: Biology and Infection*. (New York: Plenum Press)
23. Dummer, J.S., White, L.T., Ho, M., Griffith, B.P., Hardesty, R.L. and Bahnson, H.T. (1985). Morbidity of cytomegalovirus infection in recipients of heart or heart–lung transplants who received cyclosporine. *J. Infect. Dis.*, **152**, 1182
24. Meyers, J.D., Flournoy, N. and Thomas, E.D. (1982). Nonbacterial pneumonia after allogeneic marrow transplantation: a review of ten years' experience. *Rev. Infect. Dis.*, **4**, 1119
25. Shepp, D.H., Danliker, P.S., Miranda, P., Burnette, T.C., Cederberg, D.M., Kirk, L.E. and Meyers, J.D. (1985). Activity of 9-[2-hydroxyl-1-(hydroxymethyl) ethoxymethyl] guanine in the treatment of cytomegalovirus pneumonia. *Ann. Intern. Med.*, **103**, 368
26. Erice, A., Jordon, M.C., Chace, B.A., Fletcher, C., Chinnock, B.J. and Balfour, H.H. Jr. (1987). Ganciclovir treatment of cytomegalovirus disease in transplant recipients and other immunocompromised hosts. *J. Am. Med. Assoc.*, **257**, 3082
27. Syndman, D.R., Werner, B.G., Heinze-Lacey, B., Berardi, V.P., Tilney, N.L., Kirkman, R.L., Milford, E.L., Cho, S.I., Bush H.L. Jr., Levey, A.S., Strom, T.B., Carpenter, C.B., Levey, R.H., Harmon, W.E., Zimmerman, C.E., Shapiro, M.E., Steinman, T., Logerfo, F., Idelson, B., Schroter, G.P.J., Levin, M.J., McIves, J., Leszczyrski, J. and Grady, G.F. (1987). Use of cytomegalovirus immune globulin to prevent cytomegalovirus disease in renal transplant recipients. *N. Engl. J. Med.*, **317**, 1049
28. Ho, M., Miller, G., Atchison, R.W., Breinig, M.K., Dummer, J.S., Andeman, W., Starzl, T.E., Eastman, R., Griffith, B.P., Hardesty, R.L., Bahnson, H.T., Hakala, T.R. and Rosenthal, J.T. (1985). Epstein–Barr virus infections and DNA hybridization studies in posttransplantation lymphoma and lymphoproliferative lesions: The role of primary infection. *J. Infect. Dis.*, **152**, 876
29. Beveridge, T., Krupp, P. and McKibbin, C. (1984). Lymphomas and lymphoproliferative lesions developing under cyclosporine therapy (Letter). *Lancet*, **1**, 788
30. Hanto, D., Frizzera, G., Gajl-Peczalska, K. and Simmons, R. (1985). Epstein–Barr virus, immunodeficiency and B-cell lymphoproliferation. *Transplantation*, **39**, 461
31. Starzl, T.E., Nalesnik, M.A., Porter, K.A., Ho, M., Iwatsuki, S., Griffith, B.P., Rosenthal, J.T., Hakala, T.R., Shaw, B.W. Jr., Hardesty, R.L. et al. (1984). Reversibility of lymphomas and lymphoproliferative lesions developing under cyclosporine-steroid therapy. *Lancet*, **1**, 583
32. Allen, M.D., Burke, C.M., McGregor, C.G.A., Baldwin, J.C., Jamieson, S.W. and Theodore, J. (1986). Steroid-responsive bronchiolitis after

human heart–lung transplantation. *J. Thorac. Cardiovasc. Surg.*, **92**, 449

33. Dummer, J.S., Bahnson, H.T., Griffith, B.P., Hardesty, R.L., Thompson, M.E. and Ho, M. (1983). Infections in patients on cyclosporine and prednisone following cardiac transplantation. *Transplant. Proc.*, **15**, 2779

34. Dummer, J.S., Ho, M., McMahon, D.K., Griffith, B.P., Hardesty, R.L., Trento, A. and Bahnson, H.T. (1987). Infectious complications in heart and heart–lung transplant recipients. *Proceedings of the 1st European Conference on Transplantation*, Venice, Italy, March 1987

35. Steffenson, D.O., Dummer, J.S., Granick, M.S., Pasculle, A.W., Griffith, B.P. and Cassell, G.H. (1987). Sternotomy infections with *Mycoplasma hominis*. *Ann. Intern. Med.*, **106**, 204

36. Bygdeman, S.M. and Mardh, P.A. (1984). Antimicrobial susceptibility and susceptibility testing of *Mycoplasma hominis*. *Sex. Trans. Dis*, **11**, 366

37. Kenny, T., Hooten, M. and Roberts, M.C. (1987). Sensitivities of *Mycoplasma hominis* and *Ureaplasma urealyticum* to quinolones. *Abstracts of the 1987 International Conference on Antimicrobial Agents and Chemotherapy*, New York

38. Griffith, B.P., Hardesty, R.L., Trento, A. and Bahnson, H.T. (1985). Asynchronous rejection of heart and lungs following cardiopulmonary transplantation. *Ann. Thorac. Surg.*, **40**, 488

39. Griffith, B.P., Durham, S.J., Hardesty, R.L., Trento, A. and Paradis, I.L. (1987). Acute rejection of the heart–lung allograft and methods of its detection. *Transplant. Proc.*, **19**, 2527

40. Novitzky, D., Cooper, D.K.C., Wicomb, W.N., Rose, A.G. and Reichart, R. (1985). Transplantation of the heart and both lungs. *S. Afr. Med. J.*, **67**, 575

41. Yousem, S.A., Burke, C.M. and Billingham, M.E. (1985). Pathologic pulmonary alterations in long-term human heart–lung transplantation. *Hum. Pathol.*, **16**, 911

42. Theodore, J., Jamieson, S.W., Burke, C.M., Reitz, B.A., Stinson, E.B., Van Kessel, A., Dawkins, K.D., Herran, J.J., Oyer, P.E., Hunt, S.A., Shumway, N.E. and Robin, E.D. (1984). Physiologic aspects of human heart–lung transplantation. *Chest*, **86**, 349

43. Burke, C.M., Theodore, J., Dawkins, K.D., Yousem, S.A., Blank, N., Billingham, M.E., Van Kessel, A., Jamieson, S.W., Oyer, P.E., Baldwin, J.C., Stinson, E.B., Shumway, N.E. and Robin, E.D. (1984). Post-transplant obliterative bronchiolitis and other late lung sequelae in human heart–lung transplantation. *Chest*, **86**, 824

44. Gryzan, S., Paradis, I.L., Zeevi, A. *et al.* (1988). Unexpectedly high incidence of *Pneumocystis carinii* infection after lung–heart transplantation: implications for lung defense and allograft survival. *Am. Rev. Respir. Dis.*, **137**, 1268

42
Physiology and Pharmacology of the Transplanted Lungs

J. THEODORE

INTRODUCTION

The lungs are an integral part of the respiratory system, which comprises a complex, highly integrated and multi-structured system performing gas exchange between the body and ambient air as its primary function. In conjunction with the cardiovascular system, the primary purpose of the respiratory system is to provide molecular O_2 to the cells of the tissues, and to remove CO_2 generated by them, in accord with cellular metabolic requirements. The lungs, as the principal sites for gas exchange, are the focal points for both the respiratory system (i.e. non-lung components) and the circulatory system, since close integration of function between both systems is required to meet the ever-changing demands of the body.

A comprehensive review of respiratory physiology is beyond the scope of this chapter, and can be found elsewhere[1-7]. In brief, respiration in man may be divided into five separate steps or processes[8]. These are:

(1) *Pulmonary ventilation*: the exchange of gases between the lungs and ambient atmosphere. Total ventilation and its distribution within the lungs are both important.

(2) *Pulmonary perfusion*: the flow and distribution of blood within the pulmonary circulation resulting in the arterialization of mixed venous blood as a result of gas exchange.

(3) *Pulmonary gas exchange*: the transfer of O_2 and CO_2 across the alveolar–capillary barriers of the lung. Optimal gas exchange is dependent upon: (a) the degree of alveolar ventilation (i.e. ventilation of alveoli perfused with blood); (b) diffusing properties of the alveolar–capillary barriers and the surface area available for gas exchange; (c) the proper matching of ventilation to blood perfusion ($\dot{V}/\dot{Q}$ ratios); and (d) the degree of shunt that is present (i.e. venous blood bypassing ventilated alveoli).

(4) *Gas transport and uptake*: the conveying of arterial blood from the left ventricle to the peripheral tissues, which extract O_2 and release CO_2 for transport back to the right heart. In addition to the cardiac output, the amounts of O_2 and CO_2 conveyed are dependent upon their gas tensions, hemoglobin, red blood cells, and other factors involved in the chemical interactions and reactions associated with O_2 and CO_2 transport in blood.

(5) *Regulation of ventilation*: the control of blood acidity–alkalinity and respiratory gas tensions (PaO_2, $PaCO_2$) by increasing or decreasing ventilation.

The extrapulmonary components (non-lung) of the respiratory system primarily involve the 'controller' and 'air pump' segments of the system which are responsible for initiating and generating, respectively, the forces required for ventilating the lungs through the contraction of the respiratory muscles (diaphragm, principal muscle). As a result, ventilation is a multifactorial process which is dependent upon the integrated function of a number of structures which include: (1) the respiratory control centers in the brain stem; (2) the central and peripheral chemoreceptors, and an extensive efferent and afferent neural network (including the autonomic system innervating the cardiopulmonary axis) which are involved in the modulation of respiratory control; (3) the phrenic (principal motor nerve) and intercostal nerves which convey the neural motor output to the respiratory muscles (diaphragm and intercostals, respectively); and (4) the chest wall which includes the thoracic cage, respiratory muscles, and the abdominal contents. In addition, the mechanical properties of the lungs and chest wall also have a significant effect on ventilation.

Ventilation is affected by chemical, humoral and neural mediators with adjustments being made according to the metabolic needs of the body (e.g. rest vs. exercise). In addition to the usual chemical mediators affecting ventilatory control (i.e. hydrogen ion, CO_2, hypoxemia), neural 'feedback' loops from receptors in peripheral tissues, including the lungs and chest wall, also have modulating effects on ventilatory output[9]. During exercise, ventilation increases in a linear fashion with CO_2 production until the onset of acidemia, at which time it rises more sharply. This relationship reflects the linking of the ventilatory response to metabolic demand in the performance of increasing levels of work during exercise.

Some of the physiologic issues that may be of concern in heart–lung or lung transplantation can be touched upon at this point, in anticipation of the forthcoming sections.

In combined heart–lung or lung transplantation, all components of the recipient's respiratory system remain essentially intact, with the exception of the allografts. Thus, in general, central ventilatory control or functioning of the respiratory 'air pump' should not be significantly impaired post-transplant. The real issue is how important are the neural 'feedback' loops from the cardiopulmonary axis on central controlling functions. What effects will lung denervation have on the control of ventilation (loss of pulmonary afferents) or cardiopulmonary denervation on the integrated responses that are required between the respiratory and circulatory systems during exercise (loss of efferents and afferents)? The other issue is how important is the central nervous system in the control of intrapulmonary function via the parasympathetic and sympathetic systems? Thus, what effect will lung denervation have on the regulation of airway function, or on the pulmonary circulation? Some insight into these questions is provided in the next sections.

PHYSIOLOGY OF THE TRANSPLANTED LUNG

Combined heart–lung transplantation in humans (i.e. 'en bloc' transplantation of both lungs and heart) has served as a unique model for defining the physiology of the transplanted lung and respiratory system. Despite cardiopulmonary denervation and the disruption of the pulmonary lymphatic and bronchial arterial systems at the time of surgery, the transplanted lungs (and heart) function sufficiently well to support the activities of normal life, providing no complications occur. Long-term pulmonary function appears to be well preserved with the maintenance of essentially normal gas exchange for extended periods of time measurable in years. In general, the overall function of the respiratory system does not appear to be adversely affected by the extensive nature of combined heart–lung transplantation[10-12].

The discussion on the physiology and pharmacology of the transplanted lung to be presented in this chapter is based primarily on studies performed on the human heart–lung transplant model. In general, any observations made on this model should be applicable to the lung function of single or double lung transplants which do not include the heart.

Pulmonary function of the transplanted lung following heart–lung transplantation

Standard measurements of pulmonary function demonstrate that function is well preserved in the transplanted lung with a tendency towards improvement with the passage of time, rather than the opposite. There are mild to moderate abnormalities of the static properties of the respiratory system, particularly in the first 6 months postoperatively. These alterations do not have major functional significance and tend to improve with time. Gas exchange is remarkably well preserved after transplantation, and this critical function remains normal for at least years after surgery[10].

Volumes and pulmonary statics

The most significant alteration of pulmonary function that arises following heart–lung transplantation is the development of a mild to moderate restrictive ventilatory defect. This is associated with significant reductions in all lung volumes, as compared to predicted normal values, with the exception of residual volume (RV) and functional residual capacity (FRC), which remain essentially normal[10].

The reduction in volumes appears to be primarily related to a decrease in inspiratory capacity (IC) as a result of alterations of the chest wall produced at surgery. Under these conditions, determinations of the pressure–volume characteristics of the lung indicate that the elastic properties of the transplanted lung are normal[13]. The reductions in total lung capacity (TLC) that are present correlate highly with reductions in maximum inspiratory pressure and transpulmonary pressure. These findings implicate chest wall factors as the source of the restrictive defect. In particular, they suggest reductions in the generation of inspiratory forces which could result from a variety of causes including post-surgical mechanical factors, alterations of length–tension relationships of the respiratory muscles due to geometric alterations of the chest wall, or muscular weakness *per se*, among others[13].

Pulmonary dynamics

Pulmonary dynamic function is essentially normal in the transplanted lung. Although there is a greater degree of variability among the various flow parameters measured in the lung, the flow resistive forces in the airways are normal as determined by measurements of specific airway conductance. Reductions in flow that are present are usually related to significant decreases in lung volumes or are parameters which are highly effort dependent (e.g. peak expiratory flow rates, or maximum expiratory flow rate). Effort independent flow parameters which are volume related or volume corrected are usually normal[10].

Early recognition of discordant decreases in flow rates that are not completely accounted for by reductions in volume is imperative since this may be the first indication of obstructive airway disease. The most sensitive parameter in this respect is a decrease in the FEF_{25-75} (forced expiratory flow rate at points between 25 and 75% of the forced vital capacity). The early detection of obstructive airway disease is important since it may represent the first manifestation of obliterative bronchiolitis, the major complication of the long-term transplanted lung[11,14,15].

The maximal voluntary ventilation (MVV) is well preserved following transplantation, with no significant differences found between pre- and post-transplant values for MVV. This clearly indicates that the ventilatory capacity of the respiratory system is not significantly altered as a result of transplantation. The MVV usually found post-transplant reflects a ventilatory capacity which is more than adequate for meeting the ventilatory requirements of exercise[10,12].

Distribution of ventilation, diffusing capacity, and arterial blood gases

In terms of standard measurements of pulmonary function at rest, gas exchange in the transplanted lung remains normal in the uncomplicated state. In this context, the distribution of ventilation within the lung, and the lung diffusing capacity for carbon monoxide (DCO) are normal. In the early post-transplant period (i.e. within 3 months), DCO tends to be reduced towards borderline low-normal values, primarily as a result of low hemoglobin concentrations that are frequently present. DCO improves towards more normal values with the passage of time[10].

The arterial blood gases confirm the ability of the transplanted lungs to sustain normal gas exchange. The average of mean values ($\pm$ SD) for arterial PO_2 and PCO_2 taken over a 3-year period are 90.0 ± 7.3 torr and 35.2 ± 2.8 torr (mmHg), respectively. Although the $PaCO_2$ indicates mild alveolar hyperventilation, the calculated alveolar-arterial O_2 difference is essentially normal[10,11].

Long-term pulmonary function

Serial pulmonary function measurements were obtained on ten long-term survivors with heart–lung transplants who remained free of complications and returned to normal life. Functional indices were obtained in the immediate post-transplant period and at yearly intervals up to 3 years after operation. The restrictive ventilatory defect present in the early postoperative period persisted, but showed no evidence of progression. All other parameters remained essentially normal[11].

These results demonstrate that the transplanted lung is capable of essentially normal function over a long time, providing that it remains uncomplicated.

Dynamic functions at rest and exercise following heart–lung transplantation

Post-transplant studies performed under dynamic conditions of exercise provide a more rigorous assessment of function than is possible from standard measurements of pulmonary function alone. Integrated functions of the heart and lungs can be maximally stressed under conditions of exercise, which can be used to define any limitations that may exist.

The transplanted lungs, together with the respiratory system, respond appropriately to the demands of increasing levels of exercise despite denervation of the cardiopulmonary axis. At maximum exercise, pulmonary gas exchange and ventilation are normal, and the limiting factors during exercise are not pulmonary, but circulatory in nature[12].

Functional parameters assessing gas exchange, ventilation and circulatory capacity were measured in 16 heart–lung transplanted patients at rest and during increasing levels of constant work-rate treadmill exercise to tolerance. The results of measurements obtained during rest and maximum exercise are summarized below.

Arterial blood gases

Post-transplant blood gases showed normal oxygenation of arterial blood during both rest and exercise. At maximum exercise, the mean arterial PO_2 was 98.9 ± 1.8 (SE) torr with a mean alveolar–arterial gradient of 18.3 ± 1.7 torr.

Alveolar hyperventilation was present at rest, as reflected by a $PaCO_2$ of 32.1 ± 0.9 torr. The $PaCO_2$ at maximum exercise was slightly less and not significantly different from the resting value.

Composition of the arterial blood gases during maximum exercise can be used as an index for determining the efficiency of pulmonary gas exchange. Under these conditions, the transplanted lungs are capable of essentially normal gas exchange. This would indicate that the integrating function required for matching ventilation and perfusion (i.e. maintenance of proper $\dot{V}/\dot{Q}$ relations) is intrapulmonary and autoregulatory in nature, and that an external nerve supply is not a crucial requirement for regulating gas exchange within the lung.

Ventilation

Post-transplant resting ventilation was mildly to moderately increased with increases in minute ventilation ($\dot{V}_E$), alveolar ventilation, and the ventilatory equivalents for CO_2 and O_2.

Minute ventilation ($\dot{V}_E$) increased appropriately with increasing levels of exercise. At maximum exercise, the ventilatory equivalents for CO_2 and O_2 were slightly less, though not significantly different from those values obtained at rest. This indicates that the rise in $\dot{V}_E$ with maximum exercise over resting $\dot{V}_E$ was appropriate for the O_2 consumed and the increased work performed. The mean $\dot{V}_E$/MVV ratio ($\dot{V}_E$/maximum voluntary ventilation) was 0.34 ± 0.04 (SE) during maximum exercise, which is well below the upper limit of 0.7, indicating that a substantial ventilatory reserve still remained[12].

The control of ventilation during exercise is also normal in heart–lung transplant recipients. Although limitations of this nature may have been a concern prior to human heart–lung transplantation[16], the results of these studies indicate that this is not the case. The ventilatory response to increasing levels of submaximal exercise, defined as the slope of minute ventilation over carbon dioxide production ($\dot{V}_E/\dot{V}CO_2$), was found not be significantly different in heart–lung transplanted patients from that found in heart transplanted patients and normals[17]. Since heart–lung transplantation results in denervation of the cardiopulmonary axis, the normal nature of post-transplant ventilation also suggests that pulmonary neural reflexes may play a relatively minor role in the control of ventilation with exercise in normals as well[17].

Circulatory capacity

Cardiac and circulatory function associated with the denervated transplanted heart are discussed in Chapter 13, and will not be covered in detail. Suffice it to say, cardiac function in heart–lung transplants is not significantly different from that in heart transplants alone. In exercise physiology, O_2 consumption ($\dot{V}O_2$), heart rate, O_2-pulse, and blood lactates are useful indices for approximating the limitations of the circulation in conjunction with defining exercise capacity. Measurements of these parameters at maximal exercise can be used to qualitatively estimate circulatory capacity.

Post-transplant resting parameters are not essentially different from what would ordinarily be expected, except for the modest increase in heart rate that is associated with cardiac denervation[12].

Post-transplant exercise is significantly improved over pretransplant exercise in patients who had undergone heart–lung transplantation for pulmonary hypertension, primarily as a result of an improved circulation[12]. Although significantly improved, circulatory limitations may still persist post-transplant, as judged by $\dot{V}O_2$, heart rate, and O_2-pulse values that were attainable at maximum levels of exercise. At approximately 8 weeks post-transplant, the $\dot{V}O_2$ was $39.3 \pm 2.6\%$ (SE); heart rate $68.1 \pm 2.5\%$ and O_2-pulse $57.4 \pm 2.5\%$ of predicted values at maximum exercise. These values tend to be somewhat higher by 6 months post-transplant[12]. These limitations of exercise present in heart–lung transplanted patients are in keeping with previous observations made in heart transplanted subjects who were studied hemodynamically by cardiac catheterization during supine exercise[18] and also by progressive incremental exercise to exhaustion on a bicycle[19].

Long-term exercise

After transplantation, long-term follow-up exercise studies have been performed comparing the effects of time on maximal $\dot{V}O_2$, heart rate, O_2-pulse, ventilation, and arterial blood gases. Although the circulatory parameters tended to be somewhat greater at 6 months than at 8 weeks post-transplant, the maximal values for all parameters were essentially unchanged for periods of time up to 2 years following transplantation.

In the absence of complications producing intrinsic graft injury, long-term cardiopulmonary dynamic function during exercise is well maintained for at least 2 years following heart–lung transplantation. Gas exchange and ventilation at maximum exercise are maintained at essentially normal levels. Circulatory limitations persist, but without significant trends in either direction, i.e. worsening or improving.

Several factors are present in post-transplant patients which can limit exercise capacity and maximum $\dot{V}O_2$, and, as a result, directly influence qualitative estimates of circulatory capacity. These may lead to underestimates of 'true' circulatory capacity by limiting exercise performance. Factors potentially limiting post-transplant exercise include cardiac denervation, chronic anemia, physical deconditioning, and, in a significant number of cases, systemic hypertension as a result of cyclosporine effects on the kidney.

In summary, the results of studies described here clearly indicate that the integrated functions of the transplanted heart and lungs are well maintained with exercise. Although circulatory limitations may persist, the allografts perform sufficiently well to sustain the activities of normal life.

Denervated lung

Studies aimed at defining the physiology of the denervated human lung are still in the preliminary stages, although a considerable amount of information from animal work has been available for years. New insights into control mechanisms regulating airway function, the pulmonary circulation, and the control of ventilation have been derived from studies on the denervated lungs of heart–lung transplanted subjects. Some of the effects of lung denervation on respiratory function have already been discussed. Other aspects will be briefly commented on here and in the section on the pharmacology of the transplanted lung.

Airway regulation in the transplanted lung

The central regulation of airway tone is primarily mediated through the bronchoconstrictor activity of parasympathetic efferents on bronchial smooth muscle. Despite denervation, however, in general, airway tone and function do not appear to be particularly altered in the transplanted lung since measurements of airway resistance, specific conductance, and dynamic function are essentially normal under baseline conditions[10].

Under specific experimental conditions, however, new findings have been made in the transplanted lung which may provide new insights into control mechanisms regulating airway responsiveness and function. These include the following:

The airways of the transplanted lungs are hyper-responsive to methacholine inhalation[20]. The degrees of bronchial hyperresponsiveness to methacholine are similar to that present in bronchial asthma. However, patients with heart–lung transplants have none of the clinical manifestations of bronchial asthma. It is speculated that post-transplant bronchial hyper-responsiveness could result from hypersensitive muscarinic receptors deprived of tonic vagal stimulation, or from a modification of the third nervous system (i.e. non-adrenergic, non-cholinergic system) which normally inhibits bronchial smooth muscle tone, as a result of lung denervation[20].

The second finding of significance is the loss of a specific airway reflex which is normally present, i.e. following induced bronchoconstriction, the bronchodilatory response associated with deep inspiration is absent in the transplanted lung[21].

These findings appear to be unique to the transplanted lung and, most likely, represent expressions of lung denervation[20,21].

Regulation of the pulmonary circulation in the transplanted lung

Heart–lung transplantation does not appear to adversely affect the pulmonary circulation. Pulmonary hemodynamics, at rest, remain normal for extended periods of time measurable in years post-transplant[22]. Hypoxic pulmonary vasoconstriction persists in the transplanted lung, suggesting that this response does not depend on an intact neural supply to the pulmonary vasculature and is locally mediated within the lung vasculature itself[23].

Neural regulation of ventilation

Overall, the control of ventilation appears to be virtually intact and normal in heart–lung transplanted subjects, despite lung denervation. As previously discussed, the ventilatory response to submaximal exercise in these patients is similar to that found in normals[16].

Summary: overall effect of lung denervation

The integrated functions of the respiratory system appear to be operationally intact and, at least grossly, unaffected by the denervation of the lungs. The integrated responses between the pulmonary and circulatory systems during exercise are grossly intact. The ventilatory response to increasing levels of exercise is normal; ventilation is not limiting to exercise with a sufficient ventilatory reserve at maximum exercise, and gas exchange is normal, indicating that $\dot{V}/\dot{Q}$ relationships are well maintained during exercise. In the latter, it is clear that the function of matching ventilation with perfusion for the purpose of optimizing gas exchange in the lung is not dependent upon an intact external nerve supply.

Unilateral lung transplantation

Unilateral lung transplants perform sufficiently well to support the activities of daily life in selected cases. Pulmonary function and exercise are significantly improved following unilateral lung transplantation in patients with pulmonary fibrosis[24,25]. Overall pulmonary function (i.e. the combined functioning of the diseased fibrosed lung and the unilateral transplanted lung) in these patients showed significant improvement in total lung capacity, the timed forced expiratory volumes, lung diffusing capacity for carbon monoxide, and the arterial blood gases. The arterial blood gases were at essentially normal values. Exercise was improved as demonstrated by timed walking tests and the maintenance of O_2 saturations of greater than 90% during exercise.

The unilateral lung transplant is suited for patients with pulmonary fibrosis with an essentially normal heart[24]. Physiologically, it is unsuited for patients with emphysema or those with combined cardiopulmonary disease where the heart is significantly impaired. Clinically, single lung transplants are also unsuited for those with bilateral pulmonary sepsis. In unilateral lung transplantation for emphysema, function of the transplanted lung is compromised by the emphysematous lung. The loss of elastic recoil in the latter leads to progressive air trapping (and distention) in the native lung and a shift of the mediastinum toward the transplanted side[22]. This leads to $\dot{V}/\dot{Q}$ mismatching and compromised gas exchange. Adequate post-transplant pulmonary physiology requires bilateral lung transplantation in patients with emphysema[24,26].

PHARMACOLOGY OF THE TRANSPLANTED LUNG

Pharmacologic studies in the human transplanted lung are few, and information on the related pharmacology remains limited at this stage. It is expected however, that significant advances will be made in this area as more patients with lung transplants become available in the future. Although a considerable body of pharmacologic knowledge currently exists on respiratory and non-respiratory functions of the lung[27], these observations derived from animals and non-transplanted humans, will not be discussed here. Comment will be confined only to studies performed on the denervated transplanted lung of humans.

Recent work has been primarily aimed at defining the nature of control mechanisms that regulate airway function and responsiveness in the denervated human lung following heart–lung transplantation.

Airway hyper-responsiveness to methacholine inhalation was presented earlier as a manifestation of denervation in the transplanted lung[20]. The prior inhalation of ipratropium bromide (atropine-like substance) inhibits the bronchoconstrictor response to methacholine inhalation, indicating that the post-transplant bronchial hyper-responsiveness to methacholine is mediated through muscarinic receptors since ipratropium bromide exerts its inhibitory effect at the muscarinic receptor site. This also indicates that the bronchial hyper-responsiveness to methacholine is not a non-specific response[28].

Ipratropium bromide inhalation also produces increases in specific airway conductance and FEV_1, indicating bronchodilation. This suggests the presence of some degree of 'tone' in the airways despite lung denervation[28].

The inhalation of propranolol, a β-blocker, does not produce significant changes in specific airway conductance. This lack of response provides additional evidence that post-transplant bronchial hyper-responsiveness and the bronchial hyper-responsiveness associated with asthma are mechanistically different. Clinical asthma is frequently exacerbated by the use of β-blockers in asthmatic patients. Clinical asthma has not been a feature of the transplanted lung[20,28].

Salbutamol, a β_2 agonist, produces a rise in FEV_1 and specific airway conductance, indicating a positive bronchodilator response when maximal doses are used[28].

These studies, at best, represent the early stages for defining the pharmacology of the transplanted denervated lung in humans. Practically, the early clinical experience with lung transplanted patients has not as yet revealed any major alterations of drug effects on the lungs in ordinary use. This may change as more experience with these patients is obtained.

COMMENT

It should be emphasized that the functional and pharmacologic studies presented in this chapter represent post-transplant lung function at its best when the transplanted lungs were essentially free of complications. Although the lungs function at essentially normal levels, it is important to emphasize that late complications have occurred in approximately 50% of the long-term survivors. Obliterative bronchiolitis represents the complication of most concern and, at present, is the greatest threat to long-term survival following transplantation. Severe obstructive airway disease rapidly develops with the onset of obliterative bronchiolitis, and, if unchecked, can lead to a rapid and fatal downhill course[11,14,15]. Thus, careful observation of airway function is of the utmost importance in the management of lung transplanted patients.

References

1. Comroe, J.H. (1974). *Physiology of Respiration*. 2nd ed. (Chicago: Year Book Medical Publishers)
2. West, J.B. (1974). *Respiratory Physiology*. (Baltimore: Williams & Wilkins)
3. Murray, J.F. (1976). *The Normal Lung*. (Philadelphia: W.B. Saunders)
4. Bouhuys, A. (1977). *The Physiology of Breathing*. (New York: Grune & Stratton)
5. Gong, H., Jr. and Drage, C.W. (eds.) (1982). *The Respiratory System. A Core Curriculum*. (Norwalk, USA: Appleton–Century-Crofts)
6. Cherniack, R.M. and Cherniack, L. (1983). Basic considerations. In *Respiration in Health and Disease*, 3rd ed. p.7 (Philadelphia: W.B. Saunders)
7. Fishman, A.P. (section editor) (1985, 1986, 1987). *Handbook of Physiology. Section 3, The Respiratory System*. Vol. I–IV. American Physiological Society. (Bethesda: Waverly Press, Inc.)
8. Luce, J.M., Tyler, M.L. and Pierson, D.J. (1984). *Intensive Respiratory Care*. (Philadelphia: W.B. Saunders)
9. Donohue, J.F. (1982). Control of ventilation. In Gong, H., Jr. and Drage, C.W. (eds.) *The Respiratory System. A Core Curriculum*. p. 95. (Norwalk, USA: Appleton-Century-Crofts)
10. Theodore, J., Jamieson, S.W., Burke, C.M., Reitz, B.A., Stinson, E.B., Van Kessel, A., Dawkins, K.D., Herran, J.J., Oyer, P.E., Hunt, S.A., Shumway, N.E. and Robin, E.D. (1984). Physiologic aspects of human heart–lung transplantation: pulmonary function status of the post-transplanted lung. *Chest*, **86**, 349
11. Burke, C.M., Theodore, J., Baldwin, J.C., Tazelaar, H.D., Morris, A.J.R., McGregor, C.G.A., Shumway, N.E., Robin, E.D. and Jamieson, S.W. (1986). Twenty-eight cases of human heart–lung transplantation. *Lancet*, **1**, 517
12. Theodore, J., Morris, A.J., Burke, C.M., Glanville, A.R., Van Kessel, A., Baldwin, J.C., Stinson, E.B., Shumway, N.E. and Robin, E.D. (1987). Cardiopulmonary function at maximum tolerable constant work rate exercise following human heart–lung transplantation. *Chest*, **92**, 433
13. Glanville, A.R., Theodore, J., Harvey, J. and Robin, E.D. (1988). Elastic behavior of the transplanted lung: exponential analysis of static pressure–volume relationships. *Am. Rev. Respir. Dis.*, **137**, 308
14. Burke, C.M., Theodore, J., Dawkins, K.D., Yousem, S.A., Blank, N., Billingham, M.E., Van Kessel, A., Jamieson, S.W., Oyer, P.E., Baldwin, J.C., Stinson, E.B., Shumway, N.E. and Robin, E.D. (1984). Post-transplant obliterative bronchiolitis and other late lung sequelae in human heart–lung transplantation. *Chest*, **86**, 824
15. Glanville, A.R., Baldwin, J.C., Burke, C.M., Theodore, J. and Robin, E.D. (1987). Obliterative bronchiolitis after heart–lung transplantation: apparent arrest by augmented immunosuppression. *Ann. Intern. Med.*, **107**, 300
16. Nakae, S., Webb, W.R., Theodorides, T. and Sugg, W.L. (1967).

Respiratory function following cardiopulmonary denervation in dog, cat, and monkey. *Surg. Gynecol. Obstet.*, **125**, 1285
17. Theodore, J., Robin, E.D., Morris, A.J.R., Burke, C.M., Jamieson, S.W., Van Kessel, A., Stinson, E.B. and Shumway, N.E. (1986). Augmented ventilatory response to exercise in pulmonary hypertension. *Chest*, **89**, 39
18. Stinson, E.B., Griepp, R.B., Schroeder, J.S., Dong, E. and Shumway, N.E. (1972). Hemodynamic observations one and two years after cardiac transplantation in man. *Circulation*, **45**, 1183
19. Savin, W.M., Haskell, W.L., Schroeder, J.S. and Stinson, E.B. (1980). Cardiorespiratory responses of cardiac transplant patients to graded symptom-limited exercise. *Circulation*, **62**, 55
20. Glanville, A.R., Burke, C.M., Theodore, J., Baldwin, J.C., Harvey, J. Van Kessel, A. and Robin, E.D. (1987). Bronchial hyper-responsiveness after human cardiopulmonary transplantation. *Clin. Sci.*, **73**, 299
21. Glanville, A.R., Yeend, R.A., Theodore, J. and Robin, E.D. (1988). The effect of single respiratory maneuvers on specific airway conductance in heart–lung transplant recipients. *Clin. Sci.*, **74**, 311
22. Glanville, A.R., Burke, C.M., Hunt, S.A., Baldwin, J.C. and Theodore, J. (1986). Long-term pulmonary hemodynamics in human heart–lung transplant recipients. *Chest*, **89** Suppl., 512S
23. Robin, E.D., Theodore, J., Burke, C.M., Oesterle, S.N., Fowler, M.B., Jamieson, S.W., Baldwin, J.C., Morris, A.J., Hunt, S.A., Van Kessel, A., Stinson, E.B. and Shumway, N.E. (1987). Hypoxic pulmonary vasoconstriction persists in the human transplanted lung. *Clin. Sci.*, **72**, 283
24. Toronto Lung Transplant Group (1986). Unilateral lung transplantation for pulmonary fibrosis. *N. Engl. J. Med.*, **314**, 1140
25. Cooper, J.D., Pearson, F.G., Patterson, G.A., Todd, T.R.J., Ginsberg, R.J., Goldberg, M. and DeMajo, W.A.P. (1987). Technique of successful lung transplantation in humans. *J. Thorac. Cardiovasc. Surg.*, **93**, 173
26. Patterson, G.A., Cooper, J.D., Dark, J.H., Jones, M.T. and Toronto Lung Transplant Group (1988). Experimental and clinical double lung transplantation. *J. Thorac. Cardiovasc. Surg.*, **95**, 70
27. Hollinger, M.A. (1985). *Respiratory Pharmacology and Toxicology.* (Philadelphia: W.B. Saunders)
28. Glanville, A.R., Theodore, J., Baldwin, J.C. and Robin, E.D. (1990). Bronchial responsiveness after human cardiopulmonary transplantation. In press

43
Diagnosis and Management of Bronchiolitis Obliterans (Chronic Rejection): Retransplantation

R.S. BONSER, R.Y. TARAZI AND S.W. JAMIESON

INTRODUCTION

The detailed features of chronic rejection following heart–lung transplantation are as yet inadequately defined. Any discussion of these late complications requires an understanding of the physiology of the heart–lung bloc after implantation, and the factors that may superimpose changes in these variables. This chapter will attempt to outline the cardiac and pulmonary changes that can occur in the later period following transplantation, and current thoughts on chronic rejection and other late sequelae.

HEMODYNAMIC CHANGES FOLLOWING HEART–LUNG TRANSPLANTATION

Hemodynamic evaluation of well-rehabilitated long-term survivors of heart–lung transplantation has demonstrated that normal pulmonary arterial pressure, pulmonary vascular resistance, cardiac output, and left ventricular function are possible at 1 and 2 years postoperatively[1,2]. Exercise may manifest some circulatory limitations, but effort tolerance is maintained[3,4]. However, increasing pulmonary artery pressure and pulmonary vascular resistance have developed in some patients, who had previously had excellent hemodynamic function documented late after transplantation[2]. This development of pulmonary arterial obstruction occurs in parallel with changes in airway morphology.

Even after an initial good functional result, increasing exertional dyspnea may rapidly progress from normal ventilation to the need for assisted ventilation over a period of a few weeks[5]. In association with severe irreversible airway changes, cardiac catheterization demonstrates pulmonary hypertension. Pulmonary arteriography reveals pruning of the distal pulmonary vessels, consistent with obliterative pulmonary artery changes[2].

The cardiac circulation is also affected, and coronary angiography may show evidence of diffuse coronary artery disease[6]. In one such case, successful retransplantation was performed and histological examination of the explanted heart demonstrated severe triple vessel graft atherosclerosis[2]. Deaths have occurred as early as 14 months following transplantation as a result of myocardial ischemia from atherosclerosis[7]. This diffuse proliferative graft atherosclerosis leads to peripheral, as well as proximal, vessel occlusion. Coronary arteriography in these patients may fail to demonstrate irregularities of the coronary arteries clearly because of the diffuse and concentric nature of graft atherosclerosis. Recurrence of primary pulmonary hypertension has not been demonstrated in heart–lung transplant recipients.

PULMONARY FUNCTION FOLLOWING TRANSPLANTATION

Following heart–lung transplantation, the transplanted lungs are capable of sustaining normal gas exchange, which improves over the first 6 months[8] (Chapter 42). Subsequently, gas exchange remains normal unless late complications supervene[9]. A mild-to-moderate restrictive ventilatory defect occurs after transplantation, with a reduced total lung capacity and forced vital capacity, and is probably related to chest wall rigidity following surgery rather than intrinsic lung disease[8]. This restrictive ventilatory defect tends to improve in the initial year following transplantation, with static lung volumes approaching normal values after 2 years[10]. Early after surgery, effort-dependent flow rates fall, before returning to pretransplantation values about 1 year after surgery. Diffusion capacity of the lungs does not appear to change significantly following transplantation[11]. Bronchial tone and the vasoconstrictor response to hypoxia following transplantation are retained[12,13].

OBLITERATIVE AIRWAY CHANGES FOLLOWING TRANSPLANTATION

Introduction

A substantial proportion of late survivors have developed airflow obstruction as a result of obliterative bronchiolitis[14,15]. In the Stanford series, five of 14 long-term initial survivors developed obstructive lung lesions[14]. Additional increasing restrictive changes were seen in 60% of those affected. These alterations in lung function have been associated with an obliterative bronchiolitis on biopsy. Other patients have developed recurrent pulmonary infections, pleural fibrosis, and bronchiectasis. More recently, the Stanford group has reported a 50% incidence of obstructive changes in the late survivors following heart–lung transplantation[5]. Six of the initial long-term survivors have subsequently died of pulmonary failure. No correlation between late pulmonary sequelae and organ ischemic time has been demonstrated.

Clinical features of airway obstruction

The clinical course of these patients is similar to that of patients with chronic obstructive airway disease, but the time scale is telescoped into a period of months rather than years. Initially cough, productive of mucopurulent sputum, develops[14]. Recurrent pulmonary infections are common. Increasing dyspnea on exertion occurs, and the patient's course may follow a relentless decline unless pharmacological intervention is successful. Alternatively, patients may remain relatively stable, albeit with a degree of dyspnea of effort and a slow deterioration of pulmonary function tests[5,11]; they remain apparently clinically well, apart from periodic respiratory tract infections, for many months after the initial diagnosis of airway obstruction. The reasons for this discrepancy in the rate of decline of pulmonary function between patients remains obscure. In contrast to chronic bronchial asthma, the dyspnea is not paroxysmal, cannot be related to precipitating factors, except intercurrent infections, and is not reversible by bronchodilator therapy.

The majority of patients with post-transplant obliterative lung lesions have suffered an episode of lower respiratory tract infection weeks or months prior to the appearance of progressive dyspnea[14]. These infections, diagnosed on the basis of fever, purulent sputum, and radiographic changes, may be sputum and bronchoscopic-aspirate culture negative, although they have generally improved with culture-directed or empirical antibiotics[16].

Investigations

Chest radiography, tomograms, and computerized tomographic scanning may reveal peribronchial and interstitial infiltrates, with variable pleural thickening, in the presence of obstructive lesions[6]. Micronodular opacities, predominantly in lower zones, are occasionally present. The infiltrative changes are more prominent than those seen in chronic obstructive airway disease.

Pulmonary function tests reveal a progressive reduction in lung function superimposed on the restrictive changes common to most patients with heart–lung transplantation[15,11] (Chapter 42). Forced vital capacity (FVC) and the forced expiratory volume in 1 second (FEV_1) fall in parallel, with the fall in the flow-dependent FEV_1 being more pronounced, leading to an obstructive ventilatory defect[14]. In contrast to other forms of chronic obstructive lung disease, total lung capacity falls rather than increases, indicating that air trapping does not occur.

More sensitive indices of flow, such as (1) the ratio of the forced expiratory flow at 50% of FVC (FEF_{50}) and FVC (FEF_{50}/FVC), and (2) the mean forced expiratory flow between 25% and 75% of vital capacity (FEF_{25-75}), are more markedly reduced, reflecting the obstructive process. Helium equilibration times are only minimally abnormal because of the reduction in total lung capacity, and are nearer normal than those seen in classical chronic obstructive airway disease. Diffusing capacity for carbon monoxide, initially depressed in the early post-transplant period, becomes more modestly depressed with the onset of obstruction.

Arterial hypoxemia, and depressed alveolar–arterial oxygen gradients are found uniformly, and hypocapnia rather than carbon dioxide retention occurs[15]. The hypoxemia may lead to pulmonary vasoconstriction and elevated pulmonary vascular resistance, as the vasoconstrictor response to hypoxemia is retained in transplanted lungs despite denervation[13].

The most sensitive parameters for defining the changes of obliterative lung disease are the mean mid-expiratory flow (FEF_{25-75}), specific conductances (SG_{aw}), arterial oxygen tension, and alveolar–arterial oxygen gradients. Less sensitive indices include the flow-volume loop, FEV_1, the ratio of FEV_1/FVC, and peak expiratory flow rates, all of which are more commonly used indices of obstruction.

The role of bronchoalveolar lavage in postoperative graft intolerance surveillance

The possible eventual contribution of bronchoalveolar lavage (BAL) in the diagnosis and management of late complications following transplantation remains unknown[11]. It is clearly useful in the diagnosis of bacterial, viral, fungal, and protozoal lung infections in the immunocompromised host[17] (Chapter 41). As such, it is almost automatically required in the diagnostic evaluation of the late postoperative pulmonary infiltrate following lung or heart–lung transplantation. Analysis of the cellular content of BAL fluid can provide additional information regarding a number of conditions, and it could be anticipated that the study of cells obtained from the donor lung could provide information regarding the presence or absence of pulmonary rejection.

Early after heart–lung transplantation BAL aspirates reveal greater overall cell numbers than those seen in normal lung, but with a similar fractional distribution of cell types[18]. During both early rejection episodes and infection, absolute neutrophil counts in BAL rise, and the relative number of pulmonary macrophages decreases[19]. However, although cell numbers are persistently abnormal during the early postoperative period, changes in both absolute numbers and relative fractions of different cell types do not differentiate between the presence of rejection and infection or their absence[20].

The phenotypic make-up of lymphocytes obtained during BAL changes during the first few months after transplantation[21]. Early after transplant, lymphocytes and macrophages within the lung demonstrate major histocompatibility antigens of both donor and recipient. After 1 month, the vast majority of the cell population is of recipient phenotype, and after 3 months all cells are recipient in origin[22].

Functional evaluation of retrieved recipient lymphocytes has also been unhelpful in the diagnosis of rejection[23]. T-lymphocytes, activated to respond to donor-specific HLA antigens, can be demonstrated in BAL fluid, but their appearance does not seem necessarily indicative of rejection in human or animal studies[24,25]. In animal studies, although cell counts and differential cannot differentiate between infection and rejection, they are helpful in distinguishing these two phenomena from transplanted lungs suffering from neither infection nor rejection[26]. In addition, enhanced neutrophil chemiluminescence activity may aid identification of the infected group. Clearly further work in this area is required if BAL is to become a useful technique in rejection surveillance.

Pathology of obliterative airway disease

This topic is discussed fully in Chapter 40. Only a brief summary will be given here.

Animal studies have suggested that long-term survival following heart–lung autotransplantation is possible without the occurrence of late pulmonary histological abnormalities[27]. This would suggest that denervation and loss of lymphatic drainage do not (*per se*) affect long-term function or histology[27–29]. In primate heart–lung allotransplantation, however, morphological changes do occur in both pulmonary vasculature and small airways[27], though the airways were secondarily involved by interstitial scarring thought to be unrelated to rejection. Focal and sometimes diffuse interstitial fibrosis can be seen, with mesothelial invasion of the lung parenchyma and pleural fibrosis; in addition, fibrosis of the alveolar septa, and intimal proliferation of the muscular arterioles have been detected. With the exception of the vascular changes, however, these features are not thought to be related to a rejection reaction.

(These changes are different from those of acute unmodified pulmonary rejection, which is characterized by perivascular (predominantly perivenular) and interstitial mononuclear infiltrates in combination with perivascular and interstitial edema[30]. In acute pulmonary rejection, extracellular fibrinous exudates are also seen with eventual hemorrhagic necrosis of the graft and loss of alveolar architectural configuration[31].)

Studies of human lung tissue following heart–lung transplantation in patients who developed airways obstruction have demonstrated varying degrees of bronchiolitis obliterans associated with mucus plugging and obstructive changes in the distal airways[16]. The bronchiolitis has been described as affecting all lobes, although it may be patchy in distribution, both within a lobe and between lobes.

The earliest histological changes consist of ulcerated bronchiolar epithelium, with necrotic epithelial and polymorphonuclear cells enmeshed in mucus within the airway lumen. Other bronchioles may show the lumen plugged with foamy fat-laden histiocytes indicative of proximal obstruction. More organized mucopolysaccharide-laden Masson bodies may form onion-skin-appearing plugs within the airway lumen, associated with epithelial thinning and squamous metaplasia. At the base of these plugs, there is interruption of the basal elastic layer of the bronchiolar wall. These changes progress, leading to submucosal scars lined by cuboidal epithelium and scar tissue replacing part of the bronchiolar smooth muscle wall, interruption of the elastic lamina, and eventual total replacement of bronchioles with scar tissue. An inconsistent mononuclear cell infiltrate may be seen. Different patients may show different degrees of obstructive changes in bronchiolitis obliterans. Focal pleural fibrosis is also seen, extending into interlobular septa without acute inflammatory changes.

In association with these changes, arteriosclerotic changes in the walls of the muscular pulmonary arterioles are a constant feature, consisting of a concentric fibroelastosis of the intimal surface and muscular hypertrophy. This diffuse concentric pattern contrasts the uneven, eccentrically located changes of age-related atherosclerosis in systemic vessels. (Cholesterol clefts and erosion of the arterial wall and elastic lamina are not seen.) Parallel changes are observed in the coronary circulation of the affected cases, with severe concentric intimal thickening observed. Waxy intimal thickening may also be seen in pulmonary venules.

Clinical course

Once a substantial deterioration in airflow rates has occurred, spontaneous improvement does not occur[5]. An inexorable decline of pulmonary function is seen over a varying time period of weeks or months[14]. Late in the natural history of the disease, no response to augmentation of corticosteroids has been seen, but, if instituted early enough, high dose prednisone therapy has been associated with a marked improvement in both symptomatology and pulmonary function tests[9,32]. Relapses may occur, however, though again these may be steroid-responsive. No demonstration of histological reversal has been documented.

Management

Following heart–lung transplantation the close surveillance of infection and graft intolerance must continue late into the postoperative course. Serial pulmonary function tests, including FEF_{25-75}, SG_{aw}, arterial blood oxygen tension, and alveolar–arterial oxygen gradients are followed; a 10% deterioration in any of these variables is regarded with suspicion, especially if a change in two or more is seen in a consistent direction.

Once suspected, the chest radiograph is reviewed to detect infiltrates due to infection. In airway obstruction due to bronchiolitis obliterans, the chest radiograph may be normal. Bronchoscopy is performed in order to exclude infection, and bronchial and transbronchial biopsies are taken for histological analysis. If bronchiolitis is confirmed, high-dose oral prednisone therapy, initially 100 mg/day, is commenced, gradually tapering to 30 mg/day, at which level it is held for at least 1 month before again tapering to pre-obstructive steroid dosing. Pulmonary function tests are repeated frequently to document anticipated reversal. Close surveillance for infection during this period of increased immunosuppression is maintained and cyclosporine levels are optimized. There is no evidence that this phenomenon can be improved or reversed by the use of bronchodilators, or aggressive chest physiotherapy, although both of these may be necessary in the treatment of an acute infectious exacerbation[9].

In cases detected during the chronic phase, or if augmented immunosuppression fails, a continued decline can be anticipated and consideration must be given to retransplantation, though this may be contraindicated by the presence of associated systemic disease. As the fibrotic changes of obliterative bronchiolitis have been consistently associated with parallel changes of intimal proliferation of the coronary arteries, investigation of the coronary circulation, including arteriography, is also necessary. The detection of diffuse graft atherosclerosis and, more significantly, near-occlusion of major coronary arteries will aid in the decision of whether to offer retransplantation. Certainly myocardial infarction and myocardial failure have been noted as preterminal events in patients succumbing late after heart–lung transplantation[7].

Etiology of bronchiolitis obliterans and other changes

Bronchiolitis obliterans is a non-specific finding of airway injury associated with toxic fume inhalation, infection, and in association with connective tissue disorders; in some cases its etiology is unknown[33]. There are a number of reasons why heart–lung transplantation may result in bronchiolitis obliterans unrelated to rejection.

Factors favoring a non-rejection etiology of bronchiolitis obliterans

Patients with post-transplant bronchiolitis obliterans have uniformly experienced repeated respiratory tract infections of both bacterial and viral origin[14,32]. Impaired immunological response to these infections may lead to progressive airway scarring and obstruction. This impaired response is contributed to by both immunosuppression and abnormalities of mucus clearance by the ciliary carpet. A vicious cycle commences, further damage due to chronic inflammation leading to squamous metaplasia. Denervation of donor bronchi leads to an absence of the cough reflex below the carina. If coughing cannot be excited by material in the lower airways, self-generated pulmonary toilet is lost and mucus accumulates, increasing the risk of secondary bacterial contamination.

Interruption of the bronchial arterial supply may also lead to some impairment of the capacity to combat infection[34]. The secreted mucus from the bronchial tree of heart–lung transplant patients appears more viscid and more difficult to expectorate than normal sputum, a further possible factor predisposing to repeated infection. Subclinical airway damage due to aspiration, in the presence of peripheral denervation, may also contribute. The clinical picture of bronchiolitis obliterans seems to occur primarily in those patients suffering from repeated respiratory infections with purulent sputum and chronic post-nasal drainage[32]. In addition, alongside the changes of bronchiolitis obliterans, focal bronchial pneumonia has been seen in some specimens, and viral and fungal pathogens have been identified[16].

Inadequate preservation of the lung during storage prior to transplantation may also play a role in the development of late morphological changes. Pleural fibrosis, obstructive and emphysematous changes have been noted in canine lung autografts more than 6 years after transplantation[35]. Bronchiolitis obliterans has been identified in canine autografts after inadequate 24-hour preservation[36].

Progression of the disease is associated with bronchiectasis. The distribution of lesions is somewhat different from those seen in acute pulmonary rejection in both human and animal studies. This anatomical discrepancy is a feature against bronchiolitis obliterans being a rejection phenomenon. In acute rejection, infiltrates appear to be predominantly perivascular, with subsequent alveolar exudates and infiltration noted in advanced stages[31]. Special staining and electromicroscopic studies have failed to identify immune complex or complement deposits in these areas of airway destruction[16]. This would tend to argue against significant humoral rejection phenomena occurring, at least in the late changes of post-transplant bronchiolitis obliterans.

The known fibroblastic effects of cyclosporine may interplay with these secondary infective phenomena in the process of airway damage[37]. It can also be anticipated that some fibrosis may be secondary to inadequate lung preservation and prolonged ischemia at the time of implantation.

Factors favoring an etiology of chronic rejection

In keeping with bronchiolitis obliterans being a result of chronic rejection is its occurrence in parallel with vascular changes. Concentric intimal proliferation of the coronary arteries in heart transplant patients has long been held to be a manifestation of chronic rejection[38]. Similar changes are seen in renal transplants, leading to a progressive endarteritis obliterans and renal sclerosis[39].

In the heart-lung transplant patient succumbing to airway disease, coronary disease has been a constant feature. In addition, similar accelerated intimal hyperplasia is seen in the elastic and muscular pulmonary arterioles, and intimal thickening is seen in the pulmonary venules[16]. Perivenular infiltrates are seen in acute pulmonary rejection, and thus the changes observed in heart-lung transplant patients may represent a subclinical chronic rejection phenomenon. A further feature of these changes is that they have tended to occur in patients with suboptimal immunosuppression, and that at least symptomatic and physiological improvement occurs with augmented immunosuppression in the early stages of the disease[14]. Another factor supporting the rejection theory is the presence of infiltrates compatible with acute rejection in some, but not all, of the histological specimens reviewed.

The changes of bronchiolitis obliterans are not seen following primate heart-lung autotransplantation, and thus the role of denervation, bronchial artery ligation, and lymphatic division would not seem to play a primary role[27]. Primate heart-lung autotransplants, however, do not receive cyclosporine, which has been associated with fibroproliferative reactions in both heart and kidney recipients[40]. Although a contribution of cyclosporine cannot be disproved, a major role is unlikely, as heart and kidney transplant recipients do not show any tendency to develop bronchiolitis obliterans or interstitial pulmonary fibrosis, even after many years of follow-up. In addition, the vascular changes cannot be attributed to cyclosporine, as these occur in heart transplant recipients treated with conventional immunosuppression.

Bronchiolitis obliterans has also been seen in bone marrow transplant recipients, but not other solid organ grafts, and is thought to be an expression of graft-versus-host disease[41,42]. Although the lung is a large source of lymphoid tissue, graft-versus-host disease is unlikely in heart-lung transplantation, especially as all detectable lymphocytes are of recipient origin within 3 months of transplantation[22]. More likely is the converse, host-versus-graft reaction, namely, rejection.

Although the anatomical discrepancy of the sites of histological changes in acute rejection and post-transplant bronchiolitis obliterans is puzzling, this does not exclude the possibility of chronic low-grade rejection occurring throughout the lung parenchyma without evident cellular infiltrates. Interestingly, experimental studies in rats undergoing lung allotransplantation without immunosuppression have also found obliterative airway changes[43]. More proximal bronchial injury has also been noted, with bronchiolar epithelial ulceration. No difference in the incidence of post-transplant bronchiolitis obliterans has been noted between patients with different primary diseases before transplantation, and it does not appear that 'primary' pulmonary hypertension can reappear following transplantation.

RETRANSPLANTATION

Progressive deterioration of graft function following heart-lung transplantation must lead to the question of retransplantation in affected individuals. Successful retransplantation has been performed following heart-lung transplantation, and the operative details are similar to the primary procedure. The recipient operation is again performed via a median sternotomy, and careful attention is directed to the protection of the phrenic nerves, which may be involved in postoperative adhesions. The heart and lungs are removed separately. Dense pleural adhesions may be present and should be divided by cautery, taking care not to enter any potential foci of infection within the lung. Meticulous hemostasis is, of course, equally important in secondary as in primary operations.

The first reported successful retransplantation procedure was performed by the senior author in 1984 at Stanford[44]. Initial heart-lung transplantation had been performed in 1981; the early postoperative course was marred by a systemic cytomegalovirus infection. Subsequently the patient remained well, apart from a single episode of right upper lobe chest infection, for 36 months. At this time, the patient presented with progressive dyspnea and chest radiographic changes suggestive of bronchiolitis obliterans. Endomyocardial biopsy was normal, but pulmonary function tests revealed a marked obstructive and restrictive ventilatory defect. At cardiac catheterization, pulmonary vascular resistance was noted to be elevated and pulmonary arteriography showed small vessel occlusion and peripheral pruning. Selective coronary angiography, normal 1 year previously, demonstrated diffuse triple vessel disease. Bronchiolitis obliterans was confirmed by open lung biopsy.

The patient's clinical condition deteriorated rapidly, and he required reintubation and assisted ventilation. No improvement was noted after treatment with steroids, bronchodilators, and antibiotics. After 2 months of mechanical ventilation, donor organs became available and successful retransplantation was performed. Postoperative rehabilitation was entirely satisfactory. Examination of the explanted organs revealed severe coronary artery disease, but normal myocardium histologically, and bronchiolitis obliterans.

Probably the most difficult aspect of retransplantation is recipient selection. The current scarcity of suitable donors already greatly limits the application of heart–lung transplantation in patients with primary disease. As always in transplantation, the best result, and thus the best use of scarce donor organs, can be anticipated in young recipients without concurrent systemic disease who are thus likely to have the best chance of early survival and successful rehabilitation. Selection of candidates for retransplantation must take into account the scarcity of the precious commodity of donor organs.

COMMENT

Clinical heart–lung transplantation, although no longer an experimental form of treatment, is still in its infancy. Excellent rehabilitation can be expected in the medium-term following transplantation, leading to a vastly improved quality of life[45,46]. Further experience and research will hopefully further define the long-term sequelae after transplantation, both in terms of causation and management.

On balance, we have tended to regard post-transplant bronchiolitis obliterans as a consequence of chronic rejection, with secondary infective phenomena superimposed. The relative contribution of various possible factors, such as inadequate preservation and early acute rejection, to late airway disease must await clarification.

Of concern is the relatively high incidence of late sequelae in long-term survivors. Because of this, the results of heart–lung transplantation in all units must now be carefully examined to obtain the maximum information regarding these late phenomena.

References

1. Dawkins, K.D., Hunt, S.A., Jamieson, S.W., Theodore, J., Oyer, P.E., Stinson, E.B. and Shumway, N.E. (1984). Heart–lung transplantation for pulmonary vascular disease: follow-up hemodynamic data. *J. Am. Coll. Cardiol.*, **3**, 596
2. Dawkins, K.D., Jamieson, S.W., Hunt, S.A., Baldwin, J.C., Burke, C.M., Morris, A., Billingham, H.E., Theodore, J., Oyer, P.E. and Stinson, E.B. (1985). Long-term results, hemodynamics and complications after combined heart and lung transplantation. *Circulation*, **71**, 912
3. Theodore, J., Burke, C., Dawkins, K., Jamieson, S.W., Stinson, E.B., Van Kessel, A., Shumway, N.E. and Robin, E.D. (1984). Circulatory versus respiratory limitations to exercise before and after human heart–lung transplantation. *J. Am. Coll. Cardiol.*, **3**, 509
4. Herran, J.J., Theodore, J., Van Kessel, A., Reitz, B., Jamieson, S., Stinson, E. and Robin, E.D. (1984). Appropriate ventilatory response to exercise in human heart–lung transplantation. *Clin. Res.*, **31**, 417A
5. Burke, C.M., Baldwin, J.C., Morris, A.J., Shumway, N.E., Theodore, J., Tazelaar, H.D., McGregor, C., Robin, E.D. and Jamieson, S.W. (1987). Twenty-eight cases of human heart–lung transplantation. *Lancet*, **1**, 517
6. Dawkins, K.D., Burke, C.M., Baldwin, J.C., Theodore, J. and Jamieson, S.W. (1984). Long-term complications of combined heart and lung transplantation. *Circulation*, **70**, II 690
7. Morris, A.J.R., Burke, C.M., Dawkins, K.D., Yousem, S., Billingham, H., McGregor, C.G., Baldwin, J.C., Blank, N., Jamieson, S. and Theodore, J. (1985). Late clinical results of heart–lung transplantation. *Am. Rev. Respir. Dis.*, **131**, A87
8. Theodore, J., Jamieson, S.W., Burke, C.M., Reitz, B.A., Stinson, E.B., Van Kessel, A., Dawkins, K.D., Herran, J.J., Oyer, P.E., Hunt, S.A., Shumway, N.E. and Robin, E.D. (1984). Physiological aspects of human heart–lung transplantation: pulmonary function status of the post-transplanted lung. *Chest*, **86**, 349
9. Burke, C.M., Morris, A.J., Dawkins, K.D., Yousem, S., Blank, N., McGregor, C., Baldwin, J.C., Theodore, J. and Jamieson, S.W. (1985). Obliterative bronchiolitis and chronic pulmonary rejection. *J. Heart Transplant*, **4**, 144
10. Dawkins, K.D. and Jamieson, S.W. (1986). Pulmonary function of the transplanted lung. *Ann. Rev. Med.*, **37**, 263
11. Griffith, B.P., Hardesty, R.C., Trento, A., Paradis, I.L., Duquesnoy, R.J., Zeevi, A., Dauber, J.H., Dummer, J.S., Thompson, M.E., Gryzan, S. and Bahnson, H.T. (1987). Heart–lung transplantation: lessons learned and future hopes. *Ann. Thorac. Surg.*, **43**, 6
12. Theodore, J., Reitz, B., Jamieson, S., Herran, J.J., Van Kessel, A., Stinson, E. and Robin, E.D. (1983). Persistence of bronchial tone in human transplanted lung. *Clin. Res.*, **31**, 514A
13. Robin, E.D., Theodore, J. and Burke, C.M. (1987). Hypoxic pulmonary vasoconstriction persists in the human transplanted lung. *Clin. Sci.*, **72**, 283
14. Burke, C.M., Theodore, J., Dawkins, K.D., Yousem, S.A., Blank, N., Billingham, M.E., Van Kessel, A., Jamieson, S.W., Oyer, P.E., Baldwin, J.C., Stinson, E.B., Shumway, N.E. and Robin, E.D. (1984). Post-transplant obliterative bronchiolitis and other late lung sequelae in human heart–lung transplantation. *Chest*, **86**, 824
15. Burke, C.M., Morris, A.J.R., Dawkins, K.D., McGregor, C.G., Yousem, S.A., Allen, M., Theodore, J., Harvey, J., Billingham, M.E., Oyer, P.E., Stinson, E.B., Baldwin, J.C., Shumway, N.E. and Jamieson, S.W. (1985). Late airflow obstruction in heart–lung transplantation recipients. *J. Heart Transplant.*, **4**, 437
16. Yousem, S.A., Burke, C.M. and Billingham, M.E. (1985). Pathologic pulmonary alterations in long-term human heart–lung transplantation. *Hum. Pathol.*, **16**, 911
17. Reynolds, H.Y. (1987). Bronchoalveolar lavage. *Am. Rev. Respir. Dis.*, **135**, 250
18. Gryzan, S., Paradis, I.R., Dauber, J.H., Hardesty, R.L. and Griffith,

B.P. (1985). The role of bronchoalveolar lavage (BAL) in monitoring patients after heart–lung transplantation (H/L Tx). *J. Heart Transplant.*, **4**, 134

19. Gryzan, S., Paradis, I.R., Griffith, B., Hardesty, R. and Dauber, J. (1985). Bronchoalveolar lavage cell profile after heart–lung transplantation (H/L Tx). *Chest*, **88**, 35
20. Gryzan, S., Paradis, I.L., Hardesty, R.L., Griffith, B.P. and Dauber, J.H. (1985). Bronchoalveolar lavage in heart–lung transplantation. *J. Heart Transplant.*, **4**, 414
21. Paradis, I.L., Marrari, M., Zeevi, A., Duquesnoy, R., Griffith, B.P., Hardesty, R.L. and Dauber, J.H. (1985). The transition of lung lavage cells from donor to recipient phenotype after heart–lung transplantation. *J. Heart Transplant.*, **4**, 138
22. Paradis, I.L., Marrari, M., Zeevi, A., Duquesnoy, R.J., Griffith, B.P., Hardesty, R.L. and Dauber, J.H. (1985). HLA phenotype of lung lavage cells following heart–lung transplantation. *J. Heart Transplant.*, **4**, 422
23. Duquesnoy, F.J., Zeevi, A., Fung, J., Paradis, I., Dauber, J., Griffith, B. and Hardesty, R.L. (1985). Functional characterization of lymphocytes in bronchoalveolar lavages from heart–lung transplant patients. *J. Heart Transplant.*, **4**, 135
24. Zeevi, A., Fung, J.J., Paradis, I.L., Dauber, J.H., Griffith, B.P., Hardesty, R.L. and Duquesnoy, R.J. (1985). Lymphocytes of bronchoalveolar lavages from heart–lung transplant recipients. *J. Heart Transplant.*, **4**, 417
25. Kirby, J.A., Reader, J.A. and Pepper, J.R. (1986). Lung transplantation: effect of cyclosporin-A on the frequency of cytolytic lymphocytes recovered from blood and the bronchoalveolar space. *J. Heart Transplant.*, **5**, 33
26. Hoefter, E., Reichenspurner, H., Krombach, F., Kemkes, B.M., Fiehl, E., Kugler, C., Ertel, W., Osterholzer, G., Konig, G., Gokel, J.M. and Hammer, C. (1987). Morphology and function of free lung cells following combined hetero-orthotopic heart–lung transplantation in the dog. *Transplant. Proc.*, **19**, 1045
27. Haverich, A., Dawkins, K.D., Baldwin, J.C., Reitz, B.A., Billingham, M.E. and Jamieson, S.W. (1985). Long-term cardiac and pulmonary histology in primates following combined heart and lung transplantation. *Transplantation*, **39**, 356
28. Castaneda, A.R., Zamora, R., Schmidt-Habelman, P., Hornung, J., Murphy, W., Ponto, D. and Moller, J.H. (1972). Cardiopulmonary autotransplantation in primates (baboons): late functional results. *Surgery*, **72**, 1064
29. Dawkins, K.D., Haverich, A., Derby, G.C., Scott, W.C., Reitz, B.A., Stinson, E.B., Jamieson, S.W. and Shumway, N.E. (1985). Long-term hemodynamics following combined heart and lung transplantation in primates. *J. Thorac. Cardiovasc. Surg.*, **89**, 55
30. Veith, F.J. and Hagstrom, J. (1972). Alveolar manifestations of rejection: an important cause of the poor results with human lung transplantation. *Ann. Surg.*, **175**, 336
31. Veith, F.J., Montefusco, C., Kamholz, S.L. and Mollenkopf, F.P. (1983). Lung transplantation. *J. Heart Transplant.*, **2**, 155
32. Allen, M.D., Burke, C.M., McGregor, C.G.A., Baldwin, J.C., Jamieson, S.W. and Theodore, J. (1986). Steroid-responsive bronchiolitis after human heart–lung transplantation. *J. Thorac. Cardiovasc. Surg.*, **92**, 449
33. Epler, G. and Colby, T. (1983). The spectrum of bronchiolitis obliterans. *Chest*, **83**, 161
34. Deffenbach, M.E., Charon, N.B., Lakshminarayan, S. and Butler, J. (1987). The bronchial circulation: small, but a vital attribute to the lung. *Am. Rev. Respir. Dis.*, **135**, 463
35. Garzon, A.A., Goldstein, S., Okadigwe, C.I., Paley, N.B. and Minkowitz, S. (1977). Hypothermic lung preservation functions, six or more years later. *Ann. Surg.*, **186**, 711
36. Hino, K., Grogan, J.B. and Hardy, J.D. (1968). Viability of stored lungs. *Transplantation*, **6**, 25
37. Cohen, R.G., Hoyt, G., Billingham, M.E., Bieber, C.P., Jamieson, S.W. and Shumway, N.E. (1984). Myocardial fibrosis due to cyclosporin in rat heterotopic heart transplantation. *Heart Transplant.*, **3**, 355
38. Billingham, M.E. (1987). Cardiac transplant atherosclerosis. *Transplant. Proc.*, **19**, 19
39. Porter, K. (1974). Renal transplantation. In Hepinstall, R.H. (ed.) *Pathology of the Kidney*. (Boston: Little, Brown)
40. Karch, S.B. and Billingham, M.E. (1985). Cyclosporin-induced myocardial fibrosis: a unique controlled case report. *Heart Transplant.*, **4**, 210
41. Ralph, D.D., Springmeyer, S.C., Sullivan, K.M., Haekman, R.C., Storb, R. and Thomas, E.D. (1984). Rapidly progressive air flow obstruction in marrow transplant recipients: possible association between obliterative bronchiolitis and chronic graft-versus-host disease. *Am. Rev. Respir. Dis.*, **129**, 641
42. Wyatt, S.E., Nunn, P., Hows, J.M., Yin, J., Hayes, M.C., Catovsky, D., Gordon-Smith, E.C., Hughes, J.M., Goldman, J.M. and Galton, S. (1984). Airways obstruction associated with graft-versus-host disease after bone marrow transplantation. *Thorax*, **39**, 887
43. Tazelaar, H.D., Prop, J., Nieuwenhuis, P., Billingham, M.E. and Wildevuur, C.R.H. (1987). Obliterative bronchiolitis in the transplanted rat lung. *Transplant. Proc.*, **19**, 1052
44. Jamieson, S.W., Dawkins, K.D., Burke, C., Baldwin, J.W., Yousem, S., Billingham, M.E., Hunt, S.A., Reitz, B.A. Theodore, J., Oyer, P.E., Stinson, E.B. and Shumway, N.E. (1985). Late results of combined heart–lung transplantation. *Transplant. Proc.*, **17**, 212
45. Starnes, V.A. and Jamieson, S.W. (1986). Current status of heart and lung transplantation. *World J. Surg.*, **10**, 442
46. Yacoub, M.H., Banner, N.R., Gibson, S., Thakkar, S.A. and Khaghani, A. (1987). A quantitative assessment of the quality of life after combined heart–lung transplantation. *J. Am. Coll. Cardiol.*, **9**, 30A

44
Results of Heart–Lung Transplantation and Factors Influencing Survival

D.L. MODRY

CLINICAL BACKGROUND

Combined heart–lung transplantation was first performed in 1968, but by the end of 1971 only three procedures had been performed, with the longest survival being 23 days[1-3] (Chapter 33).

No further heart–lung transplantation procedures were performed until March 1981, when Reitz, Shumway and colleagues, stimulated by laboratory successes in primates[4] and by the improved results of clinical cardiac transplantation with cyclosporine, performed the first clinically successful combined heart and lung transplantation procedure; the 45-year-old patient remained well for over 5 years until she met an untimely accidental death in May 1986[5].

One year elapsed before another center, Hopital La Pitie in Paris, followed the Stanford lead[6]. By September 1985, 14 transplantation centers had performed heart–lung transplants[6]. A total of 110 patients, 54 female and 56 male, had undergone 112 procedures, with two patients undergoing retransplantation[7,8]. By December 31, 1987, the Registry of the International Society for Heart Transplantation harbored information on 373 patients transplanted in 36 centers throughout the world (Figure 44.1)[9]; 20 centers accounted for 151 of the transplants in the USA alone. By the end of 1988, the total of reported cases had risen to 501[10]. The age range of the patients extends from the infant (2 months) to 57 years (Figure 44.2), with a mean of 29 years. Of the recipients, 59% have been female, and 41% male.

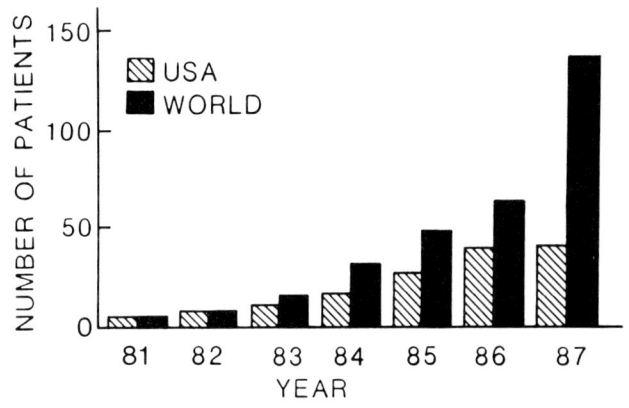

Figure 44.1 Number of heart–lung transplants performed in the USA and worldwide between 1981 and 1987 (International Society for Heart Transplantation (ISHT) Registry, 1988). In 1988, 200 patients underwent this procedure worldwide

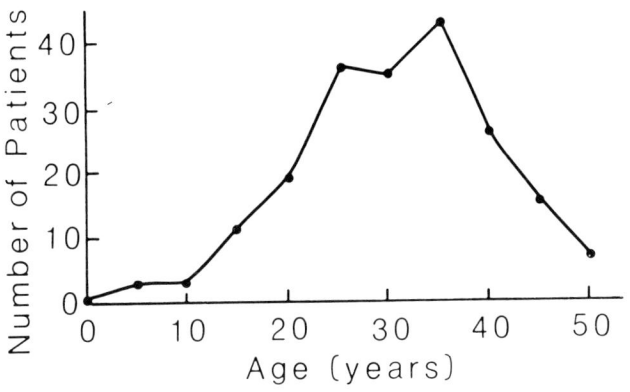

Figure 44.2 Ages of patients undergoing heart–lung transplantation (ISHT Registry, 1988)

INDICATIONS FOR HEART–LUNG TRANSPLANTATION

The underlying pathology necessitating transplantation has been most commonly primary pulmonary hypertension or congenital heart disease associated with the Eisenmenger syndrome. Table 44.1 lists the most common indications leading to heart–lung transplantation to-date. A most interesting group of patients, those with primary lung parenchymal disease, has accounted for only a small proportion of the total number of recipients, but this group represents a vast reservoir of potential candidates[6,11]. Pathology

Table 44.1 Underlying conditions for which heart–lung transplantation was performed in 415 patients*

Pathology	% of total
Primary pulmonary hypertension	39
Eisenmenger syndrome	24
Congenital heart disease	13
Pulmonary parenchymal disease	13
Cystic fibrosis	8
Cardiomyopathy	3
	100

*(Source: Heck, C. F., Shumway, S. J. and Kaye, M. P.[10])

necessitating heart–lung transplantation has included: valvular heart disease with pulmonary hypertension, multiple pulmonary emboli, emphysema, α_1 antitrypsin deficiency, cystic fibrosis, bronchiectasis, eosinophilic granuloma, fibrosing alveolitis, histiocytosis X, primary pulmonary fibrosis, pulmonary asbestosis, pulmonary lymphangiolyomyomatosis, pulmonary staphylococcus infection, pulmonary sarcoidosis, and chronic rejection of the lung in a previously transplanted patient.

Heart–lung, single lung, or double lung transplantation – the dilemma

The ultimate role of combined heart–lung transplantation in the management of patients with primary parenchymal disease, primary pulmonary hypertension, or easily correctable congenital heart disease (e.g. PDA or ASD) with Eisenmenger syndrome remains uncertain, but in patients where heart function is well-preserved (i.e. normal left ventricular function and a right ventricular ejection fraction greater than 25%), there are several reasons why unilateral or double lung transplantation may prove to be a preferable alternative[12]. With hyperinflated pulmonary disease (emphysema) or bilateral pulmonary infection (e.g. bronchiectasis, cystic fibrosis) associated with *normal* cardiac function, it remains to be proven whether or not combined heart–lung transplantation is a superior procedure to double lung transplantation[12].

If only the right ventricle is compromised pretransplant, there is evidence accumulating that right ventricular function can improve dramatically following unilateral or double lung transplantation[12], negating the need for transplantation of the heart as well as the lungs. Retention of the native heart allows for the maintenance of normal neural control of cardiac function. Furthermore, the native heart is not at risk of developing accelerated coronary atherosclerosis (Chapter 19). Retention of the contralateral lung and native heart in patients with pulmonary fibrosis and/or primary pulmonary hypertension also maintains carinal and bronchial (in the non-transplanted lung) innervation, with better preservation of the cough reflex[13].

One early advantage of heart–lung transplantation no longer holds true. Initially, it was thought that endomyocardial biopsy could be used to monitor the immunological status of the lungs as well as that of the heart[5]. Use of the heart as a monitor for lung rejection, however, has proven to be of little value since lung rejection almost always antedates cardiac rejection[14,15]. Unfortunately, an easy, reliable diagnostic test for lung rejection remains elusive.

Given the marked shortage of suitable donors for lung, double lung, or heart–lung transplantation, it seems prudent to use donors in the most economic way possible. For example, if unilateral lung transplantation is equally effective in the palliation of symptoms and extension of life in patients with pulmonary fibrosis, yet avoids the higher operative mortality and late sequelae that have been noted following heart–lung transplantation, then it makes sense to perform the lesser procedure[11,13]. Furthermore, the opposite lung and the heart of the donor can benefit two other recipients[12]. At the present time, however, experience with single and double lung transplantation is limited (Section III), and the advantages and disadvantages of these procedures over heart–lung transplantation remain uncertain.

Another option at the time of heart–lung transplantation in a patient with a normal, or near-normal, native heart is its donation to a second recipient, a procedure performed initially and independently by both Reitz and Yacoub, and termed the 'domino transplant'. Further studies will be required to determine which combination of procedures is optimal. If healing of the tracheal anastomosis proves to be dependent, at least to a certain extent, on coronary–bronchial collaterals[16], which can clearly play no role when double lung transplantation is performed, and if omental wrapping does not prove to ensure satisfactory healing of this anastomosis, then heart–lung transplantation (with the use of the recipient's own heart in a second recipient) could prove safer.

For patients with irreversible combined heart and lung dysfunction, it is clear that the combined procedure is essential, although heart and unilateral lung transplantation may be another possible option if the airways are otherwise normal[17].

SURVIVAL AND CAUSES OF DEATH

Thirty-day mortality for patients undergoing heart–lung transplantation during 1988 was 19%[10], which was an improvement on previous years (23% in 1985, 26% in 1987).

Presently, actuarial survival following combined heart and lung transplantation is 70% at 2 months, falling to approximately 62% by 24 months (Figure 44.3)[9,10]. There has been a 10–15% improvement in survival since 1985 when compared to the period 1981–85. This likely reflects better selection of both donor and recipient, associated with increased operative experience[8,9]. The significant early

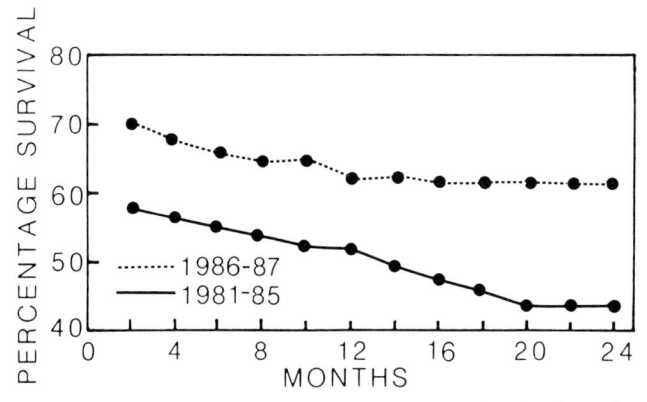

Figure 44.3 Actuarial 2-year survival of patients undergoing heart–lung transplantation between (1) 1981 and 1985, and (2) 1986 and 1987 (ISHT Registry, 1988)

mortality of approximately 30% in the first 2 months indicates the steep learning curves of the surgical procedure itself and of the early postoperative care, which, in regard to degree of difficulty is at least an order of magnitude greater than that for heart transplantation.

Table 44.2 indicates the causes of death in 51 of 112 patients transplanted worldwide between March 1981 and September 1985[6].

Early mortality

The early causes of death relate primarily to (1) hemorrhage, (2) acute respiratory failure, possibly related to inadequate lung storage or significant donor–recipient size mismatch, (3) early cardiac dysfunction, again probably related to inadequate storage, (4) multi-system organ failure associated with perioperative bleeding and infection, (5) acute rejection, (6) cerebral edema, (7) tracheal dehiscence, (8) renal failure, (9) myocardial infarction, and (10) tracheo-aortic fistula.

Table 44.2 Causes of death in 51 of 112 recipients following heart–lung transplantation*

Infection	19
Multi-system organ failure ± postoperative bleeding	15
Acute respiratory failure	5
Tracheal dehiscence	2
Cerebral edema ± infection	2
Renal failure	2
Myocardial infarction	1
Tracheo-aortic fistula	1
Respiratory failure (donor–recipient size mismatch)	1
Respiratory failure (chronic rejection)	1
Hepatic failure	1
Lymphoma	1
Total	51

*(Source: Modry, D. L. and Kaye, M. P.[6])

Late mortality

Late deaths have generally been due to (1) infection, (2) chronic rejection of the heart (graft atherosclerosis) (Chapter 19), (3) bronchiolitis obliterans (Chapter 43), (4) hepatic failure, or (5) lymphoma (Chapter 21).

Infection is the leading cause of mortality, accounting for 48% of early deaths and 73% of late deaths[10] (Chapter 41). Acute rejection is the next most common factor, resulting in approximately 20% of both early and late deaths.

MAJOR FACTORS INFLUENCING SURVIVAL

The following factors adversely affect short and long-term survival.

Selection of the recipient

The timing of recipient selection is frequently difficult due to the fact that patients with end-stage combined heart and lung disease often remain in a stable but compromised status for long periods, able to derive a modicum of satisfactory life quality[18]. Survival in 27 patients with primary pulmonary hypertension referred for heart–lung transplantation, but who died without transplantation, was 50.3 ± 52.5 months (median 37 months), with a symptom duration of 68.4 ± 57.5 months (median 64 months)[18]. The only pretransplant variables that seemed to correlate inversely with survival in this group were low cardiac output and elevated right atrial and mean pulmonary artery pressures[18].

Therefore, given the significant early mortality associated with heart–lung transplantation, many potential years of 'useful existence' may be lost by too early an acceptance for transplantation. On the other hand, fatal pulmonary hemorrhage or arrhythmia may supervene at any unpredictable time. Furthermore, accepting candidates too late in the course of their illness may also lead to poor early survival rates. Although it is now possible to transplant the kidney or liver along with the heart and lungs[19], most centers do not transplant patients with severely compromised hepatic or renal dysfunction[7].

Previous significant intrathoracic surgery which has caused extensive adhesion formation also mitigates against good early results. Excessive hemorrhage may occur during excision of the native organs, requiring large transfusions which in turn may lead to respiratory and multi-system failure[8,20].

Selection of the donor

Unfortunately, as a consequence of trauma, aspiration, pneumonia, or pulmonary edema, only approximately

10–15% of potential donors are suitable for donation[21]. (Donors of heart–lung allografts tend to be slightly younger than those of hearts, with more than 50% being under the age of 20 years[10]). Acceptance of donors with partially compromised heart and/or lung function may lead to early primary graft failure. Although not common practice, donors with mild pulmonary infiltrates, atelectasis, or edema may be converted, on occasion, from unsuitable to suitable donors by judicious fluid management, hemodynamic support, pulmonary physiotherapy, postural drainage, endotracheal suctioning, and antibiotic administration.

Until physicians preserve the integrity of all organ systems in the brain-injured individual, there will continue to be a shortage of suitable heart–lung and lung donors. Considerable efforts will be required to prevent and reverse adverse pulmonary changes for there to be any meaningful increase in the numbers of heart–lung donors.

Successful methods of long-term lung preservation remain elusive, which further limits donor supply as referring physicians and families are reluctant to allow transport of the body. Although limited success with autoperfusion[22,23], hypothermic perfusion on cardiopulmonary bypass[24], and flush cooling techniques[20,25] has been achieved for periods up to 3–4 hours, these techniques have not been uniformly reliable in ensuring immediate lung function after longer preservation periods (Chapter 35).

Prostacycline infusion for 10 minutes prior to explantation of dog lungs flush-cooled with EuroCollins solution conferred significant improvement on early postoperative graft function as determined by improved PaO_2 and survival and some decrease in pulmonary vascular resistance[26]. Similar clinical studies with PGE_1 (25–100 $\mu g/kg$ per min), infused for 15 minutes before and during infusion with modified EuroCollins solution, led to more rapid cooling of the lungs, with a significant decrease in peak inspiratory pressures (29 vs. 33 mmHg post-transplant, $p < 0.01$), a tendency to less 'reimplantation response', and a reduced alveolar–arterial O_2 gradient[27].

Technical factors

The most important technical consideration is the potential for bleeding from severe vascular adhesions (from previous thoracic surgery or inflammation), or from the presence of large bronchial collaterals, especially in recipient candidates with Eisenmenger syndrome[8,20].

A second important technical complication is tracheal disruption from impaired healing of the anastomosis. Many advocate wrapping the tracheal anastomosis with omentum[8], as the omentum seems to have the unique property of providing almost immediate supplementary revascularization to the anastomotic site. Moreover, where tracheal disruption has occurred in the presence of encircling omentum, the omentum has allowed containment of the leak and eventual healing with stenosis, which may subsequently be managed by dilation and intralumenal silastic stenting[12] (Chapter 52).

Pulmonary edema and the 'reimplantation response'

Pulmonary edema, hypoxia, and corresponding bilateral roentgenographic pulmonary infiltrates occurring within the first 24 hours after operation are almost certainly due to lung injury acquired during the preservation period, and may relate to (1) inadequate storage, (2) excessive intravascular fluid (especially crystalloid, causing a fall in blood oncotic pressure and an increase in hydrostatic pressure, predisposing to pulmonary edema), (3) rough handling of the lungs, (4) unrecognized interstitial pneumonitis, and (5) lymphatic interruption.

Reitz *et al.* originally described the 'reimplantation response' (hypoxia with radiological evidence of diffuse interstitial pulmonary infiltrates) as a process unrelated to rejection[5]. According to these authors, this process occurred and resolved between the first and third weeks post-transplant. However, current evidence points to the clearing of such infiltrates shortly after the initiation of steroids on about the 14th postoperative day[8]. Others, who commence low-dose steroids earlier in the post-transplant period, have not observed this problem. The resolution and prevention of the 'reimplantation response' with steroids points to an immunological basis.

DIFFERENTIATION BETWEEN INFECTION AND REJECTION

Failure to distinguish accurately between acute rejection and infection may lead to catastrophic errors in treatment. The occurrence of pulmonary infiltrates on the chest radiograph always presents the dilemma of distinguishing between rejection and infection. Although it was initially thought that heart and lung rejection occurred in a synchronous fashion, which would have allowed transvenous endomyocardial biopsy to be used to monitor the immunological status of the graft[5], it is now known that heart and lung rejection is usually asynchronous, with lung rejection usually preceding heart rejection[14,15,28].

Presently, since there is no absolutely reliable method of determining lung rejection, it is frequently a diagnosis of exclusion. By ruling out infection, and observing a favorable physiological and radiological response to the administration of anti-rejection therapy, oftentimes the diagnosis of rejection can be made[7,8]. Although Wallwork and his colleagues have demonstrated the utility of transbronchial lung biopsies in the differentiation of rejection from infection (Chapter 38), confirmation of the validity of this technique must await further information from Papworth and other centers.

RELATIONSHIP BETWEEN IMMUNOSUPPRESSIVE THERAPY POLICY AND INFECTION

Excessive immunosuppressive therapy is probably the most important factor leading to the most common cause of death following heart–lung transplantation, namely infection[6-8]. Inadequate immunosuppression, on the other hand, is likely the most important factor leading to late death from chronic rejection or bronchiolitis obliterans[29,30].

Whereas the Pittsburgh group has had a 42% operative/early mortality, mainly from infection (particularly *Pneumocystis carinii*), they have not had a major problem with bronchiolitis obliterans. The early (up to 1 year) survival at Stanford is 70%, reflecting fewer infection-related deaths, but Stanford has also experienced a much higher incidence of bronchiolitis obliterans. One might conclude that the Pittsburgh physicians have over-immunosuppressed their patients early post-transplant, leading to a higher incidence of infection, and that those at Stanford have under-immunosuppressed their patients, leading to a higher incidence of bronchiolitis obliterans. Undoubtedly, prophylactic antibiotic cover should prevent the early pneumocystis infections seen at Pittsburgh, with expectation of improvement in both early and long-term survival.

The high morbidity and mortality associated with primary cytomegalovirus (CMV) infection in CMV-seronegative recipients of organs from CMV-seropositive donors has caused some centers to match donor and recipient for CMV status, and other centers to administer CMV hyperimmune globulin prophylactically. Presently, Stanford is investigating the prophylactic administration of the viricidal drug dihydroxypropoxymethylguanine (DHPG, Syntex Ltd.) in CMV-seronegative recipients of hearts from CMV-seropositive donors.

The colonization of airways, particularly by resistant pathogens in patients with cystic fibrosis or bronchiectasis, was thought initially to mandate against heart–lung transplantation in some cases. However, removal of the site of sepsis and source of organisms with the native lungs, followed by combined heart and lung transplantation, has been rewarded with excellent results in several patients to date. Interestingly, although native lungs in patients with cystic fibrosis have abnormally large negative potential differences across nasal and lower airway epithelium, lungs transplanted in such patients are not associated with an electrochemical defect[31].

That both early and late rejection (cellular and humoral) and infection still occur, along with hypertension and renal dysfunction secondary to cyclosporine toxicity[32], necessitates further strenuous efforts to improve our ability to control the immune system and eliminate unwanted drug side-effects.

LATE LUNG FUNCTION AND QUALITY OF LIFE

In 20 patients discharged from Stanford Medical Center following heart–lung transplantation for primary pulmonary hypertension or Eisenmenger syndrome, 1-year follow-up demonstrated a mean PaO_2 of 86.9 ± 9 mmHg, and a mean $PaCO_2$ of 35.6 ± 4 mmHg. Cardiac catheterization at 1 year revealed a mean pulmonary artery pressure of 9 mmHg, which did not change significantly in five patients at 2 years. However, one patient at 3 years had developed such an increase in pulmonary vascular resistance that retransplantation was required[20].

Excellent lung function and quality of life can also be expected in patients undergoing heart–lung transplantation for chronic end-stage lung disease, as demonstrated in six of seven late survivors reported by the Papworth group[25]. FEV_1 improved progressively in all of the survivors to 75–150% of the predicted normal, compared to an FEV_1 of only 11–22% noted before operation. All six patients were fit to return to work 3–6 months post-transplant, and three did so.

Obliterative bronchiolitis does not seem to occur with the same vengeance in patients in whom transplantation was performed for chronic lung disease, as in patients transplanted for pulmonary vascular disease[11,20,29], but differences may be related to the immunosuppressive therapy rather than to patient selection[30,33]. That augmentation of immunosuppression may arrest the obliterative bronchiolitis process points to an underlying rejection etiology[31] (Chapter 43).

COMMENT

It is clear that heart–lung transplantation can be performed successfully in patients with end-stage heart and lung dysfunction, and that excellent pulmonary physiology and quality of life can be achieved. In selected patients, unilateral and double lung transplantation may provide some advantages over heart and lung transplantation.

The long-term outlook for heart and lung transplantation is guardedly optimistic. Present problems include (1) the identification of suitable donors, (2) the education of donor management teams on the prevention and reversal of adverse pulmonary pathology, (3) the need to develop a simple and reliable preservation method to ensure organ preservation for at least 12–24 hours, (4) the need to develop simple non-invasive and reliable methods to diagnose lung and heart rejection, and (5) improvements in control of the immune system to prevent the development of rejection, infection, and bronchiolitis obliterans.

That third party insurance carriers are now funding cardiac transplantation in most centers in Canada and the United States underscores the widely-held belief in the therapeutic and rehabilitative value of the procedure. Although heart–lung transplantation is still considered experimental, those individuals who have survived the operative procedure and who have been fortunate enough not to develop obliterative bronchiolitis, have, in general, enjoyed a return to a healthy, productive life.

References

1. Cooley, D. A., Bloodwell, R. D., Hallman, G. L., Nora, J. J., Harrison, G. M. and Leachman, R. D. (1969). Organ transplantation for advanced cardiopulmonary disease. *Ann. Thorac. Surg.*, **8**, 30
2. Lillehei, C. W. (1970). Discussion of Wildevuur, C.R.H. and Benfield, J.R. A review of 23 human lung transplantations by 20 surgeons. *Ann. Thorac. Surg.*, **9**, 489
3. Barnard, C. N. and Cooper, D. K. C. (1981). Clinical transplantation of the heart: a review of 13 years personal experience. *J. R. Soc. Med.*, **74**, 670
4. Reitz, B. A., Burton, N. A., Jamieson, S. W., Bieber, C. P., Pennock, J. L., Stinson, E. B. and Shumway, N. E. (1980). Heart and lung transplantation, autotransplantation and allotransplantation in primates with extended survival. *J. Thorac. Cardiovasc. Surg.*, **80**, 360
5. Reitz, B. A., Wallwork, J., Hunt, S. A., Pennock, J. L., Billingham, M. E., Oyer, P. E., Stinson, E. B. and Shumway, N. E. (1982). Heart–lung transplantation: successful therapy for patients with pulmonary vascular disease. *N. Engl. J. Med.*, **306**, 557
6. Modry, D. L. and Kaye, M. P. (1986). Heart and heart/lung transplantation. The Canadian and world experience from December 1967–September 1985. *Can. J. Surg.*, **29**, 275
7. Starnes, V. A. and Jamieson, S. W. (1986). Current status of heart and lung transplantation. *World J. Surg.*, **10**, 442
8. Griffith, B. P., Hardesty, R. L., Trento, A., Paradis, I. C., Duquesnoy, R. L., Zeevi, A., Dauber, J. H., Dummer, J. S., Thompson, M. E., Gryzan, S. and Bahnson, H. T. (1987). Heart–lung transplantation: lessons learned and future hopes. *Ann. Thorac. Surg.*, **43**, 6
9. Fragomeni, L. S. and Kaye, M. P. (1988). The Registry of the International Society for Heart Transplantation: fifth official report – 1988. *J. Heart Transplant.*, **7**, 249
10. Heck, C. F., Shumway, S. J. and Kaye, M. P. (1989). The Registry of the International Society for Heart Transplantation: sixth official report – 1989. *J. Heart Transplant.*, **8**, 271
11. Penketh, A., Higenbottam, T., Hakim, M. and Wallwork, J. (1987). Heart and lung transplantation in patients with end-stage lung disease. *Br. Med. J.*, **295**, 311
12. Cooper, J. D. (1984). Lung transplant symposium, Toronto, March 28–29, 1988. *Chest*, **86**, 824
13. Toronto Lung Transplant Group (1986). Unilateral lung transplantation for pulmonary fibrosis. *N. Engl. J. Med.*, **314**, 1140
14. Scott, W. C., Haverich, A., Billingham, M. E., Dawkins, K. D. and Jamieson, S. W. (1984). Lethal rejection of the lung without significant cardiac rejection in primate heart–lung allotransplants. *J. Heart Transplant.*, **4**, 33
15. McGregor, C. G. A., Baldwin, J. C., Jamieson, S. W., Burke, C. M., Oyer, P. E., Stinson, E. B., Shumway, N. E., Billingham, M. E. and Yousem, S. A. (1985). Isolated pulmonary rejection after combined heart–lung transplantation. *J. Thorac. Cardiovasc. Surg.*, **90**, 623
16. Guthaner, D. F., Wexler, L., Sadeghi, A. M., Blank, N. E. and Reitz, B. A. (1983). Revascularization of tracheal anastomosis following heart–lung transplantation. *Invest. Radiol.*, **18**, 500
17. Cooley, D. A., Frazier, O. H., Macris, M. P. and Duncan, J. M. (1987). Heterotopic heart–single lung transplantation: report of a new technique. *J. Heart. Transplant.*, **6**, 112
18. Glanville, A. R., Burke, CC. M., Theodore, J. and Robin, E. D. (1987). Primary pulmonary hypertension. Length of survival in patients referred for heart–lung transplantation. *Chest*, **91**, 675
19. Wallwork, J., Williams, R. and Calne, R. Y. (1987). Transplantation of liver, heart and lungs for primary biliary cirrhosis and primary pulmonary hypertension. *Lancet*, **2**, 182
20. Jamieson, S. W. and Ogunnaike, H. O. (1986). Cardiopulmonary transplantation. *Surg. Clin. North Am.*, **66**, 491
21. Harjula, A., Baldwin, J. C., Starnes, V. A., Stinson, E. B., Oyer, P. E., Jamieson, S. W. and Shumway, N. E. (1987). Proper donor selection for heart–lung transplantation: the Stanford experience. *J. Thorac. Cardiovasc. Surg.*, **94**, 874
22. Hardesty, R. L. and Griffith, B. P. (1987). Autoperfusion of the heart and lungs for preservation during distant procurement. *J. Thorac. Cardiovasc. Surg.*, **93**, 11
23. Adachi, H., Fraser, C. D., Kontos, G. J., Borkon, A. M., Hutchins, C. M., Galloway, E., Brawn, J., Reitz, B. A. and Baumgartner, W. A. (1987). Autoperfused working heart–lung preparation versus hypothermic cardiopulmonary preservation for transplantation. *J. Heart. Transplant.*, **6**, 253
24. Kontos, G. J., Adachi, H., Borkon, A. M., Cameron, D. E., Baumgartner, W. A., Hutchins, G. M., Brawn, J. and Reitz, B. A. (1987). A no-flush, core-cooling technique for successful cardiopulmonary preservation in heart–lung transplantation. *J. Thorac. Cardiovasc. Surg.*, **94**, 836
25. Hakim, M., Higenbottam, T., Bethune, D., Cory-Pearce, R., English, T. A. H., Kneeshaw, J., Wells, F. C. and Wallwork, J. (1988). Selection and procurement of combined heart and lung grafts for transplantation. *J. Thorac. Cardiovasc. Surg.*, **95**, 474
26. Jurmann, M. J., Dammenhayn, L., Schafers, H. J., Wahlers, T., Fieguth, H. G. and Haverich, A. (1987). Prostacyclin as an additive to single crystalloid flush: improved pulmonary preservation in heart–lung transplantation. *Transplant. Proc.*, **19**, 4103
27. Harjula, A. L. J., Baldwin, J. C., Stinson, E. B., Oyer, P. E. and Shumway, N. E. (1987). Clinical heart–lung preservation with prostaglandin E-1. *Transplant. Proc.*, **19**, 4101
28. Wahlers, T., Khaghani, A., Martin, M., Banner, N. and Yacoub, M. (1987). Frequency of acute heart and lung rejection after heart–lung transplantation. *Transplant. Proc.*, **19**, 3537
29. Burke, C. M. Theodore, J., Dawkins, K. D., Yousem, S. A., Blank, N., Billingham, M. E., Van Kessel, A., Jamieson, S. W., Oyer, P. E., Baldwin, J. C., Stinson, E. B., Shumway, N. E. and Robin, E. (1984). Post-transplant obliterative bronchiolitis and other late lung sequelae in human heart–lung transplantation. *Chest*, **86**, 824
30. Burke, C. M., Glanville, A. R., Theodore, J. and Robin, E. D. (1987). Hypotheses: lung immunogenicity, rejection and obliterative bronchiolitis. *Chest*, **92**, 547
31. Alton, F. W., Batten, J., Hodson, M., Wallwork, H., Higenbottam, T. and Geddes, D. M. (1987). Absence of electrochemical defect of cystic fibrosis in transplanted lungs. *Lancet*, **1**, 1026
32. Imoto, E. M., Glanville, A. R., Baldwin, J. C. and Theodore, J. (1987). Kidney function in heart–lung transplantation recipients: the effect of low dose cyclosporine therapy. *J. Heart, Transplant.*, **6**, 204
33. Glanville, J., Baldwin, J. C., Burke, C. M., Theodore, J. and Robin, E. D. (1987). Obliterative bronchiolitis after heart–lung transplantation: apparent arrest by augmented immunosuppression. *Ann. Intern. Med.*, **107**, 300

Section III

Single and double lung transplantation

45
Experimental Background and Early Clinical Experience

J.D. HARDY

INTRODUCTION

Early developmental studies of lung transplantation will be reviewed briefly, as well as the first lung allotransplant in man. In addition, the first 22 clinical lung allotransplants are tabulated (Table 45.1).

Genesis

Experimental lung transplantation was begun at least in the 1940s[1] and perhaps even before then. Many investigators entered the field, but limited space allows acknowledgement of only a few[2-11]. In our laboratories at the University of Mississippi, Webb and associates[12] began canine heart–lung transplantations in the late 1950s, which led ultimately to the first heart transplantation in man in 1964[13]. In parallel studies, my group transplanted the single lung[14] and, later, both lungs at the same operation, primarily in dogs and monkeys.

Meanwhile, two clinical cases brought special focus and immediacy to our laboratory lung transplantation program. These patients had each represented a circumstance in which, if a single lung could be transplanted into a patient who was in potentially temporary, but surely otherwise fatal, hypoxia, then the patient might later survive on his contralateral lung even if the allograft had to be removed. The first patient (1960) was a man with small bowel obstruction who vomited as anesthesia was being induced, with resulting massive bilateral pulmonary aspiration; he died of hypoxia several days later. If it had been possible

Table 45.1 Early experience with clinical lung transplantation

Investigator (year)	Indications for transplantation	Length of survival (days)	Cause of death
(1) Hardy et al. (1963)	Carcinoma/emphysema	18	Renal failure
(2) Magovern and Yates (1963)	Emphysema/cor pulmonale	7	Pneumonia
(3) Shinoi et al. (1965)	Bronchiectasis*	18 (lobe removed)	Patient survived
(4) Neville (1965)	Carcinoma	< 1	Pulmonary edema
(5) White et al. (1965)	Silicosis	7	Pneumonia
(6) Tsuji (1966)	Unknown*	Unknown	Unknown
(7) Morris and Gago (1967)	Pulmonary hypertension*	< 1	Hemorrhagic congestion
(8) Bucherl (1967)	Acute exposure hydrochloric acid	< 1	Cardiac arrest
(9) Bucherl (1967)	Trauma	2	Unknown
(10) Hayata (1967)	Bronchiectasis*	Status of lobe unknown	Patient survived
(11) Matthews et al. (1968)	Paraquat poisoning	13	Paraquat poisoning
(12) Haglin (1968)	Carcinoma	< 1	Bleeding diathesis
(13) Beall (1968)	Emphysema	26	Viral pneumonia
(14) Hallman (1968)	Emphysema	4	Atelectasis
(15) Derom et al. (1968)	Silicosis	10 months	Patient survived
(16) Hardy (1969)	Emphysema	28	Pneumonia
(17) Veith (1969)	Carcinoma/emphysema	8	Pneumonia
(18) Ross (1969)	Emphysema	10	Pneumonia
(19) Beall et al. (1969)	Emphysema	10	Pneumonia with abscess
(20) Vanderhoeft (1969)	COPD	11	Uncertain
(21) Kahn (1969)	COPD	4	Unknown
(22) Haglin (1970)	COPD†	11	Infection? rejection

*One lobe only transplanted; †both lungs transplanted; COPD = chronic obstructive airways disease

to transplant a single functioning lung, to provide time for the patient's own remaining lung to clear, the transplant could have been removed later if rejected. Azathioprine and steroids for immunosuppression were already in use in our kidney transplant patients.

The second patient (1962) was a 73-year-old man with extensive bilateral alveolar carcinoma of the lungs. Already severely dyspneic, he sustained a spontaneous left pneumothorax that soon proved fatal. Here again, a situation presented in which a lung transplant might have prolonged life.

The younger first patient – with a benign condition – might have been considered as having been 'morally assaulted' by a lung transplant (since conceivably he might have survived without the risk of a lung transplant). In the instance of the second patient, with imminently fatal hypoxia and no other effective treatment available for the extensive bilateral malignant pulmonary infiltration, the only major ethical objections to lung transplantation might have been that there was (1) no precedent, (2) no guarantee that a lung allograft would function in the new human host and prolong comfortable life, and (3) that in any event such an 'experiment' was not justified because of his dismal cancer prognosis.

However, by this time we had transplanted lungs in several hundred animals, and good early function of a transplanted lung(s) had been well-established; this finding had also been demonstrated by research groups elsewhere. I was now satisfied in my own mind that either of these two clinical circumstances – massive bilateral pulmonary aspiration or extensive pulmonary cancer with hypoxia – would likely present again, as would terminal respiratory insufficiency due to emphysema or pulmonary fibrosis. Therefore, we believed we should press on with our laboratory work so as to be prepared if and when such a clinical need arose again. Webb and I cleared the prospect of a clinical lung transplant with the officials of the University of Mississippi Medical Center.

EXPERIMENTAL STUDIES

Lung reimplantation

Operative technique

A wide variety of questions confronted lung transplant groups in the late 1950s and early 1960s. To begin with, a consistently dependable autotransplant (reimplant) operative technique had to be developed and mastered by the lung transplant team in each laboratory. This achievement of consistently successful reimplantation was important because it was desirable to establish first the functional characteristics of the *autotransplanted* lung, before moving on to the *allotransplanted* lung, the function of which was certain to be influenced adversely by the allograft immunological rejection process. Appropriate transoperative and postoperative management of the animal was also important, in order to achieve statistically valid results.

Our own experimental investigations[14–21] will be briefly reviewed.

Initially the pulmonary veins were anastomosed individually, but soon, and preferably, a left atrial cuff containing all four ostia of the pulmonary veins was anastomosed to the atrium of the recipient, thus reducing the incidence of stenosis and thrombosis of the pulmonary veins. The pulmonary artery caused little problem, but it was anticipated that stricture of the bronchial anastomosis would commonly occur. This did occur occasionally, and some animals did exhibit bronchial necrosis and fistula. On the whole, however, bronchial problems were less frequent than expected, even though no effort was made to anastomose the bronchial arteries. In subsequent experimental and human lung allotransplants, healing of bronchial (or tracheal) anastomoses was found to be problematic when corticosteroids were included in the early post-transplant immunosuppressive regimen.

Function of the reimplanted lung

The successfully reimplanted lung was studied variously by auscultation, chest radiography, arterial blood gases, bronchoscopy and bronchography, bronchospirometry, isotope scans, pulmonary arteriography (angiocardiography), and by immediate or subsequent ligation of the pulmonary artery to the opposite (unoperated) lung[14–16]. Extensive gross anatomical and microscopic studies were also performed. Ligation of the pulmonary artery to the contralateral lung (instead of performing contralateral pneumonectomy) preserved more nearly the normal pulmonary respiratory reflexes, which afforded much more effective pulmonary ventilatory mechanics than those observed later when both lungs were reimplanted at the same operation.

When, in later experiments, neural connections were severed completely by bilateral lung reimplantation, the animal usually exhibited a slow and deep pattern of respiration and, although commonly able to survive the operation, overall respiratory efficiency was much impaired. Microscopic studies demonstrated vagal nerve degeneration, and the Hering–Breuer reflex was abolished in the reimplanted lung. However, within weeks, early nerve regeneration was demonstrated microscopically, and in chronic dogs studied months or years later, the Hering–Breuer reflex was commonly found to have returned.

The respiratory efficiency of the single reimplanted lung, where respiratory reflexes were essentially normal because of the 'normal' contralateral lung, was good initially, but then declined over the following 7–10 days to about one-half the normal level; thereafter, it gradually improved to regain a low normal level of respiratory efficiency at approximately 2 weeks. Large numbers of animals were studied in the investigation of this decline–recovery pattern. Structures of the pulmonary hilum – pulmonary artery, bronchial arteries, nerves, bronchus, pulmonary veins, lymphatics – were divided individually in various series of animals, to determine the effect on pulmonary function. Suffice it to say that definitive conclusions were hard to come by, but a positive temporal correlation was demonstrated between impaired function and the time required for regeneration of the lymphatics[19]. Regeneration of pulmonary lymphatics following lung reimplantation (and allotransplantation, if the animal were adequately immunosuppressed) could be demonstrated across the bronchial anastomosis by 7–12 days. The ischemia and hypoxia to which the lung was subjected during reimplantation were other potentially significant factors.

In puppies, it was found that the reimplanted lung grew in both size and function[20].

Many studies were directed toward short-term cold storage and also longer cold hyperbaric oxygen storage of the lung, with either delayed reimplantation (occasionally) or, later, allotransplantation of the preserved lung. However, these efforts resulted in only limited extension of the safe storage time.

Lung allotransplantation

The large number of lung reimplantation experiments paved the way for similar anatomical and functional studies of lung allotransplants[17,18]. In brief, it was found in a substantial series that in the untreated dog the allotransplant was rejected in an average of approximately 7 days. In contrast, immunosuppressive therapy, consisting of various regimens involving azathioprine, prednisone, and mediastinal radiation, produced an average allograft survival of approximately 35 days. In some instances, animals that had undergone unilateral or single-operation bilateral lung allotransplantation lived many months. In the process of rejection, the normal lung anatomical structure was replaced by disordered architecture and necrosis. In the occasional animal, the rejected and necrotic lung became encased in protective fibrin and fibrous tissue, permitting long survival of the host.

THE FIRST LUNG TRANSPLANT IN MAN

Following approximately 7 years of lung transplant research involving hundreds of animals, Webb and I obtained permission from the University of Mississippi Medical Center administration to perform a lung transplant in a human patient should the need and the appropriate set of ethical circumstances arise, as noted above. The principal criteria set for selecting a recipient were as follows:

(1) The patient must have a probably fatal disease, so that in the event untoward results were encountered, his life would not have been materially shortened;

(2) There must be a reasonable possibility that the patient would benefit from the lung transplant;

(3) The removal of the patient's own lung must not result in the sacrifice of a significant amount of his own functioning lung tissue;

(4) Transplantation of the left lung had been found to be somewhat simpler technically than transplantation of the right, and thus it was elected to initiate the clinical phase of the work by transplanting a left lung.

The recipient

On April 15, 1963, a 58-year-old man with carcinoma of the left lung and dyspnea at rest from emphysema was admitted to the University of Mississippi Hospital. He had borderline renal failure, secondary to long-standing chronic glomerulonephritis. Details of diagnosis, general evaluation, ethical considerations, and other matters were published at the time[21]. Suffice it to say here that the four pre-set criteria for a potential lung transplant recipient were essentially fulfilled.

There followed a period during which antibiotics were administered in an attempt to clear the pneumonitis distal to the obstructing carcinoma of the left main bronchus. This was only partially successful. The indications for *left pneumonectomy* were the apparently localized carcinoma of the left main stem bronchus and the persistent sepsis distal to this obstructing lesion. The indication for *lung transplantation* was that, already dyspneic on even mild exertion, it was considered vital to replace even the very limited function being provided by the left upper lobe.

The donor

At approximately 7.30 p.m. on June 11, 1963, a patient entered the emergency room of University Hospital in shock and pulmonary edema secondary to massive myocardial infarction. All resuscitative efforts failed, and the family members permitted autopsy and donation of the left lung for transplantation.

The operation

The organ was transplanted into the left hemithorax of the recipient with only moderate difficulty, caused by the prior and persisting infection and the fact that the hilar carcinoma had invaded surrounding tissues more extensively than had been detected preoperatively[21]. Blood samples taken from the transplant pulmonary artery and vein demonstrated immediate excellent respiratory function of the transplant, as reflected in the pulmonary venous versus pulmonary arterial blood gases. This effective function continued during the 18 days he lived.

Postoperative course

Immunosuppression was with azathioprine, prednisone, and mediastinal radiation. Unfortunately, his renal function declined steadily postoperatively, and this major problem, plus infection and the preoperative state of general debility due to the extensive cancer, caused his death.

Postmortem studies

Gross examination of the transplanted lung revealed a well-ventilated organ, with patent anastomoses. A small defect in the membranous portion of the transplant bronchus had been noted at bronchoscopy postoperatively, but this defect was found to have been sealed off by the inflammatory reaction in surrounding tissues. Arteriograms demonstrated excellent patency of the pulmonary vasculature. Microscopy disclosed virtually no evidence of allograft rejection[21].

Comment

This first case had demonstrated the technical feasibility of clinical lung transplantation. The transplant had functioned immediately and for the duration of the patient's life. There had been little or no rejection of the allograft under the immunosuppressive regimen administered – plus perhaps some degree of immunosuppression attributable to the gradual renal decompensation. It was concluded that clinical lung transplantation would eventually offer an effective form of management for otherwise terminal respiratory insufficiency.

SUBSEQUENT EARLY CLINICAL EXPERIENCE

By 1970, 22 known human lung allotransplants had been performed (Table 45.1)[22], and two more as units of heart–lung transplants (Chapter 33)[22]. The early results were disappointing but, with the advent of cyclosporine for improved immunosuppression, heart–lung transplant units later exhibited not only better heart transplant survival but better survival of the lungs as well. Finally, truly long-term survival after single lung transplantation was achieved by Joel Cooper (Figure 45.1) and his colleagues in Toronto, the first such operation being performed on November 7, 1983. With this source of encouragement, the clinical transplantation of one or both lungs is now poised for widespread and successful application[23].

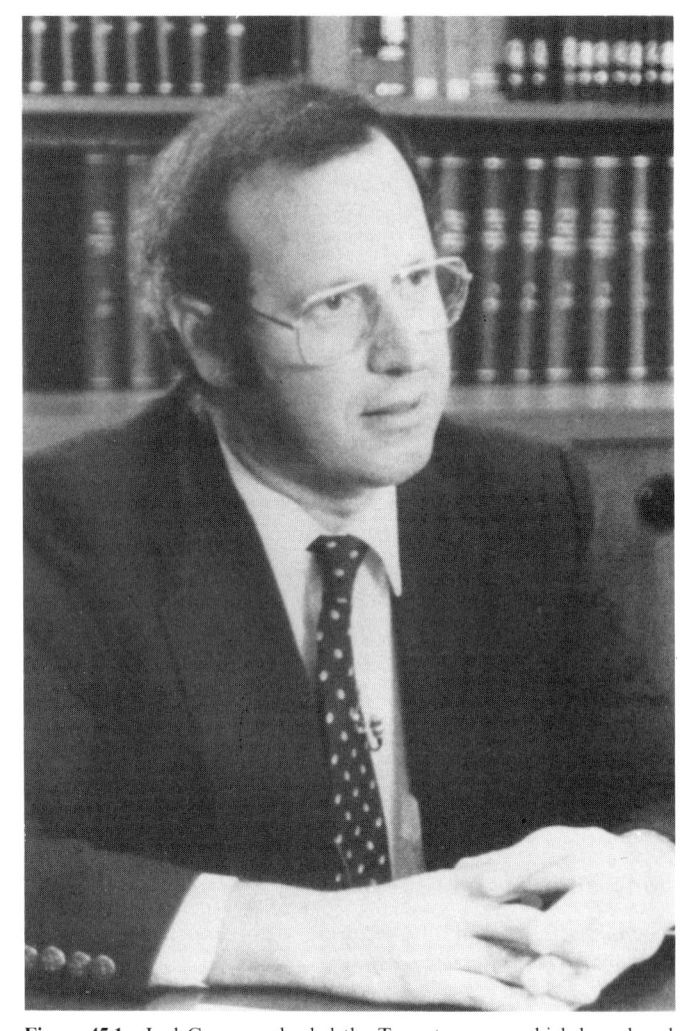

Figure 45.1 Joel Cooper, who led the Toronto group which has played a leading role in the establishment of single lung transplantation

References

1. Demikhov, V.P. (1962). *Experimental Transplantation of Vital Organs.* (Translated from Russian by Basil Haigh). p. 129. (New York: Consultants Bureau)
2. Blumenstock, D.A. and Kahn, D.R. (1961). Replantation and transplantation of the canine lung. *J. Surg. Res.*, **1**, 40
3. Barnes, B.A., Flax, M.H., Burke, J.F. and Barr, G. (1963). Experimental pulmonary homograft in the dog. I. Morphological studies. *Transplantation*, **1**, 351
4. Hardin, C.A., Kittle, C.F. and Schafer, P.W. (1952). Preliminary observations on homologous lung transplants in dogs. *Surg. Forum*, **3**, 374
5. Juvenelle, A.A., Citret, C., Wiles, C.E., Jr. and Stewart, J.B. (1951). Pneumonectomy with replantation of the lung in the dog for physiologic study. *J. Thoracic. Surg.*, **21**, 111
6. Metras, H. (1950). Note preliminaire sur greffe totale du poumon chez

le chien. *Comp. Renal Acad. Sci.*, **231**, 1176
7. Neptune, W.B., Redondo, H. and Bailey, C.P. (1952). Experimental lung transplantation. *Surg. Forum*, **3**, 379
8. Nigro, S.L., Reiman, A.F., Fry, W.A., Mock, L.F. and Adams, W.E. (1961). Alterations in cardiopulmonary physiology following autotransplantation of the lung. *Surg. Forum*, **12**, 56
9. Portin, B.A., Rasmussen, G.S., Stewart, J.D. and Andersen, M.N. (1960). Physiologic and anatomic studies thirty-five months after successful replantation of lung. *J. Thoracic. Cardiovasc. Surg.*, **39**, 380
10. Staudacher, V.E., Bellinazzo, P. and Pulin, A. (1950). Primary results in attempts at autoplastic reimplants and homoplastic transplants of pulmonary lobes. *Chirurgia*, **5**, 223
11. Yeh, T.J., Ellison, L.T. and Ellison, R.G. (1962). Functional evaluation of the autotransplanted lung in the dog. *Am. Rev. Respir. Dis.*, **86**, 791
12. Webb, W.R. and Howard, H.S. (1957). Cardiopulmonary transplantation. *Surg. Forum*, **8**, 313
13. Hardy, J.D., Chavez, C.M., Kurrus, F.D., Neely, W.A., Eraslan, S., Turner, M.D., Fabian, L.W. and Labecki, T.D. (1964). Heart transplantation in man. Developmental studies and report of a case. *J. Am. Med. Assoc.*, **188**, 1132
14. Alican, F. and Hardy, J.D. (1963). Lung reimplantation: effect on respiratory pattern and function. *J. Am. Med. Assoc.*, **183**, 849
15. Howard, H.S. and Webb, W.R. (1958). Respiratory paralysis following pulmonary denervation. *Surg. Forum*, **8**, 466
16. Eraslan, S., Hardy, J.D. and Elliott, R.L. (1966). Lung replantation: respiratory reflexes, vagal integrity, and lung function in chronic dogs. *J. Surg. Res.*, **6**, 383
17. Hardy, J.D., Eraslan, S. and Dalton, M.L., Jr. (1963). Autotransplantation and homotransplantation of the lung: further studies. *J. Thorac. Cardiovasc. Surg.*, **46**, 606
18. Hardy, J.D., Eraslan, S., Dalton, M.L., Jr., Alican, F. and Turner, M.D. (1963). Re-implantation and homotransplantation of the lung: laboratory studies and clinical potential. *Ann. Surg.*, **157**, 707
19. Eraslan, S., Turner, M.D. and Hardy, J.D. (1964). Lymphatic regeneration following lung reimplantation in dogs. *Surgery*, **56**, 970
20. Webb, W.R., Unal, M., Cook, W.A., Eraslan, S. and Hardy, J.D. (1965). Growth and function of the transplanted lung in puppies. *Clin. Res.*, **13**, 49
21. Hardy, J.D., Webb, W.R., Dalton, M.L., Jr. and Walker, G.R., Jr. (1963). Lung homotransplantation in man: report of the initial case. *J. Am. Med. Assoc.*, **186**, 1065
22. Hardy, J.D. (1971). Lung transplantation. In Hardy, J.D. (ed.) *Human Organ Support and Replacement*, p. 272 (Table 12-I). (Springfield: Charles C. Thomas)
23. Cooper, J.D. (1987). Lung transplantation: a new era. (Editorial). *Ann. Thorac. Surg.*, **44**, 447

46
Indications, Selection and Management of the Recipient

A.E. FROST, R.F. GROSSMAN AND J.R. MAURER

SINGLE LUNG TRANSPLANTATION

Single lung transplantation has been attempted in humans since 1963, but it was uniformly unsuccessful until the early 1980s (Chapter 45). These poor early results could be attributed to several factors, including technical problems resulting in bronchial dehiscence, poor donor lung preservation, infection, and inadequate immunosuppression. Probably equally important in the early failures was the selection of inappropriate patients. Most of those transplanted were desperately ill, debilitated patients with end-stage obstructive lung disease and malignancy.

The development of the omentopexy surgical technique which facilitated bronchial healing, and the avoidance of early postoperative corticosteroid administration, successfully addressed the problem of bronchial dehiscence. This, together with improvements in immunosuppressive therapy, infection control, and even in organ preservation, set the stage for successful lung transplantation.

Patient selection

To solve the patient selection problem, we felt it imperative to choose transplant candidates who had exhausted all avenues of medical therapy, yet who were still sufficiently functional to survive surgery. Accordingly, candidates for single lung transplantation at the University of Toronto must have the characteristics and meet the criteria outlined below.

Pulmonary fibrosis

Only patients with diseases in which the end-stage lung is poorly compliant have been accepted for unilateral transplant. We have shown that patients preferentially ventilate and perfuse the more normally compliant donor lung when their remaining native lung is fibrotic. It is not clear that this would happen if the underlying disease were one in which the end-stage lung had either normal or increased compliance. Some of the underlying diseases in patients eligible for unilateral transplantation include idiopathic pulmonary fibrosis, sarcoidosis, some occupational lung disease, and chronic extrinsic allergic alveolitis (Table 46.1).

Age less than 60 years

Initially, a maximum age of 50 was set for patients admitted to the Toronto program, modeled after the successful Stanford heart–lung transplant program. However, because many patients with fibrotic lung diseases do not become end-stage until the sixth decade, and because our initial patient had done well at age 58, we increased the limit to 60. Because of the incidence of coronary artery disease in this age group, however, we do require all males between ages 50 and 60, and all postmenopausal females in this age group, to have coronary arteriography before undergoing formal assessment.

Life expectancy less than 18 months

Lung transplantation is reserved for patients who have progressive disease in spite of maximal medical therapy. Because of limited donor supply and limited experience in this area of transplantation, we feel it should be reserved

Table 46.1 Indications for single lung transplantation

(1)	Idiopathic pulmonary fibrosis
(2)	Hypersensitivity pneumonitis
(3)	Occupational fibrotic lung disease
(4)	Drug/toxin-induced fibrotic lung disease
(5)	Sarcoidosis
(6)	Scleroderma
(7)	Other fibrotic lung disease (individually assessed)

for patients who have a short projected life span. Though it is sometimes difficult to judge possible life span in patients with fibrotic disease, a reasonably accurate prediction can be made using pulmonary function studies, exercise tolerance, supplemental oxygen requirements, and the rate of progression of the disease over the preceding 12–24 months. The preoperative pulmonary function of our successfully transplanted patients is listed in Table 46.2. All patients were oxygen-dependent at rest and exercise. All similar patients accepted for transplantation, but in whom a donor lung was not found, succumbed to their disease within 1 year.

Absence of systemic illness with end organ damage

All patients undergoing transplantation are committed to lifelong immunosuppressive therapy. Among the side-effects of these drugs – particularly cyclosporine and azathioprine – are renal and hepatic toxicity. Thus, it is necessary to choose patients who do not have pre-existing disease of these organs in order to avoid organ failure. Of less critical importance, but still of some concern, are patients with allergy to sulfonamides, as all patients receive prophylaxis against *Pneumocystis carinii* with trimethoprim-sulphamethoxazole post-transplant. This problem may be solved by the recent introduction of aerosolized pentamidine, both in the prophylaxis and treatment of pneumocystis.

The association of pulmonary fibrosis with active systemic disease, such as rheumatoid arthritis, dermatomyositis, or systemic lupus erythematosus, is of sufficient concern to preclude transplantation. In general, the unpredictability of these disorders, as well as the major limitations placed on the patient's rehabilitation potential by any associated musculoskeletal disorder, increase the risk of morbidity and mortality at transplant. Patients with scleroderma and severe pulmonary fibrosis might be accepted if there were no evidence of renal involvement, and other manifestations of scleroderma were mild.

Table 46.2 Lung function prior to single lung transplantation in patients at the University of Toronto

Test	Mean ± SD
Total lung capacity (liters)	2.9 ± 0.4
(% predicted)	(46.0 ± 7.0)
FVC	1.8 ± 0.1
(% predicted)	(44.0 ± 5.0)
FEV_1/FVC % predicted	122.0 ± 5.0
DLCO	6.9 ± 0.1
(% predicted)	(37.0 ± 4.0)

FEV_1 = forced expiratory volume in 1 second (in liters); FVC = forced vital capacity (in liters); DLCO = diffusing capacity for carbon monoxide (in ml min^{-1} mmHg^{-1})

Prefer no previous major abdominal surgery

The revascularization of the bronchial anastomosis is achieved via an omentopexy. This tissue is ideal for this purpose because it is large, easily manipulated, and has an excellent vascular supply and lymphatic drainage. However, in some types of abdominal surgery, for example gastric surgery, the omentum may be removed, traumatized, or adherent to other abdominal structures. This makes it unavailable for anastomotic revascularization. Generally, lower abdominal surgery and cholecystectomy leave the omentum intact. Should a patient not have an intact omentum, yet otherwise be an ideal candidate for lung transplantation, it is theoretically possible to use intercostal muscle flaps or pericardium.

Right ventricular ejection fraction > 25%

All patients with end-stage fibrotic lung disease have some degree of right ventricular dysfunction secondary to elevated pulmonary artery pressures. It is not clear what degree of right heart dysfunction is compatible with operative survival and subsequent recovery of right heart function. Three of our 15 unilateral transplant patients required partial cardiopulmonary bypass during surgery. Although cardiopulmonary bypass may be a routine procedure, it adds a considerable risk to transplant surgery, and its necessity may remove a patient from consideration of transplantation. For example, patients with extensive pleural disease or previous thoracotomies can be transplanted. If anticoagulation is required for cardiopulmonary bypass, however, these patients have a much higher risk of exsanguinating intraoperatively.

Using a right ventricular first-pass ejection fraction cut-off of around 25%, we have essentially eliminated all patients who have clinical evidence of right heart failure. Questions remain both as to the best method of assessing right heart function, and to defining the limits of the right heart's vulnerability. We have recently begun a series of invasive studies in selected patients pre- and post-transplant to try and answer these questions.

In addition to our right heart criteria, we require that patients have normal left ventricular function on radionuclide and echocardiographic studies.

Non-steroid-dependent

Studies by our surgical team in the 1970s showed impaired anastomotic healing in dogs treated with steroids[1]. Because it is critical that the anastomosis heal well in the first two postoperative weeks, we have carefully avoided choosing steroid-dependent patients. Paradoxically, however, since we require that our candidates have failed usual medical therapy, nearly all of them have had a course of steroid therapy. A potential candidate is often referred when his illness is progressing despite ongoing steroid use. We require that the drug be tapered and discontinued under the supervision of the referring physician before the patient undergoes formal assessment. Tapering of steroid therapy can be associated with disease exacerbation; when this occurs, we suggest trying the patient on an alternate therapy, like cyclophosphamide, which does not have a demonstrated effect on wound healing.

Adequate nutrition

Obese and cachectic patients present different problems which may influence the surgical outcome, but both have potentially negative effects. The obese patient presents mechanical problems at surgery, an increased risk of postoperative complications, and is more difficult to nurse. The cachectic, poorly conditioned patient may have problems with healing, predisposition to infection, and be generally weak and slow to extubate and mobilize. To prevent these problems, in most cases our patients have been required to be within 10–15 kilograms of their ideal body weight. In shorter patients, the leeway has been slightly less, and in taller patients, slightly more. In most cases in which a potential candidate has not initially met our weight requirements, he or she has been able to achieve the goal weight, and has been accepted for assessment.

Ambulatory and motivated

Patients who are bedridden and deconditioned are poor surgical risks. We have required that all candidates for our program not only be ambulatory, but that they participate in a regular preoperative rehabilitation program (see pre-transplant management). This selects those patients who are motivated as well as ambulatory. The ability to walk from 50 to 100 feet (25–30 meters) (with as much supplemental oxygen as required) is necessary for a patient to be considered ambulatory.

No major psychiatric, drug abuse problems

The stress of transplantation – particularly the waiting and perioperative period – on patients and families should not be underestimated. During these times, psychiatric disorders or inappropriate coping strategies, e.g. drug abuse, from the patient's past may surface. Furthermore, some of the drugs, e.g. steroids, that are used postoperatively may precipitate recurrence of previous psychiatric disorders. Since it is essential that transplant patients be completely compliant with medication and other treatment plans, this can present major obstacles to optimal lung graft survival and, ultimately, patient survival.

Adequate psychosocial support

It is essential that a family member or other designated person be available to offer ongoing support. Not only does the transplant candidate need emotional support, he also needs help with the usual activities of daily life, e.g. shopping, transportation.

Our criteria have been designed to select those end-stage patients who would have the highest likelihood of surviving the rigors of transplant surgery. This excludes large groups of patients with fibrotic disease, whose potential to undergo lung transplant successfully is not yet known (Table 46.3). Some of these groups include patients (1) with normally or highly compliant lungs at the end-stage of their disease, (2) who are ventilator-dependent, e.g. post adult respiratory distress syndrome, (3) who can be tapered to small doses of steroids, but are unable to be completely weaned from them.

ADDENDUM

Clinical experience gained since this chapter was written would suggest that patients with emphysema and primary pulmonary hypertension are suitable candidates for single lung transplantation. Patients with correctable congenital cardiac defects and secondary pulmonary vascular disease may prove suitable for simultaneous correction of the cardiac defect and single lung transplantation on occasions, though experience of this therapy for Eisenmenger syndrome is to date very limited.

DOUBLE LUNG TRANSPLANTATION

The Toronto Double Lung Transplant Program started performing double lung transplants in November, 1986.

Patient selection

The unique criteria for patients considered in this program are listed below.

End-stage lung disease characterized by increased compliance or end-stage bronchiectasis (chronic infection)

Unilateral lung transplantation is inappropriate in patients with chronic infection because any infection remaining

Table 46.3 Contraindications for single lung transplantation

(1)	Advanced age
(2)	Coronary artery disease
(3)	Severe right heart failure
(4)	Steroid dependence
(5)	Pulmonary sepsis
(6)	Malignancy
(7)	Ventilator dependence

following transplantation will almost certainly involve the donor lung. The role of unilateral transplantation has not yet been determined in patients with highly compliant lungs, e.g. emphysematous lungs. Our group has felt that it is likely a patient will tend to ventilate a highly compliant native lung in preference to a normally compliant donor lung. In this type of patient, we are also concerned about the possibility of progressive air trapping compromising the donor lung. For those reasons, we developed the technique of double lung transplantation.

Some of the underlying diseases that are considered eligible for double lung transplant include α_1-antitrypsin emphysema, idiopathic emphysema, bronchiolitis obliterans, eosinophilic granuloma, lymphangioleiomyomatosis, cystic fibrosis, and idiopathic bronchiectasis (Table 46.4).

Several groups have been performing heart–lung transplants for these patients. In the majority of such patients heart function is well-preserved, and the cardiac component of the transplant is unnecessary. The transplanted heart is subject to its own unique complications, such as rejection and accelerated atherosclerosis[2]. Moreover, the denervated heart does not respond normally to exercise. Finally, up to 50% of heart–lung transplant recipients have developed bronchiolitis obliterans, whereas none of our single or double lung recipients has shown progressive airway obstruction, with follow-up periods in excess of 4 years[3]. While it may be premature to claim that the transplanted heart is responsible for this phenomenon, prudence would dictate that the heart should not be transplanted if it is not necessary.

Age less than 50 years

An arbitrary age limit of 50 has been set for patients considered for double lung transplantation. Many more potential candidates in this category reach the end-stage of their disease before the sixth decade; therefore, the number of good candidates easily outstrips the number of donors without including older patients. Nevertheless, occasionally excellent candidates in their early fifties are referred to us and, as the number of successful surgeries increases, the age limits will likely become more flexible. Should this happen, however, coronary arteriography would likely become a prerequisite to formal assessment.

No surgical violation of the pleural space

Double lung transplant patients require cardiopulmonary bypass with anticoagulation. Extensive pleural adhesions due to pleurodesis, previous thoracotomies, or inflammation have been shown in heart–lung transplantation to result in excessive, and often fatal, perioperative hemorrhage. It is unlikely that double lung patients with a similar background would fare any differently.

The remainder of the criteria for potential double lung transplant recipients are similar to those for patients being assessed for single lung transplantation.

IN-HOSPITAL ASSESSMENT: ALL POTENTIAL LUNG RECIPIENTS

The second phase of patient selection is the in-hospital assessment. Patients who meet the stated criteria are admitted for a 10–14-day stay during which a series of evaluations is carried out. The potential candidates meet the primary consultants who will participate in postoperative care. They also have detailed psychiatric and nutritional assessments.

Pulmonary assessment

The degree of pulmonary compromise is evaluated with routine pulmonary function studies (Table 46.5), a compliance curve, and an exercise tolerance assessment using the 6-minute walk and Modified Bruce Protocol. During studies, patients undergo constant oximeter monitoring of oxygen saturation. Quantitative ventilation–perfusion scans are done, and are particularly useful to the surgical team in unilateral transplant candidates if there is a large discrepancy in perfusion or ventilation to one lung. Additional studies include gallium scans and computerized tomogram

Table 46.4 Indications for double lung transplantation*

(1) Obstructive lung disease
   (a) emphysema
   (b) α_1-antitrypsin deficiency
   (c) familial emphysema
   (d) bronchiolitis obliterans
(2) Septic lung disease
   (a) cystic fibrosis
   (b) bronchiectasis
(3) Eosinophilic granuloma
(4) Lymphangioleiomyomatosis

*See addendum, p. 365

Table 46.5 Lung function prior to double lung transplantation in patients at the University of Toronto

Test	Mean $\pm$ SD
Total lung capacity (liters)	7.3 $\pm$ 0.5
(% predicted)	(143.0 $\pm$ 23.6)
FVC	1.6 $\pm$ 0.5
(% predicted)	(50.7 $\pm$ 24.7)
FEV$_1$	0.6 $\pm$ 0.2
(% predicted)	(22.3 $\pm$ 9.6)
DLCO	5.4 $\pm$ 1.2
(% predicted)	(21.0 $\pm$ 2.5)

Abbreviations as for Table 46.2

scans to assess the degrees of pleural and parenchymal disease.

Cardiac assessment

Cardiac evaluation has primarily been non-invasive by using 2D echocardiograms with Doppler assessment of pulmonary artery pressure, and by using radionuclide studies. In our experience, the most accurate measure of right ventricular function on radionuclide studies is the first-pass value. A first-pass right ventricular ejection fraction more than or equal to 25% is the value used to determine whether patients meet the requirement for candidacy. The nuclide equilibrium rest and exercise data for the left ventricle are used in conjunction with echo data to determine function of the left ventricle. Normal left ventricular function is necessary.

Because it has been unclear how accurate non-invasive studies are in predicting cardiac function in this population, our group has recently initiated a series of pre- and postoperative invasive studies using Swan–Ganz catheterization. The information from this protocol will hopefully allow us to design the most useful non-invasive approach.

Other organ system assessment

Renal and hepatic functions are assessed via blood chemistries and creatinine clearance. The patient's clotting system and platelet function are tested, and the cytomegalovirus antibody titer is obtained.

Nutritional assessment

This includes caloric counts, skin fold measurements, and reviews of serum iron indices and serum protein/albumin measurements. Appropriate counseling is part of this assessment. Patients may be required to approach their ideal body weight before becoming active transplant candidates. For patients with cystic fibrosis, the ability to absorb cyclosporine is documented preoperatively.

Psychosocial assessment

Finally, detailed psychiatric, psychological, and social assessments are made. These are aimed primarily at determining the strength of the patient's coping mechanisms, and those of his family or support person, and identifying areas in which problems are likely to arise.

Following formal assessment, the data obtained are presented at a meeting of the executive committee of the Toronto Lung Transplant Group, and a decision is made regarding the person's candidacy.

PRETRANSPLANT MANAGEMENT

The time between acceptance and transplant is a particularly stressful time for patient and family. Not only is the patient living in a strange city, he is coping with the demands of increasing debility, and is constantly aware that at any time he may be called in for transplantation. A program to maintain such a patient in as good a condition as possible, and to help him cope with stresses, has been in place since 1985.

The main component of this program is rehabilitation. Under the direction of two physiotherapists, patients come as outpatients to our center two or three times per week, and participate in a formal rehabilitation program. This includes treadmill walking, stationary bicycling, and lifting of small weights. We have been able to show a significant improvement in exercise capability of these end-stage patients from the time of their entrance into the program until they undergo transplant. A second facet of the preoperative management is a support group which, under the direction of the psychosocial staff, meets only once a week and is attended by transplant candidates and their families or other support persons. The third component of care is a transplant clinic for preoperative candidates and patients who have undergone transplant. A pretransplant patient attends once a month, and his current status is reviewed by resident and staff physician.

Every 3 months, patients undergo routine reassessments. Cardiac function is closely monitored with two-dimensional echocardiography and gated radionuclide angiography. If right or left ventricular function falls below our agreed guidelines, the patient is removed from the transplant list and referred to a heart–lung transplant center. Renal, hepatic, and hematological indices are also reassessed periodically every 2–4 months.

As donor availability remains the main limiting factor to any successful transplant program, delays in transplantation are inevitable. The average wait is approximately 6 months; up to 30% of candidates die while awaiting transplantation.

All patients accepted for transplantation are informed that steroids or mechanical ventilation will not be employed in their management, and that initiation of either immediately eliminates them from candidacy for transplantation. Patients may recover from episodes of acute respiratory failure and, as long as they return to their premorbid condition, may once again be considered for transplantation.

COMMENT

Strict adherence to the selection criteria and careful preoperative management and reassessment have yielded encouraging results and long-term survival following both single and double lung transplantation (Chapter 53). Refinement of selection techniques for both candidates and donors should result in further improvement in perioperative and long-term survival.

Acknowledgements

The work presented in this chapter was supported in part by the Lung Association, Metro Toronto and York Region.

References

1. Lima, O., Cooper, J.D., Peters, W.J., Ayabe, H., Townsend, E., Luk, S.C. and Goldberg, M. (1981). Effects of methylprednisolone and azathioprine on bronchial healing following lung transplantation. *J. Thorac. Cardiovasc. Surg.*, **82**, 211
2. McGregor, C.G.A., Jamieson, S.W., Oyer, P.E., Baldwin, J.C., Modry, D.L., Hunt, S.A., Billingham, M.E., Miller, J.L., Gamberg, P.L., Stinson, E.B. and Shumway, N.E. (1984). Heart transplantation at Stanford. *J. Heart Transplant.*, **4**, 31
3. Starnes, V.A. and Jamieson, S.W. (1986). Current status of heart and lung transplantation. *World J. Surg.*, **10**, 442

47
Selection of the Donor: Excision and Storage of the Lungs

T.R. TODD

INTRODUCTION

The expansion of organ transplantation over the last 10 years has led to an increasing shortage of suitable organs[1]. In an effort to meet this need, centralized registries of urgent potential recipients were developed to ensure access to donors at distant sites. This program was able to expand as improved means of donor organ preservation were formulated. However, the demand for organ donors has exceeded the supply despite an intense educational campaign aimed at both the public and the profession. As a result, the maximum number of transplantable organs must be retrieved from every available donor.

In order to achieve this maximum number, and with lung transplantation particularly in mind, the following points deserve consideration:

(1) Assessment and selection of the donor lungs,
(2) Maintenance of selected donors,
(3) Excision and preservation of donor organs.

ASSESSMENT AND SELECTION OF THE DONOR LUNGS

There are several reasons why the lungs of brain-dead donors might not be suitable for transplantation.

Firstly, the precipitating cause of brain death may have led to significant pulmonary parenchymal or bronchial damage. Trauma is the commonest cause of brain death in an otherwise healthy young person, and thus the presence of pulmonary contusion or bronchial trauma must be considered. In addition, the aspiration of gastric contents is a frequent accompaniment of a depressed level of consciousness. As intracranial pressure rises, neurogenic pulmonary edema may be seen.

Secondly, these patients have all undergone tracheal intubation for the purpose of mechanical ventilatory support. They have been cared for in intensive care units where the presence of highly-resistant bacteria leads to colonization of the respiratory tract in half the patients within 3 days[2]. As a result, the early onset of Gram-negative pneumonia is a well-recognized feature in brain-dead subjects. In our experience, this pulmonary infection is rapidly progressive.

These factors underscore the importance of careful assessment of potential lung donors. The portable chest radiograph supplies useful information provided that the technique employed yields a film of good quality. If a portable film taken in the intensive care unit is inadequately exposed, subtle pulmonary infiltrates may not be visualized clearly. Radiographs of questionable quality should be repeated. A localized infiltrate should be of particular concern as this most likely represents pneumonitis rather than pulmonary edema. In the author's experience, the area of involvement will rapidly increase in size, and this will usually preclude donation of the lungs. On occasion, infiltrates will disappear or stabilize, emphasizing the importance of repeated radiographic assessment. When the infiltrate involves only one lung, the contralateral lung may be used for transplantation, provided the gas exchange is satisfactory. The presence of pulmonary edema demands a trial of diuresis (see below). If the clinical diagnosis of edema is correct, the radiographic appearances and gas exchange may improve sufficiently to allow for lung donation.

Arterial blood gases are measured with the subject receiving a fraction of inspired oxygen (FiO_2) of 1.0 (100% O_2) and a positive end-expiratory pressure (PEEP) of $5 \, cmH_2O$. Under these circumstances, the partial pressure of oxygen should be maintained above 300 torr (mmHg). All of the donor lungs in the Toronto experience ($n = 31$) have been selected using these criteria. Blood gases are repeated every 30 minutes while awaiting donor organ extraction to ensure continued suitability.

Bronchoscopy is undertaken routinely. Aspirates are processed bacteriologically, and both donor and recipient receive antimicrobial agents based on the initial Gram stain.

Few bronchoscopic findings will preclude the use of the donor lungs. In one subject, however, we have seen an intense bronchitis, with sloughing of the bronchial mucosa, which precluded use of the organs. In a second, aspirated teeth were removed from segmental bronchi before the lungs were excised.

The lungs are the only organs which are transplanted into a relatively rigid cavity. 'Relatively rigid' is indeed the correct adjective as the primary disease process will have altered the volume and shape of the thoracic cage. In pulmonary fibrosis, lung volumes will be smaller than those predicted for the patient's age, size, and weight. The diaphragms are high and the rib spaces compressed. In emphysema, α_1-antitrypsin deficiency, and bronchiectasis, lung volumes are increased, resulting in low diaphragms and large intercostal spaces. These factors must be considered in the selection of the appropriate donor. It is thus imperative to assess the thoracic volume accurately in both recipient and donor. We routinely measure the horizontal diameter (at the level of the highest hemidiaphragm), and the vertical dimension of each hemithorax (apex to diaphragmatic dome) on the chest radiograph (see also Chapters 34-36 and 38).

It is difficult to predict accurately the correct donor lung dimensions appropriate for the individual recipient. However, in cases of pulmonary fibrosis and contracted lung volume, it is important to select donor lungs that are (by the measurements noted above) larger than the recipient dimensions. When the recipient has expanded lung volumes, a smaller donor is appropriate. At present, there are no precise guidelines for determining how much larger or smaller these dimensions ought to be. In the Toronto experience, we have followed these principles, but have ensured that donor dimensions do not differ from those of the recipient by more than 5 cm in either direction.

The diaphragm and chest wall readily conform to the size of the new donor lungs. A decrease in lung volume in a double lung recipient is quickly accompanied by a more normal diaphragmatic contour and a reduction in the size of the intercostal spaces. On the other hand, a significant increase in thoracic volume will be noted on the chest radiograph after single lung transplantation for pulmonary fibrosis.

The limits of acceptable discrepancy and size have yet to be determined; when exceeded, innovations may be required. In one of our single lung transplant recipients, the donor lung was clearly excessively large. A portion of the donor lung was excised with a stapling device. Fortunately, preoperative appreciation of this potential size problem led to the decision to undertake transplantation on the left side in the belief that diaphragmatic descent would be greater.

MAINTENANCE OF THE DONOR

There are a few features of donor maintenance that are important only when lung donation is considered. As noted above, frequent chest radiographic and blood gas assessments are important. Diuresis may be important in lung donors to prevent or treat pulmonary edema. In our experience, this has not interfered with the subsequent function of donated renal grafts. Fluid restriction is maintained as long as urine output is adequate ($>$ 50 ml/h). Diabetes insipidus is usually controlled with desmopressin (DDAVP), as this drug has little effect on portal blood flow[3], an important consideration when the liver is to be transplanted also.

β-adrenergic infusions of dopamine may help support blood pressure and renal perfusion, thus reducing the need for fluid administration. Following brain death, hemodynamic instability is common, particularly when the interval between declaration of brain death and organ extraction is prolonged. As a result, these patients may receive large quantities of intravenous fluid as preload and peripheral vascular resistance may be low. When a predisposition to capillary leak occurs, the accumulation of extravascular lung water is directly proportional to preload. In addition, an impairment in cardiac contractility has been described in experimental models of brain death[4], and, in our own experience, has been seen in 20-25% of declared organ donors. The administration of an inotrope is therefore of potential importance. If larger (alpha) doses of dopamine are required ($>$ 6 μg/kg per min), we prefer to use phenylephrine to prevent depletion of cardiac dopaminergic receptors[5].

EXCISION AND PRESERVATION OF THE DONOR LUNGS

The techniques of excision of either one lung or both lungs (as described below) are invariably influenced by the need to preserve and excise the heart also for transplantation into a second recipient. If the two recipients (of heart, and lung, respectively) are at the same center, then the heart-lung bloc may be excised as a single unit (as described in Chapter 35), transported as such, and the final dissection carried out at the recipient center. If the two donated organs are to be transported to different centers, then the heart may be excised before removal of the lung(s); it is this technique that will be described in this chapter.

A bronchus blocker[6] is inserted through the larynx alongside the endotracheal tube and, under bronchoscopic control, is positioned in the left main stem bronchus. (Later in the procedure, the bronchus blocker will be inflated to bring about atelectasis of the left lung.)

A median sternotomy is performed. The pericardium is opened widely with lateral extensions inferiorly. Superiorly, the pericardium is incised to the origin of the innominate (brachiocephalic) artery. The superior vena cava is mobilized immediately caudal to the azygos vein and encircled with a relatively thick silk ligature. Similarly, the inferior vena cava is dissected and encircled. The ascending aorta and arch are also freed circumferentially, this dissection continuing distally to allow identification and division of the ligamentum arteriosum.

With the aorta retracted to the left and the superior vena cava to the right, the posterior pericardium overlying the distal trachea is incised. The trachea is mobilized as high above the carina as possible (at least five rings), usually at the level of the innominate artery, and a tape placed around it. No dissection should take place between this latter point and the tracheal carina except laterally against the aortic arch itself. The tissue anterior to the trachea at this level is not disturbed.

Below the tracheal carina, the anterior and inferior margins of the right pulmonary artery are identified. The main pulmonary artery is separated from the ascending aorta and encircled with the umbilical tape. The bifurcation of the artery is noted.

Both pleural spaces are opened over a modest distance so that the surgeon can be assured that no pleural adhesions are present. The lungs are inspected.

A purse-string suture is placed in the ascending aorta for insertion of a standard cardioplegic catheter. At this point, the procedure is frequently interrupted to allow the liver and/or kidney surgical team(s) to complete preparation of these organs.

Approximately 10 minutes prior to venous inflow occlusion, the anesthesiologist is asked to disconnect the ventilator momentarily and open the airway to atmosphere. The bronchus blocker is inflated, and ventilation of the right lung resumed while the left lung becomes completely atelectatic. This is performed for both single and double lung extraction, so that the left lung can be externally cooled as efficiently as possible. (This is not undertaken if perfusion of the lungs is to be carried out.)

Single lung excision (left)

The superior vena cava is divided between ligatures placed inferior (caudal) to the azygos vein. A clamp is placed on the inferior vena cava at the level of the diaphragm. After allowing the heart to beat 5–6 times and empty, the aorta is clamped and infusion of cardioplegic solution commenced (1 liter of cold hyperkalemic crystalloid solution over 3 minutes).

Venting of the right heart is accomplished by transecting the inferior vena cava above the clamp. The left heart is vented by an incision in the right pulmonary veins. The pericardial and pleural cavities are filled with cold Collins' solution at 4 °C.

Once cardioplegia is obtained, the aortic cannula is removed and the aorta divided at that level. The main pulmonary artery is then divided to ensure adequate cuffs for both cardiac and pulmonary transplantation. The proximal aorta and pulmonary artery are then retracted inferiorly. Posterior dissection is continued inferior to the right pulmonary artery, entering the posterior pericardial recess at this level (Figure 47.1). The incision in the pericardium is extended laterally to the superior pulmonary veins on each side. At this point, the heart is held in place by the pulmonary veins only.

The right pulmonary veins are then divided (Figure 47.2), and an incision is made in the left atrium half the distance between the confluence of the left pulmonary veins and the coronary sinus (Figure 47.2, inset), care being taken to leave a cuff of left atrium in the region of the circumflex artery. The incision in the left atrium is completed in a circumferential fashion, preserving a cuff of left atrium around the left pulmonary veins. (The heart is then free to be transported and transplanted.)

With the heart removed, the left and right pleura and pericardium are divided inferiorly to the level of the inferior pulmonary ligaments, which are also divided. The inferior incisions in the pericardium are joined posteriorly so that the pericardium is completely separated from the diaphragm. Similarly, the pericardium and phrenic nerves are divided superiorly on both sides down to the hila.

Traction is placed on the trachea, and the endotracheal tube and bronchus blocker are removed. The trachea is clamped and divided proximal (cephalad) to the clamp. Using the tracheal clamp for traction, the mediastinum is dissected posteriorly beyond the carina and out to the right hilum. The assistant then lifts the right lung out of the chest and the surgeon divides all the posterior attachments against the esophagus. The posterior dissection is continued to the

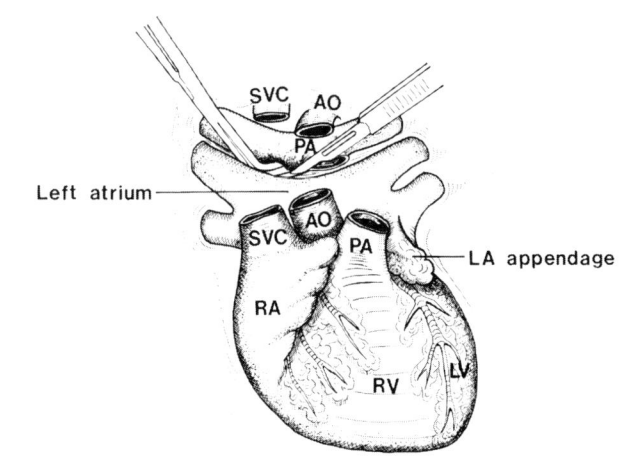

Figure 47.1 Prior excision of the heart (for transplantation into Recipient A) before mobilization and excision of the left lung (for transplantation into Recipient B). The posterior pericardial recess inferior to the right pulmonary artery and superior to the left atrium is opened

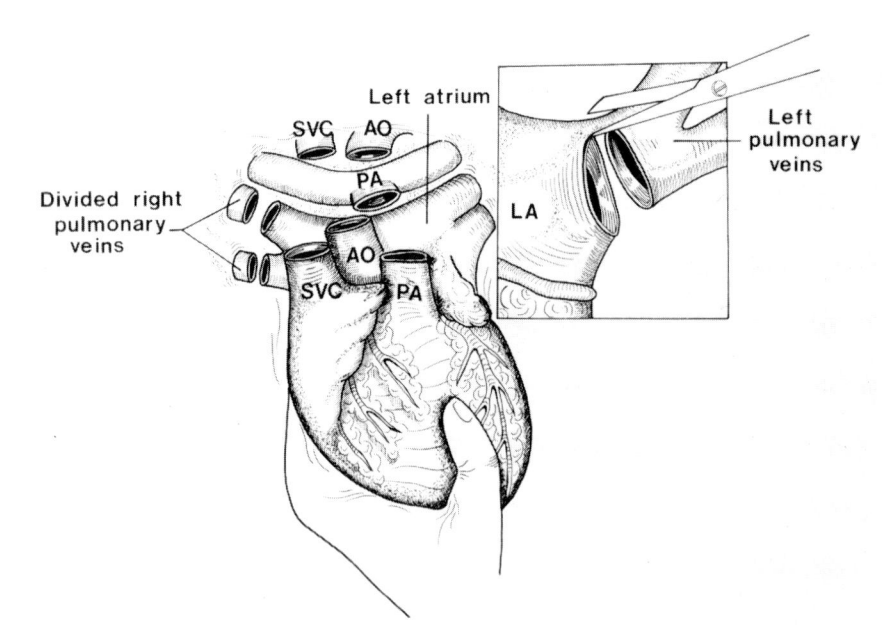

THE TRANSPLANTATION AND REPLACEMENT OF THORACIC ORGANS

Figure 47.2 Prior excision of the heart (for transplantation into Recipient A) before mobilization and excision of the left lung (for transplantation into Recipient B). The right pulmonary veins have been divided. The heart is divided from the left lung (inset) preserving a generous cuff of left atrium with the left pulmonary veins. The left atrium is divided half the distance between the confluence of the left pulmonary veins and the coronary sinus

left, anterior to the descending aorta and posterior to the left hilum. With a hand placed behind the left lung, the mediastinal pleura on the left is easily identified and incised. This latter part of the procedure is facilitated by steady traction on the tracheal clamp and right lung. The trachea is stapled closed to prevent flooding of the airway prior to immersion of the graft in a bag of Collins' solution.

Double lung excision

When extracting lungs for double lung transplantation, dissection of the interatrial groove is undertaken on the right side prior to cardioplegic arrest of the heart (Figure 47.3). This provides visualization of 1–3 cm of left atrial wall proximal (antero-medial) to the right pulmonary veins. This will be required to provide a satisfactory left atrial cuff for the double lung graft while leaving a margin of left atrium for cardiac transplantation.

During extraction, venting of the left heart is accomplished by amputation of the left atrial appendage (Figure 47.4, inset). Care must be taken to ensure that the pulmonary artery is divided at right angles (as it runs superiorly and posterolaterally to the left). An oblique incision may divide the posterior wall at the level of its bifurcation, making the subsequent pulmonary artery anastomosis for the double lung transplantation difficult. Proximal division may dam-

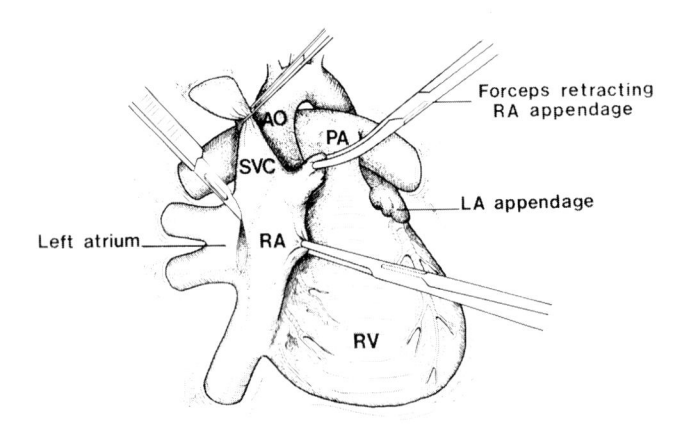

Figure 47.3 When double lung transplantation is planned (for Recipient Y), before excision of the heart (for Recipient X) it is essential to develop the interatrial groove on the right side

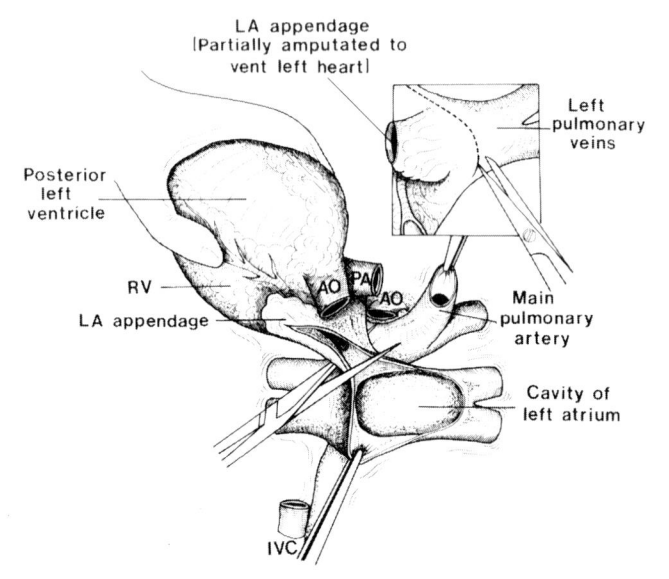

Figure 47.4 Division of the left atrium to allow double lung transplantation (in Recipient Y) as well as a cardiac transplantation (in Recipient X). Note the initial incision in the left atrium (inset). Note also the generous left atrial cuff provided by the opening of the interatrial groove on the right side

age the pulmonary valve. At this point, the incision into the posterior pericardium inferior to the right pulmonary artery is carried out as described previously (Figure 47.1).

For a double lung graft, the right pulmonary veins are left intact and an incision is made in the left atrium between the confluence of the left pulmonary veins and the coronary sinus (Figure 47.4, inset). With traction on the heart, the incision is continued superiorly and inferiorly and then to the right, preserving a cuff of left atrium between and around the orifices of both right and left pulmonary veins (Figure 47.4). The last cut in the atrium is guided by, and made through, the prior dissection of the interatrial groove. In this manner, the right atrium remains intact, and yet a satisfactory cuff of left atrium is retained around the orifices of the right pulmonary veins. At this point, the surgeon should be able to visualize the open main pulmonary artery and a generous cuff of left atrium joining and surrounding both sets of pulmonary veins (Figure 47.5). Removal of the double lung bloc then proceeds, as described for single lung extraction (above) (Figure 47.6).

Preservation of pulmonary grafts

Flushing of the lung is not an essential feature of pulmonary graft preservation. In fact, in the Toronto series only three of the first 24 lung transplants (14 single and 10 double) were performed using a flushing technique. In all other cases the left lung was made atelectatic (as described above) and both pleural spaces were filled with ice-cold (4 °C) Collins' solution at the commencement of cardioplegia. The excised lungs were then transported, immersed in ice-cold Collins' solution in a heavy plastic bag. Two further bags were placed about the graft, before placing it in a cooler full of ice. The triple bagging was felt necessary to avoid a cold burn of the lung during its transportation to the recipient hospital. An acceptable preservation was achieved with this

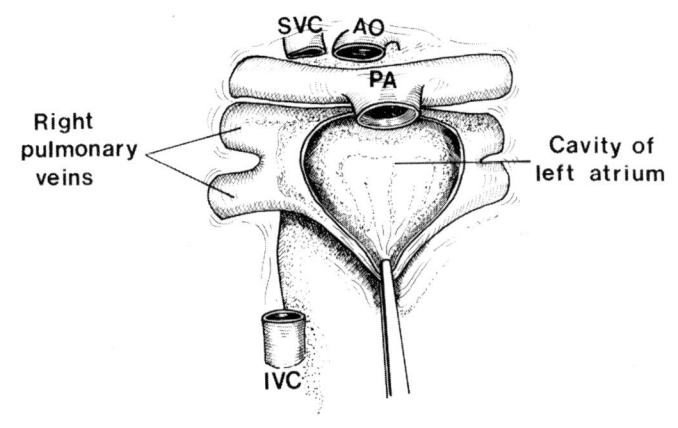

Figure 47.5 Excision of the heart (for transplantation into Recipient X) has been completed, and the structures remaining can be clearly seen. The double lung bloc (including pulmonary arteries, pulmonary veins and posterior left atrium) can now be mobilized and excised for transplantation into Recipient Y

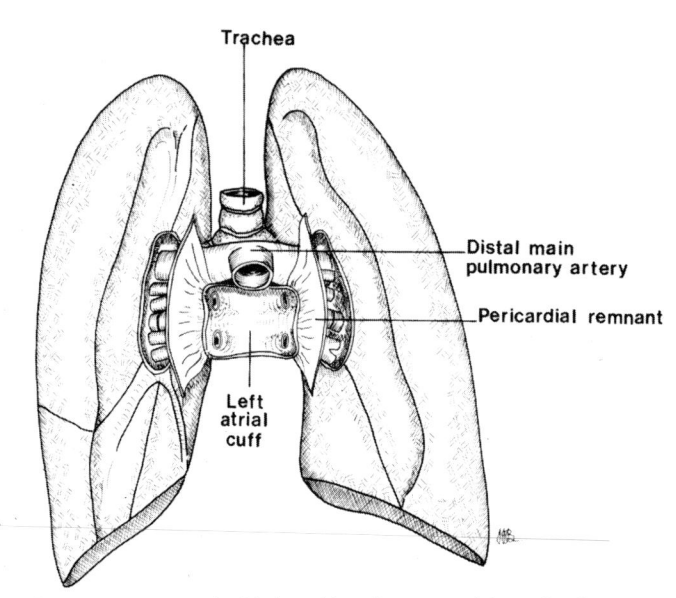

Figure 47.6 Donor double-lung bloc after removal from the chest

technique. Ischemic times up to $5\frac{1}{2}$ hours were obtained with satisfactory pulmonary function post-transplant.

Lately, we have begun to employ a flush technique of the lungs (at the time of infusion of cardioplegic solution) before extraction. This was considered an important feature in the original description of heart–lung transplantation by Jamieson et al.[7], and there is compelling experimental evidence that ischemic times may be lengthened. Several technical and qualitative points require comment. Effective flushing must be undertaken with a large cannula (14 French) inserted through an arteriotomy in the pulmonary artery. Accurate placement of the incision is essential, particularly if both a donor heart and a double lung graft are sought. Both the cardiac and pulmonary transplant teams require a portion of main pulmonary artery, and thus the incision should be made transversely at the level of eventual division of this vessel. Two liters of solution are infused into a low-pressure system over 10 minutes; flushing must be completed by the time the team is ready to excise the heart. Control of the flushing pressure must be assured to avoid damage to the pulmonary endothelium; infusion pressure should be monitored throughout, and maintained below 30 cmH$_2$O.

Controversy exists over the composition of the infusate. There is general agreement that the solution should be cold (4 °C), and that it should be preceded by a bolus injection of 500 μg of prostaglandin (PGE$_1$). The latter is a powerful pulmonary vasodilator, and is given to ensure that even distribution of the infusate is achieved throughout the lungs and excessive pressure is avoided. If a pulmonary infusion is an integral part of the preservation technique, atelectasis should be avoided. Instead, the lungs should be gently ventilated with room air to avoid alveolar collapse and subsequent increase in pulmonary artery pressure.

There is experimental evidence to support the use of (1) Collins' solution, (2) Figimora's solution, or (3) the University of Wisconsin (UW) solution as the pulmonary perfusate. The relative benefits of each must await clinical trials and further comparative animal research. Assessment of the effects of the addition of various chemicals to the perfusate is still in an experimental stage. Verapamil deserves special mention as repeated demonstrations of its preservation potential in animal models have been documented[8].

COMMENT

We have performed 15 simultaneous extractions of heart and lungs for two separate recipients. Technical problems with implantation have been minimal.

One cardiac implant was made difficult as a commissure of the pulmonary valve had been damaged during division of the pulmonary artery; appropriate intraoperative repair successfully corrected the problem. The pulmonary artery anastomosis of a double lung implant was hampered by an oblique incision of the donor pulmonary artery, which transgressed the bifurcation on the right side; a satisfactory implantation was, however, performed.

These experiences emphasize the fact that division of the pulmonary artery must be perpendicular and carefully placed to avoid the pulmonary valve, yet must provide a distal cuff for double lung transplantation. Traction on the pulmonary artery, using umbilical tape placed about it, distorts the wall of the vessel, and should be avoided. For single lung transplantation, division of the artery at its bifurcation is satisfactory. However, division beyond that point (i.e. distally or closer to the hilum) is not advisable since preservation of the wide bifurcation area may be utilized to anastomose a small donor artery to a much larger recipient artery which has been dilated from pulmonary hypertension.

It is of paramount importance that the initial incision in the left atrium be performed as described earlier to ensure that a satisfactory anterior cuff of atrium remains with the pulmonary veins on the left side. Care must be exercised when commencing the left atrial incision on the left side to ensure that it is not continued too far posteriorly. Once the incision on the anterior wall of the atrium on the left side has reached the superior and inferior margins of the pulmonary veins it should be directed abruptly to the right. Only in this way will an adequate posterior cuff of atrium be provided for the double lung graft.

When a double lung graft is to be taken, an additional important feature is the dissection of the interatrial groove, which is best performed with the heart distended with blood before the administration of cardioplegic agent. This dissection, however, can be performed after cardioplegic arrest if traction is placed on the divided inferior and superior venae cavae.

References

1. Grebenik, C.R. and Hinds, C.J. (1987). Management of the multiple organ donor. *Br. J. Hosp. Med.*, **38**, 62
2. Johanson, W.B., Pierce, A.K., Sanford, J.P. and Thomas, G.D. (1972). Nosocomial respiratory infections with Gram negative bacilli. The significance of colonization of the respiratory tract. *Ann. Intern. Med.*, **77**, 701
3. Richardson, D.W. and Robinson, A.G. (1985). Desmopressin, *Ann. Intern. Med.*, **103**, 228
4. Burt, J.M. and Copeland, J.G. (1986). Myocardial function after preservation for twenty-four hours. *J. Thorac. Cardiovasc. Surg.*, **92**, 238
5. Goldberg, L.I. (1974). Dopamine: clinical use of an endogenous catecholamine. *N. Engl. J. Med.*, **291**, 707
6. Ginsberg, R.J. (1981). New techniques for one-lung anesthesia using an endobronchial blocker. *J. Thorac. Cardiovasc. Surg.*, **82**, 542
7. Jamieson, S.W., Stinson, E.B., Oyer, P.E., Baldwin, J.C. and Shumway, N.E. (1974). Operative technique for heart–lung transplantation. *J. Thorac. Cardiovasc. Surg.*, **87**, 930
8. Hacida, M. and Morton, D.L. (1988). The protection of ischemic lung with verapamil and hydralazine. *J. Thorac. Cardiovasc. Surg.*, **95**, 178

48
Anesthesia for Single Lung Transplantation
W.A.P. DEMAJO

INTRODUCTION

The intraoperative anesthesia management of single lung transplant patients, except for those aspects that relate to placement of femoral arteriovenous partial bypass, does not involve techniques or manipulations that differ from standard thoracic anesthetic practice. Patients presenting for consideration of lung transplantation have deteriorated to the point that they require continuing oxygen to maintain adequate saturation at rest; they desaturate on exercise, and have pulmonary hypertension with or without right ventricular dysfunction. The primary consideration in these patients is whether they should undergo single or double lung transplantation, or lung–heart transplantation. Those considered for single lung transplantation are patients who have adequate right and left ventricular function, whose lung condition is fibrotic in nature with diminished lung volumes, and who do not have chronic pulmonary infection (Chapter 46).

The most critical part of the operation is the clamping of the pulmonary artery of the lung to be removed, because of the effect this has on right ventricular function. Three of a total of 15 patients required arteriovenous bypass intraoperatively, because of right ventricular failure on clamping of the pulmonary artery.

At the time of writing, the Toronto Lung Transplant group has performed 15 single lung transplants since 1983; nine patients are alive, ranging in survival time from 5 years to 6 months. (These results are updated in Chapter 53.) Of the six patients who died, three could not be weaned from mechanical ventilation and had multiple system organ failure. One patient died from a lymphomatous complication, another developed *Pneumocystis carinii* infection and gradually lapsed into respiratory failure, whilst the sixth patient died from a myocardial infarction 10 days after operation.

This paper will be restricted primarily to a discussion of the anesthetic management of single lung transplantation. Details of the operation are described elsewhere[1] (Chapter 49). Data were divided and analysed for two groups – those who required arteriovenous bypass (B group) and those who did not (non-bypass (NB) group).

SELECTION OF PATIENTS

This topic is discussed fully in Chapter 46. Consideration will be given only to those aspects of special interest to the anesthesiologist. The patient is assessed with regard to the possible need for arteriovenous bypass during the transplant operation. The investigations undertaken are: (1) pulmonary function tests, (2) hemodynamic assessment, consisting of (a) radionuclide angiographic scans of right and left ventricular function, (b) two-dimensional echo/Doppler study to assess cardiac function and pulmonary artery systolic pressure, (3) exercise testing, (4) radionuclide pulmonary perfusion scan.

Pulmonary function tests

These patients have severe restrictive lung disease (Table 48.1). In those tested to date, reductions were noted in lung volumes (total lung capacity (TLC) and forced vital capacity (FVC)), the forced expiratory volume in 1 second (FEV_1), and diffusion capacity (DLCO). There was also an increase in air flow at high lung volume and a raised FEV_1/FVC ratio. The only patient who proved an exception was TB (Table 48.1), who had eosinophilic granulomatous disease, and presented with normal TLC, FVC, FEV_1, but a reduction in DLCO.

Hemodynamic assessment

The cardiac and hemodynamic status of each patient is assessed using various modalities. General cardiac status is evaluated using two-dimensional echocardiography, while in those over the age of 50 years ventricular and coronary angiography are performed. Radionuclide angiographic scans are obtained utilizing first-pass measurements of right and left ventricular ejection fractions[2], and also gated equilibrium scans at rest and on exercise to a maximum work load of 200 kpm. If the coronary arteriography and left ventricular ejection fraction prove normal, and the right ventricular ejection fraction is greater than 20%, the patient

Table 48.1 Pretransplant pulmonary function tests

Group	TLC (%pred) (l)	FVC (%pred) (l)	FEV$_1$ (%pred) (l/s)	V$_{50}$ (%pred) (l/s)	DCO (%pred) (ml min^{-1} mmHg^{-1})	Po$_2$ (mmHg)	Pco$_2$ (mmHg)
Non-bypass (NB)							
TH	3.0 (55%)	1.6 (47%)	1.4 (58%)	7.6 (224%)	7.4 (37%)	50	40
MA	1.5 (26%)	1.0 (33%)	1.0 (33%)	4.1 (105%)	6.8 (52%)	54	56
JH	3.5 (48%)	2.1 (43%)	1.7 (46%)	3.0 (61%)	5.0 (21%)	56	37
DL	3.0 (48%)	1.9 (48%)	1.7 (59%)	5.0 (125%)	9.4 (44%)	70	40
RJ	3.8 (63%)	2.9 (78%)	2.2 (81%)	2.0 (54%)	6.5 (26%)	50	34
MD	1.8 (23%)	1.1 (19%)	1.1 (24%)	4.4 (77%)	6.8 (30%)	60	42
RR	3.5 (50%)	2.5 (51%)	2.2 (59%)	6.2 (127%)	5.9 (29%)	58	41
PG	3.2 (47%)	0.9 (30%)	0.89 (35%)	2.5 (83%)	ND	61	35
YM	ND	2.1 (50%)	1.6 (51%)	7.1 (169%)	ND	61	38
DS	ND	1.9 (42%)	1.7 (52%)	5.2 (118%)	ND	50	43
PR	ND	2.0 (50%)	1.6 (57%)	2.8 (70%)	ND	51	40
TB	6.8 (90%)	5.1 (113%)	4.0 (125%)	5.8 (129%)	7.9 (28%)	55	28
Bypass (B)							
GN	3.9 (60%)	2.3 (52%)	1.7 (52%)	1.9 (43%)	11.7 (42%)	32	43
WM	ND	2.1 (49%)	1.9 (61%)	7.1 (165%)	ND	47	26
JB	ND	3.8 (75%)	2.9 (78%)	3.3 (65%)	ND	38	29

TLC = total lung capacity; FVC = forced vital capacity; FEV$_1$ = forced expiratory volume in 1 second; VSO = flow at 50% vital capacity; DCO = diffusing capacity for carbon monoxide; Po$_2$ = partial pressure of oxygen in arterial blood; Pco$_2$ = partial pressure of carbon dioxide in arterial blood; (%pred) = percentage of predicted

is considered a suitable candidate for single lung transplantation.

Pulmonary and cardiac hemodynamic measurements, and responsiveness to pulmonary arterial vasodilators, were initially obtained in all patients being assessed for single lung transplant. Due to the development of severe respiratory dysfunction, with radiological changes consistent with pulmonary edema, and because of a belief that no additional useful information was being obtained, these investigations were discontinued. At the present time, an assessment of pulmonary artery systolic pressure is obtained by Doppler echo measurement. All patients have their pulmonary and systemic hemodynamic function (i.e. cardiac output, pulmonary and systemic vascular resistance, central venous and pulmonary capillary wedge pressures) assessed both immediately before and during operation. These data are presented here.

Exercise testing

All patients undergo a training program to help in respiratory muscle training and improvement in nutrition. Their exercise competence is assessed using the Modified Bruce Protocol[3]. The majority of patients seen to date could not complete even stage 0 of the protocol, and it was realized that a valid and useful level of exercise was 1 mph at 4° gradient on a treadmill for 3 minutes (Table 48.2).

The exercise stress test is carried out with the patient receiving optimal concentrations of oxygen via a nasal prong, the level of oxygen required having been assessed at preliminary exercise sessions. During the exercise test the patient's oxygen saturation is continuously monitored, and the test is terminated if this falls below 85%, or if the heart rate is > 125 bpm or if dysrhythmias occur.

Table 48.2 Arterial oxygen saturation on exercise*

Group	O$_2$ required (l/min)	% saturation Rest	% saturation Exercise
Non-bypass (NB)			
TH	5	96	ND
MA	1	93	91 (3 min)
JH	4	97	90 (8 min)
DL	2	98	91 (5 min)
RJ	7	97	85 (3 min)
MD	1	96	91 (5 min)
RR	3	95	89 (3 min)
PG	4	99	90 (3 min)
YM	7	98	83 (3 min)
DS	3	98	90 (5 min)
PR	6	97	91 (3 min)
TB	6	95	86 (3 min)
Bypass (B)			
GN	5	97	83 (3 min)
WM	8	94	85 (30 s)
JB	9	90	80 (30 s)

*Treadmill 1 mph 4° gradient

Radionuclide pulmonary perfusion scan

The relative distribution of blood flow in both lungs is quantified using technetium-99 (Tc-99) DTPA in the standard ways. The results of the test are utilized, in conjunction with surgical considerations, in deciding which lung should be transplanted.

PREOPERATIVE PREPARATION

When an organ donor becomes available, the patient is admitted to the intensive care unit. This facilitates the insertion of a large bore peripheral intravenous line, central venous pressure and arterial lines, and a pulmonary artery catheter. Positioning of the pulmonary artery catheter is confirmed by radiography, and biochemical and hemodynamic data are acquired. In two patients in our series (TH and JH), who were scheduled for a right lung transplant, the catheter had to be positioned in the left pulmonary artery; this was successfully achieved by placing the patient with the left chest up as the catheter was advanced from the right ventricle.

The anesthetic equipment is prepared whilst waiting to take the recipient to the operating room. The equipment used in monitoring and management is: (1) constant flow generator anesthetic ventilating machine with humidifier, (2) oxygen, medical air, (3) systemic and pulmonary artery pressure monitoring equipment, (4) cardiac output machine, (5) pulse oximeter, (6) end-tidal CO_2 monitor, (7) warming blanket, and intravenous fluid warmer, (8) fully primed bypass machine with oxygenator, (9) endotracheal tubes and 14 French Fogarty venous catheter (American Hospital Supply model # 62-080-8).

The drugs required are also prepared and consist of: (1) narcotic analgesics (Fentanyl), (2) sodium thiopentone, (3) isoflurane inhalation gas, (4) succinylcholine and/or pancuronium, (5) dopamine, nitroglycerine, and norepinephrine set up separately in continuous infusion systems.

INTRAOPERATIVE MANAGEMENT

The most important aspects of the operation from the anesthesiologist's point of view are oxygenation and ventilation, and the ability of the heart to maintain adequate function during the period when only one lung is ventilated and perfused (following clamping of the pulmonary artery and collapse of the lung that is being removed).

The patient is anesthetized with high-dose fentanyl (5–10 µg/kg) and incremental doses (25 mg) of sodium thiopentone. Muscular paralysis is achieved with succinylcholine and/or pancuronium. If the right lung is to be transplanted, the patient is intubated with a Robertshaw double-lumen endobronchial tube.

In 13 of our 15 cases, however, the left lung has been transplanted. In these cases, a Fogarty venous catheter is inserted into the trachea, after which the trachea is intubated with a single-lumen endotracheal tube. The patient is connected to the ventilator and to the end-tidal CO_2 monitor, and ventilated with 100% oxygen with a tidal volume of 8–10 ml/kg at a frequency of 12–20 breaths per minute. The final settings are determined following blood gas analysis. The end-tidal CO_2 monitor provides inaccurate data at this stage due to high dead-space ventilation[4]. The Fogarty venous catheter is next positioned in the left main bronchus, about 2 cm from the carina, under direct bronchoscopic control. The balloon of the catheter is inflated with a volume adequate to achieve blockage of the bronchus. The balloon is deflated, and the operation proceeds. The patient's status is monitored by blood gas and hemodynamic measurements.

None of our patients to date has had any hemodynamic instability on induction of anesthesia; ventilation and oxygenation have been satisfactory in all cases. Maintenance of anesthesia is with supplemental fentanyl only, or the addition of diazepam and isoflurane; ventilation is with oxygen or an oxygen/air mixture as required.

Arteriovenous bypass

The most significant decision that has to be made after anesthetizing the patient is whether femoral arteriovenous partial bypass may be required. If so, the femoral vessels on the side contralateral to the side of the thoracotomy are exposed and prepared for possible cannulation later. This decision is based both on the findings of preoperative investigation and the response during one lung ventilation of PaO_2, pulmonary artery pressures, and cardiac index. Thus, during the first stage of the operation, the lung to be removed is collapsed for 15 minutes, and changes in pulmonary artery pressures, cardiac index, and blood gases are monitored, and compared with the values obtained on two-lung ventilation.

In our series to date, the femoral vessels were exposed in those patients who (1) had a preoperative mean pulmonary artery pressure > 35 mmHg, which, on one-lung ventilation, rose to > 40 mmHg and/or (2) had a cardiac index preoperatively, or during one-lung ventilation, of ≤ 2.0 l/min per square meter in the absence of inotropic support and/or pulmonary vasodilator therapy. In addition, if the arterial oxygen saturation during one-lung ventilation fell to < 85% on an FiO_2 of 1 (100% O_2), the vessels were likewise exposed.

The final decision on whether to place the patient on bypass, however, is made at the time of clamping of the pulmonary artery. Hemodynamic parameters and arterial and mixed venous gases are monitored at this time. In our series, if the patient's cardiac index was ≤ 2.0 l/min per square meter and/or the mixed venous oxygen saturation was < 60%, a nitroglycerine (4–12 mg/h) and/or dopamine (3.5–12 µg/kg per min) infusion was begun, depending on the systemic blood pressure. If the arterial oxygen saturation were less than 90% on FiO_2 1 or, with the use of nitroglycerine and/or dopamine, the patient's cardiac index remained less than 2.0 l/min per square meter and/or mixed venous saturation less than 60%, the patient was placed on bypass. Exposure of the femoral vessels was carried out in 11 patients who had the necessary hemodynamic criteria; one also demonstrated a fall in O_2 saturation to < 85% on one-lung ventilation.

Only three patients, however, required arteriovenous bypass. Analysis of their preoperative data (Table 48.3)

Table 48.3 Preoperative blood gas, pulmonary hemodynamic, and radionuclide angiographic data on patients undergoing single lung transplantation

	Non-bypass (NB) group	Bypass (B) group	Statistical significance (NB vs. B)
Blood gases (on room air)			
$P\text{O}_2$ (mmHg)	56.3 ± 6.0	39.0 ± 7.5	$p < 0.001$
$P\text{CO}_2$ (mmHg)	40.5 ± 5.8	31.5 ± 7.7	NS
Pulmonary artery pressure (mmHg)			
Systolic	44.1 ± 8.0	59.6 ± 4.9	$p < 0.01$
Diastolic	23.4 ± 5.5	35.0 ± 7.8	$p < 0.01$
Mean	30.9 ± 5.6	45.3 ± 2.0	$p < 0.001$
Pulmonary vascular resistance (dynes s cm^{-5})	261.5 ± 83.3	546.3 ± 172.0	$p < 0.001$
Radionuclide angiography			
First pass	32.3 ± 6.5%	32.6 ± 12%	NS
Equilibrium at rest	30.0 ± 3.16%	26.0 ± 12%	NS
Equilibrium on exercise	29.0 ± 3.0%	24.0 ± 13%	NS

indicated statistically significant differences (when compared to the NB group) in respect of arterial $P\text{O}_2$ when breathing room air, systolic, diastolic, and mean pulmonary artery pressures, as well as pulmonary vascular resistance. The radionuclide angiographic scans on first pass or equilibrium at rest showed no predictive value.

The B group, on clamping of the pulmonary artery and with inotropic support, had a cardiac index of 1.23 ± 0.351 compared to that of the NB group of 2.9 ± 0.596, a significant difference at $p < 0.001$ on t test analysis. The B group had a lower exercise tolerance and/or desaturated to < 85%, while, in the NB group, all completed the 3-minute exercise test and maintained a saturation > 85% (except for YM, who desaturated to 83%).

Ventilation

No significant difficulties were encountered during two-lung or one-lung ventilation. The alveolar–arterial oxygen (A–aDO_2) gradient during two-lung ventilation on $F\text{iO}_2$ of 1 averaged 220 ± 35 mmHg (Figure 48.1). Although it increased to 523 ± 52 mmHg during one-lung ventilation, while perfusion was still present in the lung to be transplanted, there were only two patients (GN and JB) in whom arterial O_2 saturation was < 90%. After the pulmonary artery was clamped, the A–aDO_2 improved dramatically (mean 210 ± 22 mmHg) in all patients except GN and JB. These patients required bypass for completion of this operation. WM, the third member of the B group, had an arterial O_2 saturation of 94% on collapsing the lung, and an A–aDO_2 of 323 mmHg on clamping the pulmonary artery.

The peak airway pressure during two-lung ventilation was a mean of 41 ± 3 cmH$_2$O, while minute ventilation to maintain a $P\text{CO}_2$ of 50 mmHg was 10.4 ± 1.8 l/min. During one-lung ventilation, the peak airway pressure increased

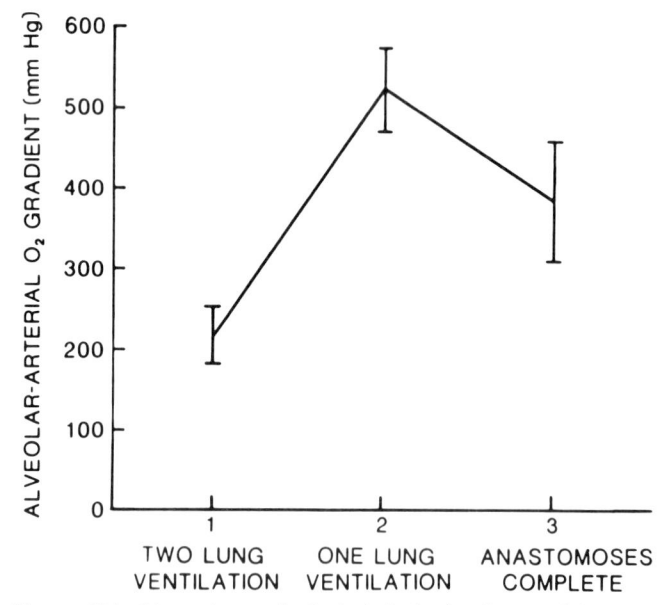

Figure 48.1 Mean (± standard deviation) alveolar–arterial oxygen (A–aDO_2) gradients in 15 patients during single lung transplantation

(52 ± 4.5 cmH$_2$O), and minute ventilation requirements likewise increased (12.5 ± 4.5 l/min).

Following establishment of the anastomoses, and unclamping of both bronchus and pulmonary artery, the peak airway pressure reverted to normal and the A–aDO_2 averaged 385 ± 75 mmHg. In the first five cases, the pulmonary artery was unclamped before the bronchial anastomosis was completed. This resulted in a shunt being established that caused a marked increase in A–aDO_2; this practice was subsequently changed so that all anastomoses are now completed before unclamping.

At the end of the procedure, the double-lumen endotracheal tube is changed to a single-lumen tube, and, in the cases where it is used, the Fogarty blocker is removed. The patient is transferred to the intensive care unit.

COMMENT

Patients with fibrotic lung disease are considered suitable candidates for single lung transplantation. Our data indicate that certain patients are more likely to require arteriovenous bypass. The preoperative arterial Po_2 on room air, the mean pulmonary artery pressure, and pulmonary vascular resistance may be significant in predicting the need for bypass. The ejection fraction of the right ventricle, as measured by scintigraphy, has not been found to be a useful parameter in this respect. The ability of the patient to exercise at 1 mph at a 4° gradient on a treadmill for 3 minutes, and maintain an arterial O_2 saturation $\geq 85\%$, may also be a useful indicator that arteriovenous bypass will not be necessary.

The support of right ventricular function in patients subjected to an acute or chronic increase in right ventricular afterload is a field that requires additional research. The literature is not conclusive as to which agents, inotropic and/or vasodilator, are best in sustaining right ventricular function either in the face of long-standing pulmonary hypertension or when there is acute cor pulmonale due to a sudden increase in pulmonary vascular resistance. Vasodilation of the pulmonary vasculature, thereby decreasing right ventricular afterload, does not seem to be the only determinant of right ventricular function.

The use of nitroglycerine or nitroprusside, potent pulmonary vasodilators, has been shown to improve contractility of the overloaded right ventricle in chronic pulmonary hypertension[5]. However, Rosenberg et al.[6], using isoproterenol in experimental pulmonary embolism, reported 100% mortality, possibly due to decreased myocardial perfusion secondary to a decrease in mean arterial pressure. In contrast, Molloy et al.[7] demonstrated a significant improvement in survival rate by the use of norepinephrine infusion in experimental pulmonary embolism in anesthetized, ventilated dogs.

In clinical studies of shock due to pulmonary embolism, Jardin et al.[8] reported the use of dobutamine, and showed significant decreases in right atrial pressure and pulmonary and systemic vascular resistances, without any changes in mean arterial and pulmonary pressures. Bourdarias et al.[9], using dopamine in the same clinical setting, showed increases in mean arterial pressure, cardiac index, and heart rate, in addition to a significant rise in mean pulmonary artery pressure. Dopamine causes a greater increase in systemic blood pressure than comparable doses of dobutamine[10].

In the management of the patients undergoing lung transplantation, the clinical goals dictating the choice of agents were reductions in (1) pulmonary artery pressure and (2) resistance, whilst (3) maintaining systemic arterial pressure. A combination of dopamine and nitroglycerine was thought to be best to achieve these goals.

References

1. Toronto Lung Transplant Group (1986). Unilateral lung transplantation for pulmonary fibrosis. *N. Engl. J. Med.*, **314**, 1140
2. Maddahi, J., Berman, D.S., Matsuoka, D.T., Waxman, A.D., Stankus, K.E., Forrester, J.S. and Swan, H.J.C. (1979). A new technique for assessing right ventricular ejection fraction using rapid multiple-gated equilibrium cardiac blood pool scintigraphy. *Circulation*, **60**, 581
3. Bruce, R.A. (1971). Exercise testing of patients with coronary heart disease. Principles and normal standards for evaluation. *Ann. Clin. Res.*, **3**, 323
4. Nunn, J.F. and Hill, D.W. (1960). Respiratory dead space and arterial to end-tidal CO_2 tension difference in anaesthetized man. *J. Appl. Physiol.*, **15**, 383
5. Konstam, M.A., Salem, D.N., Isner, J.M., Zile, M.R., Kahn, P.C., Bonin, J.D., Cohen, S.R. and Levine, H.J. (1984). Vasodilator effect on right ventricular function in congestive heart failure and pulmonary hypertension: end-systolic pressure – volume relation. *Am. J. Cardiol.*, **54**, 132
6. Rosenberg, J.C., Hussain, R. and Lenaghan, R. (1971). Isoproterenol and norepinephrine therapy for pulmonary embolism. *J. Thorac. Cardiovasc. Surg.*, **62**, 144
7. Molloy, W., Girling, L., Schick, V., Lee, K.Y. and Prewitt, R.M. (1984). What is the most appropriate treatment for shock complicating massive pulmonary embolism? *Am. Rev. Respir. Dis.*, **129**, 63A
8. Jardin, F., Genevray, B., Brun-Ney, D. and Margairaz, A. (1985). Dobutamine: a hemodynamic evaluation in pulmonary embolism shock. *Crit. Care Med.*, **13**, 1009
9. Bourdarias, J.P., Dubourg, O., Gueret, P., Ferrier, A. and Bardet, J. (1983). Inotropic agents in treatment of cardiogenic shock. *Pharmacol. Ther.*, **22**, 53
10. Stoner, J.D., Bolen, J.L. and Harrison, D.C. (1977). Comparison of dobutamine and dopamine in the treatment of severe heart failure. *Br. Heart J.*, **39**, 536

49
Surgical Technique of Single Lung Transplantation

J.D. COOPER

CHOICE OF SIDE

Unilateral lung transplantation can be performed on either side, though we have favored the left side, when possible, for several technical reasons[1]. The right pulmonary veins enter the left atrium very close to the interatrial groove, making it somewhat more difficult to place an atrial clamp proximal to the veins on this side. On the left side, placement of the clamp is easily accomplished.

For the same anatomic reason, separate extraction of the donor heart is technically somewhat easier when the left lung is to be used for transplantation (Chapter 47). As the heart is removed, it is relatively easy to leave a cuff of left atrium surrounding the left pulmonary veins, while maintaining adequate left atrium with the heart for cardiac transplantation. When the left atrium is to be shared with the right lung, the division of the left atrium requires more precision. In this situation, dissection of the interatrial groove prior to cardiac excision provides a greater margin of left atrium between the right pulmonary veins and the junction of the right and left atria.

If, however, the recipient has previously undergone major thoracotomy or pleurodesis on the left side, then a right lung transplant would be indicated.

ONE LUNG ANESTHESIA AND CARDIOPULMONARY BYPASS (see also Chapter 48)

Most lung transplants can be performed without the use of cardiopulmonary bypass (CPB), though such bypass is always available in the operating room on a standby basis. The transplant procedure is performed using one lung anesthesia, details of which are described in Chapter 48.

For a left lung transplant, a bronchus-blocking balloon (Fogarty # 14 venous occlusion catheter) is advanced into the distal trachea, and a standard endotracheal tube is inserted alongside it. Using the flexible bronchoscope through the endotracheal tube, the balloon catheter is directed into the left main bronchus and temporarily inflated to determine the volume necessary to produce complete bronchial occlusion. The balloon is then deflated for later use.

For a right lung transplant, a left-sided double-lumen Robertshaw tube is utilized for the one-lung anesthesia.

PREPARATION OF OMENTAL PEDICLE

The recipient procedure is begun with the patient in the supine position. The abdomen and the inguinal region on the side of the proposed transplant are prepared and draped. Through a small upper midline abdominal incision, the omentum is mobilized from the transverse colon (Chapter 37), which generally provides sufficient length of omentum to reach the hilum of the lung without difficulty. A retrosternal tunnel is created just behind the xiphisternum, and the apex of the omental pedicle positioned there for later withdrawal into the chest. The abdomen is then closed.

During the dissection of the omentum, a trial of one lung anesthesia is instituted (Chapter 48). If this is poorly tolerated, indicating the likely need for CPB, then the femoral vessels on the side of the proposed thoracotomy can be prepared at the same time as the omental dissection. After closure of the abdominal wound, and the groin incision if there is one, the patient is turned to the lateral thoracotomy position, and the chest, abdomen, and groin area are prepared and draped.

LATERAL THORACOTOMY

Upon entering the chest, any adhesions are divided, using cautery wherever possible. The proximal pulmonary artery is dissected free and encircled intrapericardially. On the left side, this is facilitated by division of the ligamentum arteriosum. On the right, exposure of the proximal pulmonary artery is facilitated by division of the azygos vein and forward retraction of the superior vena cava. A vascular clamp is temporarily placed on the proximal pulmonary artery to determine whether or not CPB will be required. If the patient's vital signs, oxygenation, and pulmonary artery pressure remain stable, then CPB can likely be avoided. After the trial period of pulmonary artery clamping, the clamp is removed, and the remainder of the lung dissection is performed. The pulmonary veins are isolated lateral to the pericardium. The main bronchus is encircled just proximal to the upper lobe bronchus, care being taken to preserve bronchial blood supply by avoiding unnecessary dissection of tissue from around the bronchus.

Excision of the recipient lung

Once this hilar mobilization has been completed, CPB is instituted if necessary. Cardiopulmonary bypass, if utilized, is partial veno–arterial bypass through the femoral vessels at a flow rate of 2–3 l/min. Once the transplanted lung has been sutured in place, CPB can be discontinued.

In either case, a vascular clamp is replaced on the pulmonary artery, and the lung is extracted (Figure 49.1). The first branch of the pulmonary artery is divided between ligatures, and the pulmonary artery divided just distal to this point. This provides a long segment of recipient pulmonary artery which can subsequently be trimmed back if necessary. The divided first branch of the pulmonary artery also acts as a marker, and thus later helps position the donor and recipient pulmonary arteries accurately at the time of anastomosis.

The two pulmonary veins are divided between ligatures close to the hilum of the lung. Using one lung anesthesia, the main bronchus is divided just proximal to the upper lobe bronchus.

Following excision of the lung, the pericardium is opened circumferentially around the stumps of the pulmonary veins. A vascular clamp is placed on the left atrium, care being taken not to impinge on the contralateral pulmonary veins (Figure 49.1). If a right lung transplant is being performed, it may be necessary to dissect into the interatrial groove for a short distance to allow satisfactory placement of the vascular clamp on the left atrium.

The previously placed ligatures on the stumps of the pulmonary veins are then removed, and an incision made between the two veins to create a single opening surrounded by a suitable atrial cuff (Figure 49.1).

Insertion of donor lung

The previously-prepared donor lung (Figures 49.2 and 49.3 and Chapter 47) is then positioned posteriorly in the chest. The left atrial anastomosis is performed first (Figure 49.4). The posterior wall suture line is performed from in front, using a continuous 3-0 polypropylene suture interrupted at the superior and inferior corners. The anterior wall of the atrial anastomosis is then completed. The donor and recipient pulmonary arteries are trimmed, if necessary, lined up appropriately, and anastomosed, using a continuous 5-0 polypropylene suture, interrupted at each end (Figure 49.5). The posterior wall anastomosis is performed initially, followed by the anterior suture line; this suture is left untied to permit back-bleeding to the lung when the atrial clamp is removed.

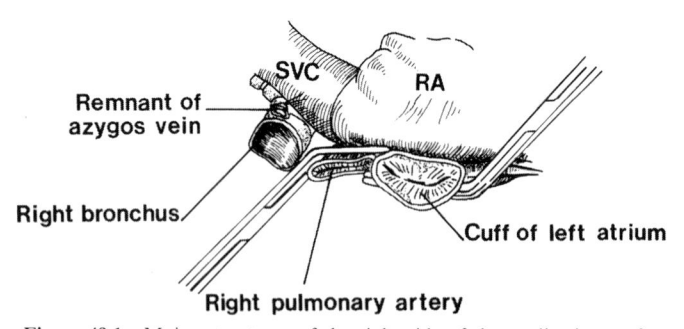

Figure 49.1 Major structures of the right side of the mediastinum after excision of the recipient lung. The right bronchus has been divided. The right pulmonary artery and left atrium have been individually clamped and divided

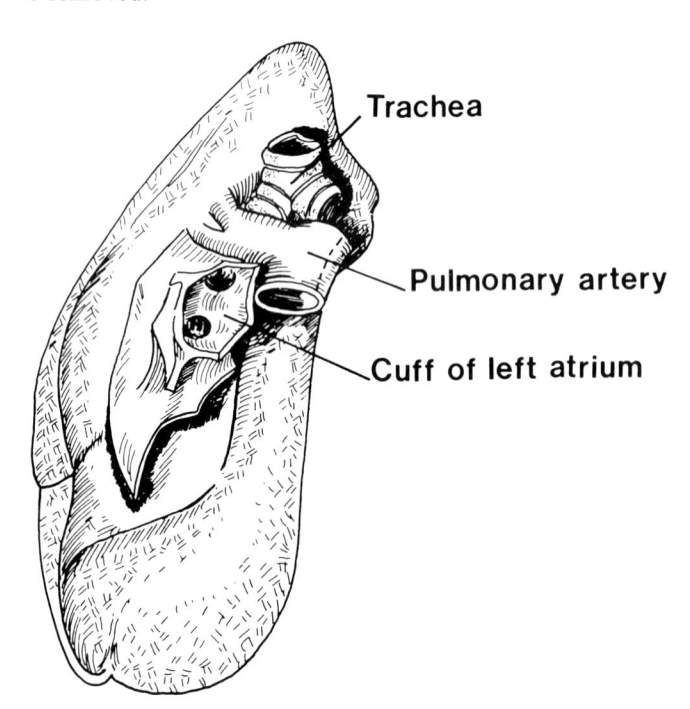

Figure 49.2 Preparation of donor lung (right). A short segment of trachea and left bronchus remain *in situ*, as does a short segment of main pulmonary artery

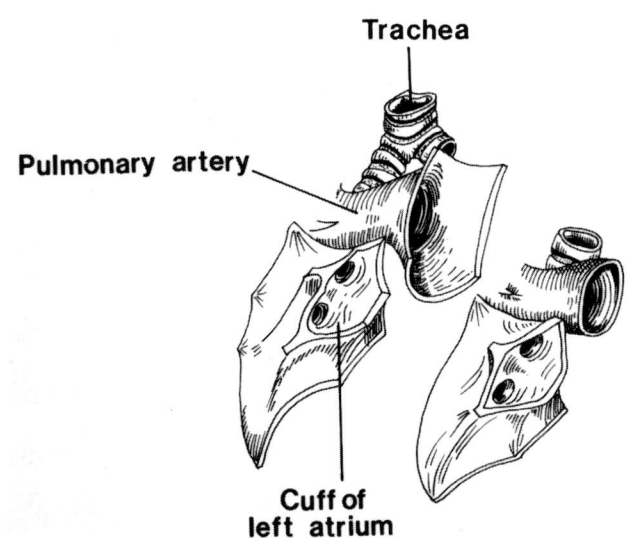

Figure 49.3 Further steps in the preparation of the right donor lung. The main pulmonary artery has been opened longitudinally to give a large cuff of pulmonary artery tissue. This is cut back to the desired length. The remnants of trachea and left bronchus have been excised

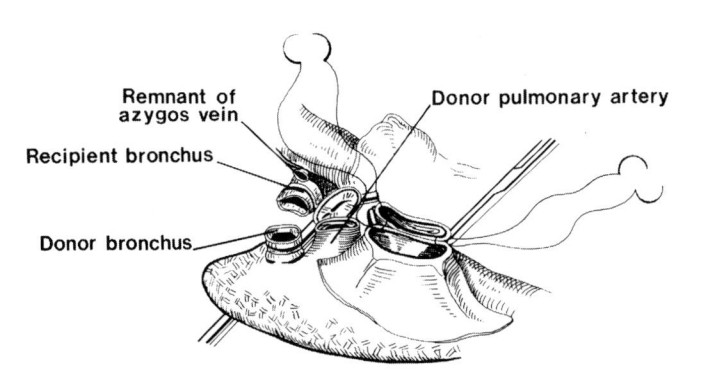

Figure 49.4 The donor lung has been placed in the right pleural cavity, and the left atrial anastomosis is in progress, beginning with the posterior wall

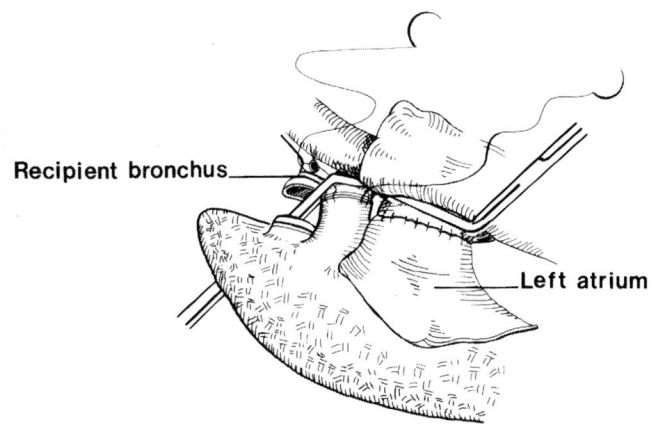

Figure 49.5 The left atrial anastomosis has been completed, and the pulmonary artery anastomosis is in progress

Positioning of omental pedicle

The omentum is withdrawn from its retrosternal position, and passed posteriorly to the hilum of the lung; the apex of the omentum is passed around the bronchial anastomosis, and sutured to itself to completely encircle the bronchial suture line. A large flap of donor pericardium remains attached to the hilum of the transplanted lung; this free edge of pericardium is loosely tacked to the omentum, providing an alternate route for collateral circulation to develop through the pericardium and into the hilum of the lung. A fiberoptic bronchoscope is inserted through the endotracheal tube, and any blood or secretions suctioned from the left lung. The bronchial anastomosis is carefully inspected to ensure that the tissues and suture line have a satisfactory appearance.

Two chest tubes are placed (apical and basal), and the chest is closed in standard fashion.

Prior to removing the vascular clamps, however, the bronchial anastomosis is performed. We utilize interrupted 4-0 absorbable sutures, with the knots placed externally wherever possible. The cartilaginous portion of the anastomosis is completed first, followed by the membranous portion. The lung is gently inflated to test for air leaks at the site of the bronchial anastomosis.

The left atrial clamp is then gradually released. Backbleeding should occur through the untied pulmonary artery suture line. This may be aided by gentle inflation of the lung. When back-bleeding has occurred, or after 3–5 minutes when no back-bleeding has occurred, the pulmonary artery clamp is momentarily released to flush the pulmonary artery. The pulmonary artery anastomosis suture is then tied, and the pulmonary clamp removed completely, restoring circulation to the transplanted lung.

COMMENT

The average blood loss has been one unit of blood. If CPB is required during the operation, bleeding has generally not been a problem, even when there have been dense adhesions between the recipient lung and the chest wall, as almost all dissection is performed prior to the administration of heparin.

Reference

1. Cooper, J.D., Pearson, F.G., Patterson, G.A., Todd, T.R.J., Ginsberg, R.J., Goldberg, M. and Demajo, W.A.P. (1987). Technique of successful lung transplantation in humans. *J. Thorac. Cardiovasc. Surg.*, **93**, 173

50
Surgical Technique of Double Lung Transplantation

J.D. COOPER AND G.A. PATTERSON

INTRODUCTION

Our success with unilateral lung transplantation stimulated our interest in providing transplants for patients with end-stage lung disease not deemed appropriate for unilateral transplant (Chapter 46). This included patients with end-stage lung disease secondary to emphysema and to bilateral sepsis, such as cystic fibrosis. In the case of emphysema, we were concerned that unilateral lung transplantation would lead to over-inflation of the contralateral lung, with mediastinal shift and restricted ventilation to the transplanted lung. With bilateral sepsis, the remaining lung would serve as a focus for contamination of the transplanted lung.

Initially, we explored the use of combined heart–lung transplantation for such patients. We soon realized however, that, in most cases, cardiac function was adequate, and that, theoretically at least, excision and replacement of both lungs would be a preferable procedure. We therefore developed an operation for simultaneous bilateral lung transplantation[1], based on the heart–lung transplant procedure. This operation involves only three anastomoses, namely between the two tracheae, the main (common) pulmonary arteries, and the left atria.

The concept of simultaneous en bloc bilateral pulmonary transplantation was demonstrated in dogs by Vanderhoeft and co-workers in 1972[2]. That procedure, however, was performed through a right thoracotomy, and was not suitable for clinical use. The technique we have employed utilized a median sternotomy, bilateral pneumonectomy, and implantation of the double-lung bloc[1,3].

EXCISION OF THE DONOR LUNG (see also Chapter 47)

The donor extraction procedure generally involves initial removal of the heart for separate cardiac transplantation, followed by removal of the double–lung bloc (Chapter 47). Prior to the cardiac extraction, the interatrial groove is dissected for a short distance to provide an extra margin of left atrial wall between the right pulmonary veins and attachment of the right atrium. Following division of the superior and inferior venae cavae, the aorta and the main pulmonary artery, the left atrium is divided in such a fashion as to leave a cuff of left atrium surrounding the orifices of the four pulmonary veins, while maintaining an adequate margin of left atrium on the heart for cardiac transplantation (Chapter 47). After the heart has been removed, the trachea is stapled and divided at its mid-point. The two lungs are then removed from the chest (Figure 47.6), together with most of the pericardium, and immersed in cold (4°C) Collins' solution for preservation.

THE RECIPIENT OPERATION

A standard endotracheal tube is utilized with the patient in the supine position.

Preparation of the omental pedicle

A median sternotomy is performed, with the incision extending into the upper abdomen. The omentum is mobilized from the transverse colon to provide a pedicle long enough to reach to the trachea (Chapter 37). A small transverse opening is made in the central portion of the diaphragm halfway between the esophageal hiatus and the xiphisternum. Through this opening, the omentum will later be passed into the posterior mediastinum.

Initial thoracic dissection

The aorta and pulmonary artery are encircled. The venae cavae are isolated and encircled. The right pulmonary artery is isolated and encircled between the superior vena cava and aorta. Both pleural spaces are inspected; pleural adhesions are divided, using cautery whenever possible.

Initiation of cardiopulmonary bypass

Superior and inferior vena caval cannulae, inserted through the right atrium, and a standard aortic cannula are placed (Figure 50.1). Cardiopulmonary bypass (CPB) is instituted. The aorta is not cross-clamped at this point; the heart remains beating. The tourniquets around the superior and inferior venae cavae are left loose to allow blood returning from the coronary sinus to be drained through the cannulae. A right ventricular drain (vent) is inserted through the right atrium to prevent distension of the right ventricle (Figure 50.1).

Bilateral pneumonectomy

The left pulmonary veins are isolated within the pericardium and stapled closed (Figures 50.1 and 50.2). The left pulmonary artery is similarly isolated, either medial or lateral to the pericardium, and stapled. The pulmonary artery and veins are divided lateral to the previously-placed staples (Figure 50.1). The left main bronchus is divided between staple lines, and the left lung is removed from the left pleural cavity.

A pleuropericardial window is created at the site where the pulmonary veins came through the pericardium. This opening is extended superiorly and inferiorly parallel and posterior to the left phrenic nerve, care being taken not to injure the nerve. (The donor left lung will subsequently be inserted through this opening.)

The right pulmonary veins are encircled within the pericardium and stapled closed (Figures 50.1 and 50.2). The

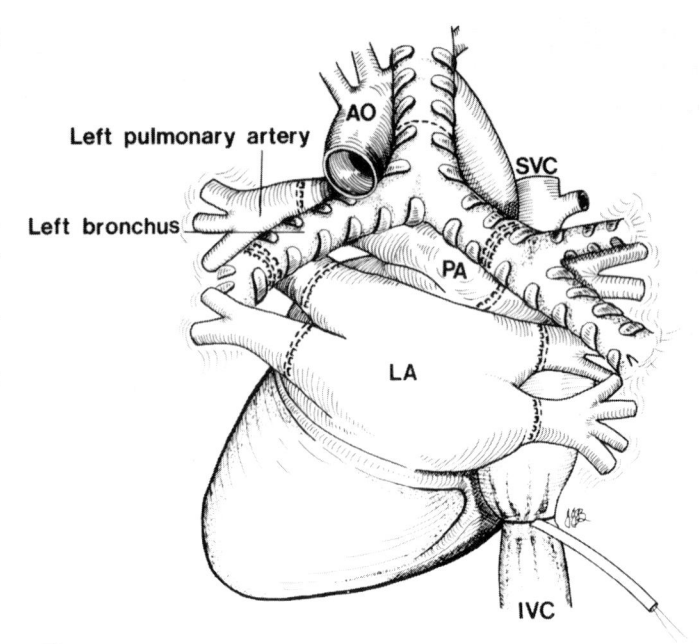

Figure 50.2 Posterior view of trachea, bronchi, and heart to show staple lines of bronchi, pulmonary arteries and pulmonary veins. The future site of division of the trachea is indicated. (SVC = superior vena cava; IVC = inferior vena cava; AO = aorta; PA = pulmonary artery; LA = left atrium)

right pulmonary artery is stapled closed at the point where it has been previously mobilized between the superior vena cava and the aorta (Figure 50.2). The right lung is then excised through the pleural space, with division of the pulmonary artery and veins lateral to the pericardium (Figure 50.1), and of the right main bronchus between staple lines (Figure 50.2).

A right pleuropericardial window is then created by enlarging the opening through which the pulmonary veins

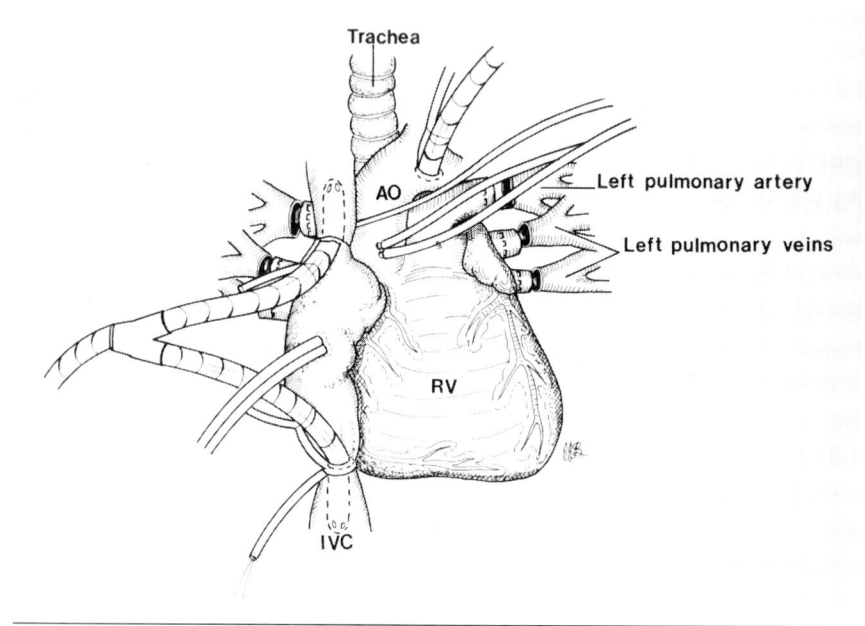

Figure 50.1 Cardiopulmonary bypass has been initiated in the recipient following cannulation of the aorta (AO), and superior and inferior (IVC) venae cavae. A cardioplegic cannula has been placed in the ascending aorta. A right ventricular drain (vent) has been inserted into the right atrium to prevent distension of the right ventricle (RV). The pulmonary veins and arteries on each side have been stapled and divided outside the pericardium

pass. This window is more difficult to create than on the left side, as it lies posterior to the superior and inferior venae cavae, which restrict visualization. If necessary, the azygos vein can be divided so that this pleuropericardial window can be extended superiorly.

The bronchial stumps and distal trachea are then dissected free and removed. This can be performed either through the right pleural space, by grasping the right main bronchus and drawing the carina into the pleural space, or through the mediastinum between the aorta and superior vena cava. The trachea is divided distally (Figure 50.2).

Both lungs have now been removed together with the distal trachea and bronchi (Figure 50.3). The remnants of the pulmonary arteries and veins, however, remain *in situ*.

Positioning of omental pedicle

The posterior pericardial attachments behind the heart are divided so that a hand can be passed freely upward behind the heart, into the superior mediastinum anterior to the esophagus. The omentum is then brought through the diaphragmatic fenestration, passed posterior to the heart, and placed behind the distal portion of the trachea.

Insertion of donor lungs

The donor graft is then placed behind the heart (Figure 50.4). The donor trachea is drawn up behind the heart, into the superior mediastinum. As this maneuver is being performed, each lung is directed through its respective pleuropericardial window into the pleural space (Figure 50.4).

Tracheal anastomosis

The recipient trachea has already been divided two rings above the carina, and the distal trachea and bronchial stumps discarded. The donor trachea is also divided 1–2 rings above the carina. An end-to-end anastomosis is constructed between donor and recipient tracheas (Figure 50.5), using a running monofilament suture for the membranous portion and interrupted absorbable sutures for the cartilaginous portion. The lungs are gently inflated to test for air leaks at the site of anastomosis.

Aortic cross-clamping

Up to this point the aorta has not been cross-clamped and the heart has continued to beat with core temperature reduced to 32°C. Following completion of the tracheal anastomosis, however, the aorta is cross-clamped, and cardioplegic solution delivered through the aortic root to arrest the heart. As there is no further coronary sinus return, the tourniquets can be snugged around the caval cannulae, and suction on the right ventricular drain discontinued.

Anastomosis of left atrium

The apex of the heart is elevated and rotated towards the right (Figures 50.4 and 50.6), exposing the back of the recipient left atrium (which, up to this point, is completely intact, with each of the pulmonary venous stumps stapled closed). The stumps of the left pulmonary veins are now excised, creating a left atriotomy (Figure 50.4). This is extended by division of the posterior wall of the left atrium

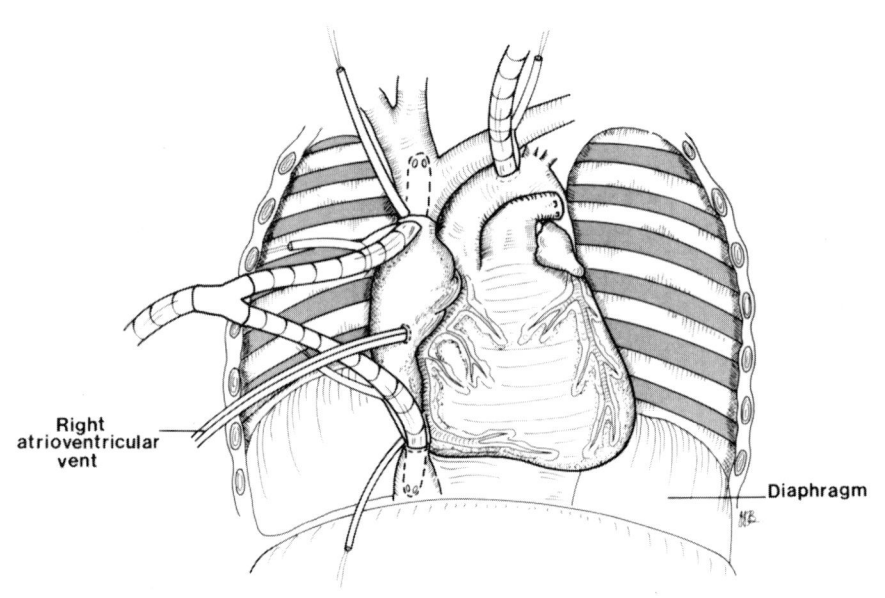

Figure 50.3 Recipient chest cavity after excision of the two lungs

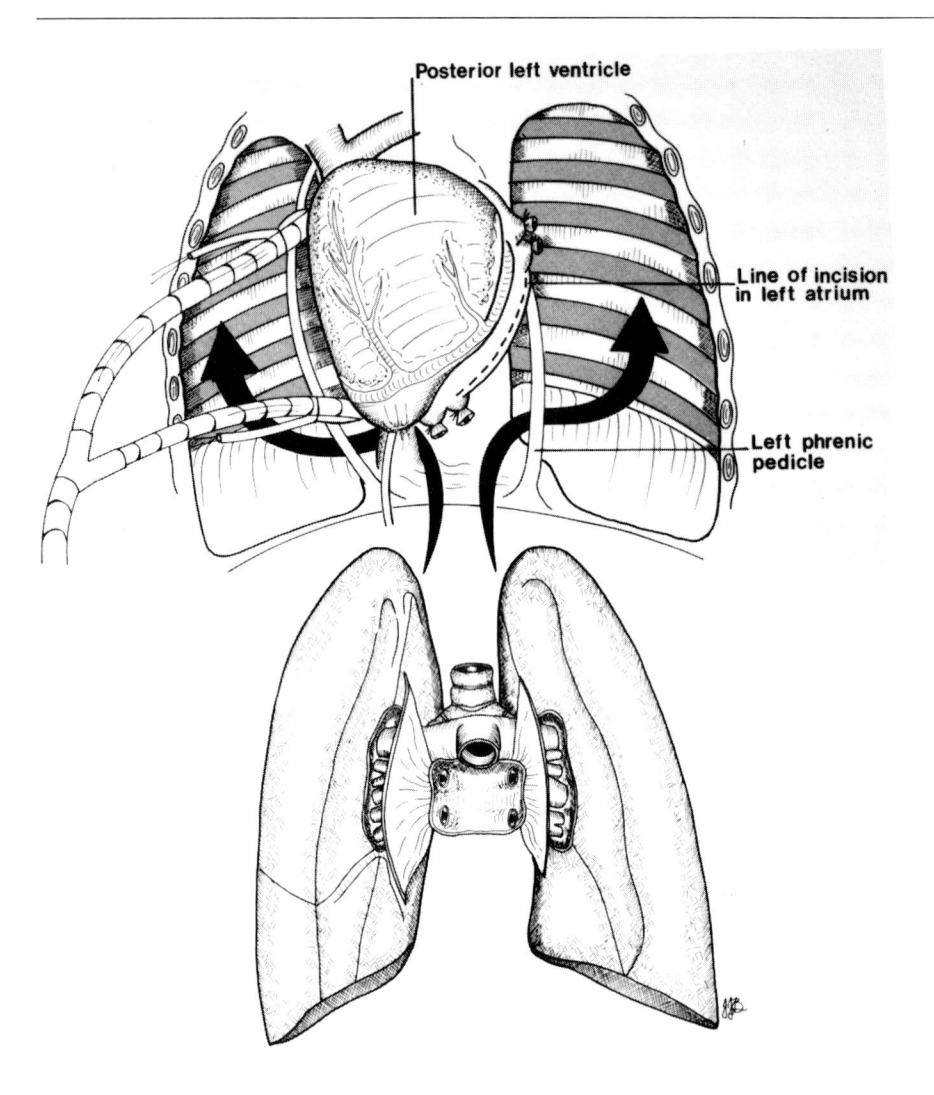

Figure 50.4 Demonstration of insertion of the double-lung bloc into the recipient chest. The donor trachea and pulmonary artery are passed posterior to the recipient heart into the superior mediastinum. The right lung is passed posterior to the right atrium and right phrenic neurovascular pedicle into the right pleural cavity, and the left lung is passed posterior to the left neurovascular pedicle into the left pleural cavity. The future line of incision in the recipient left atrium to allow anastomosis of the two left atria is indicated (adapted from Bonser, R.S. et al.[4])

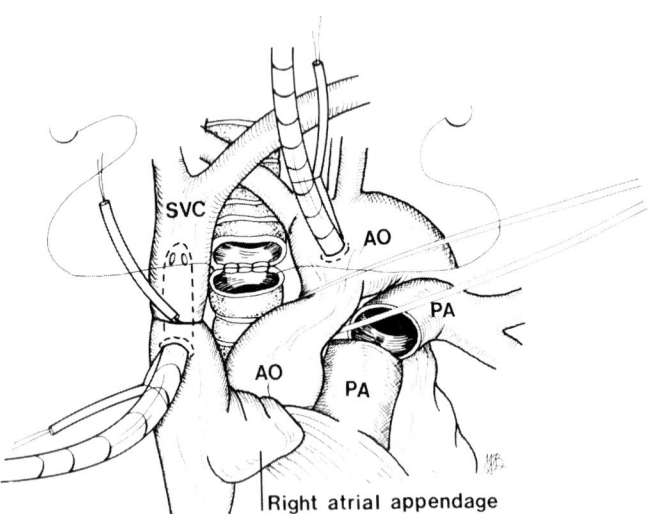

Figure 50.5 The ascending aorta has been retracted to the left to expose the site of tracheal anastomosis. This anastomosis is in progress. (The previously positioned omentum, which lies posterior to the site of anastomosis, is not shown)

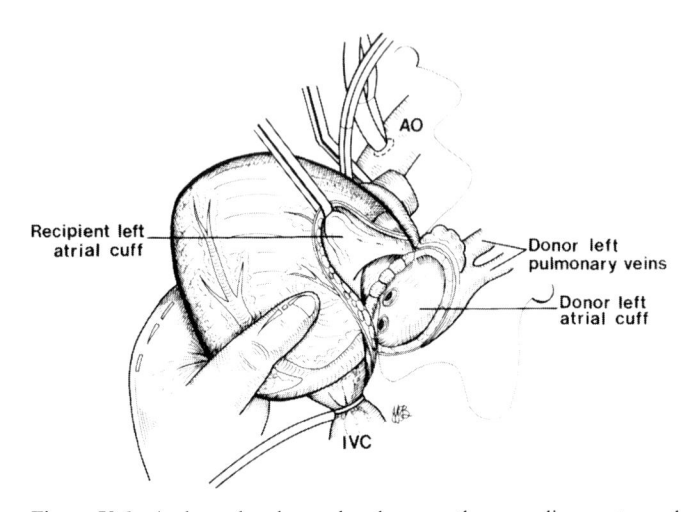

Figure 50.6 A clamp has been placed across the ascending aorta, and cardioplegic solution has been infused. The recipient heart has been lifted up and to the right, and the anastomosis of the two left atria is in progress

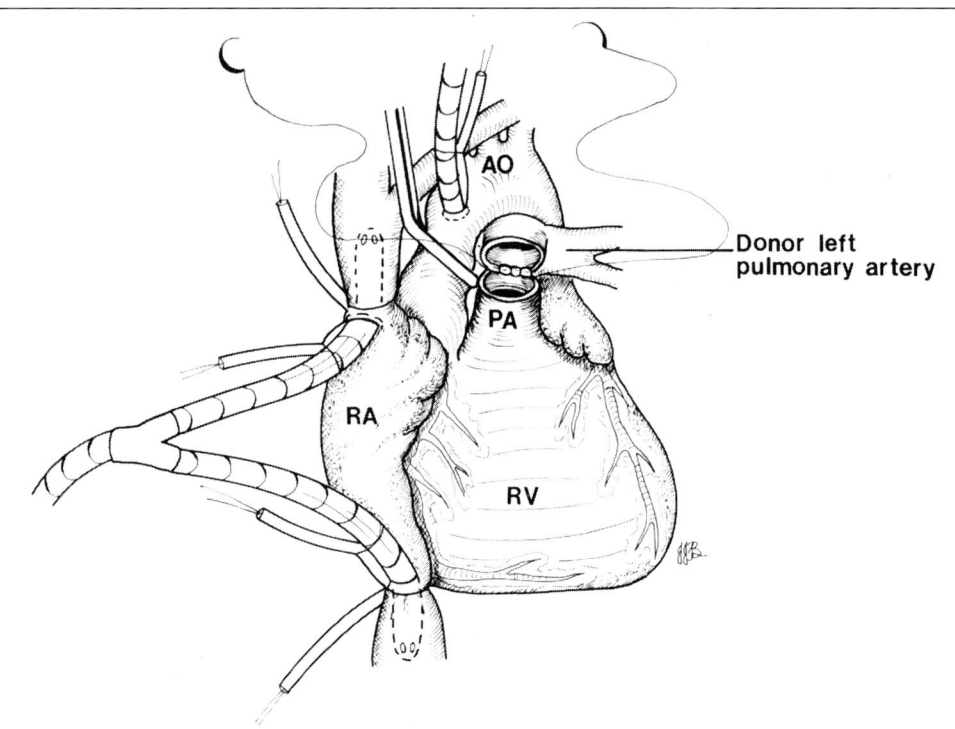

Figure 50.7 The pulmonary artery anastomosis is being performed

towards the right pulmonary veins, creating an atrial cuff which is anastomosed to the donor atrial cuff, using a running monofilament suture (Figure 50.6). The anastomosis is performed with the surgeon standing at the left side of the table. The suture line is begun at the far (right) side of the atrial cuff. Following completion of the atrial suture line, the heart is returned to its normal position.

Anastomosis of pulmonary arteries

The recipient common pulmonary artery is now transected just proximal to its bifurcation; it is not necessary to excise the bifurcation or the right or left pulmonary artery stumps. An end-to-end anastomosis is constructed between donor and recipient pulmonary arteries to complete the transplant procedure (Figure 50.7).

Positioning of omental pedicle

Finally, the omentum is wrapped completely around the tracheal anastomosis and tacked to itself to prevent displacement (Chapter 37).

Closure

Four drains are inserted, two (apical and basal) in each pleural cavity. The sternum is closed. Fiberoptic bronchoscopy is performed through the endotracheal tube to suction out any blood or secretions in the bronchial tree, and to inspect the tracheal anastomosis.

References

1. Patterson, G.A., Cooper, J.D., Goldman, B., Weisel, R.D., Pearson, F.G., Waters, P.F., Todd, T.R., Scully, H., Goldberg, M. and Ginsberg, R.J. (1988). Technique of successful clinical double-lung transplantation. Ann. Thorac. Surg., 43, 626
2. Vanderhoeft, P., Dubois, A., Lauvau, N., de Francquen, P.H., Carpentier, Y., Rocmans, P., Nelson, R., Kaufman, S., Brickman, L., Gyhra, A. and Ectors, P. (1972). Block allotransplantation of both lungs with pulmonary trunk and left atrium in dogs. Thorax, 27, 415
3. Dark, J.H., Patterson, G.A., Al-Jilaihawi, A.N., Hsu, H., Egan, T. and Cooper, J.D. (1986). Experimental en bloc double-lung transplantation. Ann. Thorac. Surg., 42, 394
4. Bonser, R.S., Fragomeni, L.S., Kriett, J.M., Kaye, M.P. and Jamieson, S.W. (1988). Technique of clinical double-lung transplantation. J. Heart Transplant., 7, 298

ADDENDUM

Since this chapter was written, both authors have independently modified the procedure considerably. The technique as described is no longer employed. Instead, the chest is opened by bilateral thoracotomy with transverse sternotomy, and sequential bilateral single lung transplantation is performed with or without partial cardiopulmonary bypass without cardioplegia.

51
Postoperative Management
C.G.A. McGREGOR

INTRODUCTION

This chapter will concentrate on the routine postoperative care of the single lung transplant recipient, and will avoid topics covered in other chapters, such as immunosuppressive therapy and postoperative complications, except where a specific alternative management philosophy exists.

Much of the postoperative management of patients undergoing double lung transplantation is similar to that following heart–lung transplantation, and will not be duplicated here. The postoperative care of the patient who has undergone single lung transplantation is somewhat different in that (1) left or right thoracotomy, rather than median sternotomy, is performed, (2) cardiopulmonary bypass is generally not utilized, and (3) the contralateral native diseased lung remains *in situ*. Whatever the technique of lung transplantation used, however, the problems of lung preservation, diagnosis of pulmonary rejection and infection, and obliterative bronchiolitis, exist. In this chapter, only those aspects peculiar to single lung transplantation will be elaborated upon. As the indications for single lung transplantation expand to include, for example, pulmonary hypertension, postoperative management will clearly be modified.

Postoperative management can be conveniently divided into two phases – (1) the early intensive therapy period, and (2) the medium and pre-discharge period (stepdown and general ward). The mean stay in the intensive care unit in the first 11 patients in the Toronto series and in our own smaller series of single lung transplants was 9.5 days and 7 days respectively; the mean hospital stay was 41 days in both series[1,2].

EARLY POSTOPERATIVE PERIOD

As for much of cardiothoracic surgery, the relative difficulty of immediate postoperative care is largely dictated by the events that occurred in the operating room. If a good donor lung is obtained and preserved well, and the operative procedure is technically uncomplicated, then the early management of the single lung transplant recipient is relatively straightforward.

No consensus exists regarding the effectiveness of reverse barrier nursing in the care of the transplant recipient (Chapter 17), but many accept that reverse isolation in the early postoperative period is helpful in minimizing traffic of personnel, and impresses on both staff and visitors the risk of transmitting infection and the importance of maintaining strict hygienic standards. After the first few days, if the patient is in a stable condition, the level of reverse barrier nursing can be safely reduced; this minimizes the patient's feelings of claustrophobia and emotional separation, reduces costs, and facilitates nursing and medical management. However, an individual nurse should not combine care of a transplant patient with that of an infected patient, and continuing strict adherence to hand washing, in particular, is essential[3].

In the immediate postoperative period, two nurses are generally required to perform the extensive duties that are necessary. Standard intensive care monitoring of vital signs is carried out. Experienced resident medical presence is mandatory. Frequent clinical examination is important. Early signs of rejection or infection can be subtle, but, if elicited, can allow timely investigation and therapy. It has been our practice for the senior medical team (surgeon, anesthesiologist, respiratory physician, infectious disease specialist) to meet at least twice daily to review in depth the patient's condition; this allows for the results of investigations to be noted, management to be optimized, and provides continuity of care, as well as serving as a forum for communication and education of the staff involved. This proactive approach results in the timely introduction of measures that prevent the development of complications and emergency problems.

Ventilatory management

A standard volume-cycled mechanical ventilator is adequate for ventilation of most single lung recipients. In rare circumstances, high frequency ventilation and membrane oxygenation may prove helpful.

The aim of mechanical ventilation is to achieve adequate oxygenation of the patient ($PaO_2 > 80$ torr (mmHg)) at the lowest possible inspired oxygen concentration ($FiO_2 < 0.6$) and the lowest possible peak airway pressure ($< 30\,cmH_2O$). Measures to achieve these ends include:

(1) Optimization of ventilatory rate, inspiratory time, and tidal volume, to achieve the same minute ventilation.

(2) The use of positive end expiratory pressure (PEEP)) $\leqslant$ 4–6 cmH_2O. Greater levels of PEEP may be necessary to achieve adequate oxygenation in the presence of compromised lung function, but are clearly undesirable for prolonged periods in view of a potentially deleterious effect on bronchial healing.

(3) Adequate pulmonary toilet. A soft endotracheal suction catheter is introduced into the lower trachea 2-hourly, or more frequently if secretions are copious. Aggressive endotracheal suction with a rigid catheter in the region of the bronchial anastomosis should be avoided. Excessive hyperinflation by 'hand bagging' before endotracheal suction should also be avoided to minimize stress on the anastomosis. If there are significant secretions that cannot be aspirated, or lobar collapse develops, then fiberoptic bronchoscopy should be carried out; with care, it is possible to traverse the bronchial anastomosis. Throughout the period of mechanical ventilation, and after extubation, active respiratory therapy, including vibration and percussion, is given 4-hourly.

(4) Maintenance of the lowest left atrial pressure compatible with satisfactory hemodynamics, preferably maintaining the pulmonary arterial diastolic pressure lower than 12 torr (see also Hemodynamic management below). This aims to minimize the propensity for pulmonary edema in the preserved, transplanted lung.

(5) Avoidance of pleural fluid collection by continuous suction (at $-20\,cmH_2O$) of apical and basal chest tubes inserted at the time of transplantation.

Many single lung transplant recipients can be extubated within 1–3 days of operation, but some require more prolonged periods of ventilation. Before weaning, the following criteria should be met:

(1) The patient's mental status should be satisfactory. He should be easily rousable, and have satisfactory cough and gag reflexes.

(2) Blood gas parameters must include
 (a) $PaO_2 > 75$ torr, with an $FiO_2 < 0.5$, a $PaCO_2 < 40$ torr, and PEEP $< 6\,cmH_2O$;
 (b) a vital capacity $> 10\,ml/kg$;
 (c) a peak inspiratory pressure force $> -25\,cmH_2O$;
 (d) the demonstrated ability of the patient to resume adequate spontaneous ventilation during a progressive decrease in assisted ventilation.

(3) Acceptable chest radiographic appearances. In the presence of diffuse opacification of the lung in a patient with marginal blood gases, ventilation should be continued until improvement is seen.

(4) Stable hemodynamics, including stable cardiac rhythm and acceptable hemodynamic parameters without heavy inotropic therapy.

(5) Good muscle strength, reflected by adequate chest excursion. Pain may prevent satisfactory chest movement; the insertion of a lumbar epidural catheter for postoperative pain management is helpful, unless cardiopulmonary bypass has been used, in which case this technique of analgesia is probably contraindicated.

(6) Satisfactory acid base status. Significant metabolic alkalosis should be corrected prior to weaning.

(7) Acceptable fluid balance. In particular, the patient should not be fluid overloaded; diuresis may be indicated prior to weaning.

Once an adequate level of oxygenation with an FiO_2 equal or less than 0.5 is achieved, a standard weaning protocol can be used. For example, the ventilator is switched from assist control to an intermittent mandatory ventilation (IMV) of 8 breaths/minute. If the patient remains comfortable with acceptable blood gases, then the rate is further decreased to 4 breaths/minute, and the patient is subsequently extubated.

In patients with early impairment of donor lung function, from use of a suboptimal donor or inadequate pulmonary preservation (Figure 51.1), weaning first requires improvement in the patient's overall clinical status. This allows a gradual increase in spontaneous ventilatory work with concomitant decrease in ventilatory assistance. Intravenous nutrition may be required if this period is prolonged, as well as control of any volume overload and/or sepsis. Even though ventilator-dependent, suitable physical activity should be encouraged. The patient's psychological status should be maintained as near normal as possible, with avoidance of sleep deprivation and depression. The rehabilitation process (see later) is begun at this time, and is tailored to the general state of the patient. Continuity of expert care is essential in such cases. The overall philosophy is to increase the periods of active respiratory movement by alternating these with periods of muscle rest, usually entailing an assist control mode of ventilation at night. Gradually, periods off the ventilator are increased until ventilation can be discontinued permanently.

In the Toronto series of single lung transplants, the duration of ventilatory support ranged from 3 to 10 days,

POSTOPERATIVE MANAGEMENT

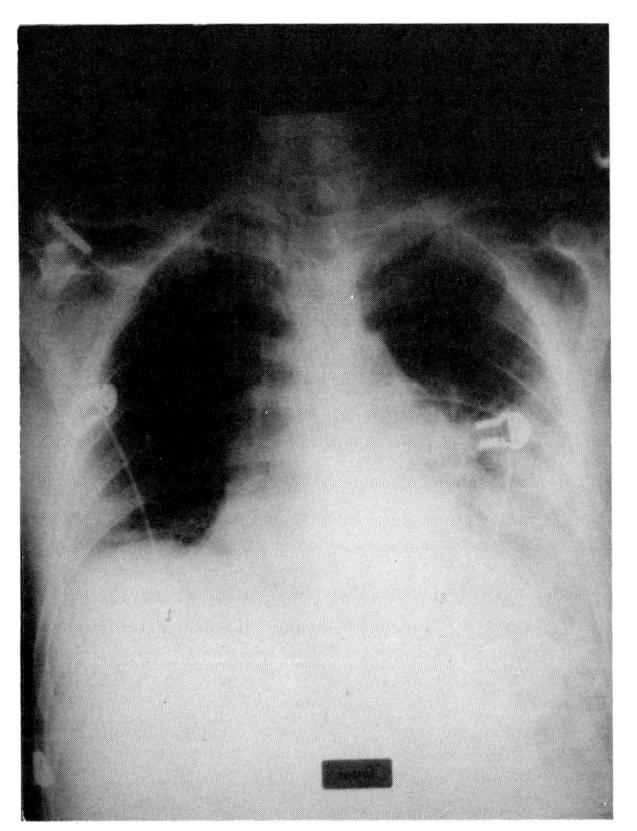

Figure 51.1 Anteroposterior chest radiograph of patient taken 48 hours after single left lung transplantation. The left lung opacification was believed to result from inadequate donor lung preservation

with a mean of 5.5 days. A number of patients required reintubation, sometimes on more than one occasion. The periods of ventilation required in our series of three patients were 12 hours, 36 hours, and 4 days, respectively.

After extubation, a close-fitting mask delivering 40% or 70% O_2 is applied, and blood gases monitored 30 minutes later, and then at hourly or 2-hourly intervals until the patient's respiratory status is clearly satisfactory. Continuous ear or finger oximetry for SaO_2 is carried out. Chest radiographs are taken at 8-hourly intervals throughout the first postoperative week. Four-hourly chest physiotherapy, with breathing exercises and vibration or percussion therapy, is provided to help prevent atelectasis. Pulse oximetry and heart rate should be monitored during respiratory therapy, and any deterioration in these parameters reported to the physician. Bronchodilator therapy is not employed routinely. The patient is given guidance in the use of incentive spirometry with one of the many commercially available devices, and encouraged to perform this therapy for 2–5 minutes of every waking hour.

Hemodynamic management

Continuous invasive hemodynamic monitoring is essential until the patient is established off the ventilator. An arterial line, a Foley urinary catheter, and either two central venous lines or a triple lumen central venous catheter are utilized. Additionally, Swan–Ganz catheterization is helpful; if anxiety exists regarding trauma to the pulmonary arterial anastomosis, the catheter can be passed into the contralateral lung under the surgeon's control in the operating room before the chest is closed.

It is optimal to maintain the central venous pressure $\leqslant 10$ torr, and the mean arterial pressure $\geqslant 70$ torr; maintenance of an adequate blood pressure may be important in ensuring satisfactory blood supply to the ischemic bronchus. To achieve these hemodynamic parameters, it is often necessary to use a dopamine infusion at 2–5 µg/kg per min. In the presence of normal renal function, it is rarely necessary to use diuretics to maintain urine output > 0.5 ml/kg per hour. Concomitant vasodilator therapy (sodium nitroprusside) may be used to optimize cardiac function. More powerful pulmonary vasodilator therapy (PGE_1 or PGI_2) may be helpful if pulmonary artery pressures remain high, with resultant right heart failure; this problem is most acutely faced, however, during the period of one-lung ventilation that is necessary as the donor lung is being implanted[4] (Chapter 48).

As cardiopulmonary bypass is rarely required for single lung transplantation, postoperative bleeding is usually minimal. The mean and maximum operative blood requirements for the first 11 recipients in the Toronto series were 1 and 2 units respectively[1]. Transfusion is indicated if the hematocrit falls below 30%. It is important that anesthesiologists and internists recognize that cardiopulmonary bypass has not been employed, and that fluid overloading must be avoided.

Immunosuppressive therapy

Triple immunosuppressive drug therapy is employed following single lung transplantation (see also Chapters 12 and 38). Oral corticosteroid therapy is withheld for the first 7–21 days to avoid its deleterious effect on bronchial healing; during this period, prophylactic ATG or OKT3 therapy is utilized[5]. As the patient has been subjected to a limited laparotomy for mobilization of the omentum, it may be several days before bowel activity returns; carefully titrated intravenous cyclosporine therapy may be required during this time. A nasogastric tube, placed at the time of surgery, is left *in situ* until bowel sounds have returned; if it is wished to avoid intravenous cyclosporine, this tube can be used for administration of cyclosporine during this period. Azathioprine can be administered intravenously until bowel function is re-established.

The administration of antithymocyte or antilymphocyte globulin, or OKT3, may result in an anaphylactic reaction, and so pretreatment with hydrocortisone, an antipyretic, and an antihistamine is indicated. Should a mild or moderate anaphylactic reaction occur, the infusion of the cytolytic agent should be stopped, the premedication repeated, and the infusion recommenced 30 minutes later at half the rate. If a severe reaction occurs, then standard resuscitation measures should be taken, including the administration of epinephrine.

Acute rejection episodes are treated with intravenous methylprednisolone pulse therapy (10 mg/kg per day) for 3 days.

Anticoagulation

In the Toronto series, an intravenous infusion of heparin and dipyridamole has been administered in the early postoperative period in order to minimize the risk of anastomotic thrombosis[6]. We have not utilized any specific anticoagulation in our own small series, and believe it is unnecessary. The use of subcutaneous heparin for prophylaxis of deep venous thrombosis seems appropriate for the patient who is unable to be mobilized in the early postoperative period.

Infectious disease management

The presence in the donor trachea of heavy bacterial or fungal growth, or of large numbers of neutrophils, increases morbidity and mortality after heart–lung transplantation[7]. Material obtained from the airways of the donor lung at the time of harvest is routinely sent for bacteriological examination; when the results are known, routine antibiotic prophylaxis must be modified accordingly. Invasive tubes and lines, with the exception of the central venous line, are removed as soon as possible; the chest drains and Foley catheter are usually removed 1–2 days after operation, and the arterial line 24 hours after extubation. Narrow spectrum antibiotic prophylaxis (nafcillin or floxacillin, 1 g i.v. every 6 hours) for wound and line infection is given until this time. We have given metronidazole therapy (500 mg i.v. every 8 hours) for the first 3 weeks to minimize potential anaerobic infection around the 'ischemic' bronchial anastomosis.

Our own approach to prevention of infection is aggressive. When the patient is able to take oral medication, prophylactic acyclovir therapy (200–400 mg orally 4 times a day) is begun for a 3-month period in an attempt to reduce the incidence of herpes, cytomegalovirus (CMV)[8], and Epstein–Barr virus infections, the latter of which may be implicated in the development of lymphoma. Nystatin mouthwash (5 ml) is given 4 times a day, and, in women, a nystatin pessary daily. Prophylactic cotrimoxazole therapy (1 double strength tablet daily) is administered for 6 months to prevent pneumocystis and nocardial infections, as well as toxoplasmosis in sero-mismatched patients. When the patient is allergic to sulfa drugs, pyramethamine (25 mg orally daily) is given for 3 months. Early and aggressive pursuit of any infective process to determine its microbiological cause is carried out; this may necessitate bronchoscopy and bronchoalveolar lavage.

In a CMV-negative recipient who received an organ from a CMV-positive donor, CMV hyperimmune globulin (1 ml/kg) is given on days 1, 7, 14, 28, 49, 70 and 91. Passive immunization with CMV hyperimmune globulin has been shown to be effective in diminishing the frequency and severity of CMV diseases in seronegative mismatched recipients of renal[9] and cardiac allografts[10]. In such a CMV 'mismatch', prophylactic i.v. ganciclovir therapy is substituted for acyclovir for the first 3 weeks.

Investigations

Chest radiography is performed 3 times a day for 1 week, twice a day for a further week, and daily thereafter, as well as when clinically indicated. A baseline ventilation-perfusion (V/Q) scan is performed, as well as daily spirometry. When the patient is able to visit the pulmonary laboratory, full pulmonary function tests are carried out weekly. Unlike the Toronto group, we have not found V/Q scans helpful in the diagnosis of rejection. They do, however, provide interesting physiological information, such as by demonstrating a shift in ventilation to the transplanted lung with time (Figure 51.2).

Daily investigations include a complete blood count, T-cell subsets (if OKT3 or ATG are being used), basic blood tests of renal function and metabolism (urea, creatinine, glucose and electrolytes), and cyclosporine level. A general blood chemistry panel is monitored twice a week.

Routine surveillance specimens of urine, throat, sputum, and endotracheal secretions (if intubated), are cultured for bacteria and fungi twice a week. Blood and urine are cultured for CMV weekly. Toxoplasma, cryptococcal, and CMV serologies are monitored weekly.

Diagnosis of implantation response, rejection, and infection

The nature of any new pulmonary opacification seen on the chest radiograph may be suggested by the time of its occurrence in relation to the transplantation procedure. Opacification developing in the first few days after transplantation is most likely related to an implantation response resulting from preservation–reperfusion injury and/or division of lymphatics (Figure 51.1) (Chapter 35). Rejection is possible at this early stage, but is more common after the first 4–5 days. Thereafter, the clinical features and radiographic appearances of rejection and infection can be indistinguishable. Pulmonary rejection may develop over a

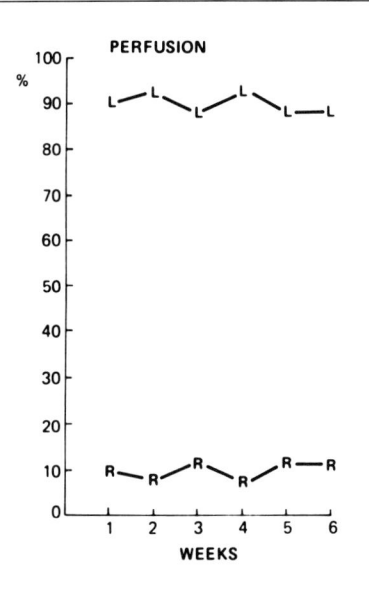

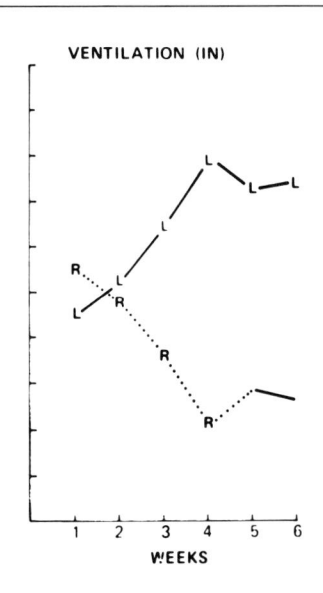

Figure 51.2 Ventilation and perfusion of left (L) and right (R) lungs after single left lung transplantation. Ventilation (and perfusion) of each lung, recorded at weekly intervals, is expressed as a percentage of the total

short time period (hours), but, if diagnosed early, can resolve in an equally short period (Figures 51.3A, B and C).

In the investigation of any new respiratory sign or symptom, or any significant change in a physiological or radiographic parameter, we maintain an aggressive approach with regard to bronchoscopy and bronchoalveolar lavage (BAL). After BAL of the 'opacified' area of lung, four transbronchial biopsies are obtained by fiberoptic bronchoscopy using alligator forceps under local anesthesia (with an anesthesiologist in attendance) and fluoroscopic control (Figure 51.4). Alligator forceps provide a 3–4 mm^3 specimen. Ideally, biopsies should contain the three pulmonary anatomical elements – bronchiolar epithelium, alveolus, and blood vessel (Chapter 40). Bronchoscopy also allows inspection of the bronchial anastomosis.

BAL specimens are stained and cultured according to a standard 'immunocompromised host protocol', which includes investigation for bacteria, legionella, nocardia, mycobacteria, fungi, viruses, and pneumocystis. Biopsies undergo rapid histological processing.

Transbronchial biopsy has been shown to be of value in the diagnosis of unsuspected pulmonary rejection and infection, and also provides information on the development of obliterative bronchiolitis after heart–lung transplantation[11,12] (Chapter 38). We therefore perform this procedure on a routine basis at the time of hospital discharge, and at 4 months and 1 year after transplantation. It is now known that obliterative bronchiolitis can occur after single lung transplantation[2].

MEDIUM AND PREDISCHARGE PERIOD

Monitoring

The indications for transfer from the Intensive Care Unit to a Stepdown Unit will vary between institutions. It is psychologically preferable for a patient to leave the Intensive Care Unit as soon as he/she no longer requires this level of care. The decision to transfer a patient may be influenced by the availability of monitoring facilities in the Stepdown Unit.

It has been our practice to monitor the patient continuously by electrocardiographic telemetry as well as by ear or finger pulse oximetry. (Pulse oximetric telemetric monitoring should be available in the near future, and will allow greatly increased mobility of the patient.) Non-invasive blood pressure monitoring is also helpful. At this stage of postoperative care, the patient will be in the early phase of mobilization; most invasive monitoring lines will have been removed, but it has been our practice to maintain a central venous line to provide vascular access in an emergency and to allow blood sampling without needle stick. The disadvantages of this policy, however, are the risks of line sepsis and air embolism (see also Chapter 52). Careful nursing practice should avoid the latter complication. In our experience, the risk of line infection is minimized by three measures: (1) meticulous daily change of dressing, (2) the line is changed to a separate site each week, and (3) the line is flushed with sodium metabisulfite solution (0.05%) after any venous sample has been taken[13].

Rehabilitation

A preoperative rehabilitation program (as described in Chapter 46) is extremely important, not only in optimizing the condition of the potential single lung transplant recipient, but also by preparing him for postoperative rehabilitation, which is integral to the successful outcome of the transplant. The goals of a postoperative rehabilitation program include: (1) improvement and maintenance of efficient breathing; (2) musculoskeletal reconditioning; (3) improvement in the maintenance of aerobic capacity, and of body posture and

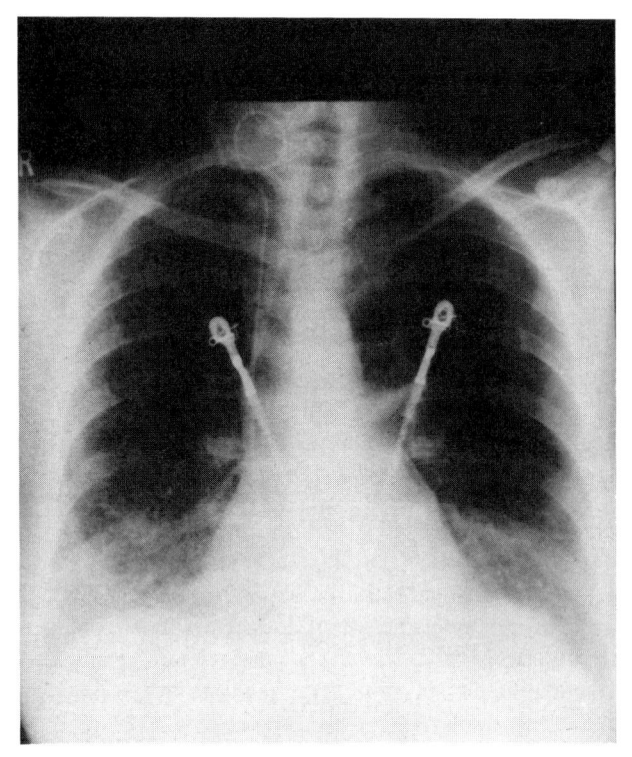

Figure 51.3A Posteroanterior chest radiograph taken (in the morning) 10 days after single left lung transplantation

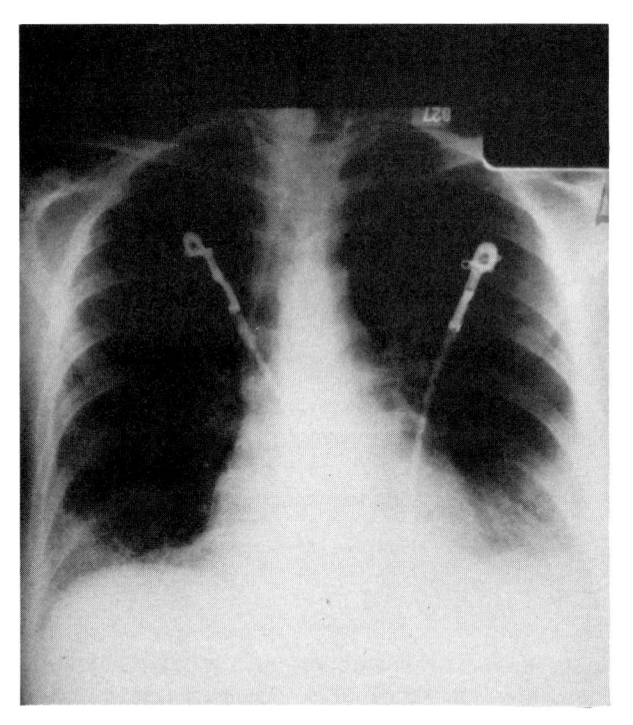

Figure 51.3B Chest radiograph (taken later the same day) showing a left basal pulmonary infiltrate and effusion, which was associated with fever, pleuritic pain, and a pleural rub

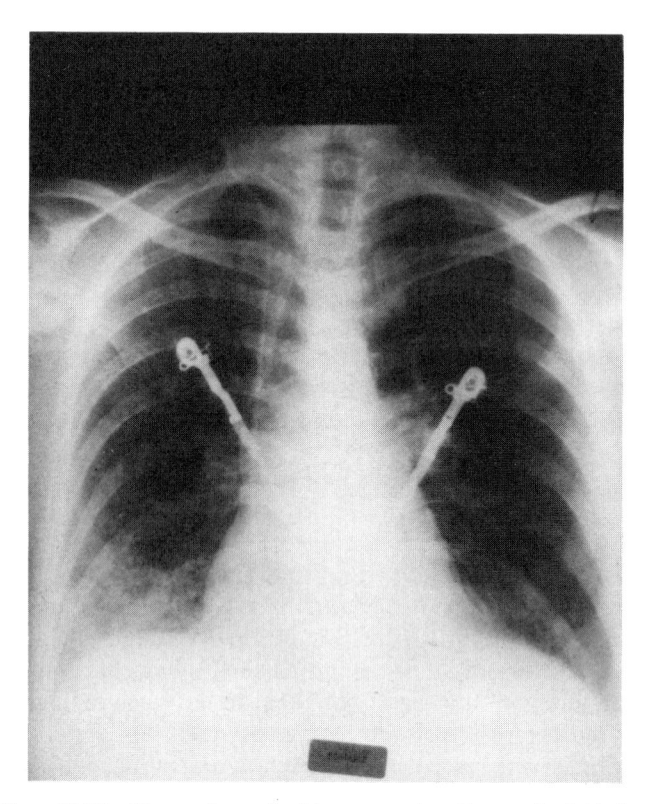

Figure 51.3C Chest radiograph of the same patient 6 hours after initiating antirejection therapy, demonstrating marked clearing of the left lower zone opacification

neuromuscular relaxation (see also Chapter 28).

By promoting physical self-reliance, attainment of these goals results in decreased anxiety and depression, and also assists in the process of retraining for an independent existence. As patients vary considerably in their physical status at the time of transplantation, it is necessary to provide an accelerated as well as a standard program. A standard program is necessary in the patient who has lost considerable muscle mass; this may result from enforced inactivity or represent the cachexia that develops secondary to advanced pulmonary disease. An accelerated program is indicated in the patient who is relatively fit.

The patient is treated twice a day, and is allowed to progress in a sequential fashion to the next stage of exercise when he has satisfactorily completed two consecutive treatments at the previous level. Continued measurement of oxygen saturation is essential during exercise; oxygen therapy should be adjusted to maintain the oxygen saturation of the blood greater than 90% (Figure 51.5).

In the event of a rejection or infectious episode, activity is modified accordingly. In the presence of severe rejection, only gentle passive movements are continued. With moderate rejection, activity can be maintained, but not increased. With mild rejection, progress can be continued as per protocol.

Our own protocol includes five levels of activity, with

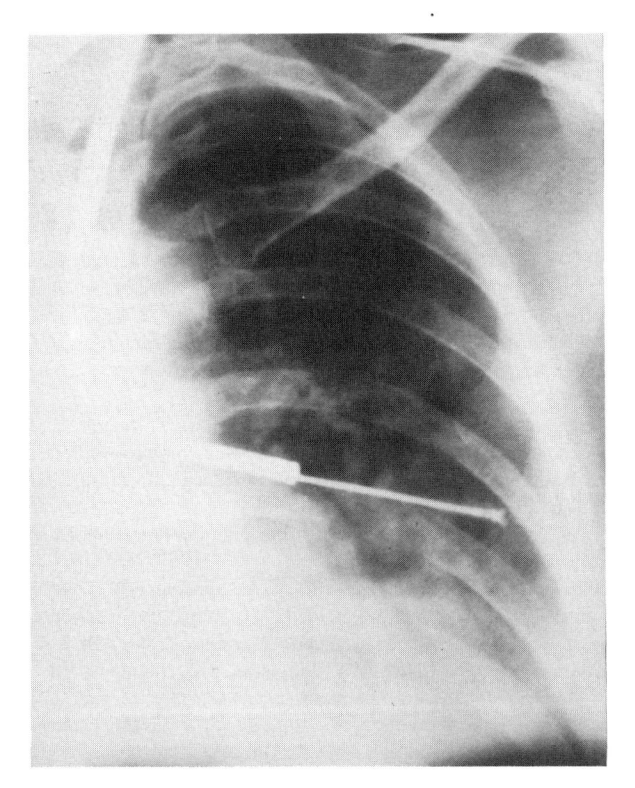

Figure 51.4 Fluoroscopic appearance of a transbronchial biopsy being taken, using alligator forceps directed through a fiberoptic bronchoscope

documentation of changes in heart rate, respiratory rate, blood pressure, and oxygen saturation, and of the development of any symptoms. Indications for cessation of a specific activity include: (1) a heart rate response > 30–40 beats above the resting rate, (2) a respiratory rate > 30/minute, or (3) an oxygen saturation persistently < 90%.

Education

As with all solid organ transplants, a successful long-term result will be more likely if each patient takes a degree of personal responsibility for his or her own health care. This can be achieved only by the methodical education of the patient. This should include relevant information on (1) transplantation in general, (2) lung transplantation in particular, (3) medications, (4) nutrition, and guidelines on (5) exercise and activity, (6) personal health surveillance, and (7) medical follow-up care. Information should also be provided on how the patient can obtain the appropriate medical care should problems arise. Basic knowledge of (8) the immune system, (9) the problems of pulmonary rejection and infection, and (10) the potential long-term complications of lung transplantation should be discussed. The patient should be made aware of the symptoms and signs of these complications so that he can refer himself early for medical care, which may be crucial if the process is to be fully reversed.

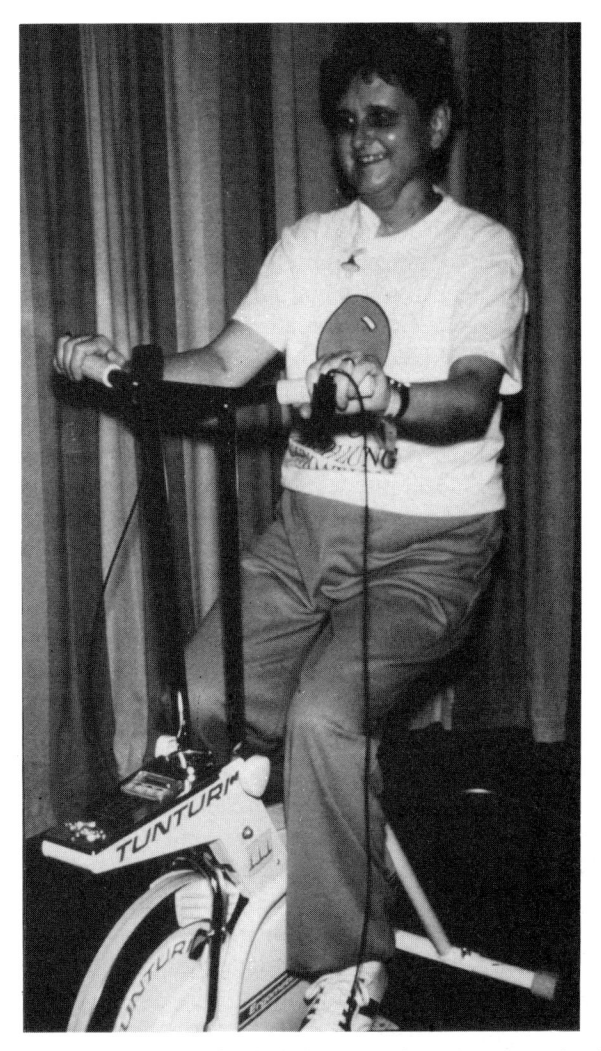

Figure 51.5 A recipient of a single lung transplant, shown 2 weeks after surgery, participating in a postoperative exercise program. Continuous monitoring of oxygen saturation is provided by finger oximetry

Detailed advice regarding discharge medications should include: (1) dose of drug, (2) method of administration, (3) potential side-effects, and (4) the reason it is prescribed. Medications discussed should include cyclosporine, azathioprine, corticosteroids, antihypertensive agents, and diuretics.

Practical nutritional advice is essential as most patients will be receiving corticosteroid therapy, which can act as an appetite stimulant as well as lead to metabolic changes that predispose to obesity. Such advice should include: (1) appropriate calorie intake, (2) food preferences, and (3) food intake patterns. Basic principles include: (1) modification of the fat content of the diet, and (2) calorie control, to achieve and maintain desired body weight (see also Chapter 27).

After discharge from hospital, the patient will continue to participate in a medically supervised and monitored pulmonary rehabilitation program, but specific guidelines are required for the patient to exercise on his own. The importance of a continuing exercise program and of the promotion of mental and physical well-being should be emphasized. A regular schedule of moderate exercise will increase stamina, strength, and endurance, will assist in the handling of stress, and lead to improved relaxation and easier weight control. Patients should recognize that, when they accepted the transplantation option, they made a long-term commitment to rehabilitation. Guidance to the patient regarding personal and recreational and sexual pursuits should also be proffered.

The transplant recipient should be given an outline of his future outpatient care. When the recipient resides a long distance from the transplant center, arrangements should be made with a local physician to share the long-term care. Close cooperation and communication between patient, family, home physician, and transplant team is essential, both to achieve full rehabilitation and to detect potential complications at the earliest opportunity.

A record book is given to the patient in which he is instructed to record daily the medications he has taken, his temperature, pulse rate, weight, and incentive spirometry performance, and any new symptoms he has developed. When the transplant physician sees the patient, he will record the results of examination and investigations in another part of the record book.

The patient should be instructed to avoid individuals with any infection, crowded theaters, stores, and restaurants, particularly in the early postoperative weeks. Avoiding construction sites or other dust-laden atmosphere is also prudent.

Clinic visits are arranged initially twice a week, subsequently once a week, and after 6 months reduced to a frequency of once per month. The patient is advised to report to the physician any new symptom or sign, e.g. fever, breathlessness, or a decrease in spirometry performance. Specific instructions regarding preparation for transbronchial biopsy are necessary. Finally, it is important for a member of the transplant team to be available to the patient or his local physician at all times for discussion, reassurance, and advice.

References

1. Toronto Lung Transplant Group (1988). Experience with single lung transplantation for pulmonary fibrosis. *J. Am. Med. Assoc.*, **259**, 2258
2. McGregor, C.G.A., Dark, J.H., Hilton, C.J., Freeman, R., Conacher, I.D. and Corris, P.A. (1989). Early results of single lung transplantation in patients with end-stage pulmonary fibrosis. *J. Thorac. Cardiovasc. Surg.*, **98**, 350
3. Holt, L., Freeman, R., Gould, K., McGregor, C.G.A. and Dark, J. (1989). Is reverse barrier nursing necessary for the cardiopulmonary transplant patient? (Abstract). *J. Heart Transplant.*, **8**, 84
4. Conacher, I.D., McNally, B., Choudhry, A.K. and McGregor, C.G.A. (1988). Anaesthesia for isolated lung transplantation. *Br. J. Anaesth.*, **60**, 588
5. Lima, O., Cooper, J.D., Peters, W.J., Ayabe, H., Townsend, E., Luk, S.C. and Goldberg, M. (1981). Effects of methylprednisolone and azathioprine on bronchial healing following lung autotransplantation. *J. Thorac. Cardiovasc. Surg.*, **82**, 211
6. Glynn, M.F.X. (1988). Modulation of coagulation. *Proceedings Seminar Lung Transplantation*, Toronto
6. Harjula, A., Baldwin, J.C., Starnes, V.A., Stinson, E.B., Oyer, P.E., Jamieson, S.W. and Shumway, N.E. (1987). Proper donor selection for heart–lung transplantation. *J. Thorac. Cardiovasc. Surg.*, **94**, 874
8. Balfour, H.H., Jr., Chace, B.A., Stapleton, J.T., Simmons, R.L. and Fryd, D.S. (1989). A randomized, placebo-controlled trial of oral acyclovir for the prevention of cytomegalovirus disease in recipients of renal allografts. *N. Engl. J. Med.*, **310**, 1381
9. Snydman, D.R., Werner, B.G., Heinze-Lacey, B., Berardi, V.P., Tilney, N.L., Kirkman, R.L., Milford, E.L., Cho, S.I., Bush, H.L. and Levey, A.S. (1987). Use of cytomegalovirus immune globulin to prevent cytomegalovirus disease in renal transplant recipients. *N. Engl. J. Med.*, **317**, 1049
10. Schafers, H.J., Milbradt, H., Flik, J., Wahlers, Th., Fieguth, H.G. and Haverich, A. (1988). Hyperimmuneglobulin for cytomegalovirus prophylaxis following heart transplantation. *Clin. Transplant.*, **2**, 51
11. Berry, G., Tazelaar, H., Billingham, M.D., Starnes, V. and Sibley, R. (1989). Transbronchial biopsies in heart–lung transplant patients. (Abstract) *Modern Path.*, **2**, 9A
12. Yousem, S.A., Paradis, I.L., Dauber, J.H. and Griffith, B.P. (1989). Efficacy of transbronchial lung biopsy in the diagnosis of bronchiolitis obliterans in heart–lung transplant recipients. *Transplantation*, **47**, 893
13. Freeman, R., Holden, M.P., Lyon, R. and Hjersing, N. (1982). Addition of sodium metabisulphite to left atrial catheter infusates as a means of preventing bacterial colonization of the catheter tip. *Thorax*, **37**, 142

52
Complications

G.A. PATTERSON

INTRODUCTION

In the 20 years preceding our first successful single lung transplant in 1983, there were approximately 45 such procedures performed worldwide without success (Chapter 45). We have now experienced success with single lung[1,2] and double lung[3] transplantation. Given the past history of lung transplantation, it is not surprising that this success has been accompanied by significant morbidity and mortality.

To date we have restricted the application of single lung transplants to those patients with pulmonary fibrosis (Chapter 46). We have performed 17 such procedures with four operative deaths and three late deaths. During the past 2 years we have employed double lung transplantation in patients with end-stage obstructive and septic lung disease, who have no clinical evidence of right ventricular failure (Chapter 46). There have been three postoperative deaths; no late deaths have occurred as yet.

The following discussion will outline our experience with complications of single and double lung transplantation under the broad categories of (1) intraoperative, (2) early, and (3) late complications. These patients are, of course, subject to all the general risks of organ transplantation, but in this chapter only those complications which are peculiar to isolated lung transplantation will be reviewed in detail.

INTRAOPERATIVE COMPLICATIONS

Ventilation

Induction

The anesthetic management of patients undergoing single lung transplantation has been discussed fully in Chapter 48. It can be emphasized, however, that the initiation of anesthesia and establishment of endotracheal positive pressure ventilation is hazardous. All patients subjected to single or double lung transplantation have required constant oxygen supplementation, often at high flow rates. It is critical that their oxygen supplementation be continued, and intubation expeditiously carried out, with the benefit of full hemodynamic monitoring.

Patients with obstructive lung disease present a particular problem during initiation of positive pressure ventilation. Indiscriminate application of positive pressure ventilation can result in air trapping, increased lung volume, and increased intrathoracic pressure, with resultant decreased venous return and cardiac output. We have experienced such a sequence of events in a patient who suffered a cardiac arrest following anesthetic induction for combined heart–lung transplantation. In patients with obstructive lung disease, institution of positive pressure ventilation must be carried out with the utmost care. Careful monitoring of airway pressure and systemic blood pressure is essential.

Maintenance

In general, the maintenance of satisfactory oxygenation and ventilation is not particularly difficult. However, single lung transplant recipients may pose a problem with regard to oxygenation at certain points during the operative procedure. It is our usual practice to perform single lung transplantation with the benefit of independent lung ventilation, made possible by a left-sided Robertshaw tube for right lung transplants, or an endobronchial blocking catheter for left lung transplants. If the initial dissection in the recipient (for pneumonectomy) is carried out with the lung deflated, a significant shunt may occur, which can produce severe hypoxemia. The shunt will be eliminated, of course, by clamping the ipsilateral pulmonary artery. This should, therefore, be performed early during the procedure if a significant shunt is present.

If the bronchial anastomosis has not already been performed, a shunt may occur after removal of the vascular clamps and restoration of pulmonary artery flow to the transplanted lung. In recent cases, therefore, we have completed the bronchial anastomosis before releasing the vascular clamps.

Cardiopulmonary bypass (CPB) is clearly required for all double lung transplants. At the time of writing, of our single lung transplants, four have been conducted with the benefit of partial femoral arteriovenous bypass (Chapter 48). In three of these patients, CPB was instituted because it was impossible to maintain satisfactory oxygenation on one lung. In one other patient with severe pulmonary hypertension, CPB was instituted because clamping of the ipsilateral pulmonary artery produced right ventricular distension and marked elevation of central venous pressure. In general, establishment of adequate venous drainage to maintain right heart decompression has been readily achieved by a single inferior vena caval cannula. In one instance a separate right atrioventricular vent was required to ensure satisfactory right heart decompression.

EARLY COMPLICATIONS

Hemorrhage

In our series to date, there has been no instance of postoperative hemorrhage requiring re-exploration following single lung transplantation. There are two explanations for this. The excellent exposure of the pleural space achieved through a generous posterolateral thoracotomy makes careful inspection of the entire operative field possible. Meticulous hemostasis can be achieved prior to chest closure. In addition, without the need for systemic heparinization and CPB for the majority of single lung transplants, significant hemorrhage should not occur.

Following double lung transplantation, however, we have had two patients who required re-exploration for hemorrhage. Both were bleeding from arteries in the posterior mediastinum, a difficult area to visualize following graft placement. In both cases hemorrhage was controlled by a second operative intervention.

The risk of hemorrhage is greater in patients who have undergone previous thoracotomy or trans-sternal operation[4]. Very few candidates for bilateral lung transplantation have extensive pleural scarring, the usual etiology of which is previous surgery. Careful investigation and the elimination of those who have such scarring, however, is essential if successful results are to be obtained. Routine use of computerized tomographic scanning in patients with bronchiectasis and cystic fibrosis has allowed more accurate assessment of pleural scarring, and has improved the selection of patients undergoing transplantation.

Previous surgery or the presence of pleural fibrosis does not influence our selection of patients requiring single lung transplantation. However, to minimize the difficulty of the dissection, we would elect to perform the transplant on the unaffected side.

Hypotension

Hypotension may, of course, result from blood loss, but we have also experienced prolonged decreased systemic vascular resistance in all patients undergoing double lung transplantation, despite adequate filling pressures, and normal or increased cardiac output and ventricular function. This peripheral vasodilation generally persists for 4–5 days, and during this time inotropic support is required. The etiology of this phenomenon remains uncertain, but may relate to a lack of angiotensin-converting enzyme in the donor lungs immediately following transplantation.

Poor graft function

While most lung transplant recipients show quite good immediate graft function, on several occasions we have seen a marked deterioration in function within the first 24 hours. Fortunately, this has usually proved to be a transient event, and has not been a significant clinical problem following double lung transplantation. Whether it occurs more frequently following single lung transplantation because cardiac output is preferentially delivered to the transplanted lung is not known.

Several possible explanations for this deterioration in function exist. The most likely is poor preservation of the graft. The longest ischemic period to which a single donor lung has been subjected is $5\frac{1}{2}$ hours, and significant early graft dysfunction was documented in this case. On the other hand, patients who have had relatively short ischemic times have also experienced difficulty with early graft function (Figures 52.1A and B). Until recently we did not employ vasodilators and pulmonary artery flush prior to donor lung extraction, but relied solely on topical hypothermia, with the lung immersed in EuroCollins solution (at 4°C). Other transplant centers have used different techniques for heart–lung graft preservation[5] (Chapter 35). Athough we have recently begun flushing the donor lung with EuroCollins at 4°C after the intravenous administration of prostaglandin E_1, we have not observed any major improvement in immediate graft function.

The interruption of the pulmonary lymphatic drainage is another possible etiology, although it is difficult to understand why the transected lymphatics do not drain into the pleural space at the hilum of the lung. Acute rejection is also an unlikely cause as these patients demonstrate a radiographic clearing of the infiltrate and improved oxygenation (on a lower inspired oxygen concentration) by application of positive end-expiratory pressure and diuresis.

Acute rejection

Clinical episodes of rejection are common following isolated lung transplantation; all of our patients have had at least

COMPLICATIONS

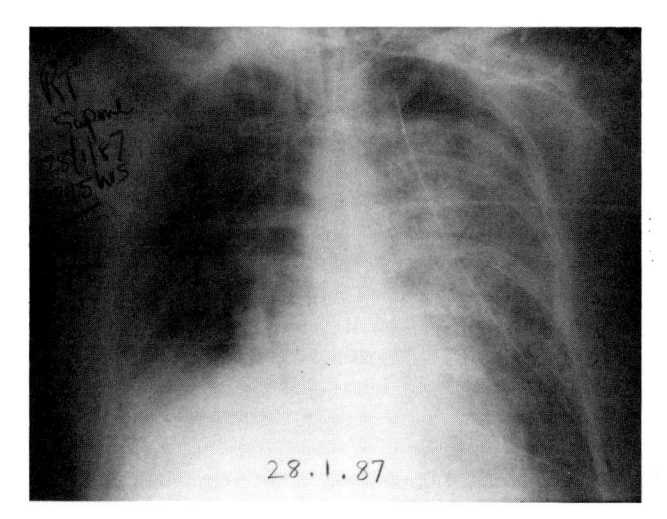

Figure 52.1A Anteroposterior chest roentgenogram showing a diffuse alveolar pattern associated with hypoxemia on the second day following left lung transplantation. The donor lung ischemic time was less than 3 hours

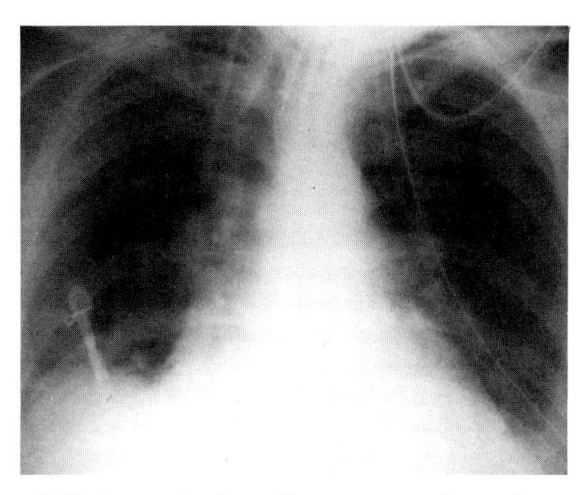

Figure 52.1B Improved radiographic appearance and gas exchange were noted by the sixth postoperative day. The patient had received positive end-expiratory pressure ventilation and vigorous diuresis only

one such episode. Unfortunately, the diagnosis of rejection has proved difficult. We have traditionally relied on clinical parameters to make this diagnosis. Patients typically experience a feeling of malaise, with moderate dyspnea. A low-grade fever is commonly present, as is a moderate elevation in white blood cell count. The chest radiograph generally demonstrates an alveolar pattern with blurring of the pericardial shadow at the hilum, or indeed a frank hilar 'flare' (Figure 52.2A). The PaO_2 is decreased. This clinical picture most typically occurs between the fifth and seventh postoperative day. Patients often have several rejection episodes spaced days or weeks apart. Each is treated by intravenous bolus methylprednisolone (10–15 mg/kg) on 3 successive days (Figure 52.2B).

Some centers have considerable experience with other, more objective, modalities in the diagnosis of rejection. Bronchoalveolar lavage[6], bronchial biopsy (Figure 52.3), transbronchial biopsy[7], and open lung biopsy (Figure 52.4) have all been used to improve the objectivity and accuracy of the diagnosis of rejection. We are gaining experience with these investigational techniques, but continue to rely heavily on the clinical features of rejection. Generally, patients respond to a single dose of methylprednisolone within 6 or 8 hours, at which time one is able to determine whether the diagnosis was correct.

Prolonged ventilation

A prolonged requirement (greater than 7 days) for mechanical ventilation is common following isolated lung transplan-

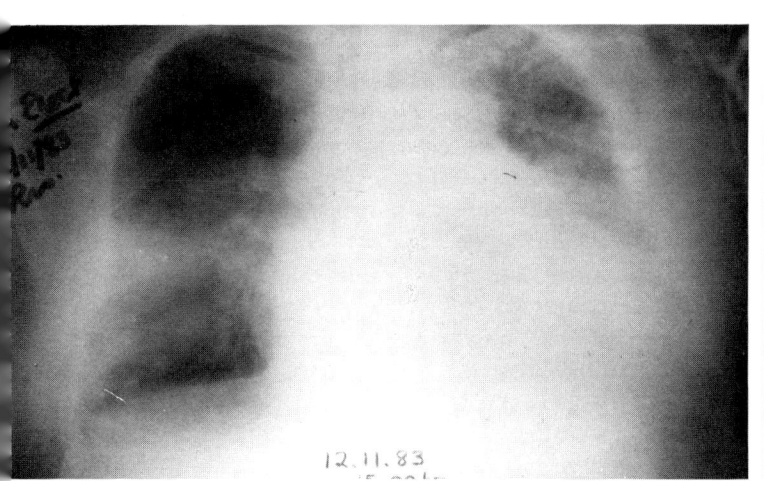

Figure 52.2A Anteroposterior chest roentgenogram from a patient with clinical features of acute rejection 5 days following right lung transplantation. Note the alveolar infiltrate and blurring of the right heart border

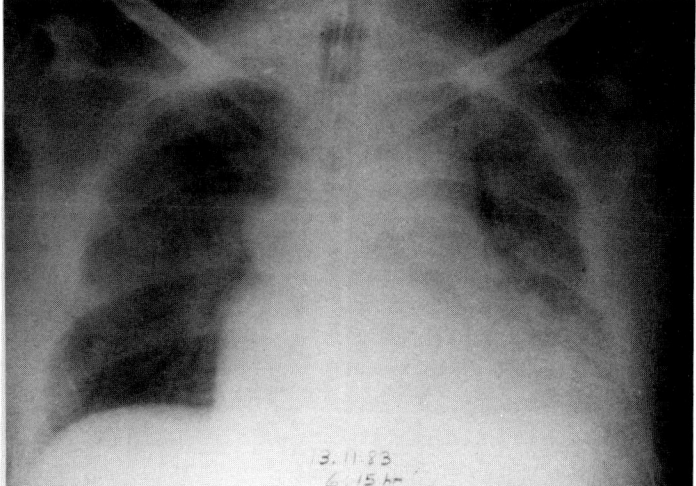

Figure 52.2B Marked resolution of the infiltrate is apparent 15 hours following the administration of 1 g methylprednisolone intravenously

401

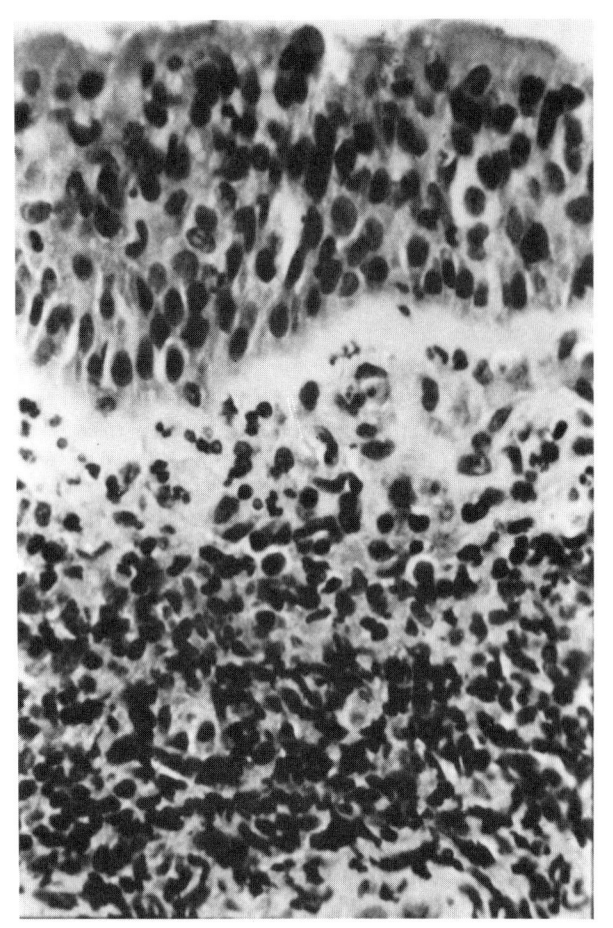

Figure 52.3 A bronchial biopsy from a patient with a clinical acute rejection episode. The extensive submucosal lymphocytic infiltrate resolved with augmentation of immunosuppressive therapy including intravenous methylprednisolone

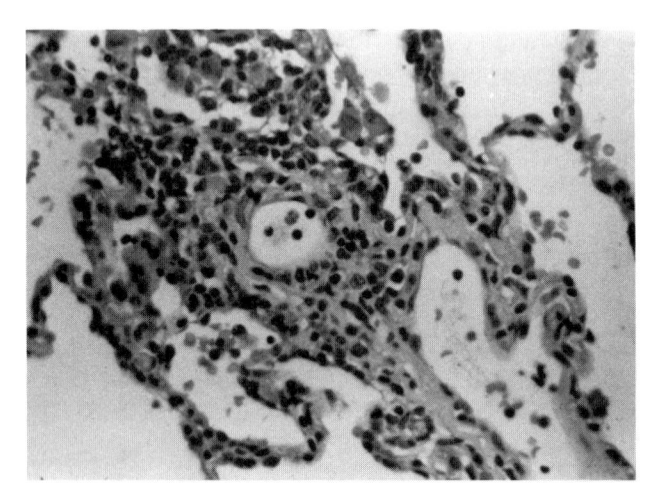

Figure 52.4 An operative lung biopsy from a patient with an undiagnosed pulmonary infiltrate on chest radiograph. The perivascular lymphocytic infiltrate is typical of lung rejection

tation. Four of our single lung recipients required ventilation for extended periods of time. Two of these four patients subsequently died, and two survived (one requiring tracheostomy) and are currently well. Among double lung recipients, five required prolonged ventilation; three died and two are currently well.

The pathogenesis of respiratory failure in these patients was varied, and included pneumonia (bacterial or viral), acute rejection, and adult respiratory distress syndrome resulting from sepsis. One patient received a single lung graft from a seemingly normal donor whose contralateral discarded lung showed histologic evidence of pulmonary hypertension. The recipient demonstrated persistent ventilation–perfusion mismatching as a result of decreased perfusion to the transplanted lung, and remained ventilator-dependent until his death from multisystem organ failure 5 weeks post-transplant.

Airway necrosis

Bronchial (or tracheal) wall necrosis was a common occurrence in early (pre-cyclosporine) clinical lung transplantation (Chapter 45). With the introduction of cyclosporine as the mainstay of immunosuppression, and thus the opportunity to avoid the use of corticosteroids in the early post-transplant period, healing of the bronchial anastomosis has become more reliable. In addition, the anastomotic omentopexy (Chapter 37), which we use routinely for both single and double lung transplantation, has provided a source of collateral circulation to the donor bronchus, and also provides protection against mediastinal sepsis should partial dehiscence occur.

We have observed two instances of bronchial disruption following single lung transplantation. The first patient experienced a partial disruption and developed a mediastinal cavity. With the omentum in place, this cavity eventually closed by granulation, leaving the patient with a chronic stricture which has been treated effectively by transbronchoscopic placement of an endobronchial silastic stent. The second patient experienced a bronchial dehiscence while requiring mechanical ventilation for multi-system organ failure 5 weeks following his transplant.

Predictably, airway necrosis has been a greater problem following double lung transplantation. The long donor airway, disconnected from its own arterial supply, is at increased risk of undergoing necrosis. Four instances of complete or partial airway necrosis have been documented. In three patients, necrosis extended from the tracheal anastomosis to the lobar bronchi bilaterally; two of these developed large mediastinal cavities at the site of airway separation (Figure 52.5), ultimately progressing to fatal tracheopulmonary artery fistulae.

Partial airway necrosis developed in one patient in the

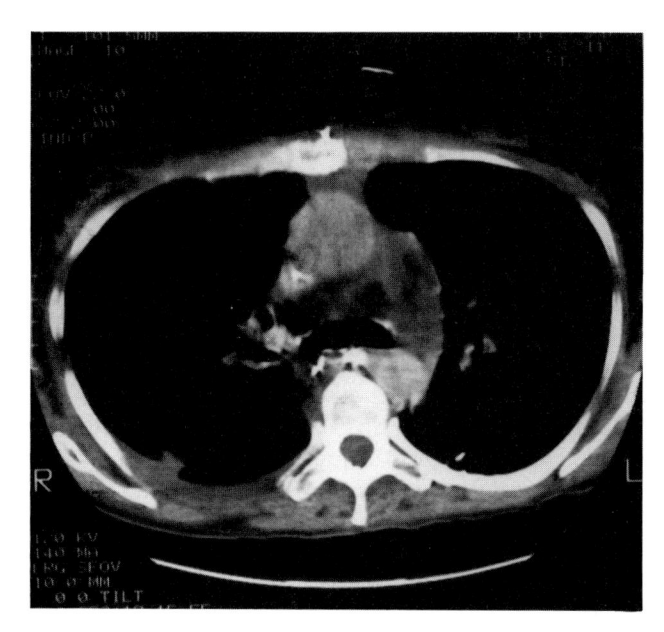

Figure 52.5 A computerized axial tomogram of the chest of a patient 2 weeks following double lung transplantation. Tracheobronchial necrosis was apparent endoscopically. The mediastinal cavity can be visualized anterolateral to the origin of the right main bronchus

anterolateral wall of the donor trachea. This defect healed by secondary intention, leaving the patient with a tracheal stricture, managed satisfactorily by endobronchial placement of a bifurcation stent (Figure 52.6). One further patient was retransplanted by heart–lung transplantation prior to actual dehiscence of his airway; in our urgency, we were forced to use a suboptimal heart–lung graft which never functioned adequately, and the patient died 2 days later.

Airway complications are likely to remain a problem following lung transplantation. The airway survives for the first several days by retrograde collateral flow from the pulmonary arterial circulation to the bronchial arterial circulation[8]. It is quite likely that a number of factors such as postoperative hypotension, poor lung preservation, rejection, or parenchymal infection, may result in a marked reduction in this retrograde collateral circulation and expose the long length of donor airway to ischemic necrosis. Whether prolonged mechanical ventilation with positive pressure and positive end-expiratory pressure contributes towards the development of necrosis is not known. It is likely, however, that the underlying condition(s) for which mechanical ventilation is required is more important in contributing to the interruption of the bronchial circulation than mechanical ventilation itself.

Infection

Lung transplant recipients are at risk of parenchymal infection during the early postoperative period. A variety

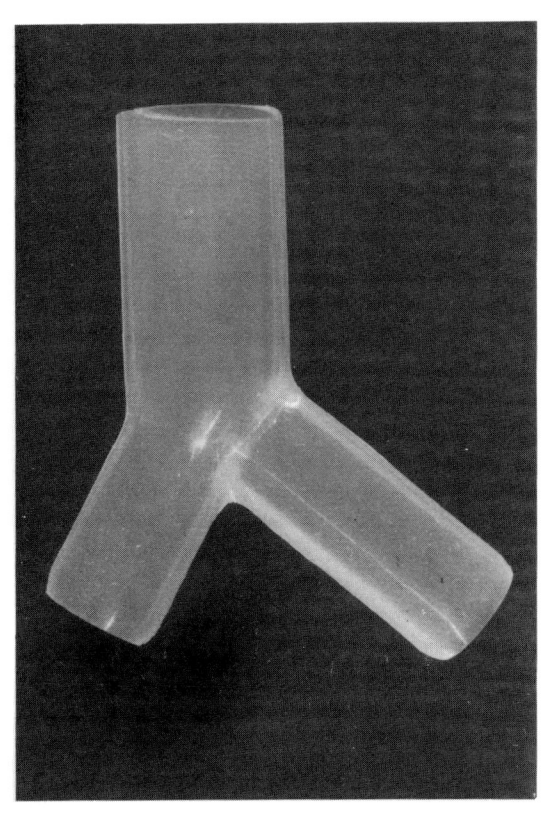

Figure 52.6 The silastic bifurcation stent used in three recipients of double lung transplants. The limbs of the stent can be easily trimmed to the desired length. The stent is placed over a 6 mm rigid bronchoscope. The stent is well tolerated by the patient, and kept patent and clean by twice daily use of N-acetylcysteine inhalation

of organisms are commonly isolated from the donor and/or recipient airways. It is our usual practice to employ antibiotics for those organisms cultured from the recipient or donor lung at the time of transplantation. In patients with negative cultures from both donor and recipient, we have elected to administer a second generation cephalosporin as prophylaxis for several days. Nonetheless, we have experienced significant bacterial infection in several patients. A progressive Gram-negative pneumonia proved fatal, as did an early viral pneumonia.

We have had only one instance of a cytomegalovirus (CMV) pneumonia occurring during the early postoperative period, and this was treated successfully. We employ prophylactic acyclovir and CMV hyperimmune globulin in CMV-negative recipients receiving CMV-positive donor lungs.

Psychiatric

Our program has benefitted from a close working relationship with the psychiatric staff in our institution, who have identified postoperative delirium in several patients undergoing lung transplantation[9]. We have subsequently instituted a program of prophylactic low-dose haloperidol

(1–2 mg intravenously 4–6 hourly). This has markedly reduced the incidence of delirium, and has resulted in more rapid weaning from mechanical ventilation and earlier discharge from the Intensive Care Unit.

Air embolism

Venous air embolism has occurred in three of our single lung transplant recipients, on each occasion associated with manipulation of a central venous line. Patients with pulmonary fibrosis and marked restrictive lung disease are capable of generating significant negative intrathoracic pressure.

One patient suffered air embolism during the preoperative insertion of a Swan–Ganz catheter; several hours later, during the conduct of a single lung transplant, which until that point in time had been fairly uneventful, the patient developed all of the manifestations of air embolism, including pulmonary edema and severe hypoxemia. Another experienced a venous air embolus during change of a central line several days after operation; this necessitated reinstitution of mechanical ventilation until the pulmonary edema had resolved. One final patient experienced a fatal air embolus minutes after removal of a central venous line on the tenth postoperative day.

LATE COMPLICATIONS

Airway stenosis

We have observed late airway stenosis following both single and double lung transplantation. A recipient of a single lung, whose airway initially healed without problem, developed a stenosis at the bronchial anastomosis which became manifest 3 months post-transplant. She has subsequently been managed by bronchial dilation and placement of an endobronchial silastic stent.

Two patients have developed late tracheobronchial stenosis following double lung transplantation. In both, initial airway healing was excellent, with no evidence of ischemia or dehiscence. However, both presented between 3 and 4 months later with symptoms of dyspnea and decreased measured flow rates. At bronchoscopy, a circumferential stricture was noted at the site of the tracheal anastomosis, as was a circumferential web-like stricture 1 cm distal to the origin of the left main bronchus. These latter strictures contained no cartilaginous supportive tissue.

We postulate that such strictures are ischemic in origin, and occur in a watershed zone between the retrograde pulmonary artery–bronchial artery circulation and the antegrade collateral circulation arising from the tracheal omentopexy. This, of course, does not explain the late development of the tracheal component of the stricture. Management by rigid bronchoscopic dilation and placement of silastic endobronchial bifurcation stents has been successful in both cases.

Infection

Lung transplant recipients remain at risk from a variety of parenchymal pulmonary infections. We have observed a small number of Gram-negative and Gram-positive parenchymal infections many months after transplantation. A good response has been obtained from appropriate antibiotic therapy. *Pneumocystis carinii* pneumonia and CMV pneumonia have both contributed to death many months after transplantation in recipients of single lungs. Two of our patients have developed disseminated herpes zoster infections late after transplantation, but both responded well to acyclovir therapy. A double lung recipient developed *Mycobacterium hominis* infection many months after transplantation and remains on triple antituberculous drug therapy.

Lymphoproliferative disorders

While not a specific complication of lung transplantation, a number of hematologic complications has occurred. The most significant was a B-cell lymphoma which developed in a young man 5 months after single lung transplantation. The Pittsburgh Group[10] has reported resolution of such lymphoproliferative disorders following withdrawal of immunosuppressive drug therapy. Unfortunately, reduction of immunosuppressive therapy had no effect in this patient, and, although he underwent intensive chemotherapy and contralateral pneumonectomy, his tumor progressed rapidly, and he died with disseminated disease within a month of the initiation of therapy.

Chronic rejection

Persistent chronic rejection has been a problem in only one patient (Figures 52.7 and 52.8). The diagnosis was confirmed by histological examination of two open lung biopsies performed several months apart. While there was evidence of perivascular and peribronchial inflammation in these biopsies, there was no histological evidence of airway obstruction even in the later biopsy. Augmentation of immunosuppression has not improved his clinical course, and he is currently awaiting retransplantation. As yet we have not observed clinical or histological bronchiolitis obliterans in any patient following isolated lung transplantation (as we and other groups have observed following combined heart–lung transplantation).

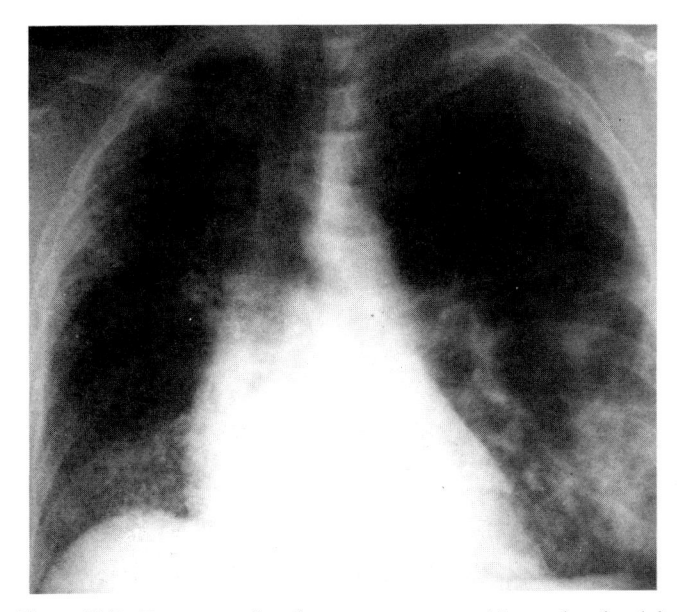

Figure 52.7 Posteroanterior chest roentgenogram 15 months after left lung transplantation. The diffuse lower lobe infiltrate (and deteriorating gas exchange) prompted open lung biopsy of the affected area on two occasions. Histological examination of both biopsies showed features consistent with chronic rejection without airway obstruction

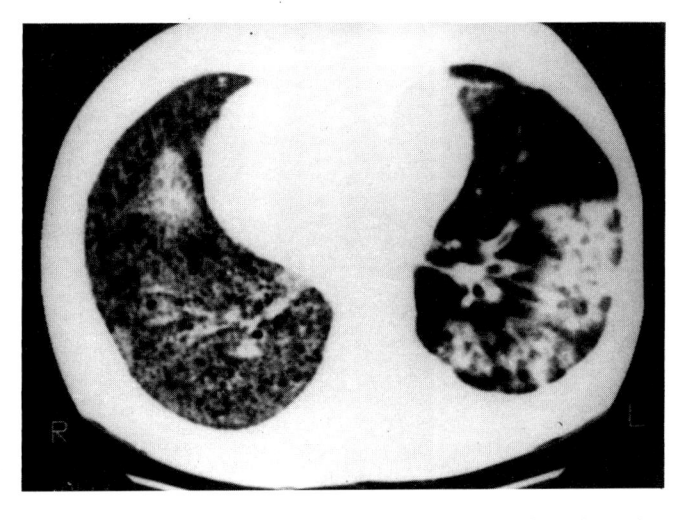

Figure 52.8 A computerized axial tomogram of the chest from the patient whose chest roentgenogram is shown in Figure 52.7. Note the patchy consolidation of the left lower lobe and the severe fibrosis and 'honeycombing' in the native right lung

COMMENT

Despite the success of our clinical lung transplant program, we have had major complications resulting in significant mortality and morbidity. A significant contributory factor, however, may be the advanced state of the underlying disease process at the time of transplantation in our recipients, all of whom were judged likely to die within a year if transplantation were not performed.

References

1. The Toronto Lung Transplant Group (1986). Unilateral lung transplantation for pulmonary fibrosis. *N. Engl. J. Med.*, **314**, 1140
2. The Toronto Lung Transplant Group (1988). Experience with single lung transplantation for pulmonary fibrosis. *J. Am. Med. Assoc.*, **259**, 2258
3. Patterson, G.A., Cooper, J.D., Goldman, B., Wiesel, R.D., Pearson, F.G., Waters, P.F., Todd, T.R., Scully, H., Goldberg, M. and Ginsberg, R.J. (1988). Technique of successful clinical double lung transplantation. *Ann. Thorac. Surg.*, **45**, 626
4. Griffith, B.P., Hardesty, R.L., Trento, A., Paradis, I.J., Duquesnoy, R.J., Zeevi, A., Dauber, J.H., Dummer, J.S., Thompson, M.E., Gryzan, S. and Bahnson, H.T. (1987). Heart–lung transplantation: lessons learned and future hopes. *Ann. Thorac. Surg.*, **43**, 6
5. Harjula, A., Baldwin, J.C., Starnes, V.A., Stinson, E.B., Oyer, P.E., Jamieson, S.W. and Shumway, N.E. (1987). Proper donor selection for heart–lung transplantation. *J. Thorac. Cardiovasc. Surg.*, **94**, 874
6. Paradis, I.L., Zeevi, A., Duquesnoy, R., Griffith, B.P., Hardesty, R.L., Kormos, R., Yousem, S. and Dauber, J.H. (1988). Immunologic risk factors for human chronic lung rejection. *Am. Rev. Respir. Dis.*, **137**, 46
7. Higenbottam, T.W., Stewart, S., Penketh, A. and Wallwork, J. (1987). Diagnosis of lung rejection and opportunistic infection by transbronchial lung biopsy. *Transplant. Proc.*, **19**, 3777
8. Ladowski, J.S., Hardesty, R.L. and Griffith, B.P. (1984). Pulmonary artery blood supply to the supracarinal trachea. *J. Heart Transplant.*, **4**, 40
9. Craven, J.L. and the Toronto Lung Transplant Group (1990). Postoperative organic mental syndromes in lung transplant recipients. *J. Heart Transplant.*, In press
10. Starzl, T.E., Nalesnic, M.A., Porter, K.A., Ho, M., Iwatsuki, S., Griffith, B.P., Rosenthal, J.T., Hakala, T.R., Shaw, B.W. Jr., Hardesty, R.L., Atchison, R.W., Jaffe, R. and Bahnson, H.T. (1984). Reversibility of lymphomas and lymphoproliferative lesions developing under cyclosporin–steroid therapy. *Lancet*, **1**, 583

53
Results of Lung Transplantation

D.K.C. COOPER, G.A. PATTERSON AND J.D. COOPER

INTRODUCTION

Lung transplantation remains in its formative stages; there is still little experience worldwide, and few reported series. Information regarding lung transplantation is beginning to be accumulated by the International Society for Heart Transplantation Registry[1]. To date, the Registry has received data on 33 single and 18 double lung transplant patients. Patient age ranged from 8 to 45 years, with a mean of 26 years. Of these, 61% were male. Mean donor age has been 27 years, with a range from 14 to 48 years.

The actuarial survival for the 51 patients was 70% at 1 month and 54% at 1 year (Figure 53.1).

To date, the only individual group with significant experience is the Toronto Lung Transplant Group[2-7].

SINGLE LUNG TRANSPLANTATION

Between November 1983 and June 1988, 16 single lung transplants were performed at the Toronto General Hospital[2], the first being on 7th November, 1983[3]. There were four in-hospital deaths. There were no deaths related to bronchial complications. Of the 12 surviving patients, two developed late bronchial stenosis, which were both managed by dilation and endoscopic implantation of a silicone stent. The longest survivor remains alive and well over 5 years since transplantation.

Of the first 11 cases, of which more detailed information is available[4], there were two early deaths – from inadequate donor lung function in one case, and from unrelated air embolism through a central venous cannula in the other. Ventilatory support in the other nine patients was required for 3–10 days (mean 5.5 days), the patients' stay in the intensive care unit was for a mean of 9.5 days, supplemental oxygen was required for up to 21 days, and hospital stay was for a mean of 41 days.

In this group, there were two late deaths at 7 and 18 months from persistent pulmonary rejection, in one case associated with the presence of antibodies in the recipient against donor lymphocytes (positive lymphocytotoxic crossmatch), which was not known until after the operation had been performed. However, there was no evidence of bronchiolitis obliterans found at autopsy in either case, contrary to the experience with the combined heart–lung transplant. One of the remaining survivors died at 8 months from a lymphoma.

Vital capacity, forced expiratory volume in 1 second, and diffusing capacity of carbon monoxide are all considerably improved in the surviving patients, and the PaO_2 on room air 3 months after transplantation was in excess of 85 mmHg. Lung perfusion scans demonstrated that blood flow to the transplanted lung increased with time, from a mean of 66% at 7 days after surgery to 72% at 3 weeks.

Seven of the nine long-term survivors have normal bronchoscopic findings. Two patients developed complications of the airway. In one, stenosis of the bronchial anastomosis developed at 3 months and has required endoscopic placement of a short silicone rubber stent into the left main bronchus; this has been in place for over 3 years without further complication. A second patient, who

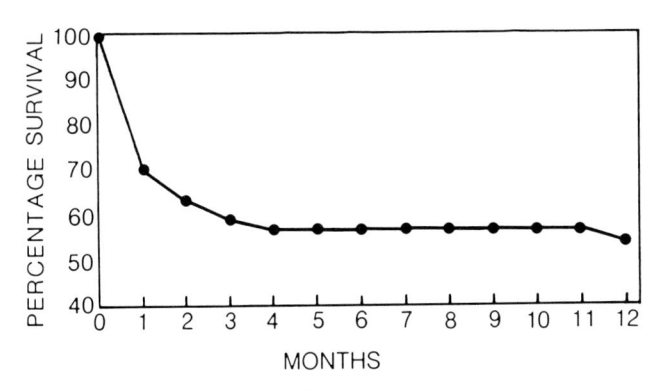

Figure 53.1 Actuarial survival of patients undergoing single or double lung transplantation as reported to the International Society for Heart Transplantation Registry (Heck *et al.*[1])

had received a prolonged course of bolus methylprednisolone therapy for rejection episodes, developed necrosis and dehiscence of the medial half of the bronchial anastomosis 3 weeks after transplantation. This did not become apparent clinically, presumably because the omental flap surrounding the anastomosis had sealed off the area. A silicone stent was placed in the bronchus and remained in place until the patient died from persistent pulmonary rejection at 18 months.

DOUBLE LUNG TRANSPLANTATION

The first patient who underwent this procedure (on 26 November, 1986) at Toronto General Hospital[5] remains alive and well over 3 years later, though she developed a stenosis of the left main bronchus which has been stented with a Y-shaped prosthesis inserted endoscopically. Eight of the first nine patients survived and were discharged home from hospital, though there have been a number of complications[2,6,7]. Of the total number of patients, 25% have died of tracheal complications, and 20% have developed airway stenosis.

More detailed information has been reported on the first six patients to undergo this procedure[6,7]. In this group, operative time averaged 5 hours, with total cardiopulmonary bypass time ranging from 149 to 217 minutes, and aortic cross-clamp time from 33 to 52 minutes. After operation, in all patients there was a decrease in right ventricular volume and increase in ejection fraction as a result of a decrease in right ventricular afterload. Adequate postoperative gas exchange was uniformly present.

Of the initial nine double lung recipients in the Toronto experience, one died of airway necrosis which involved the trachea and main bronchi, and was apparent by the second postoperative day. Its occurrence was almost certainly related to the presence of a low perfusion pressure after being weaned from cardiopulmonary bypass, requiring massive vasoconstrictor drug support. Retransplantation, using a less-than-ideal heart–lung donor block, was attempted on the 11th postoperative day, but inadequate donor function was obtained and the patient died 2 days later.

Two other recipients developed late stenosis of the distal trachea, which also involved the left main bronchus in one of the patients. Both were treated satisfactorily with a bifurcation silicone prosthesis which was inserted endoscopically[2]. One patient died of a pseudomonas pneumonia 10 months after transplant. At the present time, seven of the original nine double lung transplant recipients remain alive and well from 12 to 27 months following transplantation.

COMMENT

The Toronto group believes that several factors have been important in obtaining successth these two operative procedures These include (1) strict criteria for selecting transplant recipients, (2) a structured and vigorous preoperative rehabilitation program that increases the patient's exercise performance and his ability to withstand the rigors of the transplant procedure and the early postoperative course, (3) the use of the omentum to protect and revascularize the bronchial anastomosis, and (4) the avoidance of routine corticosteroid therapy in the initial 2–3 weeks.

At the present time, the Toronto group favors the single lung transplant for patients with pulmonary fibrosis, double lung transplantation for those with emphysema or cystic fibrosis when right ventricular function is preserved, and combined heart–lung transplantation for patients who have a combination of pulmonary hypertension and irreversible right-sided heart failure. In recent months, success has been reported from several centers with single lung transplantation for emphysema. Whether single or double lung transplantation may eventually prove successful in patients with primary pulmonary hypertension who have not yet developed irreversible right-sided heart failure remains uncertain. Single or double lung transplantation has the great advantage of allowing the donor heart to be used in a second recipient.

Selection of patients for double lung transplantation, in particular, can be difficult, especially with regard to assessment of right ventricular function. This group believes that a patient in whom right ventricular contractility is preserved, despite a low ejection fraction induced by right ventricular dilation, will have an excellent result following double lung transplantation. Those in whom right ventricular fibrosis or persistent right ventricular dysfunction has been documented would not be suitable for this procedure.

Assurance of an adequate tracheal blood supply in all patients undergoing double lung transplantation clearly remains a significant problem. A low early post-transplant perfusion pressure is likely to be a contributing factor towards an inadequate tracheal blood supply, as may be the use of vasconstrictor drugs, but the absence of the bronchial artery circulation is thought to be important, as may be the absence of tracheo-bronchial collaterals that arise from the coronary network; further experimental work may indicate the incorporation of a technique for directly reconnecting the bronchial artery circulation at the time of transplantation. An alternative approach, namely bilateral single lung transplantation with anastomoses of the airway at the bronchial level, has recently given encouraging results and may prove the technique of choice.

Several more years' experience is required before the role of single and double lung transplantation can be fully evaluated for end-stage lung disease. In the meantime, however, it is hoped that these new procedures will play an important role in providing a therapeutic option for patients with terminal pulmonary parenchymal pathology. The initial results would suggest that there is a definite role for single lung transplantation in patients with pulmonary fibrosis. Whether the problems at present inherent in double lung transplantation can be overcome remains less certain, but it is hoped that they can. The procedure may then be preferred to heart–lung transplantation in carefully selected patients, and will allow the donor heart to be used in a second recipient.

References

1. Heck, C.F., Shumway, S.J. and Kaye, M.P. (1989). The Registry of the International Society for Heart Transplantation: sixth official report – 1989. *J. Heart Transplant.*, **8**, 271
2. Cooper, J.D. (1989). Lung transplantation. *Ann. Thorac. Surg.*, **47**, 28
3. The Toronto Lung Transplant Group (1986). Unilateral lung transplantation for pulmonary fibrosis. *N. Engl. J. Med.*, **314**, 1140
4. The Toronto Lung Transplant Group (1988). Experience with single-lung transplantation for pulmonary fibrosis. *J. Am. Med. Assoc.*, **259**, 2258
5. Patterson, G.A., Cooper, J.D., Dark, J.H., Jones, M.T. and The Toronto Lung Transplant Group (1988). Experimental and clinical double lung transplantation. *J. Thorac. Cardiovasc. Surg.*, **95**, 70
6. Patterson, G.A., Cooper, J.D., Goldman, B., Weisel, R.D., Pearson, F.G., Waters, P.F., Todd, T.R., Scully, H., Goldberg, M. and Ginsberg, R.J. (1988). Technique of successful clinical double-lung transplantation. *Ann. Thorac. Surg.*, **45**, 626
7. Cooper, J.D., Patterson, G.A., Grossman, R., Maurer, J. and The Toronto Lung Transplant Group (1989). Double-lung transplant for advanced chronic obstructive lung disease. *Am. Rev. Resp. Dis.*, **139**, 303

Section IV

The role of mechanical support devices in cardiac transplantation

54
Indications and Selection of Cardiac Support Device

D.G. PENNINGTON AND M.T. SWARTZ

INTRODUCTION

Approximately 20% of patients awaiting cardiac transplantation die before a donor heart is located[1]. These patients may benefit from mechanical circulatory support as a temporary measure until a donor heart is found. Circulatory support systems comprise a broad range of devices, from simple roller pumps to electrically-powered implantable hearts. It is becoming increasingly clear that there are specific indications for each type of device. Major cardiac centers performing transplantation may require access to more than one form of device so that the most suitable can be used for each individual patient.

INDICATIONS AND PATIENT SELECTION

Patient selection is the most important factor relating to survival[2]. The generally accepted hemodynamic criteria for application of an assist device are shown in Table 54.1. Patients who meet these hemodynamic criteria should be excluded if they have renal failure (blood urea nitrogen greater than 100 mg/dl (35.5 mmol/l) and serum creatinine greater than 5.0 mg/dl (440 μmol/l)), sepsis, neurologic deficit, or any other condition that would preclude cardiac transplantation. In general, younger patients make better candidates for the use of such devices, and those over 60 years should probably be excluded.

Although patients in cardiogenic shock after open heart surgery or following acute myocardial infarction may be suitable candidates for temporary assist by such a device (when myocardial recovery is anticipated), this chapter will concentrate only on those patients who are being supported as a bridge to cardiac transplantation.

AVAILABLE DEVICES (Table 54.2)

External centrifugal pumps

External pumps are positioned outside the body and connect to the cardiac chambers by cannulae. Centrifugal pumps rely on centrifugal force to propel blood through non-occlusive pump heads, and therefore are generally non-traumatic, though hemolysis may become a problem if the device is used for more than a few days. They do not provide pulsatile flow, though this is not essential. Frequently, the centrifugal pump is used in collaboration with an intra-

Table 54.1 Criteria for insertion of cardiac assist device

(1)	Cardiac index < 1.8–2.0 l/min per m²
(2)	Systolic blood pressure < 90 mmHg (or mean arterial < 60 mmHg)
(3)	Left atrial (or pulmonary capillary wedge) and/or right atrial pressure > 20–25 mmHg
(4)	Urine output < 20 ml/hour (in adults)
(5)	Systemic vascular resistance > 2100 dynes s cm⁻⁵
(6)	Trial of volume infusion, maximal pharmacologic (vasopressor and vasodilator) support, and intra-aortic balloon counterpulsation (if vascular access permits) without adequate improvement of ventricular function
(7)	Other signs of poor perfusion (e.g. metabolic acidosis, decreased mentation) may be present
(8)	If the cardiac assist device is intended as a bridge to transplantation, then clearly the patient must be acceptable as a candidate for cardiac transplantation

Table 54.2 Available devices

Centrifugal pumps
  Biomedicus
  Sarns-Centrimed

External pulsatile VADS
  Thoratec
  Symbion
  Abiomed

ECMO
  Bard System
  Datascope ECMO (Phillips)
  St. Louis University System

Internal electrical LVAS
  Novacor

Orthotopic biventricular replacement device (TAH)
  Symbion Jarvik-7

---

aortic balloon pump (which may have been inserted previously), which provides a pulse.

Left heart support is accomplished by cannulae in the left atrium or left ventricle, with infusion into the aorta. Right heart support is accomplished by cannulae in the right atrium and pulmonary artery. These devices have three major limitations: (1) the need for anticoagulants, (2) the slight tendency to hemolyze at high flows, and (3), in general, they can be used only for periods of up to 7–10 days, although successful support for 30 days has been documented[3]. These limitations make them most suitable for short-term use in patients whose myocardium is expected to recover within a few days.

Of the devices available, the Biomedicus centrifugal pump has had wide application as a ventricular support device for periods of several days (Chapter 55). It can be connected to the patient by various cannula systems that have not been standardized. Some investigators have used it without anticoagulants[4], while others have employed a continuous heparin infusion as soon as bleeding has been controlled[5]. The device is easy to insert and can be used for left or right heart support.

The Sarns-Centrimed pump requires anticoagulation therapy and functions in a manner similar to the Biomedicus pump.

Pulsatile external ventricular assist devices

Pulsatile external ventricular assist devices (VADs) are pneumatically driven, sac-type, external pumps that lie on the abdomen or chest wall, and are connected to the patient by cannulae placed in the left or right side of the heart. The Pierce–Donachy (Thoratec) VAD is the most commonly used (Chapter 56). It does not require anticoagulation with heparin if used for less than 1 week, and, at high flow rates, is relatively safe in terms of thromboembolism. At lower flow rates (less than 3 l/min), or when the device is to be used for longer than 1 week, anticoagulation is recommended[6]. Sites of cannulation are the same as for the centrifugal pumps, although left ventricular cannulation is preferred in patients with large dilated left ventricles. We prefer atrial cannulation in patients with small left ventricles. One pump can be employed to support the left (LVAD) or right (RVAD) ventricle, or two pumps can be inserted to provide biventricular (BVAD) support. It may be difficult to insert such a device in patients with a heavily calcified ascending aorta and in small patients whose cardiac chambers are not large enough to receive the cannulae. This type of device allows the patient a moderate degree of mobility. When compared with the external centrifugal pumps, external pulsatile VADs are better suited for the longer periods of circulatory support that may be necessary in successfully bridging a patient to transplantation[6,7].

Extracorporeal membrane oxygenation

Extracorporeal membrane oxygenation (ECMO) is designed to provide temporary ventricular support for patients in severe cardiogenic shock or oxygenation for those with pulmonary failure[8]. The system consists of a membrane oxygenator connected to a heat exchanger and a roller pump or centrifugal pump system. The pump can be connected to the patient by femoral cannulae, which are placed in the proximal and distal artery and vein, or it can be inserted through a sternotomy to provide right atrial to aortic bypass. Continual heparinization and constant surveillance by a cardiopulmonary perfusionist are essential, whereas the centrifugal pump or VAD can be managed largely by the nursing staff. ECMO is best suited for use as an acute resuscitative measure as the system can be set up quickly. There is generally a high complication rate (e.g. bleeding) if used for more than 48 hours.

Electrically-powered implantable left ventricular assist systems

Left ventricular assist systems (LVAS) are being developed for permanent implantation, but several have been adapted for temporary use. The Novacor system consists of a balanced solenoid energy converter, dual pusher plate sac-type blood pump (Figure 54.1), and a microprocessor-based control/monitoring console. Electrical energy is converted to mechanical energy that is used to eject blood from the smooth-surfaced blood pump. Conduits connecting the pump to the heart allow blood flow from the left ventricular apex through the pump to the ascending aorta. For temporary use, an external electrical driveline is brought out through the abdominal wall to provide a power source and an air vent. The device can be synchronized to the patient's own ventricular function. Its limitations are (1) it requires anticoagulation, (2) it can only be connected to the left

CARDIAC SUPPORT DEVICES

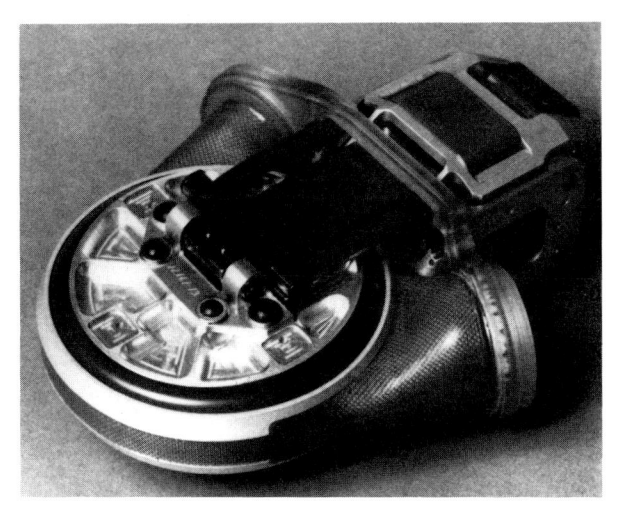

Figure 54.1 Unencapsulated Novacor left ventricular assist device

ventricular apex and is therefore not appropriate for left or right atrial use, and (3) if severe right ventricular failure occurs, another type of pump is required to support the right ventricle; this latter limitation is a major disadvantage of the system. In spite of this limitation, it has been very effective in maintaining patients for long periods (up to 90 days) prior to cardiac transplantation[7].

Orthotopic biventricular replacement prosthesis – the total artificial heart (TAH)

The Symbion Jarvik TAH consists of pneumatic sac-type biventricular prosthetic devices that can be sutured to the atria (Chapter 57). It requires the use of continuous anticoagulation and platelet-deaggregating drugs. Prolonged use has been associated with a moderately high incidence of thromboembolic complications[9] and mediastinitis[10]. It allows mobility of the patient awaiting a donor heart, and may be indicated in patients with irreversible biventricular injury, or in patients with thrombus in the ventricles.

PATIENT CATEGORIES

Postcardiotomy ventricular failure

If there is any possibility that the damaged myocardium may recover, an external VAD for left, right, or both sides is indicated. If recovery is not expected, due to either extensive previous myocardial damage or a large perioperative myocardial infarction[11], a BVAD or TAH may be indicated. Alternatively, if the patient has only isolated left ventricular failure, a LVAS may be implanted. A centrifugal pump should only be used if recovery is expected within a short period of time (less than 7 days), and transplantation is not expected to be necessary. ECMO is contraindicated in most adult postcardiotomy heart failure patients, and should be used only as a resuscitative technique.

Acute myocardial infarction

Rapid resuscitation and support can be obtained using femoro-femoral ECMO. This allows time for full assessment to insure that the patient is a suitable candidate for cardiac transplantation. Once stabilized with ECMO, another system, such as a VAD, LVAS, or TAH, can be inserted.

Deteriorating patients already awaiting transplantation

Patients in whom sudden deterioration occurs with the development of cardiogenic shock can be immediately stabilized and resuscitated with an ECMO circuit, which provides time for further evaluation of the candidate. ECMO is necessary if pharmacological agents and intra-aortic balloon pumping are unsuccessful and the patient is rapidly deteriorating. If ECMO has been initiated in a patient with irreversible heart failure, and it subsequently becomes clear that the patient is not a cardiac transplant candidate, the patient should not be transferred to another device.

Deteriorating patients with severe biventricular failure may be supported with a BVAD or a TAH. The BVADs have the advantage that they can be withdrawn if recovery of the heart occurs (though this is unlikely in patients awaiting transplantation). The TAH has the advantage of having been designed for long-term use. If left ventricular failure alone has occurred, the LVAS is preferable, since the device is designed for long-term use, and offers the theoretical advantage of allowing for heart recovery.

CLINICAL RESULTS AT ST. LOUIS UNIVERSITY

Experience over the last 10 years at St. Louis University has shown that survival of postcardiotomy patients supported with Thoratec VADs is 37%[6]. Survival in adults following ECMO or centrifugal pump support is poor. However, many of these patients were not candidates for the more sophisticated devices because of older age or vital organ dysfunction. We now recognize the inappropriateness of ECMO for postcardiotomy adult patients.

Cardiac transplantation has been performed in ten patients who were supported with various devices (ECMO, $n = 2$; Pierce–Donachy VAD, $n = 6$; Novacor LVAS, $n = 2$). Both patients supported pretransplant by ECMO died, and we now believe that ECMO should not be continued for more than 24 hours in cardiac transplant candidates; after this period of time another device should be used. The remaining eight patients had successful transplants, and proved the effectiveness of the devices used.

Our success with the Pierce–Donachy Thoratec VAD encourages us to continue the use of this system. Many patients, however, require long periods of support, and may be better served by the implantable devices, though we have supported two patients with BVADs for 75 and 81 days respectively, before successful cardiac transplantation.

COMMENT

More than one device will be needed in almost every center carrying out cardiac transplantation. An acute resuscitative device such as femoro-femoral ECMO is essential to salvage patients with cardiogenic shock following acute myocardial infarction. Some type of external device that can be implanted in postcardiotomy patients, such as the Thoratec VAD, is also essential. Centrifugal pumps, though less satisfactory for long-term support, may also play a role in this patient group. In patients who are definitely awaiting cardiac transplantation, and who may require support for several weeks or months, an implantable LVAS or TAH may be preferable. Further experience in the use of mechanical assist devices and the TAH, such as that presented in the following four chapters, will help to clarify the role of each type of support system in the care of patients being assessed for and awaiting cardiac transplantation.

References

1. Copeland, J.G., Emery, R.W., Levinson, M.M., Copeland, J., McAleer, M.J. and Riley, J.E (1985). The role of mechanical support and transplantation in treatment of patients with end-stage cardiomyopathy. *Circulation*, **72**, (Cardiovascular Surgery Suppl. 2), 7
2. Pennington, D.G. and Swartz, M.T (1988). Selection of circulatory support devices. *Heart Failure*, **4**, 5
3. Golding, L.A.R., Stewart, R.W., Sinkewich, M., Smith, W. and Cosgrove, D.M. (1988). Nonpulsatile ventricular assist bridging to transplantation. *Trans. Am. Soc. Artif. Intern. Organs.*, **34**, 476
4. Park, S.B., Liebler, G.A., Burkholder, J.A., Maher, T.D., Benckart, D.H., Magovern, G.J. Jr., Christlieb, I.Y., Kao, R.L. and Magovern, G.J. Sr. (1986). Mechanical support of the failing heart. *Ann. Thorac. Surg.*, **42**, 627
5. Pennington, D.G., Merjavy, J.P., Codd, J.E., Swartz, M.T. and Willman, V.L. (1985). Temporary mechanical support of patients with profound ventricular failure. In Unger, F. (ed.) *Assisted Circulation 2*. (New York: Academic Press)
6. Pennington, D.G., Kanter, K.R., McBride, L.R. *et al.* (1988). Seven years experience with the Pierce Donachy ventricular assist device. *J. Thorac. Cardiovasc. Surg.*, **96**, 901
7. Pennington, D.G., McBride, L.R., Kanter, K.R. *et al.* (1989). Bridging to cardiac transplantation with circulatory support devices. *J. Heart Transplant.*, **8**, 116
8. Pennington, D.G., Merjavy, J.P., Codd, J.E., Swartz, M.T., Miller, L.L. and Williams, G.A. (1984). Extracorporeal membrane oxygenation for patients with cardiogenic shock. *Circulation*, **70** (3, part 2), I, 130
9. Joyce, L.B., Johnson, K.E., Pierce, W.S., Devries, W.C., Semb, B.K.H., Copeland, J.G., Griffith, B.P., Cooley, D.A., Frazier, O.H., Cabrol, C., Keon, W.J., Unger, F., Bucherl, E.S. and Wolner, E. (1986). Summary of world experience with clinical use of total artificial hearts as heart support devices. *J. Heart Transplant.*, **5**, 229
10. Griffith, B.P., Kormos, R.L., Hardesty, R.L., Armitage, J.M. and Dummer, J.S. (1988). The artificial heart: infection-related morbidity and its effect on transplantation. *Ann. Thorac. Surg.*, **45**, 409
11. Pennington, D.G., McBride, L.R., Kanter, K.R., Swartz, M.T., Lagunoff, D., Palmer, D., Martin, T. and Miller, L.W. (1988). The effect of perioperative myocardial infarction on survival of postcardiotomy patients supported with ventricular assist devices. *Circulation*, **78**, 110

ADDENDUM

The Food and Drug Administration has recently withdrawn permission for use of the Jarvik-7 artificial heart in the USA. The reasons for this are not yet certain, and whether the ban will be temporary or permanent also remains unknown.

55
Non-pulsatile Centrifugal Pumps

R.M. BOLMAN III

EXPERIMENTAL BACKGROUND AND EARLY CLINICAL EXPERIENCE

Within a few years of the introduction of cardiopulmonary bypass (CPB) as a life support technique, which made possible a surgical attack on cardiac lesions, investigators began exploring varied applications of this technology for circulatory support of desperately ill patients. In 1962, Dennis and his colleagues demonstrated experimentally that left heart bypass resulted in reduction of the oxygen utilization of the myocardium[1]. Spencer et al. reported in 1965 a series of four patients requiring assisted circulation following cardiac surgery[2]. CPB was employed to provide circulatory assistance in these patients and, although none survived, the ability of prolonged bypass to improve tissue perfusion and reduce atrial filling pressures was encouraging and proved quite provocative to subsequent investigators.

In the late 1960s and early 1970s, attention was turned to the application of intra-aortic balloon counterpulsation in the salvage of the failing myocardium. It remained clear, however, that this method was inadequate in certain patients who had sustained severe temporary or permanent damage to the heart. Pennington et al., in experiments in dogs with normal hearts, as well as in dogs with myocardial infarction, estimated that left ventricular peak systolic pressure and oxygen consumption could be reduced approximately 50% with effective left heart bypass, utilizing a non-pulsatile perfusion system[3]. Pennington applied the non-pulsatile centrifugal pump as a ventricular assist device clinically, and two of his first six patients were able to be weaned from the device, though they did not leave the hospital[4]. Golding et al. also described a patient who was supported after operation by a centrifugal pump, and was weaned after 5½ days; this patient eventually succumbed, but the system functioned adequately[5].

During the same era, the centrifugal pump had initial applications in CPB for open heart surgery. The constrained force vortex pump (BioPump) was compared with the conventional roller pump with respect to microemboli production. The intensity of the embolic activity from the BioPump appeared to be less than the roller pump, both at baseline levels of flow and at times when the inflow and outflow sides of the pumps were partially occluded. Thus, the BioPump was established as a reliable circulatory support device during periods of cardiopulmonary bypass[6].

Magovern et al. employed the BioPump as a left heart assist device in animal studies[7]. Attempts were initially made to coat the tubing and connectors with either a graphite benzalkonium chloride-heparin solution or a tridodecylmethyl ammonium chloride (TDMAC) solution. There were complications with both of these solutions which led to this group adopting the policy of no systemic heparinization and no pretreatment of the system components. Dogs supported up to 24 hours with left heart assistance demonstrated no excessive bleeding, and no evidence of thromboembolic sequelae was observed at autopsy. Coagulation factors remained unaffected. Longer term experiments in sheep, utilizing left heart assistance for 14–22 days, were associated with some thromboembolic phenomena, leading to the policy of changing the pump head every 2–3 days during long-term assistance. The animal experiments revealed the following findings: (1) inflow obstruction was not observed; (2) low serum hemoglobin levels attested to the atraumatic manner of blood flow; (3) anticoagulation was not required when the BioPump was run at 2–3000 rpm for periods up to 2 weeks[7].

Armed with this experimental information, Magovern and his group began applying the BioPump clinically in 1980. Between 1980 and 1985, 41 patients with postcardiotomy ventricular failure required left (LVA), right (RVA), or bi (BVA) ventricular assistance. Attempts were made to maintain the flow at 2 l/min per m² or higher, and the median sternotomy wound was either left open, covered with sterile towels, or only the skin was approximated. The length of assist ranged from 2 to 186 hours.

Thirteen of these 41 patients were long-term survivors of circulatory support. Ten were supported with LVA, one with RVA, and two with BVA. The authors note that in the last year of their study, survival increased to 46% overall, compared to 25% in previous years. This is attributed to increasing experience and the willingness to employ BVA when LVA or RVA alone were not adequate. In addition, earlier institution of assist was felt to have contributed significantly to these improving results. The marked simplicity of application of this commercially available pump, employed without anticoagulation, added greatly to its appeal for the support of postcardiotomy cardiac failure[8]. These authors have also demonstrated the versatility of the BioPump by employing it for circulatory support during resection or repair of traumatic tears or dissections, as well as of acquired aneurysms of the thoracic aorta.

Other groups have also reported favorable experiences with the BioPump as an assist device. Dembitsky et al. recently reported their experience with the centrifugal pump as an RVA in patients with severe right ventricular failure following cardiac surgical procedures[9]. Four of six patients were weaned from the device and one is a long-term survivor. Golding recently utilized the BioPump as a ventricular assist device for as long as 31 days (Golding, L., unpublished). Frazier has suggested several technical modifications which may allow an increase in the period of safe support with this device (Frazier, O.H., unpublished). He describes cannulation of the ventricle as opposed to the left or right atrium. He also employs complete closure of the sternum in the interest of early mobilization of the patient.

Magovern and his colleagues have studied BVA with centrifugal pumps in a previously fatal canine model[10]. This model of normothermic ischemia is generally fatal with standard resuscitative measures. After 24 hours of BVA with the centrifugal pump, seven of ten dogs survived and had cardiac outputs not significantly different from controls. Thus, the centrifugal pump has demonstrated its utility in a variety of clinical circumstances; this versatile device can provide safe and reliable support for up to 4 weeks in the hands of an experienced team. With the advent of cardiac transplantation as a therapeutic modality for patients with end-stage heart disease, the centrifugal pump has seemed the logical, readily available and inexpensive support system to apply to those patients requiring pretransplant mechanical support.

PATIENT SELECTION

Ventricular assistance can be employed in the support of patients in one of three general categories. Within these categories certain hemodynamic characteristics serve to describe individuals who are candidates for this form of support; these characteristics have been detailed in Chapter 54 (Table 54.1).

The first category of patient in whom this may occur is the patient who has sustained a massive myocardial infarction with cardiogenic shock. Secondly, individuals on the transplant waiting list may suffer further deterioration of their cardiac status, with the onset of cardiogenic shock refractory to conventional measures. Finally, patients undergoing routine cardiac surgical procedures may suffer perioperative myocardial damage and it may prove impossible to wean them from CPB support. With the appropriate techniques and experience, the centrifugal pump can be successfully applied in support of each of these three categories of patients.

INSERTION OF CENTRIFUGAL PUMP

The centrifugal pump system employed in these three categories of patient has been the BioPump (Bio-Medicus model 540, Bio-Console model BP-80, BioPump, Bio-Medicus, Eden Prairie, MN, USA) (Figure 55.1).

For LVA, left atrial to aortic bypass is employed. A 36 French right-angled cannula (Polystan A/S, Ballerup, Denmark) is inserted in the roof of the left atrium at its junction with the right superior pulmonary vein, with the cannula tip directed to the middle of the left atrium, as previously described by our group[11]. Aortic cannulation is performed low in the ascending aorta with a standard aortic root cannula. The cannulae are held in place with purse-string sutures, and secured with Rummel tourniquets.

For RVA, the above described right-angled venous cannula is placed in the right atrium (through a purse-string suture placed inferiorly in the right atrial wall) such that the tip of the cannula can be directed through the tricuspid valve. A standard arterial cannula is placed in the proximal pulmonary artery.

For BVA, cannulation is as described above for LVA and RVA in combination. For institution of extracorporeal

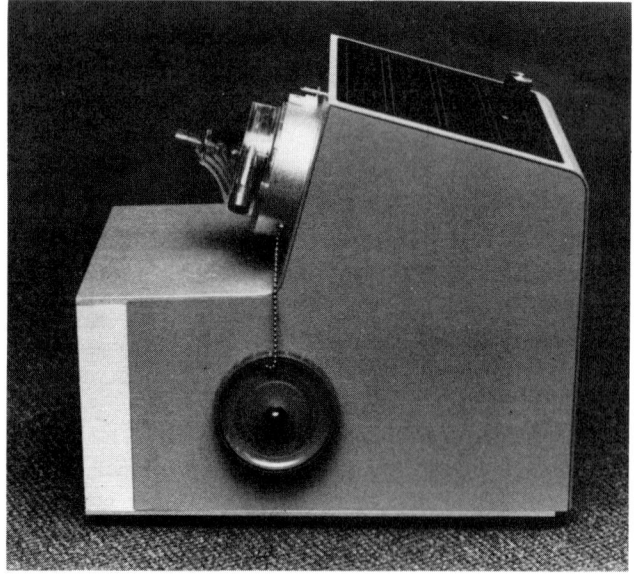

Figure 55.1 The BioPump console with centrifugal pump head in place

membrane oxygenation (ECMO), right atrial to aortic bypass is utilized, with cannulation as described above. In patients supported with the BioPump in any of these configurations, the cannulae have been brought out through the median sternotomy incision, with the sternum left open and the skin closed; in two patients, however, a sternal retractor remained in place, with an adhesive dressing over retractor and cannulae.

PATIENT MANAGEMENT

In the operating theater, heparin is reversed with protamine to effect hemostasis. Once in the intensive care unit, when mediastinal drainage is acceptably low, continuous heparin infusion is instituted to achieve an activated clotting time between 150 and 200 seconds for individuals on LVA, RVA or BVA, and between 250 and 400 seconds for individuals requiring ECMO. Patients are maintained on broad spectrum antibacterial therapy during the period of circulatory support.

Meticulous reverse isolation is employed by all staff and family having contact with the patient to avoid contamination of drive lines, incisions, and other support lines. This is performed in an attempt to limit contamination of the patient prior to the time of transplantation and the institution of immunosuppressive therapy. All dressings are changed daily using a sterile technique.

In order to assess suitability for transplantation, these patients are allowed to awaken from anesthesia. Adequacy of neurological function must be assured, since not infrequently periods of cardiac arrest and profound hypotension have occurred at some point prior to or during the institution of circulatory support. Renal and hepatic function and infection status are also carefully surveyed. Individual patients are assessed from the standpoint of potential recovery of ventricular function, and must demonstrate no signs of recovery. It is important to emphasize that patients placed on circulatory support must meet conventional criteria for transplantation prior to initiating a search for a donor heart.

CARDIAC TRANSPLANTATION

At the time of orthotopic transplantation, the patient is placed on CPB via an aortic cannula high in the ascending aorta. The superior vena cava is cannulated either directly or via the posterior right atrium with a 32 French right-angled cannula (Polystan A/S, Ballerup, Denmark). The inferior vena cava is cannulated via a 36 French right-angled cannula inserted through a posteriorly and inferiorly placed purse-string in the right atrium. As CPB is initiated, the centrifugal pump or pumps are turned off. Orthotopic transplantation proceeds in routine fashion following excision of the diseased recipient organ (Chapter 10).

Before closure, the surgical field is thoroughly irrigated with antibiotic solution. Meticulous wound care is required after operation. Wound sepsis is a serious potential complication.

ASPECTS OF PERIOPERATIVE AND POST-TRANSPLANT MANAGEMENT

Immunosuppression is initiated with triple therapy, consisting of cyclosporine, azathioprine and prednisone. This regimen, introduced in 1983, has yielded excellent results with respect to rates of rejection- and infection-free survival[12-14]. Perioperative antibiotic prophylaxis, consisting of vancomycin for 48 hours and a cephalosporin until all invasive lines are removed, is administered. Specific infectious complications are treated according to the organism identified. All patients receive mycostatin orally and by nasal inhalation for the first 3 months, and are maintained on trimethoprim sulfa prophylaxis indefinitely. Patients seronegative for cytomegalovirus (CMV) prior to transplantation receive exclusively CMV-negative blood and blood products; all patients receive CMV hyperimmune globulin (Conti, R., University of Minnesota) at 1 week and 1 month post-transplant as passive prophylaxis.

RESULTS OF TRANSPLANTATION IN PATIENTS ON CIRCULATORY SUPPORT

Since January, 1985, the Heart Transplant Program at Washington University School of Medicine, St. Louis, has performed 94 heart transplants in 91 patients. Twenty-two patients (24% of the total) required mechanical support of respiration or circulation prior to transplantation. For the purposes of this review, attention will be focused only on the nine patients supported with the BioPump as LVA, BVA or ECMO.

These patients ranged in age from 16 to 57 years with a mean of 42 years (Table 55.1). Two-thirds (six patients) had ischemic heart disease; this compares with a 50% incidence of coronary artery disease in our series as a whole. One patient had aortic insufficiency, one cardiomyopathy, and one Wolff–Parkinson–White (WPW) syndrome with associated cardiomyopathy. Further details of the patients, device insertion and flows, and outcome are outlined in Table 55.1.

Results of left ventricular assistance

Six patients required LVA (Table 55.1). In two instances, the BioPump was inserted without the use of CPB. Both these individuals had sustained massive myocardial infarctions and were in cardiogenic shock. The device was

Table 55.1 Details of nine patients requiring BioPump support before cardiac transplantation

Age (years)	Cardiac diagnosis	Type and period (days) of support	CPB for insertion	Flow rate (l/min) range (mean)	Outcome
57	Periop. MI during redo CABG	LVA (2)	yes	1.0–2.5 (2.3)	OHT, alive
45	Periop. MI, cardiac arrest after CABG	LVA (1)	yes	2.0–4.0 (3.0)	OHT, alive
41	Periop. MI, cardiac arrest after CABG	BVA (1.5)	yes	3.5–4.5 (4.0)	OHT, alive
44	MI, cardiogenic shock	LVA (1)	no	1.5–2.5 (2.0)	Expired on device
48	MI, cardiogenic shock	LVA (0.5)	no	1.5–3.5 (2.0)	OHT, alive
46	MI, cardiogenic shock	LVA (3)	no	2.0–5.0 (3.5)	OHT, alive
16	Postcardiotomy pump failure (WPW, CM)	BVA (4)	yes	3.0–5.0 (4.0)	CVA on device
45	Postcardiotomy pump failure (AVR x 3)	LVA (1.5)	yes	2.2–4.3 (4.0)	OHT, died (17 months)
32	Right ventricular failure, cardiac arrest after OHT	ECMO (1.5)	no	3.0–5.0 (4.0)	OHT, alive
Mean 42		Mean 1.6 days		Mean 3.2 l/min	

CPB = cardiopulmonary bypass; MI = myocardial infarction; CABG = coronary artery bypass grafting; WPW = Wolff–Parkinson–White syndrome; CM = cardiomyopathy; AVR = aortic valve replacement; OHT = orthotopic heart transplant; LVA = left ventricular assist; BVA = biventricular assist; ECMO = extracorporeal membrane oxygenator; CVA = cerebrovascular accident

inserted via a 36 French right-angled cannula placed in the roof of the left atrium just posterior to the interatrial groove, with routine aortic cannulation as previously described by our group[11]. Five of the six patients were adequately resuscitated on the device and determined to be suitable candidates for cardiac transplantation by virtue of return of neurologic function and stable extracardiac organ function. All five were successfully transplanted within 12 hours to 3 days; all are long-term survivors, except for one who expired at 17 months post-transplant from a cerebral hemorrhage. In the sixth patient, LVA proved inadequate due to the presence of significant right ventricular failure; he expired before additional measures could be instituted.

Results of biventricular assistance

Two patients were supported with biventricular BioPump devices (Table 55.1). One was successfully supported for 36 hours and transplanted, and is a long-term survivor. The second suffered a cerebrovascular accident on the fourth day of BioPump support, and was declared brain-dead.

Results of extracorporeal membrane oxygenation

One patient required ECMO utilizing the BioPump (Table 55.1). This 32-year-old man had undergone orthotopic heart transplantation for cardiomyopathy, and developed acute right ventricular decompensation and cardiac arrest several hours later. He was taken to the operating room with his chest open and receiving internal cardiac massage, and was placed on ECMO without the use of CPB. He regained neurologic function and was deemed a suitable candidate for retransplantation. A second donor organ was located 36 hours later, and he is a long-term survivor of transplantation, although he has mild neurologic residue attributable to his prolonged cardiac arrest.

Long-term outcome after transplantation

Seven of these nine desperately ill individuals were deemed suitable candidates for transplantation while being maintained on circulatory support. All seven were successfully transplanted and proved long-term survivors of transplantation, though one developed alcoholic pancreatitis and suffered an intracerebral hemorrhage and expired 17 months post-transplant. The actuarial survival in this group is 100% at 3, 6 and 12 months, and 71% at 24 months. Six of the seven patients (86%) have been rehabilitated to their premorbid activity.

COMPLICATIONS

The complications which have occurred in these nine patients are listed in Table 55.2. Four of the nine (44%) experienced complications while on the device prior to transplantation. One expired on LVA from inadequate circulatory support. Two developed neurologic damage as a result of cardiac arrest before the institution of circulatory support and one whilst being supported.

Post-transplant, three of seven (42%) developed complications. Enterobacter septicemia occurred in one and was

Table 55.2 Complications of circulatory support with the non-pulsatile centrifugal pump

	n	%
Pretransplant		
Inadequate circulatory support (died on device)	1	11
Cerebrovascular accident		
prior to device insertion	2	22
on device (died)	1	11
Total	4	44
Post-transplant		
Sepsis	1	14
Adult respiratory distress syndrome	1	14
Superficial wound dehiscence	1	14
Total	3	42

successfully treated. Another developed severe adult respiratory distress syndrome and a superficial wound dehiscence, both of which were managed successfully.

Thus, there were seven complications in nine patients for a complication rate of 77%. This constitutes a high rate of complication, though fortunately, post-transplant, none proved fatal.

When the patient has suffered a cerebrovascular accident from poor perfusion prior to ventricular assist, neurological assessment may prove extremely difficult. After insertion of the device, and before proceeding to transplantation, the surgeon should, at the very least, ascertain that the patient has regained consciousness and can move all extremities on command.

Incidence of acute rejection

Among the seven patients successfully transplanted, only three demonstrated any evidence of rejection during the first 3 months. This is an incidence of 0.42 episodes/patient, and is comparable to the incidence of rejection observed in our total patient experience.

COMMENT

In appropriately selected individuals, heart transplantation has been demonstrated to be an effective modality for increasing longevity and improving the quality of life. Many patients who are candidates for transplantation die while on the waiting list for transplant because of the current and ongoing shortage of available donors. Other patients develop severe myocardial damage, either as a result of myocardial infarction or during attempted surgical correction of a cardiac lesion. Replacement of the heart becomes their sole option for survival. Previously, these patients would have died without benefit of heart replacement, and many still do. A fortunate few, however, as in the current series, develop their catastrophic illness in a setting where capabilities for both mechanical circulatory support and heart transplantation are present.

The ventricular assist device has found increasing application in support of patients with cardiogenic shock prior to transplantation. The non-pulsatile centrifugal pump is a readily available, inexpensive device which can be inserted and managed by anyone trained in cardiothoracic surgery. The device can be inserted without the need for CPB and attendant heparinization (four of nine cases in our small series), and some groups advocate that no maintenance anticoagulation is required. As increasing numbers of hospitals become involved with cardiac transplantation, circulatory support will be invoked more frequently in the support of critically ill patients prior to the availability of a donor organ. Clearly, the non-pulsatile centrifugal pump offers the most simple form of support currently available.

Hill has reported that 25 patients have been supported prior to transplant with the BioPump (Hill, D., unpublished). Sixteen (69%) were transplanted, and ten (62.5%) were discharged from hospital. In our series, nine patients were supported with the intention to transplant, of whom seven (77%) were transplanted, and all were long-term survivors.

With certain investigators now reporting success with longer term support utilizing the BioPump, this becomes an even more attractive modality for the support of desperately ill individuals awaiting transplantation. Clearly, this device has earned a place in the armamentarium of circulatory support for the foreseeable future.

References

1. Dennis, C., Hall, D.P., Moreno, J.R. and Senning, A. (1962). Reduction of the oxygen utilization of the heart by left heart bypass. *Circ. Res.*, **10**, 298
2. Spencer, F.C., Eiseman, B., Trinkle, J.K. and Rossi, N.P. (1965). Assisted circulation for cardiac failure following intracardiac surgery with cardiopulmonary bypass. *J. Thorac. Cardiovasc. Surg.*, **49**, 56
3. Pennington, D.G., Hahn, J.W., Standever, J.W., Vitale, T.J., Morton, P.E. and Willman, V.L. (1979). Hemodynamic effects of a centrifugal LVAD in dogs with acute myocardial infarction and interventricular shunt. *Surg. Forum*, **30**, 231
4. Pennington, D.G. (1980). Clinical experience with a centrifugal pump ventricular assist device. *USA–USSR Joint Symposium on Circulatory Assistance and the Artificial Heart.* NIH 80-2032, July
5. Golding, L.R., Groves, L.K., Peter, M., Jacobs, G., Sukalac, R., Nose, Y. and Loop, F.D. (1980). Initial clinical experience with a new temporary left ventricular assist device. *Ann. Thorac. Surg.*, **29**, 66
6. Mandl, J.P. (1977). Comparison of emboli production between a constrained force vortex anticoagulants for postoperative left ventricular assist. *Proc. Am. Soc. Extracorporeal Technology*, **5**, 27
7. Magovern, G.J., Park, S.B. and Maher, T.D. (1985). Use of a centrifugal pump without anticoagulants for postoperative left ventricular assist. *World J. Surg.*, **9**, 25
8. Park, S.B., Liebler, G.A, Burkholder, J.A., Maher, T.D., Benckart, D.H., Magovern, J.G. Jr., Christlieb, I.Y., Kao, R.L. and Magovern, G.J. (1986). Mechanical support of the failing heart. *Ann. Thorac. Surg.*, **42**, 627
9. Dembitsky, W.P., Daily, P.O., Raney, A.A., Moores, W.Y. and Joyo, C.I. (1986). Temporary extracorporeal support of the right ventricle. *J. Thorac. Cardiovasc. Surg.*, **91**, 518
10. Magovern, G.J., Christlieb, I.Y., Kao, R.L., Leiber, G.A., Park, S.B., Burkholder, J.A., Maher, T.D., Benckart, D.H. and Magovern, G.J. (1987). Recovery of the failing canine heart with biventricular support in a previously fatal experimental model. *J. Thorac. Cardiovasc. Surg.*, **94**, 656
11. Bolman, R.M., Spray, T.L., Cox, J.L., Kouchoukos, N., Cance, C., Saffitz, J., Genton, R.E. and Eisen, H. (1987). Heart transplantation in patients requiring preoperative mechanical support. *J. Heart Transplant.*, **6**, 273
12. Bolman, R.M., Elick, B., Olivari, M.T., Ring, W.S. and Arentzen, C. (1985). Improved immunosuppression for cardiac transplantation. *J. Heart Transplant.*, **4**, 315
13. Bolman, R.M., Olivari, M.T., Sibley, R., Saffitz, J., Spardaro, J., Cance, C. and Elick, B. (1987). Current results with triple therapy for heart transplantation. *Transplant. Proc.*, **19**, 2490
14. Bolman, R.M., Cance, C., Spray, T., Genton, R., Weiss, C., Saffitz, J. and Eisen, H. (1988). The changing face of cardiac transplantation: Washington University Program 1985–1987. *Ann. Thorac. Surg.*, **45**, 192

56
Pulsatile Ventricular Assist Devices
P.K. DAVIS, W.E. PAE, Jr. AND W.S. PIERCE

INTRODUCTION

During the past 10 years, cardiac transplantation has become an accepted and more commonplace therapy for end-stage cardiomyopathy in selected patients. Increased interest and improved results, however, have led to a progressive rise in the number of centers and procedures, so that the availability of donor organs has become a problem. Under the current organ procurement system, it is unlikely that more than 1100 transplants per year will be performed in this country[1]. Unfortunately, the number of patients requiring transplantation is much higher, and approximately 20% of those patients accepted as candidates for cardiac transplantation die before a donor organ can be obtained[2].

The standard methods used to support the failing heart, such as administration of inotropic drugs, afterload reduction, and intra-aortic balloon (IAB) counterpulsation, can support many potential candidates. In some patients, however, ventricular failure is refractory to these measures, and more aggressive forms of circulatory support are necessary. Clinical evidence is accumulating which suggests that temporary ventricular assistance is an acceptable way to support the systemic and, at times, the pulmonary circulation in patients whose hemodynamic condition deteriorates while awaiting cardiac transplantation[3-6]. Cardiac transplantation and temporary ventricular support, therefore, appear to have complementary roles in salvaging certain critically ill patients who are transplant candidates.

In this chapter we shall discuss the historical development of ventricular assist devices, describe the types of pulsatile devices which have been used clinically, outline operative techniques, and discuss the application of ventricular assistance in bridge to transplant. No attempt will be made to discuss all the devices under development; rather we will concentrate on those which have received clinical use, with the Pierce-Donachy pump as a prototype. The non-pulsatile systems, which are designed for cardiopulmonary bypass, that have been used for ventricular assistance are discussed elsewhere (Chapters 54 and 55).

EARLY CLINICAL EXPERIENCE

Temporary ventricular assistance was first clinically described by Stuckey and his associates in 1957; they reported the survival of a patient in cardiogenic shock, secondary to an acute myocardial infarction, after temporary support by total conventional cardiopulmonary bypass[7]. Efforts to use left heart bypass for the support of patients with profound cardiogenic shock, secondary to massive acute myocardial infarction, continued throughout the early 1960s. Despite favorable experimental results, patient survival in clinical trials was exceedingly poor[8].

Clinical use of a ventricular assist device to support patients who could not be weaned from cardiopulmonary bypass after cardiac surgery was first attempted in 1963 by DeBakey's group[9]. In 1965, Spencer *et al.* described the first successful use of left ventricular assistance, in the form of left atrial to femoral bypass, in a patient for 6 hours following intracardiac surgery[10]. DeBakey developed an early pneumatic ventricular assist device, and reported long-term patient survival when he subsequently updated his clinical experience in 1971[11]. During the decade that followed, a number of groups reported varying survival rates in small series of patients using different types of mechanical circulatory assist pumps.

In the late 1970s, both Norman and his group at the Texas Heart Institute, and Bernhard and his associates at Boston Children's Hospital began clinical trials of pneumatic assist devices developed independently[12]. Although the concept of temporary ventricular assistance was reinforced by several patients who were weaned from the device, long-term patient survival was poor in both series[13,14]. A roller pump system was employed with better short- and long-term results by Litwak and associates, at Mount Sinai, and Rose *et al.* at New York University[15,16]. In 1978, Golding and colleagues of the Cleveland Clinic reported experience with the Medtronic centrifugal pump (Medtronic Inc., Minneapolis, Minnesota, USA)[17]. Magovern and co-workers later reported the use of a centrifugal pump designed by Biomedicus (Biomedicus Inc., Minnetonka, Minnesota,

USA) with minimal anticoagulation[18]. In 1981, our center (Pennsylvania State University) reported excellent recovery of myocardial function with the use of the Pierce–Donachy pneumatic device in patients with postcardiotomy cardiogenic shock[19]. Pennington et al. at St. Louis University later confirmed these results[20].

BRIDGE TO TRANSPLANTATION

Temporary support of the circulation with intra-aortic balloon pump (IABP) counterpulsation, followed by cardiac transplantation, was first reported by Reemtsma and associates in 1978[21]. That same year the use of a ventricular assist device as a bridge to transplantation was described by Norman and his associates at the Texas Heart Institute[22]. A 21-year-old man who could not be weaned from cardiopulmonary bypass after valvular surgery was supported for 6 days with a Thermedics pneumatic left ventricular assist device (Thermedics Inc., Waltham, Massachusetts, USA), followed by combined heart and kidney transplantation. The patient died of multi-organ failure 14 days after allografting. In 1984, Pennington reported his initial experience with an extracorporeal membrane oxygenation circuit consisting of a Scimed membrane lung (Scimed Inc., Minneapolis, Minnesota, USA) and the Biomedicus centrifugal pump in a bridge-to-transplant application[23,24]. Zumbro and colleagues reported early bridge application of a roller pump system in a single patient in 1985[25]. Despite the fact that these devices appeared to provide adequate circulatory support, in all cases the patients died after transplantation.

The first bridge-to-transplant procedure resulting in long-term survival was reported by Portner and colleagues at Stanford University in 1985[26]. A 51-year-old man with ischemic cardiomyopathy was supported for 8 days by an electrically powered Novacor ventricular assist device (Novacor Medical Corp., Oakland, California, USA) prior to undergoing transplantation. Hill and associates at the Pacific Medical Center in San Francisco reported the first successful bridge procedure using the Thoratec (Thoratec Laboratories Corp., Berkeley, California, USA) version of the Pierce–Donachy ventricular assist device[5]. Since that publication, several groups have reported successful bridge application of this device[27]. Over the past 2 years a progressive increase in the number of bridge procedures has occurred, utilizing a variety of devices for ventricular support.

TYPES OF VENTRICULAR ASSIST DEVICES

Pierce–Donachy ventricular assist device

The Pierce–Donachy ventricular assist device consists of a flexible segmented polyurethane blood sac, which is seamfree and has a highly polished surface, enclosed within a rigid polysulfone case (Figure 56.1). The inner chamber of the case is in the shape of an oblate spheroid. A flexible diaphragm transects the frontal plane of the outer case and separates the air port from the thin-walled blood sac. Bjork–Shiley 70° concavo-convex Delrin inlet and outlet valves (Shiley Laboratories, Irvine, California, USA) provide unidirectional flow. The device is placed paracorporeally on the anterior abdominal wall, and is connected to an external pneumatic power unit by polyvinyl chloride tubing which is approximately 2 m in length. The pumping action is created by pulses of compressed carbon dioxide introduced between the pump housing and the flexible diaphragm, periodically displacing the diaphragm and emptying the valved blood sac. The stroke volume of the device is 70 ml.

For left ventricular assistance, blood can be removed from either the left atrium or ventricle, using a segmented polyurethane cannula, and returned to the ascending aorta

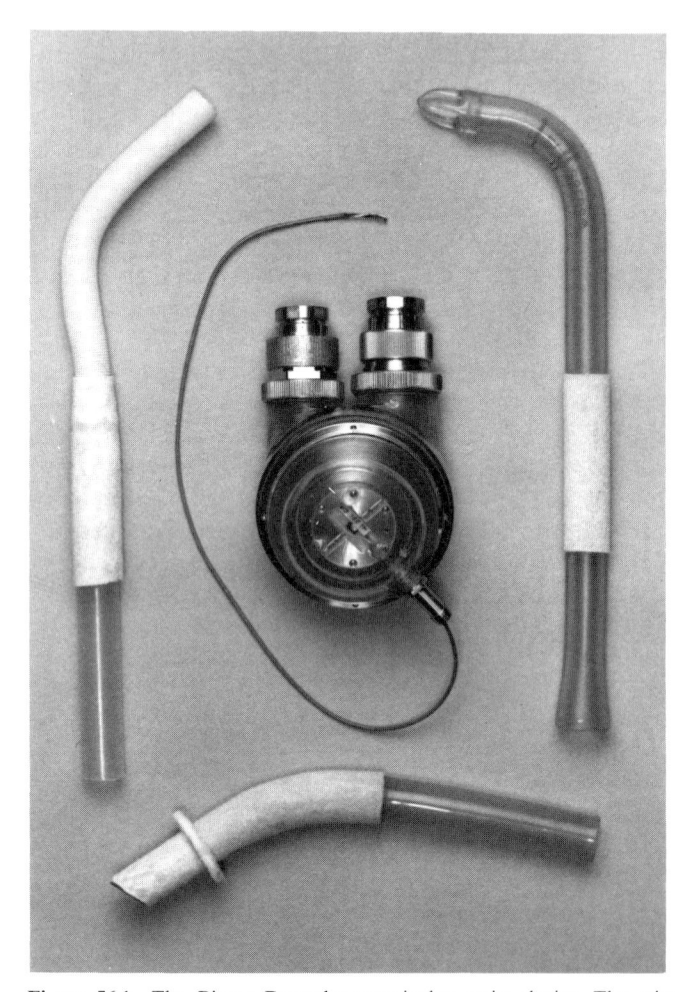

Figure 56.1 The Pierce–Donachy ventricular assist device. The wire exiting the case is attached to a Hall-effect proximity switch that indicates complete pump filling. The outflow composite cannula (left) and the atrial inflow cannula (right) can be used for either left or right ventricular assistance. The cannula below the pump can be used for ventricular cannulation in certain bridge-to-transplant applications

using a composite segmented polyurethane–Dacron graft (Figure 56.2). Right ventricular assistance is instituted by cannulation of the right atrium to withdraw blood, which is then returned to the pulmonary artery via the outflow composite graft. Two pumps may be employed if biventricular assistance is necessary. The cannulae traverse the diaphragm and exit the skin below the costal margin in the same manner as mediastinal drainage tubes.

The pump can operate in either the automatic or manual mode. In the automatic mode, pump systole is initiated when a Hall-effect proximity switch, located between the diaphragm and the outer case, senses when the blood sac is full. This allows the pump to run in a full-to-empty mode which provides maximum washout of the blood sac, thereby decreasing the possibility of thrombus formation. Observation of the pump, or analysis of the air-line pressure curve, can verify complete emptying. No effort is made to synchronize the pump systole and the QRS of the

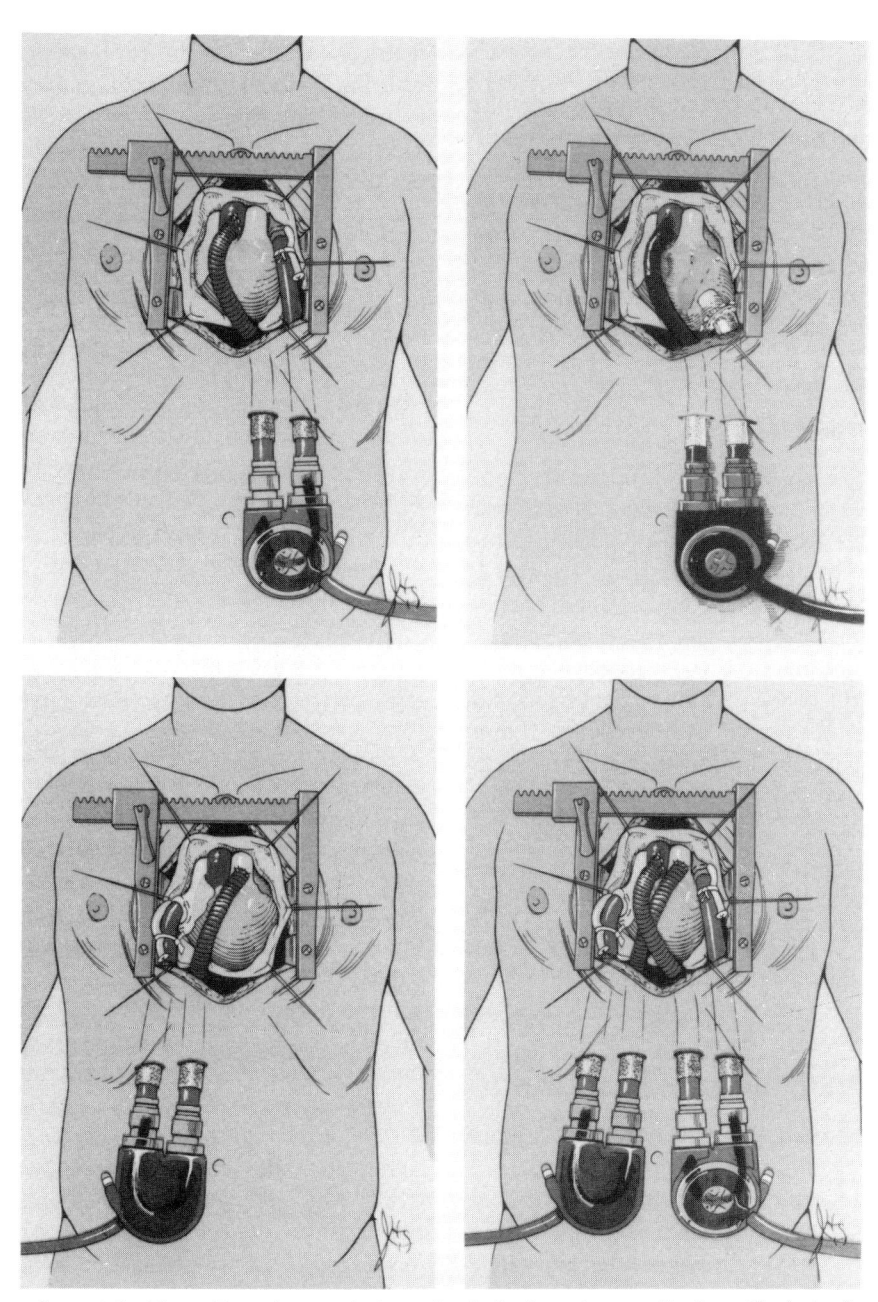

Figure 56.2 Illustrations of the Pierce–Donachy ventricular assist device in various applications. Clockwise from top left: (A) left ventricular assistance with atrial inflow cannulation and blood return to the ascending aorta; (B) left ventricular assistance with ventricular inflow cannulation; (C) biventricular assistance with left and right atrial cannulation; (D) right ventricular assistance with right atrial inflow cannulation and blood return to the pulmonary artery

electrocardiogram. In the manual mode, the pump rate can be set at any desired value.

Thermedics ventricular assist device

The Thermedics left ventricular assist device is a pusher-plate blood pump which has been used for bridge-to-transplant application at the Texas Heart Institute. The Thermedics Corporation is developing a permanent device which is to be electrically powered, but the device as used clinically has been pneumatically powered by an external console. The pump is designed to be placed in a preperitoneal pocket in the abdomen. The inflow and outflow cannulae are 20 mm Dacron grafts, each with a glutaraldehyde-preserved porcine bioprosthetic valve to provide unidirectional flow. The pump inlet cannula drains blood from the left ventricular apex and the outlet cannula returns blood to the ascending aorta. The maximum stroke volume is 85 ml[28]. This device requires ventricular cannulation, and has not been adapted for right ventricular assistance.

Novacor ventricular assist device

The Novacor Corporation is working towards the development of a permanent implantable left ventricular assist device, but the device has been used clinically in bridge-to-transplant procedures. The system is electrically powered, and consists of a microprocessor-controlled solenoid energy converter with a dual pusher-plate, sac-type, blood pump. The pump is designed to be placed in a preperitoneal pocket of the left upper quadrant of the abdomen. Unidirectional flow through the pump is ensured by the use of 21 mm Carpentier–Edwards porcine bioprostheses (American Edwards Laboratories, Santa Ana, California, USA). The pump inflow cannula passes through the diaphragm, and drains blood from the left ventricular apex. The pump outlet cannula is anastomosed to the supraceliac aorta or ascending aorta. The nominal maximum stroke volume is 83 ml[29]. This system, like the Thermedics device, has not been adapted for right ventricular support.

INDICATIONS FOR VENTRICULAR ASSISTANCE

Hardesty et al. have reported that the results of cardiac transplantation in mortally ill patients requiring circulatory support with IAB counterpulsation compare favorably with the results obtained for patients who do not require aggressive hemodynamic support[30]. Ventricular assistance for those transplant candidates whose condition deteriorates further may be desirable[4]. In the present climate of relative donor organ unavailability, the temptation to provide circulatory support to deteriorating patients, especially those with multi-system organ failure who are not transplant candidates, in the hope that they might become candidates, must be resisted. This approach may lead to a lingering pool of patients who never become transplant candidates, or worse, on whom donor organs are wasted with a minimal chance of survival.

The absolute number of patients who might truly benefit from ventricular assistance is uncertain. At our institution, between February, 1984 and January, 1988, 52 patients were selected for orthotopic heart transplantation. During this period, eight of the 52 patients died waiting for a donor heart. To ameliorate this problem, in July of 1985 we began utilizing temporary ventricular support to provide a bridge to transplantation.

The hemodynamic criteria used at our institution for deciding when to implement ventricular assistance in patients who are hemodynamically unstable are very similar to those detailed in Chapter 54 (Table 54.1). To be selected, patients must demonstrate ongoing hemodynamic instability, as evidenced by a pulmonary capillary wedge pressure or left atrial pressure of greater than 25 mmHg, systolic blood pressure less than 90 mmHg, and cardiac index less than 1.8 l/min per square meter, coupled with evidence of poor renal perfusion, with urine output less than 20 ml per hour. Full resuscitative efforts must be undertaken, including volume infusion, pharmacological support, and IAB, without adequate improvement of systemic perfusion. Most importantly, the patient must have no contraindication to transplantation.

VENTRICULAR ASSIST PUMP IMPLANTATION

A median sternotomy provides the optimal exposure for assist pump placement. The patient is most often placed on cardiopulmonary bypass using standard cannulation. We have felt that these patients have such poor cardiac reserve that they would not otherwise tolerate the procedure. Recently we have successfully implanted biventricular assist pumps, using atrial cannulation, without cardiopulmonary bypass. A similar procedure has been performed in Europe[31]. Further clinical trials are necessary to determine the place of this technique in assist pump implantation, but our experience has been encouraging.

A patent foramen ovale must be searched out and closed if only a left ventricular assist device is being placed. A significant number of patients have a patent foramen ovale, which is not clinically significant when the proper relationship between right and left atrial pressures exists. When a left ventricular assist device is placed, the right atrial pressure may remain elevated and greater than the left atrial pressure if there is right ventricular dysfunction. This atrial pressure gradient can lead to significant right-to-left shunting across the foramen and profound hypoxemia[32].

Initially, we utilized left ventricular apex cannulation for pump inflow in bridge-to-transplant patients in an effort to provide maximum ventricular decompression and preservation of the atrial tissue for the transplant procedure[33]. Because of excellent clinical performance of the pump in postcardiotomy, cardiogenic shock patients with atrial cannulation, and technical problems with ventricular cannulation, we have recently favored the atrial route in bridge applications. Hemodynamic performance of the device in these cases has been similar to ventricular cannulations, and there has been no difficulty with the subsequent transplant procedure.

The outflow graft is sutured as low as possible to the ascending aorta in order to allow its excision with recipient cardiectomy. The cannulae are brought out below the costal margin, and the pump placed paracorporeally as previously described. Pumping is gradually initiated after the pump has been de-aired, and the patient is weaned from cardiopulmonary bypass. It is important not to employ diastolic vacuum to aid in filling of the blood sac until the chest is closed and mediastinal drainage begun, because air can be drawn through the suture lines around the cannulae, leading to air embolism.

Frequently, small amounts of dopamine or isoproterenol are necessary to improve right ventricular performance after a left ventricular assist pump has been placed. Although right ventricular failure may be profound, it is often not recognized until a left device has been placed[34]. In our experience, if the patient demonstrates preoperative clinical signs of right ventricular decompensation, such as ascites, elevated central venous pressure, and borderline high pulmonary resistance, it is likely that biventricular assistance will be necessary. Further clinical research is necessary to demonstrate reliable preoperative determinants of biventricular failure so that the appropriate operation may be planned. Certainly, after left pump placement, if the cardiac index remains less than 1.8 l/min per square meter and right atrial pressures exceed 20 mmHg, with left atrial pressures less than 15 mmHg, right ventricular assistance will also be required. A second assist pump is placed with the pump inflow cannula in the right atrium and the outflow graft sutured to the pulmonary artery (Figure 56.2).

POSTOPERATIVE MANAGEMENT OF PATIENTS WITH VENTRICULAR ASSISTANCE

Monitoring

Except for regulation of assist pumping, postoperative care is similar to that given to any seriously ill cardiac patient in the intensive care unit. Pumping is adjusted to maintain a cardiac index between 2.2 and 3.0 l/min per square meter, usually in a full-to-empty mode. A left atrial line is routinely placed at the time of surgery, and is extremely useful in regulating pumping in the first 48 hours. Careful evaluation of the pneumatic waveform not only gives an excellent indication of the device's performance, but can also be correlated with the left atrial and aortic pressures[35,36]. This is especially useful later in the patient's course when invasive monitoring lines have been removed.

In the absence of biventricular assistance, the limiting factor in left ventricular assist pump output is right ventricular function. With the careful addition of diastolic vacuum to a properly positioned inflow cannula, the left heart can usually be completely decompressed. In our experience, maintenance of the left atrial pressure between 10 and 15 mmHg provides the best balance between optimal pump output and pulmonary function.

Infectious complications

One of the major concerns surrounding the use of mechanical circulatory assistance is that of septic complications. This is of special concern in the bridge patient who must ultimately undergo chronic immunosuppression. Accordingly every effort must be made to minimize and discontinue mechanical ventilation, invasive monitoring, and access catheters at the earliest possible point in the patient's course. Although these patients often require hyperalimentation, enteral feeding should be used whenever possible. The percutaneous pneumatic drive lines are cleaned daily with alcohol, coated with an iodine-based ointment and dressed sterilely. Serious infectious complications are a risk of ventricular assistance, but with appropriate care these patients can undergo transplantation and subsequent long-term immunosuppression with excellent results.

Thromboembolism

A second area of concern is the risk of thromboembolism. The most important elements in preventing thrombus formation in the blood sac, or on the prosthetic valves, are system design and pump flow rates. While these factors may be sufficient to prevent thromboembolic complications, clinical use of the device has most often included some type of anticoagulation. Agents to decrease platelet adhesiveness, such as dipyridamole or low molecular weight dextran, were most often employed in our early experience.

Recently, because of bleeding after the transplant procedure in patients receiving platelet-active drugs, we have been using a continuous infusion of heparin to maintain an activated clotting time of approximately 150–250 seconds. The heparin infusion is initiated postoperatively after the mediastinal tube drainage has decreased to 50 ml per hour. This can be converted to low-dose warfarin sodium therapy if the wait for a donor organ becomes lengthy. Further clinical experience will help to determine the optimum anticoagulation regime for these patients, and whether anticoagulation is necessary.

Transplant status

As stated previously, it is important to ensure an appropriate distribution of donor organs. Accordingly, we do not list patients with mechanical circulatory assistance for transplantation until they have recovered all organ functions and are acceptable candidates for transplantation. If a complication occurs, such as renal failure or sepsis, it must completely resolve before the patient is once again considered for transplantation.

RESULTS OF BRIDGE APPLICATION OF VENTRICULAR ASSISTANCE

Since July of 1985, nine patients at our institution have undergone ventricular assist pump placement as a bridge to cardiac transplantation (Table 56.1). Three patients required biventricular assistance because of profound right and left ventricular failure. Five patients ultimately underwent cardiac transplantation after being supported for an average of 16 days. Three patients went on to achieve long-term survival without cardiac or non-cardiac disability. The first of these patients is alive and well 30 months after transplantation and is active as a homemaker. The second is 1 year post-transplant and has returned to college. The third, also alive and well 12 months after transplantation, is undergoing occupational therapy in preparation for return to work in several months.

Two patients underwent transplantation but did not survive. One developed a *Pseudomonas aeruginosa* urinary tract infection, and the same organism was cultured from the tip of a Swan–Ganz catheter. Despite aggressive appropriate antibiotic therapy the patient died 27 days post-transplantation of *Pseudomonas aeruginosa* sepsis. A patient who required biventricular assistance was supported for 7 days and was in excellent condition at the time of allograft placement. Unexplained low systemic vascular resistance developed postoperatively, and the patient died of graft failure on the fourth day after transplantation. Autopsy revealed no evidence of a septic focus, nor were any positive cultures obtained during the period of mechanical support.

Four of the nine patients died prior to transplantation. One developed a severe *Enterobacter aerogenes* pneumonia, secondary to the aspiration of gastric contents, and died of overwhelming sepsis after 12 days of support. Another, who had recently suffered a severe myocardial infarction involving the left ventricular apex, died after 7 hours of support from uncontrollable hemorrhage from the left ventricular apex cannulation site. Two of the patients requiring biventricular assist pumps died prior to allografting. Both patients, supported less than 36 hours, developed difficulty with unexplained low systemic vascular resistance.

COMMENT

These results demonstrate that paracorporeal assist pumping can be used successfully to support selected patients who decompensate hemodynamically while awaiting transplantation. At the present time the optimal system of mechanical circulatory assistance which should be used to support hemodynamically unstable transplant candidates is uncertain. Those patients with severe isolated left ventricular failure refractory to IAB counterpulsation may benefit from left ventricular assistance. Further clinical trials are necessary, however, to determine those patients who will require biventricular support preoperatively, and to demonstrate whether biventricular assist pump placement or total artificial heart implantation is best for such patients.

The use of mechanical circulatory assistance as a bridge to cardiac transplantation is a new field, and a period of clinical investigation is necessary before patient benefit can adequately be assessed. Bridge procedures cannot increase the total number of transplants performed in this country, but ultimately the type of patient undergoing allograft placement may be altered[37,38]. With so many patients who require transplantation, and the current problem of donor organ scarcity, the aggressive use of ventricular assistance in attempting to salvage patients must be carefully justified. As the bridge-to-transplant procedure evolves, comparison of the results after transplant in these patients with the

Table 56.1 Staged cardiac transplant application of the Pierce–Donachy ventricular assist pump: complications and outcome

Patient	Complications	Transplanted	Outcome
1 (LVAD)	Cannula site infection	yes	Alive at 28 months
2 (LVAD)	Catheter sepsis	yes	Died postop. day 27
3 (LVAD)	CVA, Candida aortitis	yes	Alive at 12 months
4 (LVAD)	None	yes	Alive at 12 months
5 (LVAD)	Hemorrhage from vent. cannulation site	no	Died LVAD 7 hours
6 (BVAD)	Pneumonia, sepsis	no	Died BVAD day 12
7 (BVAD)	Low systemic vascular resistance	no	Died BVAD day 2
8 (BVAD)	Low systemic vascular resistance	no	Died BVAD 4 hours
9 (BVAD)	None: BVAD placed without cardiopulmonary bypass	yes	Died postop. day 4 donor heart failure

Abbreviations: LVAD = left ventricular assist device; BVAD: biventricular assist device

results in less critically ill patients will serve to provide future guidelines.

References

1. Evans, R.W., Manninen, D.L., Garrison, L.P., Jr. and Maier, A.M. (1986). Donor availability as the primary determinant of the future of heart transplantation. *J. Am. Med. Assoc.*, **255**, 1892
2. Copeland, J.G., Emery, R.W., Levinson, M.M., Copeland, J., McAleer, M.J. and Riley, J.E. (1985). The role of mechanical support and transplantation in treatment of patients with end-stage cardiomyopathy. *Circulation*, **72**, II-7
3. Pennock, J.L., Wisman, C.B. and Pierce, W.S. (1982). Mechanical support of the circulation prior to cardiac transplantation. *Heart Transplant.*, **1**, 299
4. Pennock, J.L., Pierce, W.S, Campbell, D.B., Pae, W.E., Davis,D., Hensley, F.A., Richenbacher, W.E. and Waldhausen, J.A. (1986). Mechanical support of the circulation followed by cardiac transplantation. *J. Thorac. Cardiovasc. Surg.*, **92**, 994
5. Hill, J.D., Farrar, D.J., Hershon, J.J., Compton, P.G., Avery, G.J., Levin, B.S. and Brent, B.N. (1986). Use of a prosthetic ventricle as a bridge to cardiac transplantation for postinfarction cardiogenic shock. *N. Engl. J. Med.*, **314**, 626
6. Oaks, T.E., Pae, W.E., Rosenberg, G., Pennock, J.L. and Pierce, W.S. (1987). The use of a paracorporeal ventricular assist device as a bridge to cardiac transplantation. *Am. Soc. Artif. Intern. Organs Trans.*, **33**, 408
7. Stuckey, J.H., Newman, M.N., Dennis, C., Berg, E.H., Goodman, S.E., Fries, C.C., Karlson, K.E., Blumenfeld, M., Weitzner, S.W., Binder, L.S. and Winston, A. (1957). The use of the heart–lung machine in selected cases of acute myocardial infarction. *Surg. Forum*, **8**, 342
8. Dennis, C., Carlens, E., Senning, A., Hall, D.P., Moreno, J.R., Cappelletti, R.R. and Wesolowski, S.A. (1962). Clinical use of a cannula for left heart bypass without thoracotomy; experimental protection against fibrillation by left heart bypass. *Ann. Surg.*, **156**, 623
9. Liotta, D., Hall, C.W., Henly, W.S., Cooley, D.A., Crawford, E.S. and DeBakey, M.E. (1963). Prolonged assisted circulation during and after cardiac or aortic surgery: prolonged partial left ventricular bypass by means of intracorporeal circulation. *Am. J. Cardiol.*, **12**, 399
10. Spencer, F.C., Eiseman, B., Trinkle, J.K. and Rossi, N.P. (1965). Assisted circulation for cardiac failure following intracardiac surgery with cardiopulmonary bypass. *J. Thorac. Cardiovasc. Surg.*, **49**, 56
11. DeBakey, M.E. (1971). Left ventricular bypass pump for cardiac assistance. *Am. J. Cardiol.*, **27**, 3
12. Norman, J.C. and Bernhard, W.F. (1975). Criteia, protocols and reporting forms for initial left ventricular assist device clinical trials. *Cardiovasc. Dis.*, **2**, 438
13. Bernhard, W.F., Schoen, F.J., Poirier, V. and Carr, J. A temporary ventricular assist device for patients exhibiting intractable postcardiotomy shock. In Unger, F. (ed.) *Assisted Circulation*, Vol. 2, p. 49. (New York: Springer-Verlag)
14. Norman, J.C. (1979). ALVAD: 1979. Precedence, potentials, prospects and problems. *Proc. Int. Soc. Artif. Organs*, **2**, 407
15. Litwak, R.S., Koffsky, R.M., Jurado, R.A., Mitchell, B.A. and King, P. (1975). A decade of experience with a left heart assist device in patients undergoing open intracardiac operation. *World J. Surg.*, **9**, 18
16. Rose, D.M., Colvin, S.B., Culliford, A.T., Cunningham, J.N., Adams, P.X., Glassman, E., Isom, O.W. and Spencer, F.C. (1982). Long-term survival with partial left heart bypass following perioperative myocardial infarction and shock. *J. Thorac. Cardiovasc.Surg.*, **83**, 483
17. Golding, L.R., Groves, L.K., Peter, M., Jacobs, G., Sukalac, R., Nose', Y. and Loop, F.D. (1978). Initial clinical experience with a new temporary left ventricular assist device. *Ann. Thorac. Surg.*, **29**, 66
18. Magovern, G.J., Park, S.B. and Maher, T.D. (1985). Use of a centrifugal pump without anticoagulants for post-operative left ventricular assist. *World J. Surg.*, **9**, 25
19. Pierce, W.S., Parr, G.V.S., Myers, J.L., Pae, W.S., Bull, A.P. and Waldhausen, J.A. (1981). Ventricular assist pumping in patients with cardiogenic shock after cardiac operations. *N. Engl. J. Med.*, **305**, 1606
20. Pennington, D.G., Samuels, L.D., Williams, G., Palmer, D., Swartz, M.T., Codd, J.E., Merjavy, J.P., Lagunoff, D. and Joist, J.H. (1985). Experience with the Pierce–Donachy ventricular assist device in postcardiotomy patients with cardiogenic shock. *World J. Surg.*, **9**, 37
21. Reemtsma, K., Drusin, R., Edie, R., Bregman, D., Dobelle, W. and Hardy, M. (1978). Cardiac transplantation for patients requiring mechanical circulatory support. *N. Engl. J. Med.*, **298**, 670
22. Norman, J.C., Cooley, D.A., Kagan, V.D., Keats, A.S., Massin, E.K., Solis, R.T., Luper, W.E., Brook, M.I., Klima, T., Frazier, O.H., Hacker, J., Duncan, J.M., Dacso, C.C., Winston, D.S. and Reul, G.J. (1978). Total support of the circulation of a patient with post-cardiotomy stone-heart syndrome by a partial artificial heart (ALVAD) for five days followed by heart and kidney transplantation. *Lancet*, **1**, 1125
23. Pennington, D.G., Merjavy, J.P., Codd, J.E., Swartz, M.T., Miller, L.L. and Williams, G.A. (1984). Extracorporeal membrane oxygenation for patients with cardiogenic shock. *Cardiovascular Surg.* 1983. *Circulation*, **70**, I-130
24. Pennington, D.G., Codd, J.E., Merjavy, J.P., Swartz, M.T., Kaiser, G.C., Barner, H.B. and Willman, V.L. (1983). The expanded use of ventricular bypass systems for severe cardiac failure and as a bridge to cardiac transplantation. *Heart Transplant.*, **3**, 38
25. Zumbro, G.L., Shearer, G., Kitchens, W.R. and Galloway, R.F. (1985). Mechanical assistance for biventricular failure following coronary bypass operation and heart transplantation. *J. Heart Transplant.*, **4**, 248
26. Portner, P.M., Oyer, P.E., McGregor, C.G., Baldwin, J.C., Ream, A.K., Wyner, J., Zusman, D.R. and Shumway, N.E. (1985). First human use of an electrically implantable ventricular assist system. *Artif. Organs*, **9**(A), 36
27. Pae, W.E. and Pierce, W.S. (1987). Combined registry for the clinical use of mechanical ventricular assist pumps and the total artificial heart: first official report – 1987. *J. Heart Transplant.*, **6**, 68
28. Frazier, O.H. (1986). The Texas Heart Institute experience with assist devices. Presented at a symposium on *Heart Assist Devices – Heart Replacement*, Baltimore, Maryland, September 12–13
29. Portner, P.M., Oyer, P.E., Jassawalla, J.S. et al. (1984). A totally implantable ventricular assist device for end-stage disease. In Unger, F. (ed.) *Assisted Circulation*, Vol. 2, pp. 115–41. (New York: Springer-Verlag)
30. Hardesty, R.L., Griffith, B.P., Trento, A., Thompson, M.E., Ferson, P.F. and Bahnson, H.T. (1986). Mortally ill patients and excellent survival following cardiac transplantation. *Ann. Thorac. Surg.*, **41**, 126
31. Carpentier, A., Perier, P., Brugger, J.P., Dreyfus, G., Meli, M., Hahn, C.H., Benasson, D., Guibourt, P., Mollin, B., Dubost, C., Berthier, B., Abry, B., Odermatt, R., Schahmaneche, L., Tournay, D., Guillemain, R., Fabiani, J.N. and Gay, J. (1986). Heterotopic artificial heart as a bridge to cardiac transplantation. *Lancet*, **2**, 97
32. Magovern, J.A., Pae, W.E., Richenbacher, W.E. and Pierce, W.S. (1986). The importance of a patent foramen ovale in left ventricular assist pumping. *Trans. Am. Soc. Artif. Intern. Organs*, **32**, 449
33. Pennock, J.L., Pae, W.E., Pierce, W.S. and Waldhausen, J.A. (1979). Reduction of myocardial infarct size: comparison between left atrial and left ventricular bypass. *Circulation*, **59**, 275
34. Pierce, W.S. (1979). Clinical left ventricular bypass: problems of pump inflow obstruction and right ventricular failure. *Trans. Am. Soc. Artif. Intern. Organs*, **2**, 1
35. Coleman, S.J., Bornhorst, W.J., LaFarge, C.G. and Carr, J.G. (1972). Pneumatic waveform diagnostics of implanted ventricular assist pumps. *Trans. Am. Soc. Artif. Intern Organs*, **18**, 176
36. Rosenberg, G., Landis, D.L., Phillips, W.M., Stallsmith, J. and Pierce,

W.S. (1978). Determining arterial pressure, left atrial pressure, and cardiac output from the left pneumatic drive line of the total artificial heart. *Trans. Am. Soc. Artif. Intern. Organs*, **24**, 341
37. Relman, A.S. (1986). Artificial hearts – permanent and temporary. *N. Engl. J. Med.*, **314**, 644
38. Annas, G.J. (1985). No cheers for temporary artificial hearts. *Hastings Cent. Rep.*, **15**, 27

57
Total Artificial Hearts
E. SOLIS, C. MUNERETTO AND C. CABROL

EXPERIMENTAL BACKGROUND

The first attempt to utilize a total artificial heart (TAH) was by Demikhov (Figure 33.1), who removed a dog's heart and replaced it with a mechanical device[1]. His original plan was to maintain an artificial circulation, so that the organs from a cadaver could be used for transplantation[1].

Twenty years later, W. Kolff (Figure 60.3) and Akutsu obtained the first animal survival (90 minutes) using two artificial blood pumps made of polyvinyl chloride[2]. In the following years, Kolff and his colleagues experimented with a solenoid-driven electrohydraulic heart[3], and with roller type and pendulum-type artificial hearts[4] (Chapter 59). The advent of pneumatic driving systems was in the early 1960s. Modifications were introduced to control the pressure and diastolic vacuum generated by the pneumatic ventricles.

In 1964, Pierce, at Penn State University, developed a new substance, the biomer. This has been used as the major component of the membrane of the TAH, and has reduced the problems originating at the interface between the blood and the artificial ventricle[5]. At the same time, the Division of Artificial Organs at the University of Utah developed a control system for the TAH. In 1971, they designed the first artificial heart in which the cardiac output improved as a response to increased atrial pressure (Starling's response of a pneumatic artificial heart)[6].

EARLY CLINICAL EXPERIENCE

Clinical experience dates from 1969 when Cooley (Figure 60.1) first utilized a TAH as a bridge to transplantation[7]. He implanted a pneumatically-driven TAH (Liotta) in a patient who could not be weaned from cardiopulmonary bypass. This patient underwent heart transplantation after 64 hours of total mechanical support, but died 2 days later from infection. In 1982, DeVries (Figure 60.2) performed the first permanent TAH (JARVIK 7, Symbion Inc.) implantation on his patient, Barney Clark, who lived 112 days[8] (Chapter 60).

The first successful use of the TAH (JARVIK 7) as a bridge to transplantation was in August, 1985[9]. Since then, more than 80 implantations have been carried out worldwide (Table 57.1), establishing the TAH as a clinical reality. As approximately 86% of the TAHs implanted have been of the JARVIK 7 design, this chapter will concentrate attention on this type of mechanical heart.

PATIENT SELECTION

A successful bridge-to-transplant procedure includes four important steps:

(1) Adequate selection of a recipient with irreversible myocardial failure, but with no irreversible dysfunction of any other major organ or other major contraindication.

(2) Implantation of a device that successfully supports the circulation, thus improving secondary organ function, without producing or increasing morbidity.

(3) Replacement of the device with an allograft.

(4) Discharge of the patient from hospital with minimal or no morbidity.

If these steps can be successfully achieved, there are three major groups who could benefit from the use of the TAH as a bridge to transplantation: (1) patients in chronic end-stage cardiac failure who have already been selected for transplantation and are awaiting a donor heart; (2) patients who develop acute, potentially terminal, heart failure at a time when a suitable donor organ is not available; (3) postcardiotomy patients who cannot be weaned from pump-oxygenator support. Our clinical TAH program at Hopital La Pitie in Paris was started in 1986 to help these three groups of patients. In our experience, patient selection and preoperative assessment are the most important determinants in patient survival after implantation of a TAH.

In addition to the routine clinical assessment of any

Table 57.1 World experience in the application of the total artificial heart (TAH) as a 'bridge to transplant' (as of November 1, 1987)

	Number of implants	Device	Transplanted	Alive
Hopital La Pitie, Paris, France	27	18 Jarvik 7-100	12	7
		9 Jarvik 7-70		
University of Pittsburgh, USA	15	3 Jarvik 7-100	13	9
		12 Jarvik 7-70		
University of Arizona, USA	6	1 Phoenix	4	3
		1 Jarvik 7-100		
		4 Jarvik 7-70		
University of Ottawa, Canada	5 (4 pts.)	1 Jarvik 7-100	4	3
		4 Jarvik 7-70		
Texas Heart Institute, Houston, USA	4	1 Liotta (1969)	1	0
		1 Akutsu (1981)	1	0
		1 Jarvik 7-100		
		1 Jarvik 7-70	1	1
Minneapolis Heart Institute, USA	4	4 Jarvik 7-70	4	3
Universities of Salzburg and Vienna, Austria (Unger and Wolner)	5	4 Unger	2	0
		1 Berlin		
Karolinska Institute, Stockholm, Sweden	2	Jarvik 7-70	2	2
Midwest Heart Surgical Institute, Milwaukee, USA	3	Jarvik 7-70	2	2
University of Berlin, West Germany	3	Berlin	0	0
Penn State University, USA	2	Penn State	1	1 (on TAH)
Papworth Hospital, Cambridge, UK	1	Jarvik 7-100	1	1
University of Florida, USA	1	Jarvik 7-70	1	0
Hopital Henri Mondor, Paris, France	1	Jarvik 7-70	1	0
Mercy Medical Center, Des Moines, USA	1	Jarvik 7	1	0
Sharp Memorial Hospital, San Diego, USA	1	Jarvik 7-70	1	1

patient undergoing major cardiac surgery, special consideration has to be given to five crucial points.

The thoracic dimensions

The preoperative evaluation of the chest size of the patient is primarily subjective, as there is no solely objective way to make this assessment. Following a multi-institutional cooperative study, Jarvik concluded that the combination of body surface area (BSA) and thoracic anteroposterior depth, measured by computerized tomographic scan at the level of the 10th thoracic vertebra, can be used to select the correct prosthesis[10]. In patients with a BSA less than $2 m^2$, the JARVIK 7-70 ml TAH will provide a cardiac index sufficient for bridge-to-transplant application. If the BSA is greater than $2 m^2$, the JARVIK 7-100 ml should be used.

Thoracic depth at the level of T10 (DT10) was found to be the most important measurement in deciding where the TAH should be implanted. Patients in whom a JARVIK 7-100 is to be implanted (based on $BSA > 2 m^2$) should have a DT10 greater than 13–14 cm to allow for medial positioning of the TAH. Patients in whom a JARVIK 7-70 is to be implanted in a medial location should have a DT10 greater than 11–12 cm. In patients with a DT10 less than these diameters, lateral positioning of the prosthesis will allow better function. We believe, however, that lateral positioning of the TAH can contribute to compression of the left lung, with an increased risk of pulmonary infection. At our institution, all implantations (28 patients) have been performed in medial positions (Figures 57.1A and 1B), with only one mismatch between the size of the TAH and that of the thorax.

The dimensions of the pericardial cavity may also be important for positioning a TAH. J. Kolff drew attention to difficulty in implanting the JARVIK 7-100 in a patient with a normal heart size and pericardial space[11]. It is our impression that a patient with a small DT10, but who has a dilated heart and pericardium, can receive a JARVIK 7-100 without complications.

Renal function

Preoperative renal function is critical to the survival of patients receiving a TAH. It is therefore essential to evaluate carefully the degree of permanent injury produced in the kidney prior to the implantation. Our preoperative studies include measurement of blood urea, total proteins, calcium and uric acid, urinary electrolytes and creatinine clearance, as well as urine microscopy and culture. Plasma aldosterone level and renin activity will be measured if the patient's condition permits, especially in patients with chronic heart disease. Daily determinations of creatinine clearance, fractional excretion of sodium, serum and urine osmolality, serum potassium, magnesium, calcium and phosphorus are obtained.

Respiratory function

Pulmonary function is vulnerable and critical. It is vulnerable because rapid changes in systemic and pulmonary

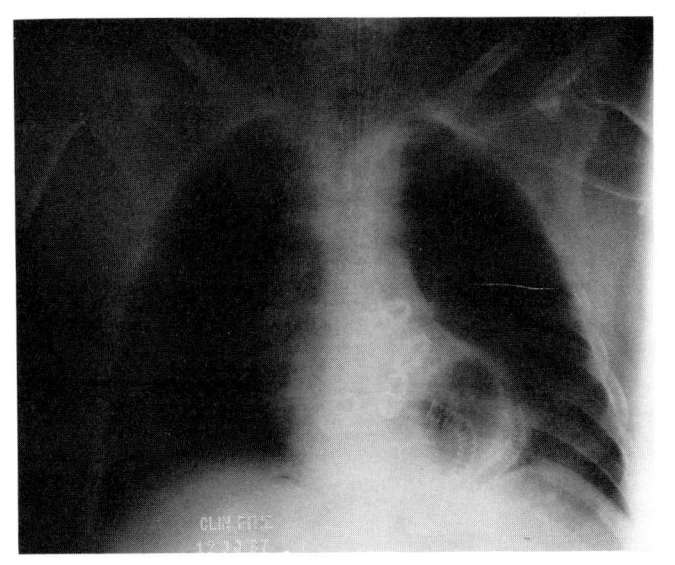

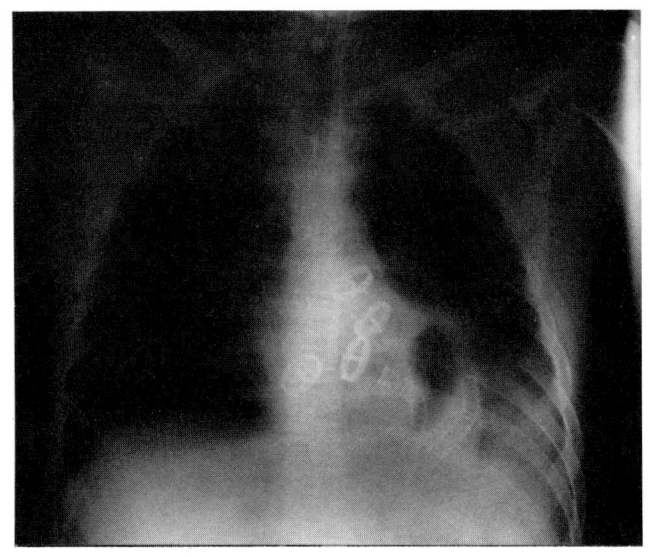

Figure 57.1 Plain posteroanterior chest radiographs of a patient with a JARVIK 7-100 ml TAH implanted in the medial position. Images show the air chambers of the artificial ventricles in the systolic (left) and mid-diastolic (right) positions. The TAH fits easily into the pericardial space

resistance increase left atrial pressure, producing pulmonary edema within a few minutes. It is critical because pulmonary failure with prolonged intubation predisposes to infection and increases mortality. Simple pulmonary function tests, such as blood gases and spirometry, are determined to obtain base-line figures. If the clinical status of the patient permits, full pulmonary function studies are performed.

Coagulation

Preoperative coagulation is evaluated by measuring the functional status of the platelets, thrombin formation and its regulatory pathways, and the fibrinolytic system; our protocol is summarized in Table 57.2.

Suitability for transplantation

Finally, but no less important, it is necessary to be certain that the patient will be acceptable for subsequent cardiac transplantation. Therefore, all of the examinations and investigations necessary to confirm this point must be carried out.

An assessment of the cumulative risks anticipated from careful studies of the patient's thoracic dimensions, renal, pulmonary, and coagulation functions, and transplant status, will indicate whether or not the TAH should be implanted.

SURGICAL TECHNIQUES

Medial positioning of the TAH

Through a median sternotomy, the pericardium is opened widely from the ascending aorta to the diaphragm. To

Table 57.2 Coagulation monitoring check list at Hopital La Pitie

Platelet function
Platelet aggregation to ADP, epinephrine, collagen and arachidonic acid by Born method
Platelet count
Platelet aggregate evaluation by Wu–Hoak method
Ivy–Borchgrevink bleeding time
Platelet factor 4 (PF-4)
Betathromboglobulin (BTG)

Thrombin formation and its regulatory pathways
Prothrombin time (PT)
Activated partial thromboplastin time (APTT)
Fibrinogen titration*
Recalcified whole blood thromboelastography (wbTEG)*
Plasma and serum antithrombin III (AT III) titration (estimate of antithrombin potential index (API) as: API = plasma AT III − serum AT III)
Plasma and serum factor X titration
Fibrinopeptides A (FpA)
Raby's transference test in thromboelastography*

Fibrinolytic system
Fibrinogen degradation products (FDP)
Alpha-2-antiplasmin (α-2-AP)

*Tests that evaluate one or more systems
NB All systems related to coagulation are systematically monitored (1) preoperatively, (2) 30 minutes after protamine neutralization, and (3) once each day after implantation when the patient is in a stable condition. These parameters are evaluated 2 or 3 times a day if there is a serious deterioration in the patient's condition

reduce the length of cardiopulmonary bypass (CPB), we prefer to place the ventricular drivelines before the CPB cannulae (Figure 57.2).

To accomplish the appropriate placement and positioning of the drivelines, the left border of the divided sternum is retracted to the left, and the pericardial incision is extended horizontally along the diaphragm. The diaphragmatic insertions into the posterior xiphoid and sternum are freed to obtain adequate access to the left side of the thorax and abdomen.

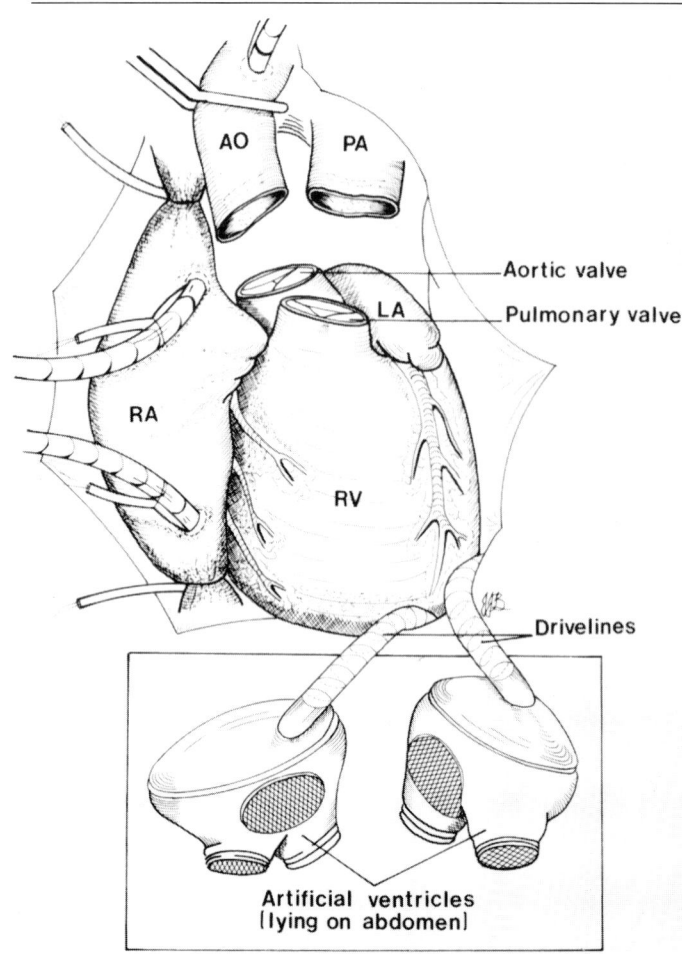

Figure 57.2 Surgical technique of TAH implantation. The aorta and pulmonary artery have been transected just above their respective valves. Note the two artificial ventricles protected by a drape

is introduced through the subcutaneous tunnel into the pericardial cavity and attached to the tape, permitting the drivelines to be pulled through the tunnel without damaging the internal surface. The felt cuff of each sheath is trimmed to 5 mm in width, to be placed later at the level of the subcutaneous tissue. The two artificial ventricles are covered, and stored on the upper portion of the abdomen (Figure 57.2).

CPB is established using two right-angled caval cannulae for venous drainage, inserted anteriorly through the right atrium, and an arterial inflow cannula, inserted into the ascending aorta (Figure 57.2). The posterior segment of the right atrium is preserved intact to facilitate subsequent cardiac transplantation. Two electrodes are inserted in the anterior wall of the right ventricle, and the heart is electrically fibrillated; the caval tapes are tightened and the aorta is cross-clamped.

Heart excision

The pulmonary artery and the aorta are transected just above their respective valves (Figure 57.2), and separated from each other to facilitate the subsequent anastomoses. The right ventricle is sectioned 2 cm in length below the right atrioventricular groove (Figure 57.3). Through this

Two horizontal skin incisions (2 cm long) are made in the left upper quadrant of the abdomen in the mammary line, 8 cm below the costal margin. Then, through the sternotomy, the left rectus abdominis muscle is mobilized. A tunnel is created, from inside-out, through the subcutaneous tissue from the skin incision to the pericardial cavity. The surgeon avoids opening the peritoneal cavity, and leaves the posterior fascia of the muscle intact. The tunnel needs to be large enough to permit the easy passage of the index finger.

While this dissection is being accomplished, the felt and silicone sheaths to be used for passing the drivelines through the abdominal wall are prepared. The internal surfaces are saturated with a silicone lubricant, permitting easy passage of each driveline through its respective sheath. Also at this stage, the function of the artificial ventricles should be carefully checked.

To avoid contamination of the internal surface of the drivelines with blood or fat when they are placed in position, we use a piece of latex rubber (obtained from a surgical glove) to protect the distal end of the driveline. Umbilical tape is tied around the inferior end of the felt sheaths, around the drivelines, and the latex finger. A strong clamp

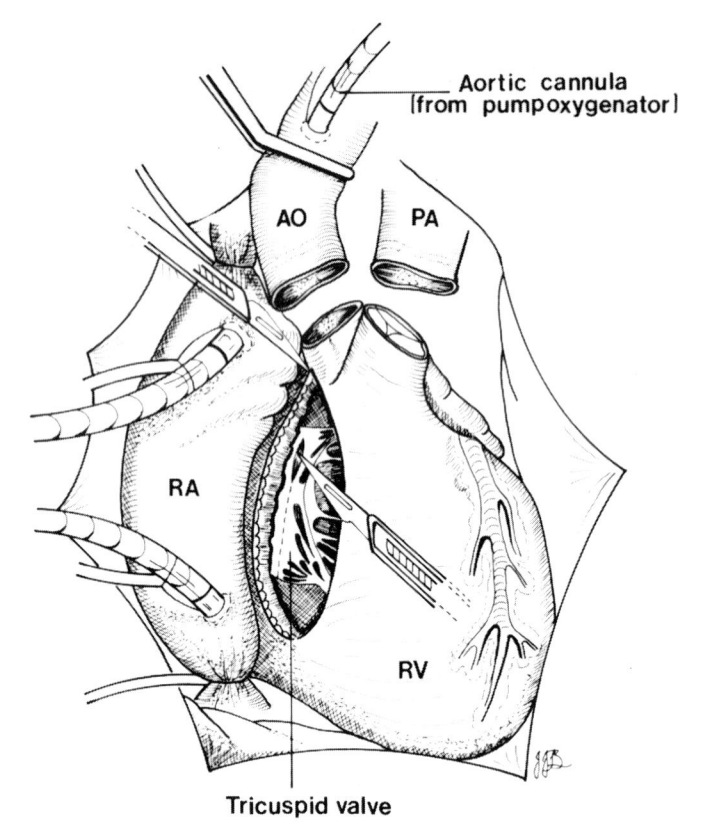

Figure 57.3 The right ventricle has been sectioned 2 cm below the right atrioventricular groove. Through this incision, the internal anatomy of the right ventricle and tricuspid valve can be seen. The tricuspid valve is excised, leaving a cuff attached to the annulus

aperture, the internal surface of the right ventricle and the tricuspid valve are visualized. Under direct vision, the ventricular incision is continued, staying 5–8 mm away from the tricuspid annulus. The tricuspid valve leaflets are sectioned 2–3 mm away from their insertion into the annulus. The interventricular septum is opened through an incision made 3–4 mm in front of the tricuspid annulus (Figure 57.4). This maneuver allows the surgeon to visualize the mitral valve, and to continue the dissection of the left ventricular wall, staying 3–4 mm from the mitral annulus (Figure 57.4).

The root of the aorta is opened longitudinally, continuing the incision into the left ventricular cavity (Figures 57.4 and 57.5). The left ventricle is now opened like a book, and the mitral valve is excised, leaving a thin strip around the annulus (Figure 57.5). The excision of the left ventricle is now completed by dividing its lateral wall, staying 4–5 mm away from the mitral orifice, and taking care not to enter the left atrium; to avoid this, the root of the aorta is preserved.

The coronary sinus ostium is closed with a 4-0 polypropylene suture, and the venous coronary sinus in the left atrioventricular groove is ligated (Figure 57.5).

Implantation of pulmonary, aortic, and atrial connectors

The two atrial prosthetic cuffs are trimmed identically, to within 2–3 mm from the orifices. The formation of a blind sac between the connectors and the atrial cavity will thus be avoided, and the area in which thrombus formation may occur will be reduced.

The anastomosis between these cuffs and the atrioventricular remnants is started using a 3-0 polypropylene double-running suture, beginning in the cephalic portion of the septum. The first stitch is introduced through the right cuff, across the septum, and through the left cuff. The double anastomosis line in the atrial septum is performed with a simple running suture, joining the two cuffs to the entire thickness of the septum. The lateral portion of the right cuff is then sutured with a simple running suture of 3-0 polypropylene, taking the muscle, the tricuspid annulus, and the cuff. A second simple running suture is used to secure the fat and connective tissue of the groove to the cuff to reinforce the previous suture.

The left cuff is sutured identically to the right one. The adequacy of these anastomoses is tested by the injection under pressure of saline solution mixed with blood, using the test plugs provided (Figure 57.6). If leaks are present, the anastomosis will be supplemented with interrupted sutures and with the use of gelatine resorcin formol adhesive (GRF) (Figure 57.6).

The aortic and pulmonary grafts (7 cm long) are sutured end-to-end to their respective vessels with a 5-0 polypropylene running suture (Figure 57.7). The suture lines are tested and sealed, as described for the atrial cuffs.

A catheter to measure the left atrial pressure is placed through the right superior pulmonary vein under direct vision to ensure correct length and positioning (Figure 57.8).

Connection of the TAH

Small marks are placed on the atrial cuff, respective major vessel (aorta or pulmonary artery), and on the respective artificial ventricle, to prevent anatomical distortion when the ventricle is connected, and to ensure a satisfactory position (Figure 57.8). The artificial ventricles are attached with the aid of the 'quick connectors' to their respective cuffs. The left ventricle is connected first (Figure 57.8),

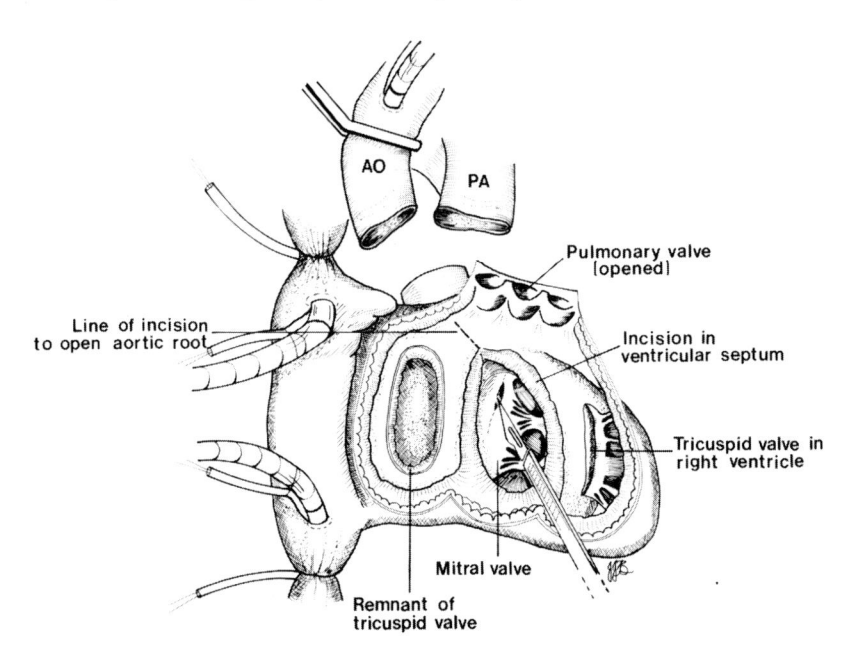

Figure 57.4 The intraventricular septum has been divided, allowing visualization of the mitral valve, which is excised. The outflow tract of the right ventricle has been opened up, exposing the three cusps of the pulmonary valve. The line of incision to open the aortic valve is indicated

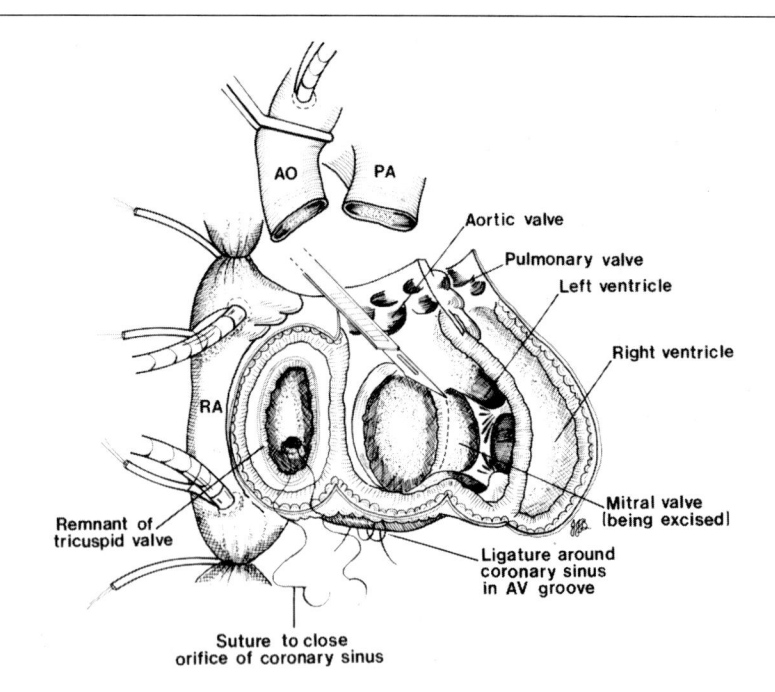

THE TRANSPLANTATION AND REPLACEMENT OF THORACIC ORGANS

Figure 57.5 The aortic root has been opened longitudinally, exposing the aortic valve, the incision being extended into the left ventricle. The left ventricle has been opened like a book, and the mitral valve is being excised, leaving a cuff of 3–4 mm attached to the mitral annulus. The coronary sinus ostium in the right atrium is closed with a suture, and the coronary sinus in the left atrioventricular groove is ligated

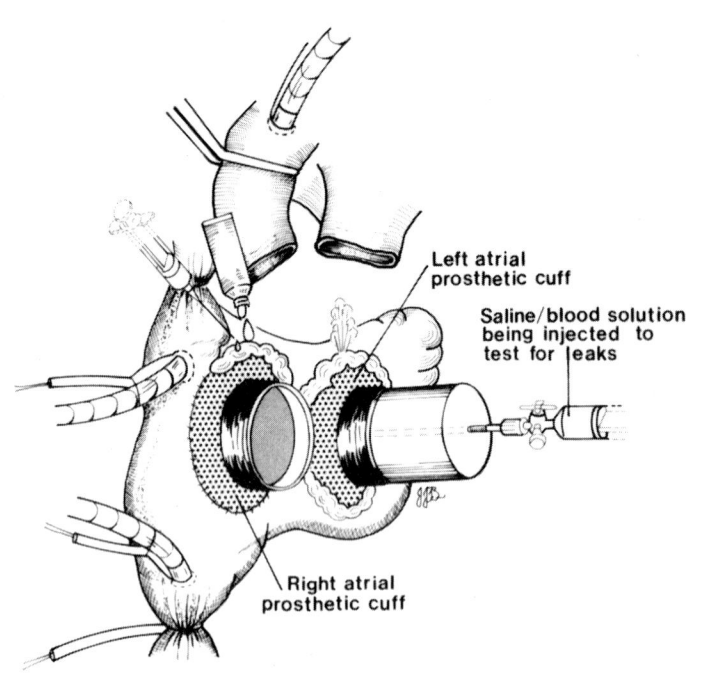

Figure 57.6 The ventricles have been removed, and the two atrial prosthetic cuffs have been sutured in position. The hermeticity of these suture lines is tested, using the test plugs provided; if leaks are present, the suture line will be supplemented by interrupted sutures and by the application of gelatine resorcin formol adhesive (GRF)

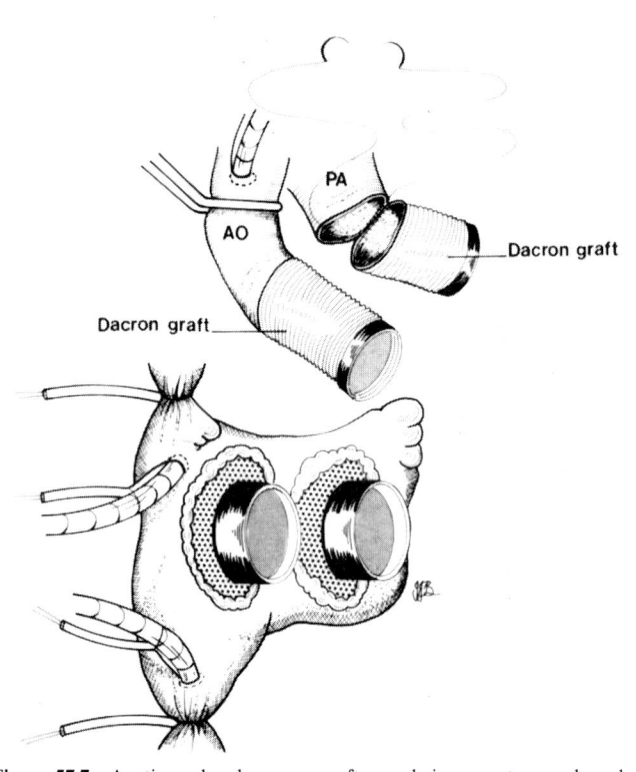

Figure 57.7 Aortic and pulmonary grafts are being anastomosed, end-to-end with 5-0 polypropylene running sutures

clamping both the atrial and arterial cuffs with two strong clamps (on each side of the mark), and sliding the artificial ventricle into the correct position.

All residual air is evacuated from the aortic root through a vent, and from the aortic graft by needle aspiration (Figure 57.9). The air in the chamber of the artificial ventricle is evacuated through a vent port designed specifically for this purpose (Figure 57.9). When all of the air has been evacuated, the aspiration needle is removed from the vent port, which is clamped and securely tied to prevent the introduction of air or leaking. Pumping through the left artificial ventricle is now begun, avoiding left atrial pressures greater than 9 mmHg.

The right ventricle is connected (as described for the left),

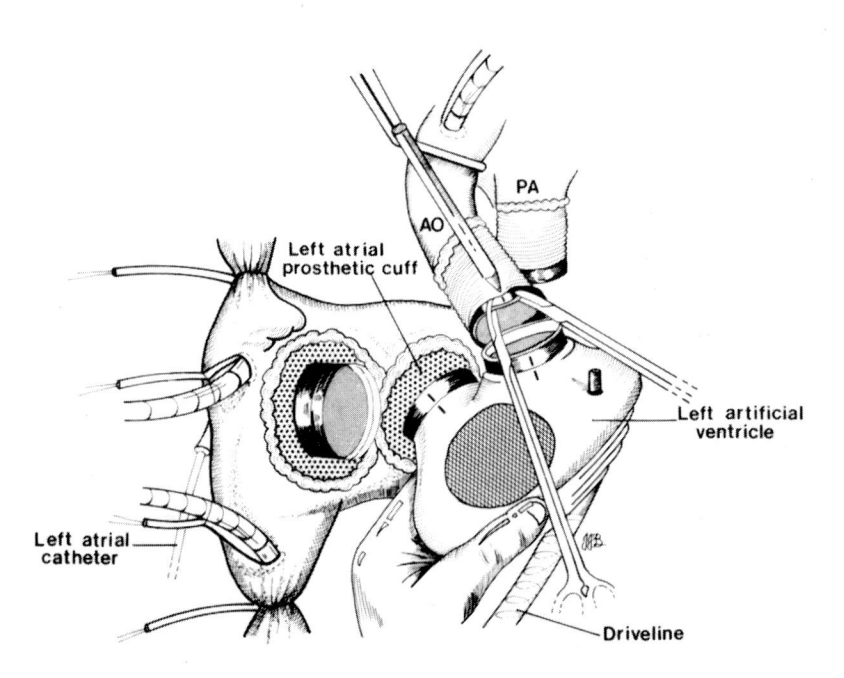

Figure 57.8 The artificial left ventricle has been attached with the aid of the 'quick connection' to its respective (left atrial) ring. A small mark is used to assure proper alignment to prevent anatomical distortion. The aortic connection is in progress

and is carefully de-aired before pumping is started. It is extremely important to locate both ventricles as far to the left as possible to prevent obstruction of the venous return to the artificial heart (Figure 57.10).

When the output of the artificial ventricles is adequate, reflected by a left atrial pressure of 8–9 mmHg and a systemic pressure of 100–120 mmHg, CPB is discontinued. A catheter to measure pulmonary artery pressure is placed. The aortic vent and CPB cannulae are removed, pericardial blood is aspirated, and all the suture lines are carefully inspected to assure hemostasis. The positions of the drivelines are adjusted. The internal silicone sheath is fixed with the felt sheath, and hermeticity is secured with two wires around the drivelines and by the application of silicone adhesive. Both driveline sheaths are secured to the skin with interrupted sutures of 2-0 polyester.

Two drains are inserted above and below the TAH, and the sternotomy is closed in the usual manner. It is important to confirm that the closure does not modify the hemodynamic status of the patient. Radiographic views of a TAH implanted in the medial position are represented in Figures 57.1A and 1B.

Figure 57.9 Residual air is evacuated from the aortic root through a vent and from the aortic graft by needle aspiration. The air in the chamber of the artificial ventricle is evacuated through a vent port designed specially for this purpose

Lateral positioning of the TAH

We have implanted 28 TAH with the above technique. There was one mismatch in size between TAH and thorax in a patient who could not be weaned from CPB support after an orthotopic transplant failed to function adequately. We were not able to close the sternum. Retrospectively, it might have been possible to insert the TAH in a lateral position in this patient.

For this rare situation, the left pericardium is widely excised to within 2 cm of the phrenic nerve. The left ventricle is placed deep and quite far to the left, permitting the right ventricle to lie anterior to it, mostly to the left of the sternum. The exit of the drivelines is accomplished through an intercostal space. A longer aortic graft and, in some cases, special trimming of the atrial cuffs may be necessary[10].

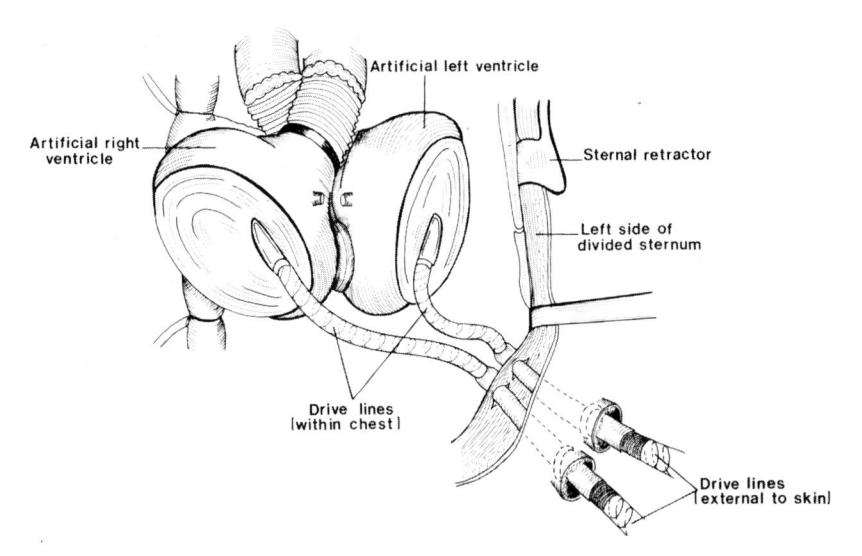

Figure 57.10 Before closure of the chest, the position of the drivelines is adjusted

TAH removal before orthotopic heart transplantation

The median sternotomy is re-opened. Generally, the TAH is surrounded by clots that should be washed thoroughly. CPB is established with two right-angled caval cannulae for venous drainage, inserted through the right atrium as posterior as possible, and an arterial inflow line inserted into the ascending aorta (Figure 57.11). As CPB is initiated, the TAH is stopped. The aortic exit of the left ventricle is immediately disconnected to avoid distention of the left atrium. The atrial and arterial connections of the right ventricle are then disconnected, followed by the atrial connection of the left side.

To prepare the patient for transplantation, the pulmonary artery and aorta are transected just above the suture lines of the Dacron grafts (Figure 57.11). The right and left atrial walls are transected posterior to the suture lines and to the two atrial appendages.

Standard techniques are then used for orthotopic heart transplantation (Chapter 10).

POSTOPERATIVE CARE

A patient with a TAH is not entirely different from any patient after cardiac surgery. Management involves four major areas:

(1) Coagulation/anticoagulation control.

(2) Clinical status – general, peripheral circulation, urinary output, blood gases, etc.

(3) Hemodynamic monitoring – continuous monitoring of arterial, central venous, left atrial, and pulmonary artery pressures.

(4) Drive unit – control of TAH parameters (COMDU).

In our opinion, after TAH implantation, the patient should be kept in strict isolation. A minimal number of personnel should have access to him. Before entering the patient's room, all personnel must wash their hands, and put on cap, mask, boots and sterile gown. It is important to minimize the number of machines and other objects that are taken in and out of the room. In our hospital, the doors of such rooms are made of glass, enabling the bed to be placed in such a position to allow radiographs to be taken from outside the room. Chest radiographs are obtained

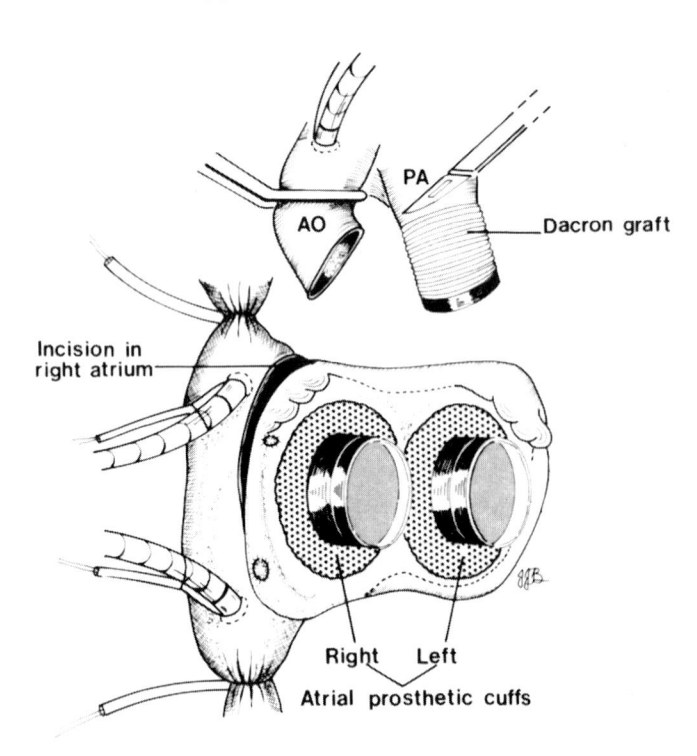

Figure 57.11 To prepare for insertion of an orthotopic allograft, the aorta and pulmonary artery are transected just above the anastomoses of the Dacron grafts. The right and left atrial walls are transected just posterior to the cuff anastomotic lines and to the atrial appendages

every 12 hours in the early postoperative period. A nurse or a doctor is always with the patient, who is routinely examined every 6 hours.

Coagulation/anticoagulation control

Coagulation-related problems in patients supported by TAH are due to interaction between the blood and the TAH. Coagulation is a dynamic system represented by a group of agonist and antagonist forces that either increase or decrease clot formation (Figure 57.12). Under TAH support, blood stability is altered by (1) the presence of four mechanical valves, (2) a large interface between foreign material and blood, and (3) the presence of localized turbulent blood flow in a patient with a poor general status, secondary to hemodynamic failure. The coagulation problems (bleeding or thromboembolism) that result from this complex TAH/blood interaction require systematic investigation and therapy in each individual patient if implantation is to be brought to a successful conclusion.

The perioperative coagulation investigation protocol (developed by J.C. Bellon and J. Szefner) utilized in our hospital is summarized in Table 57.2[12].

Control of coagulation in patients supported over long periods by a permanent TAH presented major clinical problems, including fatal hemorrhage and major disabling thromboemboli[13] (Chapter 58). Coagulation control in patients with a temporary TAH has been more successful, with a lower incidence of complications[13-15]. Multiple anticoagulation protocols have been used, but the great majority of centers involved in this field are using heparin in association with a platelet inhibitor (acetyl salicylic acid or dipyridamole)[16].

Our treatment protocol is summarized in Table 57.3[15].

Heparin neutralization

We systematically neutralize the heparin given at operation with a dose of protamine sulfate equal to 60% of the heparin administered for CPB.

Table 57.3 Anticoagulation regimen used during TAH implantation at Hopital La Pitie*

Heparin	1000–5000 i.v./day
Dipyridamole	150–300 mg/6 hours
Acetyl salicylic acid	50 mg/day
Aprotinin	1 000 000 PI/U i.v. + 4000 PI/U per minute
Pentoxyphylline	400 mg/day
Ticlopidine	250 mg/2–3 days
Fresh plasma AT III Blood cell concentrates	According to the evaluation of the patient's state

*Frequent modifications are required, depending on the patient's condition

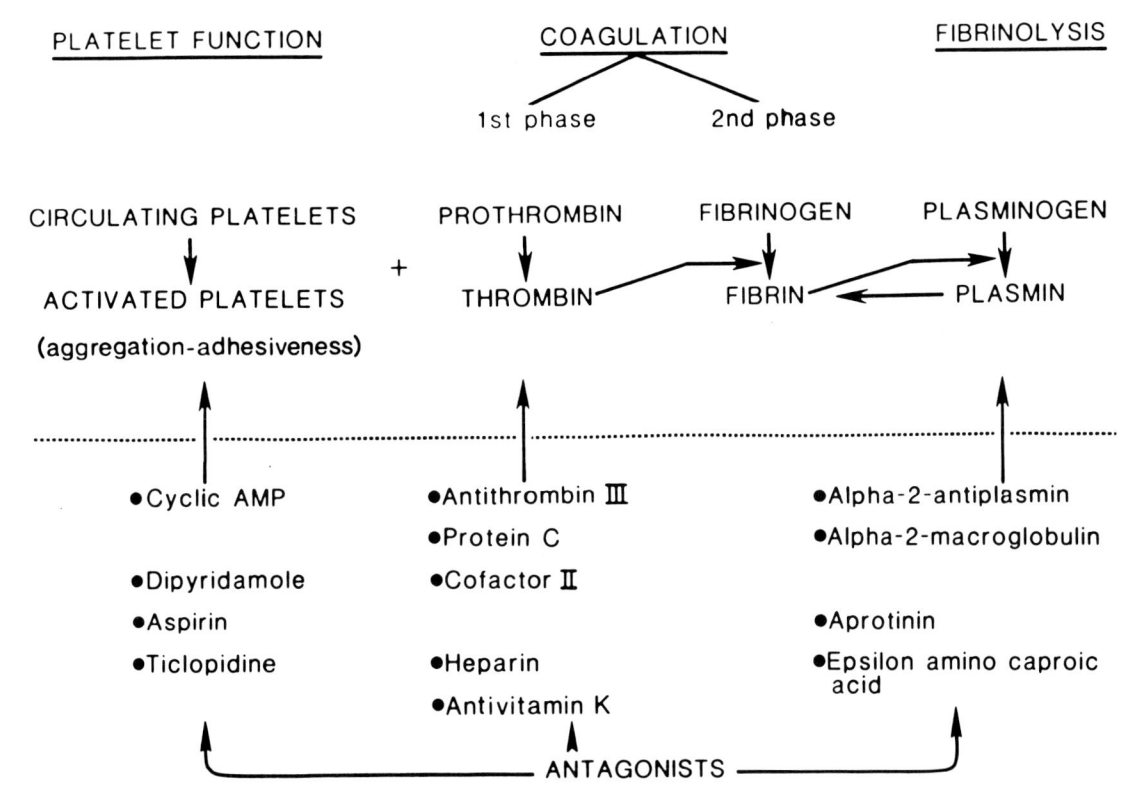

Figure 57.12 Diagrammatic representation of the hemostatic process. Agonist and antagonist forces will increase or reduce the possibilities of clot formation

Platelet aggregation

Exaggerated platelet activity, as evidenced by (1) hyperaggregability *in vitro* and (2) an increase in the plasma levels of platelet factor 4 and betathromboglobulin, is corrected by dipyridamole (150–300 mg i.v. every 6 hours) as a platelet-stabilizer; its inhibitory action takes place at the level of the phosphodiesterase, increasing cyclic AMP at the platelet level[12]. When the platelet aggregation curves and the platelet proteins return to normal, demonstrating recovery of platelet function, we give acetyl salicylic acid (ASA) (50 mg/day) as an anti-platelet drug (beginning usually on the 3rd or 4th postoperative day).

To decrease platelet adhesiveness, evidenced by a Wu–Hoak coefficient greater than 1 unit and a normal Ivy–Borchgrevink bleeding time, we use ticlopidine in a dose adjusted to maintain the Ivy–Borchgrevink bleeding time at about 20 minutes (usually 250 mg every 2 days).

Coagulation

To normalize the coagulation process, evaluated by Raby's transference test, plasma and serum factor X titration, and plasma and serum antithrombin III titration (API), we use low doses of heparin (10–50 mg/day) in continuous infusion.

Fibrinolytic system

If a fibrinolytic process is evidenced by (1) the decrease of alpha-2 antiplasmin, (2) an increase of fibrin degradation products, and (3) a decrease of plasmatic fibrinogen, we use aprotinin (Kunitz inhibitor), given in an initial i.v. bolus of 1 000 000 PI/units, followed by 4000 PI/units i.v. per minute in a continuous infusion until the laboratory data are normalized.

No clinical thromboembolic events or major bleeding complications were seen in 28 implantations in which this protocol was used. On examination of the TAH, only small fibrin deposits in the inflow portion of the artificial ventricle and along the suture lines of the atrial cuff connectors were seen.

Hemodynamic status

The functional status of the pneumatic TAH is evaluated non-invasively, based on the air flow curves (Figure 57.13). From these data on cardiac output, filling volume, and whether filling is complete or incomplete, and relative atrial pressure, the volemic state of patient and malfunction of drive mechanism or prosthetic valves can be analyzed.

During the early postoperative period, correct hemodynamic balance should be obtained. Systemic, pulmonary, and atrial pressures are kept within therapeutic ranges by regulation of the machine and/or by i.v. infusion. It is important to drive both ventricles with a filling volume of 70–80% of full capacity, so that they operate on the steep portion of Starling's curve, with the possibility of adjusting the cardiac output by pre- and post-load changes.

Left atrial pressures greater than 15 mmHg must be avoided to reduce the risk of pulmonary edema. Right atrial pressures are maintained as low as possible to avoid renal venous hypertension that may cause a low glomerular filtration rate. Atrial pressures may be reduced by the use of diastolic vacuum, vasodilators, or by decreasing systolic/diastolic duration. We believe a cardiac output of 5–6 l/min is effective in the great majority of patients, but, in some, a moderate degree of overperfusion will improve kidney function. Increased resistance with systemic and/or pulmonary hypertension is treated using vasodilators. We prefer sodium nitroprusside in the early postoperative period to increase glomerular filtration and urine output.

Decreased systemic vascular resistance with hypotension, indicated by an overdrive status of the left ventricle, can be corrected by the administration of alpha-adrenergic drugs. Serious hypotension during TAH support, however, has a poor prognostic value, and strongly suggests generalized sepsis with circulatory collapse.

Renal status

Renal failure may occur following implantation of a TAH, especially in patients with pre-existing renal dysfunction. In the patient with postoperative renal failure, adequate renal perfusion must be maintained.

We currently begin the protection of the kidney in the operating room by avoiding low perfusion pressures during CPB, by utilizing a membrane oxygenator to reduce hemolysis, and by maintaining a good urinary output throughout the surgical procedure.

After implantation of the TAH, the driving parameters should be controlled to improve glomerular filtration rate and to optimize blood urea nitrogen (BUN), creatinine, and urine excretion. Every effort should be made to maintain the urine output greater than 2 ml/kg per hour during the first 36 hours, with the use of albumin, furosemide, and filling volume control. Sodium nitroprusside may help to increase glomerular filtration rate. PCO_2 levels should be maintained at normal values in order to avoid renal damage, and moderate urine alkalinization helps to protect the kidney in the presence of oliguria. Ultrafiltration can be effective in patients with serious hemodilution and/or massive edema.

In patients with compromised renal function, nephrotoxic drugs are avoided. Those drugs excreted by the kidney are adjusted to appropriate dosages. Metabolic encephalopathy, acidosis, hyperkalemia, hypercalcemia, hypermagnesemia, hypernatremia, and hyperphosphatemia are indications for dialysis.

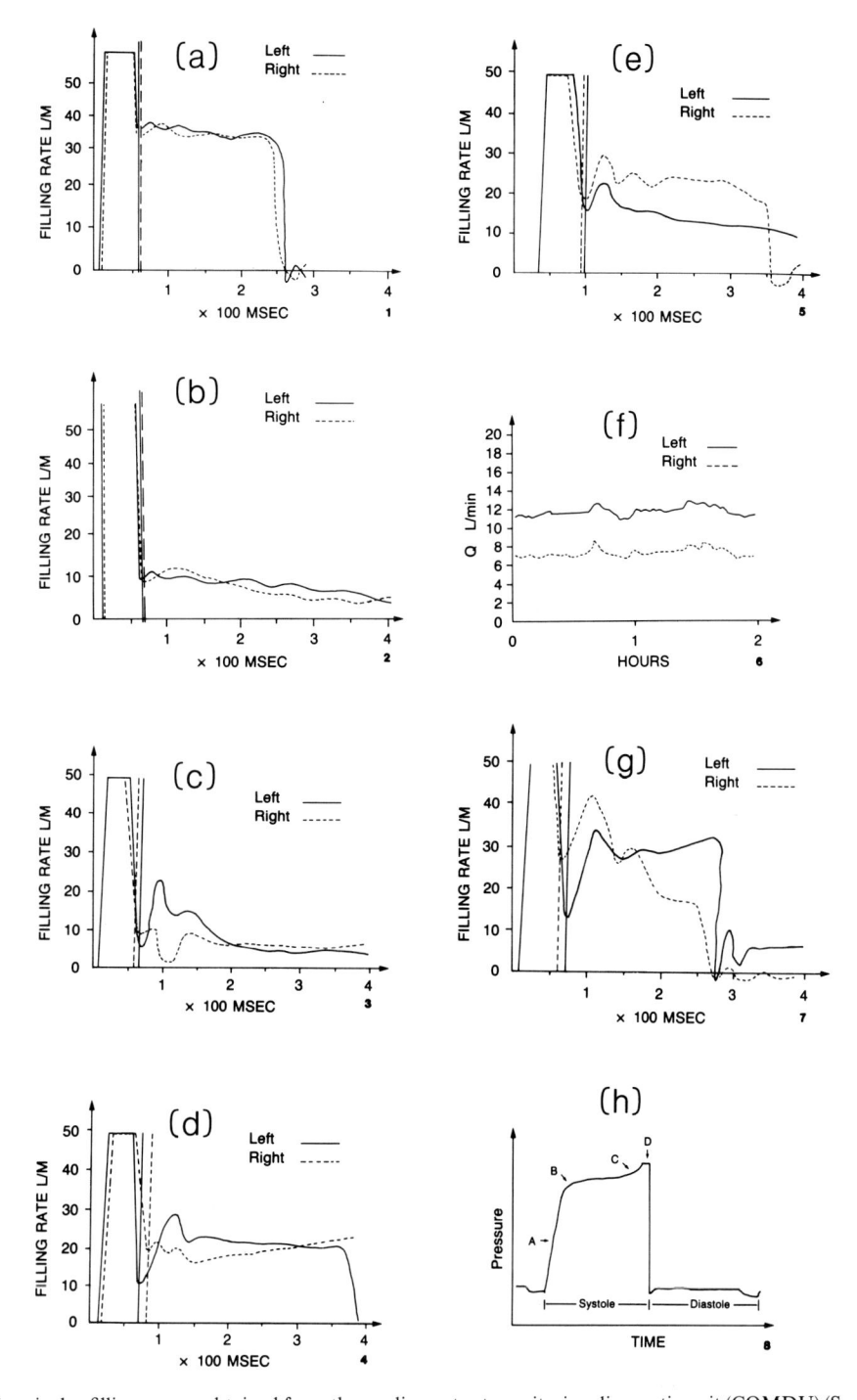

Figure 57.13 Ventricular filling curves obtained from the cardiac output monitoring diagnostic unit (COMDU) (Symbion Inc.). During diastole, the blood enters the artificial ventricle passively. An equal volume of air is displaced and expulsed out of the artificial ventricle. This air is quantified and integrated by the console to give a cardiac output, which is derived from the filling rates per ventricle (l/min) over a millisecond time interval multiplied by the heart rate.

The air flow curves provide information on various conditions: (a) hypervolemia, (b) hypovolemia, (c) malposition of the right ventricle, (d) underdriven left ventricle, (e) valve regurgitation, (f) imbalance due to valve regurgitation, (g) air between diaphragm layers, (h) drive pressure wave form, which is used to determine mechanical functional status of the TAH: (A) isovolumetric contraction; (B) ejection phase; (C) increase in pressure indicating that all of the blood has been ejected from the ventricle; (D) plateau indicating that the activation pressure set in the console was obtained before the end of systole, and that complete emptying of the artificial ventricle has occurred

Respiratory status

The patient arrives in the intensive care unit intubated. Whenever possible, extubation is planned within 24 hours, with sedation and ventilator settings gradually changed to meet this goal. This period allows for adequate rewarming, assurance of hemodynamic stability, and the initiation of a spontaneous diuresis, before full awakening and extubation.

Ventilatory rate must be adjusted to maintain normocarbia. Arterial blood gas measurements are obtained immediately after arrival in the intensive care unit and 15 minutes after each ventilator adjustment, or at least every 2 hours until the patient has stabilized. After the rewarming period, arterial blood gas measurements are rarely required more frequently than every 4 hours.

The inspired oxygen concentration is gradually reduced, allowing the patient to maintain a Po_2 of at least 80 mmHg. Ventilator rate is gradually decreased as the patient awakens. Extubation is usually performed in the awake, non-acidotic patient, with a Po_2 of at least 80 mmHg and a Pco_2 of 35–40 mmHg on continuous positive airway pressure on a Fio_2 of 40%.

Intensive physiotherapy is needed to prevent atelectasis and to keep the airways clear of secretions. Postural drainage aided by chest vibration, tracheobronchial lavage, hyperinflation by manual Ambu bagging, and suction of secretions should be carried out every 3 hours. Specimens from the tracheobronchial aspirate should be sent for culture to detect early infection.

After extubation, most patients can cooperate with respiratory exercises to prevent atelectasis. Chest physiotherapy with percussion vibration and postural drainage is continued, especially in patients with heavy secretions or persistent atelectasis. Prolonged intubation may be required in patients with pulmonary edema, acute renal failure, or diminished cerebral function.

Nutritional status

Adequate nutritional support of these patients is essential in the postoperative period (Chapter 27). When perfusion and oxygen transport are restored followed TAH implantation, the response to tissue demand will produce a rapid turnover in substrates; peripheral oxidation of fat may be accelerated, as well as fat mobilization secondary to catecholamine excess. This increase in caloric needs will also produce accelerated protein breakdown, causing skeletal muscle wasting. This induced metabolic state predisposes to multiple organ failure and infection. It should be corrected by early food administration or, when necessary, by parenteral nutrition. We should emphasize that malnutrition plays an important role in the genesis of multiple organ failure and infection.

CLINICAL RESULTS

The world results in the use of TAH as a bridge to transplantation are summarized in Table 57.4. Overall, 62% of the patients treated with a TAH were successfully supported and received a heart transplant. Of these, 69% remain alive and well after transplantation.

The underlying cardiac pathology for which implantation of the TAH was necessary is summarized in Table 57.5. Ischemic heart disease and idiopathic cardiomyopathy have been the indication in more than 80% of the cases to date.

Factors influencing outcome of TAH support

In our experience, there are three main factors to be taken into consideration if good results are to be obtained from TAH implantation: (1) age, (2) chronicity of the underlying disease, and (3) the time that has elapsed between the onset of sudden cardiac failure and the introduction of mechanical support. We have learned that patients in a chronic terminal state, with multiple organ dysfunction, are too weak to withstand such a major procedure.

The influences of age and duration of the disease on outcome are shown in Figures 57.14–57.16. Figure 57.14 reflects the influence of age alone. Of TAH patients younger than 40 years, 82% were transplanted, with 63% remaining long-term survivors. The results in older patients were far less successful. When severe heart failure developed within the month before implantation of the TAH, this was considered acute decompensation (Figure 57.15). In this group, patients younger than 40 years had both a greater chance of surviving to transplantation and improved long-term survival when compared with older patients. This difference was even greater in the chronic decompensation group (Figure 57.16), in which the mortality of patients older than 40 years on mechanical support was 100%. In

Table 57.4 World results of implantation of the TAH as a bridge to transplantation

	Number of patients (%)
Died during mechanical support	32 (38)
Transplanted	51 (62)
died	16 (31)
alive	35 (69)
Total	83 (100)

Table 57.5 Underlying cardiac pathology necessitating TAH implantation

Etiology	%
Ischemic	44
Idiopathic cardiomyopathy	38
Acute viral cardiomyopathy (myocarditis)	8
Valvular cardiomyopathy	5
Others	5

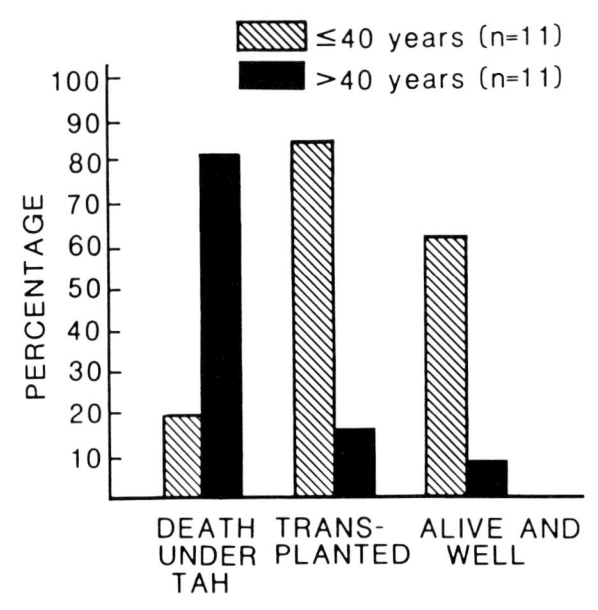

Figure 57.14 Influence of age on survival of patients with TAH support. (Four patients with acute rejection after transplantation were not included in this analysis.) One patient > 40 years of age remains on mechanical support in critical condition

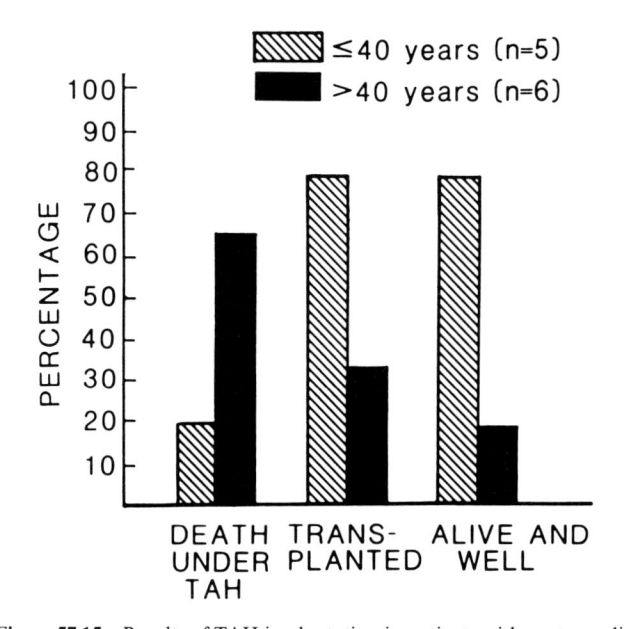

Figure 57.15 Results of TAH implantation in patients with acute cardiac decompensation in relation to age. (One patient > 40 years of age remains on mechanical support in critical condition)

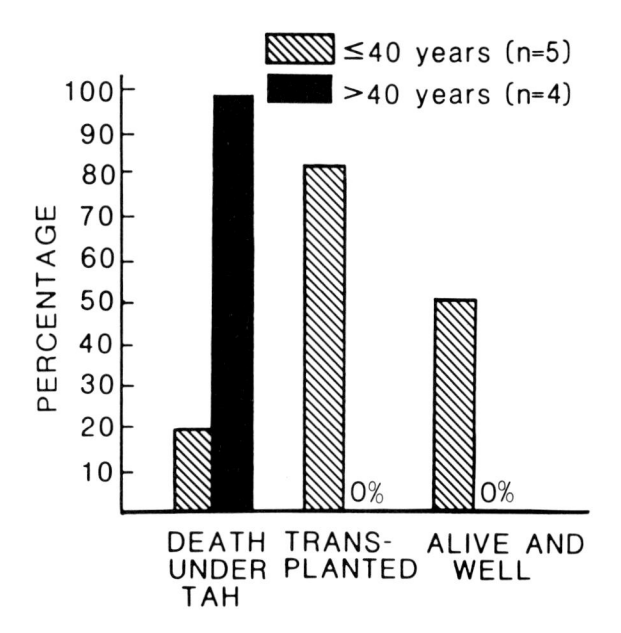

Figure 57.16 Results of TAH implantation in patients with chronic cardiac decompensation in relation to age. (Four patients with acute rejection after transplantation were not included in this analysis)

comparison, younger patients had an 80% success of being transplanted, with 75% of these long-term survivors.

Infection and multiple organ failure are the main causes of morbidity and mortality in patients on TAH support. Sixty percent of our patients died from infectious complications, reflecting the problems relating to the complex management of such patients, all of whom require multiple intravenous and pressure monitoring lines, and frequently prolonged ventilatory support. Pulmonary infections accounted for 44%, 11% originated in the urinary tract, and in 33% the origin was uncertain. In one patient, the infection appeared to be associated with the drivelines. Some patients had documented infection sites before TAH implantation, and this was most likely the source of the subsequent sepsis.

The use of a TAH *after* transplantation in patients with acute or chronic rejection has been reported, with generally poor results[15-20]. All of these patents required a long period of hospitalization, complicated by infection. Almost all died under mechanical support or at subsequent transplantation. All such patients in our series (four patients) died whilst on TAH support from septic complications. In general, these patients are poor candidates for TAH implantation.

Results of transplantation in TAH patients

Early infection after transplantation occurred in 45% of our patients, was successfully resolved in 60% of these, but proved fatal in 40%. Pre-existing infection is therefore an important risk factor in patients who will be immunosuppressed. Overall, 64% of our transplanted patients are alive and well, with a mean follow-up time of 257 days.

COMMENT

The implantation of a TAH carries several potential risks, among them bleeding, infection, thromboembolic phenomena, and multiple organ failure.

In our experience, thromboembolic complications have not been a problem, because of the rigorous control of coagulation to which these patients are subjected. Similarly, perioperative bleeding has been moderate, in spite of severe coagulopathies and prolonged CPB in some cases; the use of gelatin resorcin formol glue to seal the anastomotic sites has been of great help.

Hemolysis was initially a great concern, based on the theoretical concepts of red cell membrane fragility induced by the four mechanical valves, the exposure of the blood elements to a large surface area of foreign material, high dp/dt, and fast TAH rate. Based on the world's reported data[21], as well as our own[15], it seems that the modification made in the pneumatic drive system, to deliver compressed air at a lower dp/dt, has been enough to reduce hemolysis dramatically to insignificant levels.

The most difficult question to answer is whether a patient has developed irreversible damage of one or several organs. The majority of patients have developed some degree of renal, hepatic and/or pulmonary insufficiency, secondary to heart failure. Although many recover from their multiple organ failure following TAH implantation, it is clear that there is a point where the degree of organ failure becomes irreversible, despite correction of the hemodynamics. The highest probability for a successful outcome lies in a young subject in whom sudden cardiac failure has occurred, because the organs have suffered limited damage of short duration, and therefore probably have better reserves to reverse this insult.

We would emphasize the importance of not transplanting a patient until his condition has improved and stabilized. A transplanted heart will not perform better than a mechanical heart, and any hope that the patient will improve after transplantation is ill-founded. It is therefore mandatory that a patient placed on TAH support be thoroughly scrutinized to try to ensure that a donor organ is not wasted in a vain and unsuccessful attempt to save the patient.

ACKNOWLEDGEMENTS

The authors wish to acknowledge the major surgical contributions to the work reviewed in this chapter by Profs. I. Gandjbakhch and A. Pavie and Dr V. Bors.

References

1. Demikhov, V.P. (1962). *Experimental Transplantation of Vital Organs*. Translated by Basil Haig. p. 212. (New York: Consultants Bureau)
2. Kolff, W.J., Akutsu, T., Dreyer, B. and Horton, H. (1959). Artificial heart in the chest and use of polyurethane for making hearts, valves and aortas. *Trans. Am. Soc. Artif. Intern. Organs*, **5**, 298
3. Akutsu, T., Houston, C.S. and Kolff, W.J. (1960). Artificial heart inside the chest, using a small electromotor. *Trans. Am. Soc. Artif. Intern. Organs*, **6**, 299
4. Akutsu, T., Seidel, W., Mirkovitch, V., Feller, J. and Kolff, W.J. (1961). An electromotor-driven pendulum type artificial heart inside the chest. *Trans. Am. Soc. Artif. Intern. Organs*, **7**, 374
5. Wright, J.I. and Nose, Y. (1970). Materials for artificial heart. *Adv. Biomed. Eng. Med. Phys.*, **3**, 295
6. Symbion Inc. (1987). Jarvik-7 total artificial heart clinical training manual. Symbion Inc.
7. Cooley, D.A., Liotta, D., Hallman, G.L., Bloodwell, R.D., Leachman, R.D. and Milam, J.D. (1969). Orthotopic cardiac prostheses for two staged cardiac replacement. *Am. J. Cardiol.*, **24**, 723
8. Devries, W.C. (1983). Total artificial heart. In Sabiston, D.C. and Spencer, F.C. (eds.) *Gibbons' Surgery of the Chest*, 4th ed. p. 1629. (Philadelphia: W.B. Saunders)
9. Levinson, M.M. (1985). Report of bridge to transplantation with total artificial heart. NHLBI Contractors Meeting, Washington, DC, December
10. Jarvik, R.K., DeVries, W.C., Semb, B.K.H., Koul, B., Copeland, J.G., Levinson, M.M., Griffith, B.P., Joyce, L.D., Cooley, D.A., Frazier, O.H., Cabrol, C. and Keon, W.J. (1986). Surgical positioning of the Jarvik-7 artificial heart. *J. Heart Transplant.*, **5**, 184
11. Kolff, J. and Deeb, C.M. (1985). Artificial heart and left ventricular assist device. *Surg. Clin. N. Am.*, **65**, 661
12. Bellon, J.L., Szefner, J. and Cabrol, C. In Fevrier, J.S. (ed.) *Coagulation et Coeur Artificiel*. (Paris: Masson)
13. Jarvik, R.K. (1987). Clinical application of the total artificial heart. In D'Alessandro, L.C. (ed.) *Heart Surgery*, 1987. (Rome: Casa Editrice Scientifica Internazionale)
14. Joyce, L.D., Pritzker, M.R., Kiser, J.C., Nicoloff, D.M., Kersten, T.E., Bon Rueden, T.J., Eales, F., Johnson, K.E., Jorgensen, C.R., Gobel, F.L. and Van Tassel, R.A. (1986). Use of the mini Jarvik-7 total artificial heart as a bridge to transplantation. *J. Heart Transplant.*, **5**, 203
15. Cabrol, C., Gandjbakhch, I., Pavie, A., Bors, V., Mestiri, T., Cabrol, A., Leger, P., Levasseur, J.P., Vaissier, E., Szefner, J., Auriol, A., Aupetit, B. and Solis, E. (1988). Total artificial heart as a bridge for transplantation: La Pitie' 1986 to 1987. *J. Heart Transplant.*, **7**, 12
16. Joyce, L.D., Johnson, K.E., Pierce, W.S., DeVries, W.C., Semb, B.K.H., Copeland, J.G., Griffith, B.P., Cooley, D.A., Frazier, O.H., Cabrol, C., Keon, W.J., Unger, F., Bucherl, E.S. and Wolner, E. (1986). Summary of the world experience with clinical use of total artificial hearts as heart support devices. *J. Heart Transplant.*, **5**, 229
17. Levinson, M.M., Smith, R.G., Cork, R., Gallo, J., Icenogle, T., Emery, R., Ott, R. and Copeland, J.G. (1986). Three recent cases of the total artificial heart before transplantation. *J. Heart Transplant.*, **5**, 215
18. Griffith, B.P., Kormos, R.L., Wei, L.M., Borovetz, H.S., Trento, A. and Hardesty, R.L. (1986). Use of the total artificial heart as an interim device: initial experience in Pittsburgh with four patients. *J. Heart Transplant.*, **5**, 210
19. Pennock, J.L., Pierce, W.S., Campbell, D.B., Pae, W.E. Jr., Davis, D., Hensley, F.A., Richenbacher, W.E. and Waldhausen, J.A. (1986). Mechanical support of the circulation followed by cardiac transplantation. *J. Thorac. Cardiovasc. Surg.*, **92**, 994
20. Loisance, D.Y., Deleuze, P., Kawasaki, K., Hillion, M.L., Binhas, M., Heurtematte, P., Tavolaro, O., Leandri, J. and Cachera, J.P. (1987). Total artificial heart as a bridge to retransplantation in acute cardiac rejection. *J. Heart Transplant.*, **6**, 281
21. Levinson, M.M., Copeland, J.G., Smith, R.G., Cork, R.C., DeVries, W.C., Mays, J.B., Griffith, B.P., Kormos, R., Joyce, L.D., Pritzker, M.R., Semb, B.K.H., Koul, B., Menkis, A.H. and Keon, W.J. (1986). Indexes of hemolysis in human recipients of the Jarvik-7 total artificial heart: a cooperative report of fifteen patients. *J. Heart Transplant.*, **5**, 236

ADDENDUM

The Food and Drug Administration has recently withdrawn permission for use of the Jarvik-7 artificial heart in the USA. The reasons for this are not yet certain, and whether the ban will be temporary or permanent also remains unknown.

58
Results of Mechanical Circulatory Support as a 'Bridge' to Cardiac Transplantation – Combined Registry Report

W.E. PAE, Jr., S.A. PARASCANDOLA, C.A. MILLER AND W.S. PIERCE

INTRODUCTION

Unfortunately, about 20% of all candidates for cardiac transplantation die before a donor organ is obtained[1]. Many can be sustained with inotropic agents and the intra-aortic balloon until cardiac transplantation can be performed[2]. For some patients, however, these forms of therapy do not provide adequate circulatory support. More aggressive means of treatment are needed. The encouraging results obtained with temporary mechanical ventricular assistance in patients with postcardiotomy cardiogenic shock have led many investigators to utilize these modalities as a 'bridge' to cardiac transplantation.

Experiences with aggressive mechanical circulatory support as a bridge to cardiac transplantation are at best sporadically or anecdotally reported in the literature, as no one institution has accumulated the large clinical experience necessary to perform appropriate statistical analyses. Multicenter clinical trials with established protocols are likewise lacking. Thus there have been insufficient data available to assess the outcome of staged transplantation and its overall impact on the availability of donor organs and ultimate survival.

Accordingly, a Combined Registry for the clinical use of mechanical ventricular assist pumps and the total artificial heart was established in 1985 under the auspices of the International Society for Heart Transplantation and the American Society for Artificial Internal Organs. The Combined Registry is computerized to allow statistical manipulation of the database. Data from worldwide centers are consolidated and summarized, allowing comparison of clinical results. The participants are provided easy access to this information, and results from special analyses are available to Registry participants at their request. Overall and yearly results are reported annually at the meetings of the societies. The following report details information submitted to the Combined Registry since its inception[3,4].

DATABASE AND RESULTS

Through December 1988, a total of 44 centers (21 in the United States and 23 elsewhere) have contributed patient data to the Combined Registry. Many centers have been kind enough to provide data on implants prior to 1985. This has been encouraged to ensure completeness of the database. The current database is comprised of 219 patients, ranging from 7 to 64 years of age (Table 58.1). Males predominate, and are older than their female counterparts.

The number of mechanical implants for staged cardiac transplantation has grown exponentially since 1984 (Figure 58.1). In the majority of patients, biventricular support with either a paracorporeal biventricular assist device (BVAD) or a total artificial heart (TAH) has been utilized.

The indications for staged orthotopic cardiac transplantation included hemodynamic deterioration before transplantation in 197 patients, and acute rejection of an ortho-

Table 58.1 Patients undergoing circulatory support for bridge-to-cardiac transplantation: distribution by age and sex

	All years	1988
Total number of implants	219	46
Males		
Age ($\pm$ SEM) (years)	179 (82%)	42 (91%)
	43 ($\pm$ 0.9)	44 ($\pm$ 2)
Range	11–64	17–63
Females		
Age ($\pm$ SEM) (years)	40 (18%)	4 (9%)
	33 ($\pm$ 2)	20 ($\pm$ 4)
Range	7–59	13–26

SEM = standard error of the mean

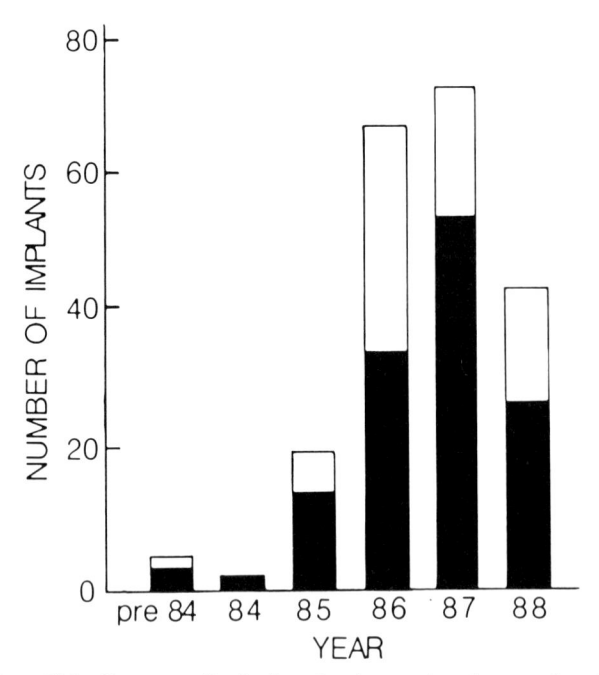

Figure 58.1 Frequency distribution of patients undergoing staged cardiac transplantation by year. Dark, solid bars indicate ventricular assist devices; open bars indicate total artificial hearts (Combined Registry Report, 1988)

Table 58.3 Number of days of circulatory support in patients undergoing staged cardiac transplantation

	LVAD	RVAD	BVAD	TAH
All years				
Mean ($\pm$ SEM)	14.1 ($\pm$ 0.3)	3.0 ($\pm$ 2.0)	9.0 ($\pm$ 0.2)	25.5 ($\pm$ 0.8)
Range	0–90	1–5	0–83	0–396
1988				
Mean ($\pm$ SEM)	21.4 ($\pm$ 1.6)	N/A	20.1 ($\pm$ 1.7)	19.1 ($\pm$ 2.0)
Range	0–71	N/A	0–83	1–135

LVAD = left ventricular assist device; RVAD = right ventricular assist device; BVAD = biventricular assist device (extracorporeal); TAH = total artificial heart; N/A = not applicable

topically transplanted heart in the remaining 22 patients. Of the latter group, 15 (68%) were able to be retransplanted, and of these six (40%) were ultimately discharged from hospital.

Although not included in the database of 219 patients, 24 patients were reported to a separate area of the Combined Registry devoted to the analysis of circulatory support for postcardiotomy cardiogenic shock. These 24 patients exhibited immediate donor organ failure and refractory cardiogenic shock not secondary to acute rejection. Nine of the 24 patients (38%) were weaned from circulatory support, and four of the nine were hospital survivors. This overall survival of 17% is somewhat lower than that reported in postcardiotomy cardiogenic shock following non-transplant procedures[5].

Circulatory support has been provided prior to transplantation for a wide range of time periods (Tables 58.2 and 58.3). The longest period of support (396 days) has been provided with a TAH (Table 58.3). In 1988, there was no significant difference in the duration of support between those patients with a successful outcome versus those with an unsuccessful outcome. However, the overall experience would indicate shorter durations of support are associated with a more favorable outcome. In 1988, duration of circulatory support was not related to the type of support employed (ventricular assist device(s) versus artificial heart). Nonetheless, the overall experience indicates a shorter duration of use when ventricular assist device(s) are employed. Rates of subsequent transplantation and hospital discharge were independent of ventricular assist pump type (pneumatic vs. centrifugal vs. electric) (Table 58.4).

The results of staged cardiac transplantation through 1988, and for 1988 alone, are summarized in Tables 58.5

Table 58.4 Outcome of staged cardiac transplantation based on ventricular assist pump type

Type	Number of patients	Transplanted (%)	Transplanted/ discharged from hospital (%)
Pneumatic	82	58 (71%)	43 (74%)
Centrifugal	36	22 (61%)	15 (68%)
Electric	21	13 (62%)	9 (69%)
Totals	139	93 (67%)	67 (72%)

Table 58.5 Overall results of bridge to transplantation (as of December 31, 1988)

System	Number of patients	Transplanted (%)	Transplanted/ discharged from hospital (%)
LVAD	58	41 (71%)	31 (76%)
RVAD	2	1 (50%)	1 (100%)
BVAD	82	57 (70%)	38 (67%)
TAH	77	60 (78%)	29 (48%)
Totals	219	159 (73%)	99 (62%)

Abbreviations as for Table 58.3

Table 58.2 Number of days of circulatory support and clinical outcome in patients awaiting cardiac transplantation ($n = 219$)

	All patients	Not transplanted	Transplanted	Transplanted/discharged from hospital
All years				
Mean ($\pm$ SEM)	16.1 ($\pm$ 2.6)	23.7 ($\pm$ 8.0)	13.2 ($\pm$ 2.0)	11.5 ($\pm$ 1.7)
Range	0–396	1–396	0–246	0–90
1988				
Mean ($\pm$ SEM)	20.1 ($\pm$ 4.0)	20.2 ($\pm$ 10.9)	20.9 ($\pm$ 3.9)	16.4 ($\pm$ 4.0)
Range	0–135	0–135	0–83	1–83

Table 58.6 Results of bridge to transplantation – 1988 only

System	Number of patients	Transplanted (%)	Transplanted/ discharged from hospital (%)
LVAD	14	10 (71%)	6 (60%)
RVAD	0	0 (0%)	0 (0%)
BVAD	15	10 (67%)	9 (90%)
TAH	17	14 (82%)	10 (71%)
Totals	46	34 (74%)	25 (74%)

Abbreviations as for Table 58.3

and 58.6. The overall hospital discharge was 45% (99/219) for all 219 patients receiving circulatory support for staged cardiac transplantation (all indications) (Table 58.5). Seventy-three percent (159/219) were transplanted, and 99 of these (62%) were discharged from the hospital. The 30-day mortality following transplantation was 25%. The rates of transplantation were not dependent upon the type of support employed. Approximately 71%, 70%, and 78% of patients bridged with univentricular, biventricular, or TAH devices respectively underwent subsequent transplantation.

Following transplantation, 76% of patients receiving univentricular support, 67% receiving biventricular support, and 48% receiving TAH support, were discharged from hospital. The difference in hospital discharge rates between those supported by a TAH and those supported by a ventricular assist device is approaching statistical significance ($p < 0.07$ by generalized Wilcoxon analysis).

In 1988, a total of 46 patients was reported to the Combined Registry as undergoing staged cardiac transplantation (Table 58.6). Seventy-four percent (34/46) underwent subsequent transplantation, and 25/34 patients (74%) were hospital discharges, giving an overall hospital discharge rate of 54% (25/46). Results with the TAH improved, with 14/17 (82%) implanted going on to transplantation, and 10/14 patients (71%) surviving to be discharged.

Based on long-term follow-up, the Kaplan–Meier survival estimate for all patients undergoing circulatory support is 61.9% at 2 years following transplantation (Figure 58.2). This is in contrast to the 79.6% actuarial survival of patients undergoing orthotopic cardiac transplantation without prior mechanical support[6]. When Kaplan–Meier survival estimates are prepared for each type of mechanical support, the 2-year post-transplant survival differences between the groups do not approach statistical significance at present.

Complications precluding transplantation after establishment of mechanical circulatory support are listed in Table 58.7; many patients had more than one complication. All of the listed complications except infection were powerful univariate predictors of not receiving a subsequent transplant. When these complications were entered into a stepwise logistic regression analysis, renal failure, persistent biventricular failure, and a neurological event (in order of decreasing importance) impacted significantly in a negative fashion on future transplantation. There was no significant

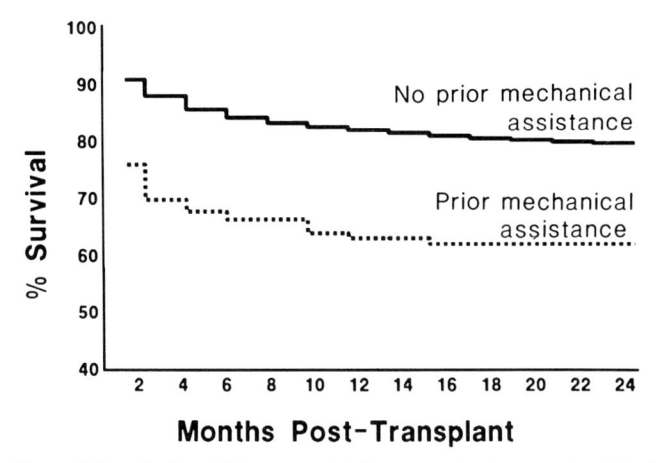

Figure 58.2 Kaplan–Meier actuarial 2-year survival curves for (1) all patients undergoing cardiac transplantation after a period of mechanical support (bridging by ventricular assist device or total artificial heart) (lower curve); and for (2) all patients undergoing cardiac transplantation who did not require prior mechanical support (upper curve) (Combined Registry Report, 1988)

Table 58.7 Complications precluding transplantation (all years)* ($n = 60$ patients)

	Number of patients		
Complication	VAD (%) ($n = 20$)	BVAD (%) ($n = 23$)	TAH (%) ($n = 17$)
Bleeding	6 (30%)	7 (30%)	6 (35%)
Biventricular failure	11 (55%)	8 (34%)	—
Renal failure	6 (30%)	4 (17%)	7 (41%)
Respiratory failure	5 (25%)	6 (26%)	5 (29%)
Infection	5 (25%)	5 (22%)	6 (35%)
Neurologic	2 (10%)	3 (13%)	3 (18%)
Multisystem failure	0 (0%)	1 (4%)	3 (18%)

*Based on the Combined Registry Report, 1988[4]. A single patient may have had more than one complication.
Abbreviations as for Table 58.3

difference in complications by type of support.

Table 58.8 illustrates the factors contributing to death following transplantation, and again any given patient may have had more than one causative factor. Univariate analysis would indicate that bleeding, renal failure, persistent respiratory failure, infection, poor cardiac output, and a neurological event negatively impacted on hospital discharge. When variables were entered into a stepwise logistic regression analysis, renal failure, infection, and bleeding were significant predictors of in-hospital death. Causes of death occurring later than 30 days parallel those in a standard transplant population (Chapter 31).

COMMENT

Patients who decompensate hemodynamically while awaiting cardiac transplantation can be effectively supported by a paracorporeal assist pump system or a TAH. The number of such implants is steadily increasing; the lower absolute

Table 58.8 Factors contributing to death following staged cardiac transplantation (all years)*

Factor	Deaths occurring < 30 days VAD (%) (n = 8)	BVAD (%) (n = 13)	TAH (%) (n = 19)	Deaths occurring > 30 days All patients (%) (n = 11)
Infection	3 (38%)	2 (15%)	7 (37%)	5 (45%)
Ventricular failure	3 (38%)	5 (38%)	3 (16%)	—
Bleeding	3 (38%)	2 (15%)	5 (26%)	—
Renal failure	4 (50%)	1 (8%)	3 (16%)	1 (9%)
Rejection	0 (0%)	3 (23%)	5 (26%)	3 (27%)
Respiratory failure	2 (25%)	3 (23%)	2 (11%)	—
Neurologic/multisystem	1 (13%)	1 (8%)	4 (21%)	—
Medical non-compliance	—	—	—	2 (18%)

*Based on the Combined Registry Report, 1988[4]. A single patient may have had more than one factor contributing to his/her death. Abbreviations as for Table 58.3

figures for 1988 almost certainly reflect the lag period in reporting to the Combined Registry.

In 1987, more than twice as many patients received biventricular support by paracorporeal BVAD than by a TAH (69% vs. 31%). This may be due to a number of factors: (1) ventricular assist pumps are currently more accessible than is the TAH; (2) there is potential for weaning a patient from biventricular assistance; (3) in some cases, biventricular support can be established without cardiopulmonary bypass; (4) thoracic size does not limit paracorporeal support; and (5) some patients subsequently develop right heart failure, necessitating biventricular paracorporeal support. Further studies will be required to determine prospectively the need for univentricular versus biventricular support, as well as to clarify which is the optimal device when biventricular support is necessary.

As evidenced in Table 58.2, the period of circulatory support varied widely. In any single patient, the period of support that will be required is unpredictable; this underscores the importance of utilizing a device with short, intermediate, or long-term support capabilities.

Incomplete follow-up data may preclude accurate conclusions regarding the effect of prior circulatory support on long-term survival following transplantation. Current data would indicate that survival is significantly reduced in this group of patients compared with those who require no prior mechanical support[6] (Chapter 31). In a selected series utilizing a specific pneumatic device, however, a 1-year survival of 92% was reported[7]. Survival may, therefore, be dependent to a certain extent on the specific device as well as the type of support. At present, the numbers of each type of device utilized and reported to the Combined Registry are too small to afford accurate statistical analyses. However, it presently appears that the post-transplant 2-year survival appears equivalent for all types of support.

Many patients had more than one complication during mechanical support, and although many can be attributed to the patient's critical condition before implantation, a number must be considered device-related, especially hemorrhage, neurological events, infection, and hemolysis. Bleeding, infection, and renal failure are common complications, and significantly influence progress to transplantation and survival. Further efforts to prevent and successfully treat such complications may enhance survival.

In summary, analysis of data at this time would indicate similar results regardless of the type of pump utilized for mechanical support. Overall results following transplantation are reasonable and, in the future, may approach those achieved in patients who have not required prior mechanical assistance. Hopefully, as devices, patient selection, and management can improve, complications precluding subsequent transplantation and hospital discharge will be minimized, and overall survival increased.

The members of the Combined Registry hope that data acquisition will continue to improve, enabling objective analysis of results, and comparison of staged transplantation with that of 'routine' cardiac transplantation in a valid statistical fashion. As such clinical trials continue, the influence of bridged cardiac transplantation on the availability of donor hearts will be better defined, enabling limited resources to be utilized to their fullest potential.

Acknowledgement

We acknowledge Ms. Mary J. Bartholomew for assistance with the statistical analyses.

(Investigators working in this area, who are not already participating in the Combined Registry of the Societies, are encouraged to contribute to the Registry. Inquiries may be directed to: Walter E. Pae, Jr., MD, Associate Professor, or William S. Pierce, MD, Professor and Chief, Division of Artificial Organs, The Milton S. Hershey Medical Center, The Pennsylvania State University, PO Box 850, 500 University Drive, Hershey, PA 17033. Telephone: (717)-531-8328/8329).

References

1. Copeland, J.G., Emery, R.W., Levinson, M.M., Copeland, J., McAleer, M.J. and Riley, J.E. (1985). The role of mechanical support and

transplantation in treatment of patients with end-stage cardiomyopathy. *Circulation*, (Suppl. 2), **72**, 7
2. Hardesty, R.L., Griffith, B.P., Trento, A., Thompson, M.E., Ferson, P.F. and Bahnson, H.T. (1986). Mortally ill patients and excellent survival following cardiac transplantation. *Ann. Thorac. Surg.*, **41**, 126
3. Pae, W.E. and Pierce, W.S. (1989). Combined Registry for the clinical use of mechanical ventricular assist pumps and the total artificial heart: second official report – 1987. *J. Heart Transplant.*, **8**, 1
4. Pae, W.E., Miller, C.A. and Pierce, W.S. (1989). Combined Registry for the clinical use of mechanical ventricular assist pumps and the total artificial heart: third official report – 1988. *J. Heart Transplant.*, **8**, 277
5. Pae, W.E. (1987). Temporary ventricular support: current indications and results. *Trans. Am. Soc. Artif. Intern. Organs*, **32**, 4
6. Solis, E. and Kaye, M.P. (1986). The Registry of the International Society for Heart Transplantation: third official report – June 1986. *J. Heart Transplant.*, **5**, 2
7. Farrar, D.J., Hill, J.D., Gray, L. A., Pennington, D.G. McBride, L.R., Pierce, W.S., Pae, W.E., Glenville, B., Ross, D., Galbriath, T.A. and Zumbro, G.L. (1988). Heterotopic prosthetic ventricles as a bridge to cardiac transplantation: a multi-center study in 29 patients. *N. Engl. J. Med.*, **318**, 333

Section V

Permanent cardiac replacement by the total artificial heart

59
Experimental Background and Current Problems
W.J. KOLFF

INTRODUCTION

Many surgeons have now seen the rapid improvement of a dying patient following the implantation of a total artificial heart (TAH). The secondary organ failures, such as renal, liver, and lung failure, if caused by cardiac insufficiency, disappear within hours or days. The edematous patient may even become dehydrated, and improved liver function may render the dosage of anticoagulant ineffective. As increasing numbers of patients are supported by artificial hearts as a bridge to transplantation, and as an ever increasing number of them awaits a suitable donor heart, eventually such patients will ask to be sent home with the device. Thus, slowly but steadily, the permanent TAH will take its place among the methods of accepted treatment for end-stage cardiac failure.

Salisbury mentioned the artificial heart in his Presidential address to the American Society for Artificial Internal Organs (ASAIO) in 1957. In the Western world, the first TAH was implanted by Akutsu and the author in December of that year in an anesthetized dog that survived for 90 minutes[1].

In this chapter, certain selected aspects in the development of the TAH will be discussed, as will problems that still complicate the long-term use of such devices.

SOURCES OF ENERGY

A number of different sources of energy has been used experimentally to power artificial hearts. The pneumatically-powered TAH is today in vogue.

Pneumatic (compressed air)

While we were struggling with electrohydraulic and mechanically driven artificial hearts[2,3], Kirby and Hiller of the National Aeronautics and Space Energy (NASA) suggested the use of compressed air as a source of energy for a drive system outside the body. They proceeded to build a most sophisticated drive system for us which would respond to physiological needs[3-5]. The pressure curve of the driving air could be altered at will, and the percentage systole/diastole could be changed, or was automatically regulated, depending on the rate. The system was, however, extremely complex to manage, and stimulated personal efforts to try to develop the simplest possible drive system outside the chest and the simplest blood pumps inside the chest.

The result was the Detroit Driver (made by the Detroit Coil Company in Michigan), distributed by the National Institutes of Health (NIH) free of charge to laboratories interested in artificial hearts[3,6]. When larger artificial hearts were developed for larger experimental animals, Kwan-Gett enlarged the size of the valves[7].

Air-driven systems have been maligned more than they deserve, particularly with regard to their size and mass. The large weight of the drive system used in the first patient to receive a permanent TAH, Barney Clark, comprised compressed air cylinders for redundancy, two drive systems instead of one (also for redundancy), and recording equipment. The drive system can be greatly simplified; we have demonstrated, for example, that, with a minor change, the drive system of the Datascope intra-aortic balloon pump can be adapted to drive a TAH[8]. In contradistinction to the intra-aortic balloon pump, synchronization with the natural heart is, of course, not required.

The basic design of a pneumatically-powered TAH is illustrated in Figure 59.1, which is based on the Philadelphia TAH (Figure 59.2)[9]. The implantable portion of the Philadelphia TAH is comprised of two rigid ventricular chambers. The volume within each chamber is divided by a flexible diaphragm, separating the chamber into compartments for blood and air. When the blood chamber is completely filled, the air chamber is empty. Introduction of pressurized air into the air chamber causes the ejection of blood from the

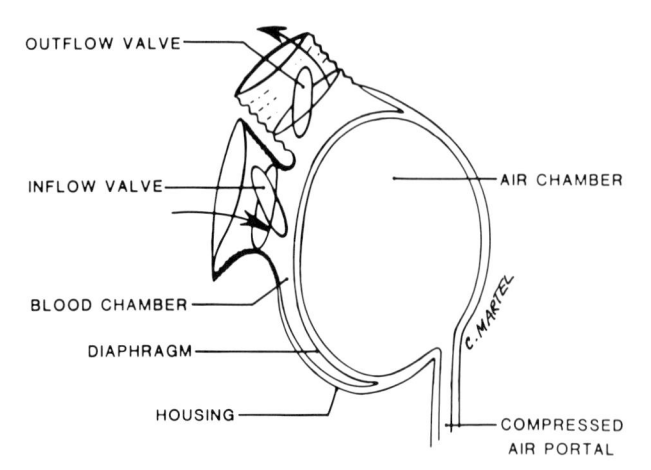

Figure 59.1 Diagram of basic design of the Philadelphia total artificial heart (TAH) (after Kolff, J. et al.[9])

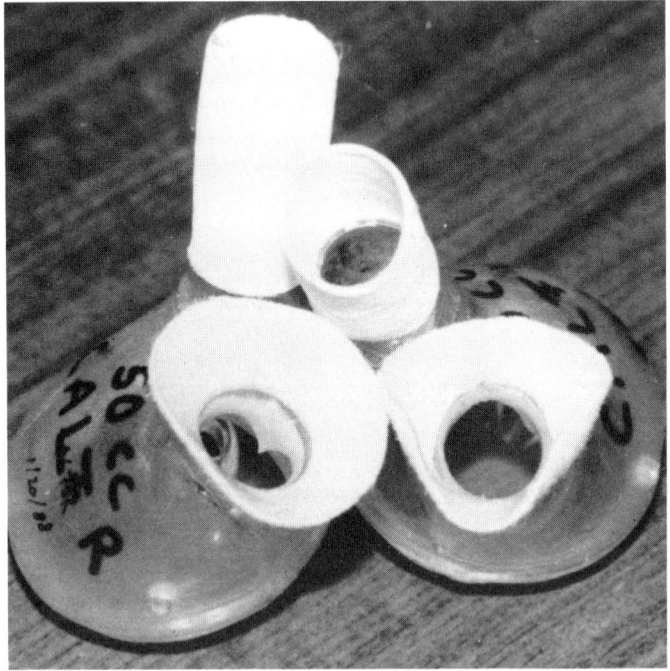

Figure 59.2 The 'Philadelphia' TAH has no connectors (quick-connects). The atriaKolff, J. et al.[9])

assume that the ventricle is completely emptied with each stroke, this also represents the stroke volume. If multiplied by rate, the cardiac output of both right and left sides can be measured with an accuracy of 10% without need for transducers inside the chest. The COMDU only considers the inflow volume, and does not automatically compensate for regurgitation or other losses. The shape of the curve, however, gives valuable information regarding (1) whether or not the ventricle is sufficiently filled, (2) the presence of a broken valve, or (3) air between the diaphragms, and (4) 'valving' (occlusion of the airline entry point into the ventricle by a distended diaphragm).

Portable air-drive systems

Portable air-drive systems situated outside the chest have some obvious advantages: (1) they are small and no heavier than the oxygen tank that many people with emphysema walk around with; (2) the system can be replaced, reducing the demand on durability; (3) they can be repaired without opening the chest; (4) their batteries, which can run for 6–8 hours, can be recharged or replaced. (Leif Stenberg, a patient in Stockholm, Sweden (Figure 59.3), walked with this drive system to a restaurant, served himself four times at the smorgasbord table, and sent a telegram to the United States saying, 'I am the happiest man in Europe.')

The portable drive system used by Leif Stenberg was designed and built by Heimes[12], who has recently built a newer version which provides continuous readouts of cardiac output and pressures and can be connected to recorders (Figure 59.4). Another portable drive system has been built by Affeld and his associates in Berlin[13].

Electrohydraulic

The first electrohydraulic heart was built by Norton, together with my laboratory personnel, in 1962[3] (Figure 59.5). Five mechanically coordinated electromagnets compressed hydraulic fluid, which bathed both right and left ventricles. The important principle that not only mechanical energy, but also heat, is conveyed by the hydraulic fluid, was established. The heat radiates into the blood, and the body serves as a radiator.

Another electrohydraulic pump utilizes a small electric motor which can be reversed within 14 thousandths of a second from a top speed of 12 000 revolutions in one direction to top speed in the other direction. Small turbine blades on the rotor propel hydraulic fluid from left to right. The switch-over can be accomplished by back electromotive force; sensors for venous pressure should and can be avoided.

The difference in cardiac output between the left and right ventricle is considerable and must be provided for. In calves, we have seen it to be 2 l/min. There are at least two sources for the difference in cardiac output: (1) the bronchial

ventricle, and removal of air allows the blood compartment to fill once again. The air conduits, or drivelines, connect the ventricles with the external control console via the chest wall; the console provides the pneumatic driving energy. The Philadelphia TAH driver has a gentle dp/dt. The pneumatic drive source was designed to produce a gentle, pulsatile, pumping action that closes the inflow valve before the more powerful ejection phase occurs[8,9].

Air-driven artificial hearts can be monitored with the COMDU (Cardiac Output Monitor and Diagnostic Unit), which incorporates a flow meter in the driveline. Usually only the diastolic flow of air is recorded[10,11]. The amount of air that leaves the artificial heart during diastole is equal to the amount of blood that enters the ventricle and, if we

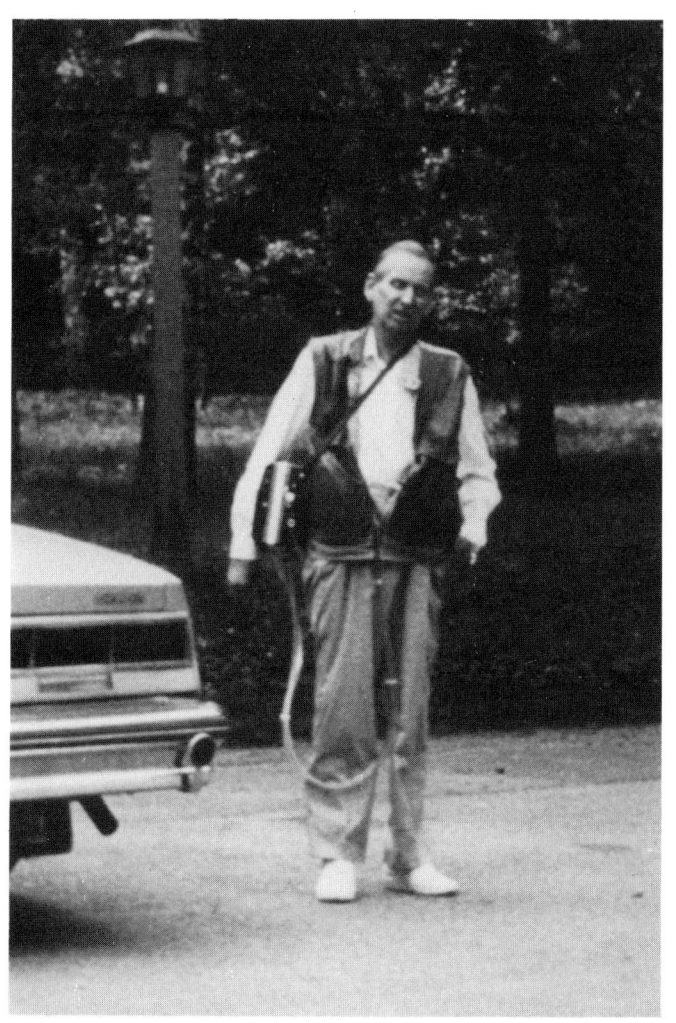

EXPERIMENTAL BACKGROUND AND CURRENT PROBLEMS

Figure 59.3 Leif Stenberg with his portable drive system

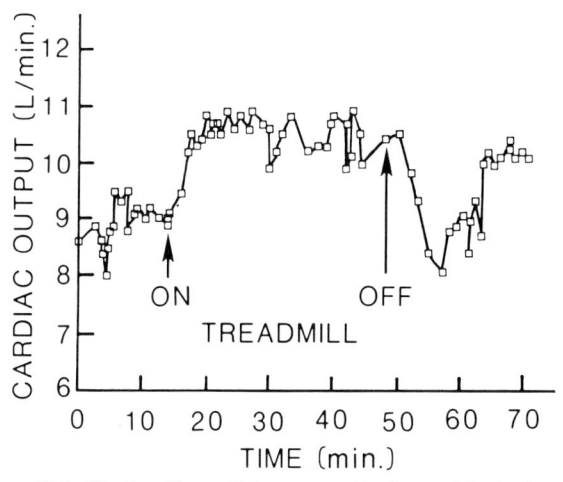

Figure 59.4 Tracing (from Heimes portable heart driver) shows the cardiac output of a calf, 'Albert', 50 days after implantation of a TAH. Before the animal is on the treadmill, the cardiac output is about 9 l/min. During exercise, the cardiac output automatically increases to 10.5 l/min. When the treadmill is stopped, the cardiac output falls to 8 l/min within minutes. The rise 10 minutes later occurs when the animal walks off the treadmill back to its cage

circulation, which comes from the left side and returns to the left side, and (2) the higher pressures on the left side, which result in greater regurgitation through valves and increased loss by distension of the ventricle.

(There is some additional loss in an air-driven system due to the compressibility of the driving air, but it becomes important only when the volume of the driving air is large.)

In the electrohydraulic heart, the difference between right and left cardiac output can be compensated by creating a leak in the right side so that part of the blood which is pumped out returns during diastole. If the pulmonary artery valve is purposely made insufficient, during a long diastole a large backflow from the pulmonary artery will occur; during a short diastole a smaller backflow will occur. This allows regulation of imbalance by varying the ratio between systole and diastole[28]. An unfortunate consequence is that, since the right and left ventricles are hydraulically coupled, a longer diastole on the right side results in a longer systole on the left, and we need a relatively longer diastole for adequate filling.

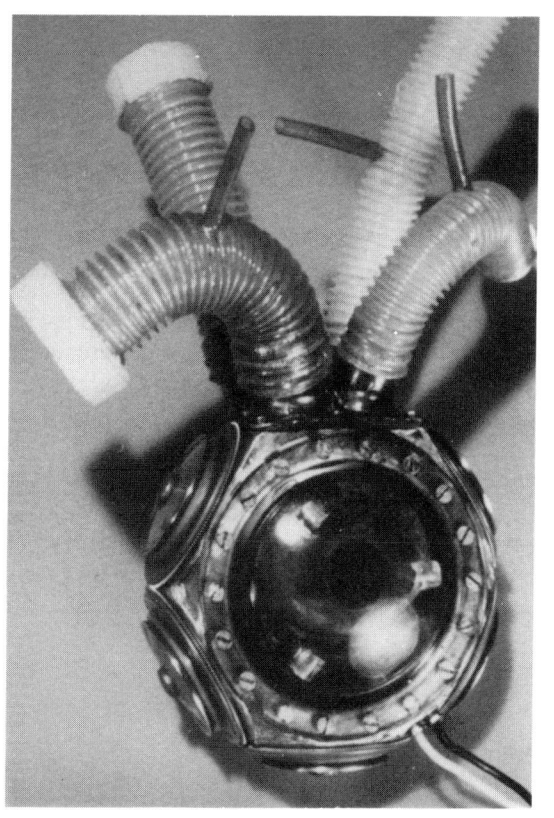

Figure 59.5 Five solenoids are arranged in a rosette. When energized, they compress a hydraulic fluid that is within the housing. On the top of the artificial heart one sees the atria, the pulmonary artery, and the aorta. These vessels are made of corrugated polyurethane so they can be bent without kinking

There is another solution, which is not a compensation with blood but with the driving fluid. This can easily be accomplished if a small extension for the driving fluid is provided on the right side (Figure 59.6). During systole, part of the hydraulic fluid goes into the extension, not into the right ventricle, the volume being controlled possibly by electromagnets. The magnet is closed during right-sided diastole when pressure is minimal. It can be kept closed with a very small current during systole.

Alternatively, one can decouple the right and left sides making them quite independent, and then provide a compliance sack for each ventricle during diastole. It has been well substantiated by Nose's laboratory[14] and others, that compliance sacks covered with fibrils can maintain their flexibility for years.

Atomic energy

The first totally implanted TAH was actually built for the Atomic Energy Commission between 1971 and 1974[15]. An atomically-driven motor fueled by plutonium 238 (built by North American Phillips) was placed in the abdomen, and a flexible driveline passed through the diaphragm to the artificial heart. The mechanical drive was built by Westinghouse, and our laboratory built the blood-handling mechanism (called the soft-shell artificial heart). Atomically-driven artificial hearts are not being pursued at present from a fear of radiation hazard. For the same reason, atomically-driven pacemakers have also disappeared from the market.

Electricity

Using an electric motor (instead of the Sterling hot air engine driven by atomic energy), a calf was maintained alive in a reasonable condition for 35 days[16]. This record for a mechanically driven pump, achieved in 1975, stood for almost 10 years, until it was broken by Pierce's group in Hershey, Pennsylvania[17] (Chapter 56).

With improved batteries and methods to transfer energy through the intact skin, atomic sources of energy are no longer necessary. Pusher-plate hearts have been brought to a considerable degree of sophistication and reliability, yet remain heavy and cumbersome[18]. Novacor's pusher-plate has been used to power a left ventricular assist device in man. If the drive system is mounted between the ventricles and moves back and forth, as in the pendulum heart[19], the space required by the system is smaller. (The most elegant pusher-plate drive system to date has been bulit by Heimes in Aachen, Germany (unpublished).

REGULATION OF CARDIAC OUTPUT

Starling's law of the heart assumes that the innervation of the pulmonary and peripheral systemic vascular systems is intact, and that if each ventricle (of the TAH) pumps out all of the blood that is delivered to it, the natural regulating systems of the body will suitably adjust pulmonary and peripheral systemic arterial pressures. Thus, when the venous or atrial pressure rises, our artificial ventricle is more fully filled, and automatically pumps out more blood. This also ensures a balance between the pulmonary and systemic circulations.

One might anticipate that, if the right heart delivers more blood to the left side, then the left heart will pump out more; consequently, the right side would pump out more, and so on. Fortunately, this does not happen – neither in a mock circulation nor in the experimental animal.

An air-driven TAH usually vents into the atmosphere, but if one applies a small amount of suction during diastole, Starling's curves shift to the left. This simple system requires heart valves that offer little resistance, and pumping diaphragms or sacks that are thin so that they can move easily; with a heavy diaphragm, other methods must be used.

The most sensitive, purely mechanical application of Starling's law is possible with a TAH that incorporates anti-vacuum bellows[20] (Figure 59.7).

If one has a non-thinking, reciprocating drive system, Starling's law can be accommodated by making part of the ventricle collapsible, but not distensible (Figure 59.8). If not enough blood is available during diastole, then part of the ventricle simply collapses; during the next stroke, only that amount of blood that fills the non-collapsed ventricle is pumped out[16].

PROBLEMS WITH ARTIFICIAL HEARTS

Placement within the chest

The major problem in the development of the TAH has been to design it so that it would fit satisfactorily within the chest. My personal design was of a flat 'pancake' TAH (Figure 59.9). A calf, in which this heart was inserted, was the first calf that did not show an increase in venous pressure over a period of time[21]. I asked Robert Jarvik to redesign the heart, which later became the Jarvik III. The dimensions

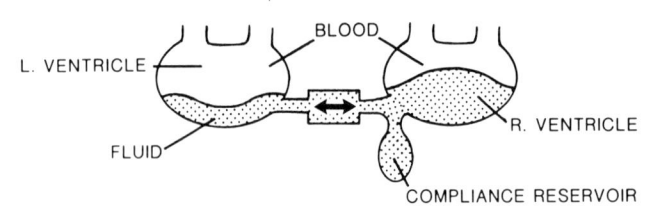

Figure 59.6 Diagram of electrohydraulic heart. A reversible pump moves fluid (not blood) from left to right and vice versa. Some of the fluid can be diverted to a compliance reservoir to reduce the stroke volume of the right ventricle

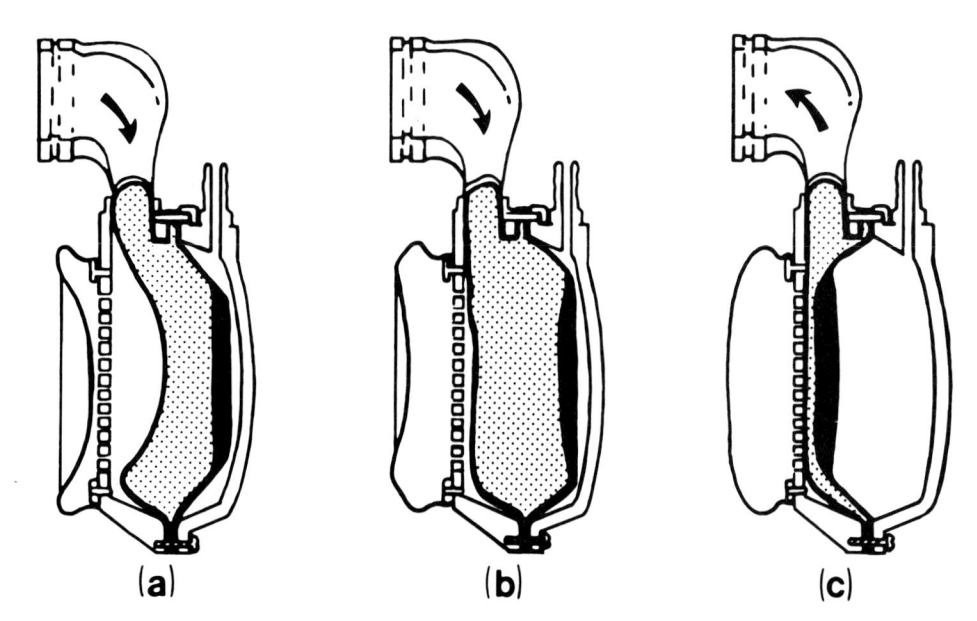

Figure 59.7 Diagram of an artificial heart (TAH) with anti-vacuum bellows. If a simple reciprocating pump is used to drive a TAH with compressed air or fluid, then undue suction might be generated during diastole if there is insufficient blood available to fill the ventricle. The *left* cross-sectional diagram (a) demonstrates what happens if not enough blood is available. The left wall of the ventricle, which is supported by a screen, is sucked into the ventricle, and the bellows on the outside are drawn inward. The *middle* diagram (b) shows what happens if there is enough blood to fill the ventricle during diastole. The ventricle is entirely filled, and the left side of the ventricular wall remains against the screen. The *right* diagram (c) shows what happens during systole. The ventricle is compressed so that the blood is expelled. The screen provides support for the flexible left side of the ventricle

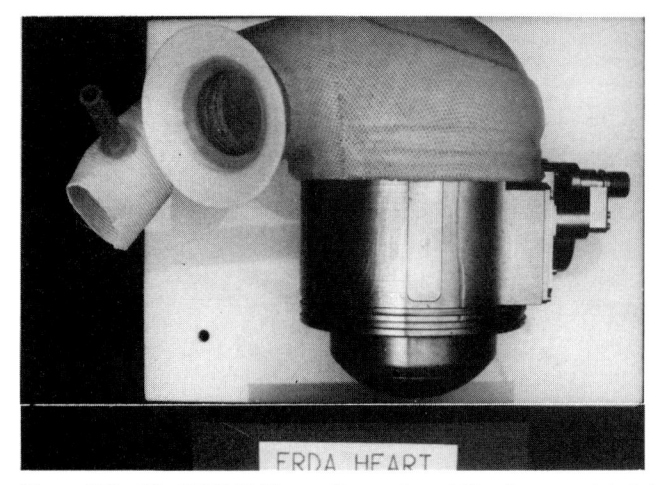

Figure 59.8 The 'ERDA' (Energy Research and Development Administration) heart. Only one ventricle is shown. The blood ventricle has a collapsible part (top of the figure). The drive shaft is to the far right. Blood handling parts are made of silastic

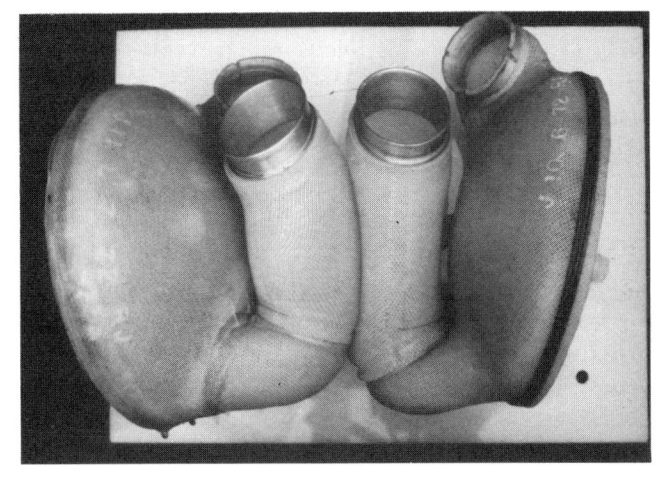

Figure 59.9 In the 'pancake' artificial heart the ventricles lie against the ribcage, thus leaving the area between sternum and vertebral column available for the connections to the atria, aorta, and pulmonary artery

were such that it would fit inside a calf's chest without compromising the venous return of the right and left atria. In the course of developing a larger heart with a larger cardiac output, the Jarvik VII heart was developed, and was the heart implanted in Barney Clark in 1982[22,23] (Chapter 60).

Before the first clinical implantation, Jack Kolff demonstrated convincingly (in brain-dead cadavers) that it was preferable to place the left ventricle more to the left, or the right ventricle more to the right, so that the narrow space between the sternum and the vertebral column was not overcrowded[24]. During the implantation in Barney Clark, the pericardium on the left was slit to allow space for the left ventricle.

To facilitate positioning of the TAH, with its rather rigid driveline, in the chest, the surgeon can experiment with a dummy ventricle (Figure 59.10), which has the exact size of the ventricle to be implanted. When he has determined the best possible location, he can use a flexible driveline to plan the point of exit from the chest. He then feeds the rigid

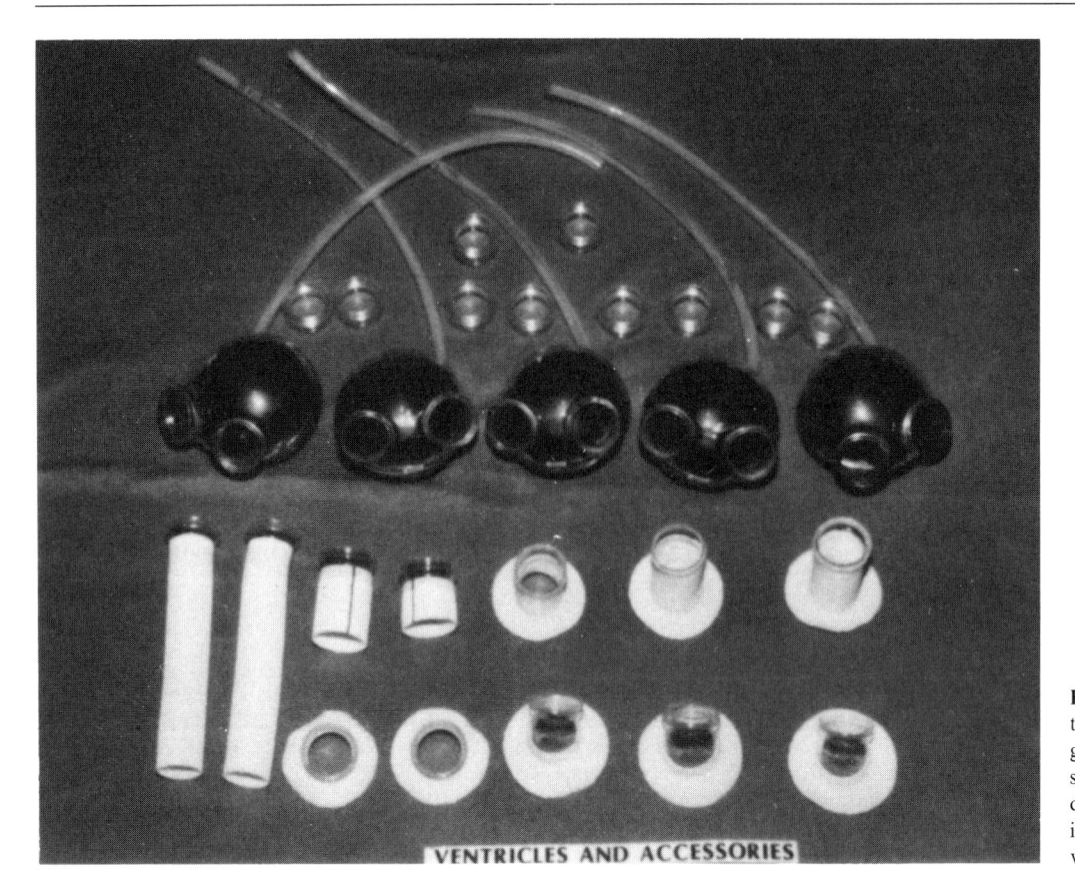

Figure 59.10 Set of dummy ventricles and accessories that the surgeon may use to estimate ideal size and position in the chest. The drivelines are not connected. There is a choice of atria and shape of ventricles

driveline through the incision, and the artificial ventricle will fit satisfactorily in place.

Thromboemboli

Of the first six patients who received the Jarvik-type TAH, five had thromboemboli. The unfortunate alternative to such thromboemboli is hemorrhage from anticoagulant therapy. Thrombus formation is most common: (1) on the suture lines, (2) in the connectors (so-called quick-connects), (3) around the valves, and (4) at the junction between the diaphragm and the housing (DH junction)[25-27].

Finding a small thrombus in a crevice in the TAH is not necessarily a bad omen; it should be considered as part of the natural repairing process of the body. Sooner or later the equilibrium between thrombus-producing and thrombus-removing factors will be established, and a small thrombus in a crevice may be smoothed off at the surface and even overgrown with endothelium.

Jack Kolff has suggested doing away with the quick connect system used heretofore in nearly all TAH implants. The left atrium, left ventricle, and aorta are now manufactured in one piece, as are the right atrium, right ventricle, and pulmonary artery (Figure 59.2). The surgeon can now sew in (on the operating table) the valve of his choice; St. Jude, Bjork–Shiley, or Hall-Kaster valves can be used. If he is particularly concerned with the risk of thrombosis, he can sew in tissue or polyurethane valves (Figure 59.11).

A promising and compact solution has been suggested by Olsen and his associates[29]; it consists of axial flow pumps magnetically suspended in the bloodstream, thus negating the need for bearings, which are notorious for causing thromboemboli.

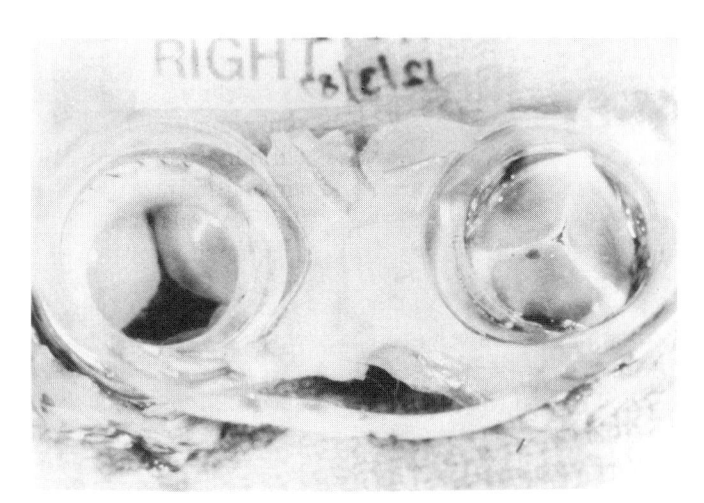

Figure 59.11 Polyurethane valves, with sewing cuffs removed, 28 days after implantation in a TAH. One leaflet of the inflow valve has been cut out for study. The leaflets were clear of thrombus except for one small speck

In general, to avoid thrombus formation in the TAH or in the patient's atria, one of two approaches can be used.

The first is the use of a rough intima, accepting that fibrin formation will occur, but trusting that it will not be dislodged as emboli. This rough intima can consist of (1) small titanium balls[30], or, on moving diaphragms, of (2) Dacron fibrils firmly anchored with a second layer of polyurethane, or (3) of a facsimile of the Dacron fibrils but consisting of the same kind of polyurethane (as used by the Thermedics device). Rough intimas can be successfully coated with what Nose has called 'a biolyzed surface', which basically is pure gelatine cross-linked with glutaraldehyde[14]. This highly hydrophylic surface has proved very successful.

The second – and, to date, more popular – approach is to use smooth, elastomer surfaces[31]. (Smooth intimas are used by Symbion, the Berlin group, Thoratec, Cardiac Systems, and Abiomed.) For a long time it was believed that air-dried polyurethane was to be preferred, though this is probably not so. The ideal is for thrombus never to form, and therefore embolization never to take place, but this ideal is rarely achieved. Jack Kolff's group in Philadelphia has demonstrated that there is basically no difference when one looks with the scanning electron microscope at the smooth intima of a TAH implanted for 2, 10, or 30 days (J. Kolff, unpublished). This suggests that small thrombi are formed all the time, but are then dissolved. This appears to be harmless, as long as the thrombi do not become too large.

The treatment of the smooth intima with heparin, prostaglandin, heparin–prostaglandin compound, albumin, or albumin IgG is aimed to make the smooth surface even less thrombogenic. At present, there is competition between two concepts: (1) incorporating the substances in the polyurethane so that they leach out, which, of course, results in a limited active life, or (2) grafting them on to the surface. It has been well-substantiated that if heparin, for example, is grafted to the surface with a long chain of carbon atoms, so that the heparin can wave back and forth in the bloodstream, it provides high protection against thrombus formation[32–34].

The inertness of smooth surfaces can be further enhanced by coating them with pyrolytic carbon[35,36]. The pyrolytic carbon surface may be the most inert surface known to man. Coating the inert surface with compounds in which water is incorporated (hydrophilic coating), such as is used in contact lenses, is another possibility. Owen (at the Biosouth Research Institute in New Orleans) is using polyhydroxyethylene oxide acrylate to coat artificial hearts for our group at the present time.

Infection

It is believed that even a small thrombus may be a place where bacteria can proliferate; the number of local infections (often around the valves of the TAH) seen in experimental animals is high. Once a vegetative bacterial endocarditis has developed, it is usually impossible to ascertain whether or not its origin was a pre-existing thrombus. Recently, Gristina has ascertained that bacteria, which are innocuous while circulating, will proliferate and become clinically significant when they find a surface on which to settle (e.g. elastomers). Indeed, specific bacteria appear to have a preference for specific elastomers, and other bacteria for other elastomers[37]. The possibility of making the surface of the elastomer less attractive to bacteria is one of the challenges of the future. It may possibly be achieved with antibiotics or antiseptic agents, as long as they are not damaging to the blood components.

Aging of polyurethane

For many reasons, polyurethanes are the easiest and most desirable material with which to make artificial hearts and artificial heart valves, but *all polyurethanes age*. A TAH which has been in a mock circulation for many years shows brittleness of the diaphragm. We have therefore returned to the use of silicones, which do not age. The newer silicones (e.g. silastic HP 100) are stronger than those used around 1970, have a greatly reduced tendency to tear, and can be reinforced with fibers, such as carbon fibers, if needed.

FINANCIAL CONSIDERATIONS

An air-driven TAH need not be exorbitantly expensive. The production of a TAH by vacuum-forming techniques requires only simple molds, and is a rapid process compared to that of solution-casting. (Cardiac Systems Inc. (1027 Conshohocken Road, Conshohocken, PA 19428, USA) has a license from the University of Utah for the production of such TAHs, and Food and Drug Administration approval is pending.)

Neither need the drive system be expensive. One such system at our center (a slightly modified two-cylinder gasoline engine driven by an electric motor) costs less than $1000, and has been pumping every night for 6 months to test hearts and valves for durability. Other more sophisticated reciprocating pumps, which can be regulated, were designed by Norton and were relatively inexpensive[38]. Other types of drive systems for air-driven hearts are available for approximately $12 000. They are usually operated by solenoid-driven valves, and need a source of compressed air. Drive systems which use air-actuated valve systems, such as are commonly used in respirators and diving equipment, are extremely inexpensive, but have a tendency to drift.

If we wish to provide an inexpensive TAH, it makes no sense to incorporate four commercially available valves, knowing that their costs range between $1800 and $4200 each. During the last 2 years, therefore, we have concentrated our efforts on building elastomer valves. My co-worker, Long Sheng Yu, can do this with either the vacuum-forming or solution-casting technique, or by spraying on simple male molds. The valves can be inserted into the ventricles during production of the TAH.

COMMENT

It has been estimated that some 35 000–50 000 people per year in the United States alone will need some kind of replacement of their failing heart[39]. It is unlikely that human donor hearts will be found for more than a very small proportion of them, possibly only one in every 15–25. There is, therefore, a great incentive to persist in our efforts to develop the perfect TAH.

But can we afford the development costs, which, it is estimated, have already been in excess of $200 million in the USA alone? If we do not squander our money on SDI ('Star Wars'), there would be plenty of money in the United States to take care of its citizens in need. We must convert our military-directed industry towards peaceful goals, and our production-oriented society toward a service-oriented society. Now is the time to tell our political representatives where our priorities are.*

References

1. Akutsu, T. and Kolff, W.J. (1958). Permanent substitute for valves and hearts. *Am. Soc. Artif. Intern. Organs.*, **4**, 230
2. Kolff, W.J., Akutsu, T., Dreyer, B. and Norton, H. (1959). Artificial heart in the chest and use of polyurethane for making hearts, valves and aortas. *Am. Soc. Artif. Intern. Organs.*, **5**, 298
3. Kolff, W.J. (1969). The artificial heart: research, development or invention? *Dis. Chest.*, **56**, 314
4. Hiller, K.H., Seidel, W. and Kolff, W.J. (1963). An electronic–mechanical control for an intrathoracic artificial heart. *Am. J. Med. Electronics*, **2**, 212
5. Kolff, W.J., Hiller, K., Seidel, Moulopoulos, S., Akutsu, T., Mirkovitch, V. and Topaz, S.R. (1962). Results obtained with artificial hearts driven by the N.A.S.A. Servomechanism and the pathologic physiology of artificial hearts. *Am. Soc. Artif. Intern. Organs*, **8**, 135
6. Nose, Y. and Kolff, W.J. (1966). The intracorporeal mechanical heart. *Vasc. Dis.*, **3**, 25
7. Kwan-Gett, C., Zwart, H.H., Kralios, A.C., Kessler, T., Backman, K. and Kolff, W.J. (1970). A prosthetic heart with hemispherical ventricles designed for low hemolytic action. *Am. Soc. Artif. Intern. Organs*, **16**, 409
8. Kolff, W.J. (1988). The Tenth Hastings Lecture. Experiences and practical considerations for the future of artificial hearts and of mankind. *Artif. Organs*, **12**, 89
9. Kolff, J., Cavarocchi, N.C., Riebman, J.B., McClurken, J.B. and Jessup, M. (1988). The artificial heart: design, capabilities, and indications in the treatment of heart failure. *Heart Failure*, **4**, 13
10. Willshaw, P., Nielsen, S.D., Nanas, J., Pichel, R. and Olsen, D.B. (1984). A cardiac output monitor and diagnostic unit for pneumatically driven artificial heart. *Artif. Organs*, **8**, 215
11. Kless, H., Blumenthal, N.V., Mohnhaupt, A., Affeld, K. and Bucherl, E.S. (1974). Extracorporeal measurement of hemodynamic parameter of the artificial heart. *Eur. Soc. Artif. Organs*, **1**, 166
12. Heimes, H.P. and Klasen, F. (1982). Completely integrated wearable TAH-drive unit. *Int. J. Artif. Organs*, **5**, 157
13. Affeld, K. (1984). A redundant portable driver for the total artificial heart (Abstract) *Am. Soc. Artif. Intern. Organs*, **13**, 1
14. Kiraly, R.J. (1988). Development of an implantable left ventricular assist system. In Andrade, J. (ed.) *Artificial Organs*, VCH, Inc., New York, p. 45
15. Smith, L., Backman, K., Sandquist, G., Kolff, W.J., Schatten, K. and Kessler, T. (1974). Development on the implantation of a total nuclear-powered artificial heart system. *Am. Soc. Artif. Intern. Organs*, **20**, 732
16. Smith, L., Olsen, D.B., Sandquist, G., Crandall, E., Gentry, S. and Kolff, W.J. (1975). A totally implantable mechanical heart. *Eur. Soc. Artif. Organs*, **II**, 150
17. Rosenberg, G., Snyder, A.J., Landis, D.L., Geselowitz, D.B., Donachy, J.H. and Pierce, W.S. (1984). An electric motor-driven total artificial heart: seven months survival in the calf. *Am. Soc. Artif. Intern. Organs*, **30**, 69
18. Chen, H., Miller, P.J., Conley, M.G., Beering, F.K., Brugler, J.S., Jassawalla, J.S. and Portner, P.M. (1988). Development of an implantable, permanent electromechanical ventricular assist system. In Andrade, J. (ed.) *Artificial Organs*, VCH, Inc., New York, p. 59
19. Houston, C.S., Akutsu, T. and Kolff, W.J. (1960). Pendulum type of artificial heart within the chest: preliminary report. *Am. Heart J.*, **59**, 723
20. Norton, S.H., Akutsu, T. and Kolff, W.J. (1952). Artificial heart with anti-vacuum bellows. *Am. Soc. Artif. Intern. Organs*, **8**, 131
21. Jarvik, R., Volder, J., Olsen, D., Moulopoulos, S. and Kolff, W.J. (1974). Venous return of an artificial heart designed to prevent right heart syndrome. *Ann. Biomed. Eng.*, **2**, 335
22. Joyce, L.D., DeVries, W.C., Hastings, W.L., Olsen, D.B., Jarvik, R.K. and Kolff, W.J. (1983). Response of the human body to the first permanent implant of the Jarvik-7 total artificial heart. *Am. Soc. Artif. Intern. Organs*, **29**, 81
23. Kolff, W.J., DeVries, W.C., Joyce, L.D., Olsen, D.B., Jarvik, R.K., Nielsen, S., Hastings, L., Anderson, J. and Anderson, F. (1984). Lessons learned from Dr Barney Clark, the first patient with an artificial heart. *Prog. Artif. Organs*, **2**, 165
24. Kolff, J., Deeb, G.M., Cavarocchi, C., Riebman, J., Olsen, D.B. and Robbins, P.S. (1984). The artificial heart in human subjects. *J. Thorac. Cardiovasc. Surg.*, **87**, 825
25. Levinson, M.M., Smith, R.G., Cork, R.C., Gallo, J., Emery, R.W., Icenogle, T.B., Ott, R.A., Burns, G.L. and Copeland, J.G. (1986). Thromboembolic complications of the Jarvik-7 total artificial heart: case report. *Artif. Organs*, **10**, 236
26. Riebman, J.B., Liotta, D., Navia, J.A., Cooley, D.A., Frazier, O.H., Del Rio, P. and Quintana, O.R. (1988). Orthotopic univentricular artificial heart. In Andrade, J. (ed.) *Artificial Organs*, VCH, Inc., New York, p. 73
27. Levinson, M.M., Smith, R., Cork, R., Gallo, J., Emery, R.W., Icenogle, T.B., Ott, R.A. and Copeland, J.G. (1988). Clinical problems associated with the total artificial heart as a bridge to transplantation. In Andrade, J. (ed.) *Artificial Organs*, VCH, Inc., New York, p. 169
28. Lioi, A.P., Orth, J.L., Crump, K.R., Diffee, G., Dew, P.A., Nielsen, S.D. and Olsen, D.B. (1988). In vitro development of automatic control for the actively filled electrohydraulic heart. *Artif. Organs*, **12**, 152
29. Kolff, W.J. (1988). The future of artificial organs and of us all. In Andrade, J. (ed.) *Artificial Organs*, VCH, Inc., New York, p. 730
30. Buczak, S. (1987). Fabrication of implantable artificial heart devices

---

*Physicians for Social Responsibility, 1601 Connecticut Ave., N.W., Suite 800, Washington, D.C. 20009, USA.
International Physicians for the Prevention of Nuclear War, Inc. 225 Longwood Avenue, Boston, Massachusetts 12115, USA.

and components. Thermedics Report #1-HV-92907-6, Devices and Technology Branch, *NIH Report*, October 28

31. Farrer, D.J., Litwak, P., Lawson, J.H., Ward, R.S., White, K.A., Robinson, A.J., Rodvein, R. and Hill, J.D. (1988). *In vivo* evaluations of a new thromboresistant polyurethane for artificial heart blood pumps. *J. Thorac. Cardiovasc. Surg.*, **95**, 191

32. Jacobs, H., Okano, R., Lin, J.Y. and Kim, S.W. (1985). PGE_1–heparin conjugate releasing polymers. *J. Controlled Release*, **2**, 313

33. Kim, S.W. (1987). Platelet adhesion and prevention at blood–polymer interface. *J. Artif. Organs*, **11**, 228

34. Heyman, P.W., Cho, C.S., McRea, J.C., Olsen, D.B. and Kim, S.W. (1985). Heparinized polyurethanes: *in vitro* and *in vivo* studies. *J. Biomed. Mater. Res.*, **19**, 419

35. Paccagnella, A., Majni, G., Ottaviani, G., Arru, P., Santi, M. and Vallana, F. (1986). Properties of a new carbon film for biomedical applications. *Int. J. Artif. Organs*, **9**, 127

36. Arru, P., Santi, M., Vallana, F., Majni, G., Ottaviani, G. and Paccagnella, A. (1986). A new pyrolytic carbon film for biomedical application. Presented at the Congress *Ceramics in Biomaterials*, Milan

37. Gristina, A.G. (1987). Biomaterial-centered infection: microbial adhesion versus tissue integration. *Science*, **237**, 1588

38. Panayotopoulos, E.K., Norton, S.H., Akutsu, T. and Kolff, W.J. (1964). A special reciprocating pump to drive an artificial heart inside the chest. *J. Thorac. Cardiovasc. Surg.*, **48**, 844

39. Working Group on Mechanical Circulatory Support of the National Heart, Lung, and Blood Institute (1985). *Artificial Heart and Assist Devices: Directions, Needs, Costs, Societal and Ethical Issues*. US Dept of Health and Human Services publication (NIH) 85-2723. Bethesda, Md, Public Health Service

60
Clinical Experience

D.K.C. COOPER

INTRODUCTION

Cooley (Figure 60.1) and colleagues[1] implanted the first total artificial heart (TAH) in a human in 1969. This attempt was intended as an interim measure until a suitable human heart could be located and transplanted. This group performed a second bridge-to-transplant procedure in 1981[2,3]. Since then, the TAH has successfully served as a bridge to transplant in more than 35 patients (Chapters 57 and 58).

The first intended permanent implantation of a TAH was performed by DeVries (Figure 60.2) and his colleagues in 1982[4-8], who used the device to prolong the lives of four patients. This initial clinical experience was based to a great extent on pioneering work by Willem Kolff (Figure 60.3) and his colleagues in Utah, whose bioengineering research did much to advance the artificial heart to the point where its clinical use could be considered (Chapter 59). The clinical

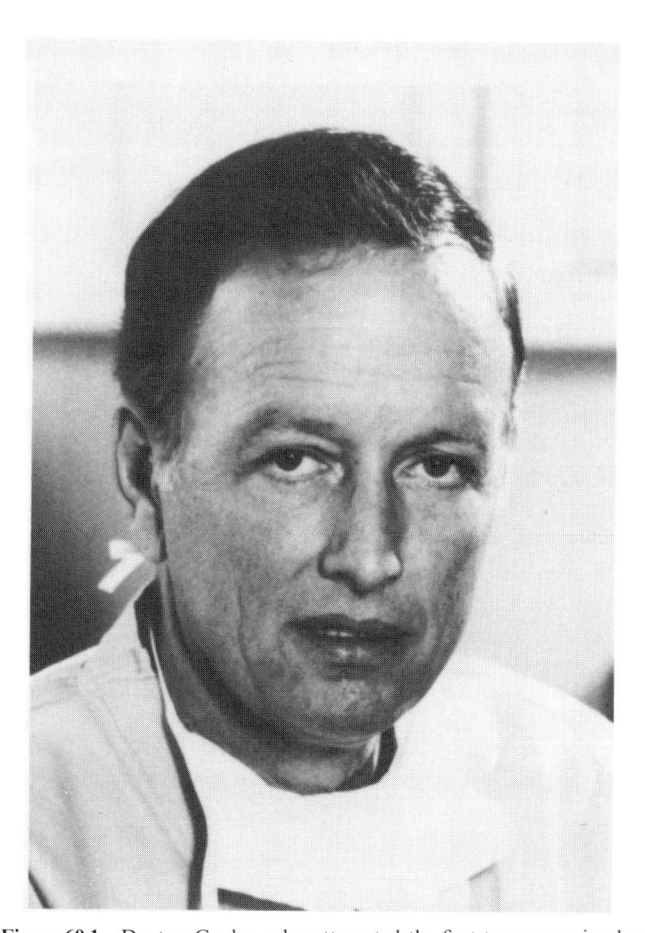

Figure 60.1 Denton Cooley, who attempted the first temporary implantation of an artificial heart (the Liotta heart) in 1969

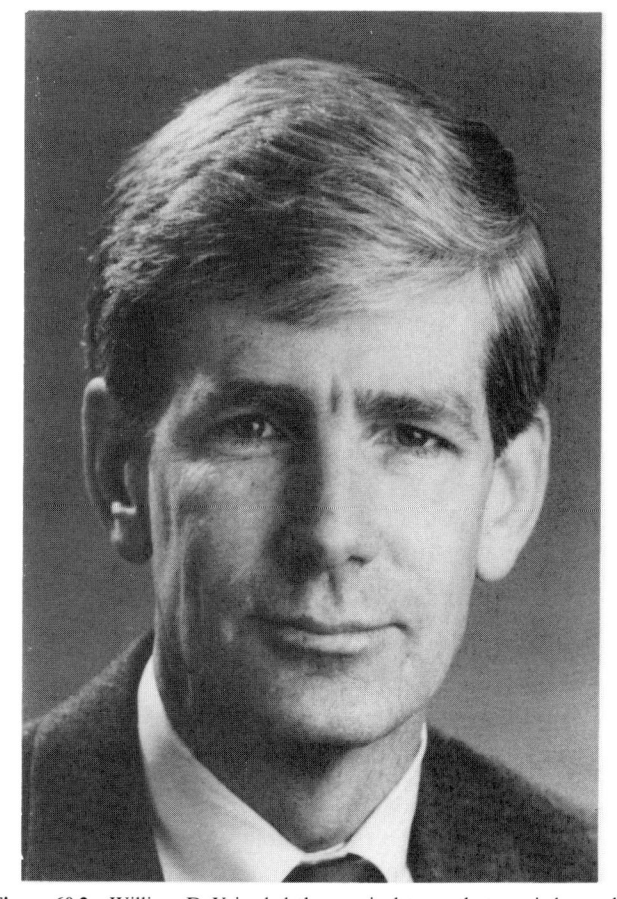

Figure 60.2 William DeVries led the surgical team that carried out the first trial of permanent replacement of the heart by an artificial device

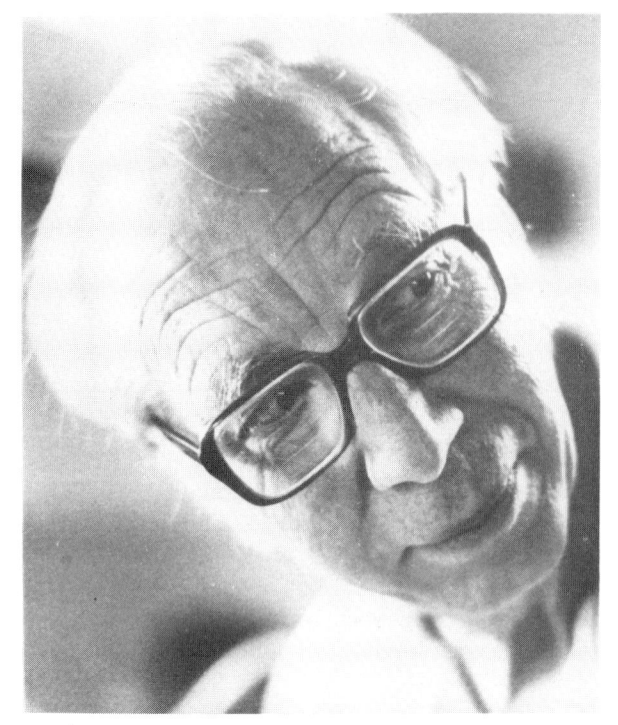

Figure 60.3 Willem Kolff, of the University of Utah, whose pioneering work contributed much to the development of the artificial heart

experience of DeVries and his colleagues (initially at the University of Utah and subsequently at Humana Hospital Audubon, Louisville) will be briefly reviewed[4-9].

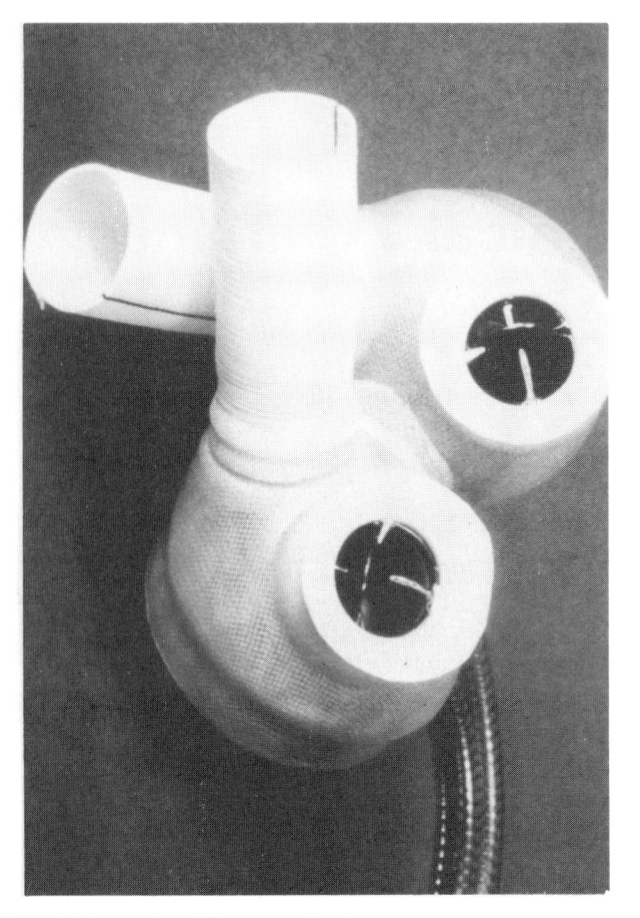

Figure 60.4 Jarvik-7-100 total artificial heart

DEVICE

The Jarvik-7-100 (Figure 60.4) TAH consists of right and left ventricles and four tilting-disk valves with anatomical communications to the atria and great vessels. Each ventricle contains a flexible diaphragm constructed of multilayered polyurethane. At the base of each ventricle is a 30-F polyvinylchloride connecting tube that is tunneled under the skin and exits the body in the left lateral abdominal area through Dacron felt skin buttons. The connecting tubes are attached to polyvinylchloride drivelines, 1.6 cm in external diameter and 2.2 m in length. The drivelines are attached to an external pneumatic pump (the Utah drive System II console, Symbion, Inc., Salt Lake City). The lines may be connected to a portable heart driver during periods of patient mobility.

The maximum stroke volume of each Jarvik-7-100 ventricle is 100 ml. The ventricles are pneumatically 'driven'. During diastole, blood fills the ventricle on the upper side of the diaphragm. During systole, air is pulsed on the underside of the diaphragm to eject the blood from the ventricle. The heart functions in response to circulatory needs (Frank–Starling law); thus, with increased venous return, stroke volume is increased without a change in heart rate (Chapter 59).

PATIENT SELECTION CRITERIA

The four potential recipients of the TAH were categorized as New York Heart Association class IV, and each had been rejected as candidates for cardiac transplantation by at least three programs. All revealed stable psychological profiles, and had strong, reliable family support systems. They were all unanimously approved by an evaluation committee, and gave informed consent.

Details of the four recipients are given in Table 60.1[8].

Table 60.1 Preimplant clinical data of the four recipients of permanent total artificial hearts

Patient	Age	Underlying cardiac pathology	Reason transplantation denied
1	61	Dilated CM COPD	Advanced age
2	54	Ischemic CM	Insulin-requiring diabetes mellitus
3	58	Dilated CM	Advanced age
4	62	Ischemic CM Mild COPD	Advanced age

CM = cardiomyopathy; COPD = chronic obstructive pulmonary disease

The first patient to undergo this procedure was the first human subject in whom the Jarvik-7-100 TAH was implanted; the operation was performed on December 1, 1982.

SURGICAL TECHNIQUE

The technique of implantation is described in Chapter 57; details have been reported by DeVries previously[9].

MONITORING

A computerized bedside monitor-terminal stored and displayed systemic and pulmonary arterial and right and left atrial pressures. A cardiac output monitoring diagnostic unit (COMDU) displayed and stored left and right filling volumes, left and right cardiac outputs, and heart rate[10]. Left and right drive pressure wave forms were also recorded. These data were stored on a tape recorder for later analysis[11,12].

CLINICAL PROGRESS

These patients lived for periods of 112, 620, 488, and 10 days respectively. The Jarvik-7-100 TAH functioned well, and hemodynamic stability was achieved in all patients[10,11]. Only one device failure was experienced – a broken mitral valve prosthesis (patient 1)[4]. Their postoperative course was, however, eventful in every case (Table 60.2), the major problems being hemorrhage, acute tubular necrosis, embolic phenomena, and infection, all of which occurred in all three long-term survivors. Detailed reports of their clinical courses have been described elsewhere[8]. Only one patient (patient 2) was able to be discharged from the hospital, this patient being able to live in an apartment close to the hospital after day 133.

Table 60.2 Chronological order of significant post-implant events and complications in patient 2*

Days	
1	TAH implanted
1	Exploration of mediastinum for bleeding
3–6	Renal failure
19	CVA (thromboembolic)
68	Neutropenia
94	CVA (hypoperfusion)
133	Discharged from hospital
150–620	Subacute bacterial endocarditis
163	CVA (hemorrhagic)
202	Changed to new Utahdrive console with low dp/dt
352	CVA (thromboembolic)
444	Liver biopsy – microabscesses
590	Feeding gastrostomy
612	Tracheostomy
620	Respiratory failure, sepsis, death

*Based on DeVries[8]
CVA = cerebrovascular accident (stroke)

Hemodynamic observations

All of the patients demonstrated a remarkable degree of autoregulated hemodynamic homeostasis for prolonged periods[12]. Patient 1 was maintained with high cardiac outputs (6–8 l/min) that were associated with the onset of seizures. In the cases of patients 2–4, cardiac outputs were initially maintained at 3–4 l/min, and, over a 7-day period, were increased and stabilized at 5–6 l/min.

The cardiac output was readily altered by elevating the heart rate[12], which was usually set initially at 50 beats/minute, and increased gradually over a 1-month period to 80 beats/minute. Systolic and diastolic blood pressures could be maintained within normal ranges with heart rate set at 75–80 beats/minute. After approximately 45 days, an autoregulation of the vascular system in response to changes in device parameters was noted in all patients. At this time, attempts to increase cardiac output by increasing heart rate led to vasodilation, resulting in a return of cardiac output to the original level. Cardiac output was extremely stable. Light exercise activities on the nonresistant exercise cycle, achieved by patients 2 and 3, were associated with an increase in cardiac output of 1–2 l/min.

Complications

Hemorrhage

All four patients required re-operation for bleeding. The surgical team's experience led them to conclude that postoperative bleeding in these anticoagulated patients should be treated by prompt re-operation rather than by repeated blood transfusion and observation.

Hemolytic anemia

All patients developed a significant hemolytic anemia. After a change in the Utah drive consoles to provide a lower dp/dt (on days 116 and 202 for patients 3 and 2, respectively), transfusion requirements decreased. This was paralleled by a fall in the lactate dehydrogenase and plasma free hemoglobin levels.

Acute renal failure

Depressed preoperative cardiac output and poor renal perfusion undoubtedly increased the risk of postoperative renal failure. Patient 4 had the greatest compromise in renal function before operation, and was the only patient to require dialysis postoperatively. The etiology of acute tubular necrosis in the early postoperative course in patients with implants was considered to be multifactorial. The combination of high transfusion requirements and postoperative hemolysis probably played a significant role, and the toxic effects of long-term aminoglycoside therapy were also considered to be a possible contributing factor.

In the light of this experience, DeVries and his colleagues believe that in future patients several therapeutic approaches could be used to prevent the development of renal failure. Patients at other centers, who received TAHs in which the low dp/dt Utah drive System II was utilized, have not developed severe renal failure[13,14]. Therefore, this drive system, or the Heimes driver, would seem preferable in the future. Improved hemostasis would minimize the need for multiple transfusions in the early postoperative period. Renal blood flow, already reduced in such patients, could be maintained by low-dose dopamine in the intraoperative period, and by the use of mannitol and furosemide at critical times.

Thromboembolism

One of the greatest concerns in the care of the TAH patient is the prevention of thromboembolism. The use of anticoagulants, however, is not without risk, and requires careful monitoring of the thrombotic and fibrinolytic systems.

In this small series, anticoagulation policy varied from patient to patient[8]. Patient 1 had no thromboembolic events, but his course was complicated by recurrent bleeding episodes. Patient 2 experienced several thromboembolic episodes, though patient 3 experienced only minor transient episodes. At autopsy, both of these patients had prominent infected thrombi (subacute bacterial endocarditis) on all of the valves of the prosthesis.

DeVries' group point out that, in assessing the thrombogenic potential of the artificial heart, several factors must be considered, including the effects of (1) activation of both the intrinsic and extrinsic pathways of the coagulation cascade, (2) activation of platelets, and of (3) the fibrinolytic system, and (4) the antithrombotic/antiplatelet regimen used. None of these systems acts in isolation; they interact with one another, as well as with other enzymes and cellular systems, such as complement and kinin. Whether the coagulation cascade proceeds to completion depends on the adequacy of the anti-thrombotic/anti-platelet regimen that is used.

As a result of the experience with these four patients, several changes were recommended in the anticoagulation protocol to be used in the future. Once hemostasis has been achieved in the surgical wound, heparin should be administered by continuous infusion; heparin kinetic studies should be employed to estimate dosage, with the goal being a partial thromboplastin time increased 50% above control. When the indwelling catheters have been removed and prophylactic antibiotics discontinued, heparin administration should be by subcutaneous injection every 8 hours.

Since the patients in this study demonstrated thromboembolic problems after the diagnosis of bacteremia, concern was expressed that subacute bacterial endocarditis accounted for some or all of the thromboembolic events, and that this would not be responsive to antithrombotic therapy. In view of this possibility, in future cases treatment of infectious problems should have the highest priority as an anti-thrombotic measure.

Infection

After TAH implantation, the blood is in continuous contact with synthetic materials; it was considered possible that blood–material interactions impacted adversely on the immune status of the recipient. Infections severely compromised these patients, necessitating multiple and long courses of antibiotics for infections caused by urinary tract, bowel, respiratory, and skin normal flora and contaminants. Many of the organisms that caused chronic problems were detected in the early postoperative period[15].

Infection arising from the drivelines, with spread to the mediastinal periprosthetic space, was the major limiting factor in long-term use of the device. Intensive antimicrobial therapy for prolonged periods seemed to suppress but not to eradicate infection, and was accompanied by the appearance of multiresistant bacterial strains. Complications of antimicrobial therapy included diarrhea secondary to overgrowth with *Clostridium difficile* in two patients[15].

The surgical group concluded that the prevention of infection needed to be of foremost importance in the future development and utilization of the artificial heart. Of particular concern for TAH development was the finding of culture-negative 'skip areas' between the prosthesis and the skin; this was believed to imply a blood-borne infectious source of origin in some cases, rather than infection ascending along the drivelines from the skin[16]. Infection could therefore be a problem even with a future device that was fully implantable.

It was concluded that the incidence of infection could possibly be reduced in future cases by (1) improved selection of patients to exclude those with a predisposition to infection, (2) perioperative antibiotic prophylaxis with the use of narrow-spectrum antibiotics whenever possible, (3) particularly careful aseptic urinary bladder catheterization, (4) the use of non-invasive hemodynamic monitoring techniques, (5) frequent surveillance cultures, (6) the use of full antithrombotic and anti-platelet therapies with the subcutaneous (rather than intravenous) administration of heparin, and (7) improved protective isolation and wound dressing procedures.

COMMENT

The complications of thromboembolism and infection were considered to be the most significant limiting factors to the use of the Jarvik-7 as a long-term cardiac replacement; it was thought that avoidance of these complications might prove difficult. Exposure of circulating blood to foreign surfaces appeared to induce changes in both humoral and cellular immunity. Such changes complicated efforts to avoid blood-borne infection of the TAH, or ascending infection along the drivelines.

Those associated with this initial clinical research program are to be commended on clarifying many of the problems that need to be overcome before permanent replacement of the heart by a mechanical device can become a totally successful and routine procedure.

References

1. Cooley, D.A., Liotta, D., Hallman, G.L., Bloodwell, R.D., Leachman, R.D. and Milam, J.D. (1969). Orthotopic cardiac prothesis for two-staged cardiac replacement. *Am. J. Cardiol.*, **24**, 723
2. Frazier, O.H., Akutsu, T. and Cooley, D.A. (1982). Total artificial heart (TAH) utilization in man. *Trans. Am. Soc. Artif. Intern. Organs*, **23**, 534
3. Cooley, D.A. (1982). Staged cardiac transplantation: report of three cases. *Heart Transplant.*, **1**, 145
4. DeVries, W.C., Anderson, J.L., Joyce, L.D., Anderson, F.L., Hammond, E.H., Jarvik, R.K. and Kolff, W.J. (1984). Clinical use of the total artificial heart. *N. Engl. J. Med.*, **310**, 273
5. Joyce, L.D., DeVries, W.C., Hastings, W.L., Olsen, D.B., Jarvik, R.K. and Kolff, W.J. (1983). Response of the human body to the first permanent implant of the Jarvik-7 total artificial heart. *Trans. Am. Soc. Artif. Intern. Organs*, **29**, 81
6. Anderson, F.L., DeVries, W.C., Anderson, J.L. and Joyce, L.D. (1984). Evaluation of total artificial heart performance in man. *Am. J. Cardiol.*, **54**, 394
7. DeVries, W.C. and Joyce, L.D. (1983). The artificial heart. *Clin. Symp.*, **35**, 1
8. DeVries, W.C. (1988). The permanent artificial heart. Four case reports. *J. Am. Med. Assoc.*, **259**, 849
9. DeVries, W.C. (1988). Surgical technique for implantation of the Jarvik-7-100 total artificial heart. *J. Am. Med. Assoc.*, **259**, 875
10. Willshaw, P., Nielsen, S.D., Nannas, H., Pichel, R. and Olsen, D.B. (1984). A cardiac output monitor and diagnostic unit for pneumatically driven artificial heart. *Artif. Organs*, **8**, 215
11. Mays, J.B., Williams, M.A., Barker, L.E., Hastings, L. and DeVries, W.C. (1986). Diagnostic monitoring and drive system management of patients with total artificial heart. *Heart Lung*, **15**, 466
12. Mays, L.B., Williams, M.A., Barker, L.E., Pfeifer, M.A., Kammerling, J.M., Jung, S. and DeVries, W.C. (1988). Clinical management of total artificial heart drive systems. *J. Am. Med. Assoc.*, **259**, 881
13. Levinson, M.M., Copeland, J.G., Smith, R.G., Cork, R.C., DeVries, W.C., Mays, J.B., Griffith, B.P., Kormos, R., Joyce, L.D., Pritzker, M.R., Semb, B.K.H., Koul, B., Menkis, A.H. and Keon, W.J. (1986). Indexes of hemolysis in human recipients of the Jarvik-7 total artificial heart: a cooperative report of 15 patients. *J. Heart Transplant.*, **5**, 236
14. Joyce, L.D., Johnson, K.E., Pierce, W.S., DeVries, W.C., Semb, B.K.H., Copeland, J.G., Griffith, B.P., Cooley, D.A., Frazier, O.H., Cabrol, C., Keon, W.J., Unger, F., Bucherl, E.S. and Wolner, E. (1986). Summary of the world experience with clinical use of total artificial hearts as heart support devices. *J. Heart Transplant.*, **3**, 229
15. Kunin, C.M., Dobbins, J.J., Melo, J.C., Levinson, M.M., Love, K., Joyce, L.D. and DeVries, W.C. (1988). Infectious complications in four long-term recipients of the Jarvik-7 artificial heart. *J. Am. Med. Assoc.*, **259**, 860
16. Dobbins, J.J., Johnson, G.S., Kunin, C.M. and DeVries, W.C. (1988). Postmortem microbiological findings of two total artificial heart recipients. *J. Am. Med. Assoc.*, **259**, 865

ADDENDUM

The Food and Drug Administration has recently withdrawn permission for use of the Jarvik-7 artificial heart in the USA. The reasons for this are not yet certain, and whether the ban will be temporary or permanent also remains unknown.

Section VI

Cardiac xenotransplantation

61
Xenotransplantation: Overview

D.K.C. COOPER

INTRODUCTION

The worldwide shortage of organ donors for purposes of transplantation would be overcome if the problems associated with xenografting could be solved. Transplant operations could be carried out on routine operating lists electively, and no potential recipient would need to die for lack of a suitable organ. Even if this ideal state of affairs could not be achieved, then at least xenografts might be used as temporary life-saving procedures whilst a suitable cardiac allograft was awaited.

'CONCORDANT' AND 'DISCORDANT' XENOGRAFTS

Calne has suggested that the response to xenografting can be divided into two major groups[1]. 'First-set cross-species grafts which are rejected at a tempo and with morphological characteristics similar to first-set allografts (acute or cellular rejection) would be one class'[1]. This type of rejection can occur when grafting is performed between closely related animal species, such as chimpanzee to man, sheep to goat, or hamster to rat. Calne has suggested that these be known as *concordant* xenografts.

'First-set cross-species grafts which are hyperacutely (or humorally) rejected, with vascular lesions similar to those observed in second-set allografts in sensitized animals would belong to the other category'[1]. Such rejection occurs predominantly when transplantation is carried out between widely disparate animal species, for example, pig to man, or cat to dog, and could be known as *discordant* xenografts. Under such circumstances hyperacute rejection closely resembles that seen when allografting is carried out in the presence of a positive lymphocytotoxic cross-match, or when ABO blood group incompatibility exists.

This suggested nomenclature is helpful, but experimental and clinical experiences have demonstrated that there are not just two distinct groups of xenograft, but gradations, in as much as an organ from one animal species, when transplanted into an animal of a different species, may in some pairs be rejected acutely and in others hyperacutely. Furthermore, features of both cellular (acute) and vascular (hyperacute) rejection can occur within the same xenografted organ[2,3].

It would therefore seem that additional nomenclature is required to define the immunological similarity or otherwise between two species. There will clearly be few truly concordant pairs, as a degree of vascular rejection is likely to be seen in many cases.

CHOICE OF A DONOR FOR MAN

If man were to be the recipient, and using presently available immunosuppressive therapy, xenografting from a 'concordant' animal species such as the chimpanzee, or possibly the baboon, would have a much greater chance of success than would a graft from a 'discordant' animal. Pioneering work in the use of primate kidneys as donor organs for man showed clearly that the closer phylogenetically the donor to man, then the longer was the donor organ survival time. Reemtsma (Figure 61.1) obtained longer survival using chimpanzee kidneys as donors[4-8] than did Starzl[9,10], or Hitchcock[11], who used baboons; rhesus monkey kidneys fared even worse[4].

Immunological similarities and differences between various primate species have been studied by Sarich[12], using micro-complement fixation, which has been shown to be a sensitive and reliable technique to measure the degree of immunological cross-reactivity between species. There were a number of considerations which led to albumin being the molecule whose evolutionary changes were studied. The very close relationships existing among all hominoid albumins, and particularly amongst the higher primates, are shown in Table 61.1.

The baboon does not grow to a size large enough to make it a suitable donor of some organs, for example the heart, for adult humans, though there may be a role for this animal as a donor for children. The rationale for baboon

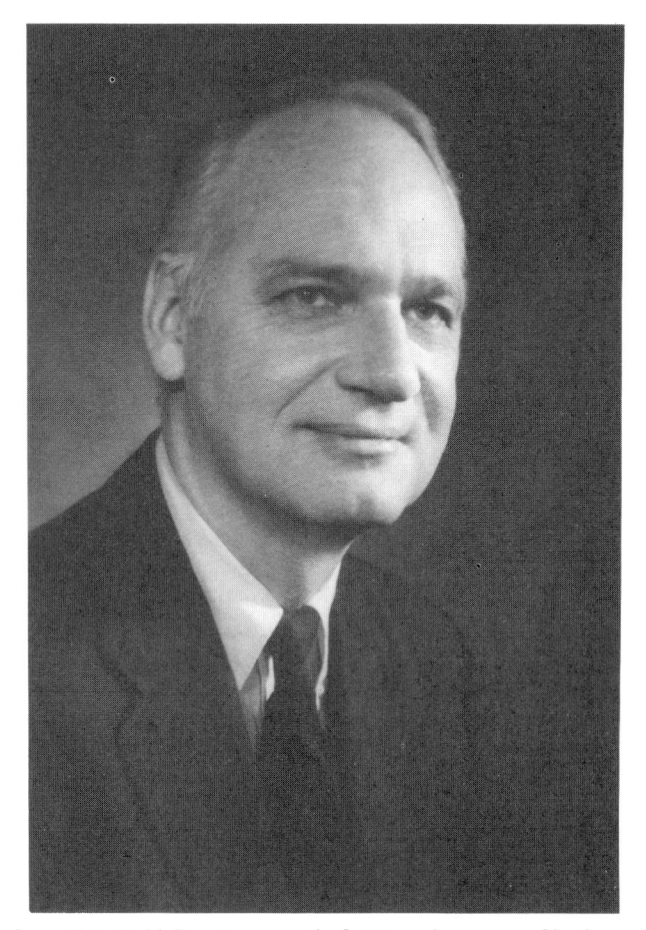

Figure 61.1 Keith Reemtsma was the first to explore xenografting in man in a scientific manner. Between 1963 and 1965, whilst at Tulane University in New Orleans, he transplanted a series of chimpanzee kidneys into patients with advanced renal failure; kidney function was obtained for periods up to 8 months

Table 61.1 Reactivity in the micro-complement fixation procedure of sera from various species with a pool of three antisera directed to human serum albumin*

Species	Index of dissimilarity
Hominoidea (man and apes)	
Homo sapiens (Man)	1.0
Pan troglodytes (Chimpanzee)	1.14
Gorilla gorilla (Gorilla)	1.09
Pongo pygmaeus (Orangutan)	1.22
Hylobates lar (Gibbon)	1.28
Symphalangus syndactylus (Gibbon)	1.30
Cercopithecoidea (Old World monkeys)	2.23–2.65
Ceboidea (New World monkeys)	2.7–5.0
Prosimii (Prosimians, e.g. lemur)	8.6–18
Non-primates	
Bos taurus (Bull)	32
Sus scrofa (Pig)	> 35

*Adapted from Sarich, V.M.[12]

transplantation in infants and small children is that few human donors can be found in this age group, selective immunoregulation is available in the form of cyclosporine with pulsed steroids and/or azathioprine, and the immature immune system of newborn infants may have less competence to reject foreign tissue[13]. There is good experimental evidence that growth of xenograft anastomoses occurs, but less conclusive evidence that it will be possible to control rejection well enough to expect even medium-term survival.

Other higher primates are, in general, endangered species, and would not be available in sufficient numbers unless extensive and costly breeding programs were initiated. Even the chimpanzee heart may not be large enough to support the circulation alone in a large human adult[14] (Chapter 1). There would, in addition, almost certainly be ethical and moral objections to the use of such animals; many of these ethical considerations have been discussed by Kaplan[15] and Veath[16]. It would appear, therefore, that xenografting between concordant species will not provide the final answer to donor supply in man.

Certain discordant animals, such as the pig or sheep, would provide organs of a suitable size and anatomy for man, but transplantation would be greatly complicated by the development of hyperacute rejection, which is not prevented or modified by the presently available immunosuppressive drugs[17,18]. The mechanism of the rapid onset (sometimes occurring within 5 minutes) of hyperacute (vascular, humoral) rejection is complex, and is discussed in Chapter 63, but appears mainly to be related to the presence of preformed species-specific (heterophile, heterospecific, xeno) antibodies (e.g. anti-pig) in the recipient. If this immunological problem could be overcome, however, such animals as the pig or sheep would provide a readily accessible, continuous supply of donor organs. Moral and ethical objections would almost certainly be few and easily overcome as such animals are, in any case, slaughtered in large numbers on a daily basis to provide food for human consumption.

One further aspect of xenogeneic organ transplantation that must be considered is whether an organ from one species of animal will metabolize and function satisfactorily in the perhaps different metabolic environment of a host animal of another species. In 1970, Calne pointed out that 'because no discordant organ grafts have functioned for long periods, we cannot answer this question'[1]. The question remains unanswered. 'Minor differences in, for example, pH or serum hormone levels .... could have profound and unfavorable effects on the function of the graft'[1].

Auchincloss, in a comprehensive and valuable recent review of xenotransplantation[19], draws attention, however, to clinical experiments in which blood from patients in hepatic failure was perfused through a pig liver and demonstrated that the pig liver has the capacity to perform at least some of the functions necessary to support human life[20–24]. Organs from animals closely related to man would seem more likely to function satisfactorily when used as xenografts. Chimpanzee and baboon kidneys, for example, can clearly function adequately in the human metabolic environment[4-11], and chimpanzee and baboon hearts have functioned satisfactorily in man until rejected[25,26] (Chapter 64). Chimpanzee livers have also shown moderate function after transplantation into man[27,28]. In Auchincloss' view, however, it is unlikely that all the enzymes and hormones that show species variation will function with equal efficiency in xenogeneic recipients[19]. 'One of the exciting side products of successful xenogeneic transplantation would be the new insights inevitably gained into the normal processes of physiology'[19].

XENOGRAFTING BETWEEN CLOSELY RELATED ANIMAL SPECIES

From an extensive review of the experimental literature, it would seem that, with regard to transplantation of organs between some closely related species, there is a very real possibility that, with the currently available immunosuppressive drugs, acute rejection can be delayed significantly. There is increasing evidence that immunosuppression with cyclosporine prolongs graft survival when xenografting is performed between two closely related animal species, such as the wolf and dog[29], fox and dog[30], hare and rabbit[31], sheep and goat[32], cynomolgus monkey and baboon[33-35] (Table 61.2). Rejection in these models appears to be primarily cellular; humoral factors, which might lead to vascular rejection, generally play a less important role, though this is not always so, as found in the closely related vervet monkey to baboon model[2,3,36,37].

Rejection between such animal species is, in general, more vigorous than when allografting is performed, and is therefore more likely to result in early graft failure from accelerated acute rejection; humoral factors would also appear to play a role in some cases. In addition, possibly rather higher doses of immunosuppressive drugs might have to be administered than would be necessary after allografting, making the recipient more susceptible to the complications of such therapy, in particular, infection.

As grafts between closely related primate species are rejected acutely in some models[33-35] but hyperacutely in others[2,3], it is difficult to predict accurately the outcome of a transplant in man using any one primate subgroup as donor. For example, cynomolgus monkey hearts inserted heterotopically into baboons are rejected by a cellular (acute) rejection response, which can be successfully overcome by combination immunosuppressive therapy using cyclosporine, azathioprine, corticosteroids, and anti-thymocyte globulin[33,34,38]. Hearts from African green (vervet) monkeys, on the other hand, transplanted into baboons, are frequently rejected hyperacutely, and survival is not greatly prolonged by combination immunosuppressive therapy[2,3], though if anti-thymocyte globulin is added to the regimen, and acute rejection episodes vigorously treated with bolus steroid therapy, some prolongation can be achieved[37]. Pretransplant total lymphoid irradiation, in collaboration with pharmacological immunosuppression, does result in longer survival of some hearts, but, in this experimental model, has been associated with a high mortality[36].

Whether pharmacological immunosuppression including cyclosporine will delay or prevent rejection of transplanted

Table 61.2 Selected results of cardiac xenografting between closely related species

Reference	Donor	Recipient	n	Immunosuppression	Periods of survival (days)
Sugimoto et al.[48]	mouse	rat	6	none	3 (mean 3)
			6	CsA	3 (mean 3)
Sugimoto et al.[48]	rat	mouse	8	none	5 (mean 5)
			7	CsA	12–21 (mean 14)
Corry and Kelley[49]	rat	mouse	11	none	5
			11	ATS	24–> 365 (mean 58)
Homan et al.[50]	hamster	rat	7	none	2–4 (median 2)
			11	CsA	5–23 (median 6)
Knechtle et al.[39]	hamster	rat	6	none	3–4 (median 4)
			8	CsA	5–6 (median 5)
			7	TLI	5–6 (median 6)
			10	TLI, CsA	5–> 100 (median > 100)
Ertel et al.[30]	fox	dog	8	CsA, CS	9–33 (mean 19)
Bailey et al.[51]	goat	lamb	5	CsA	13–72 (mean 32)
Bailey et al.[32]	lamb	newborn goat	10	CsA, AZA, CS	24–165 (mean 72)
Reemtsma et al.[38]	cynomolgus monkey	baboon	9	none	5–8 (mean 7)
			7	AZA, CsA, CS	12–154 (mean 61)
			5	AZA, CsA, CS, ATG	53–> 103 (mean 81)
Cooper et al.[2]	vervet monkey	baboon	9	none	1–18 (mean 10)
			6	CsA, AZA, CS	6–29 (mean 13)
Reichenspurner et al.[37]	vervet monkey	baboon	6	CsA, AZA, CS, ATG	25–76 (mean 43)
Cooper et al.[36]	vervet monkey	baboon	10	TLI, CsA, AZA, CS	1–> 35 (mean 17)

Abbreviations: CsA = cyclosporine; TLI = total lymphoid irradiation; CS = corticosteroids; AZA = azathioprine,; ATG = antithymocyte globulin

primate hearts in man remains uncertain, but, from early (pre-cyclosporine) clinical studies using chimpanzee kidneys in man[4-8], it would seem reasonable to expect that chimpanzee hearts will function for at least some weeks or even months or years under these circumstances. The outlook for baboon hearts, again based on early renal transplantation in man[9,11], would seem less optimistic, though function for 3 weeks has already been shown to be possible[26] (Chapter 64).

If clinical concordant xenografting is to be performed, the success of the procedure will almost certainly be increased if donor and recipient are of compatible ABO blood group. This conclusion is supported to some extent by experimental work using the vervet monkey as donor and the Chacma baboon as recipient[2,3], and by a single clinical experience[26] (Chapter 64). In the experimental studies, early hyperacute rejection (within the first 60 minutes) was not seen in those cases where ABO compatibility was present between donor and recipient, but was seen in a significant percentage of cases (three of eight) where incompatibility was present. Mean donor heart survival was also shorter in baboons receiving ABO-incompatible vervet monkey hearts. These observations were noted in both non-immunosuppressed recipients, and in recipients immunosuppressed with a combination of pharmacological agents, including cyclosporine.

The role of truly concordant xenografts in providing temporary support for patients with grossly inadequate function of important organs, such as the heart or liver, though at present uncertain, may well warrant clinical investigation within the near future. Permanent long-term function of such grafts would appear to be less likely, as almost certainly recurrent acute rejection episodes and early chronic rejection (graft arteriosclerosis) would take place, leading to relatively early graft failure.

The encouraging experimental results obtained by several groups, however, lead to some optimism in this respect (Table 61.2). Total lymphoid irradiation, although associated with morbidity and mortality in the vervet monkey to baboon model[36], was extremely successful in association with cyclosporine therapy in the hamster to rat model[39,40]. The development of new pharmacological agents, such as FK 506 (formely FR900506)[41], and 15-deoxyspergualin[37], particularly if used in low-dose combination with cyclosporine so that the toxic effects of each drug are minimized, may lead to further possibilities in this field, particularly if hyperacute rejection can be successfully prevented. 15-deoxyspergualin has been demonstrated to have an effect in preventing vascular rejection[37].

Other new approaches to immunosuppresion have also shown encouraging results. The monoclonal antibody anti-Tac, which is specific to the interleukin-2 receptor of activated T-cells, has been used in a chelated form to carry yttrium-90 to host T-cells in a xenograft model[42]. This form of yttrium-90 therapy resulted in significant prolongation of survival of heterotopic cynomolgus monkey hearts transplanted into rhesus monkeys; graft survival was extended from a mean of 6.7 days (in control experiments) to 38.4 days. Neither anti-Tac therapy alone nor when the monoclonal was used as a carrier of pseudomonas toxin was successful in prolonging cardiac graft survival longer than in control non-immunosuppressed animals.

XENOGRAFTING BETWEEN DISTANTLY RELATED SPECIES

The problem of immediate hyperacute rejection when organ transplantation is performed between discordant animals has not yet been overcome, although immunoadsorption of antibodies[18] and plasmapheresis[43] can delay this response significantly (Table 61.3). Further antibodies against the donor species, however, rapidly develop, and to date no experimental study has shown survival of transplants between such animal species in excess of a few days[18,43]. Clinical investigation using a discordant donor, therefore, is not warranted at the present time. The currently available immunosuppressive agents are not effective either in preventing development of these antibodies or in prolonging survival. Total lymphoid irradiation has not been studied fully in the discordant model, although it may hold some hope for future advances.

The effects of major blood group incompatibility between donor and recipient in discordant xenotransplantation are uncertain, but present evidence from the pig to baboon model would indicate that it has no influence on outcome[17].

XENOGRAFTS AS A BRIDGE TO ALLOTRANSPLANTATION

The use of a heterotopic or orthotopic non-human primate heart as a 'bridge' to allotransplantation would seem feasible, for, as already mentioned, it seems likely that chimpanzee hearts, in particular, will function satisfactorily for possibly weeks or months. This would allow time for a suitable human heart to be located and inserted (with removal of both the chimpanzee organ and the recipient's native heart, if it is still *in situ*).

Indeed, this was one possibility in two patients in whom auxiliary cardiac xenografts (one baboon and one chimpanzee) were implanted by Barnard and his colleagues in 1977[25] (Chapter 64).

The use of a xenograft as a bridge to allotransplantation would, therefore, seem to be indicated particularly in infants and children with complex congenital heart disease, as left ventricular assist devices and artificial hearts have not yet been developed of a size whereby they can be implanted easily in these small patients. It will probably be in this

Table 61.3 Selected results of cardiac xenografting between distantly related species

Reference	Donor	Recipient	n	Immunosuppression		Periods of survival (minutes)
Jamieson[52]	guinea pig	rat	16	none		8–14
Adachi et al.[53]	guinea pig	rat	6	none	Mean	12.2 ± 2.5
			6	cyclosporine		13.9 ± 2.9
			4	aspirin		11.5 ± 3.1
			6	cobra venom factor		40.6 ± 7.2
			6	cyclosporine and cobra venom factor		68.1 ± 11.6
			4	cobra venom factor (every 24 hours)		70.2 ± 10.6
						(hours)
Cooper et al.[18]	pig	baboon	4	none		0.75–8.0
			3	splenectomy		0.5–8.0
			5	cyclosporine and steroids		0.25–120
			7	immunoadsorption		6–120
			4	immunoadsorption, cyclosporine and steroids		8–96

field, therefore, that xenografts will be explored initially, and, in fact, the first such step has already been taken[26]. The small volume of the thoracic cavity may prohibit the insertion of an auxiliary (heterotopic) heart, and orthotopic transplantation may prove necessary. The complex abnormal anatomy of the recipient's own heart may be another factor making heterotopic transplantation difficult or impossible, again necessitating orthotopic siting of the xenograft. Re-transplantation would be performed when a suitable human donor organ became available.

An animal heart inserted as a bridge to transplantation would have some advantages over a mechanical support device, the most important and obvious being the fact that the animal heart can be totally enclosed within the thoracic cavity, thus reducing the risk of infection. There is similarly a reduced risk of thromboembolism when mechanical parts are not implanted (Section IV). If the xenograft is sited heterotopically, it would seem wise to anticoagulate patients just as it is in patients with heterotopic allografts (Chapter 23), as there remains a possibility that thrombus formation will occur in the patient's poorly contracting native right or left ventricle, and that embolism to the pulmonary or systemic circulations may take place.

Three aspects of this procedure, however, remain for discussion. The first has already been alluded to, and concerns the ethics of using an animal such as a chimpanzee for this purpose[15,16]. The use of the higher primates, with their close relationship to man, stimulates a considerable emotional response in the public, a significant percentage of whom may object to their use for this purpose. Such objections would probably be particularly vociferous if chimpanzee hearts were used in adults (as opposed to infants and children), as adequate mechanical devices for the support of adult patients with failing ventricles are readily available, and, indeed, in many cases insertion has been followed by successful allotransplantation (Section IV).

A second feature of the use of a xenograft heart as a 'bridge' has not yet been fully explored. This relates to whether the recipient will develop lymphocytotoxic antibodies to the xenograft that will also cross-react with human tissue, thus increasing the difficulty of finding a suitable human heart for subsequent definitive allotransplantation. This point has not been clarified in the experimental work which has been carried out to date, and would seem worthy of exploration. If lymphocytotoxic antibodies to chimpanzee cells, for example, develop in the recipient, and these cross-react with human donor cells, then clearly the advantages of the xenograft may be greatly diminished.

The third aspect of the implantation of a primate heart in man (whether temporary or permanent) that requires very careful consideration is the risk of transferring pathogenic agents that may result in serious infection or the development of neoplasia. Primates captured in the wild, and to a lesser extent colony-bred animals, are known to harbor a host of pathogenic agents[44], of which viruses probably represent the greatest risk to man[45,46]. This concern regarding the transfer of pathogens is reinforced by the consideration that the transfer of even a naturally mildly pathogenic agent may result in serious disease in an immunosuppressed patient. The Simian retroviruses, which include viruses related to the human immunodeficiency virus Type-1, which can cause the acquired immune deficiency syndrome (AIDS) in man (Figure 61.2), and the herpesviruses, in particular, must be considered dangerous if transferred to man.

Results of recent studies suggest that primates bred under suitable conditions of management would exhibit a lower tendency towards viral infection than do wild-caught animals[46]. The use of non-human primates as organ donors may be possible, therefore, provided that they are at least free of those infectious agents that are known to pose a serious

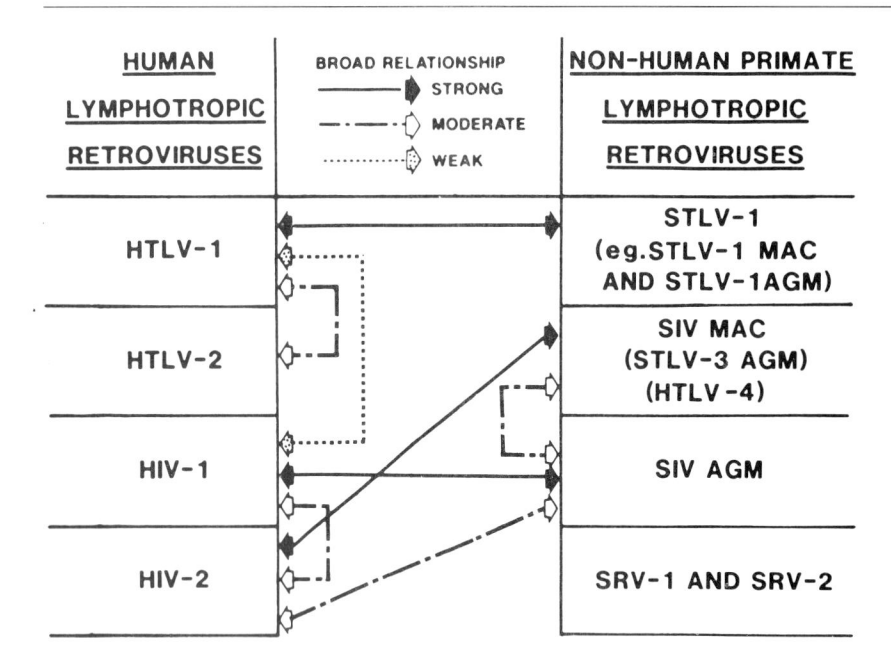

Figure 61.2 Broad immunological relationships of some lymphotropic retroviruses of humans and non-human primates. (Abbreviations: HTLV = human T-lymphotropic virus (types 1 and 2); HIV = human immunodeficiency virus (types 1 and 2); STLV = simian T-lymphotropic virus (types 1 and 2); MAC = of macaques; AGM = of African green (vervet) monkeys; SIV = simian immunodeficiency virus; SRV = simian (AIDS) retroviruses (types 1 and 2). Note: STLV-3agm (simian T-lymphotropic virus type 3) and HTLV-4 (human T-lymphotropic virus type 4) are now thought likely to be contaminants of SIVmac). (Courtesy of Dr F. Van der Riet, Cape Town)

threat to human health, eg. *Mycobacterium tuberculosis*, herpesviruses, exogenous retroviruses, and Marburg virus. In this regard, the feasibility of breeding and maintaining specified pathogen-free animals seems worthy of investigation.

COMMENT

The problem of overcoming xenograft rejection is proving more difficult than predicted by no less an authority than Sir Peter Medawar[47] who, in 1969, made the following remarks: 'A new solution is therefore called for: the use of heterografts – that is to say, of grafts transplanted from lower animals into man. Of the use of heterografts I can say only this: that in the laboratory we are achieving greater success with grafts *between* species today than we achieved with grafts *within* species 15 years ago. We shall solve the problem by using heterografts one day if we try hard enough, and maybe in less than 15 years'[47]. His optimistic prediction has unfortunately not been fulfilled.

We would, however, appear to be at the threshold of an exciting era in cardiac transplantation where the use of xenografts is explored, initially as bridging devices, particularly in infants and young children. In adults and larger children, it would seem wise to utilize the heterotopic position for xenografts when inserted as temporary assist devices. Experience gained in this area may lead to developments which allow xenografts to be used on a more permanent replacement basis.

References

1. Calne, R.Y. (1970). Organ transplantation between widely disparate species. *Transplant Proc.*, **2**, 550
2. Cooper, D.K.C., Human, P.A. and Rose, A.G. (1987). Is ABO compatibility essential in xenografting between closely related species? *Transplant Proc.*, **19**, 4437
3. Cooper, D.K.C., Human, P.A., Rose, A.G., Rees, J., Keraan, M., Reichart, B., Du Toit, E. and Oriol, R. (1989). The role of ABO blood group compatibility in heart transplantation between closely related animal species. An experimental study using the vervet monkey to baboon cardiac xenograft model. *J. Thorac. Cardiovasc. Surg.*, **97**, 447
4. Reemtsma, K., McCracken, B.H., Schlegel, J.V. and Pearl, M. (1964). Heterotransplantation of the kidney: two clinical experiences. *Science*, **143**, 700
5. Reemtsma, K., McCracken, B.H., Schlegel, J.V., Pearl, M.A., Pearce, C.W., Dewitt, C.W., Smith, P.E., Hewitt, R.L., Flinner, R.L. and Creech, O. Jr. (1964). Renal heterotransplantation in man. *Ann. Surg.*, **160**, 384
6. Reemtsma, K., McCracken, B.H., Schlegel, J.V., Pearl, M.A., Dewitt, C.W. and Creech, O. Jr. (1964). Reversal of early graft rejection after renal heterotransplantation in man. *J. Am. Med. Assoc.*, **187**, 691
7. Reemtsma, K. (1969). Heterotransplantation. *Transplant. Proc.*, **1**, 251
8. Reemtsma, K. (1969). Renal heterotransplantation from non-human primates to man. *Ann. N.Y. Acad. Sci.*, **162**, 412
9. Starzl, T.E., Marchioro, T.L., Peters, G.N., Kirkpatrick, C.H., Wilson, W.C., Porter, K.A., Rifkind, D., Ogden, D.A., Hitchcock, C.R. and Waddell, W.R. (1964). Renal heterotransplantation from baboon to man: experience with six cases. *Transplantation*, **2**, 752
10. Porter, K.A., Marchioro, T.L. and Starzl, T.E. (1965). Pathological changes in six treated baboon to man renal heterotransplantations. *Br. J. Urol.*, **37**, 274
11. Hitchcock, C.R., Kiser, J.C., Telander, R.L. and Seljeskob, E.L. (1964). Baboon renal grafts. *J. Am. Med. Assoc.*, **189**, 934
12. Sarich, V.M. (1968). The origin of the hominids: an immunological approach. In Washburn, S.L. and Jay, P.C. (eds.) *Perspectives on Human Evolution*. p. 94. (New York: Holt, Rhinehart and Winston)
13. Sade, R.M., Crawford, F.A. and Fyfe, D.A. (1986). Symposium on hypoplastic left heart syndrome. *J. Thorac. Cardiovasc. Surg.*, **91**, 937
14. Hardy, J.D., Chavez, C.M., Kurrus, F.D., Neely, W.A., Eraslan, S., Turner, M.D., Fabian, L.W. and Labecki, T.D. (1964). Heart transplantation in man: developmental studies and report of a case. *J. Am. Med. Assoc.*, **188**, 1132
15. Kaplan, A.L. (1985). Ethical issues raised by research involving xenografts. *J. Am. Med. Assoc.*, **254**, 3339

16. Veatch, R.M. (1986). The ethics of xenografts. *Transplant Proc.*, **18**, 93
17. Lexer, G., Cooper, D.K.C., Rose, A.G., Wicomb, W.N., Rees, J., Keraan, M. and Du Toit, E. (1986). Hyperacute rejection in a discordant (pig to baboon) cardiac xenograft model. *J. Heart Transplant.*, **5**, 411
18. Cooper, D.K.C., Human, P.A., Lexer, G., Rose, A.G., Rees, J., Keraan, M. and Du Toit, E. (1988). The effects of cyclosporine and antibody adsorption on pig cardiac xenograft survival in the baboon. *J. Heart Transplant.*, **7**, 238
19. Auchincloss, H. (1988). Xenogeneic transplantation. *Transplantation*, **46**, 1
20. Eiseman, B., Liem, D.S. and Raffucci, F. (1965). Heterologous liver perfusion in treatment of hepatic failure. *Ann. Surg.*, **162**, 329
21. Norman, J.C., Saravis, C.A., Brown, M.E. and McDermott, W.V. Jr. (1966). Immunochemical observations in clinical heterologous (xenogeneic) liver perfusions. *Surgery*, **60**, 179
22. Saunders, S.J., Terblanche, J., Bosman, S.C.W., Harrison, G.G., Walls, R., Hickman, R., Biebuyck, J., Dent, D., Pearce, S. and Barnard, C.N. (1968). Acute hepatic coma treated by cross-circulation with a baboon and by repeated exchange transfusions. *Lancet*, **2**, 585
23. Bosman, S.C.W., Saunders, S.J., Terblanche, J., Harrison, G.G. and Barnard, C.N. (1968). Cross-circulation between man and baboon. *Lancet*, **2** 583
24. Abouna, G.M., Ashcroft, T., Muckle, T.J., Skillen, A.W., Hull, C.J., Kirkley, J.R. and Hodson, A.W. (1970). Heterologous extracorporeal hepatic support: hemodynamic, biochemical and immunological observation. *Br. J. Surg.*, **57**, 213
25. Barnard, C.N., Wolpowitz, A. and Losman, J.G. (1977). Heterotopic cardiac transplantation with a xenograft for assistance of the left heart in cardiogenic shock after cardiopulmonary bypass. *S. Afr. Med. J.*, **52**, 1035
26. Bailey, L.L., Nehlsen-Cannarella, S.L., Concepcion, W. and Jolley, W.B. (1985). Baboon-to-human cardiac xenotransplantation in a neonate. *J. Am. Med. Assoc.*, **254**, 3321
27. Starzl, T.E. (1969). In *Experience in Hepatic Transplantation.* p. 408, (Philadelphia: W.B. Saunders)
28. Starzl, T.E. (1986). Referenced by Deodhar, S.D. Review of xenografts in organ transplantation. *Transplant. Proc.*, **18**, 83
29. Krombach, F., Hammer, C., Gebhard, F., Danko, I., Scholz, S. and Gokel, M. (1985). The effects of cyclosporin on wolf to dog kidney xenografts. *Transplant. Proc.*, **17**, 1436
30. Ertel, W., Reichenspurner, H., Hammer, C., Welz, A., Uberfuhr, P., Hemmer, W., Reichart, B., Gokel, M. and Brendel, W. (1984). Heart transplantation in closely related species: a model of humoral rejection. *Transplant. Proc.*, **16**, 1259
31. Kemp, E., Starklint, H., Larsen, S. and Kieperink, H. (1985). Cyclosporine in concordant renal hare-to-rabbit xenotransplantation: prolongation and modification of rejection, and adverse effects. *Transplant. Proc.*, **17**, 1351
32. Bailey, L.L., Jang, J., Johnson, W. and Jolley, W.B. (1985). Orthotopic cardiac xenografting in the newborn goat. *J. Thorac. Cardiovasc. Surg.*, **89**, 242
33. Sadeghi, A.M., Robbins, R.C., Smith, C.R., Kurlansky, P.A., Michler, R.E., Reemtsma, K. and Rose, E.A. (1987). Cardiac xenograft survival in baboons treated with cyclosporine in combination with conventional immunosuppression. *Transplant. Proc.*, **19**, 1149
34. Kurlansky, P.A., Sadeghi, A.M., Michler, R.E., Smith, C.R., Marboe, C.C., Thomas, W.A., Coppey, L. and Rose, E.A. (1987). Comparable survival of intra-species and cross-species primate cardiac transplants. *Transplant. Proc.*, **19**, 1067
35. Sadeghi, A.M., Robbins, R.C., Smith, C.R., Kurlansky, P.A., Michler, R.E., Reemtsma, K. and Rose, E.A. (1987). Cardiac xenotransplantation in primates. *J. Thorac. Cardiovasc. Surg.*, **93**, 809
36. Cooper, D.K.C., Human, P.A. and Reichart, B. (1987). Prolongation of cardiac xenograft (vervet monkey to baboon) function by a combination of total lymphoid irradiation and immunosuppressive drug therapy. *Transplant Proc.*, **19**, 4441
37. Reichenspurner, H., Human, P.A., Boehm, D.H., Rose, A.G., May, R., Cooper, D.K.C., Zilla, P. and Reichart, B. (1989). Optimalization of immunosuppression after xenogeneic heart transplantation in primates. *J. Heart Transplant.*, **8**, 200
38. Reemtsma, K., Pierson, R.N., Marboe, C.C., Michler, R.E., Smith, C.R., Rose, E.A. and Fenoglio, J.J. (1987). Will atherosclerosis limit clinical xenografting? *Transplant. Proc.*, **19**, 108
39. Knechtle, S.J., Halperin, E.C. and Bollinger, R.R. (1985). Cardiac xenograft survival using total lymphoid irradition and cyclosporine. *J. Heart Transplant.*, **4**, 605
40. Knechtle, S.J., Halperin, E.C. and Bollinger, R.R. (1987). Xenograft survival in two species combinations using total-lymphoid irradiation and cyclosporine. *Transplantation*, **43**, 173
41. Ochiai, T., Nakajima, K., Nagata, M., Suzuki, T., Asano, T., Uematsu, T., Goto, T., Hori, S., Kenmochi, T., Nakagoori, T. and Isono, K. (1987). Effect of a new immunosuppressive agent, FK506, on heterotopic cardiac allotransplantation in the rat. *Transplant. Proc.*, **19**, 1284
42. Cooper, M.M., Robbins, R.C., Waldmann, T.A., Gansow, O.A. and Clark, R.E. (1988). Use of anti-Tac antibody in primate cardiac xenograft transplantation. *Surg. Forum*, **39**, 353
43. Merkel, F.K., Bier, M., Beavers, C.D., Merriman, W.G., Wilson, C. and Starzl, T.E. (1971). Modification of xenograft response by selective plasmapheresis. *Transplant. Proc.*, **3** 534
44. Benirschke, K. (1986). *Primates – The Road to Self-Sustaining Populations.* (New York: Springer-Verlag)
45. Kalter, S.S. (1986). Overview of Simian viruses and recognized virus diseases and laboratory support for the diagnosis of viral infections. In Benirschke, K. (ed.) *Primates – The Road to Self-Sustaining Populations.* (New York: Springer-Verlag)
46. Van der Riet, F. De St. J., Human, P.A., Cooper, D.K.C., Reichart, B., Fincham, J.E., Kalter, S.S., Kanki, P.J., Essex, M., Madden, D.L., Laitung, M.T., Chalton, D. and Sever, J.L. Virological implications of the use of primates in xenotransplantation. *Transplant. Proc.*, **19**, 4068
47. Medawar, P. (1969). Quoted by Reemtsma, K. Heterotransplantation. *Transplant. Proc.*, **1**, 251
48. Sugimoto, K., Shelby, J. and Corry, R.J. (1985). The effect of cyclosporine on cardiac xenograft survival. *Transplantation*, **39**, 218
49. Corry, R.J. and Kelley, S.E. (1975). Survival of cardiac xenografts. *Arch. Surg.*, **110**, 1143
50. Homan, W.P., Williams, K.A., Fabre, J.W., Millard, P.R. and Morris, P.J. (1981). Prolongation of cardiac xenograft survival in rats receiving cyclosporin A. *Transplantation*, **31**, 164
51. Bailey, L., Li, Z., Lacour-Gayet, F., Perier, P., Killeen, D., Perry, J., Schmidt, C., Roost, H. and Jolley, W. (1983). Orthotopic cardiac transplantation in the cyclosporine-treated neonate. *Transplant. Proc.*, **15**, 2956
52. Jamieson, S.W. (1974). Xenograft hyperacute rejection. *Transplantation*, **17**, 533
53. Adachi, H., Rosengard, B.R., Hutchins, G.M., Hall, T.S., Borkon, A.M., Baumgartner, W.A. and Reitz, B.A. (1986). Effects of cyclosporine, aspirin, and cobra venom factor on discordant cardiac xenograft survival in rats. *Transplant. Proc.*, **19**, 1145

62
Pathology of Xenograft Rejection

A.G. ROSE

INTRODUCTION

Rejection of cardiac xenografts between closely-related species may be exclusively acute (cellular) (e.g. cynomolgus monkey to baboon) or may be due to a mixture of hyperacute (humoral, vascular) and acute (e.g. vervet monkey to baboon). Rejection of xenografts between distantly-related species (e.g. pig to baboon) is always by a hyperacute mechanism in the untreated model. Though the acute response can be delayed, or even prevented, by currently available immunosuppressive agents and techniques, hyperacute rejection has, until now, proved extremely difficult to prevent or delay. Cardiac xenografts have very occasionally been used in humans in a desperate attempt to save the life of a patient for whom no human donor heart was available[1-3] (Chapter 64). Xenogeneic (and allogeneic in sensitized hosts) cardiac transplants have been performed in a wide range of experimental animals, and have helped to further our understanding of the mechanism of hyperacute rejection[4-36] (Chapter 63).

PATHOPHYSIOLOGY

The hyperacute rejection response, which classically manifests itself within minutes or hours following transplantation, is characterized by the immediate or early failure of graft function, and is accompanied by the development of typical morphological changes (Figures 62.1–62.4). These include microvascular thrombi, endothelial cell necrosis, and widespread interstitial hemorrhages throughout the graft, accompanied by a polymorphonuclear cellular infiltration. This is in sharp contrast to acute rejection, which is relatively rarely encountered within the first 5 days after transplantation.

The reason for this difference in the rapidity of onset is believed to lie in the different mechanisms involved in these two types of rejection. Thus, acute rejection is based on the development of cellular immunity, which takes several days to develop following exposure of the recipient's immune system to the foreign antigens contained in the graft. Hyperacute rejection may be brought about by pre-existing circulating antibodies, which rapidly cross-react with the foreign antigens of the xenograft. As it is the vascular

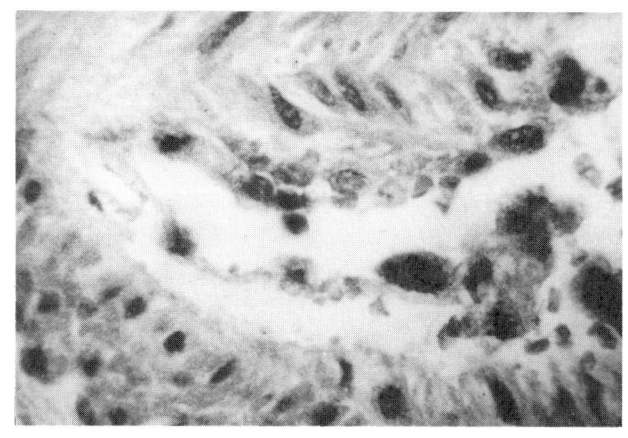

Figure 62.1 Desquamation of partially necrotic endothelial cells within a chimpanzee heart which was hyperacutely rejected on the fourth post-transplant day after being transplanted into a human patient. Mitoses within one or two endothelial cells represent attempts at regeneration (H & E, × 450)

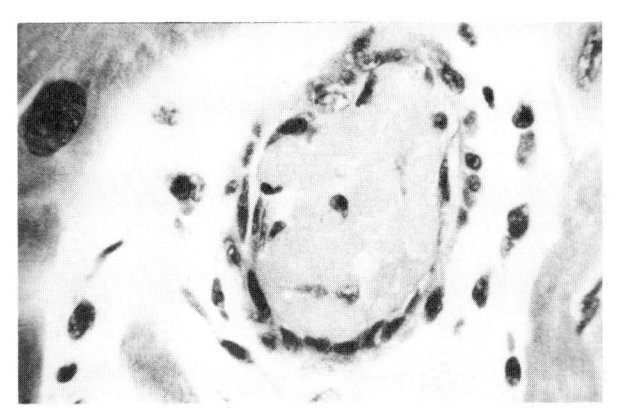

Figure 62.2 Capillary occluded by platelet-fibrin thrombus in the same hyperacutely rejected cardiac xenograft shown in Figure 62.1 (H & E, × 450)

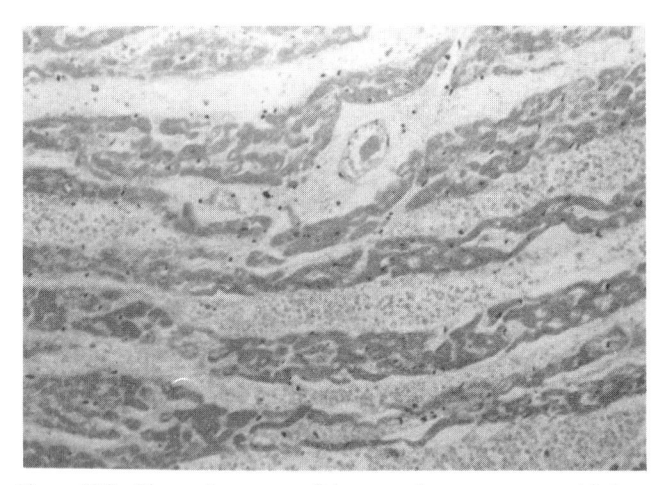

Figure 62.3 Pig cardiac xenograft in a non-immunosuppressed baboon recipient. The donor heart ceased functioning within 60 minutes, and histologically shows massive interstitial edema and hemorrhage, capillary disruption, microvascular thrombi, myocyte necrosis, and scanty cellular infiltration (H & E, × 75)

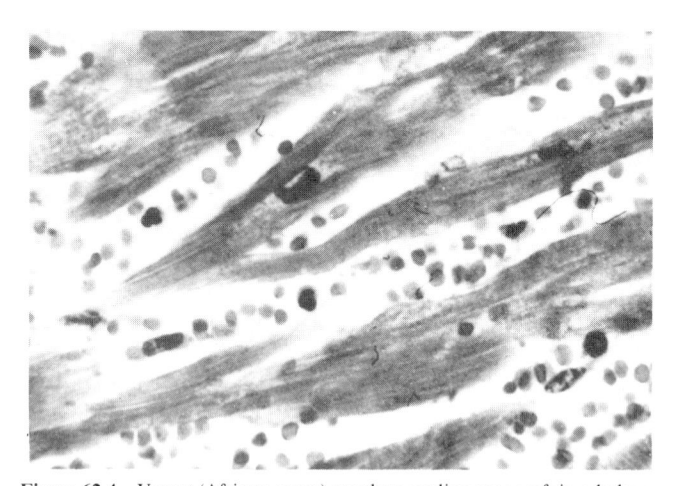

Figure 62.4 Vervet (African green) monkey cardiac xenograft in a baboon recipient shows diffuse capillary destruction with resultant massive erythrocyte extravasation and prominent interstitial edema characteristic of hyperacute rejection (H & E, × 120)

endothelium of the xenograft that comes into initial contact with the host, interacting with the host's circulating blood, it is not surprising that it is the donor organ's microcirculation that appears to undergo maximum damage during the hyperacute rejection reaction. Formation of immune complexes may lead to endothelial cell necrosis.

The ill effects of the immune damage are most apparent in the capillaries, since they are composed of only a single layer of endothelial cells resting upon a basement membrane. The formation of platelet thrombi may precede the phase of recognizable endothelial cellular damage, but the thrombosis is also believed to be triggered by the formation of immune complexes within the microcirculation of the xenograft. Widespread necrosis of capillary endothelial cells, which form the only intrinsic cellular component of the capillary, will lead to dissolution of many capillaries throughout the xenograft.

The resulting vascular obstruction and destruction rapidly lead to serious malfunction of the graft and, if the graft is not shortly removed, ischemic changes will become recognizable in the myocytes. In some instances the xenograft may become totally necrotic. The appearance of myocyte necrosis, associated with massive interstitial hemorrhage, is reminiscent of reperfusion-type myocardial infarction in patients with ischemic heart disease, or in experimental infarcts in which the heart is reperfused following a period of ischemia. The presence of these changes in a rejecting xenograft, which functioned well initially and in which preservation appeared to be adequate, should help distinguish these two pathologic processes. Identification of microvascular thrombi may also aid in identifying hyperacute rejection.

The presence of neutrophils within the xenograft has been widely emphasized as a characteristic feature of hyperacute rejection, and analogies have been drawn to the Arthus reaction, in which neutrophils are essential mediators of tissue damage. Different strains of rat have been used as a highly-reproducible and rigidly-controlled model of hyperacute cardiac allograft rejection. Forbes et al.[14], however, have presented experimental evidence to show that the absence of neutrophils from the graft produced no alteration in the characteristic pattern of vascular and myocardial damage in hyperacutely rejecting rat allografts. They concluded that neutrophils are neither essential nor specific participants in hyperacute allograft rejection in the rat model.

The initial morphological event that characterizes hyperacute rejection in rat cardiac allografts is extensive platelet aggregation throughout the vasculature of the graft, in the presence of a largely-intact endothelium (Figure 62.2). This is followed by widespread endothelial damage. Forbes and his colleagues do not exclude a possible role for neutrophils in the production of myocardial injury in the later stages of hyperacute rejection[16].

O'Regan et al.[24] in a study of C6-deficient rabbits showed that sufficiency of the sixth component of complement is required for hyperacute xenograft rejection in this model. In a study using cobra venom factor as a means of depressing recipient hemolytic C3 activity, Forbes et al.[20] further demonstrated that complement activation by graft-bound alloantibody is a critical effector mechanism of hyperacute rejection in an inbred rat model. Hyperacute rejection also proceeded in the usual fashion in cardiac allografts in a rat strain with a hereditary platelet function defect[16]. A recent report suggests that the presence of antibodies against vascular endothelial cells may be related to hyperacute rejection in human cardiac allografts[32].

HISTOPATHOLOGICAL FEATURES OF REJECTION IN CONCORDANT AND DISCORDANT XENOGRAFT MODELS

In a personal series reviewing the histopathological changes seen in 75 experimental cardiac xenografts (52 between closely related ('concordant') and 23 between distantly related ('discordant') species) in which the roles of ABO-incompatibility and concordance, and the effects of immunosuppression were evaluated[36], the following histological patterns of rejection were observed (Table 62.1). Hyperacute rejection was seen in all 23 discordant xenografts (Figure 62.3) and in 13 concordant xenografts (Figure 62.4). Acute (cellular) rejection was seen in 20 concordant xenografts, and a mixture of acute and hyperacute rejection in ten concordant xenografts (Figure 62.5). Nine concordant xenografts showed no rejection at the time of death of the recipient baboon; death was believed to result from side-effects of heavy immunosuppressive drug therapy in the majority of cases. It would appear that, if hyperacute rejection can be averted in the early period following xenotransplantation, subsequent rejection will either take the form of classical acute rejection or a less familiar mixture of acute and hyperacute rejection.

The latter mixed form of rejection appears superficially similar to severe acute rejection with interstitial hemorrhages, but the mixed rejection reaction is characterized by a lymphocytic response which does not approach the severity of that seen in severe acute rejection. The microvascular destruction is thus the dominant factor and is disproportionate to the lymphocytic infiltration. Sharma

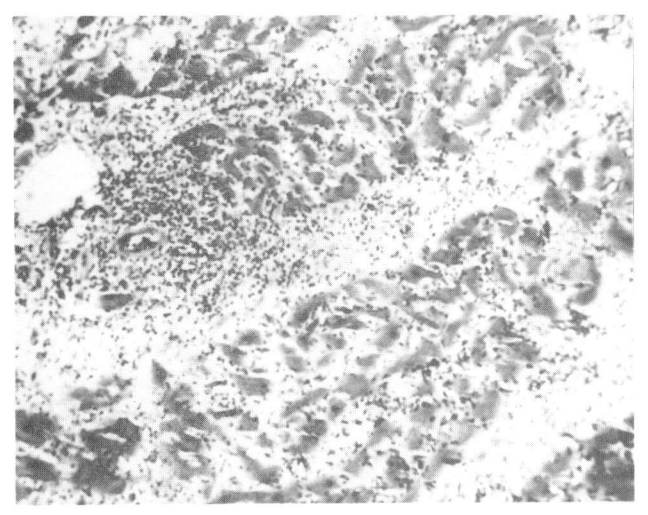

Figure 62.5 Vervet (African green) monkey cardiac xenograft in a baboon recipient demonstrating a mixture of acute rejection (indicated by moderate lymphocytic infiltration, top left) and hyperacute rejection (indicated by massive interstitial edema and erythrocytic extravasation, elsewhere) (H & E, × 56)

et al.[6] experimentally prevented hyperacute rejection in cardiac transplants performed in presensitized dogs, which were later rejected by what they regarded as primary cellular rejection. These authors made a clear separation between hyperacute and acute rejection and did not describe a mixed form. The experiments performed in our institution (University of Cape Town Medical School) show that this distinction between acute and hyperacute rejection is not always so clear-cut, and mixed forms may occur. The late onset of the hyperacute component of mixed rejection also differs from the classical concept of early-phase hyperacute rejection.

The clinical significance of the above observations is that

Table 62.1 Histopathology of rejection in heterotopic cardiac xenografts in the baboon

Group		n	None	Acute	Mixed	Hyperacute
Concordant (vervet monkey to baboon)						
(1) No IS*		9	0	0	4	5
(2) ABO incompatible, no IS		9	0	4	2	3
(3) CsA, AZA, MP		6	0	5(2)	0	1
(4) ABO incomp., CsA, AZA, MP		5	0	3(1)	1	1
(5) CsA, AZA, MP	i.v. MP	5	1(1)	3	0	1
(6) RATG, CsA, AZA, MP	therapy for	6	3(3)	2	0	1
(7) 15-DS, CsA, AZA, MP	rejection	7	4(4)	2	0	1
(8) 15-DS, CsA, MP	episodes	5	1(1)	1	3	0
Discordant (pig to baboon)						
(9) No IS		4	0	0	0	4
(10) Splenectomy		3	0	0	0	3
(11) CsA, AZA, MP		5	0	0	0	5
(12) Antibody adsorption		7	0	0	0	7
(13) Antibody adsorption, CsA, AZA, MP		4	0	0	0	4(1)

IS = immunosuppression; CsA = cyclosporine; AZA = azathioprine; MP = methylprednisolone; RATG = rabbit anti-human thymocyte globulin; 15-DS = 15-deoxyspergualin
*All concordant xenograft pairs were ABO blood group compatible except where stated
Figures in parentheses denote recipient died

the semi-quantitative scoring systems presently used to measure acute allograft rejection may have to be modified once xenografts are introduced into clinical use. Furthermore, vascular rejection may lead to graft failure at a relatively late stage after transplantation, as demonstrated by graft failure occurring as late as 21 days in the studies outlined above. The term 'hyperacute' is therefore a misnomer, and vascular or humoral rejection would be a more suitable term.

COMMENT

The successful use of animals as sources of organs for transplantation in humans awaits a solution to the problem of hyperacute rejection. If this can be overcome, then the currently available pharmacological agents may well be able to prevent or treat subsequent acute rejection that may develop. It has also been suggested, however, that accelerated atherosclerosis will eventually present a significant problem in cross-species transplantation[30], and, if this proves to be the case, the longevity of such xenografts may clearly be limited.

References

1. Hardy, J.D., Chavez, C.M., Kurrus, F.E., Neely, W.A., Webb, W.R., Eraslan, S., Turner, M.D., Fabian, L.W. and Labecki, J.D. (1964). Heart transplantation in man: development studies and report of a case. *J. Am. Med. Assoc.*, **188**, 1132
2. Barnard, C.N., Wolpowitz, A. and Losman, J.G. (1977). Heterotopic cardiac transplantation with a xenograft for assistance of the left heart in cardiogenic shock after cardiopulmonary bypass. *S. Afr. Med. J.*, **52**, 1035
3. Bailey, L.L., Nehlsen-Cannarella, S.L., Concepcion, W. and Jolley, W.B. (1985). Baboon-to-human cardiac xenotransplantation in a neonate. *J. Am. Med. Assoc.*, **254**, 3321
4. Mullerworth, M.H., Lixfield, W., Rachkewich, R.A., Goldman, B.S., Silver, M.D., Shumak, K.H. and Crookston, J.H. (1972). Hyperacute rejection of heterotopic heart allografts in dogs. *Transplantation*, **13**, 570
5. Dempster, W.J. (1973). Nature of hyperacute rejection. *Br. Med. J.*, **1**, 740
6. Sharma, H.M., Rosensweig, J., Chatterjee, S., Moore, S. and De Champlain, M.L. (1973). Platelets in hyperacute rejection of heterotopic cardiac allografts in presensitized dogs. *Am. J. Pathol.*, **70**, 155
7. Caves, P.K., Dong, E. and Morris, R.E. (1973). Hyperacute rejection of orthotopic cardiac allografts in dogs following solubilized antigen pre-treatment. *Transplantation*, **16**, 252
8. Guttmann, R.D. (1974). Genetics of acute rejection of rat cardiac allografts and a model of hyperacute rejection. *Transplantation*, **17**, 383
9. Jamieson, S.W. (1974). Xenograft hyperacute rejection. *Transplantation*, **17**, 533
10. Kuwahara, O., Kondo, Y., Kuramochi, T., Grogan, J.B., Cockrell, J.V. and Hardy, J.D. (1974). Organ specificity in hyperacute rejection of canine heart and kidney allografts. *Ann. Surg.*, **180**, 72
11. Cattell, V. and Jamieson, S.W. (1975). Hyperacute rejection of guinea-pig to rat cardiac xenografts. I. Morphology. *J. Pathol.*, **115**, 183
12. Corry, R.J. and Kelley, S.E. (1975). Survival of cardiac xenografts. Effect of antithymocyte serum and enhancing heteroantiserum. *Arch. Surg.*, **110**, 1143
13. Jamieson, S.W. (1975). Modification of the hyperacute reaction in the rat by sulphinylpyrazone. *Thromb. Diath. Haemorrh.*, **30**, 349
14. Forbes, R.D.C., Guttmann, R.D., Kuramochi, T., Klassen, J. and Knack, J. (1976). Non-essential role of neutrophils as mediators of hyperacute cardiac allograft rejection in the rat. *Lab. Invest.*, **34**, 229
15. Whittum, J.A. and Lindquist, R.R. (1977). Mechanism of cardiac allograft rejection in the inbred rat: the effect of complement depletion by cobra venom factor on hyperacute cardiac allograft rejection. *Transplantation*, **24**, 226
16. Forbes, R.D., Guttmann, R.D. and Bazin, H. (1977). Hyperacute rejection of cardiac allografts in a rat strain with a hereditary platelet function defect. *Lab. Invest.*, **37**, 158
17. Guttmann, R.D. (1977). *In vitro* correlates of rejection. I. Suppressive effect and specificity in mixed lymphocyte interaction of alloantiserum producing hyperacute rejection. *Transplant. Proc.*, **9**, 755
18. Forbes, R.D., Guttmann, R.D. and Kuramochi, T. (1977). Controlled studies of the pathogenesis of hyperacute cardiac allograft rejection in actively immunized recipients. *Transplant. Proc.*, **9**, 301
19. Guttmann, R.D. (1977). *In vitro* correlates of rejection. II. Rat mixed lymphocyte reactivity in vitro and cardiac allograft acute rejection, hyperacute or accelerated rejection, and prolongation by active immunization. *Transplantation*, **23**, 153
20. Forbes, R.D., Pinto-Blonde, M. and Guttmann, R.D. (1978). The effect of anticomplementary cobra venom factor on hyperacute rat cardiac allograft rejection. *Lab. Invest.*, **39**, 463
21. Forbes, R.D., Guttmann, R.D. and Pinto-Blonde, M. (1979). A passive transfer model of hyperacute rat cardiac allograft rejection. *Lab. Invest.*, **41**, 348
22. Guttmann, R.D. and Bazin, H. (1979). Lack of significance of allograft differences in hyperacute rejection of rat cardiac allografts. *Transplantation*, **28**, 155
23. Coleman, D.A. and Eichwald, E.J. (1978). Hyperacute rejection of allografted murine hearts and the white graft reaction. *Transplantation*, **26**, 355
24. O'Regan, C.C., Robitaille, P., Pinto-Blonde, M. and Chartrand, C. (1979). Delayed rejection of cardiac xenografts in C6-deficient rabbits. *Immunology*, **38**, 245
25. Lexer, G., Cooper, D.K.C., Rose, A.G., Wicomb, W.N., Rees, J., Keraan, M. and Du Toit, E. (1986). Hyperacute rejection in a discordant (pig to baboon) cardiac xenograft model. *J. Heart Transplant.*, **5**, 411
26. Cooper, D.K.C., Lexer, G., Rose, A.G., Rees, J., Keraan, M., Du Toit, E. and Oriol, R. (1987). Cardiac allograft survival in ABO blood group incompatible baboons. *Transplant. Proc.*, **19**, 1036
27. Lexer, G., Cooper, D.K.C., Wicomb, W.N., Rose, A.G., Rees, J., Keraan, M., Reichart, B. and Du Toit, E. (1987). Cardiac transplantation using discordant xenografts in a non-human primate model. *Transplant. Proc.*, **19**, 1153
28. Cooper, D.K.C., Human, P.A. and Reichart, B. (1987). Prolongation of cardiac xenograft (vervet monkey to baboon) function by a combination of total lymphoid irradiation and immunosuppressive drug therapy. *Transplant. Proc.*, **19**, 4441
29. Cooper, D.K.C., Human, P.A. and Rose, A.G. (1987). Is ABO compatibility essential in xenografting between closely related species? *Transplant. Proc.*, **19**, 4437
30. Reemtsma, K., Pierson, R.N., Marboe, C.C., Michler, R.E., Smith, C.R., Rose, E.A. and Fenoglio, J.J. (1987). Will atherosclerosis limit clinical xenografting? *Transplant. Proc.*, **19**, 108
31. Cooper, D.K.C., Human, P.A., Lexer, G., Rose, A.G., Rees, J., Keraan, M. and Du Toit, E. (1988). Effects of cyclosporine and antibody adsorption on pig cardiac xenograft survival in the baboon. *J. Heart Transplant.*, **7**, 238
32. Trento, A., Hardesty, R.L., Griffith, B.P., Zerbe, T., Kormos, R.L. and

Bahnson, H.T. (1988). Role of the antibody to vascular endothelial cells in hyperacute rejection in patients undergoing cardiac transplantation. *J. Thorac. Cardiovasc. Surg.*, **95**, 37

33. Cooper, D.K.C., Lexer, G., Rose, A.G., Keraan, M., Rees, J., Du Toit, E. and Oriol, R. (1988). Cardiac allotransplantation across major blood group barriers in the baboon. *J. Med. Primatol.*, **17**, 333

34. Reichenspurner, H., Human, P.A., Boehm, D.M., Cooper, D.K.C., Rose, A.G., May, R., Zilla, P. and Reichart, B. (1989). Optimalization of immunosuppression after xenogeneic heart transplantation in primates. *J. Heart Transplant.*, **8**, 200

35. Cooper, D.K.C., Human, P.A., Rose, A.G., Rees, J., Keraan, M., Reichart, B., Du Toit, E. and Oriol, R. (1989). The role of ABO blood group compatibility in heart transplantation between closely related animal species. *J. Thorac. Cardiovasc. Surg.*, **97**, 447

36. Rose, A.G., Cooper, D.K.C., Human, P.A., Reichenspurner, H. and Reichart, B. (1990). Histopathology of hyperacute rejection of the heart – experimental and clinical observations in allografts and xenografts. *J. Heart Transplant.*, In press

63
Mechanisms and Possible Management of Hyperacute (Vascular, Humoral) or Xenograft Rejection

L. MAKOWKA, R. SHAPIRO, F.A. CHAPMAN, S. QIAN, A.G. TZAKIS AND T.E. STARZL

INTRODUCTION

Hyperacute rejection (HAR) of primarily vascularized allografted organs is generally thought to be humorally mediated and has been reported to occur in ABO-incompatible patients[1,2] and in those previously sensitized by (1) a prior transplant[3], (2) as a result of multiple blood transfusions[4], or (3) secondary to pregnancy[5]. The pathogenesis of HAR for the kidney and the heart has been extensively investigated and fairly well established. The causal event is an antibody-mediated injury (IgG and IgM) to the vascular endothelium[6], which is propagated by secondary vasoconstriction[7], the recruitment of polymorphonuclear leukocytes[8] and aggregated platelets[9,10], followed by intravascular coagulation[9-11]. The combination of vasoconstriction and the platelet–leukocyte plugs leads to occlusion of the small arterioles and capillaries with resultant ischemic necrosis of the organ.

Humorally-mediated HAR due to preformed/anti-donor antibodies is also the mechanism of rejection in discordant xenografts. The entire process is pathophysiologically very similar, if not identical, to that observed in ABO blood group major incompatibility or in the presence of serum cytotoxic anti-graft antibodies[12,13]. In phylogenetically closer species (concordant), graft rejection appears more cellular in nature[14].

Therefore, HAR represents a specific and defined, but incompletely understood, entity which can be elicited in different transplant situations and in different organs. At present, HAR cannot be managed with any significant consistency, and, although it represents the greatest threat to kidney transplants, it is increasingly becoming an important consideration in cardiac and hepatic transplantation.

The rationale for elucidation of the mechanism(s) involved in HAR is two-fold. Firstly, the highly sensitized transplant patient who has developed wide-ranging antibodies could be helped. Secondly, and of major importance for the future of organ transplantation, xenotransplants could become an approach for resolving donor organ shortages, and could create a much more ordered and elective surgical specialty.

Clinical cardiac transplantation is currently limited by the supply of donor organs, and this shortage is likely to persist or even intensify in the foreseeable future. In the absence of a reliable mechanical replacement, cardiac xenotransplantation remains an important potential solution to the problem of an insufficient donor supply, especially in pediatric patients. While not yet a clinical reality, xenotransplantation is the focus of intensive laboratory research. Many of the mechanisms involved in the rejection of xenografts have been elucidated, and a number of therapeutic approaches are under evaluation. This chapter will present an overview of the field and will describe some of the new concepts of the pathophysiology and potential management direction of hyperacute (xenograft) rejection.

EXPERIMENTAL CONCORDANT CARDIAC XENOTRANSPLANTATION

Concordant xenotransplantation is performed between two species that are closely related immunologically, e.g. two different species of subhuman primates, or mouse and rat. The mechanism(s) of rejection is primarily cellular in nature and is similar to classical acute allograft rejection[14] (Chapters 14 and 15). Various combinations of concordant xenotransplants have been reported in a number of experimental models.

Homan et al. achieved significant prolongation of cardiac survival in a hamster–rat combination with the addition of cyclosporine (CsA)[15]. However, virtually toxic levels of this drug were required for an effect, suggesting its use alone may not be appropriate in a clinical setting. Knechtle and colleagues evaluated total lymphoid irradiation along with CsA in hamster–rat and rabbit–rat combinations[16]. Highly significant prolongation of cardiac graft survival (> 100 days) was evident in the first combination, though it did not prove possible to prolong survival of rabbit–rat cardiac xenografts. Here again, the choice of donor–recipient combinations was critical. While both species combinations are considered concordant, the hamster–rat combination is phylogenetically more closely related.

A heterotopic calf-to-goat model has been used with antilymphocyte serum and steroid immunosuppression[17]. Although prolongation of graft survival was achieved, many recipients died of infectious complications with functioning xenografts. Another heterotopic cardiac xenograft model has been described in subhuman primates using cynomolgus monkeys as donors and baboons as recipients[18]. Immunosuppression with cyclosporine and prednisone was used, and average graft survival was 77 days, with a range of 16–200 days.

In a study of orthotopic cardiac xenografts, newborn goats received hearts from lamb donors[19]. Of 14 recipients, ten survived for more than 24 hours; the average postoperative survival was 72 days and ranged from 24 to 165 days. Immunosuppression consisted of CsA, azathioprine, and methylprednisolone. Various other response manipulations have been studied in different animal xenograft models with some success in prolonging graft survival; therapy has included antilymphocyte globulin[20,21], selective lymphoid irradiation[22], inhibitors of the complement system[23], inhibitors of the coagulation system[24,25], and the use of pretransplant donor blood transfusion[26].

Histopathologic studies in these concordant models showed significant acute cellular and chronic rejection, with a suggestion that a humoral component was also playing a role. Thus, the immunologic issues in concordant cardiac xenotransplantation appear relatively conventional and deal primarily with cellular rejection, albeit in a highly aggressive form. The rejection process seen in concordant xenotransplantation is generally refractory to present day immunosuppression, which may suggest that the humoral component is also important in the overall scheme and must be addressed. Moreover, in the reports of successful engraftment, the infectious complications have been lethal. A better understanding of the rejection process and the contribution of the humoral component, along with more selective and less toxic immunosuppressive protocols and other pharmacologic applications, may be expected to improve graft survival.

EXPERIMENTAL DISCORDANT CARDIAC XENOTRANSPLANTATION

Discordant cardiac xenotransplantation represents an entirely different immunologic phenomenon. Species differences are sufficiently great so that preformed heterospecific antibodies are present in the recipient. Rejection occurs within minutes and is humorally mediated. The violence of the rejection process, its course, and the resultant pathology bear resemblance to the hyperacute rejection seen clinically in situations of allograft ABO mismatch or high sensitization. Although first described in kidney transplantation[1-5,27], HAR is also seen in liver[28] and cardiac[29] transplantation. Experimental studies utilizing discordant species combinations have been primarily targeted at the characterization of pathologic lesions observed in this response as well as the mechanism(s) involved. Pharmacologic intervention with conventional immunosuppression has, for the most part, been ineffective.

In a highly discordant xenograft species combination of guinea pig–rat, cardiac graft survival time was 16 minutes in untreated controls. When treatment with CsA, cyclophosphamide, or splenectomy was associated with a 1.5 plasma volume exchange, graft survival was significantly increased[30]. However, when each treatment regimen was used alone, no beneficial effect was observed. Short-term prolongation of discordant xenograft survival has also been reported following recipient pretreatment with cobra venom factor or anti-platelet agents in combination with plasma modifications[24].

Multiple administrations of cobra venom factor alone have also resulted in prolonged cardiac xenograft function. Further, Shons et al. reported that pretreatment with aspirin (80 mg/kg) extended pig–dog renal xenograft survival from 5 minutes to 21 minutes[24]. Anti-platelet agents (aspirin) have also been studied in the guinea pig–rat combination, but successful prolongation of graft survival could not be achieved[32].

Microscopic evaluation of discordant cardiac xenografts is characterized by capillary congestion and injury, massive extravascular hemorrhage, interstitial edema, ischemic myocardial contracture, and lack of interstitial white blood cell infiltration[32] (Chapter 62). Thus, one of the motivations for studying discordant xenotransplantation is to understand the mechanism(s) and pathophysiology of HAR, as well as to study various experimental manipulations that might abrogate this process.

NEW CONCEPTS IN THE MECHANISMS OF HYPERACUTE REJECTION

The HAR which occurs when transplanted organs are exposed to recipient anti-graft antibodies in the three different situations already mentioned fundamentally represents a devascularization in which small blood vessels become plugged with coagulation products and formed blood elements. While controversy remains over which antibodies are involved, and under what circumstances immediate graft dysfunction occurs, HAR must be regarded as the product of a complex immune/inflammatory reaction (Figures 63.1 and 63.2).

Following the binding of anti-graft antibody to antigen on the endothelium, all the events that occur thereafter are immunologically non-specific, namely, activation of clotting, fibrin deposition, fibrinolysis, capillary leaking[33], and the influx of inflammatory cells with their own release of mediators and consequent tissue injury. The process of HAR, like that of organ ischemia and necrosis, involves most, if not all, of the components of a typical inflammatory response[34]. Obstruction of the small arteries by the platelet–neutrophil plugs induces an accompanying ischemia in cells, which may activate the complement system by the alternate pathway.

The release of the vasoactive substances C3a and C5a results in enhanced inflammation with neutrophil margination and migration to the damaged tissue. This results in neutrophil activation, with a burst of oxygen consumption and the production of oxygen-derived free radicals, for example, via membrane-bound NAD (O)H oxidase and release of lysosomal enzymes[34]. The activation of neutrophils leads to an increase in phospholipase A_2 activity, which hydrolyzes arachidonic acid from membrane phospholipids[34].

A cascade is started which produces a large number of biologically active lipid products that include the prostaglandins, leukotrienes, and thromboxanes. Two of the more important pathophysiologic lipid mediators include leukotriene B_1, which is a very potent neutrophil chemoattractant (therefore creating a positive feedback signal to recruit more neutrophils), and thromboxane A_2, which is an extremely potent vasoconstrictor and platelet pro-aggregator[34]. It is obvious how the many arms of the inflammatory process depicted in Figures 63.1 and 63.2 are redundant and resilient, and combine to create a relentless and mutually perpetuating progression to organ destruction.

Acetyl glycerol ether phosphorylcholine, also known as platelet-activating factor (PAF) because it was initially discovered for its ability to cause potent platelet aggregation and the release of platelet granules, represents the most recently described and novel class of potent lipid autocoids[35]. It is a potent mediator of inflammatory reactions because of its broad range of biological activities (Figure 63.3). These activities contribute to the development of vascular phenomena that characterize and evoke almost all other well-known cardinal signs of acute inflammation.

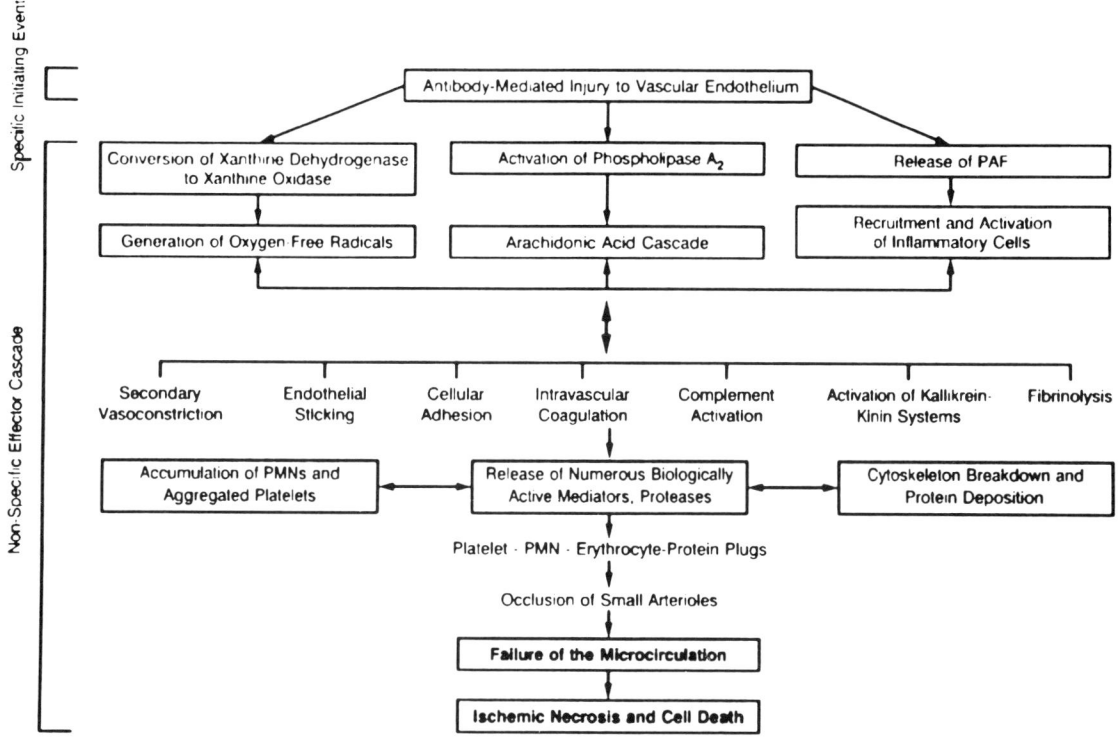

Figure 63.1 Schematic illustration of the mechanism of antibody-mediated hyperacute rejection

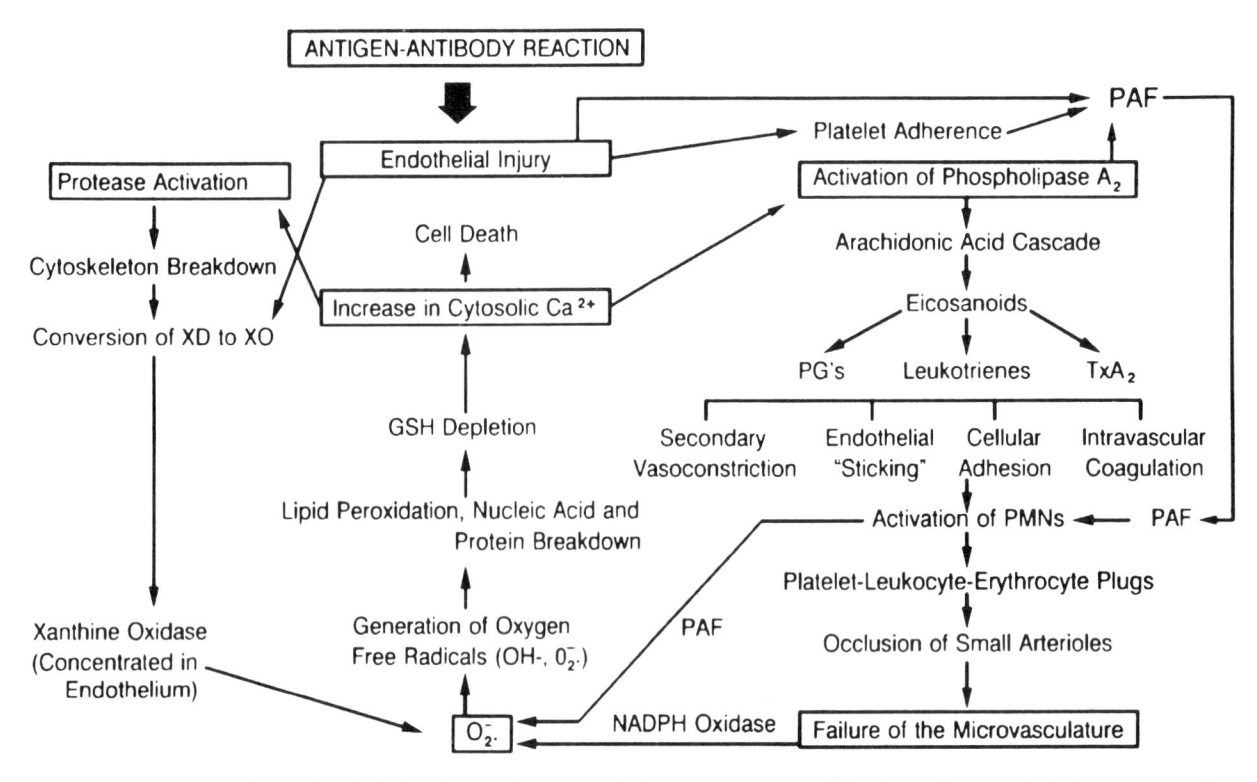

Figure 63.2 Schematic illustration depicting the complex immune/inflammatory response following antigen–antibody interaction with the endothelium of the transplanted organ

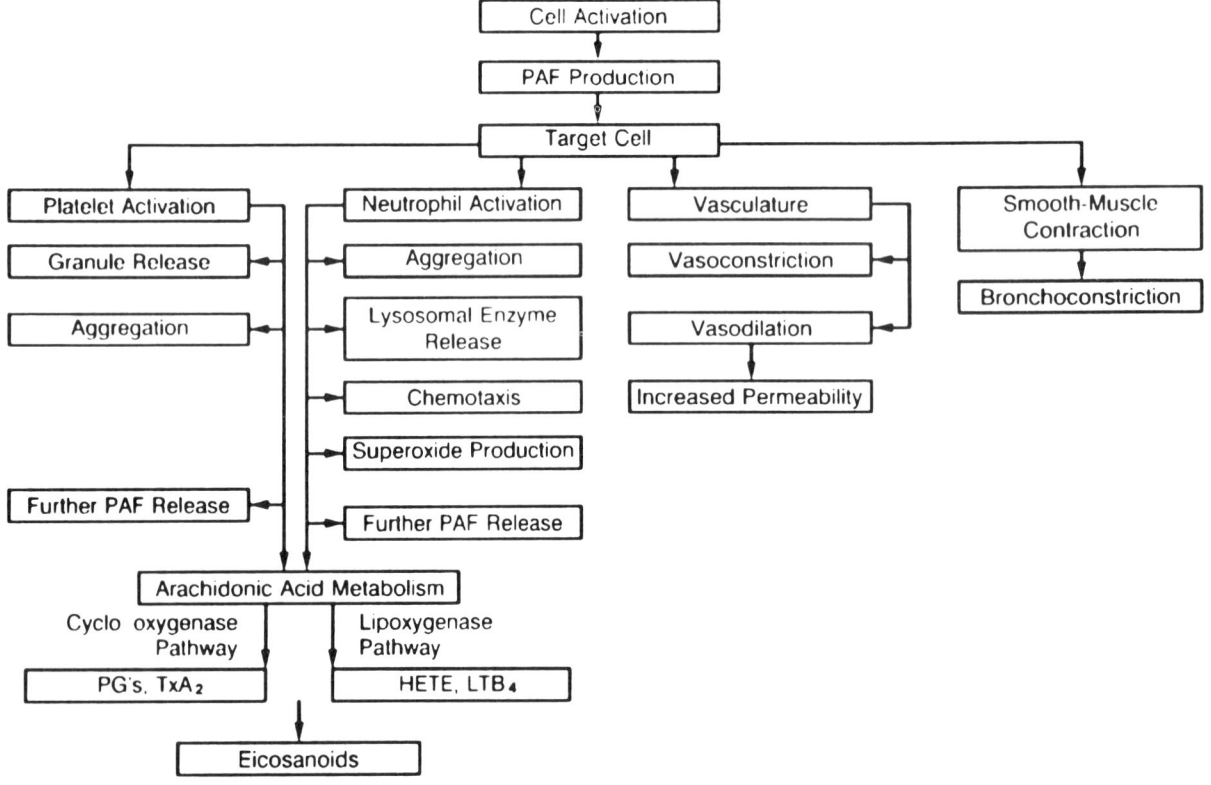

Figure 63.3 The broad range of biological activities of platelet-activating factor (PAF)

Although the precise role of PAF in immunopathologic reactions remains to be fully elucidated, all published data implicate PAF as playing a central role in the induction of tissue injury[36]. Moreover, there is already considerable evidence for the candidacy of PAF as a central and key biological mediator in the pathogenesis of humorally-mediated hyperacute allograft rejection[37,38].

In vitro studies have demonstrated that PAF is released when endothelial cells are incubated with antibody to cell surface angiotensin-converting enzyme. This has important implications for HAR, in which the specific initiating event is a transplantation antigen–antibody interaction on the endothelial surface. In a model of hyperacute renal allograft rejection in sensitized rabbits, PAF was identified in the blood effluent from the transplanted kidney, following immediate antibody and complement fixation to the endothelium of glomerular and peritubular capillaries[37].

The classical histopathologic features characteristic of HAR consist of intravascular thrombosis, interstitial hemorrhage, neutrophil and platelet accumulation, and widespread parenchymal necrosis[2,24,29,32] (Chapter 62). The time course of HAR can be variable. In its most extreme form, the sequence of events can take place within minutes. Less violent forms of HAR can progress over a period of hours or even days. Finally, the time course can vary depending upon the organ involved, as in the case of a combined liver/kidney transplant patient in which the kidney underwent hyperacute rejection within minutes of transplantation while the liver was also ultimately lost to hyperacute rejection but over 2–3 days (Starzl, T.E., manuscript submitted for publication).

SELECTED APPROACHES TO THE MANAGEMENT OF HYPERACUTE REJECTION

When one considers the multiple inflammatory effectors and events involved in the pathogenesis of HAR, it is not surprising that a successful experimental therapeutic approach has not as yet been identified. There have, however, been significant advances involving the interruption of the early events of the immunologic cascade described previously, with less successful attempts being applied to the late, end-stage events.

Initial experimentation aimed at the prevention or modulation of HAR focused predominantly on relatively non-specific agents such as aspirin, dextran, cinansersin, and trasylol[24]. The effectiveness of these agents was limited, as were the use of angiotensin-converting enzyme inhibitors and calcium channel blockers[39]. As mentioned earlier, a more specific agent, cobra venom factor, which suppresses the C3 component of the complement system, has been more effective in mitigating the inflammatory response and prolonging discordant xenograft survival[24]. Anti-platelet serum has also been used with some effect.

Newer approaches and progress in the abrogation of HAR have resulted from studies on two of the more recently recognized and characterized effector arms of the secondary response, namely PAF and the arachidonic acid cascade. Experiments in our laboratory have focused on the effect of a receptor-specific antagonist of PAF, SRI 63-441 (Sandoz Company), in both xenotransplantation and in the presensitized recipient[40,41]. Cardiac and renal graft survival was also evaluated when this antagonist was combined with immunosuppression or eicosanoids.

Experimental renal xenotransplantation

Pig-to-dog renal heterotransplantation results in a rapid and violent form of cortical necrosis and ischemic destruction of the organ, which mimics the situation in humans, and is due to preformed humoral antibodies in the recipient[9,10]. The control dogs in all of our experiments consistently demonstrated HAR of the pig kidney within a mean time of approximately 30 minutes.

The administration of SRI 63-441 (SRI) as a single agent did not result in a significant increase in graft survival. The addition of prostanoids (either PGI_2 or PGE_1) to SRI treatment resulted in a marked synergism and a significant increase in kidney survival and function. SRI and PGI_2 resulted in a greater than sixfold (217.1 ± 39.4 versus 37.4 ± 11.1 minutes, $p < 0.001$), and SRI and PEG_1 in a greater than sevenfold (268.6 ± 27.7 versus 37.2 ± 5.65 minutes, $p < 0.001$) increase in renal xenograft survival when compared with their respective controls. PGI_2 or PGE_1 infused alone as single agents had no significant effect on kidney survival.

The results for renal function paralleled those for kidney survival. SRI alone did not significantly improve renal function. The combination of SRI and PGI_2 resulted in a greater than threefold (99.5 ± 30.4 versus 29.5 ± 13.7 ml, $p < 0.05$) and of SRI and PGE_1 in a greater than 20-fold (436.2 ± 134.8 versus 21.2 ± 7.3 ml, $p < 0.02$) increase in total urine output. Neither prostanoid alone resulted in a significant increase in urine output.

When a cat–rabbit renal transplant model was utilized, recipient pretreatment with 4 mg/kg SRI i.v. prior to revascularization was able to significantly prolong xenograft survival as compared to vehicle-only treated controls (133.3 ± 8.23 versus 84.3 ± 5.26 minutes, $p < 0.002$).

Histologic sections of kidneys from animals receiving SRI showed only mild tubular vacuolization at 1 hour, compared to overt acute tubular necrosis in the control kidneys. At $1\frac{1}{2}$ hours both kidneys were similar, with at most 3% glomerular thrombosis and acute tubular necrosis.

While organ graft survival and function were extended

in these studies, HAR was not prevented. The need for a polypharmacologic approach to the treatment of HAR is clearly indicated.

Experimental cardiac allograft transplantation in the hypersensitized recipient

In a well-established model of HAR in rats[42], inbred Lewis strain (RT1$_1$) recipients were sensitized by four successive skin grafts from ACI strain (RT1a) donors. Control (vehicle only) animals consistently rejected donor cardiac grafts in a hyperacute fashion (216 ± 40.0 minutes), as depicted in Table 63.1.

Treatment of sensitized rats with SRI alone as a single intravenous bolus prior to revascularization resulted in a varied response (Table 63.1). Administration of 5 mg/kg or 10 mg/kg failed to demonstrate significant prolongation of graft survival. At a dosage of 20 mg/kg, three out of eight animals died with pulsating grafts, suggesting a certain level of drug toxicity. Significant prolongation of cardiac allograft survival was achieved, however, when animals were treated with 15 mg/kg of SRI (2475 ± 560 minutes, $p < 0.001$). In fact, nine of these hearts functioned for 2–5 days following transplantation.

Recipient animal pretreatment with multiple administrations of CsA (15 mg/kg per day commencing at 3 days prior to transplantation) either alone or in combination with SRI (at the time of transplantation) failed to exhibit an additional effect. Similarly, treatment with prostaglandin (PGE$_2$ at 3 mg/kg per day i.v.) was unsuccessful. However, the use of SRI in combination with a recently described immunosuppressive agent, FK 506[43], resulted in remarkable prolongation of graft survival, with complete abrogation of HAR in a number of cases[44].

The morphologic features of HAR, including extensive interstitial hemorrhage, occlusion of vessels by platelets, endothelial cell damage, and myocyte necrosis, were evident in all control animals (Figure 63.4). Heart allografts that functioned long-term (i.e. 2–4 days) exhibited an entirely different histologic picture. These hearts exhibited an abundant mononuclear cell infiltrate, many of which demonstrated features of blast formation (Figure 63.5). This finding was interpreted as acute cellular rejection. Typically, there was much less interstitial hemorrhage and little or no platelet plugging of vessels noted. Therefore, the use of SRI converted a picture of HAR into a setting of a very acute and aggressive, yet traditional, cellular rejection. This accounts for the potential effectiveness of and need for potent immunosuppression (i.e. FK 506).

When one considers the logic of blocking HAR at as

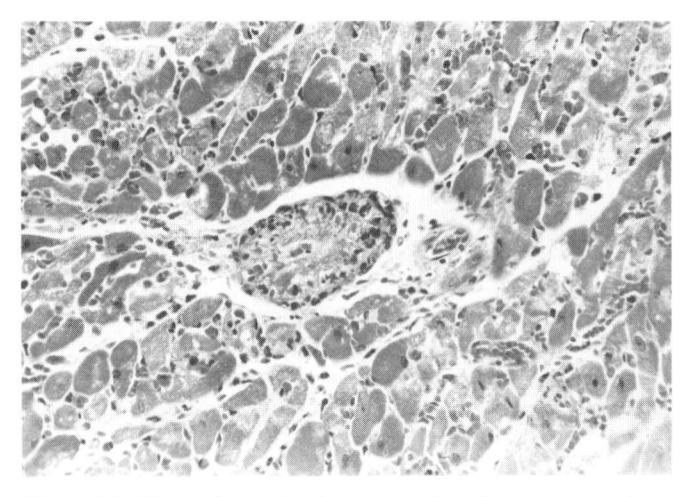

Figure 63.4 Photomicrograph of the myocardium from a heterotopic rat cardiac allograft (ACI → Lewis) previously sensitized by four successive donor skin grafts (control experiment). Note acute vasculitis and thrombosis. Slight acute inflammation can be seen in the myocardial interstitium (H & E × 290)

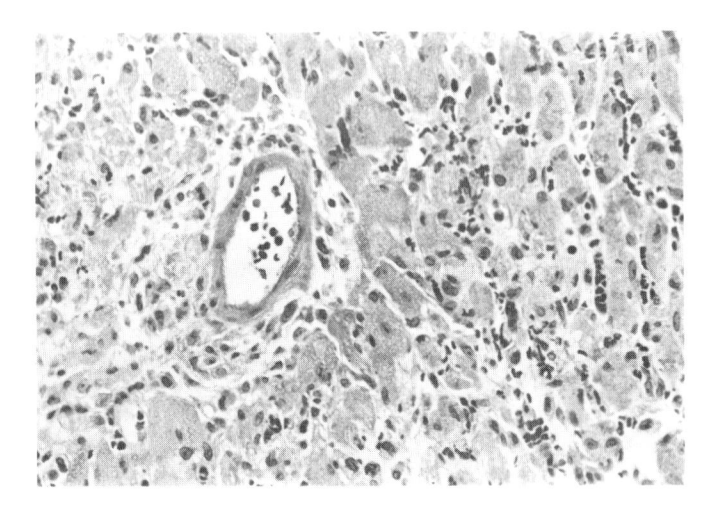

Figure 63.5 Photomicrograph of the myocardium from a heterotopic rat cardiac allograft (ACI → Lewis) previously sensitized by four successive donor skin grafts and treated with a single intravenous bolus of 15 mg/kg SRI 63-441. Note the lack of vasculitis and thrombosis. There is evidence of repair, indicating some damage to the myocardium prior to harvest. The extent of repair ranged from mild to moderate in degree (H & E × 290)

Table 63.1 The effect of SRI 63-441 on rat cardiac allograft (ACI → Lewis) survival in presensitized recipients

Group	Treatment	n	Mean graft survival time (+ SE) (minutes)	Statistical significance* (vs. Group 1)
1	Control no treatment	74	216 (40.0)	
2	SRI 63-441 5 mg/kg i.v.	4	181 (140)	NS
3	SRI 63-441 10 mg/kg i.v.	10	1270 (602)	NS
4	SRI 63-441 15 mg/kg i.v.	20	2475 (560)	$p < 0.001$
5	SRI 63-441 20 mg/kg i.v.	8	1343 (808)	NS

* t-test

early a stage as possible, the prevention of the initiating immunologic event would seem to be the ultimate goal. In this area, a new technological advance promises to have significant implications. The principle involves the ability of the Staphylococcus-A exotoxin to bind selectively the Fc receptor of IgG and IgM[45]. By attaching the Staph-A protein to a sepharose column, it is possible to run plasma over the column and subsequently adsorb the immunoglobulin[46]. Instrumentation (Citem-10, DuPont, Excorim) has been developed with two Staph-A columns in parallel; as plasma is run over one column, the other saturated column is eluted free of bound antibody. By immunoadsorbing enough plasma volume, IgG and IgM levels can be decreased tenfold (unpublished data).

In theory, sufficient immunodepletion of preformed antibodies might eliminate the endothelial antigen–antibody interaction, and thus abrogate HAR by preventing the secondary cascade. Preliminary work with Staph-A immunodepletion in a pig-to-dog xenograft model has been performed in our laboratory at the University of Pittsburgh[47], demonstrating some prolongation of graft survival (unpublished data).

Experiments along a similar line, using total plasma exchange in a guinea pig-to-rat cardiac xenograft model, have demonstrated even longer graft survival[30].

It is very likely that a combination of approaches, affecting both the immunologic and non-immunologic components of this process, will be required to achieve complete or significant elimination of HAR. Perhaps the combination of Staph-A immunodepletion, PAF inhibition with eicosanoid-mediated vasodilation, and potent new immunosuppressive regimens with such agents as FK 506 will be effective. At this point, the potential for success appears significant.

COMMENT

In this chapter we have summarized some of the data on cardiac xenotransplantation and have pointed out the issues involved and some of the problems remaining to be resolved. Cardiac xenografting is not yet a feasible clinical reality; however, research on several fronts may combine to lead to breakthroughs in the not-too-distant future.

Acknowledgements

The original research work quoted in this chapter was supported by research grants from the Veterans Administration and Project Grant AM29961 from the National Institutes of Health, Bethesda, Maryland, USA.

References

1. Starzl, T.E. (1964). *Experience in Renal Transplantation.* p. 37 and 249. (Philadelphia: W.B. Saunders)
2. Starzl, T.E., Lerner, R.A., Dixon, F.J., Groth, C.G., Brettschneider, L. and Terasaki, P.I. (1968). The Schwartzman reaction after human renal transplantation. *N. Engl. J. Med.*, **278**, 642
3. Keown, P.A. (1987). The highly sensitized patient: etiology, impact and management. *Transplant. Proc.*, **19**, 74
4. Opelz, G., Graver, B., Mickey, M.R. and Terasaki, P.I. (1981). Lymphocytotoxic antibody responses to transfusions in potential kidney transplant recipients. *Transplantation*, **32**, 177
5. Terasaki, P.I., Mickey, M.R., Yamazaki, J.N. and Vredevoe, D. (1970). Maternal-fetal incompatibility. *Transplantation*, **9**, 538
6. Busch, G.J., Martins, A.C.P., Hollenberg, N.K., Wilson, R.E. and Colman, R.W. (1975). A primate model of hyperacute renal allograft rejection. *Am. J. Pathol.*, **79**, 31
7. Klassen, J. and Milgrom, F. (1971). Studies in cortical necrosis in rabbit renal homografts. *Transplantation*, **11**, 35
8. Williams, G.M., Lee, H.M., Weymouth, R.F., Harlan, W.R. Jr., Holden, K.R., Stanley, C.M., Millington, G.A. and Hume, D.M. (1967). Studies in hyperacute and chronic renal homografts in man. *Surgery*, **62**, 204
9. Giles, G.R., Boehmig, H.J., Lilly, J., Amemiya, H., Takagi, H., Cogurg, A.J., Hathaway, W.E., Wilson, C.B., Dixon, F.J. and Starzl, T.E. (1970). Mechanism and modification of rejection of heterografts between divergent species. *Transplant. Proc.*, **2**, 522
10. Boehmig, H.J., Giles, G.R., Amemiya, H., Wilson, C.B., Coburg, A.J., Genton, T., Bunch, D.L., Dixon, F.J. and Starzl, T.E. (1971). Hyperacute rejection of renal homografts: with particular reference to coagulation changes, humoral antibodies and formed blood elements. *Transplant. Proc.*, **3**, 1105
11. Myburgh, J.A., Cohen, I., Gecetter, L., Meyers, A.M., Abrahams, C., Furman, K.I., Boldberg, B. and Van Blerk, P.J.P. (1969). Hyperacute rejection in human kidney allografts – Schwartzman or Arthus reaction? *N. Engl. J. Med.*, **281**, 131
12. Clarke, D.S., Gewurz, H., Good, R.A. and Varco, R.L. (1964). Complement fixation during homograft rejection. *Surg. Forum*, **15**, 144
13. Toth, I., Roth, E., Szmolensky, S., Pasca, S. and Torok, B. (1976). Characteristics of hyperacute rejection of swine kidney xenografts perfused with canine blood. *Int. Urol. Nephrol.*, **8**, 323
14. Deodhar, S.D. (1986). Review of xenografts in organ transplantation. *Transplant. Proc.*, **18**, 83
15. Homan, W.P., Williams, K.A., Fabre, J.W., Millard, P.R. and Morris, P.J. (1981). Prolongation of cardiac xenograft survival in rats receiving cyclosporin A. *Transplantation*, **21**, 164
16. Knechtle, S.J., Halperin, E.C. and Bollinger, R.R. (1987). Xenograft survival in two species combinations using total-lymphoid irradiation and cyclosporine. *Transplantation*, **43**, 173
17. Donawick, W.J., Shaffer, C.F., Dodd, D.C., Buchanan, J.W. and Fregin, G.F. (1971). Cardiac and skin heterograft rejection: suppression with antilymphocyte serum. *Transplant. Proc.*, **3**, 551
18. Michler, R.E., McManus, R.P., Smith, C.C., Sadeghi, A.N. and Rose, E.A. (1985). Technique for primate heterotopic cardiac xenotransplantation. *J. Med. Primatol.*, **14**, 357
19. Bailey, L.L., Jang, J., Johnson, W. and Jolley, W.B. (1985). Orthotopic cardiac xenografting in the newborn goat. *J. Thorac. Cardiovasc. Surg.*, **89**, 242
20. Corry, R.J. and Kelley, S.E. (1974). Immunological enhancement of primarily vascularized rat heart xenotransplants in rats. *Transplantation*, **18**, 503
21. Corry, R.J. and Kelley, S.E. (1975). Survival of cardiac xenografts: effects of antithymocyte serum and enhancing heteroantiserum. *Arch. Surg.*, **110**, 1143
22. Hardy, M.A., Oluwole, S., Fawwaz, R., Satake, K., Nowygrod, R. and Reemtsma, K. (1982). Selective lymphoid irradiation. II. Prolongation of cardiac xenografts and allografts in presensitized rats. *Transplantation*, **33**, 237
23. Snyder, G.B., Ballestros, E., Zarco, R.M. and Linn, B.S. (1966). Prolongation of renal xenografts by complement suppression. *Surg.*

Forum., **17**, 478
24. Shons, A.R. and Najarian, J.S. (1974). Modification of xenograft rejection by aspirin, dextran, and cinansersin: the importance of platelets in hyperacute rejection. *Transplant. Proc.*, **6**, 435
25. Jorgensen, K.A., Kemp, E., Barfort, P., Starklint, H., Larsen, S., Petersen, P.H. and Knudsen, J.B. (1983). The survival of pig to rabbit renal xenografts during inhibition of thromboxane synthesis. *Thromb. Res.*, **32**, 585
26. Kemp, E., Kemp, G., Absilgaard-Jacobsen, I.B. and Lundborg, C.J. (1977). Prolongation of survival of renal xenografts by infusion of donor blood. *Acta Pathol. Microbiol. Scand.*, **85**, 267
27. Kissmeyer-Nielsen, F., Olsen, S., Petersen, U.P. and Fjeldborg, O. (1966). Hyperacute rejection of kidney allografts associated with pre-existing humoral antibodies against donor cells. *Lancet*, **2**, 662
28. Starzl, T.E. (1969). Orthotopic heterotransplantation. In Starzl, T.E. (ed.) *Experience in Hepatic Transplantation.* p. 284. (Philadelphia: W.B. Saunders Company)
29. Weil, R., Clarke, D.R., Iwaki, Y., Porter, K.A., Koep, L.J., Paton, B.C., Terasaki, P.I. and Starzl, T.E. (1981). Hyperacute rejection of a transplanted human heart. *Transplantation*, **32**, 71
30. Van de Stadt, J., Vendeville, B., Weill, B., Crougneau, A.M., Filipponi, F., Icard, P., Renoux, M., Louvel, A. and Houssin, D. (1988). Discordant heart xenografts in the rat: additional effect of plasma exchange and cyclosporine, cyclophosphamide, or splenectomy in delaying hyperacute rejection. *Transplantaion*, **45**, 514
31. Adachi, H., Rosengard, B.R., Hutchins, G.M., Hall, T.S., Baumgartner, W.A., Borkon, A.M. and Reitz, B.A. (1987). Effects of cyclosporine, aspirin and cobra venom factor on discordant cardiac xenograft survival in rats. *Transplant. Proc.*, **19**, 1145
32. Jamieson, S.W. (1974). Xenograft hyperacute rejection. A new model. *Transplantation*, **17**, 533
33. Simpson, K.M., Bunch, D.L., Amemiya, H., Boehmig, H.J., Wilson, C.B., Dixon, F.J., Coburg, A.J., Hathaway, W.E., Giles, G.R. and Starzl, T.E. (1970). Humoral antibodies and coagulation mechanisms in the accelerated or hyperacute rejection of renal homografts in sensitized canine recipients. *Surgery*, **68**, 77
34. Simpson, P.J. and Lucchesi, B.R. (1985). Myocardial ischemia: the potential therapeutic role of prostacyclin and its analogues. In Gryglewski, R.J. and Stock, G. (eds.) *Prostacyclin and its Stable Analogue Iloprost.* p. 179. (New York: Springer-Verlag)
35. Pinckard, R.N. (1983). Platelet-activating factor. *Hosp. Prac.*, **18**, 67
36. Pinckard, R.M. (1982). The 'new' chemical mediators of inflammation. *Monogr. Path.*, **23**, 38
37. Ito, S., Camussi, G., Tetta, C., Milgrom, F. and Andres, G. (1984). Hyperacute renal allograft rejection in the rabbit: the role of platelet-activating factor and of cationic proteins derived from polymorphonuclear leukocytes and from platelets. *Lab. Invest.*, **51**, 148
38. Camussi, G., Niesen, N., Tetta, C., Saunders, R.N. and Milgrom, F. (1987). Release of platelet-activating factor from rabbit heart perfused *in vitro* by sera with transplantation alloantibodies. *Transplantation*, **44**, 113
39. Council on Scientific Affairs (1985). Xenografts: review of literature and current status. *J. Am. Med. Assoc.*, **254**, 3353
40. Makowka, L., Miller, C., Chapchap, P., Podesta, L., Pan, C., Pressley, D., Mazzaferro, V., Esquivel, C.O., Todo, S., Jaffe, R., Banner, B., Saunders, R. and Starzl, T.E. (1987). Prolongation of pig to dog renal xenograft survival by modification of the inflammatory mediator response. *Ann. Surg.*, **206**, 482
41. Makowka, L., Chapman, F., Qian, S., Pascualone, A., Sico, E., Podesta, L., Mazzaferro, V., Sher, L., Sun, H., Banner, B., Zerbe, T., Saunders, R. and Starzl, T.E. (1990). The antagonism of platelet-activating factor and hyperacute organ rejection. In Handley, D.A., Saunders, R.N., Houlihan, W.J. and Tomesch, J.C. (eds.) *Platelet Activating Factor in Endotoxin and Immune Diseases.* (New York: Marcel Dekker, Inc.) In press
42. Forbes, R.D.C., Kuramochi, T., Guttmann, R.D., Klassen, J. and Knaack, J. (1975). A controlled sequential morphologic study of hyperacute cardiac allograft rejection in the rat. *Lab. Invest.*, **33**, 280
43. Starzl, T.E., Makowka, L. and Todo, S. (1987). FK 506 a potential breakthrough in immunosuppression. *Transplant. Proc.*, **19**,1
44. Makowka, L., Chapman, F., Qian, S., Zerbe, A., Lee, P.H., Murase, N., Saunders, R., Todo, S. and Starzl, T.E. (1987). The effect of FK 506 on hyperacute rejection in presensitized rats. *Transplant. Proc.*, **19**, 79
45. Forsgren, A. and Sjoquist, J. (1966). 'Protein A' from *S. aureus*. Pseudoimmune reaction with human gamma-globulin. *J. Immunol.*, **97**, 882
46. Branda, R.F., Klausner, J.S., Miller, W.J. and Soltis, R.D. (1984). Specific removal of antibodies with an immunoadsorption system. *Transfusion*, **24**, 157
47. Shapiro, R., Scantlebury, V., Tzakis, A.G., Makowka, L., Watt, R., Oks, A., Yanaga, K., Podesta, L., Casavilla, A., Wos, S., Murray, J., Oral, A., D'Andrea, P., Banner, B. and Starzl, T.E. (1990). Immunodepletion in xenotransplantation: a model. *J. Invest. Surg.*, In press

64
Clinical Experience

D.K.C. COOPER

By the mid-1960s, the increasing success of experimental cardiac transplantation (Chapter 1), and the experience gained by Reemtsma (Figure 61.1)[1-3], Starzl[4,5] and others[6,7] in their initial attempts at renal xenotransplantation in man, led Hardy (Figure 1.9) and his colleagues to perform the first cardiac xenotransplant in man[8]. Their attempt, in 1964, to transplant the heart of a large chimpanzee into the chest of a 68-year-old man has been outlined in Chapter 1, and will not be discussed again here. Suffice it to say that the heart was too small to support the circulation adequately, and the patient died after 1 hour.

The second attempt at clinical xenotransplantation was by Cooley and his colleagues in 1968, whose transplanted a sheep heart into a 48-year-old man who had advanced coronary artery disease and whose circulatory status was deteriorating several hours after a cardiac arrest[9]. The lymphocytotoxic cross-match was positive, and the heart was immediately hyperacutely rejected. Even today, with currently available immunosuppressive agents, such an attempt using a discordant xenograft would be doomed to early failure (Chapter 61).

(Also in the late 1960s, in a hitherto unreported case in London, a pig heart was transplanted into a human recipient, but failed within minutes (Longmore, D.B., personal communication).)

The third and fourth reported attempts were in 1977, when Barnard (Figure 1.10) and his colleagues used cardiac xenografts on two emergency occasions at Groote Schuur Hospital in Cape Town[10]. On both occasions, the patient's native left ventricle failed to support the circulation when attempts were made to discontinue cardiopulmonary bypass after surgical procedures. Intra-aortic balloon pump support was unsuccessful in the first case and not available in the second. Both transplants were intended as temporary cardiac assist 'devices', to support the patient until the native ventricles recovered.

The first of these two patients received a heterotopic graft from a 30 kg baboon. This small heart proved insufficient to support the circulation in the presence of repeated attacks of ventricular fibrillation which affected the patient's own heart. The patient died some 6 hours after transplantation.

The second patient was supported successfully by a heterotopic chimpanzee heart until rejection occurred 4 days later; the recipient's own heart failed to recover sufficiently to support the circulation alone. Higher doses of immunosuppression (azathioprine, corticosteroids, and antithymocyte globulin) were used than would be the case with a human donor. Although the initial report suggested that severe acute rejection was the cause of graft failure, a recent review of the specimen by Rose has confirmed that vascular rejection was a major feature (Chapter 62). However, at the time, this experience suggested that a heterotopic transplant, using a suitable xenograft and heavy immunosuppression, might be a successful bridge to allotransplantation when there was evidence that the patient's own cardiac function would recover within 2-3 days.

The most recent experience with cardiac xenotransplantation was by Bailey et al. in 1984[11]. This group transplanted a baboon heart into a neonate who had hypoplastic left heart syndrome. With the advantage of cyclosporine in addition to other immunosuppressive therapy, the recipient survived 20 days. Death was from progressive graft necrosis, complicated by acute renal and pulmonary insufficiency. Hyperacute rejection did not occur. Autopsy findings showed only traces of cell-mediated rejection in the cardiac graft. Graft failure appeared to have resulted from a progressive humoral response, unmodified by immunosuppression.

The donor selection process in this initial baboon-to-newborn human clinical trial was concerned with the presence of preformed donor-specific lymphocytotoxic antibody, and with the degree of homology between donor and recipient tissues. The recipient was erythrocyte type O. Type O baboons are exceedingly rare, and none was available for use as a donor. Blood group matching, therefore, could not be achieved.

Anti-A and anti-B isoagglutinins to human erythrocytes and low-titered heteroagglutinins to baboon erythrocytes were present in the patient's circulation before transplantation, but disappeared afterwards. It was unclear whether the patient selectively failed to produce hemagglutinins postoperatively, or, more likely, that the hemagglutinins were immediately continuously adsorbed on to the baboon graft.

On the basis of this case and their experimental experience, in which cardiac histopathological features appeared to be those of antibody and/or complement-mediated injury despite immunosuppression, this group felt that rejection of the xenograft might have been due to ABO hemagglutinins and/or species-specific cytotoxic antibody, amongst other factors. The exact role of each type of antibody remains uncertain. It seems likely, however, that ABO antibodies and/or anti-baboon antibodies were gradually adsorbed by the graft, producing injury to the largest endothelial bed, namely the microcirculatory vessels. This phenomenon resulted in widespread microvascular lumenal narrowing. Circulatory sludging, thrombosis, cellular hypoxia, and myocyte injury and/or necrosis followed.

Though there has been continuing experimental work in this field since 1984 (Chapters 61 and 63), no further attempts at clinical cardiac xenotransplantation have been reported to date.

References

1. Reemtsma, K., McCracken, B.H., Schlegel, J.U., Pearl, M.A., Pearce, C.W., De Witt, C.W., Smith, P.E., Hewitt, R.L., Flinner, R.L. and Creech, O. (1964). Renal heterotransplantation in man. *Ann. Surg.*, **160**, 384
2. Reemtsma, K., McCracken, B.H., Schlegel, J.U., Pearl, M.A., De Witt, C.W. and Creech, O. (1964). Reversal of early graft rejection after renal heterotransplantation in man. *J. Am. Med. Assoc.*, **187**, 691
3. Reemtsma, K., McCracken, B.H., Schlegel, J.V. and Pearl, M.A. (1964). Heterotransplantation of the kidney: two clinical experiences. *Science*, **143**, 700
4. Starzl, T.E., Marchioro, T.L., Peters, G.N., Kirkpatrick, C.H., Wilson, W.E.C., Porter, K.A., Rifkind, D., Ogden, D.A., Hitchcock, C.R. and Waddell, W.R. (1964). Renal heterotransplantation from baboon to man: experience with 6 cases. *Transplantation*, **2**, 752
5. Porter, K.A., Marchioro, T.L. and Starzl, T.E. (1965). Pathological changes in 6 treated baboon to man renal heterotransplants. *Br. J. Urol.*, **37**, 274
6. Hitchcock, C.R., Kiser, J.C., Telander, R.L. and Seljeskob, E.L. (1964). Baboon renal grafts. *J. Am. Med. Assoc.*, **189**, 934
7. Ogden, D.A., Sitprija, V. and Holmes, J.H. (1965). Function of the baboon renal heterograft in man and comparison with renal homograft function. *J. Lab. Clin. Med.*, **65**, 370
8. Hardy, J.D., Kurrus, F.E., Chavez, C.M., Neely, W.A., Webb, W.R., Eraslan, S., Turner, M.D., Fabian, L.W. and Labecki, J.D. (1964). Heart transplantation in man: developmental studies and report of a case. *J. Am. Med. Assoc.*, **188**, 1132
9. Cooley, D.A., Hallman, G.L., Bloodwell, R.D., Nora, J.J. and Leachman, R.D. (1968). Human heart transplantation: experience with 12 cases. *Am. J. Cardiol.*, **22**, 804
10. Barnard, C.N., Wolpowitz, A. and Losman, J.G. (1977). Heterotopic cardiac transplantation with a xenograft for assistance of the left heart in cardiogenic shock after cardiopulmonary bypass. *S. Afr. Med. J.*, **52**, 1035
11. Bailey, L.L., Nehlsen-Cannarella, S.L., Concepcion, W. and Jolley, W.B. (1985). Baboon-to-human cardiac xenotransplantation in a neonate. *J. Am. Med. Assoc.*, **254**, 3321

Section VII

Cardiac augmentation with skeletal muscle

65
Cardiomyoplasty

G.J. MAGOVERN AND I.Y. CHRISTLIEB

INTRODUCTION

Twenty years after the first human cardiac transplantation and 5 years after the first artificial heart implant, when technological advancements in cardiac surgery seem to have reached a plateau and apparently nothing in sight can astonish the world in this field, a 50-year-old concept comes back to regain strength and to offer promise to a potentially large number of patients who are neither good candidates for transplant nor subjects for mechanical assist in its present stage of development.

De-Jesus[1], Leriche[2], and Beck[3] first used skeletal muscle both experimentally and in the clinical setting for the treatment of various myocardial pathologies, mainly those ischemic and traumatic in origin. Since then the application of muscular grafts to the central circulatory system, whether free or pedicled, innervated or denervated, paced or unpaced, has evolved into a very specific therapeutic modality. Although still in its early developmental phase, it is largely intended for long-term palliation of certain cases of ventricular dysfunction. This group of procedures which has been referred to as 'biomechanical cardiac assist' by Chiu[4], includes cardiomyoplasty and/or cardiomyopexy, and muscle-powered devices. This chapter will address only the first group since the latter are, by definition, paracardiac.

MYOCARDIAL SUBSTITUTION

Myocardial substitution can be interpreted as being anatomical, functional, or both. Anatomical substitution dates back to 1933 when Leriche proposed the use of free skeletal muscle grafts to replace infarcted areas of the human myocardium, on the basis of his experimental success with such a procedure in one dog[2]. De-Jesus appears to have been first in using skeletal muscle in a clinical case of left ventricular trauma[1]. Griffith and Bates used it in 1938 to repair an accidental perforation of the right ventricle in the course of a revascularization procedure[5]. Weinstein, in 1946, showed good fixation to the underlying myocardium, with normal muscle histology and profuse vascular anastomoses, in two of six free muscle grafts sutured on to intact myocardium in canine experiments[6].

Kantrowitz and McKinnon in 1959 took a pedicled portion of the diaphragm and wrapped it around a dog's ventricle in the direction of the long axis[7,8]. Muscular contractions were elicited by stimulating the undisturbed phrenic nerve synchronously with cardiac systole. Hemodynamic results were poor, and fatigue ensued shortly after the onset of stimulation. Four years later, Nakamura and Glenn demonstrated a hemodynamic effect *in vivo* utilizing the diaphragm[9]. They were first to point out the importance of an intact nerve supply to the graft in order to preserve contractility and avoid degeneration. Petrovsky (1966), in his article on surgical treatment of cardiac aneurysms, reports his experience with 100 cases in which he used diaphragm to reinforce the suture line and the resultant scar tissue[10]. A score of other investigators has continued to use diaphragm until very recently, for the purpose of partially replacing ventricular wall[11].

In 1966, Termet *et al.* first reported on the use of the latissimus dorsi in the form of pedicled grafts, as a more advantageous means to attempt correcting myocardial dysfunction[12]. Then came Christ and Spira (1982), who used latissimus dorsi to cover a partial thickness defect on the left ventricular wall[13]. Chachques, Carpentier and co-workers have reported on experimental 'dynamic' cardiomyoplasty by using a non-tiring stimulation of latissimus dorsi flaps[14–16], thus opening the way for the clinical application of functional as well as anatomical substitution of myocardial walls[17].

EXPERIMENTAL WORK

Several different skeletal muscles have been used in the past by many investigators in their quest to provide support to the failing ventricle. A comprehensive list should probably include diaphragm, pectoralis major, rectus abdominis, internal oblique, intercostals, sternohyoid, sternocleidomastoid, vastus lateralis, gracilis, pronator teres, and latissimus dorsi.

We have a definite preference for the latter. The use of the latissimus dorsi muscle as an artificial heart power source has been in the interest of the senior author (G.J.M.) for more than 12 years[18]. Some well known properties make the latissimus dorsi one of the most desirable skeletal muscles for myocardial substitution (Figure 65.1). Among them, (1) the architectural similarities it holds with cardiac muscle, such as the capability for bidirectional stretch as demonstrated by Sola[19], (2) its naturally large muscular mass, (3) its close proximity to the heart, (4) its neurovascular supply (thoracodorsal nerve and blood vessels), coming almost exclusively from the axillary region, and (5) the fact that it is not essential to the functioning of either chest wall or shoulder joint, resulting in few functional sequelae from its transplantation into the thoracic cavity through a window in the rib cage.

Enlisting a skeletal muscle to substitute for quantitatively or qualitatively insufficient myocardial walls would not be a reality today were it not for extensive studies by investigators in muscle physiology and in biomedical microelectronics. Amongst the first group are those who demonstrated the feasibility of transforming the so-called 'white', fast-twitch, Type-II muscular fibers, which are characterized by the strength of contraction (power) they can exert, but are subject to rapid fatigue, into the so-called 'red', slow-twitch, Type-I fibers; these are characterized by the amount of repetitive contractile work they can endure, and, are, to a large extent, resistant to fatigue from normal work. Type-II fibers are mostly glycolytic in their metabolic enzyme activity, whereas Type-I fibers depend mainly on oxidative metabolic enzymes to perform accordingly. Along with these biochemical changes, some most important histological, histochemical, immunohistochemical, and physiological characteristics of skeletal muscle also alter when subjected to prolonged periods of increased use, or training[20].

These changes can best be brought about by gradually conditioning the muscle over a period of 6–8 weeks, albeit at the expense of losing power[21], using direct (muscular fiber) or indirect (nerve) electrical stimulation[22]. The latter technique is proving promising in our own experimental laboratory (Figure 65.2). Here, the second group of investigators has played a most important role. Early attempts to stimulate skeletal muscle chronically to assist ventricular function invariably led to fatigue[23]. The use of conventional stimulators or stimulators producing measured tetanic contractions through short electrical bursts were of little or no use in long-term trials. The work of Chiu and his group at McGill University[24] opened the way to modern advances in microchip and computerized pulse generator technology, which currently permit the possibility of endless programming methods to modulate the function of striated muscle to approach that of the ventricular wall. Several experimental attempts along these lines have been the subject of key reports in the medical literature[11–13,16,19,23–28].

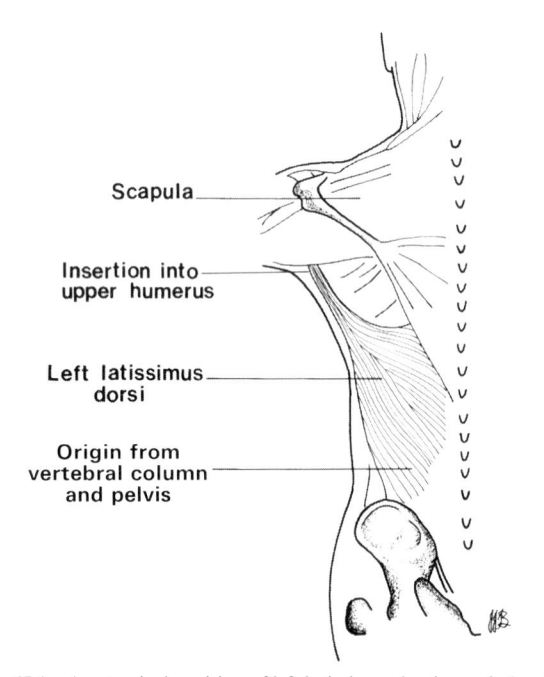

Figure 65.1 Anatomical position of left latissimus dorsi muscle (posterior view). Note the possibility of its being internalized and laid behind the heart on the posterior surface of the pericardial sac, where it will naturally wrap around the heart, joining itself anteriorly, as if molding itself in a cradle for the ventricles

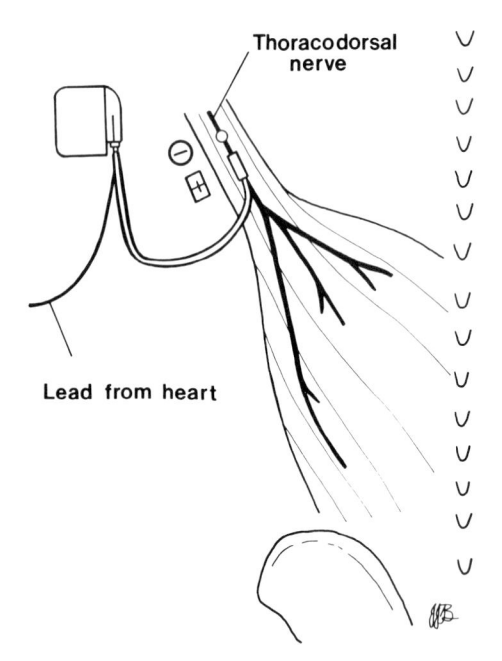

Figure 65.2 Diagram of thoracodorsal nerve stimulation, utilizing a pacemaker and a bipolar lead. The positions of the electrodes (− and +) are indicated

CLINICAL EXPERIENCE

Despite the words of Stephen Paget, who, in 1896 wrote in his book *The Surgery of the Chest*: 'Surgery of the heart has probably reached the limits set by Nature to all surgery: no new method, and no new discovery, can overcome the natural difficulties that attend a wound of the heart. It is true that "heart suture" has been vaguely proposed as a possible procedure, and has been done in animals; but I cannot find that it has ever been attempted in practice,' the clinical application of anatomical[28] and functional[29] myocardial substitution has clearly been demonstrated to be feasible.

To date, the worldwide successful clinical experience consists of ten patients who have received a dynamic cardiomyoplasty and have been followed-up long-term (30–40 months). Seven of them, including the first reported, had surgery at Broussais Hospital, University of Paris, or elsewhere, by the group of Carpentier[30]. The remaining three were part of a series of four operated in the United States by the group of Magovern[31] at Allegheny General Hospital in Pittsburgh. These patients disclaim, to some degree, Phillips' assertion in 1969 that 'the skeletal muscle could never be used to replace the heart'[32].

Surgical technique

With minor variations, the cardiomyoplasty procedure consists of dissection and internalization of the left latissimus dorsi (LD flap), with total preservation of the thoracodorsal neurovascular bundle. The LD flap is brought into the left pleural cavity through a window created by resecting a portion of the second or third rib, at which periosteal border the free tendinous end of the muscle is fixed. The heart is exposed through a median sternotomy and, if indicated, the patient is placed on cardiopulmonary bypass. Cardiac, including coronary, surgery is carried out as may be required.

Once myocardial perfusion has been reinstituted in those cases where aortic cross-clamping was used, the LD flap is brought from the left pleural cavity, positioned across the anterior wall of the left ventricle, and sutured to it with interrupted stitches in such a manner as to reinforce and further support any myocardial defect and/or the suture line following aneurysmectomy. When excisional surgery has not taken place, the LD flap is wrapped around the left ventricle from the posterior to the anterior portion of the heart (Figure 65.3), this being the cardiomyopexy procedure.

Pacing electrodes (two unipolar or one bipolar lead) are affixed to the LD flap close to the trunk and major branches of the thoracodorsal nerve. A sensing epicardial electrode is implanted on the right ventricle (we have also used endocardial leads experimentally with good results) to provide for the electric cardiac signal (either P or R wave)

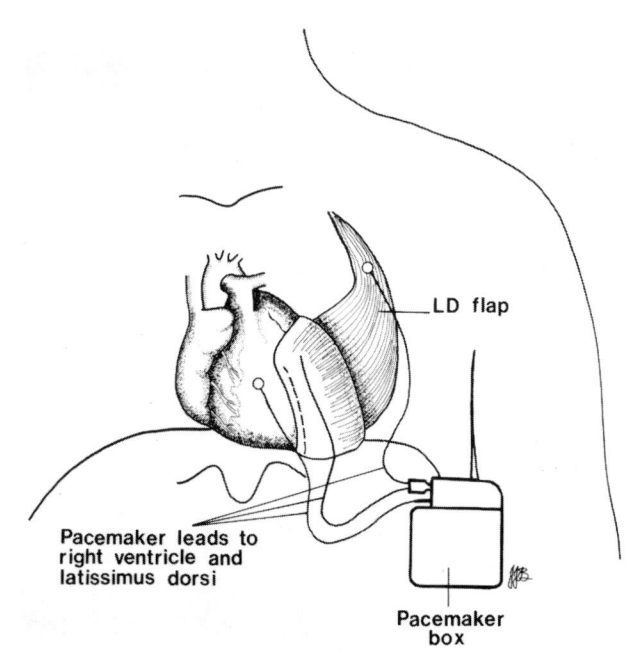

Figure 65.3 Schematic representation of cardiomyoplasty/cardiomyopexy as used in our first group of four patients. The latissimus dorsi (LD) flap, bearing two pacing electrodes, 'clings' to the anterior wall of the left ventricle, barely overlapping the left anterior descending coronary vessels. A sensing electrode is affixed to the right ventricular wall

to be conducted to the 'atrial' (cardiac) port of the pulse generator; the 'ventricular' (muscular) port is reserved for the pacing lead(s).

Programmed stimulation of the LD flap is started at or about the tenth postoperative day, at which time a gradual and progressive conditioning protocol is instituted to induce fiber transformation over a period of 35–50 days.

COMMENT

Systematic evaluation of the contribution of the muscular component to ventricular performance following cardiomyoplasty is far from being standardized. Many unavoidable differences are present among the long-term survivors, making a uniform assessment difficult at best. A protocol-controlled, standardized clinical study is in preparation by our group in compliance with Federal regulations.

If one were to use a non-invasive method for postoperative evaluation, color Doppler would be the first choice, if available, followed by the determination of left ventricular ejection fraction using either two-dimensional echo, preferably transesophageal, or MUGA scan. Utilizing the latter in our three long-term survivors[31], stimulation versus non-stimulation of the LD flap has brought improvements in ejection fraction of the magnitudes of 17% at 28 months (case 1), 32% at 13 months (case 2), and 25% at 10 months (case 4). All three cases are being stimulated with standard dual-chamber, multiprogrammable cardiac pacemakers. A

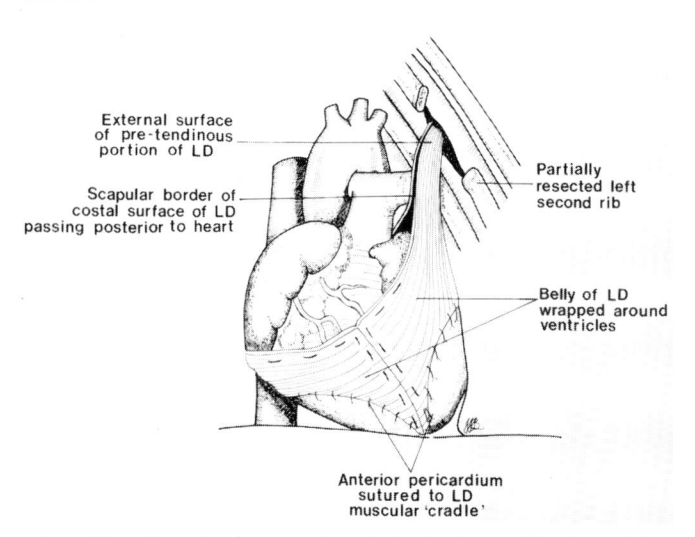

Figure 65.4 'Functional myocardial substitution' by cradling the ventricular chambers with a latissimus dorsi (LD) muscular flap, which has been mobilized and brought into the chest through the left chest wall

'burst' type implantable pulse generator is contemplated in most, if not all, of our future cases.

Our experimental work during the last 3 years has suggested improvements in the surgical technique. At present, we are working with three geometrically different methods of wrapping the LD flap around the heart. We have stated in the past[29] that this geometric orientation is, in our concept, one of the most important factors in the success of this procedure. Figure 65.4 shows the wrapping method we have been using in dogs since October, 1987. In contrast to the method depicted in Figure 65.3, the tendinous portion of the LD flap is rotated slightly clockwise (not necessary in human subjects) to allow the muscular belly that lies behind the heart to provide a cradle in the center of its costal surface for the posterior and diaphragmatic ventricular walls. The most distal part of the flap wraps around the apex, and its ventral border closes on itself to be sutured over the anterior wall of the heart. A number of fixation sutures in the ventricular side of the posterior atrioventricular groove are required to hold the flap in place.

The anteriorly-opened pericardial sac is then brought over the muscle-covered ventricular apex and tucked to the surface of the flap, avoiding constriction at the site. This will ensure permanent fixation of the heart to its original pericardiophrenic ties. Early hemodynamic studies are very encouraging, and support our current impression that this approximates closely to optimal fiber orientation of the LD flap for clinical cardiomyoplasty/cardiomyopexy procedures.

References

1. De Jesus, F.R. (1931). *Breves Consideraciones Sobre Un Caso De Herida Penetrante Del Corazon. Bol. Assoc. Med. PR*, **23**, 380
2. Leriche, R. and Fontaine, R. (1933). Essai experimental de traitement de certains infarctus du myocarde et de l'anevrisme du coeur par une greffe de muscle strie. *Bull. Soc. Nat. Chir.*, **59**, 229
3. Beck, C.S. (1935). The development of a new blood supply to the heart by operation. *Ann. Surg.*, **102**, 801
4. Chiu, R. C-J. (1986). Introduction. In Chiu, R. C-J. (ed.) *Biomechanical Cardiac Assist – Cardiomyoplasty and Muscle-powered Devices*. p. xiii. (Mount Kisco: Futura)
5. Griffith, G.C. and Bates, W. (1938). A ventricular perforation in transplanting a new blood supply. *New Int. Clin.*, **2**, 17
6. Weinstein, M. and Shafiroff, B.G. (1946). Grafts of free muscle transplants upon the myocardium. *Science*, **104**, 410
7. Kantrowitz, A. and McKinnon, W. (1959). The experimental use of the diaphragm as an auxiliary myocardium. *Surg. Forum*, **9**, 266
8. Kantrowitz, A. (1960). Functioning autogenous muscle used experimentally as an auxiliary ventricle. *Trans. Am. Soc. Artif. Int. Org.*, **6**, 305
9. Nakamura, K. and Glenn, W.L. (1964). Graft of diaphragm as a functioning substitute for myocardium. *J. Surg. Res.*, **4**, 435
10. Petrovsky, B.V. (1966). Surgical treatment of cardiac aneurysms. *J. Cardiovasc. Surg.*, **7**, 87
11. Dewar, M.L., Drinkwater, D.C. and Chiu, R.C-J. (1984). Synchronously stimulated skeletal muscle graft for myocardial repair. *J. Thorac. Cardiovasc. Surg.*, **87**, 325
12. Termet, H., Chalencon, J.L. and Estour, E. (1966). Transplantation sur le myocarde d'un muscle strie 'excite' par pace-maker. *Ann. Chir. Thorac. Cardio.*, **5**, 270
13. Christ, J. and Spira, M. (1982). Application of the latissimus dorsi muscle to the heart. *Ann. Plas. Surg.*, **8**, 118
14. Chachques, J.C., Carpentier, A. and Chavaud, S. (1984). Development of a non-tiring stimulation of the latissimus dorsi flap to replace myocardium. *Artif. Organs*, **8**, 379
15. Carpentier, A., Chachques, J.C. and Grandjean, P.A. (1985). Transformation d'un muscle squeletique par stimulation sequentielle progressive en vue de son utilisation comme substitut myocardique. *C. R. Acad. Sc. Paris*, **301**, 581
16. Chachques, J.C., Mitz, V. and Hero, M. (1985). Experimental cardioplasty using the latissimus dorsi muscle flap. *J. Cardiovasc. Surg.*, **26**, 457
17. Chachques, J.C., Grandjean, P.A. and Carpentier, A. (1986). Dynamic cardiomyoplasty: experimental cardiac wall replacement with a stimulated skeletal muscle. In Chiu, R.C-J. (ed.) *Biomechanical Cardiac Assist – Cardiomyoplasty and Muscle-powered Devices*. p. 59. (Mount Kisco: Futura)
18. Fecht, D.C., Magovern, G.J. and Dixon, C.M. (1976). Autogenous skeletal muscle as an artificial heart power source. *Med. Instrum.*, Jan/Feb
19. Sola, O.M., Dillard, D.H. and Ivey, T.D. (1981). Autotransplantation of skeletal muscle into the myocardium. *Circulation*, **71**, 341
20. Eisenberg, B.R. and Salmons, S. (1981). The reorganization of subcellular structure in muscle undergoing fast-to-slow type transformation. *Cell. Tissue Res.*, **220**, 449
21. Christlieb, I.Y., Kao, R.L. and Magovern, G.J., Jr. (1987). Correlation between fiber conversion and power in electrically stimulated *in situ* skeletal muscles. *The Physiologist*, **30**, 199
22. Armenti, F., Bitto, T. and Macoviak, J.A. (1984). Transformation of skeletal muscle for cardiac replacement. *Surg. Forum*, **35**, 258
23. Kusaba, E., Schrant, W. and Sawatani, S. (1973). A diaphragmatic graft for augmenting LV function: a feasibility study. *Trans. Am. Soc. Artif. Intern. Org.*, **19**, 251
24. Drinkwater, D., Chiu, R. C-J. and Modry, D. (1980). Cardiac assist and myocardial repair with synchronously stimulated skeletal muscle. *Surg. Forum*, **31**, 271
25. Macoviak, J.A., Stephenson, L.W. and Spielman, S. (1981). Replacement of ventricular myocardium with diaphragmatic skeletal muscle. *J. Thorac. Cardiovasc. Surg.*, **81**, 519
26. Chachques, J.C., Mitz, V. and Hero, M. (1984). Transfert d'un muscle

innerve' sur le coeur. In Magalon, G. *et al.* (eds.) *Les Lambeaux Pedicules Musculaires et Musculo-cutanes*. p. 5. (Paris: Masson)
27. Macoviak, J.A., Stephenson, L.W. and Alavi, A. (1984). Effect of electrical stimulation on diaphragmatic muscle used to enlarge right ventricle. *Surgery*, **90**, 271
28. Carpentier, A. and Chachques, J.C. (1986). The use of stimulated skeletal muscle to replace diseased human heart muscle. In Chiu, R. C-J. (ed.) *Biomechanical Cardiac Assist – Cardiomyoplasty and Muscle-powered Devices*. p. 85. (Mount Kisco: Futura)
29. Magovern, G.J., Heckler, F.R., Park, S.B. and Christlieb, I.Y. (1987). Paced latissimus dorsi used for dynamic cardiomyoplasty of left ventricular aneurysms. *Ann. Thorac. Surg.*, **44**, 379
30. Grandjean, P.A., Carpentier, A. and Chachques, J.C. (1988). Personal communication
31. Magovern, G.J., Heckler, F.R., Park, S.B., Christlieb, I.Y., Liebler, G.A., Burkholder, J.A., Maher, T.D., Benckart, D.H., Magovern, G.J., Jr. and Kuo, R.L. (1988). Paced skeletal muscle for dynamic cardiomyoplasty. *Ann. Thorac. Surg.*, **45**, 614
32. Phillips, W.L., Pallin, S. and Crastnopol, P. (1969). Diaphragm transplantation. *Angiology*, **20**, 635

66
Blood Pumps Constructed from Skeletal Muscle

C.R. BRIDGES, Jr., W.A. ANDERSON, M.A. ACKER AND L.W. STEPHENSON

INTRODUCTION

Skeletal muscle is capable of transforming chemical energy into mechanical work with extraordinary efficiency. We and others have shown that skeletal muscle has the capacity to become fatigue-resistant and adapt to new patterns of work. These changes occur when skeletal muscle is subjected to low-frequency electrical stimulation for a period of several weeks.

In laboratories worldwide, two approaches have been developed in attempts to utilize skeletal muscle to augment cardiac function. Skeletal muscle grafts have been applied directly to the beating heart in hopes of improving the collateral blood supply to ischemic myocardium and, in some cases, to directly bolster cardiac contractile function[1-11]. The other avenue of investigation has been the formation of skeletal muscle pouches or ventricles which, when stimulated to contract, provide their own pumping function.

We have fashioned pumping chambers from this transformed or 'preconditioned' muscle and demonstrated that the power output generated by these ventricular pumping chambers is sufficient to replace work done by the right ventricle or provide partial replacement or assistance of left ventricular function[12-18]. We have shown that these skeletal muscle ventricles (SMVs) can assume the function of the canine right ventricle in the circulation[19]. We have also utilized SMVs as diastolic counterpulsators in the circulation for several weeks[14,20,21].

SKELETAL MUSCLE PUMPING CHAMBERS – HISTORICAL REVIEW

Pumping chambers have been constructed from skeletal muscle by a number of investigators. The ultimate goal in these endeavors is to use these 'ventricles' to supply power for mechanical cardiac assist devices or to use them in the circulation directly as blood pumps. Skeletal muscle ventricles (SMVs) have been constructed from a variety of different muscles including the rectus abdominis, diaphragm, quadriceps femoris, pectoralis major, gluteus maximus, psoas, and latissimus dorsi. In our laboratory, SMVs have been constructed primarily from the latissimus dorsi muscle. We prefer the latissimus dorsi because of its single motor nerve, single main blood supply, ease of harvesting, minimal donor disability, and close proximity to the heart.

Kantrowitz, in 1959, wrapped the left leaf of the canine diaphragm around the descending thoracic aorta, creating a muscular tube[22,23]. The diaphragm was synchronously stimulated during diastole via the phrenic nerve. Diastolic augmentation of 15 mmHg was achieved, as well as a 26 mmHg increase in mean arterial pressure. These effects were maintained for only a few cardiac cycles, however, apparently due to muscle fatigue.

Kusserow, in 1964, was the first to use skeletal muscle as the power source for a mechanical cardiac assist device[24]. He did not construct a ventricle for this purpose, but instead used the rectus femoris in a linear configuration to exert force on a lever mechanism which served as the actuator for a bellows-type blood pump. The blood pump was connected to a hydraulic circuit which allowed calculation of flow and determination of outflow resistance. These pumps functioned in four dogs for 2–8 hours, generating flows of 600–720 ml/min against an afterload of 20 mmHg.

Spotnitz, in 1974, constructed skeletal muscle pouches from canine rectus muscle[25]. He found that their physical characteristics were similar to those of the heart as described by Frank and Starling. The transmural pressure, developed during active tension, increased as the resting wall tension (preload) was increased. The rectus muscle appeared to be less compliant than cardiac muscle. However, in his experiments with filling pressures of 50–150 mmHg, systolic pressures of greater than 500 mmHg could be obtained.

In 1975, Vachon et al. wrapped denervated pedicle grafts of diaphragm around a fluid-filled balloon pressure transducer, and allowed these ventricles to pump against a specified outflow resistance, allowing measurement of flow, power output, and isovolumetric pressure–volume relations[26]. The pouches were stimulated via stainless steel electrodes sewn into the muscle. With stimulation voltages of 30 volts, the muscle pouch generated up to 176 mmHg, the pressure decreasing proportionately with decreasing voltage. Peak pressure increased with increasing filling pressure. During these experiments, the pouches were able to generate a power output of 0.05 watts. They calculated the power output of the left and right ventricles as 0.335 watts and 0.0335 watts, respectively. Stimulation of these pouches was sustained for up to 3.5 hours.

Von Recum, Kantrowitz and co-workers in 1977 also constructed skeletal muscle pouches from diaphragm and stimulated the muscle directly[27]. In an attempt to minimize fatigue, stimulation voltages of 3–7 volts were employed. These ventricles were stimulated to contract isovolumetrically with a filling pressure of 18 mmHg. Peak pressures of approximately 60 mmHg were obtained in most experiments, and the pouches contracted continuously for up to 20 hours, although they fatigued rapidly during the initial 1–2 hours. Since the decline in pressure generation was progressive, these authors concluded that construction of an auxiliary ventricle from diaphragm was not feasible.

Juffe, in 1977, constructed pouch-like skeletal muscle pumping chambers from gluteus maximus muscle dissected free from its insertions[28]. A balloon transducer was introduced into the pouch and the muscle was stimulated via the gluteal nerve by a pacemaker. Pressures as high as 170 mmHg were recorded initially. Animals were sacrificed at regular intervals up to 26 days for histological studies. After 26 days of continuous stimulation, muscular atrophy occurred, probably as a result of nerve damage.

CONSTRUCTION OF SKELETAL MUSCLE VENTRICLES

The surgical technique for constructing a skeletal muscle ventricle is fairly straightforward[12-18]. The latissimus dorsi muscle is a large flat muscle overlying the back and flank. Its principal function is adduction of the forelimb. The muscle has attachments to the thoracic spine, the eleventh rib, the platysma, the trapezius, the teres major, the triceps, and inserts into the humerus. The blood supply comes from the thoracodorsal artery as well as numerous small arterial branches from the intercostal arteries. The thoracodorsal nerve supplies motor innervation.

The animal is anesthetized and the latissimus dorsi is mobilized through a flank incision extending from the axilla to the tip of the eleventh rib. The lesser blood supply from the overlying skin and the chest wall is divided. The attachments as mentioned above are also divided, leaving only the thoracodorsal neurovascular pedicle intact. A specially modified Medtronic pacing lead is placed around the proximal aspect of the thoracodorsal nerve. This lead is connected to a permanent implantable nerve stimulator.

The muscle is then wrapped or rolled around a previously machined Teflon mandrel of a given shape and size. The mandrel is either conically shaped when forming pouch-type ventricles, or cylindrically shaped to produce tube-type or flow-through ventricles. The mandrel also has a Teflon felt collar on one or both ends which ultimately acts as a sewing annulus. The wrapped muscle layers are sutured to each other as well as to the felt collar. The direction of the wrap is always such that the neurovascular pedicle is on the outside. Generally $1\frac{1}{2}$–$2\frac{1}{2}$ muscle wraps are obtained. The skeletal muscle ventricle can be placed inside the thoracic cavity or left on the chest wall under the skin and subcutaneous tissue. The skeletal muscle ventricle is sutured to the surrounding tissues to prevent migration or kinking of the pedicle. The subcutaneous tissue and skin are then closed over the SMV.

The skeletal muscle ventricle is allowed to rest for a 3-week vascular delay period. Although the neurovascular pedicle supplies an adequate blood supply to prevent immediate muscle necrosis at the time of mobilization, division of the blood supply from the intercostal arteries during construction renders the muscle relatively ischemic. Immediately following skeletal muscle ventricular construction, the distal half of the muscle is unable to increase its blood flow in response to the increased demands of exercise. A 3-week vascular delay period, however, allows for recovery of resting and exercise-induced increases in blood flow[29]. Using radiolabelled microspheres, Mannion et al. demonstrated that all layers of a skeletal muscle ventricle receive substantial blood flow following the vascular delay period while the ventricles are pumping in the circulation[16].

SKELETAL MUSCLE VENTRICLE PRECONDITIONING

Skeletal muscle can be divided into two basic types, one of which has relatively fatigue-resistant properties. Slow-twitch (Type I) fibers are characterized by prolonged contraction time, a large mitochondrial volume, aerobic metabolism even under prolonged periods of stimulation, and a specific complement of 'slow' contractile proteins. Muscles composed of predominantly slow-twitch fibers are usually postural in function and fatigue slowly. Fast-twitch (Type II) fibers are characterized by brisk contraction time, a relatively small mitochondrial volume, anaerobic metabolism during stimulation, and a fast set of contractile proteins.

Typical fast muscle, such as an eye muscle, is used for quick, intense episodic activity and fatigues rapidly with prolonged stimulation.

During the past 20 years, a considerable amount of biochemical research on the adaptive capabilities of skeletal muscle has been performed. Skeletal muscle changes its physiologic, biochemical and structural characteristics in response to intense exercise and electrical stimulation. The classic experiments of Buller, Eccles and Eccles showed that the nerve was able to modulate the properties of the muscle[30,31]. In those experiments, the motor nerve of a fast-twitch muscle was switched with the motor nerve of a slow-twitch muscle. When the nerves regenerated, the fast muscle became slow and the slow muscle became fast. In 1969, Salmons and Vrbova determined that it was the pattern of stimulation of the motor nerve which governed the muscle fiber type[32]. When a fast-twitch muscle was stimulated for several weeks at 10 Hz, the fibers were converted to a uniform population of slow-twitch, fatigue-resistant type I fibers. These transformed, fatigue-resistant fibers more closely resemble cardiac muscle than ordinary type I fibers, both in terms of mitochondrial content and oxidative enzyme complements[33,34].

To understand fatigue resistance induced by chronic stimulation, we used phosphorus nuclear magnetic resonance spectroscopy to study the bioenergetics of electrically conditioned canine latissimus dorsi muscle in vivo. We found that increased resistance to fatigue is related to an increased capacity of oxidative phosphorylation, which is most likely due to increased mitochondrial volume[35]. Since the capacity for oxidative phosphorylation is increased, adenosine triphosphate (ATP) production by the muscle can match the sustained increase in ATP utilization. The decline in phosphocreatine and accumulation of adenosine diphosphate (ADP) and inorganic phosphate, which usually accompany muscle fatigue, are absent.

As in the heart, resistance to fatigue of the conditioned muscle appears to derive from a highly developed aerobic capacity that supports efficient re-cycling of ADP to ATP and prevents the accumulation of inorganic phosphate. The increased ability to utilize oxygen during isometric exercise also contributes to the fatigue resistance of electrically conditioned skeletal muscle[36]. Conditioned muscle is homogeneously slow, and cross-bridge cycling, and therefore ATP consumption, of slow-twitch fibers is significantly slower than that of fast-twitch fibers. The rate of cycling of cross-bridges determines the energy cost for the maintenance of tension, and a given isometric tension is therefore maintained with less hydrolysis of ATP, and less oxygen is consumed by electrically conditioned canine muscle than control muscle for identical isometric tension.

Mannion et al. showed that the combination of a vascular delay period and electrical preconditioning allowed construction of fatigue-resistant skeletal muscle ventricles[15].

Fatigue resistance can be achieved using 2–10 Hz continuous stimulation, or using a 25 Hz burst stimulation pattern, more suited to cardiac type work[12,32,37–41]. In addition, we have shown that skeletal muscle ventricles (SMVs) fashioned from the latissimus dorsi muscle can be rendered fatigue-resistant while performing useful work in vivo[13,14]. Thus a preconditioning period may not be absolutely necessary before these ventricles can be put to work in the circulation.

SKELETAL MUSCLE VENTRICLES *IN VIVO*

Contractility reflects the intensity of the active state of the muscle. Unlike the heart, which is an electrical and mechanical syncytium, skeletal muscle is modulated by the number and rate at which fibers are activated[42]. It has been demonstrated by Dewar and associates[43], as well as by our laboratory[15], that single electrical stimulus, resulting in a single muscle twitch, does not normally generate sufficient force to augment cardiac function. However, rapid repetitive stimuli, delivered before the muscle fiber completes its relaxation, result in mechanical summation (until fusion occurs), which thereby causes the muscle to generate substantial force[44]. The burst stimulation frequency of the SMV governs the cumulative duration of the active state of the skeletal muscle and produces an effect similar to the contractility of the heart. Increasing the burst frequency of the SMV produces more work.

Skeletal muscle ventricles in mock circulation

In earlier studies, SMVs were constructed as described above using a 17 ml cone-shaped mandrel. These SMVs underwent a 3-week vascular delay period followed by 6 weeks of electrical preconditioning. The SMVs were then connected to a totally implantable mock circulation device[12]. This device allowed control of both preload and afterload, and measurement of SMV output. No wires or tubes crossed the animal's skin barrier. The animals were able to move about freely with no apparent discomfort or physical impairment. The muscles were stimulated via the thoracodorsal nerve with a 25 Hz burst frequency (312 ms on, 812 ms off), resulting in 54 contractions per minute. These SMVs pumped continuously against an afterload of 80 mmHg with a preload of 40–50 mmHg. At the initiation of pumping, mean systolic pressure was 134 mmHg and flow was 464 ml/min. After 2 weeks of continuous pumping, systolic pressure was 104 mmHg and flow was 206 ml/min. Two SMVs pumped for 5 and 9 weeks, respectively.

In a subsequent study[13], SMVs were constructed with a vascular delay period but without preconditioning. These SMVs were connected to the mock circulation system and stimulated via the thoracodorsal nerve at a 25 Hz burst frequency, as in the previous study. Preload and afterload were again set at 40 mmHg and 80 mmHg, respectively. After 2 weeks of continuous pumping, the mean stroke work of the SMVs was 0.4×10^6 ergs. The stroke work of these SMVs was intermediate between that of the canine left and right ventricles. Two dogs continued to produce significant stroke work after 2 months. Using SMVs constructed from canine rectus abdominis muscle, Stevens and Brown measured similar heart and SMV work outputs during acute studies[45].

Skeletal muscle ventricles as arterial diastolic counterpulsators

Working in our laboratory, Mannion et al. showed that properly conditioned SMVs with a vascular delay were able to function in the circulation for up to 14 hours as diastolic counterpulsators in the descending aorta[17,18]. SMV function eventually deteriorated, however, due to anemia, hypoxia, hypotension, and other complications inherent to prolonged acute experiments of this type. The stroke work of these SMVs was 0.68×10^6 ergs after 4 hours, roughly 3 times the stroke work of the right ventricle and nearly half the left ventricular stroke work.

These acute studies documented the ability of an SMV to do useful work in the circulation, while the mock circulation studies demonstrated the ability of SMVs to function for up to 2 months pumping against physiological afterloads. Neilson, Chiu and associates showed an improvement in the subendocardial viability ratio during acute studies when SMVs were used in circulation as diastolic counterpulsators[46]. Taken together, these studies suggested that a chronic circulatory assist device could be constructed from skeletal muscle.

Acker et al.[14] subsequently constructed skeletal muscle tube ventricles (SMTVs) in five mongrel dogs. The SMTV differed from the ventricles constructed in previous experiments, since these ventricles had a cylindrical geometry with both inflow and outflow conduits as depicted in Figure 66.1. The SMTVs functioned chronically in the circulation as diastolic counterpulsators. The SMTVs were connected to the systemic circulation after a 3–4-week vascular delay period, but without electrical preconditioning. The SMTVs were stimulated to contract during diastole, generally with a synchronization ratio of 1:2 or 1:3, depending on the heart rate. A totally implantable Medtronic R-wave synchronous burst stimulator was used to activate the SMTVs via the thoracodorsal nerve. This pacemaker delivered burst stimuli at 25–85 Hz, with a burst duration of 185–240 ms and a 340-ms delay from the onset of the R-wave. These animals were tether-free and no tubes or wires crossed the skin. They moved about freely with no apparent discomfort or impairment.

Two-dimensional short-axis echocardiograms of the

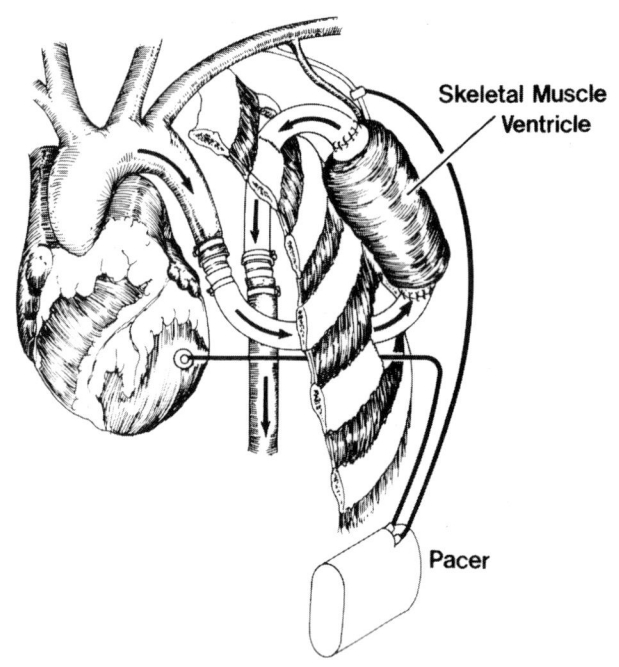

Figure 66.1 Skeletel muscle tube ventricle (SMTV) interposed into the descending aorta for use as a diastolic arterial counterpulsator. The pacemaker stimulating electrode is connected to the thoracodorsal nerve and the sensing electrode to the left ventricle

SMTV obtained from one dog after 12 days of continuous counterpulsation are shown in Figure 66.2. During these measurements, the burst frequency was altered from the chronic setting of 25 Hz to 43 Hz and then to 85 Hz. These echograms demonstrate a 70%, 90% and 100% decrease in cross-sectional area at the midpoint of the SMTV at 25 Hz, 43 Hz and 85 Hz, respectively during SMTV contraction. Pulsed Doppler blood flow just distal to the outlet end of the SMTV during a normal cardiac cycle was compared to that during an assisted cardiac cycle (SMTV contraction). The forward blood flow was 29%, 40% and 63% greater during the assisted cardiac cycle than the unassisted normal cycle at 25, 43 and 85 Hz, respectively. Arterial pressure tracings obtained from the same dog after 14 days of continuous pumping at these three burst frequencies are shown in Figure 66.3.

These SMTVs functioned in circulation for up to 11 weeks. In all animals the SMTV was functioning until termination. The longest two survivors, 5 weeks and 11 weeks, respectively, both died due to complications of renal failure. Autopsy demonstrated multiple renal and splenic infarcts, without evidence of cerebrovascular or coronary thromboembolic disease. Despite these complications, this study demonstrated for the first time that skeletal muscle could perform significant circulatory assistance for several weeks.

In a subsequent study we developed a mechanical pump that replaces a portion of the thoracic aorta and is powered by an SMV[20,21]. This mechanical pump was designed to

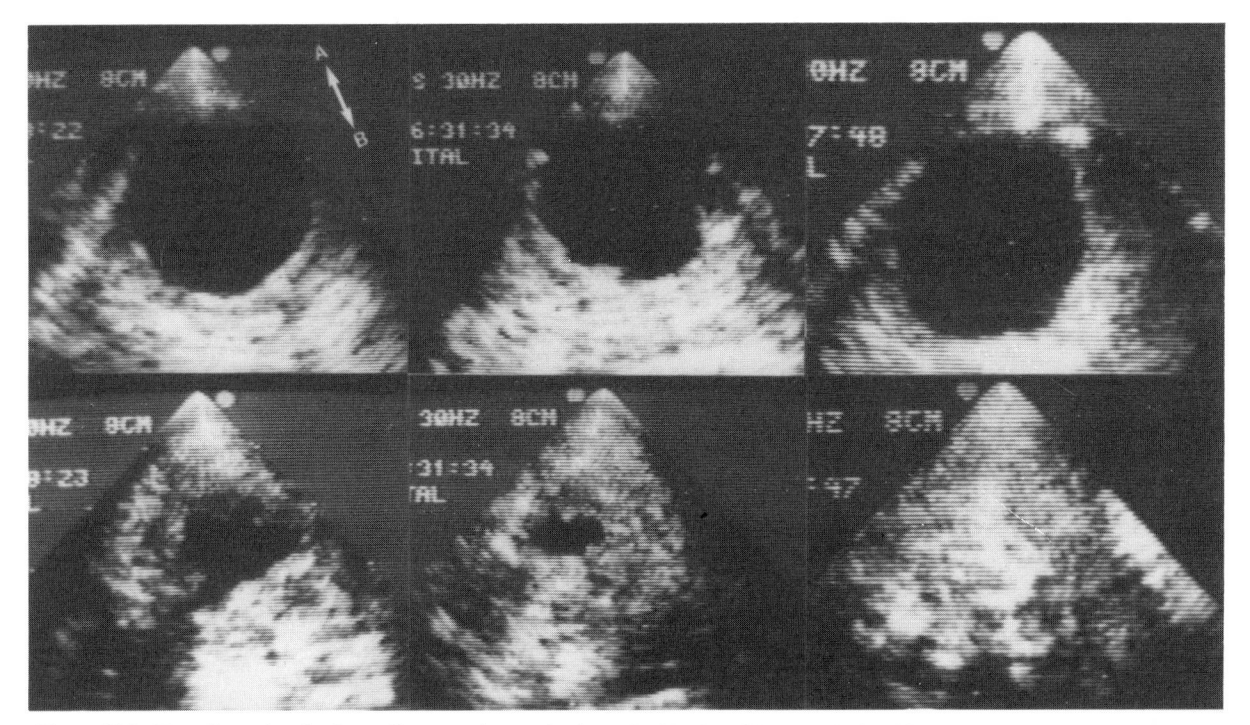

Figure 66.2 Two-dimensional echocardiogram, short axis view, of midpoint of SMTV obtained from one dog on postoperative day 12. Top row illustrates the cross-sectional area during relaxation. Bottom row illustrates the cross-sectional area during contraction. Increasing the burst frequency (25 Hz, 43 Hz, 85 Hz) leads to increasing ejection fraction

avoid thromboembolic complications by minimization of the blood–surface contact area and use of relatively thrombo-resistant polyurethane at the blood interface. The device was cylindrical with tapered ends to simplify the aortic connection (Figure 66.4). Silastic tubing connected the pump device to a polyurethane bladder inserted into the SMV. The pump device was pressurized with air. As the SMV contracted, air pressure was transferred from the SMV bladder to the pump membrane, which then evacuated blood from within the chamber. When the SMV relaxed, the descending thoracic aortic blood volume flowed directly through the pump chamber (Figure 66.4).

At the completion of this operation, the burst stimulator was activated at a burst frequency of 25 Hz, pulse duration 0.210 ms, burst duration of 240 ms, R-wave delay of 225 ms, and supramaximal voltage (4–6 volts). The stimulator delivered impulses at a ratio of 1:1, 1:2, 1:3 or 1:4 in synchrony with cardiac diastole. This ratio was dependent on the program mode selected and on the native heart rate of the animal (Mode I – 1:1 at a heart rate of less than 100 beats/min, 1:2 at a heart rate between 100 and 200 beats/min; Mode II – 1:2 at a heart rate less than 100 beats/min, 1:3 at a heart rate between 100 and 150 beats/min and 1:4 at a heart rate between 150 and 200 beats/min).

At the time of implantation, SMV intracavity pressure was $134/70 \pm 10/8$ mmHg but could be increased to $190/70 \pm 8/8$ mmHg by increasing the burst frequency to 85 Hz ($n = 4$). Aortic diastolic augmentation ranged from 31 ± 3 to 68 ± 8 mmHg, depending on the burst frequency used (25 vs. 85 Hz). Blood flows were measured in the distal thoracic aorta in one dog and were 34, 36 and 39% greater during the assisted cardiac cycle at 25, 43 and 85 Hz, respectively.

The SMVs continued to augment the aortic diastolic pressure for up to 42 days, the amount of augmentation depending on the dogs' blood pressure and the electrical burst pattern used. At the time of final measurement, SMV intracavity pressure was $126/53 \pm 10/7$ mmHg at 25 Hz and $156/52 \pm 7/6$ mmHg at 85 Hz burst frequency.

Three of the four dogs succumbed to disruption of the aorta at either the proximal or distal connection to the pump device. The other animal succumbed to a pneumonia/empyema in the left chest. None of the dogs died as a result of thromboemboli, and no thromboemboli were detected at autopsy in two of the four dogs, including the one who survived the longest.

Right heart bypass

Most recently, in acute studies, we have used skeletal muscle ventricles to totally replace the native canine right heart function[19]. SMVs were constructed in mongrel dogs, and, after a 3-week vascular delay period, these SMVs were

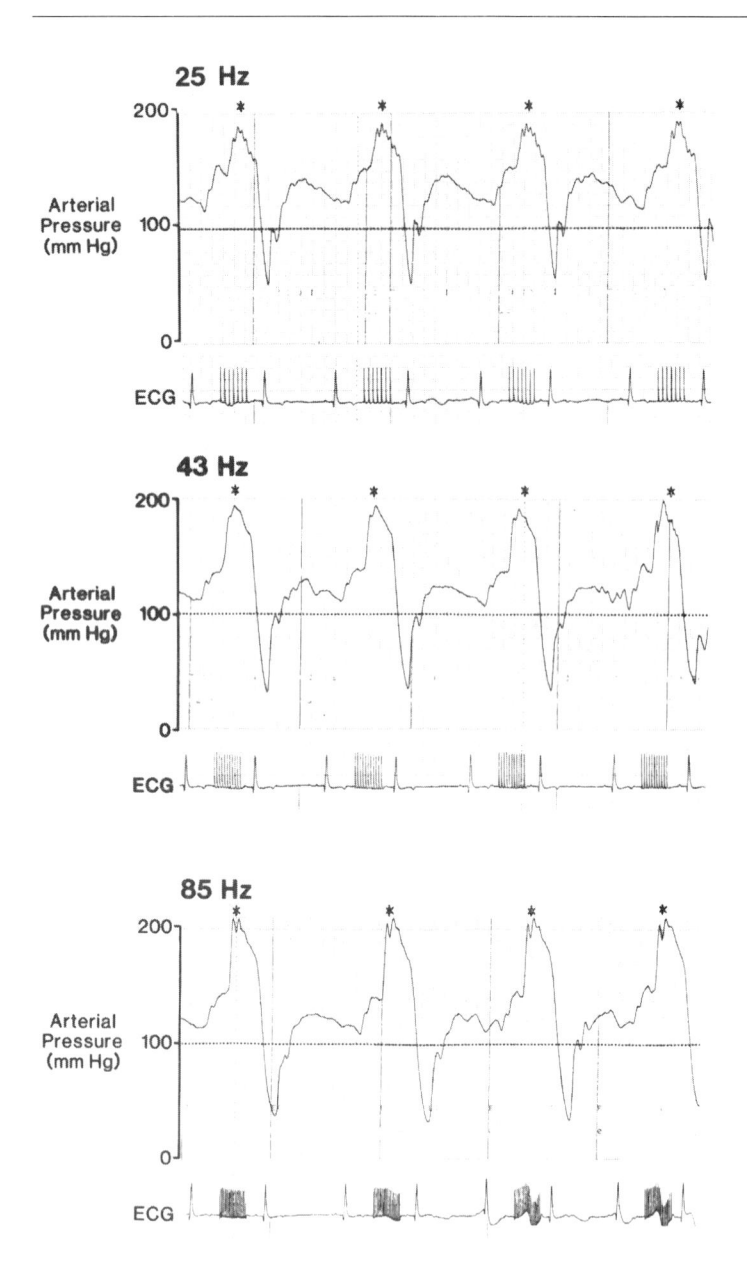

Figure 66.3 Distal aortic pressure and electrocardiogram tracings in the same dog as in Figure 66.2 on postoperative day 14 at burst frequencies of 25 Hz, 43 Hz and 85 Hz. Diastolic augmentation of 130 mmHg occurs at 85 Hz burst frequency. (*) indicates diastolic augmentation. Note corresponding superimposed burst pattern on electrocardiogram

electrically conditioned at 2 Hz for 4–6 weeks. These ventricles were constructed using large (55 ml) Teflon mandrels, resulting in higher compliance SMVs – ideally suited for low pressure work. During the second operation after electrical preconditioning, total systemic venous return was routed to these high compliance SMVs, and SMV outflow was delivered into the pulmonary artery.

These SMVs were stimulated using a synchronous burst pattern as described above and generally contracted at a rate of 1:2 with cardiac systole. An ultrasonic flow probe in the SMV outflow circuit was used to monitor cardiac (and SMV) output. Complete right heart bypass was documented by absence of flow and extreme hypotension with the SMV circuit occluded. Opening the SMV circuit allowed passive flow from the systemic venous system through the pulmonary bed, which is somewhat analogous to the physiology with the Fontan procedure. With passive flow, however, systemic systolic blood pressures were only 50–60 mmHg.

With stimulation of the SMV, systolic blood pressure increased to 100–110 mmHg and CVP decreased as well. After 2 hours of continuous pumping, SMV stroke work was 169% of normal canine right ventricular stroke work, and after 4 hours stroke work was 174% of canine right ventricular stroke work (Figure 66.5).

Total right heart bypass was accomplished in some dogs for periods of up to 8 hours, at which time the experiment was terminated. Macoviak has also studied right heart bypass in dogs using SMVs of his own design[47]. These results hold promise for patients with congenital cardiac defects associated with a single functioning ventricle such as the hypoplastic right or left heart syndromes. Development of a chronic model is currently under way.

BLOOD PUMPS FROM SKELETAL MUSCLE

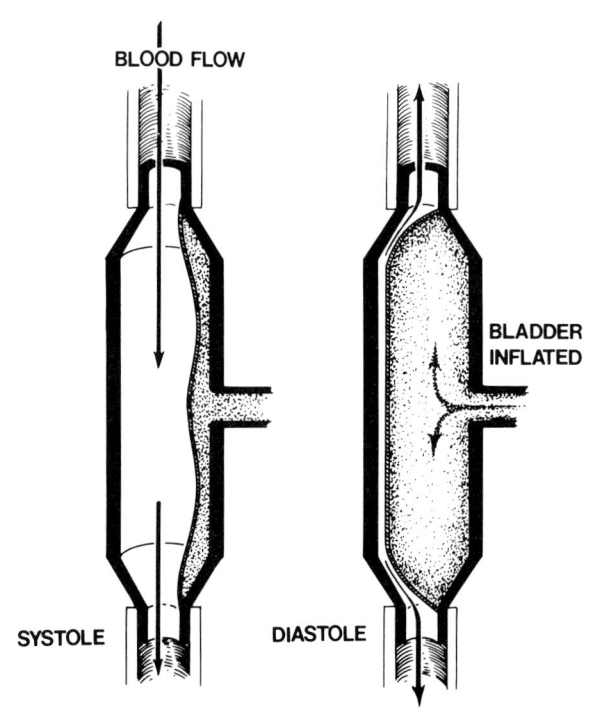

Figure 66.4 A pneumatic aortic counterpulsator device powered by a skeletal muscle ventricle (SMV). During cardiac systole, blood within the thoracic aorta flows directly through the pump device. During cardiac diastole, the SMV is stimulated to contract, transferring air pressure to the pump membrane, which then evacuates blood from within the chamber, and thus augments the aortic diastolic blood pressure

COMMENT

The extraordinary capacity of skeletal muscle to respond adaptively to an increased level of use allows construction of pumping chambers capable of performing cardiac work. Although more studies are required, potential applications of this phenomenon are enormous. Skeletal muscle pumping chambers can conceivably assist or even replace the right or left ventricle. Clinical application may improve the outlook for infants with complex congenital heart defects as well as for patients with end-stage heart failure.

Several issues must be resolved, however, before it can be determined whether muscle pumps will prove clinically feasible. We found some muscle fibrosis in chronic studies, but we do not know whether or not the fibrosis is progressive. However, in muscle *in situ* stimulated continously for 1 year, we did not observe muscle damage[38]. Finally, the means to couple SMVs to the circulation need further study, and problems of blood non-endothelial cell surface interaction, flow direction, and sites of coupling must be addressed.

Acknowledgements

Some of the research discussed in this chapter was supported by NIH Grant #HLBI 34778 and by the John Rhea Barton Research Foundation.

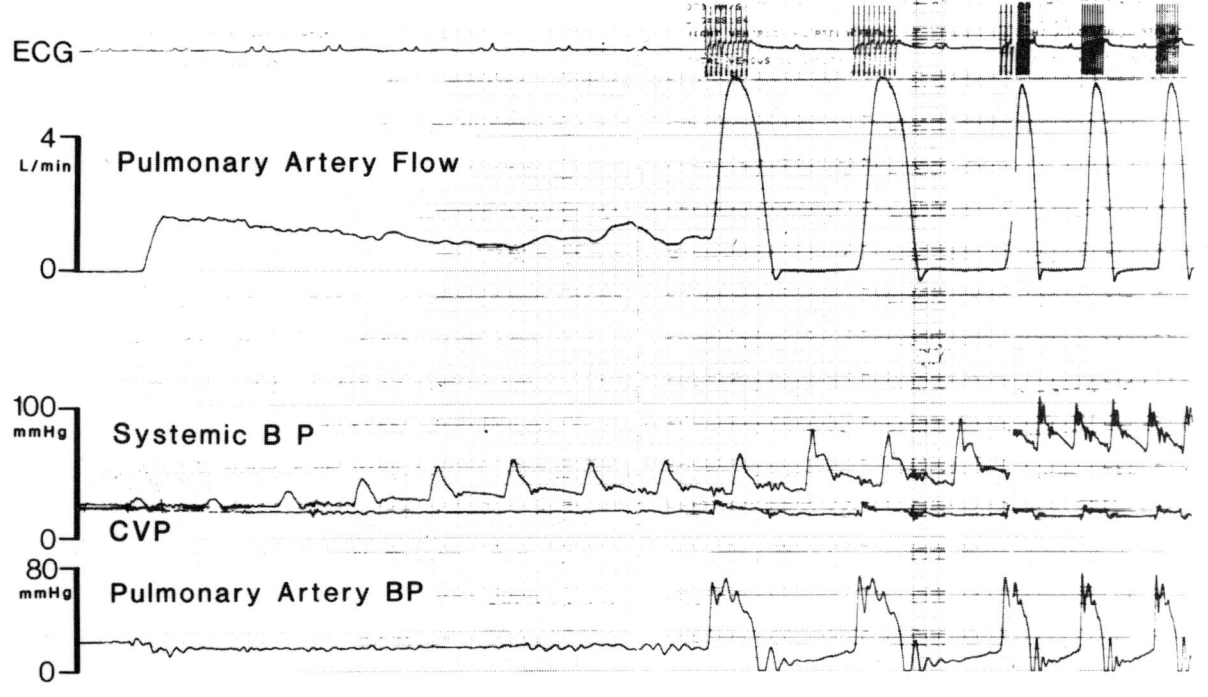

Figure 66.5 Results of total right heart bypass. From top to bottom tracings are ECG, pulmonary artery blood flow, systemic blood pressure, CVP, and pulmonary artery blood pressure. Shown from left to right are: (1) total occlusion of the SMV circuit (flow = 0); (2) open SMV circuit, SMV off (Fontan physiology); and (3) open SMV circuit, SMV on (total right heart bypass). Note that the SMV contracts at 1:2 in synchrony with the left ventricle, and generates peak flows greater than 5 l/min

References

1. Leriche, R. and Fontaine, R. (1933). Essai experimental de traitement de certains infarctus du myocarde et de l'anevrisme du coeur par une greffe de muscle strie. *Bull. Soc. Nat. Chir.*, **59**, 229
2. Beck, C.S. (1935). A new blood supply to the heart by operation. *Surg. Gynec. Obstet.*, **61**, 407
3. Petrovsky, B.V. (1961). The use of the diaphragm grafts for plastic operations in thoracic surgery. *J. Thorac. Cardiovasc. Surg.*, **41**, 348
4. Petrovsky, B.V. (1966). Surgical treatment of cardiac aneurysms. *J. Cardiovasc. Surg.* (Torino), **2**, 87
5. Macoviak, J.A., Stephenson, L.W., Spielman, S., Greenspan, A. Likoff, M., St. John-Sutton, M., Riechek, N., Rashkind, W.J. and Edmunds, L.H. Jr. (1980). Elecrophysiological and mechanical characteristics of diaphragmatic autograft used to enlarge the right ventricle. *Surg. Forum.*, **31**, 270
6. Macoviak, J.A., Stephenson, L.W., Spielman, S., Greenspan, A., Likoff, M., St. John-Sutton, M., Riechek, N., Rashkind, W.J. and Edmunds, L.H. Jr. (1981). Replacement of ventricular myocardium with diaphragmatic skeletal muscle: short-term studies. *J. Thorac. Cardiovasc. Surg.*, **81**, 519
7. Macoviak, J.A., Stephenson, L.W., Alavi, A., Kelly, A.M. and Edmunds, L.H. Jr. (1981). Effects of electrical stimulation on diaphragmatic muscle used to enlarge the right ventricle. *Surgery*, **90**, 271
8. Macoviak, J.A., Stephenson, L.W., Kelly, A., Likoff, M., Riechek, N. and Edmunds, L.H. Jr. (1981). Partial replacement of the right ventricle with a synchronously contracting diaphragmatic skeletal muscle autograft. *Proceedings of the Third Meeting of the International Society for Artificial Organs*, **5**, (Suppl. I), 550
9. Anderson, W.A., Andersen, J.S., Acker, M.A., Hammond, R.L., Chin, A.J., Douglas, P.S., Salmons, S. and Stephenson, L.W. (1988). Skeletal muscle applied to the heart: a word of caution. *Circulation*, **78**, III 180
10. Magovern, G.J., Park, S.B., Magovern, G.J. Jr, Benckart, D.H., Tullis, G., Rozar, E., Keo, R. and Christlieb, I. (1986). Latissimus dorsi as a functioning synchronously paced muscle component in the repair of a left ventricular aneurysm. *Ann. Thorac. Surg.*, **41**, 116
11. Carpentier, A. and Chachques, J.C. (1985). Myocardial substitution with a stimulated skeletal muscle: first successful clinical case. *Lancet*, **1**, 1267
12. Acker, M.A., Hammond, R.L., Mannion, J.D., Salmons, S. and Stephenson, L.W. (1986). An autologous biologic pump motor. *J. Thorac. Cardiovasc. Surg.*, **92**, 733
13. Acker, M.A., Hammond, R.L., Mannion, J.D., Salmons, S. and Stephenson, L.W. (1987). Skeletal muscle as the potential power source for a cardiovascular pump: assessment *in vivo*. *Science*, **236**, 324
14. Acker, M.A., Anderson, W.A., Hammond, R.L., Chin, .J., Buchanan, J.W., Morse, C.C., Kelly, A.M. and Stephenson, L.W. (1987). Skeletal muscle ventricles in circulation: one to eleven weeks experience. *J. Thorac. Cardiovasc. Surg.*, **94**, 163
15. Mannion, J.D., Hammond, R.L. and Stephenson, L.W. (1986). Hydraulic pouches of canine latissimus dorsi: potential for left ventricular assistance. *J. Thorac. Cardiovasc. Surg.*, **91**, 534
16. Mannion, J.D., Velchik, M.A., Acker, M., Hammond, R.L., Staum, M., Alavi, A., Duckett, S. and Stephenson, L.W. (1986). Transmural blood flow of multi-layered latissimus dorsi skeletal muscle ventricles during circulatory assistance. *Trans. Am. Soc. Artif. Intern. Organs*, **32**, 454
17. Mannion, J.D., Acker, M.A., Hammond, R.L. and Stephenson, L.W. (1986). Four-hour circulatory assistance with canine skeletal muscle ventricles. *Surg. Forum*, **37**, 211
18. Mannion, J.D., Acker, M.A., Hammond, R.L., Faltemeyer, W., Duckett, S. and Stephenson, L.W. (1987). Power output of skeletal muscle ventricles in circulation: short-term studies. *Circulation*, **76**, 155
19. Bridges, C.R., Anderson, W.A., Hammond, R.L., Andersen, J.S. and Stephenson, L.W. (1989). Functional right heart replacement with a skeletal muscle. *Circulation*, **80**, III 183
20. Anderson, W.A., Bridges, C.R., Chin, A.J., Andersen, J.S., Acker, M.A., Hammond, R.L. and Stephenson, L.W. (1988). Pneumatic aortic counterpulsator powered by skeletal muscle ventricle: 22 to 42 day experience. *Surg. Forum*, **39**, 276
21. Anderson, W.A., Bridges, C.R., Chin, A.J., Andersen, J.S., Acker, M.A., Hammond, R.L., Dimeo, F., Cahalan, P.T., Gale, D.R., Brown, W.E. and Stephenson, L.W. (1990). Long-term stimulation of skeletal muscle: its potential for tether-free biologic cardiac assist device. *Pace*, **11**, 2128
22. Kantrowitz, A. and McKinnon, W. (1959). The experimental use of the diaphragm as an auxiliary myocardium. *Surg. Forum*, **9**, 266
23. Kantrowitz, A. (1960). Functioning autogenous muscle used experimentally as an auxiliary ventricle. *Trans. Am. Soc. Artif. Intern. Organs*, **6**, 305
24. Kusserow, B.K. and Clapp, J.F. (1964). A small ventricle-type pump for prolonged perfusions: construction and initial studies including attempts to power a pump biologically with skeletal muscle. *Trans. Am. Soc. Artif. Intern. Organs*, **10**, 74
25. Spotnitz, H.M., Merker, C. and Malm, J.R. (1974). Applied physiology of the canine rectus abdominis. *Trans. Am. Soc. Artif. Intern. Organs*, **20**, 747
26. Vachon, B.R., Kunov, H. and Zingg, W. (1975). Mechanical properties of diaphragm muscles in dogs. *Med. Biol. Eng.*, **13**, 252
27. Von Recum, A., Stulc, J.P., Hamada, O., Baba, J. and Kantrowitz, A. (1977). Long-term stimulation of a diaphragm muscle pouch. *J. Surg. Res.*, **23**, 422
28. Juffe, A., Ricoy, J.R., Marquez, J., Castillo-Olivares, J.L. and Figuera, D. (1978). Cardialization: a new source of energy for circulatory assistance. *Vasc. Surg.*, **12**, 10
29. Mannion, J.D., Velchik, M., Alavi, A. and Stephenson, L.W. (1985). Blood flow in conditioned and unconditioned latissimus dorsi muscle (Abstract). *Second Vienna Muscle Symposium*, p. 28
30. Buller, A.J., Eccles, J.C. and Eccles, R.M. (1960). Differentiation of fast and slow muscles in the cat hind limb. *J. Physiol.*, **150**, 399
31. Buller, A.J., Eccles, J.C. and Eccles, R.M. (1960). Interactions between motor neurons and muscles in respect of the characteristic speeds of their responses. *J. Physiol.*, **150**, 417
32. Salmons, S. and Vrbova, G. (1969). The influence of activity on some contractile characteristics of mammalian fast and slow muscles. *J. Physiol.*, **210**, 535
33. Pette, D., Muller, W., Leisner, E. and Vrbova, G. (1976). Time dependent effects on contractile properties, fiber population, myosin light chains and enzymes of energy metabolism in intermittently and continously stimulated fast-twitch muscles of the rabbit. *Pfleugers. Arch.*, **364**, 103
34. Henry, C.G. and Lowry, O.H. (1983). Quantitative histochemistry of canine cardiac Purkinje fibers. *Am. J. Physiol.*, **245**, H824
35. Clark, B.J., Acker, M.A., Subramanian, H., McCully, K., Hammond, B., Salmons, S., Chance, B. and Stephenson, L.W. (1988). *In vivo* P-NMR spectroscopy of electrically conditioned skeletal muscle. *Am. J. Physiol.*, **254**, C258
36. Acker, M.A., Anderson, W.A., Hammond, R.L., Dimeo, F., McCullum, J., Staum, M., Velchik, M., Brown, W.E., Gale, D., Salmons, S. and Stephenson, L.W. (1987). Oxygen consumption of chronically stimulated skeletal muscle. *J. Thorac. Cardiovasc. Surg.*, **94**, 702
37. Salmons, S. and Henriksson, J. (1981). The adaptive response of skeletal muscle to increased use. *Muscle Nerve*, **4**, 94
38. Acker, M.A., Mannion, J.D., Brown, W.E., Salmons, S., Henriksson, J., Bitto, T., Gale, D.R., Hammond, R. and Stephenson, L.W. (1987). Canine diaphragm muscle after one year of continuous electrical stimulation: its potential as a myocardial substitute. *J. Appl. Physiol.*, **62**, 1264
39. Armenti, F.R., Bitto, T., Macoviak, J.A., Kelly, A.M., Chase, C.T., Hoffman, B.K., Rubenstein, N.A., St. John-Sutton, M., Edmunds, L.H. Jr. and Stephenson, L.W. (1984). Transformation of canine diaphragm to fatigue-resistant muscle by phrenic nerve stimulation. *Surg. Forum*,

35, 258
40. Macoviak, J.A., Stephenson, L.W., Armenti, F., Kelly, A.M., Alavi, A., Mackler, T., Cox, J., Palatianos, G.M. and Edmunds, L.H. Jr. (1982). Electrical conditioning of *in situ* skeletal muscle for replacement of myocardium. *J. Surg. Res.*, **32**, 429
41. Mannion, J.D., Bitto, T., Hammond, R.L., Rubenstein, N.A. and Stephenson, L.W. (1986). Histochemical and fatigue characteristics of conditioned canine latissimus dorsi muscle. *Circ. Res.*, **58**, 298
42. Johnson, E. (1979). Force-interval relationship of cardiac muscle. In Berna, R.M. (ed.) *Handbook of Physiology*, Vol. 1, Section 2, p. 475. (Bethesda: American Physiological Society)
43. Dewar, M.L., Drinkwater, D.C., Wittnich, C. and Chiu, R.C. (1984). Synchronously stimulated skeletal muscle graft for myocardial repair. *J. Thorac. Cardiovasc. Surg.*, **87**, 325
44. Carlson, F.D. and Wilkie, D.R. (1974). *Muscle Physiology*, p. 33. (Englewood: Prentice Hall)
45. Stevens, L. and Brown, J. (1986). Can non-cardiac muscle provide useful cardiac assistance? Preliminary studies of the properties of skeletal muscle. *Am. Surg.*, **52**, 423
46. Neilson, I.R., Brister, S.J., Khalafalla, A.S. and Chiu, R.C.J. (1985). Left ventricular assistance in dogs using a skeletal muscle powered device for diastolic augmentation. *J. Heart Transplant.*, **4**, 343
47. Macoviak, J.A., Stinson, E.B., Starkey, T.D., Hansen, D.E., Cahill, P.D., Miller, D.C. and Shumway, N.E. (1987). Myoventriculoplasty and neoventricle myograft cardiac augmentation to establish pulmonary blood flow: preliminary observations and feasibility studies. *J. Thorac. Cardiovasc. Surg.*, **92**, 212

Section VIII

The future of thoracic organ replacement

67
Some Ethical and Logistic Issues in Transplantation

R.W. EVANS

INTRODUCTION

Over the past several years much attention has focused on what is commonly referred to as the 'ethics of transplantation'[1-9]. Although acceptance of ethical analysis in transplantation is relatively recent, ethicists have actively contributed to medicine for many years. Today there is little question that their contributions to transplantation specifically, and medicine more generally, have been both significant, yet controversial. As medicine becomes increasingly technological, often giving rise to uncertainties over the central matter of life and death, ethicists are frequently called upon to intervene in situations where science has accomplished what it can, and morality becomes both unclear and uncertain[10-14]. In short, physicians and surgeons recognize that the dilemma of high technology in medicine includes changes in their role expectations as the providers of care to sick individuals.

Organ transplantation very poignantly illustrates what might be referred to as the 'crucible of life and death'. With the exception of living-related donor kidney transplantation, a life must end to sustain another. Most often, a personal tragedy has occurred, and an individual has been declared brain-dead. The family of the deceased is asked to consider organ donation and, upon their consent, the organs of the deceased are offered for transplantation. This, of course, will be to the delight of another individual who, in the case of heart and liver transplantation, is dying with an end-stage disease for which no treatment option other than transplantation exists.

Unfortunately, there are far fewer organs available than are needed by people on the transplant waiting list. Table 67.1 succinctly summarizes the nature of the problem as it exists in the United States today. Since not every patient in need will benefit, a wide array of ethical issues arises. Some of these are what might be referred to as 'process' issues. For example, who is the best candidate for transplant? How should transplant recipients be selected? Is it possible to

Table 67.1 The organ transplantation crucible – donor organ potential demand and supply

Transplant	Need Estimates	Number of people currently on waiting list‡	Annual supply of donor organs
Kidney (cadaveric)	13 703*	13 703	4 000
Heart	14 500†	981	1 600
Liver	9 500	552	2 000

*On dialysis awaiting transplant; † Number of people who die annually of conditions for which transplantation is indicated; ‡ United Network for Organ Sharing (Richmond, Virginia) waiting list (October, 1988)

assure that each patient is treated fairly and equitably? Should patients who have received a previous transplant be given an opportunity to receive a second or a third graft?

Some process issues are related to organ donation. For example, how can we most effectively improve the supply of donor organs without jeopardizing the moral 'fabric' of our existing organ procurement system? Should families be offered financial remuneration for the organs of a loved one? Should we approach families more aggressively concerning organ donation? Should we routinely remove organs from brain-dead cadavers without consulting the families involved?[15,16]. Clearly, one can identify a myriad of process issues that are central to the whole activity simply referred to as 'transplantation'.

Another set of issues is less concerned with the 'how to' of transplantation, but is organizational in nature. For example, we can evaluate transplantation within the broader perspective of health care. In this regard we might ask, is a disproportionate share of societal resources devoted to transplantation? Would resources committed to transplantation be better spent on preventive health care or maternal and child health care initiatives? Should ability to pay be a consideration in determining who should benefit from a transplant? Should age be a consideration in determinations of who will maximally benefit? What is the value of a human life in our society? All these issues are complex, and can hardly be dealt with in the abstract. We must surely adopt a wider perspective to appreciate the complexity of these issues[17,18].

While the foregoing distinction between process and organizational issues is useful, it is readily apparent that the two sets of issues overlap. Therefore, in the remainder of this chapter I will focus on general topics, and incorporate appropriate discussion of both the process and organization issues. The primary topics are as follows: (1) organ procurement, (2) patient selection, (3) cost and reimbursement, (4) quality of life, and (5) resource allocation.

ORGAN PROCUREMENT

In general, it is believed that there are many more potential organ donors than the procurement system is able to access. Based on our research at Battelle, we have either developed, or identified, various ranges of estimates[19-22]. These estimates are summarized in Table 67.2. Comparing these estimates with those in Table 67.1, it is evident that much remains to be done to meet the need for donor organs in the United States.

Estimates such as those in Table 67.2 have given rise to much discussion as to how we can make our procurement efforts more successful. Some people have suggested that much more could be done with organ donor cards[23]. Yet our research indicates that donor cards are an effective means by which to educate people, but relatively unproductive with respect to actual donors. Routine inquiry and required request legislation has been passed at both the state and federal levels with little real benefit realized at this time[24]. Presumed consent has been advocated, but only about 5% of the US population feels comfortable with this concept[15,16]. Others have argued that anencephalics should be considered for organ donation, but the ethical issues surrounding the definition of death seem quite formidable at this time[25]. Public education efforts could be stepped up; however, it is apparent that the public is sufficiently aware of the need for donor organs. Xenografts have some potential but, once again, significant immunological and social barriers must be overcome. Today, in light of the foregoing, much greater attention is focusing on professional education as the primary means to improve the supply of donor organs. While this is indeed a fertile area in which to concentrate our efforts, it is apparent that the task at hand is by no means easy.

Table 67.2 Potential organ donor supply estimates

Transplant	Potential donor supply estimate		
	High	Moderate	Low
Kidney	92 000	40 000	27 000
Heart	18 400	8 000	5 400
Liver	23 000	10 000	6 750

Upon surveying current efforts to enhance the supply of donor organs, ethicists would express concern that these efforts should not violate any fundamental beliefs – religious, moral or otherwise – to which people subscribe[26]. To do so may well prove counterproductive because of innate concerns people have about life and death. It is in this regard that anencephalic organ donation is viewed by many as problematic. A redefinition of death would be required to enable the routine removal of donor organs from anencephalics. This may simply be too significant a step to take at this time.

PATIENT SELECTION

The selection of transplant recipients is without a doubt the most complex issue in organ transplantation[1,3,27]. In addressing this issue, several questions immediately come to mind, including the following:

What are the proper roles of clinical and social criteria?
What role should age play?
Is quality of life an important consideration?
Is it possible to validate empirically all criteria used to select patients?
What is the appropriate timing of transplant?
Should a retransplant be performed, given that another patient will be denied a transplant?
Do the outcomes of retransplantation justify this course of action?
Is the use of an artificial device warranted to 'bridge' patients until a donor heart becomes available?
Because of complications associated with current devices, is it not likely that bridged patients will be given priority over other candidates?

The foregoing do not exhaust all the patient selection issues that transplant teams have had to address. They do, however, illustrate the *range* of issues that have been confronted.

While there are no fixed rules as to what are the right clinical and social criteria, there does appear to be a reasonable consensus within the transplant community as to what factors are key ones in the selection of patients[28-30]. Clinical criteria are of primary importance, and social criteria play a minor role. In fact, we have found that transplant teams routinely select patients according to criteria with which the public agrees. Table 67.3 summarizes the results of a national survey of the general public concerning the use of specific medical and social criteria in the selection of transplant recipients[30]. As is apparent, the public generally disagrees with the use of social criteria.

At this point in time it is difficult to validate prognostically all of the criteria used to select transplant recipients[27]. Although it is evident that certain patients are 'at risk' given

Table 67.3 Public opinion concerning the use of specific medical and social criteria in the selection of transplant recipients

	Strongly agree (%)	Agree (%)	Disagree (%)	Strongly disagree (%)	No opinion (%)
Preference should be given to younger rather than older people	10.6	46.2	28.7	2.9	11.6
Preference should be given to the sickest patients	11.6	59.5	18.4	0.9	9.7
Preference should be given to US citizens over *all* other patients	9.3	42.4	35.5	3.7	9.1
Preference should be given to those who can afford them	0.5	7.7	61.4	25.6	4.9
Preference should be given to people with a strong religious background	0.2	5.2	68.3	21.4	4.9
Preference should be given to people who do *not* drink alcohol	1.6	17.8	62.5	11.1	7.1
Preference should be given to people who are most likely to survive and benefit	17.3	66.0	10.9	0.5	5.4
Preference should be given to those who are most likely to be able to return to their usual work and/or household activities	10.2	61.7	19.6	1.2	7.3
Preference should be given to people who do *not* smoke	2.7	23.6	56.9	7.8	9.0
Preference should be given to people who live a 'healthy' lifestyle	2.8	37.9	44.8	4.5	10.0

various characteristics such as advancing age or diabetes, no firm evidence has been amassed to categorically reject patients for transplant. Even AIDS has been disputed as an absolute contraindication to transplantation.

The timing of transplant is a complicated issue[31]. While it could be argued that the sickest patients are not necessarily the best candidates for transplantation, the national organ procurement and distribution network – the United Network for Organ Sharing (UNOS) – assumes otherwise[32-34]. One could, however, reasonably argue against this policy. The sicker the patient, the more uncertain the outcome and, thus, the more likely that another patient could have benefited to a greater extent. This is an area that will require greater attention in the future.

Retransplantation raises several questions about fairness and equity[26]. While the medical and surgical team is committed to the care of all patients, the retransplanted patient seems to have an unfair advantage. For each organ a retransplant recipient receives, another patient is denied an opportunity for transplant. Over time it is likely that our policies concerning retransplantation will have to be refined, perhaps limiting individuals to no more than two transplants. This does appear to be justified clinically, as the probability of a successful transplant declines with each successive transplant.

Mechanical devices for bridging patients for cardiac transplantation seem to have fallen out of favor, perhaps as a result of the great uncertainty associated with the procurement of an acceptable heart[35-38]. While some devices have served this purpose well, and some teams have become quite successful in bridging very sick patients, the continued use of mechanical devices for this purpose is likely to be very limited in the future. It is noteworthy, nonetheless, that one major criticism of the bridging procedure – that such patients are moved to the top of the waiting list – is incorrect. Patients who are bridged are, by definition, sufficiently sick to be at the top of the list already. The mechanical device prolongs their life, it does not render them sicker and thus more worthy of heart transplant than they were previously.

There is little doubt that over the past 2 years much has been done to assure transplant candidates that they will be treated fairly and equitably by the national organ procurement and distribution system. As the policies of the United Network for Organ Sharing have been refined, patients have fewer reasons to be suspicious of the policies and procedures by which organs are procured and distributed in the United States. Fairly sophisticated distribution systems have been implemented at the local, regional, and national levels to assure that the most needy transplant candidates are given the most ready access to the donor organ procurement system. This system is a relief to the patient, the transplant team, and the health care policy makers of the United States.

COST AND REIMBURSEMENT

Heart and liver transplantation procedures are expensive according to any standard[17,18,39-42]. End-stage disease, regardless of its etiology, is expensive to treat, as is all catastrophic disease. Today, the total first year costs associated with a heart transplant can easily exceed $100 000, and a liver transplant $200 000. While many private insurers now consider heart and liver transplants to be therapeutic (no longer experimental), some public insurers, namely state Medicaid programs, have begun to reconsider their policies[42-44]. In some states, coverage has been suspended. Not surprisingly, patients without insurance, as well as those with inadequate insurance, are finding it difficult to gain admission to transplant centers. Many transplant centers now require assurance of insurance payment, or an actual down-payment, often in excess of $100 000, before a patient will be placed on the waiting list for a transplant.

For many patients, the transplant 'system' is unfair, particularly when it operates as described here. It is not unusual for patients without the necessary financial means to be denied access to a transplant. For example, several years ago the National Task Force on Organ Transplantation determined that 78% of the transplant surgeons in the United States were influenced by an individual's ability to pay when considering a patient for transplant[45]. Moreover, 38% of the surgeons surveyed said that ability to pay for immunosuppressive medications influenced their selection of cardiac transplant recipients.

Public opinion data clearly show that the general public is opposed to the use of financial criteria in the selection of transplant candidates[29,30]. Over 80% of the public agrees with the following statement: 'Medical need, not social or economic factors, should be the *only* criterion used to select transplant recipients'. Only 8.2% of the public feels that 'preference should be given to those (people) who can afford them (transplants)' (see Table 67.3). Finally, over 88% of the population is '*most* concerned that donor organs are distributed as fairly and equally as possible'. Obviously, there is absolutely no evidence that the general public will support economic discrimination when it comes to access to transplantation.

Despite their unwillingness to allow economics to play a role in the selection of transplant candidates, the public cannot ignore the significant costs associated with transplantation. One way or another we all bear the burden of higher health care costs. Either taxes are raised to help insure a growing segment of the underinsured or uninsured portion of the population, or private health care insurance premiums are increased to cover added health care costs, or both. Alternatively, private insurers can increase deductibles and co-payments as well[46]. The underlying concept here is simple; if we want increased health care benefits, we must be prepared to pay for them. While numerous attempts have been made to increase the efficiency with which health care services are delivered, in an effort to reduce total expenditures, it has become clear that such efforts have fallen short of their mark[47]. Either services must be reduced, or taxes and insurance premiums increased to cover costs. Over the past several years many major health insurance companies, including the Blue Cross and Blue Shield Association, have sustained heavy losses. As a result, this year (1989) health insurance premiums are expected to increase by an average of 30%.

Increasingly, as people are unable to afford private health insurance, the burden placed upon public insurers, primarily Medicaid programs, will become even more significant than it is already. This, of course, will lead states to cut benefits or to increase taxes, neither alternative being particularly palatable at this time. However, when push comes to shove, it is likely that certain high cost benefits may be curtailed in order to make available services that are viewed as being more cost-effective. This is basically what occurred in the State of Oregon[43]. If people object to this action, they had better be prepared to give up other non-health related services, or to pay higher taxes.

Ethically, what has been described here is rather confusing. While people may be unwilling to allow for economic discrimination, they may, in the end, have little alternative. As people recognize that both public and private insurance is a cooperative cost-sharing endeavor, they may begin to reconsider the types of coverages they believe are necessary for them, as well as other people. Perhaps the underlying ideology is best characterized by the words 'willingness to pay'[48]. If people have the resources and are willing to expend them accordingly, then transplantation is considered in the same class as cosmetic surgery, although there is one serious difference – transplantation holds the promise of saving lives, whereas cosmetic surgery has the potential to make life more appealing for oneself or others.

While this analysis may seem emotionally cold-hearted, given the altruism that underlies the transplant enterprise, there are certainly other analogies apparent within the existing health care system. For example, the quality of the health care services available to the wealthy and the poor is vastly different. The local county hospital may offer adequate health care services, but the quality and range of services available at a private institution that caters to the wealthy may be far superior to those of the county hospital. In short, not everyone has equal access or is treated equally by the complex health care delivery system that exists in the United States[49-51]. Death can conceivably be the outcome of having chosen, or been transported, to an inferior hospital for medical care.

Ultimately it seems unusual that we insist that everyone, regardless of economic status, be given equal access to transplantation when we are unable to guarantee access for all to other less sophisticated services. It would seem that we should first direct our attention to other areas in medicine where more can be accomplished. Having said this, however, I recognize that this necessarily implies that the wealthy and the insured be given priority in access to transplantation. An alternative might be to 'tax' those patients who are able to pay in order to permit some uninsured patients to have access to transplantation. For example, physicians and surgeons may *not* be allowed to charge fees for uninsured patients, or a surtax may be levied on each paying patient to create a fund for the uninsured. While in principle these options are attractive, in practice they may well be difficult to implement.

QUALITY OF LIFE

If nothing else, our limited experience with the permanent total artifical heart (TAH) has thrust upon us a new appreciation of the quality of life concept. As the media made us aware of the trials and tribulations of Barney Clark, William Schroeder, and other TAH recipients, we increasingly began to ponder when our own quality of life would be unacceptable and death a better alternative. Of course, this same question was asked of the first patients who were placed on maintenance hemodialysis. How was it that a patient could undergo 40 hours of dialysis each week and still have a will to live? Even today, during an era when medical technological developments have become increasingly advanced, we find that these same questions are contemplated. Is life worth living, and at what point will it be so compromised that the hastening of death would be attractive? In a recent report, Roberts and Kjellstrand indicate that of the 1766 hemodialysis patients they studied, 1.5% preferred death to the stress of dialysis[52].

In our many studies on the quality of life of transplant recipients, we persistently find that on subjective quality of life measures (i.e. well-being, psychological affect and life satisfaction) patients do exceptionally well[17,18,39,40,53,54]. On the objective indicators, however, patients uniformly do poorly. They often have a wide range of physical limitations, remain unemployed even though able to work, and their health status, although vastly improved since transplant, is subject to uncertainty, owing largely to chronic immunosuppression. Despite these findings, on average, transplant recipients fair well post-transplant.

What is surprising, unfortunately, is how few transplant recipients are fully aware of what their future will hold. Many view transplantation as a cure for a terminal condition, rather than a treatment that converts a terminal disease to a chronic condition. Patients often do not anticipate the limitations they will endure and are frequently inadequately informed of the rigors of immunosuppression. Many are not prepared for the occasional setbacks that may befall them as they become long-term survivors. Others have difficulty coming to grips with changes in body image that may accompany the routine administration of both corticosteroids and cyclosporine.

While the majority of patients are happy with their lives, they, perhaps, have unusual notions as to what constitutes an adequate quality of life. Each patient who has looked into 'death's eye', and survived a transplant, may in fact expect less of life than people who have not had a near-death experience. This is certainly true of patients who have survived cancer and have learnt to live each day as if it were their last. The 'little things' that used to bother them are somehow small in the grand scheme of human experience. The same is true of transplant recipients, at least initially. However, as time passes and the patient embarks upon a relatively stable post-transplant course, their expectations change. They want more out of life, and realize that they may have precious little time to accomplish their goals. Transplant recipients may become less tolerant of friends, family, and caregivers. While this may be alarming to those around the patient, it is, I think, the outcome of a new-found appreciation of life, and the very uncertainty that characterizes much of human existence.

While suicide is relatively infrequent among transplant recipients, it does occur, often in response to protracted medical complications associated with the transplant. Over time, as the side-effects of immunosuppressive drugs take their toll, patients may begin, once again, to contemplate the death experience they had previously avoided. Life may become more difficult to live as the uncertainties become more profound. Patients typically respond in several ways: (1) they may be satisfied with the periods for which their lives have been extended, (2) they may be angry that they have to face death again, and (3) they may hope that death can again be avoided.

Regardless of how it is assessed, the quality-of-life dilemma that transplant recipients face is real. Patients must be well-informed prior to transplant as to what they can expect post-transplant under ideal as well as compromised conditions. Too frequently patients are led to believe that the ideal is the norm when, in fact, this is not the case. The transplant experience can be envisioned as points along a continuum. At one end we have the ideal – the heart transplant recipient who is discharged from the hospital in 10 days without a complication or a hint of rejection. At the other end of the continuum is the patient who is hospitalized in an intensive care unit for 180 days, with many complications related to surgery as well as immunosuppression, and dies prior to discharge. The ideal patient has an excellent quality-of-life prognosis, while the patient who died prior to discharge undoubtedly had a deplorable 'quality-of-dying' experience. Hindsight would suggest that the patient who died would have been further ahead if transplantation had not been offered as a treatment alternative. This is primarily because the dying experience was protracted due to 'clinical cascade'[12].

To be sure, somewhere between these two extremes is the 'usual' transplant patient experience. The problem for the transplant community is to make the patient and his family aware of the variations that occur in the transplant experience. Transplantation is a highly unpredictable experience and, as such, the patient must have considerable social and clinical resources upon which he can draw. If the patient is not fully apprised of what to expect, an average experience could easily become an unmitigated disaster that both patient and family may regret having endured.

RESOURCE ALLOCATION

Full treatment of the resource allocation and rationing issue as it applies to transplantation is well beyond the scope of this chapter[10,11,17,55]. It is, nonetheless, important to point out that transplantation does underscore the underlying differences between the concepts of allocation and rationing. First, donor organs are essentially rationed among potential transplant candidates. Not every patient in need will get transplanted and, as a result, some patients will die. Second, the financial resources available to cover the costs associated with transplantation are, to some extent, finite, and, therefore, what constitutes the appropriate use of these resources is debated among insurers and policy analysts[55]. In short, a question of resource allocation arises. As noted previously, could the resources committed to transplantation be better used to provide other less costly, more cost-effective health care services?

The *rationing* issue has already been addressed to some extent during my discussion of the patient selection dilemma. The resource *allocation* issue has only been acknowledged superficially. In this regard, I would be remiss if I did not point out that, in the grand scheme of the resource allocation debate, transplantation has been treated unjustly[18]. Transplantation is not a weird and unusual form of treatment for patients dying with end-stage disease. In effect, transplantation should be likened to the treatment of other 'catastrophic diseases'. One can easily think of many examples of costly diseases and treatments that have not been singled out for 'negative' attention. Today, the treatment of AIDS may be the single best example of a costly condition to treat, with relatively little net benefit to the patient or society[56-61]. Medical care costs per patient over the course of the illness have been estimated to range between $23 000 and $168 000[60]. The intent here is not to be moralistic, but simply to underscore the fact that as our population ages, the prevalence of catastrophic disease will increase, as will expenditures associated with the treatment of these conditions. In 1987, 11.1% of the gross national product was devoted to health care, up from 10.7% in 1986.

If the allocation issue is as significant as many contend it is, it is unfortunate that we select for scrutiny the treatment of one or two conditions to which public resources are alleged to be diverted excessively. In this regard, one should bear in mind that transplant costs are severely constrained by the availability of donor organs[22]. Costs will be incurred only to the level that donor organs are procured and transplanted. This constraint is real, and raises another important question concerning ethics. If we are not prepared to pay for transplants, should we continue our efforts to improve (increase) the supply of donor organs? As I have observed elsewhere, people accept more readily the lack of donor organs as the reason a patient may not receive a transplant than they do the lack of funds to pay for the procedure.

Rather than single out transplantation as a major 'culprit' behind the rising cost of health care, I think we need to provide a forum for a more general discussion of the cost of medical care, the components of these costs, the role of catastrophic illness in the delivery of health care services, the opinion of the public with respect to high-cost medical care, and options available to address directly the resource allocation dilemma[62]. By limiting our attention to transplantation we, unfortunately, avoid the large issue and create problems of equity and fairness.

While some observers have argued that resource allocation and rationing decisions are not necessary, if we provide only the type and level of care the patient actually requires, I remain unpersuaded[10,11,47]. I do not think that discontinuing ineffective treatments, or eliminating those that have little or no value, will conserve sufficient resources to enable us to meet all our health care needs. Moreover, I do not believe that it is simply the overuse of little technologies that adds substantially to the cost of health care in the United States. Regardless of the explanation for the high cost of health care, the demands being placed upon the health care delivery system are considerable. It will be necessary to make difficult choices[63]. However, I think these choices must be made systematically, based upon the best available information, with an eye towards both costs and effectiveness.

Comparatively, transplantation offers benefits that are worth the costs, given other accepted forms of 'therapy' for other catastrophic conditions[17]. This is the broader perspective I alluded to at the outset of this chapter. In effect we must ask, how does transplantation fit within the grand scheme of health care? What will the future hold? Will costs increase and benefits decrease as patient selection criteria evolve? Will donor supply increase to create a resource *allocation* problem of immense proportions, while the resource *rationing* problem is minimized? These, indeed, are some of the issues of the future, all being central to the debate concerning resource constraints.

COMMENT

As medical technology has become increasingly sophisticated, the ethics associated with the practice of medicine have become a matter of much debate. This chapter has briefly considered several issues that are of significance to any discussion pertaining to the ethics of transplantation. Ethicists have offered some unique perspectives on these issues, but have, at times, been insufficiently informed about the clinical aspects of transplantation. As a result, their analyses can be misleading. Over time, however, as ethicists become more familiar with transplantation, the situation will hopefully improve. While it is unnecessary for ethicists to be a part of the team, access to a consulting ethicist may be of some benefit to the transplant team.

Unfortunately, because of their ill-defined role, and the medical profession's lack of familiarity with medical ethics, ethicists have been elevated to a status that exceeds their utility. Ethicists do not offer unequivocal solutions to the complex moral problems associated with transplantation. They simply offer an additional perspective – a perspective that often reflects the disciplinary background of the ethicist whose consultation is sought. Some ethicists have trained in philosophy, others in religious studies, and still others have a social and behavioral science background. As a result, ethicists have a variety of opinions and perspectives, and a consensus is no more likely to emerge among ethicists than among physicians and surgeons on any single issue. Moreover, because of their lack of clinical experience, many ethicists are not easily integrated into the clinical decision-making process. In fact, during clinical conferences, ethicists may be detrimental to the proceedings.

As implied here, medical ethics has significant limitations when conflict resolution is required among members of the transplant team. These limitations apply to all the issues reviewed above – organ procurement, patient selection, cost and reimbursement, quality of life, and resource allocation. To say the least, the ethical dilemmas the transplant team faces can be frightening. However, as transplantation is increasingly being forced to be publicly accountable, the satisfactory resolution of all ethical issues becomes of paramount importance. In this regard, medical ethicists may be of some help, but they will not be the savior that medicine now seeks.

References

1. Brock, D.W. (1988). Ethical issues in recipient selection for organ transplantation. In Mathieu, D. (ed.) *Organ Substitution Technology.* p. 86. (Boulder: Westview Press)
2. Caplan, A.L. (1985). Ethical issues raised by research involving xenografts. *J. Am. Med. Assoc.*, **254**, 3339
3. Caplan, A.L. (1987). Equity in the selection of recipients for cardiac transplants. *Circulation*, **75**, 10
4. Caplan, A.L. (1988). Ethical issues in the use of anencephalic infants as a source of organs and tissues for transplantation. *Transplant. Proc.*, **20** (Suppl. 5), 42
5. Kanoti, G.A. (1986). Ethical considerations in solid organ pediatric transplants. *Transplant. Proc.*, **18** (Suppl. 2), 43
6. Mathieu, D. (1988). *Organ Substitution Technology.* (Boulder: Westview Press)
7. Monaco, A.P. (1987). Problems in transplantation – ethics, education, expansion. *Transplantation*, **43**, 1
8. Simmons, R.G. and Abress, L. (1988). Ethics in organ transplantation. In Cerilli, G.J. (ed.) *Organ Transplantation and Replacement.* p. 691. (Philadelphia: J.B. Lippincott)
9. Youngner, S.J., Allen, M., Bartlett, E., Cascorbi, H.F., Hau, T., Jackson, D.L., Mahowald, M.B. and Martin, B.J. (1985). Psychosocial and ethical implications of organ retrieval. *N. Engl. J. Med.*, **313**, 321
10. Evans, R.W. (1983). Health care technology and the inevitability of resource allocation and rationing decisions. I. *J. Am. Med. Assoc.*, **249**, 2047
11. Evans, R.W. (1983). Health care technology and the inevitability of resource allocation and rationing decisions. II. *J. Am. Med. Assoc.*, **249**, 2208
12. Mold, J.W. and Stein, H.F. (1986). The cascade effect in the clinical care of patients. *N. Engl. J. Med.*, **314**, 512
13. Churchill, L.R. (1987). *Rationing Health Care in America: Perceptions and Principles of Justice.* (Notre Dame: University of Notre Dame)
14. Daniels, N. (1986). Why saying no to patients in the United States is so hard. *N. Engl. J. Med.*, **314**, 1380
15. Starzl, T.E. (1984). Implied consent for cadaveric organ donation. *J. Am. Med. Assoc.*, **251**, 1592
16. Manninen, D.L. and Evans, R.W. (1985). Public attitudes and behavior regarding organ donation. *J. Am. Med. Assoc.*, **253**, 3111
17. Evans, R.W. (1987). A catastrophic disease perspective on organ transplantation. In Ginzberg, E. (ed.) *Medicine and Society: Clinical Decisions and Societal Values.* p. 61. (Boulder: Westview Press)
18. Evans, R.W. (1986). The heart transplant dilemma. *Issues Sci. Technol.*, **2**, 91
19. Evans, R.W., Manninen, D.L., Overcast, T.D., Garrison, L.P., Jr., Yagi, J., Merriken, K. and Jonsen, A.R. (1984). *The National Heart Transplantation Study: Final Report.* (Seattle: Battelle Human Affairs Research Centers)
20. Evans, R.W., Manninen, D.L., Gersh, B.J., Hart, L.G. and Rodin, J. (1984). The need for and supply of donor hearts for transplantation. *Heart Transplant.*, **4**, 57
21. Evans, R.W. (1984). The need for and cost of liver transplantation in the U.S. (Seattle: Battelle Human Affairs Research Centers)
22. Evans, R.W., Manninen, D.L., Garrison, L.P. Jr. and Maier, A. (1986). Donor availability as the primary determinant of the future of heart transplantation. *J. Am. Med. Assoc.*, **255**, 1892
23. Overcast, T.D., Evans, R.W., Bowen, L.E., Hoe, M.M. and Livak, C.L. (1984). Problems in the identification of potential organ donors. *J. Am. Med. Assoc.*, **251**, 1559
24. Caplan, A.L. (1984). Ethical and policy issues in the procurement of cadaver organs for transplantation. *N. Engl. J. Med.*, **311**, 981
25. Harrison, M.R. (1986). Organ procurement for children: the anencephalic fetus as donor. *Lancet*, **2**, 1383
26. National Task Force on Organ Transplantation (1986). *Organ Transplantation: Issues and Recommendations.* (Rockville: Office of Organ Transplantation, Health Resources and Services Administration, Department of Health and Human Services)
27. Evans, R.W. and Yagi, J. (1986). Social and medical considerations affecting the selection of transplant recipients: the case of heart

transplantation. In Doudera, A.E. (ed.) *Legal and Ethical Aspects of Organ Transplantation.* (Ann Arbor: Health Administration Press)
28. Evans, R.W. (1987). Public perception and the realities of organ transplantation. *Mich. Hosp.*, **23**, (12),13
29. Evans, R.W. and Manninen, D.L. (1988). U.S. public opinion concerning the procurement and distribution of donor organs. *Transplant. Proc.*, **20**, 781
30. Evans, R.W. and Manninen, D.L. (1987). *Public Opinion Concerning Organ Donation, Procurement, and Distribution: Results of a National Probability Sample Survey.* (Seattle: Battelle Human Affairs Research Centers)
31. Stevenson, L.W., Donohue, B.C., Tillisch, J.H. and Schulman, B. (1987). Urgent priority transplantation: when should it be done? *J. Heart Transplant.*, **6**, 267
32. Starzl, T.E., Hakala, T.R., Tzakis, A., Gordon, R., Steiber, A., Makowka, L., Klimoski, J. and Bahnson, H.T. (1987). A multifactorial system for equitable selection of cadaver kidney recipients. *J. Am. Med. Assoc.*, **257**, 3073
33. Rapaport, F.T. (1987). A rational approach to a common goal: the equitable distribution of organs for transplantation. *J. Am. Med. Assoc.*, **257**, 3118
34. Salvatierra, O. Jr. (1988). Optimal use of organs for transplantation. *N. Engl. J. Med.*, **318**, 1329
35. Joyce, L.D., Johnson, K.E., Pierce, W.S., DeVries, W.C., Semb, B.K.H., Copeland, J.G., Griffith, B.P., Cooley, D.A., Frazier, O.H., Cabrol, C., Keon, W.J., Unger, F., Bucherl, E.S. and Wolner, E. (1986). Summary of the world experience with clinical use of total artificial hearts as heart support devices. *J. Heart Transplant*, **5**, 229
36. Griffith, B.P., Hardesty, R.L., Kormos, R.L., Trento, A., Borovetz, H.S., Thompson, M.E. and Bahnson, H.T. (1987). Temporary use of the Jarvik-7 total artificial heart before transplantation. *N. Engl. J. Med.*, **316**, 130
37. Loisance, D.Y., Deleuze, P., Kawasaki, K., Hillion, M.L., Binhas, M., Heurtematte, P., Tavolaro, O., Lenadri, J. and Cachera, J.P. (1987). Total artificial heart as a bridge to retransplantation in acute cardiac rejection. *J. Heart Transplant.*, **6**, 281
38. Pierce, W.S. (1988). Permanent heart substitution: better solutions lie ahead. *J. Am. Med. Assoc.*, **259**, 891
39. Evans, R.W. (1985). The socioeconomics of organ transplantation. *Transplant. Proc.*, **17** (Suppl. 4), 129
40. Evans, R.W. (1986). Cost effectiveness analysis of transplantation. *Surg. Clin. North Am.*, **66**, 603
41. Evans, R.W. (1987). The economics of heart transplantation. *Circulation*, **75**, 63
42. Evans, R.W. (1986). Coverage and reimbursement for heart transplantation. *Int. J. Technol. Assess. Health Care*, **2**, 425
43. Welch, H.G. and Larson, E.B. (1988). Dealing with limited resources: the Oregon decision to curtail funding for organ transplantation. *N. Engl. J. Med.*, **319**, 171
44. Welch, H.G. and Larson, E.B. (1988). Oregon's decision to curtail funding for organ transplantation. *N. Engl. J. Med.*, **319**, 1420
45. Goeken, N. (1985). *Survey on Transplantation Practices, American Society of Transplant Surgeons.* (Rockville: Office of Organ Transplantation)
46. Health Insurance Association of America (1985). *Organ Transplants and Their Implications for the Health Insurance Industry.* (Washington: Public Relations Division, HIAA)
47. Angell, M. (1985). Cost containment and the physician. *J. Am. Med. Assoc.*, **254**, 1203
48. Culyer, A.J. (1982). Assessing cost-effectiveness. In Banta, H.D. (ed.) *Resources for Health: Technology Assessment for Policy Making.* p. 107. (New York: Praeger)
49. Aday, L.A., Flemming, G.V. and Anderson, R. (1984). *Access to Medical Care in the U.S.: Who Has It, Who Doesn't?* (Chicago: Pluribus Press for the University of Chicago)
50. Iglehart, J.K. (1985). Medical care of the poor – a growing problem. *N. Engl. J. Med.*, **313**, 59
51. Iglehart, J.K. (1982). Federal policies and the poor. *N. Engl. J. Med.*, **307**, 836
52. Roberts, J.C. and Kjellstrand, C.M. (1988). Choosing death. Withdrawal from chronic dialysis without medical reason. *Acta Med. Scand.*, **223**, 181
53. Evans, R.W., Manninen, D.L., Garrison, L.P. Jr., Hart, L.G., Blagg, C.R., Gutman, R.A., Hull, A.R. and Lowrie, E.G. (1985). The quality of life of patients with end-stage renal disease. *N. Engl. J. Med.*, **312**, 553
54. Evans, R.W., Manninen, D.L., Maier, A., Garrison, L.P. Jr. and Hart, L.G. (1985). The quality of life of kidney and heart transplant recipients. *Transplant. Proc.*, **17**, 1579
55. Baily, M.A. (1988). Economic issues in organ substitution policy. In Mathieu, D. (ed.) *Organ Substitution Technology.* p. 198. (Boulder: Westview Press)
56. Scitovsky, A.A. and Rice, D.P. (1987). Estimates of the direct and indirect costs of acquired immunodeficiency syndrome in the United States, 1985, 1986 and 1991. *Public Health Rep.*, **102**, 5
57. Andrulis, D.P., Beers, V.S., Bentley, J.D. and Gage, L.S. (1987). The provision and financing of medical care of AIDS patients in U.S. public and private teaching hospitals. *J. Am. Med. Assoc.*, **258**, 1343
58. Arno, P.S. (1987). The economic impact of AIDS. *J. Am. Med. Assoc.*, **258**, 1376
59. Lafferty, W.E., Hopkins, S.G., Honey, J., Harwell, J.D., Shoemaker, P.C. and Kobayashi, J.M. (1988). Hospital charges for people with AIDS in Washington State: utilization of a statewide hospital discharge data base. *Am. J. Public Health*, **78**, 949
60. Bloom, D.E. and Carliner, C. (1988). The economic impact of AIDS in the United States. *Science*, **239**, 604
61. Scitovsky, A. (1988). The economic impact of AIDS. *Health Affairs*, **7**, 32
62. Crawshaw, R., Garland, M.J., Hines, B. and Lobitz, C. (1985). Oregon health decisions: an experiment with informed community consent. *J. Am. Med. Assoc.*, **254**, 3213
63. Cohen, B.D. (1986). *Hard Choices: Mixed Blessings of Modern Medical Technology.* (New York: Putnam's)

68
Heart and Lung Replacement: Future Perspectives

D.K.C. COOPER

INTRODUCTION

The first human-to-human heart transplant was performed 22 years ago. These last 2 decades – and, in particular, the last 10 years – have seen a rapid expansion of heart transplantation. In 1978 only a handful of centers performed this operation: today, there are over 120 centers in the United States alone. The number of patients transplanted annually has grown significantly each year since the introduction of cyclosporine, and, more recently, there has been a steady increase in activity in lung transplantation. The difficulty of obtaining suitable donor organs, which remains the major limiting factor in the number of heart transplants performed each year, may well curtail further rapid expansion, though this shortage may eventually be overcome by the use of xenografts and/or by expanded utilization of mechanical hearts.

This chapter is certainly not intended as a comprehensive review of all the possible advances that may take place in organ transplantation or in the use of cardiac mechanical devices. Certain areas of interest, however, will be briefly discussed.

WIDENING OF INDICATIONS FOR HEART TRANSPLANTATION

With the increasingly successful results of heart transplantation, this operation is slowly being offered to a wider selection of patients. The absolute contraindications for the procedure are steadily being reduced, and the operation is being recommended for patients with less advanced disease than previously; the pool of potential recipients is therefore progessively increasing.

In future years, more patients with rheumatic and congenital heart disease will almost certainly be submitted for this procedure. Patients with complex congenital deformities may undergo heart transplantation initially or, alternatively, a palliative operation to sustain life for a number of years, with subsequent heart transplantation as a secondary procedure during late childhood or early adult life. The development of Eisenmenger's syndrome may be accepted as inevitable, and a plan made at an early stage to carry out transplantation of the heart and both lungs (or possibly of a single lung, together with corrective surgery to the heart) later in the development of the child.

As the imbalance between the number of potential recipients and available donors increases, so the waiting period for suitable hearts will also increase. To offset this, patients will be placed on the transplant waiting list at an earlier stage in the progress of their myocardial disease to ensure that they do not deteriorate to an inoperable degree by the time a heart becomes available.

Expansion of heart transplantation programs to incorporate both younger and older patients will probably continue. We shall see an increasing number of neonates and infants undergoing this procedure, and possibly patients in the eighth decade of life. If the donor shortage continues, however, the ethics of transplanting patients in the older age group may be increasingly questioned.

One further, and potentially major, factor limiting the number of potential donors available to new heart transplant candidates will be the increasing number of donors required for retransplantation in patients who develop graft arteriosclerosis (chronic rejection) during the next decade.

As the skills of the surgeons and the expertise of those involved in immunosuppressive therapy increase, so there will probably be a small but steadily increasing number of patients receiving multiple organ transplants, such as heart and liver, or heart and kidney. The indications for these multiple transplants will remain relatively few, but already Starzl and his colleagues have taken an important step forward in carrying out combined heart and liver transplantation in children with errors of metabolism resulting in persistent hyperlipidemia[1,2].

During the next one or two decades, however, this expansion of the potential recipient pool may be offset to a degree by new discoveries in relation to the prevention and treatment of dilated cardiomyopathy and ischemic heart disease. At the present time, however, despite a growing awareness of the need for dietary restriction, and the increasing number of drugs which reduce serum cholesterol and triglycerides, it seems likely that a large number of patients with ischemic heart disease (and dilated cardiomyopathy) will continue to require transplantation in the foreseeable future.

In summary, unless a major breakthrough takes place in the prevention or medical treatment of coronary atheroma, there is likely to be a steady increase in the number of patients submitted for heart transplantation.

EXPANSION OF LUNG TRANSPLANTATION PROGRAMS

The recent introduction of successful single and double lung transplantation (Section III), however, has initiated a form of therapy that may show massive expansion, similar to that experienced in heart transplantation since 1980. Though the specific indications for single and double lung transplantation require further clarification, as do the contraindications, there must clearly be a large untapped pool of potential recipients with advanced lung disease who would benefit from these operative procedures.

Recent developments suggest that patients with emphysema, and even primary pulmonary vascular disease, might be successfully treated by unilateral lung transplantation rather than by heart–lung (or double lung) transplantation, as hitherto advocated. If this proves to be the case, an immense expansion in lung transplantation programs can be anticipated in the immediate future. The availability of single lungs for transplantation far exceeds that of the heart–lung block, and, furthermore, does not preclude the use of the heart in a separate recipient. The potential pool of recipients will increase further if selected cases of Eisenmenger's syndrome can be successfully treated by correction of the cardiac abnormality coupled with unilateral lung transplantation. A full assessment of the hemodynamics and respiratory physiology that result from such procedures is required before the directions to be taken in the management of both Eisenmenger's syndrome and emphysema can become clear.

Unlike the heart, however, there is no prospect at the present time of a mechanical device to replace the lung, nor is it likely that xenografted lungs will be successfully transplanted in the near future unless hyperacute rejection can be overcome. (A further, though less significant, problem is that the shape of the lungs of most of the animals that might be used as donors may not adapt well to that of the human thoracic cavity.)

POSSIBLE SOLUTIONS TO THE PROBLEM OF DONOR SUPPLY

It seems unlikely that this expansion in the number of potential recipients will be matched by a parallel increase in the supply of donors. The National Heart, Lung and Blood Institute estimates that 17 000–35 000 patients in the USA each year might be candidates for either heart transplantation or the implantation of a permanent ventricular assist device or total artificial heart[3]. At the present time, only 1500–2000 organs are potentially available annually in the USA. Aspects of this problem have been discussed in this volume by Chaffin (Chapter 5) and by Evans (Chapter 67). One further potentially important factor that might lead to a reduction in the number of available donors is the acquired immune deficiency syndrome (AIDS). If AIDS cannot be contained, and spreads to a larger percentage of the community, the number of donors acceptable for use may be seriously diminished. (Of course, the number of recipients accepted for transplantation may also be affected.)

The problem of donor supply might be overcome (1) by increasing the number of allografts available, or (2) in the case of the heart, by further advances in the design and function of permanent devices, or (3) by developing immunosuppressive techniques to allow the use of xenografts, and (4) by utilizing autologous skeletal muscle to augment the failing heart.

Allografts

Attempts to increase the supply of donors may be made by: (1) education of the public and (2) of the medical profession, particularly at the medical student level, (3) legal changes, such as the implementation of required request or, preferably, presumed consent laws, (4) widening of criteria, such as increasing the age at which donors remain acceptable (into the fifties and sixties, if coronary arteriography proves normal), and (5) accepting donors with relative contraindications, such as infection (septicemia and/or pneumonia) when the organism is known and the correct antibiotic therapy can be initiated immediately.

Of the possible legal changes, the introduction of a policy of presumed consent (in countries where this has not yet been introduced) would appear to be the most likely method of increasing the number of donors available, at least in the short-term.

Improved methods of pre-excision 'resuscitation' of the donor heart may allow hearts that today are considered unacceptable to become suitable for transplantation. This would appear to be a relatively neglected field. At the present time many hearts are abandoned as being unsuitable in view of the need for moderately high inotropic support, and little attention and research is being directed to methods of improving organ function before the heart is excised. The fact that 25% of the deaths after heart transplantation are related to inadequate donor heart function underscores and emphasizes this problem. It is hoped that research in this field will expand, and that therapies such as the administration of triiodothyronine (T3) will prove fully successful and allow a considerable expansion in the number of organs acceptable for transplantation. Similar work is required to assess whether the lungs can be pretreated to reduce ischemic damage during transportation and transplantation.

Future developments in the field of organ storage, similar to the University of Wisconsin (UW) solution, recently successfully introduced into liver transplant programs[4,5], may extend storage times to allow not only transportation of the heart over long distances[6,7], but also performance of the recipient operation as a semi-elective procedure. Prolonged storage times would also allow improved HLA matching between recipient and donor. There are already some data suggesting that matching at the B and DR loci will improve the long-term results of heart transplantation (Chapter 8). Within a few years, we may see a situation comparable to that which already exists in the realm of kidney transplantation, namely that it will be possible to distribute a heart nationally or even internationally by scheduled air services to a preselected recipient. (As countries such as Japan, with sophisticated health services, legislate laws to allow cadaveric organ donation, international exchange of organs over long distances may steadily increase.)

A similarly hitherto neglected area is whether a less-than-perfect donor heart can be improved during the storage period. It is certainly not inconceivable that continuous perfusion of a heart with a scientifically prepared solution might lead to washout of toxic products from the myocardium and replacement with molecules beneficial in stimulating physiological recovery of cells. The ischemic storage period will then become an opportunity for resuscitation of the organ.

As the ultimate destination of the organ may not be known at the time of excision from the donor, and as the distances between donor and recipient centers steadily increase, it will no longer become logistically or economically feasible for staff from the recipient center to fly to harvest the organ(s) personally. Excision and storage will become the responsibility of the transplant team situated closest to the donor center, as it is today with kidney procurement.

If transplantation could routinely be performed across the ABO blood group barrier, although the total number of hearts available would not be increased, the number of donors available to any one recipient would be significantly larger. The possibility of improved HLA matching between donor and recipient would also increase. Pioneering work in this area is progressing, and already a handful of patients has successfully received kidney grafts across this barrier[8-10].

With regards to lung transplantation, particularly in children requiring a single lung transplant, the use of a single lobe from a living related donor may prove to be another means of overcoming the shortage of donor organs in forthcoming years. The principle seems reasonable, and exploration of this field will almost certainly take place in due course.

Would the number of donor organs made available for transplantation be significantly increased if the donor's estate received a financial incentive, possibly in the form of a tax rebate or government grant? The answer to this extremely controversial question remains unknown, and will be discussed later.

Despite such possible advances, it seem likely that the supply of human hearts and lungs will always be a limiting factor to the number of transplants performed. During the next 2 decades, however, there will almost certainly be significant developments in other areas, allowing the donor shortage to be overcome. The two key areas in this respect will be (1) improvements in the mechanical heart, and (2) our ability to transplant organs from other animal species. Both of these topics have been discussed at some length in this volume, but further consideration will be given to them now.

Mechanical hearts

Use of the Jarvik-7 device as a bridge to transplantation has more than justified its development (Section IV). However, other approaches to bridging already show signs of proving superior to the total artificial hearts currently available. These include the use of ventricular assist devices, either singly or in pairs, to support one or both ventricles of a failing heart.

As the indications for heart transplantation become ever wider, and the number of candidates awaiting a donor heart ever greater, it is almost inevitable that there will be an increasing need for successful methods of bridging such patients. The use of assist devices and artificial hearts will almost certainly grow, and act as a stimulus to mechanical refinements and the development of totally new systems. One such example is the Nimbus axial flow pump that has already proved itself simple to insert and use, and successful in the short-term support of patients with a failing myocardium[11]. Temporary mechanical hearts and assist devices, however, do not increase the overall number of donors available; in fact, by prolonging survival of extremely ill patients, they actually increase the number of potential recipients competing for the same donor pool.

The presently available devices are in general unsuited for permanent implantation, and new designs are required.

'Pneumatically-powered devices' – such as the Jarvik-7 – 'now seem to be outside the mainstream of *permanent* total artifical heart development and their future use in this role will surely remain controversial'[12]. 'In contrast, the implantable electric hearts under development will overcome many of the disadvantages of the pneumatic heart and, when available, will provide an acceptable therapeutic solution for patients with end-stage heart disease who cannot have a transplant'[13].

A totally implantable device, made of biologically inert materials with surfaces that prevent thrombus formation, is clearly desirable. A long-term power source must be available, probably by means of the transfer of electrical power through the skin. Such devices as the Novacor system (Chapter 54), with further refinement, may prove to be acceptable as a long-term permanent device.

New approaches are clearly needed in this field. One of the great innovators in open-heart surgery, C.W. Lillehei, has pointed out that the greater the complexity of a problem, the greater the need for decisive simplification in solving it[14]. Lillehei believes that all of the knowledge to create a successful, fully implantable artificial heart is already available; the necessity is to pick out those portions applicable, and discard other concepts, no matter how cherished they may be.

The essentials include (1) an implanted power source, which could be either atomic energy (e.g. plutonium 238) or skeletal muscle driven by an appropriate pacemaker, (2) single biventricular drive, and (3) continuous (non-pulsatile) flow. Lillehei can find no convincing evidence that pulsatile flow is a physiologic necessity nor even advantageous. Furthermore, he sees no need for cardiac valves in such a system, and believes these can be eliminated completely; this would coincidentally eliminate several associated problems, such as blood trauma and the need for anticoagulation.

Whether these ideas might solve the problems associated with the development of a permanent artificial heart remains to be seen, but they are illustrative of a fresh approach that could only be beneficial to progress in this field.

It would seem that a completely successful device will not be available within the next few years, and that a permanent mechanical heart suitable for use in a large group of patients may not become a reality within the next decade. The potential for such devices, however, should one or more prove totally successful, is clearly enormous, and could conceivably lead to an almost complete cessation of natural biological heart transplantation activity.

Xenografts

Xenografts provide the alternative to a mechanical device with regard to the heart, and may provide the only answer for replacement of the lungs. In children, in particular, where no suitable mechanical implant is likely to be developed in the foreseeable future, and in whom the donor supply is particularly critical, xenografts may prove to be the only solution.

The potential problems related to xenografts have been discussed elsewhere in this volume (Section VI). In essence, the humoral (vascular, hyperacute) response must be overcome in all but the most closely-related primate species. Even if this can be successfully surmounted – by techniques or methods which have not yet been identified – then the cellular response remains, though it is hoped that the drug therapy available to us at present will be effective in this respect, particularly as there is some evidence that the cellular response may be less marked when discordant xenografting rather than allografting has been performed. It is also quite possible that graft arteriosclerosis (chronic rejection) will be more severe when xenografts are used[15], and this may mean that repeated retransplantation will prove necessary in any one individual patient.

Techniques that would appear to hold out some promise for preventing hyperacute rejection include pre- and post-transplantation plasmapheresis, which, with concomitant splenectomy, has already been demonstrated to allow transplantation across the ABO blood group barrier[8,9]; by removing anti-A or anti-B antibodies from the plasma, kidney transplantation can be successfully carried out in the splenectomized patient. Whether the same, or a similar, technique will allow xenotransplantation remains unknown, though work is progressing in this field in several centers.

A refinement would be the removal of only those antibodies directed against the organ donor species (e.g. anti-pig antibodies). This can be achieved by immunoadsorption, i.e. passing the potential recipient's plasma through a column of donor cells, possibly leukocytes or vascular endothelial cells, or a combination of cells, or through an entire organ, e.g. the heart. Repeated immunoadsorption by this technique, however, leads to further sensitization of the potential recipient[16]. If the anti-pig antibody titer in the recipient's blood could be maintained undetectable, or extremely low, both at the time of transplantation and for some weeks subsequently (by, for example, the administration of immunosuppressive therapy in the form of cyclosporine, cyclophosphamide, and corticosteroids), then possibly hyperacute rejection could be prevented, allowing good graft function.

Work in this area, aimed at achieving successful organ transplantation by negating the ill-effects of the presence of species-specific antibodies, will closely parallel similar work directed towards removing anti-HLA antibodies in sensitized subjects as a preliminary to successful allografting. Significant strides have already been achieved in this latter realm[17-19], and the achievement of successful allografting in previously sensitized individuals may well lead us to success in the use of xenografts.

Both plasmapheresis[17,18] and extracorporeal immunoadsorption with staphylococcal protein A[19] have been used successfully to remove HLA antibodies from the blood of highly sensitized patients needing renal transplantation. When coupled with pre- and post-transplant immunosuppressive therapy, resynthesis of the antibodies can be prevented, allowing successful renal transplantation. A modification of this technique may allow successful xenotransplantation. Work in this area has already begun[20].

The production of a xenogeneic chimera by total lymphoid irradiation and bone marrow transplantation is another possible technique that may allow organ transplantation between different animal species[21], and, though difficult to achieve in primates, is certainly worthy of further exploration.

Although these problems are considerable – and solutions are not anticipated in the immediate future – xenotransplantation may ultimately prove the solution to the supply of such organs as the liver and kidney – organs with primarily metabolic or biochemical functions, though a mechanical device may suffice with regards to the heart. Though it is conceivable that a simple means of artificially oxygenating the blood may be developed, it seems likely that the problems of lung replacement will also be best solved by xenografting.

Whether the liver and kidneys of such animals as the pig or sheep, which might be donors of organs for man, will be able to perform the metabolic activities required of the human organ(s) remains uncertain, but current evidence is that they probably will (Chapter 61). A whole new field of metabolic study will be opened up to examine how the function of the donor animal organ differs from that of the native organ in man.

Man now has the ability to create transgenic animals by, for example, the introduction of cloned foreign genes or recombinant DNA into germ lines. By this technique, human major histocompatibility complex material can be introduced into another species, and, furthermore, carried to the next and subsequent generations of this species[22-25]. At present, this work is primarily confined to rodents, but future developments in larger animals, such as the sheep or pig, may conceivably enable an animal to be 'created' that would be both anatomically suitable and immunologically 'acceptable' as a donor of organs for man. One hesitates to suggest that such a major development might take place in the next 20-year period, but such is the rapidity of the advances being made in the realm of genetic engineering that such a prospect may perhaps not be impossible.

Already, functionally rearranged Ig genes, introduced into the germ line of mice, have been shown to be correctly activated and to alter the expression of the endogenous immunoglobulin repertoire. Chicken or rabbit Ig genes in germ line configuration become rearranged in transgenic mice and form functional hybrid Ig molecules, suggesting that the production of interspecies monoclonal antibodies may be possible in genetically engineered mice. A detailed review discussing the implications of such results for our understanding of the development of the immune system has recently been published[25]. Introduction of porcine or murine Class I major histocompatibility antigens into mice showed that in both cases the foreign protein could form a functional transplantation antigen; success was not obtained, however, with a human major histocompatibility antigen.

Myocardial augmentation by somatic muscle

The use of somatic muscle to augment the myocardium is being explored (Section VII), but at the present time clinical experience is extremely limited. The various techniques being utilized have not yet been clearly demonstrated to bring about clinically significant augmentation of myocardial function. Considerable preparation of the patient is required before the muscle can be utilized to augment the myocardium, and therefore this procedure may be unsuited for those with rapidly deteriorating cardiac function. If the technique can be demonstrated to be successful beyond doubt, then it may prove valuable in the treatment of patients with extensive left ventricular aneurysms. As a form of therapy, however, in the majority of patients with global hypokinesia from end-stage ischemic heart disease or dilated cardiomyopathy, it seems unlikely that it will play a major role within the foreseeable future.

EARLY NON-INVASIVE DETECTION OF ACUTE AND CHRONIC REJECTION

Endomyocardial biopsy has been an invaluable diagnostic tool in the detection of an acute rejection episode, but remains an invasive investigation that is not popular with the majority of heart transplant patients. Efforts to find a simple non-invasive technique that negates the need for endomyocardial biopsy have so far proved less than completely successful; many such techniques have been briefly discussed in this volume (Chapter 16), and many further techniques are likely to be explored during the coming years. One prospect lies with magnetic resonance spectroscopy, which could permit biochemical analysis of the allograft. Alternatively, radioisotope labeling of immunoglobulins or cells might provide detailed information on specific aspects of the immune response.

It would indeed be a major step forward in the care of the transplant patient (heart, heart–lung, or lung recipient) if a single, inexpensive blood test, or possibly scan, could be developed that was consistently diagnostic of the onset of acute rejection. It would be essential that the test differentiated clearly between acute rejection and the presence of infection, or other immunomodulatory condition.

Of almost equal importance is the need for a simple method of demonstrating that the patient is developing coronary atheroma (or bronchiolitis obliterans), in other words, chronic rejection. Methods of detecting the development of coronary atheroma in the transplant recipient have been described in Chapter 19, but these do not always prove sensitive enough to make the diagnosis in its early stages. On occasion, the condition is found to be advanced before it is clearly demonstrated by an annual coronary arteriogram or thallium scan, and, in our own experience, these tests can prove deceptively normal only a few months before heart failure occurs.

The development of chronic rejection, be it of the heart or lung, limits the period of graft survival in the majority of recipients. Many of these patients remain acceptable for retransplantation, and, as mentioned earlier, chronic rejection is therefore proving, and will increasingly continue to prove, a serious drain on donor resources. If the diagnosis could be made at an earlier stage, there is some evidence to suggest that enhanced immunosuppressive therapy might slow up its progress, and thus maintain graft function for a longer period.

IMPROVEMENTS IN IMMUNOSUPPRESSION

Donor-specific tolerance

The ultimate aim of immune modulation is to develop donor-specific tolerance in the recipient. This has been relatively easy to achieve in the rodent, but very difficult in higher animal species. Specific immunologic unresponsiveness to organ allografts has been induced in adult rodents by treatment with donor antigens and a short course of immunosuppression with either cyclosporine or antilymphocyte serum[26-28]. The injection into the potential recipient of donor spleen and lymph node leukocytes, pretreated by ultraviolet irradiation, significantly prolongs rat cardiac allograft survival across major histocompatibility differences[29,30]. The addition of a short course of cyclosporine to such pretreatment induces donor-specific unresponsiveness that is dependent on the development of suppressor cells and possibly other suppressor factors in the host.

Total lymphoid irradiation (TLI) with or without concurrent bone marrow transplantation, however, has been successful in this respect with regard to lung transplantation in the dog[31], and to kidney transplantation in the primate[32], miniature swine[21], and in a small number of human subjects[33]. It is a complicated technique and, though it may prove to be of increasing value in the management of selected patients with renal transplants, it seems less likely that it will be used on a large scale in patients with heart transplants. Many such cardiac patients require transplantation urgently, and time may not allow for the pretransplant course of irradiation required; furthermore, some candidates would appear to be too ill to withstand the effects of such irradiation.

It should be noted that the prevention of acute rejection by immunosuppressive drug therapy may actually inhibit the development of donor-specific tolerance in TLI-treated subjects. Unless the preoperative manipulation of the immune system has been completely successful, therefore, subsequent drug therapy may jeopardize the induction of tolerance.

Bone marrow transplantation, however, in combination with other therapies or immune manipulations, is possibly the most likely mode of achieving donor-specific tolerance within the foreseeable future[34-36]. The induction of tolerance by other methods, such as the pretransplant administration of soluble antigen, has been achieved successfully in rodent species, but is certainly not at a stage of development where it could be attempted as yet in man.

The obvious alternative to attempting to induce donor-specific tolerance is the development and use of new immunosuppressive agents.

New pharmacological immunosuppressive agents

At the present time, there appears to be no definite likelihood of a new cyclosporine that is an improvement on cyclosporine A. Cyclosporine G has been demonstrated to be less nephrotoxic, but also has less immunosuppressive effect, and therefore is not anticipated to replace cyclosporine A, though it may yet prove an acceptable alternative. Analogues of cyclosporine A continue to be investigated, but advances in this field are apparently slow.

Two new pharmacological agents have been investigated in recent years, namely FK506[37-42] and 15-deoxyspergualin[43-46]. FK506, in particular, is a most potent immunosuppressive agent, being many times as potent as cyclosporine A. 15-deoxyspergualin has been shown to have an anti-B cell effect, and may therefore be effective to a certain extent against humoral rejection; in this regard, it may prove valuable in the development of therapy to overcome xenograft rejection. FK506 in combination with antithymocyte globulin has also been shown to prolong survival of xenogeneic skin grafts[42]. Both of these drugs, however, have serious toxic effects that may prove to prohibit their widespread use in clinical transplantation. They may form a basis, however, for the development of analogues that are less toxic. The use of small doses of such drugs as FK506 and 15-deoxyspergualin in combination with small doses of cyclosporine or other immunosuppressive agents, however, may provide effective immunosuppression without inducing toxicity from either cyclosporine or the new drug; further experimental work, and possibly clinical trials, would seem warranted.

Combination drug therapy

In recent years there has been an increasing trend towards multiple drug therapy in transplant patients. Many groups combine use of cyclosporine, azathioprine, and a corticosteroid, with antithymocyte globulin or OKT3 at critical periods. The next decade will probably see increasing investigation of combination drug therapy, particularly involving monoclonal antibodies, and possibly also FK506 and 15-deoxyspergualin, as well as any new agent that may become available. New agents may include IL2 inhibitors and those directed against the macrophage.

Monoclonal antibodies

Monoclonal antibodies have already been shown to be more efficient than polyclonal antibodies. Polyclonals show only an approximate 10% efficiency whereas monoclonals reach 100%. It seems likely that their use will be greatly expanded in the coming years. At present, monoclonal antibodies can be made against (1) lymphocytes (pan lymphocyte, e.g. Campath I), or (2) lymphocyte subsets (T-cell specific, e.g. OKT3), or may be (3) activation-specific or biased, e.g. anti-Tac, which is specific to the interleukin-2 receptor. All three groups appear to be equally useful in preventing rejection and in treating primary or repeated episodes of rejection. Attention has largely been directed to developing antibodies capable of ablating or compromising function of T-cells and antigen-presenting cells[47].

As more is known about the rejection response, it may be possible to develop highly specific monoclonal antibodies which block one key step. The immune response is, however, being found to be increasingly complex (Chapter 14); monoclonal antibodies against all or several lymphocyte subsets, or combinations of monoclonals against different groups of cells or receptor sites, may therefore prove preferable to those that are highly specific.

At present, most monoclonals are raised in mice, and one of their major limiting factors is the development in the patient of idiotypic anti-mouse antibodies which effectively neutralize the potency of the monoclonal, though sensitization can be minimized by concomitant therapy with low-dose azathioprine. In the future, monoclonal antibodies will almost certainly be raised in tissue culture, thereby overcoming this species antibody response. Repeated or prolonged use of the monoclonal antibody will then prove increasingly possible.

There are not yet sufficient clinical data to indicate whether monoclonal antibodies should be used in all patients as prophylaxis against rejection, or reserved only for the treatment of severe acute rejection episodes. Present evidence is that they are potent when administered in either situation. Further clinical trials will clarify their exact role.

Monoclonal antibodies may also be employed as a means of delivering toxins (or other agents) to a subset of cells (e.g. the T-cell or macrophage), thus resulting in the death of the cell. Much experimental work is already taking place in this field with such lethal agents as diphtheria and pseudomonas toxins[48-50]. In the same way, monoclonals can be used to transport radioactive materials (e.g. yttrium-90) to specific host cells, causing local cell destruction[48]. Future years may see major therapeutic strides in this form of therapy if the potential hazards can be controlled.

One further area where monoclonals may play an important future role is in regard to the prevention of hyperacute rejection, possibly by employing them to block receptor sites at key points in the complement cascade, thus aborting the chain of events that takes place during the development of hyperacute xenograft rejection.

Donor organ pretreatment

Methods aimed at reducing or masking the antigenic stimuli of the donor organ have received surprisingly little attention. Here again, monoclonal antibodies may be developed that, when administered to the donor before organ excision, or when administered during an *in vitro* organ storage phase, may 'disguise' the donor antigens to make them 'acceptable' to the recipients. Efforts here must be directed to both the passenger leukocytes and, in particular, the vascular endothelium of the donor organ.

Other immunomodulatory techniques

Possibly insufficient attention is also being paid to the materno-fetal relationship which might provide answers to important questions regarding the nature of tolerance[51-53].

Another investigational area showing promise relates to idiotypic antibodies in the recipient. Idiotypic antibodies have been demonstrated to develop in recipients against the HLA antibodies that result from heart transplantation[54,55]. Such idiotypic antibodies may contribute towards long-term acceptance of the graft, with the need for minimal immunosuppressive therapy. Methods of encouraging the development of such idiotypic antibodies may be beneficial, and clearly warrant investigation.

One aspect of immunosuppressive therapy hitherto largely ignored is its efficiency to prevent (or reverse) *chronic* rejection. The pharmacological immunosuppressive agents available to us today have proved disappointing in their inhibition of the development of chronic rejection, even when used in various combinations of multiple agents. Whether total lymphoid irradiation or the other forms of therapy discussed above will prove more successful in this respect remains unknown.

IMPROVED THERAPY FOR INFECTIOUS COMPLICATIONS

Today, infection in the immunosuppressed host remains the single most important cause of morbidity and mortality. Cytomegalovirus (CMV), in particular, is a major problem in many heart transplant programs. Though the recently-introduced drug, DHPG, is proving valuable in the treatment of patients with symptomatic CMV disease, it is not uniformly successful, and many weeks of post-transplant progress may be absorbed by the patient's fight with this life-threatening infection.

The exact role and efficacy of CMV hyperimmune globulin remains uncertain, but this therapy would appear to be valuable in reducing the incidence of CMV infection in CMV-negative patients receiving a heart from a CMV-positive donor[56]. The safety and role of prophylaxis using live human CMV vaccine remains even more questionable[57]. New drugs, such as foscarnet, are gradually being introduced, and may prove valuable.

The therapeutic armamentarium available to the transplant surgeon or physician against this and other viruses, and against fungal organisms, remains extremely limited. If heart, and lung, transplantation are to fulfill their full potential as forms of therapy for end-stage organ failure, improved methods of combatting, or preventing, such infections will be essential. It is hoped that the increasing ingenuity of the pharmaceutical industry will provide new and successful anti-viral and anti-fungal agents in the near future.

'SOCIAL REHABILITATION' OF THE TRANSPLANT PATIENT

To transplant a heart or lung and bring the patient through the first few critical weeks remains a major medical achievement that provides the recipient with an opportunity for an active life for a number of years. Yet a majority of patients find themselves unable to take full advantage of the marked improvement in their health status.

Many such patients were forced to give up their employment some time before the transplant procedure when ill health first debilitated them seriously. After transplantation, they have no job to which to return, and, in our experience, such are the prejudices and fears of their fellow men, they find it exceedingly difficult, if not impossible, to find new employment, even though their physical status would allow them to do so.

This can prove an extremely frustrating, often depressing, experience for the patient, and is itself a cause of significant emotional morbidity. The further 'education' of society to give such persons the opportunity to contribute fully to the community once again will undoubtedly take many years, but is essential if both patient and society are to benefit fully from the medical advances that have taken place, and continue to take place, in organ transplantation.

This problem is possibly more acute for patients receiving heart transplants than it is for those receiving organs such as the kidney or liver, as this former group is more likely to be considered by the prospective employer as being at high risk of collapsing or dying at work, or of being absent from work due to ill-health, than its renal or hepatic patient counterparts. The employers' anxieties encompass fear about being in someway responsible for the prospective employee's subsequent death, should it occur at work, and concern that the employee will be an economic liability both through being too frequently absent from the work place and through the high cost of medical insurance he, the employer, may be expected to pay. The problem is only just being recognized fully by medical social workers, and much more requires to be done if heart transplant recipients are to become fully productive members of the community.

SOLUTIONS REQUIRED TO CERTAIN ETHICAL AND FINANCIAL PROBLEMS

Cyclosporine has led to a significant increase in the success of transplantation of major organs, and has also simplified the management of such patients. This has enabled organ transplantation to be carried out in countries with less advanced medical systems. There are ethical differences in such countries, especially in regard to living related and unrelated renal donors[58,95]. This has led to considerable controversy, particularly with regard to the payment of unrelated donors, some of whom are fraudulently claimed as blood relations of the recipient. Such problems involve kidney transplantation only, and are clearly unlikely to relate to other organs, though payment for cadaver organs could become a similarly controversial topic.

It has already been stressed that the most important immediate problem facing the heart transplant team is the shortage of suitable donors. One possible stimulus to encourage donation would be some form of financial incentive to the family of the potential donor, though the opinions of transplant surgeons and physicians, and of the public, will clearly differ greatly with regards to this suggestion, the ramifications of which are considerable. But the medical profession surely has a duty to explore every possible reasonable avenue that might lead to an increase in the number of organs available.

Would it, in fact, be so morally wrong and unethical for the estate of a deceased to be paid a sum of money (by the State), or be allowed a tax concession, for donating organs, particularly if the sum were agreed at a national level to prevent unhealthy competition for such cadaver organs? It has been pointed out that, at the present time, in a strongly capitalist system as exists, for example, in the USA, when a potential organ becomes available surgeons receive payment for excising the organ(s) and for performing the transplant, the organ procurement agency receives a fee, attending physicians get paid, and the hospital receives an income – almost everybody, in fact, except the deceased donor and his family. Should they be the only ones who are expected to be totally altruistic?

The situation in countries with socialized medicine is clearly different, and there would appear to be a much weaker case for some form of financial inducement to be offered to the donor's family. An opinion poll of both the public and the medical profession would seem warranted, particularly in the USA.

State-supported systems not entirely different to that envisioned above, however, have already been put into practice and gained acceptance in one or two countries. In Saudi Arabia, for example, living donors of kidneys are both honored locally in various ways and rewarded by being given concessions in selected shops and functions such as major sporting events. The financial and social advantages of this scheme are not inconsiderable, and are looked upon as being a just reward for the humanitarian and socially-conscious act of voluntarily donating an organ, thus offering a fellow man a new lease of life. Can such a system of encouragement and reward be reasonably condemned? Would a similar system directed towards encouraging, honoring, and rewarding cadaveric donation be any more worthy of condemnation?

It would certainly be of great interest to see the effect of such a policy on the number of donor organs offered each year; given the great influence that financial reward undoubtedly has on the majority of mankind, my own suspicion is that the number would certainly not decline. We as physicians may well find ourselves embroiled in such a controversy within the next decade or two.

The costs of transplantation, which are considerable, and have to be met by patient, state, or other source, have also given rise to much discussion and controversy (Chapter 67), particularly in the USA, where treatment of a catastrophic illness, such as irreversible cardiac failure, may be largely dependent on the patient's ability to pay. Serious consideration has to be given to methods of ensuring that patients can receive the treatment they require, irrespective of their financial situation. The financial ability of a country to provide modern health care has become an almost universal problem, particularly as the medical profession and its colleagues in such fields as biomedical engineering are steadily expanding the investigational and therapeutic options available in the care of any one patient. Providing the finances to pay for such care is not, of course, a problem confined to the field of transplantation. The patient whose continued life is dependent on a transplant, however, provides a dramatic crystallization of the problem that can make a major impact on society. Transplantation may prove to be the field, therefore, that impresses on legislators and health care providers the need for urgent solutions to the financial problems that face such patients.

COMMENT

The past two decades have seen momentous advances in the field of the transplantation and replacement of thoracic organs. With the current pace of advance in both medical science and biomedical engineering, equally momentous strides will undoubtedly be forthcoming during the next 20 years. A solution to the problem of xenograft rejection and the development of a totally implantable mechanical heart almost certainly await those of us who will be fortunate enough to live through the next exciting era.

References

1. Starzl, T.E., Bilheimer, D.W., Bahnson, H.T., Shaw, B.W., Jr., Hardesty, R.L., Griffith, B.P., Iwatsuki, S., Zitelli, B.J., Gartner, J.C., Jr. and Malatack, J.J. (1984). Heart–liver transplantation in a patient with familial hypercholesterolemia. *Lancet*, **1**, 1382
2. Shaw, B.W., Bahnson, H.T., Hardesty, R.L., Griffith, B.P. and Starzl, T.E. (1985). Combined transplantation of the heart and liver. *Ann. Surg.*, **202**, 667
3. The Working Group on Mechanical Circulatory Support of the National Heart, Lung and Blood Institute (1985). *Artificial Heart and Assist Devices: Directions, Needs, Costs, Societal and Ethical Issues.* (Bethesda, Maryland, USA: National Heart, Lung and Blood Institute) Quoted by Lawrie, G.M.[12]
4. Kalayoglu, M., Stratta, R.J., Sollinger, H.W., Hoffman, R.M., D'Alessandro, A.M., Pirsch, J.D. and Belzer, F.O. (1989). Clinical results in liver transplantation using UW solution for extended preservation. *Transplant. Proc.*, **21**, 1342
5. Jamieson, N.V., Sundberg, R., Lindell, S., Claesson, K., Moen, J., Vreugdenhil, P.K., Wight, D.G.D., Southard, J.H. and Belzer, F.O. (1988). Preservation of the canine liver for 24–48 hours using simple cold storage using UW solution. *Transplantation*, **46**, 517
6. Wicomb, W.N., Hill, J.D., Avery, J. and Collins, G.M. (1989). Comparison of cardioplegic and UW solutions for short-term rabbit heart preservation. *Transplantation*, **47**, 733
7. Wicomb, W.N., Collins, G.M., Wood, J. and Hill, J.D: (1989). Improved cardioplegia using new perfusates. *Transplant. Proc.*, **21**, 1357
8. Alexandre, G.P.J., Squifflet, J.P., De Bruyere, M., Latinne, D., Moriau, M., Ikabu, N., Carlier, M. and Pirson, Y. (1985). Splenectomy as a pre-requisite for successful human ABO-incompatible renal transplantation. *Transplant. Proc.*, **17**, 138
9. Alexandre, G.P.J., Squifflet, J.P., De Bruyere, M., Latinne, D., Reding, R., Gianello, P., Carlier, M. and Pirson, Y. (1987). Present experiences in a series of 26 ABO-incompatible living donor renal allografts. *Transplant. Proc.*, **19**, 4538
10. Bannett, A.D., McAlack, R.F., Raja, R., Baquero, A. and Morris, M. (1987). Experiences with known ABO-mismatched renal transplants. *Transplant. Proc.*, **19**, 4543
11. Frazier, O.H., Macris, M.P., Wampler, R.K., Duncan, J.M., Sweeney, H.S., Moncrief, C.L., Parnis, S.H. and Fuqua, J.M. (1989). Treatment of cardiac allograft failure by use of an intra-aortic axial flow pump (Abstract). *J. Heart Transplant.*, **8**, 110
12. Lawrie, G.M. (1988). Permanent implantation of the Jarvik-7 total artificial heart: a clinical perspective. *J. Am. Med. Assoc.*, **259**, 892

13. Pierce, W.S. (1988). Permanent heart substitution: better solutions lie ahead. *J. Am. Med. Assoc.*, **259**, 891
14. Lillehei, C.W. (1987). Mechanical devices in cardiac surgery – past, present, and future perspectives. Lecture given at the *Second International Symposium on Cardiac Surgery*, Rome, Italy
15. Reemtsma, K., Pierson, R.N., III, Marboe, C.C., Michler, R.E., Smith, C.R., Rose, E.A. and Fenoglio, J.J., Jr. (1987). Will atherosclerosis limit clinical xenografting? *Transplant. Proc.*, **19**, 108
16. Cooper, D.K.C., Human, P.A., Lexer, G., Rose, A.G., Rees, J., Keraan, M. and Du Toit, E. (1988). Effects of cyclosporine and antibody adsorption on pig cardiac xenograft survival in the baboon. *J. Heart Transplant.*, **7**, 238
17. Taube, D.H., Williams, D.G., Cameron, J.S., Bewick, M., Ogg, C.S., Rudge, C.J., Welsh, K.I., Kennedy, L.A. and Thick, M.G. (1984). Renal transplantation after removal and prevention of resynthesis of HLA antibodies. *Lancet*, **1**, 824
18. Taube, D.H., Welsh, K.I., Kennedy, L.A., Thick, M.G., Bewick, M., Cameron, J.S., Ogg, C.S., Rudge, C.J. and Williams, D.G. (1984). Successful removal and prevention of resynthesis of anti-HLA antibodies. *Transplantation*, **37**, 254
19. Palmer, A., Taube, D., Welsh, K., Bewick, M., Gjorstrup, P. and Thick, M. (1989). Removal of anti-HLA antibodies by extracorporeal immunoadsorption to enable renal transplantation. *Lancet*, **1**, 10
20. Reding, R., Davies, H.ff.S., White, D.J.G., Wright, L.J., Marbaix, E., Alexandre, G.P.J., Squifflet, J.P. and Calne, R.Y. (1989). Effect of plasma exchange on guinea pig-to-rat heart xenografts. *Transplant. Proc.*, **21**, 534
21. Sundt, T.M., Suzuki, T., Kortz, E.O., Eckhaus, M., Gress, R.E. and Sachs, D.H. (1988). Induction of specific transplant tolerance in a large animal model by bone marrow transplantation. *Surg. Forum*, **39**, 365
22. Cuthbertson, R.A. and Klintworth, G.K. (1988). Transgenic mice – a gold mine for furthering knowledge in pathobiology. *Lab. Invest.*, **48**, 484
23. Erickson, R.P. (1988). Minireview: creating animal models of genetic disease. *Am. J. Hum. Genet.*, **43**, 582
24. Jaenisch, R. (1988). Transgenic animals. *Science*, **240**, 1468
25. Storb, U. (1987). Transgenic mice with immunoglobulin genes. *Annu. Rev. Immunol.*, **5**, 151
26. Wood, M.L. and Monaco, A. (1977). The effect of timing of skin grafts on subsequent survival in ALS-treated marrow infused mice. *Transplantation*, **23**, 78
27. Homan, W.P., Williams, K.A., Millard, P.R. and Morris, P.J. (1981). Prolongation of renal allograft survival in the rat by pretreatment with donor antigen and cyclosporine A. *Transplantation*, **31**, 423
28. Thomas, J., Carder, M., Cunningham, P., Park, K., Gonder, J. and Thomas, F. (1987). Promotion of incompatible allograft acceptance in rhesus monkeys given posttransplant antithymocyte globulin and donor bone marrow. *Transplantation*, **43**, 332
29. Oluwole, S.F., Fawwaz, R.A., Reemtsma, K. and Hardy, M.A. (1988). Permanent rat cardiac allograft survival induced by ultraviolet B-irradiated donor lymphocytes and peritransplant cyclosporine. *Surgery*, **104**, 231
30. Hardy, M.A., Oluwole, S.F. and Lau, H.T. (1988). Ultraviolet B-modified donor-specific blood transfusions and peritransplant cyclosporine in the induction of specific unresponsiveness to organ allografts. *Transplant. Proc.*, **20**, 1147
31. Blumenstock, D.A. and Alpern, H.D. (1989). Prolonged survival of allotransplanted lungs in beagles conditioned with short-term immunotherapy. *Transplant. Proc.*, **21**, 494
32. Smit, J.A., Stark, J.H. and Myburgh, J.A. (1987). Mechanisms of immunologic tolerance following total lymphoid irradiation in the baboon. *Transplant. Proc.*, **19**, 490
33. Myburgh, J.A., Meyers, A.M., Thomson, P.D., Botha, J.R., Margolius, L., Lakier, R., Smit, J.A., Stark, J.H. and Gray, C. (1989). Total lymphoid irradiation – current status. *Transplant. Proc.*, **21**, 826
34. Qin, S., Cobbold, S.P. and Waldmann, H. (1990). Induction of classical transplantation tolerance in the adult. Submitted for publication. Quoted by Waldmann, H.[45].
35. Wood, M.L. and Monaco, A.P. (1984). Induction of unresponsiveness to skin allografts in adult mice disparate at defined regions of the H-2 complex. 1. Effect of donor specific bone marrow in ALS treated mice. *Transplantation*, **37**, 3539
36. Thomas, J.M., Carver, F.M., Foil, M.B., Hall, W.R., Adams, C., Fahrenbruch, B.G. and Thomas, F.T. (1983). Renal allograft tolerance induced with ATG and donor bone marrow in outbred rhesus monkeys. *Transplantation*, **36**, 104
37. Goto, T., Kino, T., Hatanaka, H., Nishiyama, M., Okurhara, M., Kohsaka, M., Aoki, H. and Imanaka, H. (1987). Discovery of FK-506, a novel immunosuppressant isolated from *Streptomyces tsukubaensis*. *Transplant. Proc.*, **19** (Suppl. 6), 4
38. Ochiai, T., Nakajima, K., Nagata, M., Hori, S., Asano, T. and Isono, K. (1987). Studies of the induction and maintenance of long-term graft acceptance by treatment with FK-506 in heterotopic cardiac allotransplantation in rats. *Transplantation*, **44**, 734
39. Calne, R., Collier, D.St.J. and Thiru, S. (1987). Observations about FK-506 in primates. *Transplant. Proc.*, **18** (Suppl. 6), 63
40. Thiru, S., Collier, D.St.J. and Calne, R. (1987). Pathological studies in canine and baboon renal allograft recipients immunosuppressed with FK-506. *Transplant. Proc.*, **19** (Suppl. 6), 98
41. Todo, S., Ueda, Y., Demetris, J.A., Imventarza, O., Nalesnik, M., Venkataramanian, R., Makowka, L. and Starzl, T.E. (1988). Immunosuppression of canine, monkey, and baboon allografts by FK-506: with special reference to synergism with other drugs and to tolerance induction. *Surgery*, **104**, 239
42. Hsu, S., Thomas, J.M. and Thomas, F.T. (1988). Synergism of FK-506 and rabbit antithymocyte globulin in prolongation of xenografts. *Surg. Forum*, **39**, 372
43. Dickneite, G., Schorlemmer, H.U., Walter, P., Thies, J. and Sedlacek, H.H. (1988). The influence of 15-deoxyspergualin on experimental transplantation and its immunopharmacological mode of action. *Behring Inst. Mitt.*, **80**, 93
44. Niiya, S., Suzuki, S., Hayashi, R., Watanabe, H., Itoh, J. and Amemiya, H. (1989). 15-deoxyspergualin: a powerful rescue drug for rejection in canine kidney grafting. *Transplant. Proc.*, **21**, 1070
45. Suzuki, S., Kanashiro, M. and Amemiya, H. (1987). Effect of a new immunosuppressant, 15-deoxyspergualin, on heterotopic rat heart transplantation, in comparison with cyclosporine. *Transplantation*, **44**, 483
46. Reichenspurner, H., Human, P.A., Boehm, D.H., Rose, A.G., May, R., Cooper, D.K.C., Zilla, P. and Reichart, B. (1989). Optimalization of immunosuppression after xenogeneic heart transplantation in primates. *J. Heart Transplant.*, **8**, 200
47. Waldmann, H. (1988). Monoclonal antibodies for organ transplantation: prospects for the future. *Am. J. Kid. Dis.*, **11**, 154
48. Cooper, M.M., Robbins, Waldmann, T.A., Gansow, O.A. and Clark, R.E. (1988). Use of anti-Tac antibody in primate cardiac xenograft transplantation. *Surg. Forum.*, **39**, 353
49. Kirkman, R.L., Bacha, P., Barrett, L.V., Forte, S., Murphy, J.R. and Strom, T.B. (1989). Prolongation of cardiac allograft survival in murine recipients treated with a diphtheria toxin-related interleukin-2 fusion protein. *Transplantation*, **47**, 327
50. Pankewycz, O., Mackie, J., Hassarjian, R., Murphy, J.R., Strom, T.B. and Kelley, V.E. (1989). Interleukin-2-diphtheria toxin fusion protein prolongs murine islet cell engraftment. *Transplantation*, **47**, 318
51. Zuchermann, F.A. and Head, J.R. (1987). Possible mechanism of non-rejection of the feto-placental allograft: trophoblast resistance to lysis by cellular immune effectors. *Transplant. Proc.*, **19**, 554
52. Stranick, K.S., Ho, H.N., Locker, J., Kunz, H.W. and Gill, T.J. (1987). Regulation of major histocompatibility complex antigen expresson during pregnancy. *Transplant. Proc.*, **19**, 559

53. Gill, T.J. III and Wegmann, T.G. (eds.) *Immunoregulation and Fetal Survival*. (London: Oxford University Press)
54. Fenoglio, J., Ho, E., Reed, E., Rose, E., Smith, C., Reemtsma, K., Marboe, C., Hernadi, S. and Suciu-Foca, N. (1989). Anti-HLA antibodies and heart allograft survival. *Transplant. Proc.*, **21**, 807
55. Reed, E., Rouah, C., Hsu, D., Cechova, K., Rose, E., Smith, C., Reemtsma, K., King, D.W. and Suciu-Foca, N. (1989). Anti-idiotypic antibodies regulate the immune response to HLA in heart allograft recipients. *Transplant. Proc.*, **21**, 463
56. Metselaar, H.J., Velzing, J., Rothbarth, P.H., Simoons, M.L., Bos, E. and Weimar, W. (1989). Prevention of cytomegalovirus infections in CMV seronegative heart transplant recipients with specific immunoglobulins (Abstract). *J. Heart Transplant.*, **8**, 94
57. Brayman, K.L., Dafoe, D.C., Smythe, W.R., Barker, C.F., Perloff, L.J., Naji, A., Fox, I.J., Grossman, R.A., Jorkasky, D.K., Starr, S.E., Friedman, H.M. and Plotkin, S.A. (1988). Prophylaxis of serious cytomegalovirus infection in renal transplant candidates using live human cytomegalovirus vaccine. *Arch. Surg.*, **123**, 1502
58. Little, P.J., McMullin, J.P. and MacDonald, A. (1989). Live donor renal transplantation in Iraq. *Transplant. Proc.*, **21**, 1400
59. Daar, A.S. (1989). Ethical issues – a Middle East perspective. *Transplant. Proc.*, **21**, 1402

Index

ABO groups 63
acetyl glycerol ether phosphorylcholine (platelet-activating factor) 487–9
acquisition of tissue *see* donation
acute rejection, cardiac 115–38, 171–2
  diagnosis 127–36
    arterial pulse wave monitoring 131
    clinical features 127–8
    echocardiography 133
    electrocardiography 128–9
    endomyocardial biopsy 115–16, 131–3
    hematological monitoring 129
    immunological monitoring 129–31
    ^{31}P nuclear magnetic resonance imaging 135
    proton magnetic resonance imaging 135
    radiography 128
    scintigraphy 133–5
  hyperacute 111, 128, 487–91
  management 136–8
  mild episodes 136, 172
  moderately severe 136
  pathology 115–24
    immunofluorescence studies 122
    light microscope appearance 116–19, 122–4
    lymphocyte subpopulations 122
    macroscopic appearance 115
    patient receiving cyclosporine 121–2
    resolving acute rejection 120, 121 (fig)
    scoring system 119–20, 121 (fig)
acyclovir 155
AIDS-infected organ 31
airway regulation in transplanted lung 337
alloantigen 110 (fig)
allograft destruction immunobiology 109–13
  afferent limb: antigenic recognition, cell differentiation, cell proliferation 110–11
  efferent limb: antibody production, cellular infiltration 111
  Lafferty–Bach–Bachelor concept 110
allotransplantation
  cardiac 6
  pulmonary 359
alternatives to family consent 37–8
aluminum hydroxide 92
amikacin 153
amphotericin B 156 (table)
amyloidosis 15
anaerobic threshold (lactate turnpoint) 234
anaerobiosis 234–5
anesthesia 71–2
  induction 71–2
  non-cardiac surgery, patient with heart transplant 242–3
  pre-anesthesia management 71

single-lung transplantation 375–9
  arteriovenous bypass 377–8
  exercise testing 376
  hemodynamic assessment 375–6
  intraoperative management 377–8
  preoperative preparation 376–7
  pulmonary function tests 376–7
  radionuclide pulmonary perfusion scan 376
  ventilation 378
angiotensin-converting enzyme inhibitors 12, 16, 193
antiarrhythmic agents 106
antibiotic drug therapy, postoperative 91
antibody-dependent cell-mediated cytotoxicity 110 (fig), 111
antifailure therapy 16
antigen-presenting cell 109
anti-idiotypic antibody 97
antilymphocyte globulin 9, 96, 136, 137
  side effects 198
antimyosin antibodies 134
antithymocytic globulin 136, 137
  in children 215
  side effects 199
arterial blood gases following heart–lung transplantation 335
arterial pulse wave monitoring 131
aseptic necrosis of bone 196–7
aspergillosis 155–6
aspirin 92
asthma 338
atheromatous vascular disease 200
atrial natriuretic peptide 102
atropine 105
autoantibodies 66
autonomic (sympathetic) storm 43
autoperfusion (biological oxygenation) 54
autopsy findings 245–9
  adrenal glands 248
  arteries 249
  bones 248
  brain 248
  esophagus 269
  eyes 249
  kidneys 248
  liver 248
  lungs 246–7
  lymph nodes 247
  mediastinum 247
  oropharyngeal cavity 249
  pancreas 249
  recipient heart 247
  skeletal muscle 248
  small intestine 249
  spleen 247

stomach 249
veins 249
autotransplantation of heart 6
auxiliary intrathoracic pump, transplanted heart as 4–5
azathioprine 7, 9, 95, 112, 137
    nutritional problems 230
    side effects 193 (table), 195

B cell 109, 110 (fig), 111
    antibodies produced by 66, 111
B-cell stimulating factor 110 (fig)
Bell's phenomenon 21
biological oxygenation (autoperfusion) 54
Biomedicus centrifugal pump 414
Biopump 417–21
birefringence measurements 58
B-lactam agents 153
β-blocking agents 91
blood transfusion, pretransplant 67
bone marrow transplantation 529
    bronchiolitis obliterans after 345
brain death 19–26
    ancillary tests 22–3
        auditory brain-stem responses 23
        brain-stem auditory-evoked potentials 23
        carotid angiography 23
        electroencephalography 22
        evoked potentials 23
        lower esophageal contractility 23
        scalp electromyograms 22–3
        somatic evoked responses 23
        vertebral angiography 23
    brain-dead donor *see under* donor heart
    endothelial injury 110
    fluid loss 46
    minimum criteria 26
    myocyte injury 110
    relaxation of requirements 38
    spontaneous respiration testing 26
brain-stem damage, irreversible 19–20
brain-stem reflexes 21
bronchiectasis 353
bronchiolitis obliterans 310–11, 341–5, 353
    clinical features 342, 344
    etiology 310, 344–5
    investigations 342
    management 344
    pathogenesis 322
    pathology 343–6
    post-single lung transplantation 395
bronchoalveolar lavage 342–3

calcitonin 197
calcium antagonists 105–6
calcium cascade 56
    inhibition 56
calcium channel antagonists 193
candidiasis 156–7, 328–9
captopril 16, 193
cardiac allograft transplantation in hypersensitized recipient 490–1
cardiac disease, progression of 200
cardiac retrieval team equipment 36 (table)
cardiac support devices 413–29
    available 414 (table)
    'bridge' to cardiac transplantation 445–8
    electrically-powered implantable left ventricular assist systems 414–15
    extracorporeal membrane oxygenation 414
    indications 413
    insertion criteria 413 (table)
    non-pulsatile centrifugal pumps *see* non-pulsatile centrifugal pumps
    orthotopic biventricular replacement prosthesis *see* total artificial heart
    patient categories 415
    patient selection 413
    pulsatile external ventricular assist devices 414
    results 415–16
    see also specific devices
cardiomyoplasty 497–500, 527
    clinical experience 499
    experimental work 497–8
    surgical technique 499–500
    see also skeletal muscle blood pumps
cardiopulmonary bypass 72–3
cataract, lenticular 198
catecholamines 103, 105, 124
cefotaxime 154
cell-mediated rejection 110 (fig)
central α-receptor stimulation 195
cephalosporin 91, 153
certification of fact of death 27–8
ceruloplasmin 57
cervical carcinoma 187
Chaga's disease 123
childhood/infancy, cardiac transplantation in 209–16
    contraindications 210–11
    hypoplastic left heart syndrome 213–14
    immunosuppression 215
    indications 209–10
    preoperative evaluation 211–12
    pretransplant care 212
        immunization 212
        myocardial support 212
    rejection diagnosis 215–16
    surgical techniques 212–14
        cardiomyopathy 212–13
cholecystitis, acute 198
cholestipol 194
cholestyramine 92, 194
chronic rejection *see* bronchiolitis obliterans; graft arteriosclerosis
clindamycin 154
clinical death 19
clonidine 193
coccidioidomycosis 123
cold caloric tests 21–2
COMDU (Cardiac Output Monitor & Diagnostic Unit) 441 (fig), 454
complement 109
complications of heart transplantation 191–200
    hemorrhage 191
    pulmonary emboli 191–2
    systemic emboli 191–2
    technical 191
    wound infection 191
congestive heart failure 12
contraindications to heart transplantation 13–15
    active infection 13

INDEX

advanced age 14
cerebrovascular disease 14
diabetes mellitus 14
dysfunction of other organs 13–14
financial 15
malignancy 13
patient non-compliance 15
peptic ulcer 14
peripheral vascular disease 14
psychological instability 15
pulmonary infarction 14
pulmonary vascular resistance elevation 14
systemic disease 13
corneal reflex 21
corneo-mandibular reflex 21
corticosteroids 7, 9, 95–6, 112
  intravenous pulse 136–7
  side effects 193 (table), 195–9
    aseptic necrosis of bone 196–7
    delayed onset of puberty 197
    diabetes mellitus 195–6
    gastrointestinal 197–8
    growth retardation 197
    impotence 195
    increased sexual appetite 195
    lenticular cataracts 198
    multiple compression-fractures of vertebrae 197
    myopathy 90, 105
    osteoporosis 196–7
    pancreatitis 199
    psychiatric 198
cost of heart transplantation *see under* financial considerations
coumadin 92
cryptococcosis 156
Cushing's reflex 44
Cybex isokinetic dynamometer 235
cyclophosphamide 97–8, 112, 137
  side effects 200
cyclosporine 9, 14, 93–5, 112, 137
  drugs influencing blood levels/toxicity 94
  fibroblastic effects 345
  heart–both lungs transplantation 264–5
  malignancies related to 187–8
  patient receiving, pathology of acute rejection 121–2
  side effects
    hypercholesterolemia 194
    hypertension 102, 174, 192–3
    myopathy 90
    neuromuscular 194
    neurotoxicity 93, 194
    nutritional 230
    renal 93, 192
cyclosporine G 529
cystic fibrosis 304, 353
cytoimmunological monitoring 129
cytomegalic inclusion disease 123
cytomegalovirus infection 43, 96, 154–5, 246, 530
  in heart–lung transplantation 327–8
cytotoxicity 111

death, causes of, after heart transplantation 254
deferoxamine 57
denervated lung physiology 336–7
denervation effects in transplanted heart 105
denial 225

15-deoxyspergualin 528
Detroit Driver 453
diabetes mellitus 170, 195–6
digitalis 105
digoxin 105
dihydroxypropoxymethylguanine (DHPG) 155, 353, 530
diltiazem 193
dimethyl sulfoxide (DMSO) 57
dipyramidole 92
diuretics 16
diverticulosis coli 198
dobutamine 105
donations/acquisition of tissue 28–31
  authorization for removal of organs 30
  by:
    authority empowered to donate 29
    individual prior to death 28–9
    relative of deceased 29
  confidentiality 30
  donee 30
  importation/exportation 30
  malpractice 31
  purpose 29–30
  sale of tissue 30
donor heart 41–59
  age 41
  blood group 41–2
  brain-dead donor 43–8
    autonomic (sympathetic) storm effect 43
    electrocardiographic effects 43–4
    endocrine changes 45–6
    hemodynamic effects 44
    histopathological effects 44–5
    hormonal therapy 47–8
    management 46–7
    metabolic responses 45–6
    myocardial function/structure 43
    myocardial pathology 124
  cardiac disease exclusion 42
  functional evaluation 58
  infection 123
  lymphocytotoxic antibodies in recipient 42
  pretreatment 51–2
  size 41
  storage 51–9
    autoperfusion (biological oxygenation) 54
    combined hypothermia and hyperbaric oxygenation/supercooling/freezing 53
    combined hypothermia and pharmacological inhibition 53
    extracorporeal normothermic perfusion 54–5
    hypothermia 52–3
    intermediate host perfusion (parabiosis) 54
    pharmacological inhibition 53
    total body perfusion 53–4
  transferable disease exclusion 42–3
donor organ availability 33–9
  chain of communication 35 (fig)
  inadequacy 33–4
  routine enquiry/request policy 38
  sale/purchase of organs 38
donor management 46–8
  hormonal therapy 47–8
dopamine 105
drug therapy, postoperative 91–3
  antibiotics 91

anticoagulants 92
antituberculous 92
chronic rejection prevention 92
diuretics 92
dysrhythmias 91–2
hypercholesterolemia prevention 92
immunosuppressive see immunosuppressive therapy
mineral replacement 92–3
pain relief 91
peptic ulcer prevention 92
vasoactive drugs 91
dynamic functions at rest/exercise following heart–lung transplantation 335–6
arterial blood gases 335
circulatory capacity 336
long-term exercise 336
ventilation 335–6

electrocardiography 133
employment, post-transplant 225
enalapril 193
endomyocardial biopsy 115–16, 127, 131–3
complications 132–3, 192
eosinophil-neutrophil chemotactic factor 110 (fig)
epinephrine 103, 105
Epstein–Barr virus 196, 328
ERDA artificial heart 457 (fig)
ethical issues 515–18, 530–1
organ procurement 516
patient selection 516–18
quality of life 519–20
exercise, long-term, dynamic functions during 336
exercise rehabilitation 233–9
benefits 239
exercise intensity determination 237–8
hospital inpatient phase 236
immunosuppression-receiving patients 235
intensive-care unit phase 236
monitoring sessions 238–9
outpatient phase 236–7
termination criteria 237
testing 233–5
external centrifugal pumps 413–14
extracorporeal hypothermic perfusion 54–5
extracorporeal immunoadsorption 527
extracorporeal membrane oxygenation 414
extracorporeal normothermic perfusion 54

factors influencing graft survival 252–4, 257–8
ABO-compatibility 258
clinical status of recipient 257
donor age 257
donor organ ischemic period 252, 258
experience 253–4
HLA matching 258
immunosuppressive therapy 253
lymphocytotoxic cross-match 258
operative procedure, orthotopic vs heterotopic 252–3
recipient's age 252, 257
recipients' cardiac pathology 252, 257
recipient's sex 252, 257
family consent, alternatives to 37–8
Federal Task Force on Organ Donation 38
Federal Task Force on Organ Transplantation 39
financial considerations 518–19, 530–1

costs 11, 518–19
reimbursement 518–19
resource allocation 520–1
FK506 528
5-flucytosine 156 (table)
furosemide 92
future prospects 523–31
donor supply problem solutions 524–7
allografts 524–5
mechanical hearts 525–6
myocardial augmentation 527
xenografts 526–7
ethical problems 530–1
financial problems 530–1
immunosuppression 528–9
combination drug therapy 529
donor-organ pretreatment 529
donor-specific pretreatment 529
new drugs 528
infectious complications 530
lung transplantation programs 524
non-invasive detection of acute/chronic rejection 527–8

gallbladder disease 198
gallium-67 imaging 135
gas transport/exchange 333
gentamicin 153
gift relationship 220
glycerol 57
graft atherosclerosis 161–75
diagnosis 172–4
incidence 165–6
macroscopic appearance 161–2
microscopic appearance 162–6
risk factors 70–2
diabetes mellitus 170
hyperlipidemia 170
hypertension 170
male sex 170
smoking 171–2
treatment 174
graft-versus-host disease 345
grimace response 21
growth retardation in children 197
guanfacine 193

heart–lung transplantation 261–354
acute lung rejection 308–10, 316–17
immunohistochemistry 322
immunology 310
infection related 330
monitoring 311–13
pathology 308–10
phases 309 (table)
anesthesia 283–6
cardiopulmonary bypass 286
post-transplant bleeding 286
weaning from ventilation 286
cardiopulmonary preservation 278–61
autoperfusing heart–lung preparation 280
cooling by extracorporeal circulation 279–80
hypothermic flush perfusion with blood 279
hypothermic flush perfusion with crystalloid solution 278–9
re-implantation response 280–1

causes of death 351
chronic lung rejection 318–21
  infection related 330
combi-effect 307–8
contraindications 268–9
cyclosporine introduction 264–5
cystic fibrosis patient 304
donor management 274–5
donor organs excision 275–6, 277 (figs)
donor–recipient compatibility/matching 299–300
donor–recipient selection 299
donor selection 273–4
early clinical experience 265
hemodynamic changes following 341
hyperacute lung rejection 317–18
immunology 307–13
immunosuppressive therapy 300
implantation of donor organs 294–8
indications 267–8, 349–50
infections 325–31
  bacterial 327
  cytomegalovirus 328–9
  diagnosis 329–30
  donor factors 325
  Epstein–Barr virus 328
  fungal 328–9
  herpes simplex 328
  immunosuppressive policy relationship 353
  non-A, non-B hepatitis 328
  operative factors 325
  parainfluenzae virus 328
  postoperative factors 325–6
  protozoal 328
  rejection differentiation 352
  rejection relationship 330
  respiratory syncytial virus 328
  sternal wound with *M. hominis* 329
initial studies 261–3
late lung function 353
monitoring for acute lung rejection/pulmonary
    infection 301–3
  endomyocardial biopsy 303
  histological appearances 303
  transbronchial lung biopsy 302–3
open-lung biopsy 323
pathology 315–23
  other organs 322
patient assessment 269–70
patient selection 271
postoperative care 300
postoperative complications 301, 315–16
  adult respiratory distress syndrome 316
  air leak 301
  bleeding 301
  pneumothorax 301
  pulmonary edema 352
  reimplantation response 315–16
  tracheal dehiscence 316
  see also below treatment of pulmonary complications
postoperative monitoring 300–1
preoperative care 271–2
primates 264
pulmonary function following 341–2
quality of life after 353
recipient's heart as donor organ 270–1

reimplantation response 315–16, 352
single 337
single *vs* double 350
size match 274, 275 (fig)
supportive techniques advent 263–4
surgical technique of recipient operation 289–98
survival 350–1
  factors affecting 351–2
transbronchial biopsy 323
treatment of pulmonary complications 303–4
  acute rejection 303
  aspergillus infection 304
  cytomegalovirus pneumonitis 303–4
  obliterative bronchiolitis 304
  pneumocystis pneumonia 304
  pyogenic pneumonia 304
heart transplantation
  children *see* childhood
  complications *see* complications
  contraindications *see* contraindications
  early experience 3–9
  heterotopic 81–7, 203–6
    abdominal 4
    advantages/disadvantages 203 (table)
    cervical 4
    donor-heart excision/preparation 81–2
    myocardial protection of recipient/donor hearts 83
    permanent 203–6
    physiology following 103–4
    pump-oxygenation discontinuation 86
    recipient heart deterioration 104
    recipient operation 82–6
    temporary 206
    transverse section through heart 104 (fig)
  hyperacute rejection *see* hyperacute rejection
  infants *see* childhood
  maintenance of selective recipient 15–16
  orthotopic 5, 75–80
    donor heart excision 75–7
    multiple organ excision 76
    recipient operation 77–9
  patient assessment/selection 15, 217–18
  postoperative care *see* postoperative care
  psychiatric aspects *see* psychiatric aspects
  results *see* results
  selection of heart recipient 38
  when? 12–13
  which patient? 13
  see also transplanted heart
hemostatic process 439 (fig)
heparin 394
herpes simplex virus 155
high-density lipoprotein cholesterol 172
Hodgkin's disease 185
horseradish peroxidase 57
human immunodeficiency virus antibody serology 42
human leukocyte antigen system 63–6, 109
  HLA-A, B, C antigens 64
  HLA-DP, DQ, DR antigens 64–6
  see also major histocompatibility complex
Human Tissues Act (UK, 1961) 27, 28–9
hydralazine 12
hydrocortisone 7; *see also* corticosteroids
hyperacute rejection 111, 128, 487–91
  antibody-mediated 487 (fig)

management 489–91
hypercholesterolemia (hyperlipidemia) 92, 170, 194
hypertension 170
  cyclosporine-induced 102, 174
hypomagnesemia 194
hypoplastic left heart syndrome 210, 213–14
hypothalamic-pituitary dysfunction 22
hypothermia 6
hypothermic perfusion system 58

idiotypic antibodies 529
immunoglobulins
  IgE, anti-OKT3 97
  IgG 111
    anti-OKT3 97
    genes 527
  IgM 111
    anti-OKT-3 97
immunology, pretransplant 63–8
immunosuppression 6–7, 93–8, 111–13
  antilymphocyte globulin 9, 96
  antithymocyte globulin 9, 96
  azathioprine see azathioprine
  corticosteroids see corticosteroids
  cyclophosphamide 97–8, 112
  cyclosporine see cyclosporine
  factors limiting exercise 235
  graft survival influence 253
  OKT3 9, 96–7
  resting cardiac dynamics 101
  total lymphoid irradiation 113
  vincristine 97
infants see childhood
infections 143–58
  bacterial 153–4
  central nervous system 153
  donor heart 123
  fungal 155–7
  incidence 143
  nocardiosis 157
  predisposing factors 145–6, 147 (table)
  presenting features 149
  prevention 146–9
    patient care 148–9
    transplant unit 147–8
  protozoal 157–8
  pulmonary 149–52
    blood culture 149
    chest radiography 149–50
    computerized axial tomography 152
    fiberoptic bronchoscopy 150–2
    open-lung biopsy 152
    sputum examination 150
    transtracheal aspiration 150
    ultrafine needle aspiration 150
  septicemia 152–3
  site 143–5
  therapy 153–4
  type 143–5
  urinary tract 149
  viral 154–5
  see also specific infections
informed consent 12
inotropic agents 16, 105

γ-interferon (macrophage activating factor) 110 (fig), 111, 130
interleukin-1 110
interleukin-2 110, 111
  receptors 130
intermediate host perfusion (parabiosis) 54
iratropium bromide 338
isokinetic cycle ergometer 235
isometric exercise 102
isoniazid 92, 154
isoproterenol 105
isosorbide dinitrate 12

JARVIK see total artificial hearts
JARVIK-7 withdrawal 444
JARVIK-7-100 464

Kaposi's sarcoma 184, 186–7, 249
keratoacanthoma 200

lactate turnpoint (anaerobic threshold) 234
Lafferty–Bach–Batchelor concept 110
left ventricular assist systems, electrically-powered
    implantable 414–15
lip cancer 185–6
lisinopril 193
liver disease 198
lovastatin 92, 196
low density lipoprotein 172, 194
low density lipoprotein cholesterol 172, 174
lung transplantation, single/double 357–409
  allotransplantation 359
  complications 399–405
    acute rejection 400–1
    air embolism 404
    airway necrosis 402–3
    airway stenosis 404
    chronic rejection 405
    hemorrhage 400
    hypotension 400
    infection 403, 404
    intraoperative 399–400
    lymphoproliferative disorders 404–5
    poor graft function 400
    prolonged ventilation 401–2
    psychiatric 403–4
  donor lung assessment/selection 369–70
  donor lung excision 370–2
    double lung 372–3
    single lung 371–2
  donor lung presentation 373–4
  donor maintenance 370
  double lung
    donor excision 372–3
    patient selection 365–6
    results 408–9
    surgical technique 385–9
  early experience 357–60
  experimental studies 358–9
  in-hospital assessment 366–7
  pharmacology 337–8
  physiology 354–7
  post-operative management 391–8
    anticoagulation 394
    early postoperative period 391–5

education 397–8
hemodynamic 393
immunosuppression 393–4
implantation response diagnosis 394–5
infection diagnosis 395
infection management 394
investigations 394
monitoring 395
rehabilitation 395–7
rejection diagnosis 394–5
transbronchial biopsy 395, 397 (fig)
ventilation 391–3, 395 (fig)
pre-transplantation management 367
single lung 363–5
anesthesia see anesthesia
contraindications 365 (table)
donor excision 371–2
obliterative bronchiolitis after 395
patient selection 363–5
results 407–8
surgical technique 381–3
lymphocytes
activated, in vitro culture 130
fluorescent labelling 129
monoclonal antibody labelling 129
lymphocytotoxic cross-match test 66–7
lymphoid irradiation, total 112
lymphokines 110 (fig)
lymphoma 184, 186
non-Hodgkin 186

macrophage, activated 111
macrophage-activating factor (γ-interferon) 110 (fig), 111, 130
magnesium trisilicate 92
major histocompatibility complex 109–10
malignant melanoma 185
malignant neoplasia in immunocompromised patients 183–9
cyclosporine-related 187–8
de novo tumors 184–9
age of recipients 184
etiology 189
incidence 184
sex of recipients 184
treatment 188
multiple 187
pre-existing 184
transplanted malignancies 183
see also specific tumors
malpractice 31
mannitol 57
medico-legal aspects 27–31, 223–4
perioperative phase 224
mercaptopurine 7
Merkel's cell tumor 185
methacholine 337, 338
methotrexate 7
methylprednisolone 7, 95, 136
methylprednisolone sodium succinate 136
miconazole 156 (table)
β_2-microglobulin 131
mineral replacement therapy 92–3
morphine, postoperative 91
multiple organ excision 76
multiple vertebral compression fracture syndrome 196
myconazole 156 (table)

myocardium
cell metabolism 51
viability assessment 57–8

natural auxiliary heart see heart transplantation, heterotopic
National Organ Transplant Act (USA, 1984) 30, 34
natural killer cells 111
neopterin 130–1
nifedipine 106, 193
nocardiosis 157
non-A non-B hepatitis 328
non-cardiac surgery, patient with heart transplant 241–3
anesthesia 242–3
postoperative management 243
pre-operative assessment 242
non-pulsatile centrifugal pumps 417–21
complications 420–1
heart transplantation 419
insertion 418–19
patient management 419
patient selection 418
results 419–20
norepinephrine 105
North American Transplant Coordinators Organization 34, 35
Novacor 414–15, 426
nuclear magnetic resonance spectroscopy, ^{31}P 135
nutrition 227–31
drug-related problems 230
long-term care 230–1
post-transplant support 230
pretransplant assessment 227–8
pretransplant support 228–9
nystatin 156 (table)

obliterative bronchiolitis see bronchiolitis obliterans
oculo-cephalic reflex 21
OKT3 9, 96–7, 137–8
side effects 193 (table), 199
open lung biopsy 323
organ procurement agency 33
osteoporosis 92–3, 196–7
oxygen free radicals 56–7
scavengers 57

pain relief, postoperative 91
pancuronium 105
Papworth flush solution 284 (tables)
parabiosis (intermediate host perfusion) 54
paradoxical cerebral embolus 192
paradoxical vasoconstriction 173–4
penicillin 153
peptic ulcer 197–8
percutaneous transluminal coronary angioplasty 174
perineal carcinoma 184, 187
peripheral α-receptor blocking drugs 195
petriellidosis 157
Philadelphia total artificial heart 453–4
Pierce–Donachy ventilator assist device 414, 424–6, 428 (table)
plasmapheresis 527
platelet activating factor (acetyl glycerol ether phosphorylcholine) 487–9
pneumatic aortic counterpulsator device 507, 509 (fig)
pneumocystis 157–8, 246–7
pneumothorax 242
polyamine, urinary 131

postoperative care, heart transplantation 73
  boredom prevention 90–1
  drug therapy *see* drug therapy
  immediate 89–90
  infection prevention 90
  patient monitoring 89–90
  physical therapy 91
  psychological isolation prevention 90–1
  respiratory therapy 90
prazocin 193
prednisolone 95–6
prednisone 95–6, 172
  nutritional problems 230
preformed antibodies 66–7
pretransplant steps 36 (fig)
probucol 92, 194
prolactin 131
propranolol 338
propylene glycol 57
prostaglandins (eicosanoids) 91
  E_1 (PGE_1) 91
proton magnetic resonance imaging 135
psychiatric aspects, heart transplantation 217–20
  assessment 217–18
  awaiting transplant 218
  immediate postoperative period 218–19
psychiatric disorders 198
pulmonary circulation regulation in transplanted lung 337
pulmonary edema 352
pulmonary function of transplanted lung following heart–lung transplantation 334–5
  diffusing capacity 335
  distribution of ventilation 335
  long-term 335
  pulmonary dynamics 334–5
  pulmonary statics 334
  volumes 334
pulmonary gas exchange 333
pulmonary hypertension, post-heart transplantation 103
pulmonary perfusion 333
pulmonary vascular obstructive disease 211
pulmonary vascular resistance 14, 204–6
pulmonary ventilation 333
pulsatile ventricular assist devices 423–9
  'bridge' application results 428
  'bridge' transplantation 424
  complications 427–8
  implantation 426–7
  indications 426
  monitoring 427
  Novacor 414–15, 426
  Pierce–Donachy 414, 424–6, 428 (table)
  Thermedics 426
  transplant studies 428
pulse oximetric monitoring 395
pump-oxygenator 53–4
pupillary response 21
pyroninophilia 123

quality of life 353, 519–20
quinidine gluconate 106

ranitidine 92, 197
β-receptor blockers 105, 193
β-receptor stimulants 105

red blood cell, technetium-99m pyrophosphate labelled 134
red blood cell groups
  ABO 63
  Rhesus 63
reduced glutathione 57
reference of patients for heart transplantation 11–12
rehabilitation 219–20, 224–5
  exercise *see* exercise rehabilitation
reimplantation response 315–16, 352
renal xenotransplantation, experimental 489–90
reperfusion injury 55–7
  following global hypothermic ischemia 57
  prevention 57
respiration 333–4
results of heart transplantation 251–8
  causes of death 254
  donor availability 255
  overall graft survival 257
retransplantation 177–82, 345–6
  immunosuppression 181, 182
  indications 177
  patient selection 177–8
  patient with acutely rejected allograft/functioning recipient heart 180–1
  patient with heterotopic allograft 179–80
  patient with orthotopic allograft 179
  postoperative care 181
  results 181–2, 254
  timing:
    advanced chronic rejection 178–9
    intractable acute rejection 178
Rhesus group 63
rifampicin 154
right ventricular dilatation, post-heart transplantation 103

salbutamol 338
Sarcocystis species 123
Sarns Centrimed 414
Saudi Arabia, living donors of kidneys 531
scintigraphy 133–5
self-referral 217
serum sickness 199
skeletal muscle, heart augmentation *see* cardiomyoplasty; skeletal muscle blood pumps
skeletal muscle function assessment 235
skeletal muscle blood pumps 503–9
  ventricle constriction 504–5
  ventricle preconditioning 504–5
  ventricles *in vivo* 505–8
    arterial diastolic counterpulsators 506–7
    mock circulation 505–6
    right heart bypass 507–8
  see also cardiomyoplasty
skin cancer 185–6, 200
skin lesions, benign 200
smoking 170–1
social rehabilitation 530
spinal segmental reflexes 22
sternal wound infection 329
steroids *see* corticosteroids
stress management 224
suicide 198
sulphinpyrazone 92
supportive techniques advent 5–6
supraventricular arrhythmia 106

INDEX

Symbion Jarvik total artificial heart 415
sympathetic (autonomic) storm 43

taurine 57
T-cell 109, 111, 122
  cytotoxic 109, 110 (fig), 111
  helper 109, 110 (fig), 111
  suppressor 109, 110 (fig), 113
T-cell antibodies
  lymphocytotoxic 66–7
  monoclonal/polyclonal 112
terazocin 193
Thermedics ventricular assist device 426
thromboembolism 241
thromboxane A2 131
thromboxane B2 131
tissue viability tests 58
tobramycin 153
total artificial heart 415, 431–44, 453–67
  cardiac output regulation 456
  clinical experience 463–7
  coagulation/anticoagulation control 439–40
    coagulation 440
    fibrinolytic system 440
    heparin neutralization 439
    platelet aggregation 440
  complications 465
  finance 459–60
  hemodynamic observations 465
  hemodynamic status 440
  monitoring 465
  nutritional status 442
  patient selection 431–3, 464–5
  postoperative care 438–9
  problems 456–9
    infection 459
    placement within heart 456–8
    polyurethane degeneration 459
    thromboemboli 458–9
  renal status 440
  respiratory status 442
  results 442–3
    transplantation in TAH patients 443
  sources of energy 453–6
    atomic 456
    electric 456
    electrohydraulic 454–6
    pneumatic 453–4
    portable air-drive systems 454, 454 (fig)
  surgical techniques 433–8
    lateral positioning 437–8
    medial positioning 433–7
total lymphoid irradiation 528
toxoplasmosis 123, 328
tracheal dehiscence 316
transbronchial biopsy 323, 395, 397 (fig)
transferrin receptors 129
transplant centers 39
transplant coordination 35–7
  donor center 36–7
  recipient center 35–6
transplant coordinator 35
transplanted heart
  electrophysiology 104–5
  pharmacology 105–6
    antiarrhythmic agents 106
    calcium antagonists 105–6
    digoxin 105
    inotropic agents 105
    β-receptor blockers 105
  physiology 101–5
  response to exercise 102–3
  resting state 101–2
    cardiac dynamics 101
    contractility 101–2
    diastolic function 102
    heart rate 101
    humoral factors 102
    left ventricular performance 101–2
  time course of physiologic effects 103
transpulmonary gradient 206
Trichosporon beigelii (*cutaneum*) 157
triiodothyronine (T3) 91
trisodium phosphonoformate 155
tuberculosis 154, 257
type A behavior pattern 218

Uniform Anatomical Gift Act (USA, 1968) 27–8, 31, 33
unilateral lung transplantation *see* lung transplantation, single lung
United Network for Organ Sharing 34, 35

vancomycin 154
varicella zoster 155
vasodilators 105
ventilation following heart–lung transplantation 335–6
  neural 337
ventilation regulation 333
ventilation threshold 234
ventricular arrhythmias 16, 106
ventricular assist devices 255
verapamil 91, 106, 193
vestibulo-ocular reflexes 21–2
vincristine 97
vitamin C 57
vitamin E 57
viviperfusion 3
vulval carcinoma 184, 187

warts 200

xenograft, first attempt at 7–8
xenotransplantation, cardiac 471–94
  'bridge' to allotransplantation 474–6
  choice of donor for man 471–3
  clinical experience 493–4
  closely related animal species 473–4
  'concordant'/'disconcordant' xenografts 471
  distantly related species 474, 475 (table)
  experimental 'concordant' 485–6
  experimental 'disconcordant' 486
  hyperacute rejection 485–91
  rejection pathology 479–82
xenotransplantation, experimental renal 489–90

zinc depletion 230